## Animations

Animations of key nutrition concepts will help you visualize and comprehend important concepts. The animations even include quiz questions to help ensure that you are retaining the information.

Enzyme Action and the Hydrolysis of Sucrose

Glucose

Fructose

Enzyme

...accomplished, the enzyme's configuration is changed back to the original ...o monosaccharides float away, and the site becomes available for another ...cule to bind, change the enzyme's configuration, and be hydrolyzed.

Copyright © The McGraw-Hill Companies, Inc.

How Diffusion Works

Molecules dissolved in a solution are in constant random motion due to their kinetic energy. One result of this motion is that dissolved molecules become evenly distributed throughout the solution.

Copyright © The McGraw-Hill Companies, Inc.

Protein Denaturation

Protein denaturation changes the solubility of individual protein molecules, entrapping solvent water into a semisolid gel structure.

This familiar gelatin dessert actually is a good example of the process of coagulation of proteins into a three dimensional latticework that entraps water molecules to produce a semisolid gel.

## Electronic Books
### GO GREEN!

**Go Green. Save Green. McGraw-Hill eBooks.**

Green . . . it's on everybody's minds these days. It's not only about saving trees; it's also about saving money. At 55% of the bookstore price, **McGraw-Hill eBooks** are an eco-friendly and cost-saving alternative to the traditional print textbook. So, you do some good for the environment . . . and you do some good for your wallet.

Visit **www.mhhe.com/ebooks** for details.

# Eighth Edition

# Contemporary Nutrition

## Gordon M. Wardlaw

PH.D.

Formerly of Department of Human Nutrition,
College of Human Ecology
The Ohio State University

## Anne M. Smith

PH.D., R.D., L.D.

Department of Human Nutrition,
College of Human Ecology
The Ohio State University

McGraw Hill

*Connect
Learn
Succeed™*

CONTEMPORARY NUTRITION, EIGHTH EDITION

Published by McGraw-Hill, a business unit of The McGraw-Hill Companies, Inc., 1221 Avenue of the Americas, New York, NY 10020. Copyright © 2011 by The McGraw-Hill Companies, Inc. All rights reserved. Previous editions © 2009, 2006, and 2003. No part of this publication may be reproduced or distributed in any form or by any means, or stored in a database or retrieval system, without the prior written consent of The McGraw-Hill Companies, Inc., including, but not limited to, in any network or other electronic storage or transmission, or broadcast for distance learning.

Some ancillaries, including electronic and print components, may not be available to customers outside the United States.

This book is printed on acid-free paper.

1 2 3 4 5 6 7 8 9 0 WDQ/ WDQ 1 0 9 8 7 6 5 4 3 2 1 0

ISBN 978–0–07–304054–7
MHID 0–07–304054–1

Vice President, Editor-in-Chief: *Marty Lange*
Vice President, EDP: *Kimberly Meriwether David*
Executive Editor: *Colin H. Wheatley*
Director of Development: *Kristine Tibbetts*
Senior Developmental Editor: *Lynne M. Meyers*
Marketing Manager: *Amy L. Reed*
Senior Project Manager: *April R. Southwood*
Senior Production Supervisor: *Kara Kudronowicz*
Senior Media Project Manager: *Jodi K. Banowetz*
Design Coordinator: *Brenda A. Rolwes*
Cover/Interior Designer: *Ellen Pettergell*
(USE) Cover Image: *© Getty Images*
Senior Photo Research Coordinator: *John C. Leland*
Photo Research: *Mary Reeg*
Compositor: *Laserwords Private Limited*
Typeface: *10/12 Giovanni Book*
Printer: *World Color Press Inc.*

All credits appearing on page or at the end of the book are considered to be an extension of the copyright page.

**Library of Congress Cataloging-in-Publication Data**

Wardlaw, Gordon M.
  Contemporary nutrition / Gordon M. Wardlaw.—8th ed./Anne M. Smith.
    p. cm.
  Includes index.
  ISBN 978–0–07–304054–7 — ISBN 0–07–304054–1 (hard copy : alk. paper) 1. Nutrition—Textbooks.
I. Smith, Anne M., 1955- II. Title.
  QP141.W378 2011
  612.3—dc22

                                              2009030908

www.mhhe.com

# Brief Contents

**Part One** Nutrition: A Key to Health  2

  **1** What You Eat and Why  3
  **2** Guidelines for Designing a Healthy Diet  35
  **3** The Human Body: A Nutrition Perspective  81

**Part Two** Energy Nutrients and Energy Balance  122

  **4** Carbohydrates  123
  **5** Lipids  165
  **6** Proteins  209
  **7** Energy Balance and Weight Control  243

**Part Three** Vitamins, Minerals, and Water  288

  **8** Vitamins  289
  **9** Water and Minerals  347

**Part Four** Nutrition: Beyond the Nutrients  406

  **10** Nutrition: Fitness and Sports  407
  **11** Eating Disorders: Anorexia Nervosa, Bulimia Nervosa, and Other Conditions  445
  **12** Undernutrition Throughout the World  473
  **13** Safety of Our Food Supply  505

**Part Five** Nutrition: A Focus on Life Stages  540

  **14** Pregnancy and Breastfeeding  541
  **15** Nutrition from Infancy Through Adolescence  579
  **16** Nutrition During Adulthood  619

# Contents

Preface xvi

**Part One** Nutrition: A Key to Health 2

**Chapter 1** What You Eat and Why 3

Student Learning Outcomes 3

Refresh Your Memory 4

1.1 Good Health: The Nutrition Connection 4
What Is Nutrition? 4
Nutrients Come from Food 4
Why Study Nutrition? 5

1.2 Classes and Sources of Nutrients 7
Carbohydrates 7
Lipids 9
Proteins 10
Vitamins 11
Minerals 11
Water 11
Other Important Components in Food 12

1.3 Nutrient Composition of Diets and the Human Body 13

1.4 Energy Sources and Uses 14
Calories 14
Calculating Calories 15

1.5 Current State of the North American Diet and Overall Health 16
Assessing the Current North American Diet 17
Health Objectives for the United States for the Year 2010 17

1.6 Improving Our Diets 18

1.7 Why Am I So Hungry? 20
The Hypothalamus Contributes to Satiety 20
Meal Size and Composition Affect Satiety 20
Hormones Affect Satiety 21
Does Appetite Affect What We Eat? 21
Putting Hunger and Appetite into Perspective 22

Nutrition and Your Health: Eating Well in College 24

Case Study: Typical College Student 28

Summary 28

Study Questions 29

Check Your Knowledge 29

Further Readings 30

Rate Your Plate 32

**Chapter 2** Guidelines for Designing a Healthy Diet 35

Student Learning Outcomes 35

Refresh Your Memory 36

2.1 A Food Philosophy that Works 36
Variety Means Eating Many Different Foods 36
Balance Means Consuming Food From Each Group 37
Moderation Refers Mostly to Portion Size 38
Nutrient Density Focuses on Nutrient Content 39
Energy (kCAL) Density Affects Calorie Intake 39

2.2 States of Nutritional Health 40
Desirable Nutrition 41
Undernutrition 41
Overnutrition 42

2.3 How Can Your Nutritional State be Measured? 42
Analyzing Background Factors 42
Assessing Nutritional Status Using the ABCDEs 43
Recognizing the Limitations of Nutritional Assessment 44
Concern About the State of Your Nutritional Health Is Important 45

2.4 Recommendations for Healthy Eating 45
MyPyramid—A Menu-Planning Tool 45
The Mediterranean Diet Pyramid 52
Dietary Guidelines—Another Tool for Menu Planning 54

2.5 Specific Nutrient Standards and Recommendations 60
    Recommended Dietary Allowance 60
    Adequate Intake 61
    Estimated Energy Requirement 61
    Tolerable Upper Intake Level 61
    Daily Value 62
    How Should these Nutrient Standards Be Used? 62

2.6 Using the Scientific Method to Determine Nutrient Needs 62

2.7 Food Labels and Diet Planning 66
    Exceptions to Food Labeling 66
    Health Claims on Food Labels 69

2.8 Epilogue 70

Nutrition and Your Health: Evaluating Nutrition Claims and Dietary Supplements 71

Case Study: Dietary Supplements 73

Summary 74

Study Questions 74

Check Your Knowledge 75

Further Readings 75

Rate Your Plate 77

## Chapter 3 The Human Body: A Nutrition Perspective 81

Student Learning Outcomes 81

Refresh Your Memory 82

3.1 Human Physiology 82

3.2 The Cell: Structure, Function, and Metabolism 83
    Cell (Plasma) Membrane 83
    Cytoplasm 85
    Mitochondria 85
    Cell Nucleus 85
    Endoplasmic Reticulum (ER) 86
    Golgi Complex 86
    Lysosomes 86
    Peroxisomes 86
    Cell Metabolism 86

3.3 Organization of the Body 87

3.4 Cardiovascular System and Lymphatic System 87
    Cardiovascular System 88
    Lymphatic System 89

3.5 Nervous System 91

3.6 Endocrine System 93

3.7 Immune System 95
    Skin 95
    Intestinal Cells 95
    White Blood Cells 96

3.8 Digestive System 96
    Mouth 97
    Esophagus 99

    Stomach 99
    Small Intestine 100
    Large Intestine 103
    Rectum 105
    Accessory Organs 106

3.9 Urinary System 106

3.10 Storage Capabilities 107

3.11 A Closer Look at Genetics and Nutrition 108
    The Emerging Field of Nutrigenomics 108
    Nutritional Diseases with a Genetic Link 109
    Your Genetic Profile 110

Nutrition and Your Health: Common Problems with Digestion 112

Case Study: Gastroesophageal Reflux Disease 117

Summary 118

Study Questions 118

Check Your Knowledge 119

Further Readings 119

Rate Your Plate 121

## Part Two Energy Nutrients and Energy Balance 122

## Chapter 4 Carbohydrates 123

Student Learning Outcomes 123

Refresh Your Memory 124

4.1 Carbohydrates—An Introduction 124

4.2 Simple Carbohydrates 125
    Monosaccharides—Glucose, Fructose, and Galactose 126
    Disaccharides—Sucrose, Lactose, and Maltose 126

4.3 Complex Carbohydrates 128

4.4 Fiber 129

4.5 Carbohydrates in Foods 130
    Starch 131
    Fiber 131
    Nutritive Sweeteners 132
    Alternative Sweeteners 135

4.6 Making Carbohydrates Available for Body Use 136
    Digestion 137
    Absorption 138

4.7   Putting Simple Carbohydrates to Work In The Body  140
    Yielding Energy  140
    Sparing Protein from Use as an Energy Source and Preventing
       Ketosis  140
    Regulating Glucose  140
    The Glycemic Index and Glycemic Load of Carbohydrate
       Sources  142

4.8   Putting Fiber to Work  144
    Promoting Bowel Health  144
    Reducing Obesity Risk  144
    Enhancing Blood Glucose Control  145
    Reducing Cholesterol Obsorption  145

4.9   Carbohydrate Needs  145
    How Much Fiber Do We Need?  146

4.10  Health Concerns Related to Carbohydrate Intake  146
    Problems with High-Fiber Diets  146
    Problems with High-Sugar Diets  148
    Dental Caries  149

Nutrition and Your Health: Diabetes—When Blood Glucose
    Regulation Fails  151

Case Study: Problems with Milk Intake  157

Summary  157

Study Questions  158

Check Your Knowledge  158

Further Readings  159

Rate Your Plate  161

**Chapter 5** Lipids  165

Student Learning Outcomes  165

Refresh Your Memory  166

5.1   Lipids: Common Properties  166

5.2   Lipids: Main Types  167
    Fatty Acids: The Simplest Form of Lipids  167
    Triglycerides  169
    Phospholipids  170
    Sterols  170

5.3   Fats and Oils in Foods  172
    Fat Is Hidden in Some Foods  174
    Fat in Food Provides Some Satiety, Flavor, and Texture  175

Wise Use of Reduced-Fat Foods Is Important  176
    Fat Replacement Strategies for Foods  176
    Fat Rancidity Limits Shelf Life of Foods  176
    Hydrogenation of Fatty Acids in Food Production Increases *Trans*
       Fatty Acid Content  177

5.4   Making Lipids Available for Body Use  179
    Digestion  179
    Absorption  181

5.5   Carrying Lipids in the Bloodstream  181
    Dietary Fats Are Carried by Chylomicrons  182
    Other Lipoproteins Transport Lipids from the Liver to the Body
       Cells  183
    "Good" and "Bad" Cholesterol in the Bloodstream  184

5.6   Essential Functions of Fatty Acids  185
    The Essential Fatty Acids  185
    Effects of a Deficiency of Essential Fatty Acids  187

5.7   Broader Roles for Fatty Acids and Triglycerides in the
    Body  188
    Providing Energy  188
    Storing Energy for Later Use  188
    Insulating and Protecting the Body  189
    Transporting Fat-Soluble Vitamins  189

5.8   Phospholipids in the Body  189

5.9   Cholesterol in the Body  190

5.10  Recommendations for Fat Intake  190

Nutrition and Your Health: Lipids and Cardiovascular Disease  196

Case Study: Planning a Heart Healthy Diet  201

Summary  201

Study Questions  202

Check Your Knowledge  202

Further Readings  203

Rate Your Plate  205

**Chapter 6** Proteins  209

Student Learning Outcomes  209

Refresh Your Memory  210

6.1   Protein—An Introduction  210
    Amino Acids  211

6.2   Proteins—Amino Acids Bonded Together  213
    Protein Synthesis  214
    Protein Organization  215
    Denaturation of Proteins  215

6.3   Protein in Foods  216
    Protein Quality of Foods  216
    A Closer Look at Plant Sources of Proteins  218

6.4   Protein Digestion and Absorption  219
    Digestion  219
    Absorption  220

6.5   Putting Proteins to Work in the Body  221
    Producing Vital Body Structures  221
    Maintaining Fluid Balance  221

Contributing to Acid-Base Balance  222
Forming Hormones and Enzymes  222
Contributing to Immune Function  222
Forming Glucose  222
Providing Energy  223
Contributing to Satiety  223

6.6   Protein Needs  225

6.7   Does Eating a High-Protein Diet Harm You?  227

6.8   Protein-Calorie Malnutrition  228
Kwashiorkor  229
Marasmus  230

Nutrition and Your Health: Vegetarian and Plant-Based Diets  231
Case Study: Planning a Vegetarian Diet  236
Summary  236
Study Questions  237
Check Your Knowledge  237
Further Readings  238
Rate Your Plate  240

**Chapter 7** Energy Balance and Weight Control  243

Student Learning Outcomes  243
Refresh Your Memory  244

7.1   Energy Balance  245
Positive and Negative Energy Balance  245
Energy Intake  247
Energy Output  247

7.2   Determination of Energy Use by the Body  250
Direct and Indirect Calorimetry  250
Estimates of Energy Needs  250

7.3   Estimation of a Healthy Weight  251
Body Mass Index (BMI)  252
Putting Healthy Weight into Perspective  253

7.4   Energy Imbalance  254
Estimating Body Fat Content and Diagnosing Obesity  254
Using Body Fat Distribution to Further Evaluate Obesity  257

7.5   Why Some People Are Obese—Nature versus Nurture  258
How Does Nature Contribute to Obesity?  258
Does the Body Have a Set Point for Weight?  259
Does Nurture Have a Role?  260

7.6   Treatment of Overweight and Obesity  261
What to Look for in a Sound Weight-Loss Plan  261
Weight Loss in Perspective  262

7.7   Control of Calorie Intake—The Main Key to Weight Loss and Weight Maintenance  263

7.8   Regular Physical Activity—A Second Key to Weight Loss and Especially Important for Later Weight Maintenance  265

7.9   Behavior Modification—A Third Strategy for Weight Loss and Management  267
Relapse Prevention Is Important  267

Social Support Aids Behavioral Change  269
Societal Efforts to Reduce Obesity  269

7.10  Professional Help for Weight Loss  269
Medications for Weight Loss  270
Treatment of Severe Obesity  271

7.11  Treatment of Underweight  274

Nutrition and Your Health: Popular Diets—Cause for Concern  275
Case Study: Choosing a Weight-Loss Program  278
Summary  278
Study Questions  279
Check Your Knowledge  279
Further Readings  280
Rate Your Plate  282

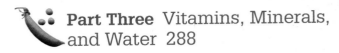

**Part Three** Vitamins, Minerals, and Water  288

**Chapter 8** Vitamins  289

Student Learning Outcomes  289
Refresh Your Memory  290

8.1   Vitamins: Vital Dietary Components  290
Have Scientists Found All the Vitamins?  291
Storage of Vitamins in the Body  291
Vitamin Toxicity  292
Preservation of Vitamins in Foods  292

8.2   The Fat-Soluble Vitamins—A, D, E, and K  293
Absorption of Fat-Soluble Vitamins  293

8.3   Vitamin A  294
Functions of Vitamin A and Carotenoids  294
Vitamin A Sources and Needs  296
Upper Level for Vitamin A  298

8.4   Vitamin D  298
Functions of Vitamin D  299
Vitamin D Sources and Needs  300
Upper Level for Vitamin D  300

8.5   Vitamin E  301
Functions of Vitamin E  302
Vitamin E Sources and Needs  303
Upper Level for Vitamin E  304

8.6    Vitamin K  305
       Functions of Vitamin K  305
       Vitamin K Sources and Needs  306

8.7    The Water-Soluble Vitamins and Choline  308
       B Vitamin Intakes of North Americans  308

8.8    Thiamin  310
       Thiamin Sources and Needs  310

8.9    Riboflavin  312
       Riboflavin Sources and Needs  312

8.10   Niacin  312
       Niacin Sources and Needs  314
       Upper Level for Niacin  314

8.11   Pantothenic Acid  315
       Pantothenic Acid Sources and Needs  316

8.12   Biotin  316
       Biotin Sources and Needs  316

8.13   Vitamin B-6  317
       Functions of Vitamin B-6  317
       Vitamin B-6 Sources and Needs  318
       Upper Level for Vitamin B-6  319

8.14   Folate  320
       Functions of Folate  320
       Folate Sources and Needs  322
       Upper Level for Folate  325

8.15   Vitamin B-12  325
       Functions of Vitamin B-12  325
       Vitamin B-12 Sources and Needs  326

8.16   Vitamin C  327
       Functions of Vitamin C  328
       Vitamin C Sources and Needs  328
       Upper Level for Vitamin C  330

8.17   Choline  330
       Choline Sources and Needs  331
       Upper Level for Choline  331

8.18   Vitamin-Like Compounds  331

Nutrition and Your Health: Dietary Supplements—Who Needs
       Them?  335

Case Study: Choosing a Dietary Supplement  339

Summary  339

Study Questions  341

Check Your Knowledge  341

Further Readings  342

Rate Your Plate  344

## Chapter 9  Water and Minerals  347

Student Learning Outcomes  347

Refresh Your Memory  348

9.1    Water  348
       Water in the Body—Intracellular and Extracellular Fluid  348
       Water Contributes to Body Temperature Regulation  349

       Water Helps Remove Waste Products  350
       Other Functions of Water  351
       How Much Water Do We Need per Day?  351
       Thirst  353
       What If the Thirst Message Is Ignored?  353
       Healthy Beverage Consumption Guidelines  353
       Is There Such a Thing as Too Much Water?  355
       Our Water Supply: Safety Issues  355
       Monitoring the Safety of Your Water  356
       Options Regarding You Water Source  356

9.2    Minerals—An Overview  356
       Mineral Bioavailability  357
       Fiber-Mineral Interactions  358
       Mineral-Mineral Interactions  358
       Vitamin-Mineral Interactions  358
       Mineral Toxicities  358

9.3    Major Minerals  359

9.4    Sodium (Na)  359
       Sodium Sources and Needs  360
       Upper Level for Sodium  361

9.5    Potassium (K)  362
       Potassium Sources and Needs  362

9.6    Chloride (Cl)  364
       Chloride Sources and Needs  364
       Upper Level for Chloride  364

9.7    Calcium (Ca)  365
       Functions of Calcium  365
       Other Possible Health Benefits of Calcium  365
       Calcium Sources and Needs  366
       Calcium Supplements  367
       Upper Level for Calcium  368

9.8    Phosphorus (P)  368
       Phosphorus Sources and Needs  369
       Upper Level for Phosphorus  370

9.9    Magnesium (Mg)  370
       Magnesium Sources and Needs  370
       Upper Level for Magnesium  372

9.10 Sulfur (S) 372

9.11 Trace Minerals—An Overview 372

9.12 Iron (Fe) 374
Absorption and Distribution of Iron 374
Functions of Iron 375
Iron Sources and Needs 375
Upper Level for Iron 377

9.13 Zinc (Zn) 378
Functions of Zinc 379
Zinc Sources and Needs 379
Upper Level for Zinc 381

9.14 Selenium (Se) 381
Selenium Sources and Needs 381
Upper Level for Selenium 382

9.15 Iodide (I) 383
Function of Iodide 383
Iodide Sources and Needs 383
Upper Level for Iodide 383

9.16 Copper (Cu) 384
Copper Sources and Needs 384
Upper Level for Copper 385

9.17 Fluoride (F) 385
Functions of Fluoride 386
Fluoride Sources and Needs 386
Upper Level for Fluoride 386

9.18 Chromium (Cr) 387
Chromium Sources and Needs 387

9.19 Manganese (Mn) 387
Upper Level for Manganese 387

9.20 Molybdenum (Mo) 388
Upper Level for Molybdenum 388

9.21 Other Trace Minerals 390

Nutrition and Your Health: Maintaining a Healthy Blood
Pressure 391

Nutrition and Your Health: Preventing Osteoporosis 394

Case Study: Giving Up Milk 399

Summary 399

Study Questions 400

Check Your Knowledge 401

Further Readings 401

Rate Your Plate 403

## Part Four Nutrition: Beyond the Nutrients 406

**Chapter 10** Nutrition: Fitness and Sports 407

Student Learning Outcomes 407

Refresh Your Memory 408

10.1 The Close Relationship Between Nutrition and
Fitness 408

10.2 Guidelines for Achieving and Maintaining Physical
Fitness 410
Aerobic Workout 411

10.3 Energy Sources for Exercising Muscles 412
Phosphocreatine Is the First Line of Defense for Resupplying ATP
in Muscles 413
Carbohydrate Fuel for Muscles 414
Fat: The Main Fuel for Prolonged Low-Intensity Activity 416
Protein: A Minor Fuel Source, Primarily for Endurance
Exercise 417

10.4 Power Food: Dietary Advice for Athletes 418
Calorie Needs 418
Carbohydrate Needs 419
Carbohydrate Loading 421
Fat Needs 422
Protein Needs 422
Vitamin and Mineral Needs 423

10.5 A Focus on Fluid Needs 425
Sports Drinks 427

10.6 Specialized Dietary Advice for Before, During, and After
Endurance Exercise 428
Replenishing Fuel During Endurance Exercise 429
Carbohydrate Intake During Recovery from Prolonged
Exercise 430

Nutrition and Your Health: Ergogenic Aids and Athletic
Performance 432

Case Study: Planning a Training Diet 434

Summary 435

Study Questions 435

Check Your Knowledge 436

Further Readings 436

Rate Your Plate 438

**Chapter 11** Eating Disorders: Anorexia Nervosa, Bulimia Nervosa, and Other Conditions 445

Student Learning Outcomes 445

Refresh Your Memory 446

11.1  From Ordered to Disordered Eating Habits 446
   Food: More than Just a Source of Nutrients 447
   Overview of Anorexia Nervosa and Bulimia Nervosa 447

11.2  A Closer Look at Anorexia Nervosa 450
   Profile of the Typical Person with Anorexia Nervosa 451
   Early Warning Signs 451
   Physical Effects of Anorexia Nervosa 452
   Treatment of Anorexia Nervosa 454

11.3  A Closer Look at Bulimia Nervosa 455
   Typical Behavior in Bulimia Nervosa 456
   Health Problems Stemming from Bulimia Nervosa 457
   Treatment of Bulimia Nervosa 457

11.4  Other Disordered Eating Patterns 459
   Binge-Eating Disorder 459
   Night Eating Syndrome 461
   Female Athlete Triad 462

11.5  Prevention of Eating Disorders 463

Nutrition and Your Health: Eating Disorder Reflections 465

Case Study: Eating Disorders—Steps to Recovery 467

Summary 467

Study Questions 468

Check Your Knowledge 468

Further Readings 469

Rate Your Plate 471


**Chapter 12** Undernutrition Throughout the World 473

Student Learning Outcomes 473

Refresh Your Memory 474

12.1  World Hunger: A Crisis on the Rise 474
   Hunger 474
   Malnutrition and Macronutrient Deficiencies 475
   Famine 475
   General Effects of Semistarvation 477

12.2  Undernutrition in the United States 478
   Helping the Hungry in the United States 478
   Socioeconomic Factors Related to Undernutrition 480
   Possible Solutions to Poverty and Hunger in the United States 481

12.3  Undernutrition in the Developing World 482
   Food/Population Ratio 483
   War and Political/Civil Unrest 484
   Rapid Depletion of Natural Resources 485
   Inadequate Shelter and Sanitation 486
   High External Debt 487

The Impact of AIDS Worldwide 488
Reducing Undernutrition in the Developing World 490

12.4  The Role of Sustainable Agriculture and Biotechnology in Worldwide Food Availability 492
   Sustainable Agriculture 492
   Biotechnology 493
   Role of the New Biotechnology in the Developing World 494
   Some Concluding Thoughts 495

Nutrition and Your Health: Undernutrition at Critical Life Stages 496

Case Study: Undernutrition During Childhood 499

Summary 499

Study Questions 500

Check Your Knowledge 500

Further Readings 501

Rate Your Plate 503


**Chapter 13** Safety of Our Food Supply 505

Student Learning Outcomes 505

Refresh Your Memory 506

13.1  Food Safety: Setting the Stage 506
   Effects of Foodborne Illness 507
   Why Is Foodborne Illness So Common? 507

13.2  Food Preservation—Past, Present, and Future 510

13.3  Foodborne Illness Caused by Microorganisms 510
   Bacteria 511
   Viruses 514
   Parasites 515

13.4  Food Additives 515
   Why Are Food Additives Used? 515
   Intentional versus Incidental Food Additives 519
   The GRAS List 519
   Are Synthetic Chemicals Always Harmful? 519
   Tests of Food Additives for Safety 520
   Approval for a New Food Additive 520

13.5  Substances that Occur Naturally in Foods and Can Cause Illness 521
   Is Caffeine a Cause for Concern? 522

13.6  Environmental Contaminants in Food 523
   Pesticides in Food 525

What Is a Pesticide? 525
Why Use Pesticides? 525
Regulation of Pesticides 526
How Safe Are Pesticides? 526
Tests of the Amounts of Pesticides in Foods 526
Personal Action 527
13.7 Food Production Choices 527
Organic Foods 528
Sustainable Agriculture 529
Locally Grown Foods 529
Community Supported Agriculture 530
Nutrition and Your Health: Preventing Foodborne Illness 531
Case Study: Preventing Foodborne Illness at Gatherings 535
Summary 535
Study Questions 536
Check Your Knowledge 536
Further Readings 537
Rate Your Plate 538

**Part Five** Nutrition: A Focus on Life Stages 540

**Chapter 14** Pregnancy and Breastfeeding 541

Student Learning Outcomes 541
Refresh Your Memory 542
14.1 Planning for Pregnancy 542
14.2 Prenatal Growth and Development 543
Early Growth—The First Trimester Is a Very Critical Time 544
Second Trimester 545
Third Trimester 546
14.3 Success in Pregnancy 546
Infant Birthweight 547
Prenatal Care and Counseling 547
Effects of Maternal Age 547
Closely Spaced and Multiple Births 548
Smoking, Medication Use, and Drug Abuse 548
Food Safety 548
Nutritional Status 548
Nutrition Assistance for Low-Income Families 549
14.4 Increased Nutrient Needs to Support Pregnancy 549
Increased Calorie Needs 550
Adequate Weight Gain 550
Increased Protein and Carbohydrate Needs 552
A Word About Lipids 552
Increased Vitamin Needs 553
Increased Mineral Needs 553
Use of Prenatal Vitamin and Mineral Supplements 554
14.5 Food Plan for Pregnant Women 555
Pregnant Vegetarians 556
14.6 Physiological Changes of Concern During Pregnancy 557
Heartburn, Constipation, and Hemorrhoids 557

Edema 558
Morning Sickness 558
Anemia 558
Gestational Diabetes 559
Pregnancy-Induced Hypertension 559
14.7 Breastfeeding 560
Ability to Breastfeed 560
Production of Human Milk 561
Let-Down Reflex 561
Nutritional Qualities of Human Milk 562
Food Plan for Women Who Breastfeed 563
Breastfeeding Today 564
Nutrition and Your Health: Preventing Birth Defects 568
Case Study: Preparing for Pregnancy 572
Summary 572
Study Questions 573
Check Your Knowledge 573
Further Readings 574
Rate Your Plate 576

**Chapter 15** Nutrition from Infancy Through Adolescence 579

Student Learning Outcomes 579
Refresh Your Memory 580
15.1 Nutrition and Child Health—An Introduction 580
15.2 Infant Growth and Nutrition Needs 580
The Growing Infant 581
Effect of Undernutrition on Growth 582
Assessment of Infant Growth and Development 582
Adipose Tissue Growth 583
Failure to Thrive 584

Infant Nutritional Needs  584
Formula Feeding for Infants  588
Feeding Technique  589
Expanding the Infant's Mealtime Choices  589
Weaning from the Breast or Bottle  592
Dietary Guidelines for Infant Feeding  592
What Not to Feed an Infant  593
Inappropriate Infant Feeding Practices  594

15.3  Preschool Children: Nutrition Concerns  595
How to Help a Child Choose Nutritious Foods  595
Childhood Feeding Problems  595
Do Children Need a Multivitamin and Mineral Supplement?  597
Nutritional Problems in Preschool Children  598

15.4  School-Age Children: Nutrition Concerns  600
Breakfast  602
Fat Intake  602
Type 2 Diabetes  603
Early Signs of Cardiovascular Disease  604
Overweight and Obesity  604

15.5  Teenage Years: Nutrition Concerns  605
Nutritional Problems and Concerns of Teens  606
Helping Teens Eat More Nutritious Foods  607
Are Teenage Snacking Practices Harmful?  607

Nutrition and Your Health: Food Allergies and Intolerances  608

Case Study: Undernutrition During Infancy  611

Summary  612

Study Questions  612

Check Your Knowledge  613

Further Readings  613

Rate Your Plate  615

## Chapter 16  Nutrition During Adulthood  619

Student Learning Outcomes  619

Refresh Your Memory  620

16.1  The Graying of North America  620

16.2  Physiological Changes During Adulthood  621
Usual and Successful Aging  623
Factors Affecting the Rate of Aging  623
Heredity  623
Lifestyle  624
Environment  624

16.3  Nutrient Needs During Adulthood  625
Defining Nutrient Needs  626
Are Adults Following Current Dietary Recommendations?  629

16.4  Factors Related to Food Intake and Nutrient Needs  629
Physiological Factors  630
Alternative Medicine and Aging  634
Psychosocial Factors  636

16.5  Nutrition Implications of Alcohol Consumption  638
How Alcoholic Beverages are Produced  639
Absorption and Metabolism of Alcohol  639
Benefits of Moderate Alcohol Use  639
Risks of Alcohol Abuse  639
Guidance Regarding Alcohol Use  642

16.6  Ensuring a Healthful Diet for the Adult Years  643
Community Nutrition Services for Older People  644

Nutrition and Your Health: Nutrition and Cancer  646

Case Study: Dietary Assistance for an Older Adult  650

Summary  650

Study Questions  651

Check Your Knowledge  651

Further Readings  652

Rate Your Plate  654


Appendix A      Solutions: Case Studies  A-1
Appendix B      Daily Values Used in Food Labels  A-10
Appendix C      Dietary Advice for Canadians  A-11
Appendix D      The Exchange System: A Helpful Menu-Planning Tool  A-23
Appendix E      Dietary Intake and Energy Expenditure Assessment  A-36
Appendix F      Chemical Structures Important in Nutrition  A-46
Appendix G      Metropolitan Life Insurance Company Height-Weight Table and Determination of Frame Size  A-51
Appendix H      Sources of Nutrition Information  A-53
Appendix I      English-Metric Conversions and Metric Units  A-57

Glossary  G-1

Credits  C-1

Index  I-1

# About the Authors

GORDON M. WARDLAW, Ph.D., has taught introductory nutrition courses to students in the Department of Human Nutrition at The Ohio State University and at other colleges and universities. Dr. Wardlaw is the author of many articles that have appeared in prominent nutrition, biology, physiology, and biochemistry journals and was the 1985 recipient of the American Dietetic Association's Mary P. Huddleson Award. Dr. Wardlaw is a member of the American Society for Nutritional Sciences and is certified as a Specialist in Human Nutrition by the American Board of Nutrition. Dr. Wardlaw is currently retired from academia.

ANNE M. SMITH, Ph.D., R.D., L.D., currently teaches nutrition majors and nonmajors at The Ohio State University and was the recipient of the 1995 Outstanding Teacher Award from the College of Human Ecology. Dr. Smith is the Director of the Didactic Program in Dietetics in the Department of Human Nutrition, College of Education and Human Ecology, of The Ohio State University and received the 2008 Outstanding Dietetic Educator Award from the Ohio Dietetic Association and the 1998 Emerging Dietetic Leader Award from the American Dietetic Association. She also was the recipient of the 2006 Outstanding Faculty Member Award from the Department of Human Nutrition for her commitment to undergraduate education in nutrition. Dr. Smith conducts research in the area of vitamin and mineral metabolism and was awarded the 1996 Departmental Research Award from the Ohio Agricultural Research and Development Center. Dr. Smith's research articles have appeared in prominent nutrition journals. She is a member of the American Nutrition Society and the American Dietetic Association.

# Preface

## Introducing the Eighth Edition

This new edition of *Contemporary Nutrition* has been revised to offer up-to-date nutrition information in a format that is easy to use. The following paragraphs showcase the new features and strengths of the eighth edition and describe content enhancements related to recent advances in nutritional science.

### Our Approach to Teaching Nutrition

Those of us who teach nutrition find it a fascinating subject. At the same time, it can be a challenge to teach nutrition because new results emerge from research studies at an incredible pace. Claims and counterclaims flourish about the need for and benefits of certain components of our diets and supplements. *Contemporary Nutrition* is a resource designed to help instructors accurately convey changing and seemingly conflicting messages to students in introductory nutrition courses. Our students commonly have misconceptions about nutrition, and many have a limited background in biology or chemistry. *Contemporary Nutrition* conveys complex scientific concepts at a level that enables undergraduate students to meaningfully apply the material we cover in class to their own lives.

### Keeping Current

The vast amount of published research is constantly reshaping our knowledge of nutritional science. As authors and teachers, we constantly search the literature to ensure that students' exposure to the study of nutrition in *Contemporary Nutrition* is reliable, accurate, and as up-to-date as this rapidly changing field allows. We emphasize recommendations published by federal agencies such as the U.S. Department of Agriculture (USDA) and the Food and Drug Administration (FDA) and professional organizations such as the American Heart Association. The eighth edition includes more integrated coverage of the 2005 Dietary Guidelines for Americans and the USDA MyPyramid. The newly released *MyPyramid for Preschoolers*, *MyPyramid for Kids*, and *Modified MyPyramid for Older Adults* have been added, as well as other recent recommendations and research findings. We continue to draw on many reputable sources to create a balanced resource for nutrition information. Each chapter contains an updated list of Further Readings as well as links to reputable nutrition and health information websites. We strive to present an objective approach to newly emerging or controversial topics so that students learn to carefully scrutinize the nutritional information they read and hear about. Several controversial topics are presented in "Making Decisions" boxes within each chapter.

### Understanding Our Audience

We have written *Contemporary Nutrition* assuming that our students have a limited background in college-level biology, chemistry, or physiology. We have been careful to include the essential science foundation needed to adequately comprehend certain topics in nutrition, such as the basic discussion of protein synthesis in Chapter 6. Scientific discussions have been written in a simple, straightforward manner.

Students enrolled in an introductory nutrition course often come from a broad range of majors and interests. We address this diversity by incorporating a thorough system of pedagogical tools, such as Learning Outcomes, critical thinking questions and the new *Concept Maps* to help them master the material. A variety of applications and case studies are included to appeal to students whose major areas of study range from business to education.

### Personalizing Nutrition

A prominent theme in nutrition today is *individuality*. This trait was even incorporated into the name of the most recent USDA food guide: "MyPyramid." Throughout *Contemporary Nutrition*, we reinforce the fact that each person responds differently to nutrients. Not all of us, for example, find that saturated fat

---

"*Contemporary Nutrition (is)* an outstanding introductory nutrition textbook. . . . It's very readable and the quality of the information is excellent.

*Karen Schuster, Florida Community College of Jacksonville*

in our diet raises our blood cholesterol values above recommended standards. The text's discussions do not assume that all students are alike. Chapter content and features, such as Making Decisions, Critical Thinking, Nutrition and Your Health, Case Studies, and Rate Your Plate, repeatedly ask students to learn more about themselves and their health status and to use their new knowledge to improve their health.

After reading this textbook, students will be better equipped to understand how the nutrition information coming from all directions—whether on food packages, Internet sites, or the evening news; in popular magazines and newspapers; or from government agencies—applies to them. Our goal is for students to understand that their knowledge of nutrition will allow them to evaluate and personalize nutrition information, rather than to follow every guideline issued for an entire population. We emphasize that a population consists of individuals with varying genetic and cultural backgrounds, and these individuals will have varying responses to diet. The section "A Closer Look at Genetics and Nutrition" (Chapter 3) has been greatly expanded and includes new information on genetic testing and the new area of study called *epigenetics.*

As a final note on bringing nutrition down to a personal level, the book covers topics of particular interest to college students such as popular weight-loss diets, eating disorders, dietary supplements, vegetarianism, and sports nutrition. These topics are introduced in the section "Eating Well in College" in Chapter 1. Regardless of topic, the overall emphasis remains the same—the importance of understanding one's food choices and modifying one's diet to best meet personal needs.

## Organization

The eighth edition of *Contemporary Nutrition* remains organized into five parts that reflect major topics typically covered in an introductory nutrition course:

| | |
|---|---|
| Part One | Nutrition: A Key to Health |
| Part Two | The Energy Nutrients and Energy Balance |
| Part Three | Vitamins, Minerals, and Water |
| Part Four | Nutrition: Beyond the Nutrients |
| Part Five | Nutrition: A Focus on Life Stages |

Although most frequently used in semester-long courses, the text's organization allows instructors to omit parts or chapters to fit the needs of quarter-length courses. For example, Part Five, Focus on the Life Stages, can be easily omitted from an introductory course. In addition, chapters are written in such a way that each can function independently so that instructors can cover the material in the order that best fits their particular course needs.

## New Illustrations and Photos Enhance the Learning Experience

We believe the more a textbook can engage readers, the more effective will be their learning experience. Carefully crafted illustrations that are closely supported by textual explanations are key to creating a dynamic learning tool. With that in mind, the eighth edition of *Contemporary Nutrition* features a totally revamped art and photo program. Over 100 new or highly modified diagrams and 200 new photos were incorporated to better convey complex scientific concepts and to provide up-to-date, real-life examples. We have also refreshed the illustrations with a more modern style and brighter colors to appeal to today's students. The dynamic new art makes *Contemporary Nutrition* the most thoroughly illustrated and visually appealing introductory textbook on the market.

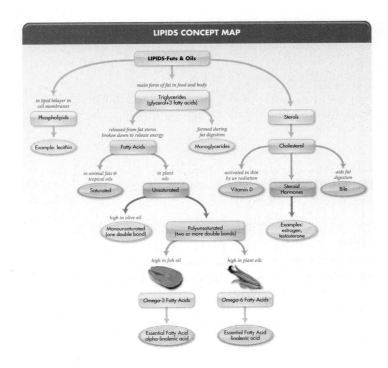

New Concept Maps for each of the macronutrients are one example of how we have used illustrations to help students grasp the interrelatedness of complex concepts. These concept maps provide students with an overall framework for understanding the characteristics and functions of the carbohydrates, lipids, and proteins, respectively.

"Besides good, research-based information, it has colorful interesting photographs, good tables and charts, interesting special topics, good case study topics for discussion. . . . , I am very impressed with it."

*Linda D. DeTurk, North Platte Community College*

## Chapter-by-Chapter Revisions

In response to feedback from instructors using this and other introductory nutrition texts, we have streamlined and refined the content to better meet the needs of today's students. The following list highlights just some of the changes in the eighth edition of *Contemporary Nutrition*. For those planning to update their class notes based on the new edition, please contact your McGraw-Hill representative for a more detailed list of changes.

## Chapter 1: What You Eat and Why

▶ Table 1-2 has been updated to provide current (2008) statistics from the CDCP on the leading causes of death in the United States.

▶ An update on the scheduled release of Healthy People 2020 objectives is included.

▶ A new chart illustrates the dramatic change in the percentage of food dollars spent by American households for food consumed at and away from home.

▶ "Nutrition and Your Health: Eating Well in College" has been updated and includes a new table of "Calorie traps for college students."

## Chapter 2: Guidelines for Designing a Healthy Diet

▶ The updated (2009) Mediterranean Diet Pyramid has been included under Recommendations for Healthy Eating.

▶ Presentation of the Dietary Guidelines now includes recommendations for specific population groups as well as the key recommendations for the general public.

▶ Discussion of the 2008 Physical Activity Guidelines for Americans is now included as a margin note to complement the Dietary Guidelines.

▶ The chapter culminates with "Nutrition and Your Health: Evaluating Nutrition Claims and Dietary Supplements" and the Case Study on Dietary Supplements, which both provide suggestions for healthful and logical nutrition decisions.

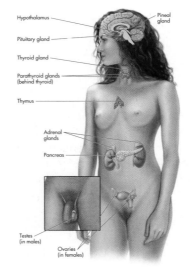

## Chapter 3: The Human Body: A Nutrition Perspective

▶ More emphasis has been given to nutrition and genetics in this edition. "A Closer Look at Genetics and Nutrition" now includes a discussion of *epigenetics* as well as nutrigenomics. "Personalized nutrition" is discussed in the Making Decisions box, and an expanded discussion of genetic testing is included under "Genetic Profile."

▶ The chapter concludes with "Nutrition and Your Health: Common Problems with Digestion" and the Case Study on Gastroesophageal Reflux Disease. Figure 3-24 is a new illustration of Gastroesophageal Reflux Disease.

## Chapter 4: Carbohydrates

▶ New Carbohydrate Concept map summarizes the characteristics and functions of the simple and complex carbohydrates.

▶ The discussion of "Alternative Sweeteners" has been expanded to include an explanation of the Acceptable Daily Intake (ADI) guideline for safe consumption of sweeteners. Information about Stevia, the sweetener recently added to the Generally Recognized As Safe (GRAS) list, is also included.

▶ New Making Decisions box provides answers to the question, "Are you pre-diabetic?"

## Chapter 5: Lipids

▶ New Lipid Concept Map illustrates the characteristics and functions of the fats and oils.

▶ Discussion of the Acceptable Macronutrient Distribution Range for fat is now included.

▶ Figure 5-11 is a new illustration of the role of bile acids in the digestion and absorption of large fat globules.

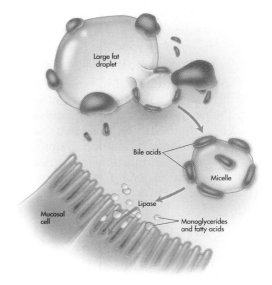

▶ The chapter concludes with a new Rate Your Plate activity enabling students to answer the question "Is Your Diet High in Saturated and Trans Fat?"

## Chapter 6: Proteins

▶ More attention has been given to the effectiveness of high-protein weight-loss diets in the section on protein's role in "Contributing to Satiety."

▶ Table 6-2 illustrates the protein content of new sample menus containing 1,600 kcal and 2,000 kcal.

▶ Protein functions are now summarized in the new Protein Concept Map.

## Chapter 7: Energy Balance and Weight Control

▶ The increase in obesity since 1990 is now illustrated in Figure 7-1 using the CDC Behavioral Risk Factor Surveillance System maps from 1990, 1998, and 2007.

▶ The section on "Estimating Body Fat Content and Diagnosing Obesity" now includes a discussion of body composition monitors, better known as body fat calculators.

▶ The "Nutrition and Your Health: Popular Diets—Cause for Concern" has been revised to include an up-to-date Summary of Popular Diet Approaches to Weight Control (Table 7-6) as well as discussion of the results of recent diet studies.

## Chapter 8: Vitamins

▶ The availability of freshly harvested fruits and vegetables from food cooperatives, Community Supported Agriculture, and farmers' markets has been emphasized in the section on "Preservation of Vitamins in Food."

▶ An expanded discussion of the safety and monitoring of the vitamin A analog, isotretinoin, is included with information about iPLEDGE, the mandatory distribution program.

▶ The nutritional advantage of whole grains is illustrated in a new figure comparing whole wheat to white bread and brown to white rice.

▶ Figure 8-36 provides a new summary of the functions of the fat-soluble and water-soluble vitamins.

## Chapter 9: Water and Minerals

▶ The water content of foods is now depicted graphically in Figure 9-3 and related to the MyPyramid food groups.

▶ A new graphic illustrates sodium sources in the American diet.

▶ Daily Values have been added to all of the Food Sources tables.

▶ Figure 9-29 has been enhanced with illustrations of women with and without osteoporosis.

## Chapter 10: Nutrition: Fitness and Sports

▶ The *Exercise Is Medicine* initiative spearheaded by the American College of Sports Medicine is now discussed and recommended as a resource for incorporating fitness goals into routine medical care.

▶ Figure 10-2 is a new illustration of the effect of age in predicting maximum heart rate (MHR).

▶ "Nutrition and Your Health: Ergogenic Aids and Athletic Performance" has been updated to include information on consumer spending on sports nutrition supplements.

## Chapter 11: Eating Disorders: Anorexia Nervosa, Bulimia Nervosa, and Other Conditions

▶ Discussion of the link between disordered eating behaviors and substance abuse has been added as a margin note.

▶ The Critical Thinking scenario is expanded to discuss what parents should do if they suspect an eating disorder.

## Chapter 12: Undernutrition Throughout the World

▶ The content of this chapter has been greatly revised with an expanded discussion of the relationships among food insecurity, homelessness, hunger, and malnutrition.

▶ The impact of the American Recovery and Reinvestment Act of 2009 on federally subsidized nutrition programs is discussed. Updates to the Food Stamp Program, now called the Supplemental Nutrition Assistance Program (SNAP), are also included.

▶ The global impact of HIV/AIDS is now illustrated in Figure 12-4, which depicts the adult prevalence of HIV infection in countries worldwide.

▶ The section on Food Availability has been revised to include *sustainable agriculture* as a major topic as well as updated content on biotechnology.

## Chapter 13: Safety of Our Food Supply

▶ The chapter has been revised to focus on safety of food. Safety of our water supply has been moved to Chapter 9, Water and Minerals.

▶ A completely new section, "Food Production Choices," has been added and includes significant discussion of organic foods, sustainable agriculture, locally grown foods, and community-supported agriculture.

▶ Table 13-1 has been updated to include information on recent outbreaks of foodborne illness.

▶ Students are asked to take "A Closer Look at Organic Foods" in the new Rate Your Plate activity.

## Chapter 14: Pregnancy and Breastfeeding

▶ "Staying Active During Pregnancy" is the focus of a new Making Decisions.

▶ A new link to *MyPyramid for Pregnancy and Breastfeeding* encourages the reader to generate recommendations for each trimester.

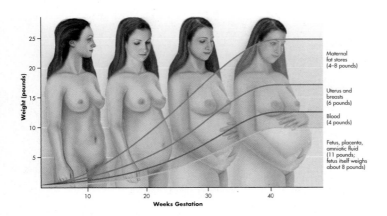

## Chapter 15: Nutrition from Infancy Through Adolescence

▶ Information about bisphenol A (BPA) use in baby bottles is included in a new margin note.

▶ Readers are directed to the *MyPyramid for Preschoolers* and the *Start Healthy, Stay Healthy* websites for resources for planning age-appropriate meals and snacks. The new *MyPyramid for Children* is included as Figure 15-3.

▶ Nutrition Problems for Preschool Children has been updated with a discussion of *autism* and nutrient-based theories concerning its cause and treatment, as well as *lead poisoning.*

▶ Healthy snack ideas for school-age children have been expanded and the key nutrients (iron, zinc, calcium, vitamin C, and fiber) provided by them have been highlighted in Table 15-4.

## Chapter 16: Nutrition During Adulthood

▶ *Sarcopenia* has been added to the discussion of "Factors Related to Food Intake and Nutrient Needs."

▶ "Nutrition Interventions for Arthritis" has been added as a Making Decisions box.

▶ The *Modified MyPyramid for Older Adults* is discussed and illustrated in Figure 16-5.

## SPECIAL ACKNOWLEDGMENTS

Writing a textbook requires much energy and constant support. We are indebted to several individuals for their creative abilities and generous interest in the production of this book. First, our deepest gratitude to our editor Lynne Meyers, whose patience and encouragement has been fantastic. She and her staff at McGraw-Hill have guided and assisted us through every phase of the revision and facilitated the beautiful enhancements to the art design of this edition. This edition is also much improved by the written contributions of Angela Collene, M.S., R.D. We thank her for always being ready at a moment's notice and for assistance in updating several chapters. We also thank Doug Lance and Tim Hickey for their frequent updates regarding media coverage of nutrition topics. Finally, we are grateful to April Southwood and her staff for the meticulous coordination of the many production efforts needed to produce the very appealing yet accurate eighth edition.

## THANK YOU TO REVIEWERS

Our goal is to provide students and educators with the most accurate, up-to-date, and useful textbook possible. As with earlier editions, the quality of the eighth edition of *Contemporary Nutrition* is largely dependent on the thorough, professional assistance of nutrition educators from academic institutions across the nation. We are indebted to these colleagues who reviewed the seventh edition, evaluated new material for the eighth edition, participated in instructional symposia, and responded to surveys. The advice and suggestions from these colleagues have been used in every chapter and have resulted in a textbook that is current and inviting.

*Darlene E. Berryman*
Ohio University

*Dawn D. Brown*
Cuesta College

*Victoria Pachero*
Pasadena City College

*Sue Carol Carr*
Patrick Henry Community College

*Prithiva Chanmugam*
Louisiana State University, Baton Rouge

*Linda D. DeTurk*
North Platte Community College

*Alyce D. Fly*
Indiana University

*Deborah Forman*
California State University Northridge

*Bernard L. Frye*
University of Texas at Arlington

*Art Gilbert*
University of California Santa Barbara

*Melissa Davis Gutschall*
Radford University

*Dea Hanson Baxter*
Georgia State University

*Nancy Harris*
East Carolina University

*Kimberly Heidal*
East Carolina University

*Karen Israel*
Anne Arundel Community College

*Janine Jensen*
Tulsa Community College

*Glenn D. Johnson*
Los Angeles Trade Tech College

*Lee-Ellen C. Kirkhorn*
University of Wisconsin–Eau Claire

*Teresa Marcus*
Chattanooga State Technical Community College

*Molly M. Michelman*
University of Nevada, Las Vegas

*Owen Murphy*
University of Colorado

*Cheryl L. Neudauer*
Minneapolis Community and Technical College

*Jen Nickelson*
University of North Florida

*Deborah Ocken*
Seattle Central Community College

*Donna M. Pace*
Delgado Community College

*Brian A. Rash*
Our Lady of the Lake College

*Bruce Rengers*
Metropolitan State College of Denver

*Rickelle Richards*
Brigham Young University

*Beverley Roe*
Erie Community College

*Karen Schuster*
Florida Community College at Jacksonville

*Dana Sherman*
Ozarks Technical Community College

*Judy Stauter*
University of Northern Colorado

*Ellen Steinberg*
Georgia State University

*James Stevens*
Metropolitan State College of Denver

*Richard Tulley*
Louisiana State University

*Jennifer Weddig*
Metropolitan State College of Denver

*Sally E. Weerts*
University of North Florida

## A Request to Instructors Who Use *Contemporary Nutrition*

Each new edition of *Contemporary Nutrition* begins with a desire to improve and enhance our textbook with the latest in information and design. As each revision comes to an end, we are satisfied knowing we have produced an effective and dependable resource for students beginning their study of nutrition. We try our best to address the vast range of nutrition science and the new developments and controversies. As you use this book, if you find content that you question or believe warrants further attention, please contact either of us:

*Gordon M. Wardlaw, Ph.D.*
44658 Little Lake Road
Mendocino, CA 95460
Phone: (707) 937-2160
E-mail: gordonmark.wardlaw@gmail.com

*Anne M. Smith, Ph.D., R.D., L.D.*
Department of Human Nutrition
The Ohio State University
350 Campbell Hall
1787 Neil Avenue, Columbus, OH 43210
Phone: (614) 292-0715  Fax: (614) 292-8880
E-mail: smith.23@osu.edu

# Supplementary Materials

## New Animations Increase Learning

Engaging 3-D animations are available for instructor and student use. Two new animations include a helpful math tutorial to help students better understand the information on nutrition facts panels and an overview of digestion, absorption, and metabolism. In addition, more than forty of McGraw-Hill's nutrition animations are available completely embedded in PowerPoint for easy, hassle-free use in lecture.

## Outstanding Media Package

The eighth edition of *Contemporary Nutrition* comes with a brand-new, cutting-edge set of tools for you to use in the classroom.

## Incorporate Engaging Presentation Materials into Lecture

A full set of PowerPoint lectures is available for you to download and customize to fit your needs.

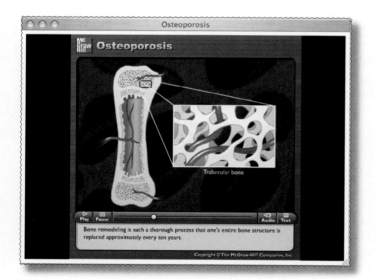

# Online Assignments and Course Management

**Connect Nutrition** is a Web-based assignment and assessment platform that gives students the means to better connect with their coursework, with their instructors, and with the important concepts that they will need to know for success now and in the future. With Connect Nutrition, instructors can deliver assignments, quizzes, and tests easily online. Students can practice important skills at their own pace and on their own schedule. With Connect Nutrition Plus, students also get 24/7 online access to a media-rich eBook to aid them in successfully completing their work, wherever and whenever they choose.

**LearnSmart's** artificially intelligent engine monitors students' knowledge level, and adaptive questioning provides appropriate content based on that level. LearnSmart helps students achieve mastery of the course material efficiently. Students learn faster and study more effectively. Learn Fast. Learn Easy. Learn Smart.

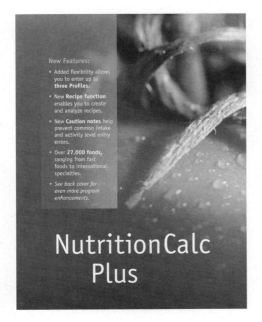

# Diet Analysis Software

**NutritionCalc Plus** is a suite of powerful dietary self-assessment tools available on CD and online. NutritionCalc Plus features approximately 27,000 foods from the ESHA Research nutrient database and a user-friendly interface that makes creating a personal diet analysis even easier. Users have the ability to add up to three profiles and to create their own recipes. The program functions are supported by detailed Help documents and helpful cautionary notes that warn the user of possible entry errors.

# CHAPTER 1 What You Eat and Why

## Student Learning Outcomes Chapter 1 is designed to allow you to:

1. Identify diet and lifestyle factors that contribute to the 10 leading causes of death in North America.
2. Define the terms *nutrition, carbohydrate, protein, lipid (fat), alcohol, vitamin, mineral, water, kilocalorie (kcal)*, and *fiber*.
3. Determine the total calories (kcal) of a food or diet using the weight and calorie content of the energy-yielding nutrients and use the basic units of the metric system to calculate percentages, such as percent of calories from fat in a diet.
4. Describe a basic plan for health promotion and disease prevention.
5. List the major characteristics of the North American diet and the food habits that often need improvement.
6. Describe how our food habits are affected by physiological processes, meal size and composition, early experiences, ethnic customs, health concerns, advertising, social class, and economics.
7. Identify food and *nutrition* issues relevant to college students.

## Chapter Outline

Student Learning Outcomes

Refresh Your Memory

1.1 Good Health: The Nutrition Connection

1.2 Classes and Sources of Nutrients

1.3 Nutrient Composition of Diets and the Human Body

1.4 Energy Sources and Uses

1.5 Current State of the North American Diet and Overall Health

1.6 Improving Our Diets

1.7 Why Am I So Hungry?

Nutrition and Your Health: Eating Well in College

Case Study: Typical College Student

Summary/Study Questions/Check Your Knowledge/Further Readings

Rate Your Plate

**ARE YOU EATING TOO MUCH SATURATED FAT, *TRANS* FAT, AND CHOLESTEROL?** Do carbohydrates in our diets cause many of our health problems? Is a high protein diet always safe and foolproof? Are some foods unsafe? Do you need to take a balanced multivitamin and mineral supplement? Should you become a vegetarian? If you have asked yourself any of these questions and are confused about what you should eat, you are not alone. Chapter 1 will help you sort out some of these issues as you are introduced to the science of nutrition.

As you begin this study of nutrition, keep this in mind. Research over the last 40 years has shown that a healthy diet—especially one rich in fruits, vegetables, and whole grains—coupled with regular prolonged, vigorous exercise and some strength-building exercise—can both prevent and treat many age-related diseases. Overall, it is clear that the nutrition aspect of the lifestyles of some (but not all) North Americans are out of balance with their metabolism and physiology. We live longer than our ancestors did, so preventing the diseases that develop during aging is a more important focus today than in the past.

What influences daily food choices? How important is taste? Appearance? Nutrition? Convenience? Cost (Value)? Celebrations (see comic below)? Do our daily food choices go on to influence long-term health? If so, to what extent? By making optimal dietary choices, we can strive to bring the goal of a long, healthy life within reach. This is the primary theme not just of Chapter 1 but throughout this book.

 **Refresh Your Memory**

As you begin your study of what you eat and why in Chapter 1, you may want to review:

- The metric system in Appendix I.

## 1.1 Good Health: The Nutrition Connection

In your lifetime, you will eat about 70,000 meals and 60 tons of food. Chapter 1 will take a close look at the general classes of nutrients supplied by this food, the role research plays in sorting out which food components are essential for the maintenance of health, and the powerful effect of dietary habits in determining overall health. Many factors influence our food choices (see the comic below) and will also be discussed in Chapter 1.

### What Is Nutrition?

*Nutrition* is the science that links foods to health and disease. It includes the processes by which the human organism ingests, digests, absorbs, transports, and excretes food substances.

### Nutrients Come from Food

**nutrients** Chemical substances in food that contribute to health, many of which are essential parts of a diet. Nutrients nourish us by providing calories to fulfill energy needs, materials for building body parts, and factors to regulate necessary chemical processes in the body.

What is the difference between food and **nutrients?** Food provides the energy (in the form of calories) as well as the materials needed to build and maintain all body cells. Nutrients are the substances obtained from food that are vital for growth and maintenance of a healthy body throughout life. For a substance to be considered an **essential nutrient,** three characteristics are needed:

- First, at least one specific biological function of the nutrient in the body must be identified.
- Second, omission of the nutrient from the diet must lead to a decline in certain biological functions, such as production of blood cells.
- Third, replacing the omitted nutrient in the diet before permanent damage occurs will restore those normal biological functions.

## Why Study Nutrition?

Nutrition is a lifestyle factor that is a key to developing and maintaining an optimal state of health for you. A poor diet and a sedentary lifestyle are known to be **risk factors** for life-threatening **chronic** diseases such as **cardiovascular (heart) disease, hypertension, diabetes,** and some forms of **cancer** (Table 1-1). Together, these and related

**essential nutrient** In nutritional terms, a substance that, when left out of a diet, leads to signs of poor health. The body either can't produce this nutrient or can't produce enough of it to meet its needs. Then, if added back to a diet before permanent damage occurs, the affected aspects of health are restored.

▲ The major health problems in North America are largely caused by a poor diet, excessive calorie intake, and not enough physical activity.

**glucose** A six-carbon sugar that exists in a ring form; found as such in blood, and in table sugar bound to fructose; also known as *dextrose*, it is one of the simple sugars.

**TABLE 1-1** Glossary Terms to Aid Your Introduction to Nutrition*

| | |
|---|---|
| Cancer | A condition characterized by uncontrolled growth of abnormal cells. |
| Cardiovascular (heart) disease | A general term that refers to any disease of the heart and circulatory system. This disease is generally characterized by the deposition of fatty material in the blood vessels (hardening of the arteries), which in turn can lead to organ damage and death. Also termed coronary heart disease (CHD), as the vessels of the heart are the primary sites of the disease. |
| Cholesterol | A waxy lipid found in all body cells; it has a structure containing multiple chemical rings. Cholesterol is found only in foods of animal origin. |
| Chronic | Long-standing, developing over time. When referring to disease, this term indicates that the disease process, once developed, is slow and lasting. A good example is cardiovascular disease. |
| Diabetes | A group of diseases characterized by high blood **glucose.** Type 1 diabetes involves insufficient or no release of the hormone insulin by the pancreas and therefore requires daily insulin therapy. Type 2 diabetes results from either insufficient release of insulin or general inability of insulin to act on certain body cells, such as muscle cells. Persons with type 2 diabetes may or may not require insulin therapy. |
| Hypertension | A condition in which blood pressure remains persistently elevated. Obesity, inactivity, alcohol intake, excess salt intake, and genetics may each contribute to the problem. |
| Kilocalorie (kcal) | Unit that describes the energy content of food. Specifically, a kilocalorie (kcal) is the heat energy needed to raise the temperature of 1000 grams (1 liter) of water 1° Celsius. Kcal refers to a 1000 calorie unit of measurement, but is commonly referred to as calories. It is a familiar term for the energy content of a food, so we will use it in this book. |
| Obesity | A condition characterized by excess body fat. |
| Osteoporosis | Decreased bone mass related to the effects of aging (including estrogen loss during menopause in women), genetic background, and poor diet. |
| Risk factor | A term used frequently when discussing the factors contributing to the development of a disease. A risk factor is an aspect of our lives— such as heredity, lifestyle choices (e.g., smoking), or nutritional habits. |

*Many bold terms are also defined in the page margins within each chapter and in the glossary at the end of this book.

▲ Many foods are rich sources of nutrients.

disorders account for two-thirds of all deaths in North America (Table 1-2). Not meeting nutrient needs in younger years makes us more likely to suffer health consequences, such as bone fractures from the disease **osteoporosis,** in later years. At the same time, taking too much of a nutrient—such as vitamin A supplement—can be harmful. Another dietary problem, drinking too much alcohol, is associated with many health problems.

U.S. government scientists have calculated that a poor diet combined with a lack of sufficient physical activity contributes to hundreds of thousands of fatal cases of cardiovascular disease, cancer, and diabetes each year among adults in the United States. Thus, the combination of poor diet and too little physical activity may be the second leading cause of death in the United States. In addition, **obesity** is considered the second leading cause of preventable death in North America (smoking is the first). Put together, obesity and smoking cause even more health problems. Obesity and chronic diseases are often preventable. The cost of prevention is a small fraction of the cost of treating these diseases. Age fast or age slowly: It is partly your choice.

**stroke** A decrease or loss in blood flow to the brain that results from a blood clot or other change in arteries in the brain. This in turn causes the death of brain tissue. Also called a *cerebrovascular accident.*

**TABLE 1-2** Fifteen Leading Causes of Death in the United States

| Rank | Cause of Death | Percent of Total Deaths |
|------|----------------|-------------------------|
| | All causes | 100 |
| 1 | Diseases of the heart (heart disease)*†# | 26.6 |
| 2 | Malignant neoplasms (cancer)*‡ | 22.8 |
| 3 | Cerebrovascular diseases (**stroke**)*†‡# | 5.9 |
| 4 | Chronic lower respiratory diseases (lung diseases)‡ | 5.3 |
| 5 | Accidents (unintentional injuries) | 4.8 |
| 6 | Diabetes mellitus* | 3.1 |
| 7 | Alzheimer's disease* | 2.9 |
| 8 | Influenza and pneumonia | 2.6 |
| 9 | Kidney disease*‡ | 1.8 |
| 10 | Blood-borne infections | 1.4 |
| 11 | Suicide | 1.3 |
| 12 | Chronic liver disease and cirrhosis† | 1.1 |
| 13 | Essential hypertension* | 1.0 |
| 14 | Parkinson's disease | 0.8 |
| 15 | Homicide | 0.7 |

From Centers for Disease Control and Prevention, *National Vital Statistics Report,* Final Data for 2005, April 24, 2008. Canadian statistics are quite similar.

*Causes of death in which diet plays a part

†Causes of death in which excessive alcohol consumption plays a part

‡Causes of death in which tobacco use plays a part

#Diseases of the heart and cerebrovascular disease are included in the more global term "cardiovascular disease."

The good news is that the increased interest in health, fitness and, nutrition shown by Americans has been associated with long-term decreasing trends for heart disease, cancer, and stroke (the three leading causes of death) that continued in 2005. Mortality from heart disease, the leading cause of death, has been declining steadily since 1980. As you gain understanding about your nutritional habits and increase your knowledge about optimal nutrition, you will have the opportunity to dramatically reduce your risk for many common health problems. For additional help, the U.S. federal government provides two websites that contain links to many sources of health and nutrition information (www.healthfinder.gov and www.nutrition.gov). Other useful sites are webmd.com and www.eatright.org.

## 1.2 Classes and Sources of Nutrients

To begin the study of nutrition, let's start with an overview of the six classes of nutrients. You are probably already familiar with the terms **carbohydrates, lipids** (fats and oils), **proteins, vitamins,** and **minerals.** These, plus **water,** make up the six classes of nutrients found in food (Table 1-3).

Nutrients can then be assigned to three functional categories: (1) those that primarily provide us with calories to meet energy needs (expressed in **kilocalories [kcal]**); (2) those important for growth, development, and maintenance; and (3) those that act to keep body functions running smoothly. Some function overlap exists among these categories. The energy-yielding nutrients, carbohydrate, fat, and protein, make up a major portion of most foods (Table 1-4).

Let's now look more closely at these six classes of nutrients.

### Carbohydrates

Chemically, carbohydrates are composed mainly of the **elements** carbon, hydrogen, and oxygen. Carbohydrates provide a major source of calories for the body, on average 4 kcal per gram. Carbohydrates can exist as simple sugars and complex carbohydrates. **Simple sugars,** frequently referred to as *sugars,* are relatively small molecules. The smallest simple sugars consist of a single sugar unit and are called monosaccharides. The sugar in your blood, glucose (also known as *blood sugar* or *dextrose*), is an example of a monosaccharide. Other simple sugars are made by joining two **monosaccharides** to form a **disaccharide.** Table sugar, sucrose, is an example of a disaccharide because it is formed from fructose and glucose (both monosaccharides). Joining many monosaccharides—often found as repeating units—forms **polysaccharides,** also known as **complex carbohydrates.** For example, plants store carbohydrates in the form of **starch,** a polysaccharide made up of hundreds of repeating glucose units.

During digestion, complex carbohydrates are broken down into single sugar molecules (such as glucose), and absorbed via **cells** lining the small intestine into the bloodstream (see Chapter 3 for more on digestion and absorption). However, the **bonds** between the sugar molecules in certain complex carbohydrates, called **fiber,** cannot be broken down by human digestive processes. Fiber passes through the small intestine undigested to provide bulk for the stool (feces) formed in the large intestine (colon).

Aside from enjoying their taste, we need sugars and other carbohydrates in our diets primarily to help satisfy the calorie needs of our body cells. Glucose, a simple sugar that the body can derive from most carbohydrates, is a major source of calories for most cells. When not enough carbohydrate is consumed to supply sufficient glucose, the body is forced to make glucose from proteins—not a healthy change. Chapter 4 focuses on carbohydrates.

**carbohydrate** A compound containing carbon, hydrogen, and oxygen atoms. Most are known as *sugars, starches,* and *fibers.*

**lipid** A compound containing much carbon and hydrogen, little oxygen, and sometimes other atoms. Lipids do not dissolve in water, and include fats, oils, and cholesterol.

**protein** Food and body compounds made of amino acids; proteins contain carbon, hydrogen, oxygen, nitrogen, and sometimes other atoms, in a specific configuration. Proteins contain the form of nitrogen most easily used by the human body.

**vitamin** Compound needed in very small amounts in the diet to help regulate and support chemical reactions in the body.

**mineral** Element used to promote chemical reactions and to form body structures.

**water** The universal solvent; chemically, $H_2O$. The body is composed of about 60% water. Water (fluid) needs are about 9 (women) or 13 (men) cups per day; needs are greater if one exercises heavily.

**kilocalorie (kcal)** Heat energy needed to raise the temperature of 1000 grams (1 L) of water 1 degree Celsius; also written as *Calories.*

**element** A substance that cannot be separated into simpler substances by chemical processes. Common elements in nutrition include carbon, oxygen, hydrogen, nitrogen, calcium, phosphorus, and iron.

**simple sugar** Monosaccharide or disaccharide in the diet.

**monosaccharide** Simple sugar, such as glucose, that is not broken down further during digestion.

**disaccharide** Class of sugars formed by the chemical bonding of two monosaccharides.

**polysaccharide** Class of complex carbohydrates containing many glucose units, from 10 to 1000 or more.

**complex carbohydrate** Carbohydrate composed of many monosaccharide molecules. Examples include glycogen, starch, and fiber.

**cell** The structural basis of plant and animal organization. Cells contain genetic material and systems for synthesizing energy-yielding compounds. Cells have the ability to take up compounds from and excrete compounds into their surroundings.

**TABLE 1-3** Essential Nutrients in the Human Diet, Their Classes* and Good Dietary Sources

Some nutrients that perform important functions can be produced by the body if they are missing from the diet. Whether these nutrients are essential is not clear-cut. For example, humans require vitamin D, but the body is capable of synthesizing its own vitamin D upon exposure of the skin to sunlight. This reduces the need for vitamin D from dietary sources among people who experience regular sun exposure (see Chapter 8).

| Class | Carbohydrate | Lipids† | Protein | Water |
|---|---|---|---|---|
| Essential Nutrients | Glucose (or a carbohydrate that yields glucose)‡ | Linoleic acid α-Linolenic acid | Amino acids | |
| Good Dietary Sources | Breads, starchy vegetables, dairy products, and fruits | Plant oils and animal fats | Meats, eggs, and beans | All beverages and fruits |

**macronutrient** A nutrient needed in gram quantities in a diet.

**micronutrient** A nutrient needed in milligram or microgram quantities in a diet.

**bond** A linkage between two atoms formed by the sharing of electrons, or attractions.

**fiber** Substances in plant foods not digested by the processes that take place in the human stomach or small intestine. These add bulk to feces. Fiber naturally found in foods is also called dietary fiber.

**TABLE 1-4** Major Functions of the Various Classes of Nutrients

| Nutrient Classes That Provide Energy | Nutrient Classes That Promote Growth, Development, and Maintenance | Nutrient Classes That Regulate Body Processes |
|---|---|---|
| Most carbohydrates | Proteins | Proteins |
| Proteins | Lipids | Some lipids |
| Most lipids | Some vitamins | Some vitamins |
| | Some minerals | Some minerals |
| | Water | Water |

Carbohydrates, proteins, lipids, and water are needed in relatively large amounts, so they are called **macronutrients.** Vitamins and minerals are needed in such small amounts in the diet that they are called **micronutrients.**

| Vitamins | | Minerals | |
|---|---|---|---|
| **Water-soluble** | **Fat-soluble** | **Major** | **Trace** |
| Thiamin | A | Calcium | Chromium |
| Riboflavin | D§ | Chloride | Copper |
| Niacin | E | Magnesium | Fluoride‖ |
| Pantothenic acid | K | Phosphorus | Iodide |
| Biotin | | Potassium | Iron |
| B-6 | | Sodium | Manganese |
| B-12 | | Sulfur | Molybdenum |
| Folate | | | Selenium |
| C | | | Zinc |

Green leafy vegetables and fruits

Dairy products, breakfast cereals, and oils

Fruits and dairy products

Fish and nuts

*This table includes nutrients for humans that are listed in the current *Dietary Reference Intakes* and related publications. Fiber could be added to the list of essential substances, but it is not a nutrient (see Chapter 4).

†The lipids listed are needed only in small amounts, about 5% to 10% of total calorie needs (see Chapter 5).

‡To prevent ketosis and thus the muscle loss that would occur if protein were used to synthesize carbohydrate (see Chapter 4).

§Sunshine on the skin also allows the body to make vitamin D for itself (see Chapter 8).

‖Primarily for dental health (see Chapter 9).

## Lipids

Lipids (mostly fats and oils) are composed primarily of the elements carbon and hydrogen; they contain fewer oxygen **atoms** than do carbohydrates. Lipids yield more calories per gram than do carbohydrates—on the average, 9 kcal per gram—because of this difference in composition. Lipids dissolve in certain solvents (e.g., ether and benzene) but not in water.

The basic structure of most lipids is the **triglyceride.** Triglycerides provide a key calorie source (e.g., **fatty acids**) for the body and are the major form of fat in foods. They are also the main form for energy storage in the body. In this book, the more

**atom** Smallest combining unit of an element, such as iron or calcium. Atoms consist of protons, neutrons, and electrons.

**triglyceride** The major form of lipid in the body and in food. It is composed of three fatty acids bonded to glycerol.

**fatty acid** Major part of most lipids; primarily composed of a chain of carbons flanked by hydrogen.

familiar terms *fats and oils* will generally be used, rather than lipids or triglycerides. Generally, fats are lipids that are solid at room temperature and oils are lipids that are liquid at room temperature.

Most lipids can be separated into two basic types—saturated fat and unsaturated fat—based on the chemical structure of their fatty acids. The presence of carbon-carbon double bonds determines whether or not the lipid is saturated and therefore solid or liquid at room temperature. Think of a double bond as a "kink" somewhere along the carbon chain of a fatty acid. Having one or more kinks limits the extent to which fatty acids can pack tightly together, and therefore how solid a mass of fatty acids can be. Saturated fats are rich in **saturated fatty acids.** These fatty acids do not contain carbon-carbon double bonds. Animal fats, such as butter or lard, are often rich in saturated fatty acids—this makes them solid at room temperature. Unsaturated fats are rich in **unsaturated fatty acids.** These fatty acids contain one or more carbon-carbon double bonds.

Plant oils, such as corn oil, tend to contain many unsaturated fatty acids—this makes them liquid at room temperature. Almost all foods contain a variety of saturated and unsaturated fatty acids. Saturated fat should be limited in our diet because it can raise blood **cholesterol.** High blood cholesterol leads to clogged arteries and can eventually lead to cardiovascular disease (see Chapter 5).

**saturated fatty acid** A fatty acid containing no carbon-carbon double bonds.

**unsaturated fatty acid** A fatty acid containing one or more carbon-carbon double bonds.

## MAKING DECISIONS

### *Trans* Fat

When liquid oil is processed to form solid fat such as margarine or shortening, unnatural lipids called *trans* fatty acids or *trans* fats can be formed. These fats are commonly found in processed foods, and especially deep-fried foods, such as doughnuts and French fries. Large amounts of *trans* fats in the diet pose certain health risks, so intake should be minimized (see Chapter 5 for details). All food labels in the United States and Canada have to list *trans* fat content. Do you still want to eat food rich in *trans* fat?

▲ Butter is an animal fat made from milk fat and is high in saturated fat.

**trans fatty acids** A form of an unsaturated fatty acid, usually a monounsaturated one when found in food, in which the hydrogens on both carbons forming that double bond lie on opposite sides of that bond, rather than on the same side, as in most natural fats. Stick margarine, shortenings, and deep fat-fried foods in general are rich sources.

**enzyme** A compound that speeds the rate of a chemical reaction but is not altered by the reaction. Almost all enzymes are proteins (some are made of genetic material).

**amino acid** The building block for proteins containing a central carbon atom with nitrogen and other atoms attached.

Certain unsaturated fatty acids are essential nutrients that must come from our diet. These key fatty acids that the body can't produce, called essential fatty acids, perform several important functions in the body: they help regulate blood pressure and play a role in the synthesis and repair of vital cell parts. However, we need only about four tablespoons of a common plant oil (such as the canola or soybean oil) each day to supply these essential fatty acids. A serving of fatty fish, such as salmon or tuna, at least twice a week is another healthy source of essential fatty acids. The unique fatty acids in these fish complement the healthy aspects of common vegetable oils. This will be explained in greater detail in Chapter 5, which focuses on lipids.

## Proteins

Like carbohydrates and fats, proteins are composed of the elements carbon, oxygen, and hydrogen. But, unlike the other energy-yielding nutrients, all proteins also contain nitrogen. Proteins are the main structural material in the body. For example, proteins constitute a major part of bone and muscle; they are also important components in blood, body cells, **enzymes**, and immune factors. Proteins can also provide calories for the body—on average, 4 kcal per gram. Typically, however, the body uses little protein for the purpose of meeting daily calorie needs. Proteins are formed when **amino acids** are bonded together. Twenty or so common amino acids are found in food; nine of these are essential nutrients for adults, and one additional amino acid is essential for infants.

Most North Americans eat about one and a half to two times as much protein as the body needs to maintain health. In a person with no evidence of cardiovascular disease, kidney disease, diabetes, or family history of colon cancer or kidney stones, this amount of extra protein in the diet is generally not harmful—it reflects the standard of living and the dietary habits of most North Americans. The excess is used for calorie needs and carbohydrate production but ultimately can contribute to storage of fat. Chapter 6 focuses on proteins.

## Vitamins

Vitamins have a variety of chemical structures and can contain the elements carbon, hydrogen, nitrogen, oxygen, phosphorus, sulfur, and others. The main function of vitamins is to enable many **chemical reactions** to occur in the body. Some of these reactions help release the energy trapped in carbohydrates, lipids, and proteins. Remember, however, that vitamins themselves contain no usable calories for the body.

The 13 vitamins are divided into two groups: four are **fat-soluble** in that they dissolve in fat (vitamins A, D, E, and K); nine are **water-soluble** in that they dissolve in water (the B vitamins and vitamin C). The two groups of vitamins have different functions and characteristics. For example, cooking destroys water-soluble vitamins much more readily than it does fat-soluble vitamins. Water-soluble vitamins are also excreted from the body much more readily than are fat-soluble vitamins. Thus, the fat-soluble vitamins, especially vitamin A, are much more likely to accumulate in excessive amounts in the body, which then can lead to toxicity. Vitamins are the focus of Chapter 8.

## Minerals

Minerals are structurally simple, **inorganic** substances, which exist as groups of one or more of the same atoms. All of the nutrients discussed so far are **organic** compounds. These terms, *inorganic* and *organic*, are based on simple chemistry concepts and have nothing to do with the term "organic foods," used to describe foods produced according to certain production standards (see Chapter 2 for use of the term organic on food labels). Inorganic substances for the most part do not contain carbon atoms.

Minerals such as sodium and potassium typically function independently in the body, whereas minerals such as calcium and phosphorus function as parts of simple mineral combinations, such as bone mineral. Because of their simple structure, minerals are not destroyed during cooking, but they can still be lost if they dissolve in the water used for cooking and that water is then discarded. Minerals are critical players in nervous system functioning, water balance, structural (e.g., skeletal) systems, and many other cellular processes, but yield no calories as such for the body.

The 16 or more essential minerals required in the diet for good health are divided into two groups: **major minerals** and **trace minerals** because dietary needs vary enormously. If daily needs are less than 100 milligrams, the mineral is classified as a trace mineral, otherwise, it is a major mineral. The dietary requirement for some trace minerals has yet to be determined. Minerals that function based on their electrical charge when dissolved in water are also called **electrolytes;** these include sodium, potassium, and chloride. Minerals are the focus of Chapter 9.

## Water

Water makes up the sixth class of nutrients. Although sometimes overlooked as a nutrient, water (chemically, $H_2O$) has numerous vital functions in the body. It acts as a **solvent** and lubricant, as a vehicle for transporting nutrients and waste, and as a medium for temperature regulation and chemical processes. For these reasons, and because the human body is approximately 60% water, the average man should consume about 3 liters—equivalent to 3000 grams or about 13 cups—of water and/or other fluids containing water every day. Women need closer to 2200 grams or about 9 cups per day.

**chemical reaction** An interaction between two chemicals that changes both chemicals.

**inorganic** Any substance lacking carbon atoms bonded to hydrogen atoms in the chemical structure.

**organic** Any substance that contains carbon atoms bonded to hydrogen atoms in the chemical structure.

**electrolytes** Substances that separate into ions in water and, in turn, are able to conduct an electrical current. These include sodium, chloride, and potassium.

**solvent** A liquid substance in which other substances dissolve.

▲ Fruits, vegetables, beans, and whole-grain breads and cereals are typically rich in phytochemicals.

Water is not only available from the obvious sources, but it is also the major component in some foods, such as many fruits and vegetables (e.g., lettuce, grapes, and melons). The body even makes some water as a by-product of **metabolism.** Water is examined in detail in Chapter 9.

## Other Important Components in Food

Another group of compounds in foods from plant sources, especially within the fruit and vegetable groups, is what scientists call **phytochemicals.** Although these plant components are not considered essential nutrients in the diet, many of these substances provide significant health benefits. Considerable research attention is focused on various phytochemicals in reducing the risk for certain diseases (e.g., cancer). Although certain phytochemicals are available as dietary supplements, research suggests that their health benefits are best obtained through the consumption of whole foods. Foods with high phytochemical content are sometimes called "superfoods" because of the health benefits they are thought to confer. There is no legal definition of the term superfood, however, and there is concern that it is being overused in marketing certain foods. Table 1-5 lists some noteworthy phytochemicals with their common food sources. Tips for boosting the phytochemical content of your diet will be discussed in Chapter 2.

**metabolism** Chemical processes in the body by which energy is provided in useful forms and vital activities are sustained.

**phytochemical** A chemical found in plants. Some phytochemicals may contribute to a reduced risk of cancer or cardiovascular disease in people who consume them regularly.

**TABLE 1-5** Food Sources of Some Phytochemical Compounds Under Study

| Phytochemical | Food Sources |
|---|---|
| Allyl sulfides/organosulfurs | Garlic, onions, leeks |
| Saponins | Garlic, onions, licorice, legumes |
| Carotenoids (e.g., lycopene) | Orange, red, yellow fruits and vegetables (egg yolks are a source as well) |
| Monoterpenes | Oranges, lemons, grapefruit |
| Capsaicin | Chili peppers |
| Lignans | Flaxseed, berries, whole grains |
| Indoles | Cruciferous vegetables (broccoli, cabbage, kale) |
| Isothiocyanates | Cruciferous vegetables, especially broccoli |
| Phytosterols | Soybeans, other legumes, cucumbers, other fruits and vegetables |
| Flavonoids | Citrus fruit, onions, apples, grapes, red wine, tea, chocolate, tomatoes |
| Isoflavones | Soybeans, other legumes |
| Catechins | Tea |
| Ellagic acid | Strawberries, raspberries, grapes, apples, bananas, nuts |
| Anthocyanosides | Red, blue, and purple plants (blueberries, eggplant) |
| Fructooligosaccharides | Onions, bananas, oranges (small amounts) |
| Resveratrol | Grapes, peanuts, red wine |

Some related compounds under study are found in animal products, such as sphingolipids (meat and dairy products) and conjugated linoleic acid (meat and cheese). These are not phytochemicals per se because they are not from plant sources, but they have been shown to have health benefits.

Chapter 1: What You Eat and Why   13

## 1.3 Nutrient Composition of Diets and the Human Body

The quantities of the various nutrients that people consume in different foods vary widely. On a daily basis we consume about 500 grams, or about 1 pound, of protein, fat, and carbohydrate. In contrast, the typical daily mineral intake totals about 20 grams (about 4 teaspoons), and the daily vitamin intake totals less than 300 milligrams (1/15 of a teaspoon). Although we require a gram or so of some minerals, such as calcium and phosphorus, we need only a few milligrams or less of other minerals each day. For example, we need about 10 milligrams of zinc per day, just a few specks of the mineral.

Figure 1-1 contrasts the relative proportions of all the major classes of nutrients in a lean man and a lean woman with the proportions of these nutrients in both a cooked steak and a baked potato. Note how the nutrient composition of the human body differs from the nutritional profiles of the foods we eat. This is because growth, development, and later maintenance of the human body are directed by the genetic material (DNA) inside body cells. This genetic blueprint determines how each cell uses the essential nutrients to perform body functions. These nutrients can come from a variety of sources. Cells are not concerned about whether available amino acids come from animal or plant sources. The carbohydrate glucose can come from sugars or starches. Thus, you really aren't what you eat. Rather, the food that you eat provides cells with basic materials to function according to the directions supplied by the genetic material (**genes**) housed in body cells. Genetics and nutrition will be discussed in Chapter 3.

**genes** A specific segment on a chromosome. Genes provide the blueprints for the production of all body proteins.

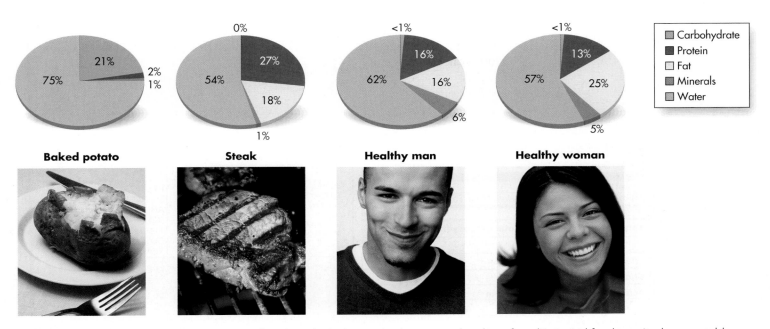

**FIGURE 1-1** ▶ The approximate proportions of nutrients in the human body compared to those found in typical foods—animal or vegetable. The amount of vitamins found in the body is negligible, and so is not shown.

Chapter 1: What You Eat and Why   13

**alcohol** Ethyl alcohol or ethanol ($CH_3CH_2OH$) is the compound in alcoholic beverages.

**compound** A group of different types of atoms bonded together in definite proportion.

**ion** An atom with an unequal number of electrons and protons. Negative ions have more electrons than protons; positive ions have more protons than electrons.

Carbohydrate
4 kcal per gram

Fat
9 kcal per gram

Protein
4 kcal per gram

Alcohol
7 kcal per gram

▲ Calorie Content of Energy Nutrients and Alcohol

# 1.4 Energy Sources and Uses

## Calories

Humans obtain the energy we need for involuntary body functions and voluntary physical activity from various calorie sources: carbohydrates, fats, and proteins. Foods generally provide more than one calorie source. Plant oils are one exception; these are 100% fat.

**Alcohol** is also a source of calories for some of us, supplying about 7 kcal per gram. It is not considered an essential nutrient, however, because it has no required function. Still, alcoholic beverages, such as beer—also rich in carbohydrate—are a contributor of calories to the diet of many adults.

The body releases the energy from the chemical bonds in carbohydrate, protein, and fat (and alcohol) into other forms of energy in order to:

- Build new **compounds.**
- Perform muscular movements.
- Promote nerve transmissions.
- Maintain **ion** balance within cells.

Chapters 7 and 10 describe how that energy is released from the chemical bonds in energy-yielding nutrients and then used by body cells to support the processes just described.

The energy in food is often expressed in terms of calories on food labels. As defined earlier, a calorie is the amount of heat energy it takes to raise the temperature of 1 gram of water 1 degree Celsius (1°C, centigrade scale). (Chapter 7 has a diagram of the bomb calorimeter that can be used to measure calories in foods.) A calorie is a tiny measure of heat, so food energy is more conveniently expressed in terms of the kilocalorie (kcal), which equals 1000 calories. (If the "c" in calories is capitalized, this also signifies kilocalories.) A kcal is the amount of heat energy it takes to raise the temperature of 1000 grams (1 liter) of water 1°C. The abbreviation *kcal* is used throughout this book. On food labels, the word *calorie* (without a capital "C") is also used loosely to mean *kilocalorie.* Any values given on food labels in calories are actually in kilocalories (Fig. 1-2). A suggested intake of 2000 calories per day on a food label is technically 2000 kcal.

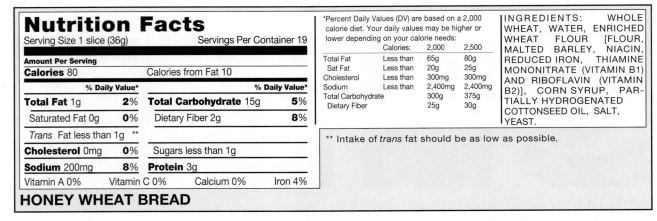

| **Nutrition Facts** | | | |
|---|---|---|---|
| Serving Size 1 slice (36g) | | Servings Per Container 19 | |
| **Amount Per Serving** | | | |
| **Calories** 80 | | Calories from Fat 10 | |
| | **% Daily Value\*** | | **% Daily Value\*** |
| **Total Fat** 1g | **2%** | **Total Carbohydrate** 15g | **5%** |
| Saturated Fat 0g | **0%** | Dietary Fiber 2g | **8%** |
| *Trans* Fat less than 1g | \*\* | | |
| **Cholesterol** 0mg | **0%** | Sugars less than 1g | |
| **Sodium** 200mg | **8%** | **Protein** 3g | |
| Vitamin A 0% | Vitamin C 0% | Calcium 0% | Iron 4% |
| **HONEY WHEAT BREAD** | | | |

\*Percent Daily Values (DV) are based on a 2,000 calorie diet. Your daily values may be higher or lower depending on your calorie needs:

| | | Calories: | 2,000 | 2,500 |
|---|---|---|---|---|
| Total Fat | Less than | | 65g | 80g |
| Sat Fat | Less than | | 20g | 25g |
| Cholesterol | Less than | | 300mg | 300mg |
| Sodium | Less than | | 2,400mg | 2,400mg |
| Total Carbohydrate | | | 300g | 375g |
| Dietary Fiber | | | 25g | 30g |

\*\* Intake of *trans* fat should be as low as possible.

INGREDIENTS: WHOLE WHEAT, WATER, ENRICHED WHEAT FLOUR [FLOUR, MALTED BARLEY, NIACIN, REDUCED IRON, THIAMINE MONONITRATE (VITAMIN B1) AND RIBOFLAVIN (VITAMIN B2)], CORN SYRUP, PARTIALLY HYDROGENATED COTTONSEED OIL, SALT, YEAST.

**FIGURE 1-2** ▶ Use the nutrient values on the Nutrition Facts label to calculate calorie content of a food. Based on carbohydrate, fat, and protein content, a serving of this food (Honey Wheat Bread) contains 81 kcal ([15 × 4] + [1 × 9] + [3 × 4] = 81). The label lists 80, suggesting that the calorie value was rounded down.

## Calculating Calories

Use the 4-9-4 estimates for the calorie content of carbohydrate, fat, and protein introduced over the last few pages to determine calorie content of a food. Consider these foods:

*1 Large Hamburger*

| | |
|---|---|
| Carbohydrate | 39 grams $\times$ 4 = 156 kcal |
| Fat | 32 grams $\times$ 9 = 288 kcal |
| Protein | 30 grams $\times$ 4 = 120 kcal |
| Alcohol | 0 grams $\times$ 7 = 0 kcal |
| **Total** | **564 kcal** |

*8-ounce Piña Colada*

| | |
|---|---|
| Carbohydrate | 57 grams $\times$ 4 = 228 kcal |
| Fat | 5 grams $\times$ 9 = 45 kcal |
| Protein | 1 grams $\times$ 4 = 4 kcal |
| Alcohol | 23 grams $\times$ 7 = 161 kcal |
| **Total** | **438 kcal** |

You can also use the 4-9-4 estimates to determine what portion of total calorie intake is contributed by the various calorie-yielding nutrients. Assume that one day you consume 290 grams of carbohydrates, 60 grams of fat, and 70 grams of protein. This consumption yields a total of 1980 kcal ([290 $\times$ 4] + [60 $\times$ 9] + [70 $\times$ 4]5 = 1980). The percentage of your total calorie intake derived from each nutrient can then be determined:

$$\text{\% of kcal as carbohydrate} = (290 \times 4) \div 1980 = 0.59 \ (\times 100 = 59\%)$$
$$\text{\% of kcal as fat} = (\ 60 \times 9) \div 1980 = 0.27 \ (\times 100 = 27\%)$$
$$\text{\% of kcal as protein} = (\ 70 \times 4) \div 1980 = 0.14 \ (\times 100 = 14\%)$$

Check your calculations by adding the percentages together. Do they total 100?

### MAKING DECISIONS

#### Percentages and the Metric System

You will use a few mathematical concepts in studying nutrition. Besides performing addition, subtraction, multiplication, and division, you need to know how to calculate percentages and convert English units of measurement to metric units.

#### Percentages

The term percent (%) refers to a part of the total when the total represents 100 parts. For example, if you earn 80% on your first nutrition examination, you will have answered the equivalent of 80 out of 100 questions correctly. This equivalent could be 8 correct answers out of 10; 80% also describes 16 of 20 (16/20 = 0.80 or 80%). The decimal form of percents is based on 100% being equal to 1.00. It is difficult to succeed in a nutrition course unless you know what a percentage means and how to calculate one. Percentages are used frequently when referring to menus and nutrient composition. The best way to master this concept is to calculate some percentages. Some examples follow:

| Question | Answer |
|---|---|
| What is 6% of 45? | 6% = 0.06 or 0.06 $\times$ 45 = 2.7 |
| What percent of 99 is 3? | 3/99 = 0.03 or 3% (0.03 $\times$ 100) |

Joe ate 15% of the adult Recommended Dietary Allowance (RDA) for iron at lunch. How many milligrams did he eat? (RDA = 8 milligrams)

$$0.15 \times 8 \text{ milligrams} = 1.2 \text{ milligrams}$$

**The Metric System**

The basic units of the metric system are the meter, which indicates length; the gram, which indicates weight; and the liter, which indicates volume. Appendix I in this textbook lists conversions from the metric system to the English system (pounds, feet, cups) and vice versa. Here is a brief summary:

A gram (g) is about 1/30 of an ounce (28 grams to the ounce).
5 grams of sugar or salt is about 1 teaspoon.
A pound (lb) weighs 454 grams.
A kilogram (kg) is 1000 grams, equivalent to 2.2 pounds.
To convert your weight to kilograms, divide it by 2.2.
A 154-pound man weighs 70 kilograms (154/2.2 = 70).
A gram can be divided into 1000 milligrams (mg) or 1,000,000 micrograms ($\mu$g or mcg).
   10 milligrams of zinc (approximately adult needs) would be a few grains of zinc.
Liters are divided into 1000 units called milliliters (ml).
One teaspoon equals about 5 milliliters (ml), 1 cup is about 240 milliliters, and 1 quart
   (4 cups) equals almost 1 liter (L) (0.946 liter to be exact).

If you plan to work in any scientific field, you will need to learn the metric system. *For now, remember that a kilogram equals 2.2 pounds, an ounce weighs 28 grams, 2.54 centimeters equals 1 inch, and a liter is almost the same as a quart.* In addition, know the fractions that the following prefixes represent: micro (1/1,000,000), milli (1/1000), centi (1/100), and kilo (1000).

### CONCEPT CHECK

Nutrition is the study of food and nutrients—their digestion, absorption, and metabolism, and their effect on health and disease. Food contains the vital nutrients essential for good health: carbohydrates, lipids (fats and oils), proteins, vitamins, minerals, and water. Nutrients have three general functions in the body: (1) to provide materials for building and maintaining the body; (2) to act as regulators for key metabolic reactions; and (3) to participate in metabolic reactions that provide the energy necessary to sustain life. A common unit of measurement for this energy is the kilocalorie (kcal). On average, carbohydrates and protein provide 4 kcal per gram of energy to the body, while lipids provide 9 kcal per gram. Although not considered a nutrient, alcohol provides about 7 kcal per gram. The other classes of nutrients do not supply calories but are essential for proper body functioning.

## 1.5 Current State of the North American Diet and Overall Health

**T**he Food and Nutrition Board of the National Academy of Sciences suggests minimizing saturated fat, *trans* fat, and cholesterol intake when putting their diet guidelines into place (see Chapter 5).

The Food and Nutrition Board (FNB) of the National Academy of Sciences advocates that 10% to 35% of calories come from protein, 45% to 65% from carbohydrate, and 20% to 35% from fat. (These standards apply to both people in the United States and Canada.) It is estimated that the calorie intakes of North American adults fall within the FNB recommendations with about 16% of their calorie intake as proteins, 50% as carbohydrates, and 33% as fats. These percentages are estimates that do not consider alcohol and vary slightly from year to year and from person to person.

Animal sources supply about two-thirds of protein intake for most North Americans; plant sources supply only about one-third. In many other parts of the world, it is just the opposite: plant proteins—from rice, beans, corn, and other grains and vegetables—dominate protein intake. About half the carbohydrate in North American diets comes from simple sugars; the other half comes from starches (such as in pastas, breads, and potatoes). About 60% of dietary fat comes from animal sources and 40% from plant sources.

## Assessing the Current North American Diet

With the aim of finding out what and when North Americans eat, federal agencies conduct surveys to collect data about food and nutrient consumption, as well as connections between diet and health. In the United States, the U.S. Department of Health and Human Services monitors food consumption with the National Health and Nutrition Examination Survey (NHANES). In Canada, this information is gathered by Health Canada in conjunction with Agriculture and Agrifood Canada.

Results from national nutrition surveys and other studies show that North Americans consume a wide variety of foods but often do not choose the right balance of foods to meet their nutrient needs. Chapter 2 will look at this situation in more detail. For now, more attention should be focused on foods rich in iron, calcium, potassium, magnesium, various B vitamins, vitamin C (especially for smokers), vitamin D, vitamin E, and fiber. Daily intake of a balanced multivitamin and mineral supplement is one strategy to help meet nutrient needs but does not make up for a poor diet, particularly for calcium, potassium, and fiber intake. Also keep in mind that taking numerous dietary supplements can lead to health problems (see Chapter 8).

Routinely, experts also recommend that we pay more attention to balancing calorie intake with needs. An excess intake of calories is usually tied to overindulgence in sugar, fat, and alcoholic beverages. African-Americans and Hispanics have a greater chance of developing hypertension than do other ethnic groups in North America and therefore may need to decrease the amount of **salt** (sodium chloride) and alcohol in their diets. These substances are two of the many factors linked to hypertension. Moderation of salt and alcohol intake—along with saturated fat, *trans* fat, cholesterol, and total calorie intake—is a recommended practice for all adults.

Many North Americans would benefit from a healthier balance of food in their diets. Moderation is the key for some foods, such as sugared soft drinks and fried foods. For other foods, such as fruits and vegetables, increased quantity and variety is warranted. Few adults currently meet the "5 to 9 a-day" recommendation promoted for total servings of vegetables and fruits.

▲ Taking numerous nutrient supplements can lead to health problems. Chapter 8 will explore the appropriate and safe use of nutrient supplements in detail.

**salt** Compound of sodium and chloride in a 40:60 ratio.

▲ Moderation in the intake of some foods, such as sugared soft drinks and fried foods, can lead to a healthier balance of food in the North American diet.

## Health Objectives for the United States for the Year 2010

Health promotion and disease prevention have been public health strategies in North America since the late 1970s. One part of this strategy is *Healthy People 2010*, a report issued in 2000 by the U.S. Department of Health and Human Services' Public Health Service. This report outlines health promotion and disease prevention objectives for the nation for the year 2010 and assigns each of the objectives to appropriate U.S. federal agencies to address. Many nutrition-related objectives are part of the overall plan (Table 1-6). The overarching goals of *Healthy People 2010* are to increase quality and years of healthy life and to eliminate health disparities. Every 10 years HHS develops a new set of objectives for promoting health and preventing disease. The Healthy People 2020 objectives are currently under development and are scheduled to be released in January 2010 along with guidance for achieving the new 10-year targets. The following Internet site provides more details on the *Healthy People* program: www.healthypeople.gov.

Another way to promote your health and prevent chronic diseases in the future is to observe the recommendations listed in Table 1-7. In total, these contribute to maximal health and prevention of disease.

▲ Many nutrition-related objectives are part of the *Healthy People 2010* report. The report outlines health promotion and disease prevention objectives for the United States for the year 2010.

**TABLE 1-6** A Sample of Nutrition-Related Objectives from *Healthy People 2010*

|  | Target | Current Estimate |
|---|---|---|
| Increase the proportion of adults at a healthy weight. | 60% | 42% |
| Reduce the proportion of overweight or obese children and adolescents. | 5% | 11% |
| Increase the proportion of persons age 2 years and older who consume: | | |
| • At least 2 daily servings of fruit. | 75% | 28% |
| • At least 3 daily servings of vegetables, with at least one-third being dark green or deep yellow vegetables. | 50% | 3% |
| • At least 6 daily servings of grain products, with at least 3 being whole grains (e.g., whole wheat bread and oatmeal). | 50% | 7% |
| • Less than 10% of calories from saturated fat. | 75% | 36% |
| • Six grams or less of salt (2400 milligrams or less of sodium) daily. | 65% | 21% |
| • Enough calcium (see DRI table for elements on inside cover of this book). | 74% | 45% |
| Reduce iron deficiency among females of childbearing age. | 7% | 11% |

Note: In later chapters, we will explore additional nutrition-related objectives, such as those addressing osteoporosis, various forms of cancer, diabetes prevention and treatment, food allergies, cardiovascular disease, low birth weight, nutrition during pregnancy, breastfeeding, eating disorders, physical activity, and alcohol use.

## 1.6 Improving Our Diets

Our cultural diversity, varied cuisines, and generally high nutritional status should be points of pride for North Americans. Today we can choose from a tremendous variety of food products, the result of continual innovation by food manufacturers.

Many dietary habits have improved during the past decade. We are eating more breakfast cereals, pizza, pasta entrees, stir-fried meats and vegetables served on rice, salads, tacos, burritos, and fajitas than ever before. Sales of whole milk are down, while in the same period sales of fat-free and 1% low-fat milk have increased. Consumption of frozen vegetables, rather than canned vegetables, is also on the rise.

A dietary objective that deserves more attention is to try to eat with others more often. Mealtime is a key social time of the day. The Japanese are ahead of us in recognizing that food's powers go beyond the realm of nutrition. Their national dietary guidelines stress the importance of eating a variety of foods, maintaining healthy weight, and moderating fat in the diet, but also advise people to make all activities pertaining to food and eating pleasurable.

Today, North Americans live longer than ever and enjoy better general health. Many also have more money and more diverse food and lifestyle choices to consider. The nutritional consequences of these trends are not fully known. Deaths from various forms of cardiovascular disease, for example, have dropped dramatically since the late 1960s, partly because of better medical care and diets. Still, if affluence leads to sedentary lifestyles and high intakes of saturated fat, *trans* fat, cholesterol, salt, and alcohol, this lifestyle pattern can lead to problems such as cardiovascular disease, hypertension, and obesity. Greater efforts are needed by the general public to lower intake of saturated fat, *trans* fat, and cholesterol intake and to improve variety in our diets. With better technology and greater choices, we can have a much better diet today than ever before—if we know what choices to make.

The goal of this book is to help you find the best path to good nutrition. Nutrition experts generally agree that there are no "good" or "bad" (i.e., "junk") foods, but some foods provide relatively few nutrients in comparison to calorie content. One's total diet is the proper focus in a nutritional evaluation. Chapter 2 will emphasize this point and show you how to balance your diet. As you reexamine

▼ A healthy diet benefits people of all ages.

**TABLE 1-7** Recommendations for Health Promotion and Disease Prevention: What Can Adults Expect from Adequate Nutrition and Good Health Habits?

### Diet

Consuming enough essential nutrients, including fiber, while moderating energy, saturated fat, trans fat, cholesterol, and alcohol intake can result in:

- Increased bone mass during childhood and adolescence
- Prevention of some adult bone loss and osteoporosis, especially in older adults
- Fewer dental caries
- Prevention of digestive problems, such as constipation
- Decreased susceptibility to some cancers
- Decreased degradation of the retina (intake of green and orange vegetables in particular)
- Lower risk of obesity and related diseases, such as type 2 diabetes and cardiovascular disease
- Reduced risk for deficiency diseases, such as cretinism (lack of iodide), scurvy (lack of vitamin C), and anemia (lack of iron, folate, or other nutrients)

### Physical Activity

Adequate, regular physical activity (at least 30 minutes on most or all days) helps reduce the risk of:

- Obesity
- Type 2 diabetes
- Cardiovascular disease
- Some adult bone loss and loss of muscle tone
- Premature aging
- Certain cancers

### Lifestyle

Minimizing alcohol intake (no more than two drinks per day for men and one drink for both women and all adults age 65 years and older) helps prevent:

- Liver disease
- Accidents

Not smoking cigarettes or cigars helps prevent:

- Lung cancer, other lung disease, kidney disease, cardiovascular disease, and degenerative eye diseases

In addition, minimum use of medication, no illicit drug use, adequate sleep (7–8 hours), adequate water and related fluid intake (9–13 cups per day), and a reduction in stress (practice better time management, relax, listen to music, have a massage, and stay physically active) provide a more complete approach to good nutrition and health. Add to this maintaining close relationships with others and a positive outlook on life. Finally, consultation with healthcare professionals on a regular basis is important. This is because early diagnosis is especially useful for controlling the damaging effects of many diseases. Prevention of disease is an important investment of one's time, including during the college years.

▲ Regular physical activity complements a healthy diet. Whether it's all at once or in segments throughout the day, ideally incorporate 30 to 60 minutes or more of such activity into your daily routine.

your nutritional habits, remember your health is largely your responsibility. Your body has a natural ability to heal itself. Offer it what it needs, and it will serve you well. Confusing and conflicting health messages hinder diet change. Nutrition science does not have all the answers, but as you will see, enough is known to help you set a path to good health and put diet-related recommendations you hear in the future into perspective.

CONCEPT CHECK

Surveys in the United States and Canada show that we generally have a variety of foods available to us. However, some of us could improve our diets by focusing on food sources rich in various vitamins, minerals, and fiber. In addition, many of us should reduce our consumption of calories, sugar, protein, saturated fat, *trans* fat, cholesterol, salt, and alcoholic beverages. These recommendations are consistent with an overall goal to attain and maintain good health.

# 1.7  Why Am I So Hungry?

Understanding what drives us to eat and what affects food choice will help you understand the complexity of factors that influence eating, especially the effects of ethnicity and social change. You can then see why foods may have different meanings to different people. In turn, this allows for greater appreciation of food habits that differ from yours.

Two drives, **hunger** and **appetite,** influence our desire to eat. These drives differ dramatically. Hunger is primarily our physical biological drive to eat and is controlled by internal body mechanisms. For example, as nutrients are digested and absorbed by the stomach and small intestine, these organs send signals to the liver and brain to reduce further food intake.

Appetite, our primarily psychological drive to eat, is affected by external food choice mechanisms, such as seeing a tempting dessert or smelling popcorn popping at the movie theater. Fulfilling either or both drives by eating sufficient food normally brings a state of **satiety,** a feeling of satisfaction that temporarily halts our desire to continue eating.

**hunger** The primarily physiological (internal) drive to find and eat food, mostly regulated by innate cues to eating.

**appetite** The primarily psychological (external) influences that encourage us to find and eat food, often in the absence of obvious hunger.

**satiety** State in which there is no longer a desire to eat; a feeling of satisfaction.

**hypothalamus** A region at the base of the brain that contains cells that play a role in the regulation of hunger, respiration, body temperature, and other body functions.

## The Hypothalamus Contributes to Satiety

The **hypothalamus,** a region of the brain, helps regulate satiety (Fig. 1-3). Imagine a game of tug-of-war in the brain: two sites in the hypothalamus—the *feeding center* and the *satiety center*—work in opposite ways to promote adequate availability of nutrients at all times. When stimulated, cells in the feeding center of the hypothalamus signal us to eat. As we eat, cells in the satiety center are stimulated, and we stop eating.

What stimulates these two centers of the hypothalamus? The amounts of macronutrients in the blood probably stimulate both the satiety and feeding centers. For example, when we haven't eaten for a while, stimulation of the feeding center signals us to eat. When the macronutrient content in the blood rises after a meal, the satiety center is stimulated and we no longer have a strong desire to seek food. (Exactly how the two are interrelated is under study.) Certain chemicals, surgery, and some cancers can destroy either center in the hypothalamus. Without satiety center activation, laboratory animals (and humans) eat their way to obesity. Without feeding center activation, the opposite happens and weight is lost.

Admittedly, this concept of a tug-of-war between the feeding and satiety centers is an oversimplification of a complex process. Overall, the entire system depends on the hypothalamus to process the signals generated by nerves in the body that are influenced in various ways by recent food intake. In reality, the hypothalamus has numerous sites crisscrossed with a network of nerves constantly receiving and passing on information about the body's nutritional state. In addition, another area of the brain, the cortex, controls conscious thought and can overcome signals from the hypothalamic hunger and satiety centers.

## Meal Size and Composition Affect Satiety

The effects of stomach expansion from food intake combined with the later intestinal absorption of nutrients during a meal likely reduce our desire to eat more food.

These actions of the **gastrointestinal (GI) tract** contribute to a feeling of satiety. In fact, a meal generally ends before significant amounts of nutrients are made available for metabolism and storage. Putting this information into practice, researchers have recently shown that bulky meals (high in fiber and water) produce much more satiety than do more concentrated meals. As the fiber and water content of the foods increase, humans experience increased satiety and thus do not seek another meal as quickly. Consider how satisfied you would feel if you ate five pieces of whole fruit versus a small serving of French fries (each yielding about 380 kcals).

## Hormones Affect Satiety

**Hormones** and hormone-like compounds in our body influence whether we eat. Hormones that increase hunger include **endorphins, ghrelin,** and **neuropeptide Y.** Those that cause satiety include **leptin** (working in conjunction with the hormone insulin), **serotonin,** and **cholecystokinin (CCK).** New research has shown how leptin, discovered in 1995, and ghrelin, discovered in 1999, work together to balance our hunger and satiety. Leptin is made by the cells that store fat, also known as **adipose tissue,** travels to the brain, stimulates the satiety center and turns off the hunger center. Ghrelin is made by the stomach and travels to the brain where it stimulates the hunger center and turns off the satiety center. High leptin levels also turn off the production of ghrelin. Problems arise when leptin levels are high over a long period, such as in obesity, which makes the satiety center insensitive to leptin. To add to the confusion, low ghrelin levels make the hunger center sensitive to ghrelin. This situation helps explain why high leptin levels in obese individuals leads to an increased sensitivity of the hunger center to low ghrelin and no decrease in hunger. Based on these mechanisms, these hormones and their mechanisms are potential targets for new weight loss drugs.

## Does Appetite Affect What We Eat?

The various feeding and satiety messages from body cells do not single-handedly determine what we eat. Almost everyone has encountered a mouthwatering dessert and devoured it, even on a full stomach. Appetite can be affected by a wide variety of external forces, such as environmental and psychological factors as well as social customs (Fig. 1-4).

We often eat because food confronts us. It smells, tastes, and looks good. We might eat because it is the right time of day, we are celebrating, or we are seeking emotional comfort to overcome the blues. After a meal, memories of pleasant tastes and feelings reinforce appetite. If stress or depression sends you to the refrigerator, you are mostly seeking comfort, not food calories. Appetite may not be a physical process, but it does influence food intake. Table 1-8 lists additional social and other related factors that influence food choices.

(a)

### Process of Satiety

Start

Flavor of food

Knowing a meal was just eaten

Influence of stomach and intestinal expansion and activity

Influence of nutrient use in the liver and related communication with the hypothalamus and other regions of the brain

Conscious thinking takes place in the brain's cortex and can overcome hunger or satiety signals

Finish

(b)

**FIGURE 1-3** ▶ The hypothalamus and satiety. (a) The hypothalamus is one important region in the brain that influences whether we eat or not. (b) The process of satiety starts with eating food and concludes with actions in the hypothalamus and other regions in the brain, such as the cortex.

---

## MAKING DECISIONS

### Satiety

Satiety associated with consuming a meal may reside primarily in our psychological frame of mind. We become accustomed to a certain amount of food at a meal. Providing less than that amount leaves us wanting more. One way to use this observation for weight-loss purposes is to train your eye to expect less food by slowly decreasing serving sizes to more appropriate amounts (see Figure 2-5 in Chapter 2 for some examples). Your appetite then readjusts as you expect less food. Keep track of what triggers your eating for a few days. Is it primarily hunger or appetite? Also, satiety regulation is not perfect; body weight can fluctuate.

**gastrointestinal (GI) tract** The main sites in the body used for digestion and absorption of nutrients. It consists of the mouth, esophagus, stomach, small intestine, large intestine, rectum, and anus. Also called the digestive tract.

**hormone** A compound secreted into the bloodstream by one type of cell that acts to control the function of another type of cell. For example, certain cells in the pancreas produce insulin, which in turn acts on muscle and other types of cells to promote uptake of nutrients from the blood.

**endorphins** Natural body tranquilizers that may be involved in the feeding response.

**ghrelin** A hormone made by the stomach that increases the desire to eat.

**neuropeptide Y** A chemical substance made in the hypothalamus that stimulates food intake. The hormone leptin inhibits neuropeptide Y production.

**leptin** A hormone made by **adipose tissue** in proportion to total fat stores in the body that influences long-term regulation of fat mass. Leptin also influences reproductive functions, as well as other body processes, such as release of the hormone insulin.

**adipose tissue** A group of fat storing cells.

**serotonin** A neurotransmitter synthesized from the amino acid tryptophan that affects mood (sense of calmness), behavior, and appetite, and induces sleep.

**cholecystokinin (CCK)** A hormone that participates in enzyme release from the pancreas, bile release from the gallbladder, and hunger regulation.

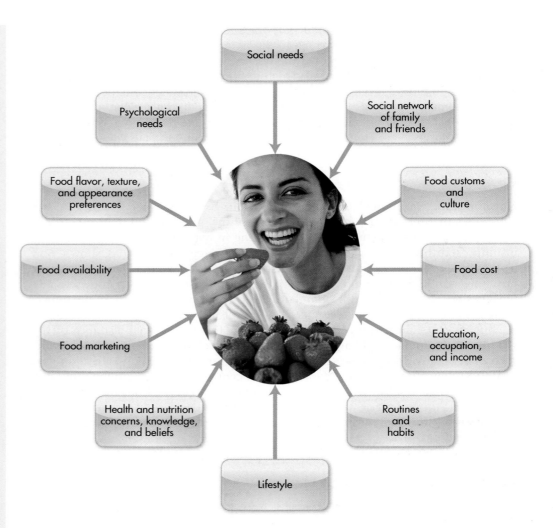

**FIGURE 1-4** ▶ Food choices are affected by many factors. Which have the greatest impact on your food choices?

## Putting Hunger and Appetite into Perspective

The next time you pick up a candy bar or ask for second helpings, remember the internal and external influences on eating behavior. Body cells (brain, stomach, small intestine, liver, and other organs), macronutrients in the blood, hormones (like leptin and ghrelin), brain chemicals (like serotonin and neuropeptide Y), and social customs all influence food intake. When food is abundant, appetite—not hunger—most likely triggers eating.

### CRITICAL THINKING

Sarah is majoring in nutrition and is well aware of the importance of a healthy diet. She has recently been analyzing her diet and is confused. She notices that she eats a great deal of high-fat foods and few fruits, vegetables, and whole grains. She also has developed a "sweet tooth." What three factors may be influencing Sarah's food choices? What advice would you give her on how to have her diet match her needs?

### CONCEPT CHECK

Hunger is the primarily physical or internal desire to find and eat food. Fulfilling it creates satiety—no further desire to eat exists. Satiety is influenced by hunger-related (internal) signals from the brain, gastrointestinal tract, liver, and other organs, as well as fiber and water content of the foods in the meal. Various hormones and hormone-like compounds also participate. Food intake is also affected by appetite-related (external) forces like social customs, time of day, flavor, appearance, texture, and being with others. Factors such as health concerns, economics, convenience, seeking emotional comfort, and social changes are also becoming important dietary determinants. North Americans probably respond more to external, appetite-related forces than to hunger-related ones in choosing when and what to eat.

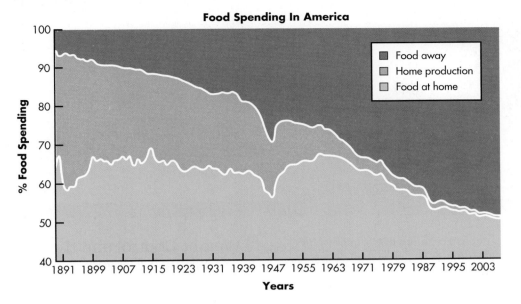

**Food Spending In America**

*Legend:*
- Food away
- Home production
- Food at home

*(Y-axis: % Food Spending, ranging 40 to 100; X-axis: Years, 1891 to 2003)*

▲ This chart shows the percentage of food spending up to 2006 for the average American household, including food purchased for consumption at home, food produced by the family for home consumption, and food consumed outside the home. Barely more than half of food eaten by Americans was consumed at home, with food eaten away from home now accounting for close to 49% of the American food dollar.

*Source:* http://www.nielsen.com/consumer_insight/issue8/ci_topline_article_VII.html

**TABLE 1-8** What Else Influences Our Food Choices?

Food means so much more to us than nourishment—it reflects much of what we think about ourselves. In the course of our lives, we spend the equivalent of 13 to 15 years eating. Beyond simple hunger and emotions, why do we choose what we eat?

- **Flavor, texture, and appearance** are the most important factors determining our food choices. Creating more flavorful foods that are both healthy and profitable is a major focus of the food industry (referred to as "better for you" products).
- **Early influences** that expose us to various people, places, and events have a continuing impact on our food choices. Many ethnic diet patterns begin as we are introduced to foods during childhood.
- **Routines and habits** are tied to some food choices. Food habits, food availability, and convenience strongly influence choices. Most of us eat from a core group of foods: About 100 basic items account for 75% of an individual's total food intake.
- **Nutrition,** or what we think of as "healthy foods," directs our food purchases. North Americans who tend to make health-related food choices are often well-educated, middle-class professionals. These same people are generally health-oriented, have active lifestyles, and focus on weight control. Consumer use of nutrition labels when making food purchases declined from 1995 to 2006. The decrease varied by population groups but was greatest for individuals 20–29 years old and those who spoke primarily Spanish.
- **Advertising** is a major media tool for capturing the food interest of the consumer. The food industry in the United States spends well over $33 billion on advertising. Some of this advertising is helpful, as it promotes the importance of food components such as calcium and fiber in our diets. However, the food industry also advertises highly sweetened cereals, cookies, cakes, and soft drinks because they bring in the greatest profits. A 2008 study by the Federal Trade Commission found that 44 major food and beverage marketers spent $1.6 billion to promote products to children and adolescents in the U.S. in 2006.
- **Restaurants** have long been a growing industry in North America. Today, about 49% of food dollars are spent on meals outside the home. Restaurant food is often calorie-dense and of poorer nutritional quality compared to foods made at home. However, in response to consumer demands, restaurants have placed healthier items on their menus and many are listing nutritional content on their menus.
- **Social changes** are leading to a general time shortage for many of us. This creates the need for convenience. Supermarkets now supply prepared meals, microwavable entrees, and various quick-prep frozen products.
- **Economics** play a minor role in our food choices. The average North American spends only about 12% of after-tax income on food (greater for low-income people). However, as income increases, so do meals eaten away from home.

Overall, daily food intake is a complicated mix of biological and social influences. The first Rate Your Plate activity in Chapter 1 asks you to keep track of what influences your food intake on a daily basis. This assessment is an important part of developing a plan to improve your diet as necessary. How do you compare to the typical North American?

# Eating Well in College

The college years are a leap into adulthood for many young adults. This is a time for freedom and a chance to make personal lifestyle decisions. Studies show that the diets and other health habits of college students are not optimal. Typically, students fall short of diet recommendations for servings of whole grains, vegetables, fruits, milk, and meat, opting instead to max out on fats, sweets, and alcohol. This information is disturbing from a public health standpoint because young adulthood is the time when many health behaviors are formed and will likely persist throughout life. With independence comes responsibility, including a responsibility to make smart food choices.

What is it about the college lifestyle that makes it so difficult to build healthy habits? Why do so many young adults gain the dreaded "freshman 15" pounds during the first months of college? How does alcohol consumption affect your waistline and academic performance? What can you do to

▼ Late-night pizza can add extra calories to the college student's daily intake.

establish healthful habits to last a lifetime? In this section we will discuss several topics and provide possible solutions to these questions and more.

## Food Choices

The college experience is exciting, but stressful. Students face changes in academic requirements, interpersonal relationships, and living environment. These stressful situations contribute to poor health behaviors. For example, take the week of midterms; during this time of writing papers and cramming for exams, balanced meals are all-too-easily replaced by high-fat and high-calorie fast-foods; convenience items; and sugary, caffeinated beverages. Physical activity is sacrificed in favor of study time.

Also consider the university environment. On campus, you are faced with a wide variety of dining choices, some healthy and some not so healthy. Dining halls, fast-food establishments, bars, and vending machines offer food 24 hours per day. While it is certainly possible to make wise food choices at each of these outlets, the temptations of convenience, taste, and value (i.e., oversized portions) may persuade the college student to select unhealthy options.

Eating is about more than just obtaining "fuel." Meals and snacks are times to socialize. You may feel pressured to eat a big lunch at noon without regard to hunger if your peers are meeting in the dining hall to catch up on class work and gossip. While chatting, it is easy to lose track of portions and to overeat. In addition, food may be a source of familiarity and comfort in a new and stressful place.

## Weight Control and the "Freshman Fifteen"

Learning to eat based on your body's hunger cues is a great way to avoid weight gain. Studies show that most college students gain weight during their first year. The "freshman fifteen" is a term used in the United States and Canada to describe the weight gained by students during their first year of college and is based on the claim that freshmen typically gain fifteen pounds. Although most students do not gain the freshman fifteen, a recent study of U.S. and Canadian college students found that students pack on 6 to 9 pounds their first year away from home. Although calorie intake does not increase significantly, dramatic increases in beer drinking and significant decreases in physical activity are key reasons for the weight gain.

There are several reasons to maintain a healthy weight. Over the long term, risk of chronic diseases goes up as weight increases. In the short term, losing excess weight can improve the way you view yourself, how others view you, and how you feel and perform. Detecting "flab" around your midsection or feeling that your clothes are getting tighter are two good indicators that you are carrying excess weight. If you determine that weight loss is necessary, with some knowledge and perseverance, you can safely lose excess pounds.

How do you go about achieving your goal? Behavioral research clearly demonstrates that setting several small, achievable goals will spur motivation. As you will learn in Chapter 7, body weight is a balancing act between calories in and calories burned. Try keeping track of your calorie

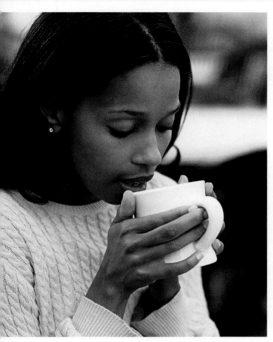

▲ Research has shown that gourmet coffee beverages, such as lattes and cappuccinos, can increase calorie consumption by about 200 kcal per day.

consumption for several days and comparing that to your energy needs, based on your age, gender, and activity level. You can use one of the equations presented in Chapter 7 or take advantage of the

▶ **Five Simple Tips to Avert the Freshman Fifteen**

- **Eat breakfast.** To rev up your metabolism include a source of protein such as an egg or low-fat yogurt, at least one serving of whole grains such as a breakfast cereal, and a fruit such as a banana.
- **Plan ahead.** Eat a balanced meal or snack every 3–4 hours
- **Limit liquid calories.** Drink water instead of high-calorie soft drinks, fruit juice, alcohol, or coffee; if you drink alcohol, limit it to 1 or 2 drinks per day
- **Stock the fridge.** Keep a stash of low-calorie, nutritious snacks, such as pretzels, light microwave popcorn, fruit (fresh, canned, or dried)
- **Exercise regularly.** Find a friend to work out with you. Experts recommend 30 minutes of moderate exercise at least 5 days a week.

interactive tools on www.mypyramid.gov to estimate your energy needs.

A healthy rate of weight loss is one to two pounds per week. Greater rates of weight loss will not likely be sustained over time. Remember that the numbers on the scale are not as important as your body composition—the amount of fat in relation to lean mass. One pound of weight loss requires a deficit of 3500 kilocalories. Thus, to lose one pound per week, you will need to cut back on food intake and/or increase your exercise routine to shift the energy balance equation by 500 kilocalories per day.

Many students skip breakfast, whether it is to save time, money, or calories. However, breakfast is the *most* important meal of the day. Starting the day off with a fortified, whole-grain breakfast cereal, skim milk, and a serving of fruit puts you on the right path for meeting recommendations for fiber, calcium, and fruit intake. Even though it may seem that a cup of coffee gets your brain going in the morning, your brain is fueled best by carbohydrates, not caffeine. In addition, studies repeatedly show that eating breakfast prevents overeating later in the day, by preventing hunger from dictating your food choices.

Calories can sneak up on the unsuspecting college student. One of the biggest contributors to weight gain is consuming several hundred calories per day in the form of sugary beverages or alcoholic beverages. One 12-ounce can of regular cola contains about 140 kcal. A 12-ounce can of regular beer has 150 kcal. In addition, a study has shown that consuming gourmet coffee beverages, such as lattes and cappuccinos increases average calorie consumption by about 200 kilocalories per day. Even fruit juices, which we perceive to be healthy, have at least 100 kcal per 8-ounce glass. Furthermore, a 24-ounce mug of a soft drink makes you feel no fuller than an equal volume of water, yet the soft drink adds 300 kcal more. A convenient stash of water is the best way to quench your thirst.

Exercise is very important to any weight loss and weight maintenance plan. It's easy to start an exercise routine, but sticking with it is the hard part. When you find yourself short on time, exercise is often

the first thing we sacrifice. To ensure your success at boosting daily activity, choose activities you enjoy such as working out with friends at the campus recreation center, participating in intramural sports, or taking an activity class like dancing. Don't forget the brisk walking to and from classes. For more information on planning an exercise program, see Chapter 10.

## Alcohol and Binge Drinking

Excessive alcohol consumption is a big problem on college campuses. Legal or not, many college students consider drinking alcohol to be a "rite of passage" into adulthood. On campuses, binge drinking—consuming five or more drinks in a row for men, or four drinks or more for women—has become an epidemic. A new level of "extreme drinking" goes far beyond binge drinking. For example, recent studies indicate that college students celebrate twenty-first birthdays with an average of 12 drinks for men and nine for women.

The statistics on the impact of binge drinking on college campuses are sobering. An estimated two of every five students on college campuses participates in binge drinking. Each year, 1400 college students between the ages of 18 and 24 die from alcohol-related unintentional injuries, including motor vehicle crashes. In addition to deaths and injuries, other problems stemming from binge drinking include unsafe sex and its consequences, long-term health problems, suicides, academic problems, legal troubles, and alcohol abuse or dependence. Thirty one percent of college students meet the criteria for a diagnosis of alcohol abuse and 6% for a diagnosis of alcohol dependence.

In addition to these dire consequences, alcohol consumption definitely contributes to weight gain—by virtue of its own calories and by way of increased food consumption at events where drinking occurs. If you choose to drink alcohol, do so in moderation—no more than two drinks per day for men or no more than one drink per day for women. For your own sake and the safety of your peers, be aware of the warning signs and dangers of alcohol poisoning shown in the margin.

## Eating Disorders

In college, the stresses of achieving academic and social success put many students, particularly women, at risk. As many as 30% of college students are at risk of developing an eating disorder. As you will learn in Chapter 11, disordered eating is a mild and short-term change in eating patterns that typically occurs in response to life stress, a desire to change appearance, or a bad habit. Sometimes, disordered eating habits may lead to an eating disorder, such as anorexia nervosa, bulimia nervosa, or binge-eating disorder. Exercise bulimia is also an eating disorder in which students obsessively work out to get rid of calories. Chapter 11 includes advice on what to do if you suspect that your roommate or friend is suffering from an eating disorder.

Starving the body also starves the brain, limiting performance in academics and beyond, and the negative consequences of disordered eating may last a lifetime. Ultimately, eating disorders do not arise from problems with food but rather from problems with self-esteem, control, and abusive relationships. Food happens to be the focus of many emotional issues. Frequently, what begins as a diet spirals into a much larger problem. Eating disorders are not just diets gone bad—they require professional intervention. Left unchecked, eating disorders lead to serious adverse effects, such as loss of menstrual periods, thinning of bones, gastrointestinal problems, kidney problems, heart abnormalities, and eventually death.

## Choosing a Vegetarian Lifestyle

During college, many students experiment with or adopt a vegetarian eating pattern. Interest in plant-based diets has been growing steadily as more research points to their health benefits. While plant-based diets can meet nutrition needs and decrease risk of many chronic diseases, they require appropriate planning at all life stages.

Protein is not typically deficient, even with a vegan diet, which contains no animal products. However, vegetarians, and especially vegans, may be at risk for deficiencies of several vitamins and minerals. Consuming a ready-to-eat breakfast cereal is an easy and inexpensive way to obtain these nutrients. See Chapter 6 for further information on food planning for vegetarians.

As interest in vegetarian meals has grown, restaurants and campus dining services have responded by offering a variety of vegetarian options. For optimal health benefits, choose foods that are baked, steamed, or stir-fried rather than deep-fried; select whole grains rather than refined carbohydrates; and consume food fortified with vitamins and minerals. Even if you do not choose to follow a plant-based diet all the time, choosing several plant-based meals each week can help with weight control and boost intake of fiber and many healthy phytochemicals.

## Fuel for Competition: Student Athletes

Students who compete in sports such as intramural and intercollegiate athletics need to consume more calories and nutrients. Despite an emphasis on a lean physique or a drive to compete at a low

▶ **The warning signs and symptoms of alcohol poisoning**

- Semiconsciousness or unconsciousness
- Slow respiration of eight or fewer breaths per minute or lapses between breaths of more than 8 seconds
- Cold, clammy, pale, or bluish skin
- Strong odor of alcohol, which usually accompanies these symptoms

Some calorie traps for college students:

| Number of calories | |
|---|---|
| Six-pack of regular beer | 900 |
| Two handfuls of almonds | 500 |
| Two handfuls of granola | 330 |
| Personal-size pizza | 500 to 600 |
| 1 cup of ice cream | 300 |
| Two handfuls of frosted cereal | 250 |

*Source:* Ann Litt, The College Student's Guide to Eating Well on Campus

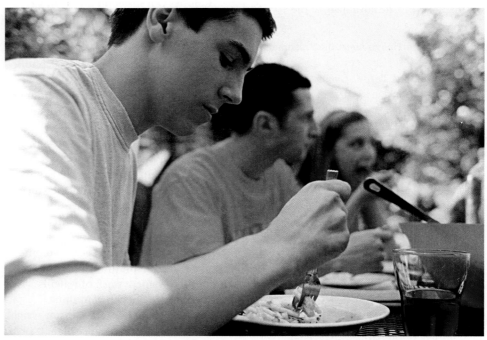

▲ Many students adopt a vegetarian diet during college. Guidelines for planning a nutritious vegetarian diet are presented in Chapter 6.

weight class, athletes at all levels must take care not to severely restrict calories, as this could impact performance and health. Muscles require adequate carbohydrates for fuel and protein for growth and repair. Fat, as well, is an important source of stored energy for use during exercise. Women who drop to low levels of body fat may become amenorrheic (cease menstruating), a condition costly to long-term bone health.

In addition to fueling the body with calories, fluids are essential for health and performance. Water is adequate for events lasting less than 60 minutes. For longer events, sports drinks are ideal because they also supply carbohydrates to fuel fatigued muscles as well as electrolytes to replenish those lost in perspiration. Intentional fluid losses to "make weight" for a competition are detrimental to health and performance.

Athletes also should take care not to be wooed by the supplement industry. Increasing food intake to meet the energy demands of athletic training is usually sufficient to also meet vitamin and mineral needs. As an exception, athletes may be at risk for iron-deficiency anemia. Consuming a balanced multivitamin and mineral supplement is adequate for most people. Individual vitamin, mineral, amino acid, or herbal supplements are not advised, in spite of the hype of supplement makers.

## Tips For Eating Well on a College Student's Budget

If you've learned one thing from college, it's that higher education can be hard on the wallet! Luckily, it is possible to eat well on campus on a budget.

If you live on campus, participate in a prepaid campus meal plan. These are generally designed to offer great food value with a variety of healthy foods. If you live off campus or have your own kitchen, plan ahead—for the day and for the week. Packing a lunch from home will save a lot of cash compared to grabbing lunch on the run and puts you more in control of healthy choices. For example, preparing a sandwich at home costs less than half as much as purchasing one at a fast-food restaurant or deli.

For those who shop for groceries, never go shopping on an empty stomach—everything will look good and you'll buy more. Also, go to the store with a list in hand and stick to it, because impulse buys tend to drain your wallet. When you shop for foods, buy store-brand foods rather than name-brand items. Make use of canned and frozen fruits and vegetables—they are just as nutritious as fresh fruits and vegetables, particularly if you choose low-sodium and low-sugar varieties. Rather than buying cartons of fruit juice, select cans of fruit juice concentrate and mix with water at home. Likewise, preparing other drinks, such as iced tea, from store-brand powder (look for sugar-free) will save over gallon jugs or vending machine containers of drinks. Canned (fruits, tuna) and dry (oatmeal) foods can be nutritious and last a long time, so you can avoid throwing out spoiled items. Finally, eggs and peanut butter are inexpensive and simple sources of protein.

## Case Study Typical College Student

Andy is like many other college students. He grew up on a quick bowl of cereal and milk for breakfast and a hamburger, French fries, and cola for lunch, either in the school cafeteria or at a local fast-food restaurant. At dinner, he generally avoided eating any of his salad or vegetables, and by 9 o'clock he was deep into bags of chips and cookies. Andy has taken most of these habits to college. He prefers coffee for breakfast and possibly a chocolate bar. Lunch is still mainly a hamburger, French fries, and cola, but pizza and tacos now alternate more frequently than when he was in high school. One thing Andy really likes about the restaurants surrounding campus is that, for less than a dollar more, he can *supersize* his meal. This helps him stretch his food dollar; searching out value meals for lunch and dinner now has become part of a typical day.

Provide some dietary advice for Andy. Start with his positive habits and then provide some constructive criticism, based on what you now know.

Answer the following questions, and check your responses in Appendix A.

1. **Start with Andy's positive habits:** What healthy choices are being made when Andy eats at local restaurants?

2. **Now provide some constructive criticisms:**
   a. What are some of the negative aspects of items available at fast-food restaurants?
   b. Why is supersizing a dangerous habit?
   c. What healthier substitutions could he make at each meal?
   d. List some healthier choices he could make at fast-food restaurants on campus.

## Summary

1. Nutrition is a lifestyle factor that is a key to developing and maintaining an optimal state of health. A poor diet and a sedentary lifestyle are known to be risk factors for life-threatening chronic diseases such as heart disease, hypertension, diabetes, and cancer. Not meeting nutrient needs in younger years makes us more likely to suffer health consequences in later years. Too much of a nutrient also can be harmful. Drinking too much alcohol is another dietary problem associated with many health problems.

2. Nutrition is the study of the food substances vital for health and the study of how the body uses these substances to promote and support growth, maintenance, and reproduction of cells. Nutrients in foods fall into six classes: (1) carbohydrates, (2) lipids (mostly fats and oils), (3) proteins, (4) vitamins, (5) minerals, and (6) water. The first three, along with alcohol, provide calories for the body to use.

3. The body transforms the energy contained in carbohydrate, protein, and fat into other forms of energy that in turn allow the body to function. Fat provides, on average, 9 kcal per gram, whereas both protein and carbohydrate provide, on average, 4 kcal per gram. Vitamins, minerals, and water do not supply calories to the body but are essential for proper body function.

4. A basic plan for health promotion and disease prevention includes eating a varied diet, performing regular physical activity, not smoking, not abusing nutrient supplements (if used), consuming adequate water and other fluids, getting enough sleep, limiting alcohol intake (if consumed), and limiting or appropriately coping with stress. The primary focus of nutrition planning should be on food, not on dietary supplements. The focus on foods to supply nutrient needs avoids the possibility of severe nutrient imbalances.

5. Results from large nutrition surveys in the United States and Canada suggest that some of us need to concentrate on consuming foods that supply more of certain vitamins, minerals, and fiber. Daily use of a balanced multivitamin and mineral supplement does not substitute for a healthy diet but does provide a strategy to address some dietary shortcomings.

6. Groups of cells in the hypothalamus and other regions in the brain affect hunger, the primarily internal desire to find and eat food. These cells monitor hormonal and nerve signals from digestive organs as well as amounts of nutrients and other substances in the blood to control satiety.

A variety of external (appetite-related) forces affect satiety. Hunger cues combine with appetite cues, such as easy availability of food, to promote food intake.

The flavor, appearance, and texture of foods primarily influence our food choices. Several other factors also help determine food habits and choices: our upbringing, various social and cultural factors, the image we want to project to others, economics, convenience, emotional state, and concerns about health.

There are no true "good" or "bad" foods, but some food choices are healthier than others. The focus should be on balancing a total diet by choosing many nutritious foods.

7. Studies show that the diets and other health habits of college students are not optimal. Students fall short of recommendations for servings of grains, vegetables, fruits, milk, and meat, opting instead for fats, sweets, and alcohol. This information is disturbing from a public health standpoint, because young adulthood is the time when many health behaviors are formed and will likely persist throughout life. Issues of particular importance on college campuses are weight control, making healthy meal choices, alcohol and binge drinking, and eating disorders.

## Study Questions

1. Name one chronic disease associated with poor nutrition habits. Now list a few corresponding risk factors.

2. Explain the concept of calories as it relates to foods. What are the values used to calculate kcals from grams of carbohydrate, fat, protein, and alcohol?

3. Identify three ways that water is used in the body.

4. Wendy's Big Bacon Classic contains 44 grams carbohydrate, 36 grams fat, and 37 grams protein. Calculate the percentage of calories derived from fat.

5. Describe two types of fat and explain why the differences are important in terms of overall health.

6. According to national nutrition surveys, which nutrients tend to be underconsumed by many North Americans? Why do you think this is the case?

7. List four health objectives for the United States for the year 2010. How would you rate yourself in each area? Why?

8. Describe the various organs and hormones that control hunger and satiety in the body. List other factors that influence our food patterns.

9. Describe how your food preferences have been shaped by the following factors:
   a. Exposure to foods at an early age
   b. Advertising (what is the newest food you have tried?)
   c. Eating out
   d. Peer pressure
   e. Economic factors

10. What products in your supermarket reflect the consumer demand for healthier foods? For convenience?

11. List five strategies to avoid weight gain during college.

## Check Your Knowledge

Answers to the following multiple choice questions are below

1. Energy-yielding nutrients include
   a. vitamins, minerals, and water.
   b. carbohydrates, proteins, and fats.
   c. trace minerals and fat-soluble vitamins.
   d. iron, vitamin C, and potassium.

2. The *essential* nutrients
   a. must be consumed at every meal.
   b. are required for infants but not adults.
   c. can be made in the body when they are needed.
   d. cannot be made by the body and therefore must be consumed to maintain health.

3. Sugars, starches, and dietary fibers are examples of
   a. proteins.     c. carbohydrates.
   b. vitamins.     d. minerals.

4. Which nutrient classes are most important in the regulation of body processes?
   a. vitamins
   b. carbohydrates
   c. minerals
   d. lipids
   e. Both a and c.

5. A kcal is a
   a. measure of heat energy.
   b. measure of fat in food.
   c. heating device.
   d. term used to describe the amount of sugar and fat in foods.

6. A food that contains 10 grams of fat would yield _____ kcal.
   a. 40          c. 90
   b. 70          d. 120

7. If you consume 300 grams of carbohydrate in a day that you consume 2400 kcal, the carbohydrates will provide _____% of your total energy intake.
   a. 12.5        c. 50
   b. 30          d. 60

8. Which of the following is true about the North American diet?

   a. Most of our protein comes from plant sources.
   b. About half of the carbohydrates come from simple sugars.
   c. Most of our fats come from plant sources.
   d. Most of our carbohydrates come from starches.

9. The _____ is a term used to describe the amount of weight college students gain during the first year of college
   a. Varsity 8
   b. Stadium 7
   c. Dormitory 12
   d. Freshman 15

10. The region of the brain that helps regulate hunger is the
   a. cortex.
   b. hypothalamus.
   c. pituitary.
   d. cerebrum.

Answer Key: 1. b, 2. d, 3. c, 4. e, 5. a, 6. c, 7. c, 8. b, 9. d, 10. b.

## Further Readings

1. Bachman JL and others: Sources of food group intakes among the US population, 2001–2002. *Journal of the American Dietetic Association* 108:804, 2008.

   *The major sources of MyPyramid food group intakes for Americans were determined for 2001–2002. Intakes of dark green and orange vegetables, legumes, and whole grains were well below recommendations. Americans were found to generally consume foods that are high in solid fats and added sugars. Foods that contributed most to the discrepancies between MyPyramid food group recommendations and actual intake were carbonated sweetened beverages, grain-based desserts, non-skim dairy products, and fatty meats. Americans do not consume the most nutrient-dense options from the food groups. Food choices appear to be affected by many factors, including the increase in eating away from home.*

2. Brown LB and others: College students can benefit by participating in a prepaid meal plan. *Journal of the American Dietetic Association,* 105:445, 2005.

   *Participation in a prepaid campus meal plan resulted in modest nutritional benefits to students through an increase in servings of foods from fruit, vegetable, and meat groups.*

3. Cordain L and others: Origins and evolution of the Western diet: health implications for the 21st century. *American Journal of Clinical Nutrition* 1:341, 2005.

   *Throughout human's existence, the number of foods rich in refined sugars, refined flours, salt, and animal fat has increased. This has resulted in a decline in diet quality for many of us in the modern world.*

4. de Graaf C and others: Biomarkers of satiation. *American Journal of Clinical Nutrition* 79:946, 2004.

   *The feeling of satiety depends on a constellation of factors, such as stomach distention; the action of various hormones, such as ghrelin; and communication between various organs and the brain. This article reviews the latest findings with regard to these and other factors affecting satiety.*

5. Edmonds MJ and others: Body weight and percent body fat increase during the transition from high school to university in females. *Journal of the American Dietetic Association* 108:1033, 2008.

   *The notion that weight gain occurs during the first year of university was studied in Canadian females making the transition from high school to university. There was a significant increase in body weight of 2.4 kg (5.28 lbs) during the first six to seven months of university. Percent body fat also increased from 23.8% to 25.6%. Although dietary energy (calorie) intake did not increase, a decrease in moderate physical activity was an important predictor of weight. Body weight, therefore, may be modified by lifestyle factors during this formative period.*

6. Federal Trade Commission: Marketing food to children and adolescents: A review of industry expenditures, activities, and self-regulation, a report to Congress. July 2008. http://www.ftc.gov/os/2008/07/P064504food-mktingreport.pdf.

   *This study by the Federal Trade Commission found that 44 major food and beverage marketers spent $1.6 billion to promote their products to children under 12 and adolescents ages 12 to 17 in the United States in 2006. The report states that food advertising to youth is dominated by advertising campaigns that combine traditional media, such as television, with previously unmeasured forms of marketing, such as packaging, instore advertising, sweepstakes, and Internet. This advertising often involves cross-promotion with a new movie or popular television program. The report calls for all food companies "to adopt and adhere to meaningful, nutrition-based standards for marketing their products to children under 12."*

7. Guenther PM and others: Diet quality of Americans in 1994–96 and 2001–02 as measured by the Healthy Eating Index-2005. Nutrition Insight 37, U.S. Department of Agriculture. December 2007. http://www.cnpp.usda.gov/Publications/NutritionInsights/Insight37.pdf

   *There was little change in the diet quality of Americans, as measured by the Health Eating Index-2005, between 1994–96 and 2001–02. HEI-2005 scores were low for the "food groups to encourage" identified in the Dietary Guidelines for Americans 2005. Although scores for Total Grains and Meat and Beans components remained at the maximum value, scores decreased for Whole Fruit, Total Vegetables, and Whole Grains. Scores improved for Milk, Oils, and Sodium but showed no significant change for Total Fruit, Dark Green and Orange Vegetables and Legumes, and Saturated Fat. These results indicate that the diet quality of Americans needs to be improved.*

8. Hoffman DY and others: Changes in body weight and fat mass of men and women in the first year of college: A study of the "freshman 15." *Journal of American College of Health.* 55:41, 2006.

   *It is commonly thought that there is a high risk of gaining 15 pounds of weight during freshman year of college. In this study, changes in body weight and percentage of body fat were measured in first-year college students. Body weight increased by an average of almost three pounds (1.3 kilograms) and body fat increased an average of 0.7%. This study, therefore, found that weight and fat gain may occur during the first year of college.*

9. Lichtenstein AH and others: Diet and lifestyle recommendations revision 2006. A scientific statement from the American Heart Association Nutrition Committee. *Circulation* 114:82, 2006.

   *The American Heart Association presents recommendations designed to reduce the risk of cardiovascular disease in the general population. Specific goals include consuming an overall healthy diet; aiming for a healthy body weight; achieving healthy targets for blood cholesterol levels, blood pressure, and blood glucose; being physically active; and avoiding the use of and exposure to tobacco products.*

10. Litt, AS: *The College Student's Guide to Eating Well on Campus.* Tulip Hill Press, Glen Echo, MD, 2005.

    *This book provides important information on how to survive and eat well during your college years and covers how to avoid and spot eating disorders.*

11. Lubin F and others: Lifestyle and ethnicity play a role in all-cause mortality. *Journal of Nutrition* 133:1180, 2003.

    *Dietary habits that reduce all-cause mortality include focusing on both high-fiber foods and those low in saturated fat and cholesterol. Positive lifestyle habits include regular physical activity and avoiding smoking and obesity.*

12. Mokdad AH and others: Actual causes of death in the United States, 2000. *Journal of the American Medical Association* 291:1238, 2004.

    *Smoking is the leading cause of preventable death in the United States, with obesity a close second. A combination of a poor diet and inactive lifestyle may account for about one third of deaths in the United States.*

13. Olshansky SJ and others: A potential decline in life expectancy in the United States in the 21st century. *The New England Journal of Medicine* 352:1138, 2005.

    *The growing problem of overweight and obesity in our society is likely to lead to more overall premature deaths. An alarming concern is that this widespread increase in body weight could result in a life expectancy of fewer years for today's children compared to their parents.*

*Reversing this trend of greater overweight and obesity is crucial.*

14. Oz D: *The Dorm Room Diet: The 8-Step Program for Creating a Healthy Lifestyle Plan that Really Works.* Newmarket Press, 2006.

    *This book is written to help students stay fit while at college. The 8-step program shows students how to stop eating out of emotional need; navigate the most common danger zones at school for unhealthy eating; get the exercise you need, even in your small dorm room; choose vitamins and supplements wisely and relax and rejuvenate amid the stress of college life.*

15. Paeratakul S and others: Fast-food consumption among U.S. adults and children: Dietary and nutrient intake profile. *Journal of the American Dietetic Association* 103:1332, 2003.

    *Regular intake of fast-food contributes a lot of fat and calories to a diet. Such foods can also crowd out more healthful foods in a diet. Regular fast-food consumers would be wise to focus on lower-fat items and greatly limit or avoid sugared soft drinks and French fries.*

16. Rutledge PC and others: 21st birthday drinking: extremely extreme. *Journal of Consulting and Clinical Psychology* 76:511, 2008.

    *A new level of extreme drinking goes beyond the four or five drinks in one sitting defined as "bingeing". At the University of Missouri, a study of 2,518 students found 34% of men and 24% of women who imbibed on their 21st birthdays drank 21 alcoholic drinks or more. The authors conclude that interventions shown to be effective with general risky drinking may prove effective in reducing 21st birthday excess.*

17. Shields DH and others: Gourmet coffee beverage consumption among college women. *Journal of the American Dietetic Association,* 104:650, 2004.

    *A significant percentage of college women were shown to consume gourmet coffee beverages which contributed additional calories and fat to their daily dietary intake.*

18. Tholin S and others: Genetic and environmental influence on eating behavior: the Swedish Young Male Twins Study. *American Journal of Clinical Nutrition* 81:564, 2005.

    *Genetics plays a distinct role in the development of eating habits, such as emotional eating or restrained eating. This may be linked to the amount of various hormones and other physiological factors that can influence eating habits.*

19. Todd JE and Variyam JN: The decline in consumer use of food nutrition labels, 1995–2006. *Economic Research Service Report.* U.S. Department of Agriculture, August 2008.

    *Consumer use of most components of nutrition labels when making food purchases declined from 1995 to 2006. Use of information about fiber and sugars did not decline over the 10-year period. The decrease varied by population groups but was greatest for individuals 20–29 years old and those who spoke primarily Spanish.*

20. Woolf K and others: Physical activity is associated with risk factors for chronic disease across adult women's life cycle. *Journal of the American Dietetic Association* 108:948, 2008.

    *The results of this study confirm that younger age and greater physical activity across the adult women's life cycle are associated with more favorable serum lipid levels; less inflammation; lower concentrations of insulin, glucose, and leptin in serum; and more favorable body composition. These factors are associated with reduced risk for several chronic diseases including cardiovascular disease, type 2 diabetes, and obesity.*

21. U.S. Department of Health and Human Services. 2008 physical activity guidelines for Americans. *www.health.gov/paguidelines*

    *Inactivity remains relatively high among American children, adolescents, and adults. These science-based guidelines are designed to help Americans aged six and older use appropriate physical activity to improve their health. The guidelines include information about the health benefits of physical activity; how to do physical activity in a manner that meets the guidelines; how to reduce the risks of activity-related injury; and how to assist others in participating regularly in physical activity.*

22. Yanover T and Sacco WP. Eating beyond satiety and body mass index. *Eating and Weight Disorders* 13:119, 2008.

    *Eating beyond satiety (EBS), snacking, night eating, and hunger were examined in undergraduate females. EBS was the strongest predictor of body mass and therefore may be a variable to target in interventions to prevent and treat overweight and obesity.*

## I. Examine Your Eating Habits More Closely

Choose one day of the week that is typical of your eating pattern. Using the first table found in Appendix E, list all foods and drinks you consumed for 24 hours. In addition, write down the approximate amounts of food you ate in units, such as cups, ounces, teaspoons, and tablespoons. After you record the amount of each food and drink consumed, indicate in the table why you chose to consume the item. Place the corresponding abbreviation in the space provided to indicate why you picked that food or drink.

| FLVR | Flavor/texture | ADV | Advertisement | PEER | Peers |
|------|----------------|------|---------------|------|-------|
| CONV | Convenience | WTCL | Weight control | NUTR | Nutritive value |
| EMO | Emotions | HUNG | Hunger | $ | Cost |
| AVA | Availability | FAM | Family/cultural | HLTH | Health |

There can be more than one reason for choosing a particular food or drink.

### Application

Ask yourself what your most frequent reason is for eating or drinking. To what degree is health or nutritive value a reason for your food choices? Should you make these higher priorities?

## II. Observe the Supermarket Explosion

Today's supermarkets carry up to 60,000 items, compared to 20,000 items 10 years ago. Think about your last grocery shopping trip and the items you purchased to eat. Following is a list of 20 newer food products added to supermarket shelves. Check the items that you have tried. Then use the key from Part I of the Rate Your Plate exercise to identify why you might have chosen these products.

_____ Prepackaged salad greens (variety packs other than iceberg lettuce) _____

_____ Gourmet salad oils (e.g., walnut, almond, olive, or sesame oil) _____

_____ Gourmet vinegars (e.g., balsamic or rice) _____

_____ Prepackaged lunch products (e.g., nacho, pizza, taco, and tortilla Lunchables) _____

_____ Precooked frozen turkey patties _____

_____ Bean soup mixes (e.g., lentil, black bean, combination bean soups) _____

_____ Microwaveable sandwiches (e.g., Hotpockets, frozen sandwiches) _____

_____ Refrigerated, precooked pasta (e.g., tortellini, fettucini) and accompanying sauces (e.g., pesto, tomato basil) _____
_____

_____ Imported grain products (e.g., risotto, farfalline, gnocchi, fusilli) _____

_____ Frozen dinners (list your favorite of any of the wide variety) _____

_____ Imported sauces for food preparation (e.g., hoisin or brown bean sauce; mandarin marinade, sesame, curry, or fire oils)
_____

_____ Bottled waters (flavored or unflavored) _____

_____ Trendy juices (e.g., draft apple cider, hurricane punch) _____

_____ Roasted and/or flavored coffees (e.g., beans, ground, or instant) _____

_____ Gourmet jelly beans and candies (e.g., gummi coca-colas or imported chocolates) _____

_____ Instant hot cereal in a bowl (add water and go!) _____

_____ "Fast-shake" pancake mix (add water, shake, and ready to cook) _____

_____ Breakfast bars (e.g., granola or fruit-flavored bars) _____

_____ Meal replacement/fitness products (e.g., "energy" bars, high-protein bars, sports drinks) _____

_____ Low-carbohydrate meat and pasta dishes _____

Finally, identify three new food products not on this list that you have seen in the past year. Discuss the appeal of these products to the North American consumer.

$1.09

# CHAPTER 2 Guidelines for Designing a Healthy Diet

## Student Learning Outcomes Chapter 2 is designed to allow you to:

1. Develop a healthy eating plan.

2. Outline the measurements used (ABCDEs) in nutrition assessment: anthropometric, biochemical, clinical, dietary, and environmental status.

3. Learn the food groupings used in MyPyramid.

4. List the Dietary Guidelines and the diseases these guidelines are designed to prevent or minimize.

5. Describe what the Recommended Dietary Allowances (RDAs) and other dietary standards represent.

6. Understand the basis of the scientific method as it is used in developing

hypotheses and theories in the field of nutrition, including the determination of nutrient needs.

7. Describe the components of the nutrition label and the various health claims and label descriptors that are allowed.

8. Identify reliable sources of nutrition information.

## Chapter Outline

Student Learning Outcomes

Refresh Your Memory

2.1 A Food Philosophy That Works

2.2 States of Nutritional Health

2.3 How Can Your Nutritional State Be Measured?

2.4 Recommendations for Healthy Eating

2.5 Specific Nutrient Standards and Recommendations

2.6 Using the Scientific Method to Determine Nutrient Needs

2.7 Food Labels and Diet Planning

2.8 Epilogue

Nutrition and Your Health: Evaluating Nutrition Claims and Dietary Supplements

Case Study: Dietary Supplements

Summary/Study Questions/Check Your Knowledge/Further Readings

Rate Your Plate

HOW MANY TIMES HAVE YOU HEARD WILD CLAIMS ABOUT HOW HEALTHFUL CERTAIN FOODS ARE FOR YOU? As consumers focus more on diet and disease, food manufacturers are asserting that their products have all sorts of health benefits. "Eat more olive oil and oat bran to lower blood cholesterol." "Drink pomegranate juice to guard your body against free radicals." Hearing these claims, you would think that food manufacturers have solutions to all of our health problems.

Advertising aside, nutrient intakes that are out of balance with our needs—such as excess calories, saturated fat, cholesterol, *trans* fat, salt, alcohol, and sugar intakes—are linked to many leading causes of death in North America. These were introduced in Chapter 1 and include obesity, hypertension, cardiovascular disease, cancer, liver disease, and type 2 diabetes. Physical inactivity is also too common. In Chapter 2, you will explore the components of a healthy diet and lifestyle—an approach that will minimize your risks of developing nutrition-related diseases. The goal is to provide you with a firm understanding of these concepts before you study the nutrients in detail.

**Refresh Your Memory**

As you begin your study of diet planning in Chapter 2, you may want to review:

- The terms in the margin in Chapter 1 and Table 1-1.

## 2.1 A Food Philosophy that Works

You may be surprised that what you should eat to minimize the risk of developing the nutrition-related diseases seen in North America is exactly what you've heard many times before: *Consume a variety of foods balanced by a moderate intake of each food.* Health professionals have recommended the same basic diet and health plan for the past 50 years: Control how much you eat, focus on the major food groups, and stay physically active. Whole-grain breads and cereals, fruits, and vegetables, as discussed in the comic in this chapter, have always been among the foods emphasized for our diet for these past 50 years.

It is disappointing, however, that according to a recent survey conducted by the American Dietetic Association, two of five people in the United States believe that following a healthful diet means completely giving up foods they enjoy. To the contrary, a healthful diet requires only some simple planning and doesn't have to mean deprivation and misery. Besides, eliminating favorite foods typically doesn't work for "dieters" in the long run. The best plan consists of learning the basics of a healthful diet—a variety and balance of foods from all food groups and moderate consumption of all foods. Monitoring total calorie intake is also important for many of us, especially if unwanted weight gain is taking place. Let's now fine-tune this advice by focusing on variety, balance, and moderation, as well as nutrient, and energy density.

▲ For the past 50 years, fruits, vegetables, and whole-grain breads and cereals have been among the foods recommended for our diet.

### Variety Means Eating Many Different Foods

Variety in your diet means choosing a number of different foods within any given food group rather than eating the "same old thing" day after day. Variety makes meals

On what do nutrition experts generally agree regarding a healthy food or diet? Why is a diet rich in fiber that includes some fish and is low in fried foods and animal fat emphasized, along with at least 30 minutes or more of physical activity on most or all days of the week? Are North Americans generally following this plan? What are the potential consequences for those who do not? Chapter 2 provides some answers.

STONE SOUP © 2007 Jan Eliot. Reprinted with permission of UNIVERSAL PRESS SYNDICATE. All rights reserved.

more interesting and helps ensure that a diet contains sufficient nutrients. A variety of foods is best because no one food meets all your nutrient needs. Meat provides protein and iron but little calcium and no vitamin C. Eggs also provide protein but little calcium because the calcium is mostly in the shell. Cow's milk contains calcium, but very little iron. None of these foods contains fiber. Thus you need a variety of foods in your diet because the required nutrients are scattered among many foods. For example, carrots—a rich source of a pigment that forms vitamin A—may be your favorite vegetable; however, if you choose carrots every day as your only vegetable source, you may miss out on the vitamin folate. Other vegetables, such as broccoli and asparagus, are rich sources of this nutrient. This concept is true of all groups of foods: fruits, vegetables, grains, and so on. Different foods within each group vary somewhat in the nutrients they contain, but they generally provide similar types of nutrients.

An added bonus of variety in the diet, especially within the fruit and vegetable groups, is the inclusion of a rich supply of the **phytochemicals.** Recall from Chapter 1 that the phytochemicals were discussed along with the nutrient classes. Many of these substances provide significant health benefits. Considerable research attention is focused on various phytochemicals in reducing the risk for certain diseases (e.g., cancer). You can't just buy a bottle of phytochemicals—they are generally available only within whole foods. Current multivitamin and mineral supplements contain few or none of these beneficial plant chemicals.

Numerous population studies show reduced cancer risk among people who regularly consume fruits and vegetables. Researchers suspect that some phytochemicals present in the fruits and vegetables block the cancer process. The cancer process and the specific roles of some phytochemicals in this regard are described in the "Nutrition and Your Health" section in Chapter 16. Some phytochemicals also have been linked to a reduced risk of cardiovascular disease. Could it be that, because humans evolved on a wide variety of plant-based foods, the body developed with a need for these phytochemicals, along with the various nutrients present, to maintain optimal health?

Foods rich in phytochemicals are now part of a family of foods referred to as **functional foods.** A functional food is a food that provides health benefits beyond those supplied by the traditional nutrients it contains. A tomato contains the phytochemical lycopene, so it can be called a functional food. You may hear this term more from the food industry in the future.

It will likely take many years for scientists to unravel the important effects of the myriad of phytochemicals in foods, and it is unlikely that all will ever be available or effective in supplement form. For this reason, leading nutrition and medical experts suggest that a diet rich in fruits, vegetables, and whole-grain breads and cereals is the most reliable way to obtain the potential benefits of phytochemicals. Some research suggests that increasing variety in a diet can lead to overeating. Thus, as one incorporates a wide variety of foods in a diet, attention to total calorie intake is also important to consider. Table 2-1 provides a number of suggestions for including more phytochemicals in your diet, as do the websites www.fruitsandveggiesmorematters .org and www.fruitsandveggiesmatter.gov.

**functional foods** Foods that provide health benefits beyond those supplied by the traditional nutrients they contain. For example, a tomato contains the phytochemical lycopene, so it can be called a functional food.

## Balance Means Consuming Food From Each Group

One way to balance your diet as you consume a variety of foods is to select foods from each of the six major food groups every day:

- Grains
- Vegetables
- Fruits
- Milk
- Meat & Beans
- Oils

▲ Focus on nutrient-rich foods as you strive to meet your nutrient needs. The more colorful the food on your plate, the greater the content of nutrients and phytochemicals.

## Critical Thinking

Andy would benefit from more variety in his diet. What are some practical tips he can use to increase his fruit and vegetable intake?

The current food guide plan, MyPyramid, is discussed later in this chapter and offers eating plans and advice to help make smart choices from each of these food groups. A dinner consisting of a bean burrito, lettuce and tomato salad with oil and vinegar dressing, a glass of milk, and an apple covers all groups.

### Moderation Refers Mostly to Portion Size

Eating in moderation requires eating moderate (i.e., small) portion sizes and planning your entire day's diet so that you don't overconsume any nutrients. For example, if you eat a bacon cheeseburger, relatively high in fat, salt, and calories, you should eat foods such as fruits and salad greens, that are less concentrated sources of these nutrients at other meals that same day. This helps balance your diet. If you prefer whole milk to low-fat or fat-free milk, reduce the fat elsewhere in your meals. Try

**TABLE 2-1** Tips for Boosting the Phytochemical Content of a Diet

- Include vegetables in main and side dishes. Add these to rice, omelets, potato salad, and pastas. Try broccoli or cauliflower florets, mushrooms, peas, carrots, corn, or peppers.

- Look for quick-to-fix grain side dishes in the supermarket. Pilafs, couscous, rice mixes, and tabbouleh are just a few that you'll find.

- Choose fruit-filled cookies, such as fig bars, instead of sugar-rich cookies. Use fresh or canned fruit as a topping for puddings, hot or cold cereal, pancakes, and frozen desserts.

- Put raisins, grapes, apple chunks, pineapples, grated carrots, zucchini, or cucumber into coleslaw, chicken salad, or tuna salad.

- Be creative at the salad bar: Try fresh spinach, leaf lettuce, red cabbage, zucchini, yellow squash, cauliflower, peas, mushrooms, or red or yellow peppers.

- Pack fresh or dried fruit for snacks away from home instead of grabbing a candy bar or going hungry.

- Add slices of cucumber, zucchini, spinach, or carrot slivers to the lettuce and tomato on your sandwiches.

- Each week try one or two vegetarian meals, such as beans and rice or pasta; vegetable stir fry; or spaghetti and tomato sauce.

- If your daily protein intake exceeds the recommended amounts, reduce the meat, fish, or poultry in casseroles, stews, and soups by one-third to one-half and add more vegetables and legumes.

- Keep a bowl of fresh vegetables in the refrigerator for snacks.

- Choose fruit or vegetable juices instead of soft drinks, and preferably 100% juice varieties.

- Substitute tea for coffee or soft drinks on a regular basis.

- Have a bowl of fresh fruit on hand.

- Switch from crisp head lettuce to leaf lettuce, such as romaine.

- Use salsa as a dip for chips in place of creamy dips.

- Choose whole-grain breakfast cereals, breads, and crackers.

- Add flavor to your plate with ginger, rosemary, basil, thyme, garlic, onions, parsley, and chives in place of salt.

- Incorporate soy products, such as tofu, soy milk, soy protein isolate, and roasted soybeans into your meals (see Chapter 6).

low-fat salad dressings, or use jam rather than butter or margarine on toast. Overall, strive to moderate serving sizes of some foods rather than eliminating these foods.

As noted in Chapter 1, many nutrition experts agree that there are no exclusively "good" or "bad" foods. Even so, many North Americans have diets that lack the foundations of a healthy food plan—variety, balance, and moderation. Consuming diets overloaded with foods high in fatty meats, fried foods, sugared soft drinks, and refined starches can result in substantial risk for nutrition-related chronic diseases.

## Nutrient Density Focuses on Nutrient Content

The **nutrient density** of a food is a characteristic used to determine its nutritional quality. Nutrient density of a food is determined by comparing its protein, vitamin, or mineral content with the amount of calories it provides. A food is said to be nutrient dense if it provides a large amount of a nutrient for a relatively small amount of calories when compared with other food sources. The higher a food's nutrient density, the better it is as a nutrient source. Comparing the nutrient density of different foods is an easy way to estimate their relative nutritional quality. Generally, nutrient density is determined with respect to individual nutrients. For example, many fruits and vegetables have a high content of vitamin C compared with their modest calorie content: That is, they are nutrient-dense foods for vitamin C. Figure 2-1 shows that fat-free milk is much more nutrient dense than sugared soft drinks for many nutrients, especially protein, vitamin A, riboflavin, and calcium.

As noted previously, menu planning should focus mainly on the total diet—not on the selection of one critical food as the key to an adequate diet. Nutrient-dense foods—such as fat-free and low-fat milk, lean meats, legumes (beans), oranges, carrots, broccoli, whole-wheat bread, and whole-grain breakfast cereals—do help balance less nutrient-dense foods—such as cookies and potato chips—which many people like to eat. The latter are often called empty-calorie foods because they tend to be high in sugar and/or fat but few other nutrients.

Eating nutrient-dense foods is especially important for people who tend to consume diets relatively low in calories. This includes some older people and those following weight-loss diets.

## Energy (KCAL) Density Affects Calorie Intake

**Energy density** is a measurement that best describes the calorie content of a food. Energy density of a food is determined by comparing the calorie (kcal) content with the weight of food. A food rich in calories but that weighs relatively little is considered energy dense. Examples include nuts; cookies; fried foods in general; and fat-free snacks, such as fat-free pretzels. Foods with low energy density include fruits, vegetables, and any food that incorporates lots of water during cooking, such as oatmeal (Table 2-2).

Researchers have shown that eating a meal with many foods of low energy density promotes satiety without contributing many calories. This is probably because we typically consume a constant weight of food at a meal, rather than a constant number of calories. How this constant weight of food is regulated is not known, but careful laboratory studies show that people consume fewer calories in a meal if most of the food choices are low in energy density, compared with foods high in energy density. Eating a diet low in energy density can aid in losing (or maintaining) weight.

Overall, foods with lots of water and fiber provide a low-energy-density contribution to a meal and help one feel full, whereas foods with high energy density must be eaten in greater amounts to contribute to fullness. This is one more reason to eat a diet rich in fruits, vegetables, and whole-grain breads and cereals, a pattern that also is typical of many ethnic diets throughout rural areas of the world.

Still, favorite foods, even if they are high in energy density, can have a place in your dietary pattern, but you will have to plan for them. For example, chocolate is a very

▲ Choosing whole-grain cereals is an excellent way to increase the nutrient content of a diet. Ideally, the cereal should have at least 3 grams of fiber per serving.

**nutrient density** The ratio derived by dividing a food's nutrient content by its calorie content. When the food's contribution to our nutrient need for that nutrient exceeds its contribution to our calorie need, the food is considered to have a favorable nutrient density.

**energy density** A comparison of the calorie (kcal) content of a food with the weight of the food. An energy-dense food is high in calories but weighs very little (e.g., potato chips), whereas a food low in energy density has few calories but weighs a lot, such as an orange.

**FIGURE 2-1** ▶ Comparison of the nutrient density of a sugared soft drink with that of fat-free (i.e., nonfat or skim) milk. Choosing a glass of fat-free milk makes a significantly greater contribution to nutrient intake than does a sugared soft drink. An easy way to determine nutrient density from this chart is to compare the lengths of the bars indicating vitamin or mineral contribution with the bar that represents calorie contribution. For the soft drink, no nutrient surpasses calorie content. Fat-free milk, in contrast, has longer nutrient bars for protein, vitamin A, the vitamins thiamin and riboflavin, and the mineral calcium than it does for calories. Including many nutrient-dense foods in your diet is a lower calorie way to meet nutrient needs.

**Percent Contribution to Adolescent Female RDAs**

Calories (kcal), Protein, Vitamin A, Vitamin C, Thiamin, Riboflavin, Niacin, Calcium, Iron

Sugared soft drink, 8 fl. oz. (1 cup)

Fat-free milk, 8 fl. oz. (1 cup)

## MAKING DECISIONS

Some people frequently choose French fries as their vegetable. What is the nutrient content of French fries? Check the food composition supplement for the vitamin C content of French fries. How many servings would you need to eat to meet vitamin C needs (75 to 95 milligrams)?

(Answer: 4 to 5 servings)

▲ Salads are low in energy density if we limit additional calories from salad dressing and especially minimize bacon bits, cheese crumbles or cubes, and croutons.

energy-dense food, but a small portion at the end of a meal can supply a satisfying finale. In addition, foods with high energy density can help people with poor appetites, such as some older people, to maintain or gain weight.

The following sections of Chapter 2 describe various states of nutritional health and provide tools and nutrient guidelines for planning healthy diets to support overall health.

### CONCEPT CHECK

Basic diet-planning concepts include consuming a variety of foods, balancing a diet by consuming foods from each of the five food groups, and moderating portion size with each food choice, so that the diet is not excessive in calories. Choosing nutrient-dense foods, such as fat-free milk, fruits, vegetables, and whole-grain breads and cereals, helps supply a diet with many nutrients but not excessive calories. Many of these foods are also rich sources of phytochemicals, supplying an even greater health benefit to the diet. Consuming foods of low energy density, such as fruits and vegetables, may also help in weight control, in that these provide satiety after a meal because of their large weight but relatively few calories.

## 2.2 States of Nutritional Health

The body's nutritional health is determined by considering the **nutritional state** of each needed nutrient. Three general categories of nutritional status are recognized: desirable nutrition, undernutrition, and overnutrition. The common term **malnutrition** can refer to either **overnutrition** or **undernutrition**. Neither state is conducive to good health. The amount of each nutrient needed to maintain a state of desirable nutrition is the basis for published dietary intake recommendations. The diet plans to meet those needs are discussed later in Chapter 2.

**TABLE 2-2** Energy Density of Common Foods (Listed in Relative Order)

| Very Low Energy Density (less than 0.6 kcal per gram) | Low Energy Density (0.6 to 1.5 kcal per gram) | Medium Energy Density (1.5 to 4 kcal per gram) | High Energy Density (greater than 4 kcal per gram) |
|---|---|---|---|
| Lettuce | Whole milk | Eggs | Graham crackers |
| Tomatoes | Oatmeal | Ham | Fat-free sandwich cookies |
| Strawberries | Cottage cheese | Pumpkin pie | Chocolate |
| Broccoli | Beans | Whole-wheat bread | Chocolate chip cookies |
| Salsa | Bananas | Bagels | Tortilla chips |
| Grapefruit | Broiled fish | White bread | Bacon |
| Fat-free milk | Fat-free yogurt | Raisins | Potato chips |
| Carrots | Ready-to-eat breakfast cereals with 1% low-fat milk | Cream cheese | Peanuts |
| Vegetable soup | | Cake with frosting | Peanut butter |
| | | Pretzels | Mayonnaise |
| | Plain baked potato | Rice cakes | Butter or margarine |
| | Cooked rice | | Vegetable oils |
| | Spaghetti noodles | | |

Data adapted from Rolls B, *The Volumetrics Eating Plan*. New York: HarperCollins, 2005.

▲ Today, soft drinks are more popular than milk, but not as beneficial to the diet. Soft drinks account for about 10% of the calorie intake of teenagers in North America and in turn contribute to generally poor calcium intakes seen in this age group.

## Desirable Nutrition

The nutritional state for a particular nutrient is desirable when body tissues have enough of the nutrient to support normal metabolic functions as well as surplus stores that can be used in times of increased need. A desirable nutritional state can be achieved by obtaining essential nutrients from a variety of foods.

## Undernutrition

Undernutrition occurs when nutrient intake does not meet nutrient needs. Any surpluses are then put to use and health begins to decline. Many nutrients are in high demand due to the constant cell loss and regeneration in the body, such as in the gastrointestinal tract. For this reason the stores of certain nutrients, including many of the B vitamins, are exhausted rapidly and therefore require a regular intake. In addition, some women in North America do not consume sufficient iron to meet monthly losses and eventually deplete their iron stores (Fig. 2-2).

Once availability of a nutrient falls sufficiently low, biochemical evidence indicates that the body's metabolic processes have slowed or stopped. At this state of deficiency there are no outward **symptoms,** thus it is termed a **subclinical** deficiency. A subclinical deficiency can go on for some time before clinicians are able to detect its effects.

Eventually clinical symptoms will develop. Clinical evidence of a nutritional deficiency; perhaps in the skin, hair, nails, tongue, or eyes, can occur within months but sometimes takes many years. Often, clinicians do not detect a problem until a deficiency produces outward symptoms, such as small areas of bruising on the skin from a vitamin C deficiency.

**nutritional state** The nutritional health of a person as determined by anthropometric measurements (height, weight, circumferences, and so on), biochemical measurements of nutrients or their by-products in blood and urine, a clinical (physical) examination, a dietary analysis, and economic evaluation; also called nutritional status.

**malnutrition** Failing health that results from long-standing dietary practices that do not coincide with nutritional needs.

**overnutrition** A state in which nutritional intake greatly exceeds the body's needs.

**undernutrition** Failing health that results from a long-standing dietary intake that is not enough to meet nutritional needs.

**symptom** A change in health status noted by the person with the problem, such as stomach pain.

**subclinical** Stage of a disease or disorder not severe enough to produce symptoms that can be detected or diagnosed.

**FIGURE 2-2 ▶** The general scheme of nutritional status. Green reflects good status, yellow marginal status, and red poor status (undernutrition or overnutrition). This general concept can be applied to all nutrients. Iron was chosen as an example because iron deficiency is the most common nutrient deficiency worldwide.

Decline in body functions associated with a decline in nutrient status. With iron deficiency, iron-containing proteins and in turn oxygen supply to body tissues is reduced. This then leads to clinical symptoms, such as fatigue upon exertion.

Adequate stores of nutrients, such as iron, and adequate blood values, such as for iron-related compounds.

Toxic damage to the body. In iron toxicity, liver cells in particular are affected.

**Undernutrition** · · · · · **Desirable Nutrition** · · · · · **Overnutrition**

## Overnutrition

Prolonged consumption of more nutrients than the body needs can lead to overnutrition. In the short run (e.g., 1 to 2 weeks), overnutrition may cause only a few symptoms, such as stomach distress from excess iron intake. But if an excess intake continues, some nutrients may accumulate to toxic amounts, which can lead to serious disease. For example, too much vitamin A during pregnancy can cause birth defects.

The most common type of overnutrition in developed nations is an excess intake of calories often leading to obesity. In the long run, outcomes of obesity include other serious diseases, such as type 2 diabetes and certain forms of cancer. Use the website shapeup.org to learn more about the importance of lifelong weight control.

For most vitamins and minerals, the gap between desirable intake and overnutrition is wide. Therefore, even if people take a typical balanced multivitamin and mineral supplement daily, they probably won't receive a harmful dose of any nutrient. The gap between desirable intake and overnutrition is smallest for vitamin A and the minerals calcium, iron, and copper. Thus, if you take nutrient supplements, keep a close eye on your total vitamin and mineral intake from both food and supplements to avoid toxicity (see Chapter 8 for further advice on use of nutrient supplements).

## 2.3 How Can Your Nutritional State be Measured?

To find out how nutritionally fit *you* are, a nutritional assessment—either whole or in part—needs to be performed (Table 2-3). Generally, this is performed by a physician, often with the aid of a registered dietitian.

### Analyzing Background Factors

Since family health history plays an important role in determining nutritional and health status, it must be carefully recorded and critically analyzed as part of a nutritional assessment. Other related background information includes: (1) a medical history, especially for any disease states or treatments that could decrease nutrient absorption or ultimate use; (2) a list of medications taken; (3) a social history (e.g., marital status, living conditions); (4) level of education to determine the degree of complexity that can be used in written materials and oral discussions; and (5) economic status to determine the ability to purchase, transport, and cook food.

▲ The most common type of overnutrition in North America is the excess intake of calories, which often leads to obesity.

**TABLE 2-3** Conducting an Evaluation of Nutritional Health

| Parameters | Example |
|---|---|
| Background | Medical history (e.g., current diseases, past surgeries, current weight, weight history, and current medications) |
| | Social history (marital status, living conditions) |
| | Family health history |
| | Education level |
| | Economic status |
| Nutritional | Anthropometric assessment: height, weight, skinfold thickness, arm muscle circumference, and other parameters |
| | Biochemical (laboratory) assessment of blood and urine: enzyme activities, concentrations of nutrients or their by-products |
| | Clinical assessment (physical examination): general appearance of skin, eyes, and tongue; rapid hair loss; sense of touch; ability to walk |
| | Dietary assessment: usual intake or record of previous days' meals |

## Assessing Nutritional Status Using the ABCDEs

In addition to background factors, four nutritional assessment categories complete the picture of nutritional status. **Anthropometric** measurements of height, weight (and weight changes), skinfold thicknesses, and body circumferences provide information about the current state of nutrition. Most measures of body composition are easy to obtain and are generally reliable. However, an in-depth examination of nutritional health is impossible without the more expensive process of **biochemical assessment.** This involves the measurement of the concentrations of nutrients and nutrient by-products in the blood, urine, and feces and of specific blood enzyme activities.

A **clinical assessment** would follow, during which a health professional would search for any physical evidence (e.g., high blood pressure) of diet-related diseases or deficiencies. Then, a close look at the person's diet (**dietary assessment**), including a record of at least the previous few days' food intake, would determine any possible problem areas. Finally, adding the **environmental assessment** (from the background analysis) provides further details about the living conditions, education level, and ability to purchase and prepare foods needed to maintain health. Now the true nutritional state of a person emerges. Taken together, these five assessments form the ABCDEs of nutritional assessment: **a**nthropometric, **b**iochemical, **c**linical, **d**ietary, and **e**nvironmental (Fig. 2-3).

<hr>

## MAKING DECISIONS

### Nutritional Assessment

A practical example using the ABCDEs for evaluating nutritional state can be illustrated in a person who chronically abuses alcohol. Upon evaluation, the physician notes:

(A) Low weight-for-height, recent 10 pound weight loss, muscle wasting in the upper body
(B) Low amounts of the vitamins thiamin and folate in the blood
(C) Psychological confusion, facial sores, and uncoordinated movement
(D) Dietary intake of little more than wine and hamburgers for the last week
(E) Currently residing in a homeless shelter; $35.00 in wallet; unemployed

Evaluation: This person needs medical attention, including nutrient repletion.

**anthropometric assessment**
Measurement of body weight and the lengths, circumferences, and thicknesses of parts of the body.

**biochemical assessment** Measurement of biochemical functions (e.g., concentrations of nutrient by-products or enzyme activities in the blood or urine) related to a nutrient's function.

**clinical assessment** Examination of general appearance of skin, eyes, and tongue; evidence of rapid hair loss; sense of touch; and ability to cough and walk.

**dietary assessment** Estimation of typical food choices relying mostly on the recounting of one's usual intake or a record of one's previous days' intake.

**environmental assessment** Includes details about living conditions, education level, and the ability of the person to purchase, transport, and cook food. The person's weekly budget for food purchases is also a key factor to consider.

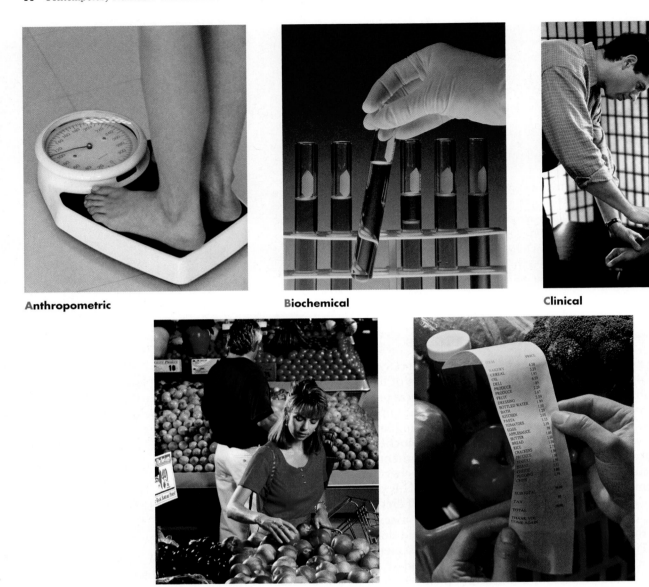

**Anthropometric**

**Biochemical**

**Clinical**

**Dietary**

**Environmental**

**FIGURE 2-3** ▶ A complete nutritional assessment includes anthropometric, biochemical, clinical, and dietary information. Environmental status adds further information, rounding out the ABCDEs of nutritional assessment.

## Recognizing the Limitations of Nutritional Assessment

A long time may elapse between the initial development of poor nutritional health and the first clinical evidence of a problem. A diet high in saturated (typically solid) fat often increases blood cholesterol, but without producing any clinical evidence for years. However, when the blood vessels become sufficiently blocked by cholesterol and other materials, chest pain during physical activity or a **heart attack** may occur. An active area of nutrition research is the development of better methods for early detection of nutrition-related problems such as heart attack risk.

Another example of a serious health condition with delayed symptoms is low bone density resulting from a calcium deficiency—a particularly relevant issue for adolescent and young adult females. Many young women do not consume the needed amount of calcium but suffer no obvious effects in their younger years. However, the bone structures of these women with low calcium intakes do not reach full potential during the years of growth, making osteoporosis more likely later in life.

**heart attack** Rapid fall in heart function caused by reduced blood flow through the heart's blood vessels. Often part of the heart dies in the process. Technically called a myocardial infarction.

Furthermore, clinical symptoms of some nutritional deficiencies—diarrhea, an inability to walk normally, and facial sores—are not very specific. These may have causes other than nutrition. The long time it takes for symptoms to develop and their potential to be vague often make it difficult to establish a link between an individual's current diet and nutritional state.

### Concern About the State of Your Nutritional Health Is Important

Table 1-7 in Chapter 1 portrayed the close relationship between nutrition and health. The good news is that people who focus on maintaining nutritional health are apt to enjoy a long, vigorous life. For example, a recent study found that women with a healthy lifestyle had a decreased risk for heart attacks (80% reduction) compared to women without such healthy practices. The healthy habits included:

- Consumed a healthy diet
  - Varied
  - Rich in fiber
  - Included some fish
  - Low in animal fat and *trans* fat
- Maintained a healthy weight
- Occasionally consumed alcohol in small amounts
- Exercised for at least 30 minutes daily
- Avoided use of tobacco

Should all adults follow this example (with optional use of alcohol)?

▲ The first evidence that one's diet is out of balance with one's physiology could be a heart attack. About 25% of heart attack victims do not survive the event.

---

#### CONCEPT CHECK

A desirable nutritional state results when the body has enough nutrients to function fully and contains stores to use in times of increased needs. When nutrient intake fails to meet body needs, undernutrition develops. Symptoms of such an inadequate nutrient intake can take months or years to develop. Overloading the body with nutrients, leading to overnutrition, is another potential problem to avoid. Nutritional state can be assessed by using anthropometric, biochemical, clinical, dietary, and economic assessments (ABCDEs).

## 2.4 Recommendations for Healthy Eating

The following sections of Chapter 2 will describe various guidelines for planning healthy diets.

### MyPyramid—A Menu-Planning Tool

Since the early twentieth century, researchers have worked to translate the science of nutrition into practical terms, so that people with no special training could estimate whether their nutritional needs were being met. The United States Department of Agriculture (USDA) simplified the recommendation by the mid-1950s to a four food-group plan: a milk group, a meat group, a fruit and vegetable group, and a bread and cereal group. In 1992 this plan was illustrated using a pyramid shape (i.e., Food Guide Pyramid).

In April 2005, USDA modified the pyramid diagram to develop their latest food guide plan, MyPyramid. Entitled "Steps to a Healthier You," MyPyramid replaces the Food Guide Pyramid and provides a more individualized approach to improving diet and lifestyle than previous food guides. Its goal is to provide advice that will help us live longer, better, and healthier lives. (Fig. 2-4) Appendix C contains Canada's Food Guide.

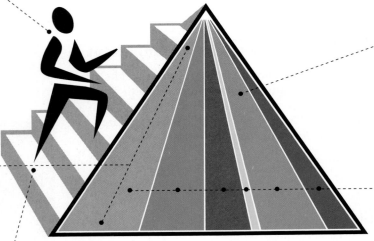

**Activity**
Activity is represented by the steps and the person climbing them, as a reminder of the importance of daily physical activity.

**Moderation**
Moderation is represented by the narrowing of each food group from bottom to top. The wider base stands for foods with little or no solid fats or added sugars. These should be selected more often. The narrower top area stands for foods containing more added sugars and solid fats. The more active you are, the more of these foods can fit into your diet.

**Personalization**
Personalization is shown by the person on the steps, the slogan, and the website. Find the kinds and amounts of food to eat each day at MyPyramid.gov.

**Proportionality**
Proportionality is shown by the different widths of the food group bands. The widths suggest how much food a person should choose from each group. The widths are just a general guide, not exact proportions. Check the website for how much is right for you.

**Variety**
Variety is symbolized by the 6 color bands representing the 5 food groups of the Pyramid and oils. This illustrates that foods from all groups are needed each day for good health.

**Gradual Improvement**
Gradual improvement is encouraged by the slogan. It suggests that individuals can benefit from taking small steps to improve their diet and lifestyle each day.

**MyPyramid.gov**
STEPS TO A HEALTHIER YOU

| Grains | Vegetables | Fruits | Oils | Milk | Meat & Beans |
|---|---|---|---|---|---|

**FIGURE 2-4** ▶ The anatomy of MyPyramid. USDA's MyPyramid symbolizes a personalized approach to healthy eating and physical activity. The symbol was designed to be simple. It was developed to remind consumers to make healthy food choices and to be active every day. In this figure, the different parts of the symbol are described.

The MyPyramid symbol represents the recommended proportion of foods from each food group (Grains, Vegetables, Fruits, Milk, Meats and Beans) to create a healthy diet. Physical activity is a new element in the pyramid.

MyPyramid is designed to illustrate personalization, gradual improvement, activity, variety, proportionality, and moderation. These concepts are explained in Figure 2-4. Consumer messages have also been developed to help us navigate MyPyramid (Fig. 2-5).

An innovative aspect of MyPyramid is the interactive technology found on MyPyramid.gov. To get the individualized advice that is the hallmark of the plan consumers need to use the website. This includes:

**MyPyramid Plan**—providing a quick estimate of what and how much food the individual should eat from the different food groups based on age, gender, and activity level.

**Inside MyPyramid**—providing in-depth information for every food group, including recommended daily amounts in commonly used measures, such as cups and ounces, with examples and everyday tips. The section also includes recommendations for choosing healthy oils, **discretionary calories,** and physical activity. This refers to the calories allowed from food choices rich in added sugars or solid fat. The overall intent is not to exceed the discretionary calorie allowance from the combination of calories from foods and beverages with calories from alcohol, added sugars, or added fats. For most of us very few discretionary calories are

**discretionary calories** The calories allowed in a diet after the person has met overall nutrition needs. This generally small amount of calories gives individuals the flexibility to consume some foods and beverages that may contain alcohol (e.g., beer and wine), added sugars (e.g., soft drinks, candy, and desserts), or added fats that are part of moderate- or high-fat foods (e.g., many snack foods).

| Grains<br>Make half your grains whole | Vegetables<br>Vary your veggies | Fruits<br>Focus on fruits | Milk<br>Get your calcium-rich foods | Meat & Beans<br>Go lean with protein |
|---|---|---|---|---|
| Eat at least 3 oz. of whole-grain cereals, breads, crackers, rice, or pasta every day<br><br>1 oz. is about 1 slice of bread; about 1 cup of breakfast cereal; or ½ cup of cooked rice, cereal, or pasta | Eat more dark-green veggies like broccoli, spinach, and other dark leafy greens<br><br>Eat more orange vegetables like carrots and sweet potatoes<br><br>Eat more dry beans and peas like pinto beans, kidney beans, and lentils | Eat a variety of fruit<br><br>Choose fresh, frozen, canned, or dried fruit<br><br>Go easy on fruit juices | Go low-fat or fat-free when you choose milk, yogurt, and other milk products<br><br>If you don't or can't consume milk, choose lactose-free products or other calcium sources such as fortified foods and beverages | Choose low-fat or lean meats and poultry<br><br>Bake it, broil it, or grill it<br><br>Vary your protein routine – choose more fish, beans, peas, nuts, and seeds |

**For a 2,000-calorie diet, you need the amounts below from each food group. To find the amounts that are right for you, go to MyPyramid.gov**

| Eat 6 oz. every day | Eat 2½ cups every day | Eat 2 cups every day | Get 3 cups every day; for kids aged 2 to 8, it's 2 | Eat 5½ oz. every day |
|---|---|---|---|---|

**Find your balance between food and physical activity**
- Be sure to stay within your daily calorie needs.
- Be physically active for at least 30 minutes most days of the week.
- About 60 minutes a day of physical activity may be needed to prevent weight gain.
- For sustaining weight loss, at least 60 to 90 minutes a day of physical activity may be required.
- Children and teenagers should be physically active for 60 minutes every day, or most days.

**Know the limits on fats, sugars, and salt (sodium)**
- Make most of your fat sources from fish, nuts, and vegetable oils.
- Limit solid fats like butter, stick margarine, shortening, and lard, as well as foods that contain these.
- Check the Nutrition Facts label to keep saturated fats, *trans* fats, and sodium low.
- Choose food and beverages low in added sugars. Added sugars contribute calories with few, if any, nutrients.

**FIGURE 2-5** ▶ These consumer messages have been developed by the USDA to help you navigate MyPyramid. The amounts shown for each food group are for a 2000 kcal diet. The amounts for other diets are shown in Table 2-4.

available in daily diet planning. See Making Decisions for an estimation of discretionary calories.

**MyPyramid Tracker**—allows the user to select from 8000 foods and 600 activities and provides more detailed information on diet quality and physical activity status by comparing a day's worth of foods eaten to the guidance provided by MyPyramid. Nutrition and physical activity messages are based on the need to maintain current weight or to lose weight.

**Start Today**—provides tips and resources that include downloadable suggestions on all the food groups and physical activity and a worksheet to track one's diet.

**W**hat about physical activity as part of MyPyramid? Physical activity is movement of the body that uses energy. Walking, gardening, briskly pushing a baby stroller, climbing the stairs, playing soccer, or dancing the night away are all examples of physical activity. For health benefits, physical activity should be moderate or vigorous and add up to at least 30 minutes on most or all days of the week.

## MAKING DECISIONS

### Discretionary Calories

Discretionary calories are estimated as follows:

| Calorie Intake (kcal) | Discretionary Calories (kcal) | Calorie Intake (kcal) | Discretionary Calories (kcal) |
|---|---|---|---|
| 1000 | 165* | 2200 | 290 |
| 1200 | 171* | 2400 | 362 |
| 1400 | 171* | 2600 | 410 |
| 1600 | 132 | 2800 | 426 |
| 1800 | 195 | 3000 | 512 |
| 2000 | 267 | 3200 | 648 |

*The amount of discretionary calories is higher for 1000–1400 kcal diets than for a 1600 kcal diet because these lower calorie diets are intended for children 2–8 years of age. Adult calorie recommendations typically start at 1600 kcal.

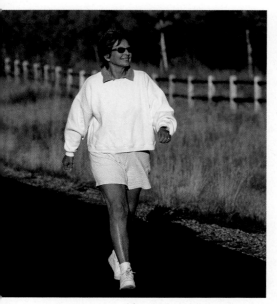

▲ Active means a lifestyle that includes physical activity equivalent to walking more than 3 miles per day at 3 to 4 miles per hour, in addition to the light physical activity associated with typical day-to-day life.

**Putting MyPyramid into Action.** To put MyPyramid into action, first you need to estimate your calorie needs (the website helps you calculate this). Figure 2-6 provides a rough guide. Overall, MyPyramid translates the latest nutrition advice into twelve separate pyramids based on calorie needs (1000 to 3200 kcal).

Once you have determined the calorie allowance appropriate for you, you can use Table 2-4 to discover how that calorie allowance corresponds to the recommended number of servings from each food group.

**What Counts as One Serving?** MyPyramid provides serving sizes of foods for the various food groups in household units. Pay close attention to the stated serving size for each choice when following MyPyramid. This helps control total calorie intake. See Figure 2-7 for a convenient guide to estimating common serving size measurements.

- **Grains:** 1 slice of bread; 1 cup of ready-to-eat breakfast cereal, or ½ cup cooked rice, pasta, or cereal counts as a 1-ounce equivalent.
- **Vegetables:** 1 cup (size of baseball) of raw or cooked vegetables or vegetable juice or 2 cups of raw leafy greens.
- **Fruits:** 1 cup of fruit or 100% fruit juice or ½ cup (size of tennis ball) of dried fruit.
- **Milk:** 1 cup of milk or yogurt, 1.5 ounces of natural cheese, or 2 ounces of processed cheese.
- **Meat & Beans:** 1 ounce of meat, poultry, or fish; 1 egg; 1 tablespoon of peanut butter; ¼ cup cooked dry beans, or ½ ounce of nuts or seeds are all 1-ounce equivalents (3 ounces of meat is size of a deck of cards).

**TABLE 2-4** MyPyramid Recommendations for Daily Food Consumption Based on Calorie Needs and Resulting in Twelve Separate Pyramids

**Daily Amount of Food From Each Group**

| Calorie Level | 1000 | 1200 | 1400 | 1600 | 1800 | 2000 | 2200 | 2400 | 2600 | 2800 | 3000 | 3200 |
|---|---|---|---|---|---|---|---|---|---|---|---|---|
| Fruits | 1 cup | 1 cup | 1.5 cups | 1.5 cups | 1.5 cups | 2 cups | 2 cups | 2 cups | 2 cups | 2.5 cups | 2.5 cups | 2.5 cups |
| Vegetables[1,2] | 1 cup | 1.5 cups | 1.5 cups | 2 cups | 2.5 cups | 2.5 cups | 3 cups | 3 cups | 3.5 cups | 3.5 cups | 4 cups | 4 cups |
| Grains[3] | 3 oz-eq | 4 oz-eq | 5 oz-eq | 5 oz-eq | 6 oz-eq | 6 oz-eq | 7 oz-eq | 8 oz-eq | 9 oz-eq | 10 oz-eq | 10 oz-eq | 10 oz-eq |
| Meat & Beans | 2 oz-eq | 3 oz-eq | 4 oz-eq | 5 oz-eq | 5 oz-eq | 5.5 oz-eq | 6 oz-eq | 6.5 oz-eq | 6.5 oz-eq | 7 oz-eq | 7 oz-eq | 7 oz-eq |
| Milk[4] | 2 cups | 2 cups | 2 cups | 3 cups | 3 cups | 3 cups | 3 cups | 3 cups | 3 cups | 3 cups | 3 cups | 3 cups |
| Oils[5] | 3 tsp | 4 tsp | 4 tsp | 5 tsp | 5 tsp | 6 tsp | 6 tsp | 7 tsp | 8 tsp | 8 tsp | 10 tsp | 11 tsp |
| Discretionary calorie allowance[6] | 165 | 171 | 171 | 132 | 195 | 267 | 290 | 362 | 410 | 426 | 512 | 648 |

oz-eq stands for ounce equivalent; tsp stands for teaspoon

[1]Vegetables are divided into five subgroups (dark green, orange, legumes, starchy, and other). Over a week's time, a variety of vegetables should be eaten, especially green and orange vegetables.

[2]Dry beans and peas can be counted *either* as vegetables (dry beans and peas subgroup), *or* in the meat & beans group. Generally, individuals who regularly eat meat, poultry, and fish would count dry beans and peas in the vegetable group. Individuals who seldom eat meat, poultry, or fish (vegetarians) would consume more dry beans and peas and count some of them in the meat & beans group until enough servings from that group are chosen for the day.

[3]At least half of the grain servings should be whole-grain varieties.

[4]Most of the milk servings should be fat-free or low-fat.

[5]Limit solid fats such as butter, stick margarine, shortening, and meat fat, as well as foods that contain these.

[6]Discretionary calories refers to food choices rich in added sugars or solid fat.

| | Calorie Range (kcal) | | |
|---|---|---|---|
| Children | Sedentary | ⟶ | Active |
| 2–3 years | 1000 | ⟶ | 1400 |
| Females | | | |
| 4–8 years | 1200 | ⟶ | 1800 |
| 9–13 | 1600 | ⟶ | 2200 |
| 14–18 | 1800 | ⟶ | 2400 |
| 19–30 | 2000 | ⟶ | 2400 |
| 31–50 | 1800 | ⟶ | 2200 |
| 51+ | 1600 | ⟶ | 2200 |
| Males | | | |
| 4–8 years | 1400 | ⟶ | 2000 |
| 9–13 | 1800 | ⟶ | 2600 |
| 14–18 | 2200 | ⟶ | 3200 |
| 19–30 | 2400 | ⟶ | 3000 |
| 31–50 | 2200 | ⟶ | 3000 |
| 51+ | 2000 | ⟶ | 2800 |

**FIGURE 2-6** ▶ Estimates of calorie needs (kcals) provided by MyPyramid.

▲ Sedentary means a lifestyle that includes only the light physical activity associated with typical day-to-day life.

**Portion sizes**

2 tbsp salad dressing, peanut butter, margarine, etc.

= 2 tbsp measure

Baked potato
Small/medium fruit
Ground or chopped food
Bagel
English muffin

= ½ to ⅔ cup measure

3 oz meat, poultry, or fish

= ½ to ¾ cup

Large apple or orange
1 cup ready-to-eat breakfast cereal

= 1 cup

**FIGURE 2-7** ▶ A golf ball, tennis ball, deck of cards, and baseball are standard-size objects that make convenient guides for judging MyPyramid serving sizes. Your hand provides an additional handy guide (for the greatest accuracy, compare your fist with a baseball, and adjust the following guides accordingly).

Fist = 1 cup
Thumb = 1 oz of cheese
Thumb tip to first Joint = 1 tsp

Palm of hand = 3 oz
Handful = 1 or 2 oz of a snack food

- **Oils:** A teaspoon of any oil from plants or fish that is liquid at room temperature counts as a serving, as do such servings of foods rich in oils (e.g., mayonnaise and soft margarine) (2 tbsp of oil is size of a golf ball).

**Menu Planning with MyPyramid** Remember the following points when using MyPyramid to plan your daily menus:

1. The guide does not apply to infants or children under 2 years of age.
2. No one food is absolutely essential to good nutrition. Each food is rich in some nutrients, but deficient in at least one essential nutrient (Table 2-5).

**TABLE 2-5** Nutrient Contributions of Groups in the MyPyramid Food Guide Plan

| Food Category | Major Nutrient Contributions |
|---|---|
| Grains | Carbohydrate<br>Vitamins such as thiamin<br>Minerals such as iron<br>Fiber* |
| Vegetables | Carbohydrate<br>Vitamins such as plant pigments that form vitamin A<br>Minerals such as magnesium<br>Fiber |
| Fruits | Carbohydrate<br>Vitamins such as folate and vitamin C<br>Minerals such as potassium<br>Fiber |
| Oils | Fat<br>Essential fatty acids<br>Vitamins such as vitamin E |
| Milk | Carbohydrate<br>Protein<br>Vitamins such as vitamin D<br>Minerals such as calcium and phosphorus |
| Meat & Beans | Protein<br>Vitamins such as vitamin B-6<br>Minerals such as iron and zinc |

*Whole-grain varieties

▲ Typical restaurant portions contain numerous servings from the individual groups in MyPyramid.

3. No one food group provides all essential nutrients in adequate amounts. Each food group makes an important, distinctive contribution to nutritional intake.
4. Variety is the key to success of MyPyramid and is first guaranteed by choosing foods from all the groups. Furthermore, one should consume a variety of foods within each group, except possibly in the milk, yogurt, and cheese group.
5. The foods within a group may vary widely with respect to nutrients and calories. For example, the calorie content of 3 ounces of baked potato is 98 kcal, whereas that of 3 ounces of potato chips is 470 kcal. With respect to vitamin C, an orange has 70 mg and an apple has 10 mg.

Overall, MyPyramid incorporates the foundations of a healthy diet: variety, balance, and moderation. The nutritional adequacy of diets planned using this tool, however, depends on selection of a variety of foods (see example in Table 2-6). In addition, vitamin E, vitamin B-6, magnesium, and zinc are nutrients sometimes low in diets based on this plan. To ensure enough of these nutrients, consider the following advice:

1. Choose primarily low-fat and fat-free items from the milk group. By reducing calorie intake in this way, you can select more items from other food groups. If milk causes intestinal gas and bloating, emphasize yogurt and cheese (see Chapter 4 for details on the problem of lactose maldigestion and lactose intolerance).
2. Include plant foods that are good sources of proteins, such as beans and nuts, at least several times a week because many are rich in vitamins (such as vitamin E), minerals (such as magnesium), and fiber.
3. For vegetables and fruits, try to include a dark green or orange vegetable for vitamin A and a vitamin C–rich fruit, such as an orange, every day. Don't focus

**TABLE 2-6** Putting the MyPyramid into Practice. This menu meets nutrient needs for all vitamins and minerals for an average adult that needs 1800 kcal. For adolescents, teenagers, and older adults add one additional serving of milk or other calcium-rich sources.

| Meal | Food Group |
| --- | --- |
| **Breakfast** | |
| 1 small orange | Fruits |
| ¾ cup Healthy Choice Low-fat Granola | Grains |
|   with ½ cup fat-free milk | Milk |
| ½ toasted, small raisin bagel | Grains |
|   with 1 tsp soft margarine | Oils |
| Optional: coffee or tea | |
| **Lunch** | |
| Turkey sandwich | |
|   2 slices whole-wheat bread | Grains |
|   2 oz turkey | Meat & Beans |
|   2 tsp mustard | |
| 1 small apple | Fruits |
| 2 oatmeal-raisin cookies (small) | Discretionary calories |
| Optional: diet soft drink | |
| **3 P.M. Study Break** | |
| 6 whole-wheat crackers | Grains |
| 1 tbsp peanut butter | Meat & Beans |
| ½ cup fat-free milk | Milk |
| **Dinner** | |
| Tossed salad | |
|   1 cup romaine lettuce | Vegetables |
|   ½ cup sliced tomatoes | Vegetables |
|   1½ tbsp Italian dressing | Oils |
|   ½ carrot, grated | Vegetables |
| 3 oz broiled salmon | Meat & Beans |
| ½ cup rice | Grains |
| ½ cup green beans | Vegetables |
|   with 1 tsp soft margarine | Oils |
| Optional: coffee or tea | |
| **Late-Night Snack** | |
| 1 cup "light" fruit yogurt | Milk |
| **Nutrient Breakdown** | |
| 1800 kcal | |
|   Carbohydrate | 56% of kcal |
|   Protein | 18% of kcal |
|   Fat | 26% of kcal |

primarily on potatoes (e.g., French fries) for your vegetable choices. Surveys show that fewer than 5% of adults eat a full serving of a dark green vegetable on any given day. Increased consumption of these foods is important because they contribute vitamins, minerals, fiber, and phytochemicals.

4. Choose whole-grain varieties of breads, cereals, rice, and pasta because they contribute vitamin E and fiber. A plate about two-thirds covered by grains, fruits, and vegetables and one-third or less covered by protein-rich foods promotes this diet advice. A daily serving of a whole-grain, ready-to-eat breakfast cereal is an excellent choice because the vitamins (such as vitamin B-6) and minerals (such as zinc) typically added to it, along with fiber, help fill in the potential gaps listed earlier.

5. Include some plant oils on a daily basis, such as those in salad dressing, and eat fish at least twice a week. This supplies you with health-promoting essential fatty acids.

## MAKING DECISIONS

### Measuring Your Portion Size

How familiar are you with serving size measurements? Common household units are listed in Appendix I with their metric equivalents. Ounces and fluid ounces differ. Ounces are a measure of weight, while fluid ounces are a measure of volume. Fluid ounces are based on the corresponding volume of water as the standard; 1 ounce of water by weight equals one fluid ounce. Any fluid more or less dense than water will yield a different number of fluid ounces per ounce of material.

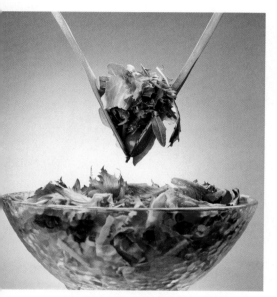

▲ Leafy green vegetables contribute many nutrients to a diet.

**Dietary Guidelines for Americans** General goals for nutrient intakes and diet composition set by the USDA and the U.S. Department of Health and Human Services.

**How Does Your Current Diet Rate?** Regularly comparing your daily food intake with MyPyramid recommendations for your age, gender, and degree of physical activity, is a relatively simple way to evaluate the quality of your overall diet. Strive to meet the recommendations. (The diet quality of most adults is low using this evaluation, especially with respect to milk, vegetables, fruits, and whole-grain breads and cereals.) If that is not possible, identify the nutrients that are low in your diet based on the nutrients found in each food group (review Table 2-5). For example, if you do not consume enough servings from the milk group, your calcium intake is most likely too low. You need to then find foods that you enjoy that supply calcium, such as calcium-fortified orange juice. Customizing MyPyramid to accommodate your food habits may seem a daunting task, but it is not difficult once you gain some additional nutrition knowledge.

**Get Going** Start putting MyPyramid into practice and use the MyTracker feature to follow your progress. Implementing even small diet and exercise changes can have positive results. Better health will likely follow as you strive to meet your nutrient needs and balance your physical activity and calorie allowance. In addition, follow the guidance from the **2005 Dietary Guidelines for Americans** regarding alcohol and sodium intake and safe food preparation.

## CONCEPT CHECK

MyPyramid translates the general needs for carbohydrate, protein, fat, vitamins, and minerals into the recommended number of daily servings from each of five major food groups and oils. It is a convenient and valuable tool for planning daily menus.

## The Mediterranean Diet Pyramid

The Mediterranean Diet Pyramid, developed by Oldways, a widely-respected non-profit "food issues think tank," is an additional consumer-friendly health-promotion tool.

The diet outlined in the Mediterranean Diet Pyramid patterns dietary data from parts of the Mediterranean region that enjoy the lowest recorded rates of chronic diseases and the highest adult life expectancy. The healthfulness of this diet pattern is supported by epidemiological and experimental nutrition research.

The Mediterranean Diet Pyramid was updated and released in 2009. The Pyramid now emphasizes the health benefits that plant foods provide by grouping these delicious and healthy foods (fruits, vegetables, grains, nuts, legumes, seeds, olives and olive oil) together. Herbs and spices were also added for reasons of both health and taste. The Pyramid also emphasizes the health benefits of eating fish and shellfish at least two times per week.

**Mediterranean Diet Pyramid**
*A contemporary approach to delicious, healthy eating*

Meats and Sweets
*Less often*

Wine
*In moderation*

Poultry and Eggs
*Moderate portions, every two days or weekly*

Cheese and Yogurt
*Moderate portions, daily to weekly*

Drink Water

Fish and Seafood
*Often, at least two times per week*

Fruits, Vegetables, Grains (mostly whole), Olive oil, Beans, Nuts, Legumes and Seeds, Herbs and Spices
*Base every meal on these foods*

Be Physically Active; Enjoy Meals with Others

Illustration by George Middleton      © 2009 Oldways Preservation and Exchange Trust      www.oldwayspt.org

▲ The Mediterranean Diet Pyramid is based on dietary patterns from the Mediterranean region that has low rates of chronic diseases and high life expectancy.

The Mediterranean Diet Pyramid is based on a historical pattern that includes the following (with several parenthetical notes adding a contemporary public health perspective). The average amounts given are in most cases intentionally nonspecific since variation is known to have been considerable within this pattern.

- An abundance of food from plant sources, including fruits and vegetables, potatoes, breads and grains, beans, nuts, and seeds.

- Emphasis on a variety of minimally processed and, wherever possible, seasonally fresh and locally grown foods (which often maximizes the health-promoting micronutrient and antioxidant content of these foods).
- Olive oil as the principal fat, replacing other fats and oils (including butter and margarine).
- Total fat ranging from less than 25% to over 35% of energy, with saturated fat no more than 7% to 8% of energy (calories).
- Daily consumption of low to moderate amounts of cheese and yogurt (low-fat and non-fat versions may be preferable).
- Weekly consumption of low to moderate amounts of fish and poultry (recent research suggests that fish be somewhat favored over poultry) and from zero to four eggs per week (including those used in cooking and baking).
- Fresh fruit as the typical daily dessert and sweets with a significant amount of sugar (often as honey) and saturated fat consumed not more than a few times per week.
- Red meat a few times per month (recent research suggests that if red meat is eaten, its consumption should be limited to a maximum of 12 to 16 ounces [340 to 450 grams] per month; where the flavor is acceptable, lean versions may be preferable).
- Regular physical activity at a level that promotes a healthy weight, fitness, and well-being.
- Moderate consumption of wine, normally with meals; about one to two glasses per day for men and one glass per day for women (from a contemporary public health perspective, wine should be considered optional and avoided when consumption would put the individual or others at risk.)

(From: Oldways Food Issues Think Tank, 266 Beacon St., Boston, MA 02116, http://www.oldwayspt.org)

## Dietary Guidelines—Another Tool for Menu Planning

MyPyramid was designed to help meet nutritional needs for carbohydrate, protein, fat, vitamins, and minerals. However, most of the major chronic "killer" diseases in North America, such as cardiovascular disease, cancer, and alcoholism, are not primarily associated with deficiencies of these nutrients. Deficiency diseases such as scurvy (vitamin C deficiency) and pellagra (niacin deficiency) are no longer common. For many North Americans, the primary dietary culprit is an overconsumption of one or more of the following: calories, saturated fat, cholesterol, *trans* fat, alcohol, and sodium (salt). Underconsumption of calcium, iron, folate and other B-vitamins, vitamin C, vitamin D, vitamin E, potassium, magnesium, and fiber is also a problem for some people.

In response to concerns regarding these killer disease patterns and poor dietary habits, the USDA and U.S. Department of Health and Human Services (DHHS) have published Dietary Guidelines for Americans (Dietary Guidelines for short) since 1980 to aid diet planning.

The latest version of the Dietary Guidelines was published in 2005 and compared to past reports, places stronger emphasis on monitoring one's calorie intake and increasing physical activity. This is because more of us are becoming overweight each year.

The 2005 report identifies 41 key recommendations, of which 23 are for the general public and 18 are for special populations. They are grouped into nine general topics:

- Adequate Nutrient Intake Within Calorie Needs
- Weight Management
- Physical Activity
- Specific Food Groups to Encourage

**A**ppendix C contains nutrient guidelines for Canadians.

**A** brochure designed for the public based on the 2005 Dietary Guidelines for Americans is entitled "Finding Your Way to a Healthier You." It communicates the major themes of the *2005 Dietary Guidelines for Americans,* but uses simpler messages and can be found at **www. healthierus.gov/dietaryguidelines.**

- Fats
- Carbohydrates
- Sodium and Potassium
- Alcoholic Beverages
- Food Safety

Figure 2-8 lists the key recommendations for the general public and for special population groups within each general topic. The advice provided refers to people two years and older.

A basic premise of the Dietary Guidelines is that nutrient needs should be met primarily through consuming foods. Foods provide an array of nutrients and other compounds that may have beneficial effects on health. Fortified foods and dietary supplements, however, are especially important for people whose typical food choices cannot meet one or more nutrient recommendations, such as for vitamin E or calcium. However, dietary supplements are not a substitute for a healthful diet.

The 2005 Dietary Guidelines for Americans (and the consumer brochure) are available at **www.healthierus.gov/dietaryguidelines**. In general the Dietary Guidelines recommend that we:

- Consume a variety of nutrient-dense foods and beverages within and among the basic food groups of MyPyramid, while choosing foods that limit the intake of saturated and *trans* fats, cholesterol, added sugars, salt, and alcohol (if used). Foods to emphasize are vegetables, fruits, legumes (beans), whole grains, and fat-free or low-fat milk or equivalent milk products.
- Maintain body weight in a healthy range by balancing calorie intake from foods and beverages with calories expended. For the latter, engage in at least 30 minutes of moderate-intensity physical activity, above usual activity, at work or home on most days of the week.
- Practice safe food handling when preparing food. This includes cleaning hands, food contact surfaces, and fruits and vegetables before preparation and cooking foods to a safe temperature to kill microorganisms.

**Practical Use of the Dietary Guidelines** The Dietary Guidelines are designed to meet nutrient needs while reducing the risk of obesity, hypertension, cardiovascular disease, type 2 diabetes, alcoholism, and foodborne illness.

The Dietary Guidelines are not difficult to implement. Table 2-7 provides examples of recommended diet changes based on the Dietary Guidelines. Despite popular misconceptions, this overall diet approach is not especially expensive. Fruits, vegetables, and low-fat and fat-free milk are no more expensive than the chips, cookies, and sugared soft drinks they should in part replace. Canned and frozen fruits and vegetables and non-fat dry milk are a few of the available lower-cost foods.

Diet recommendations for adults have been issued by other scientific groups, such as the American Heart Association, U.S. Surgeon General, National Academy of Sciences, American Cancer Society, Canadian Ministries of Health (see Appendix C), and World Health Organization. All are consistent with the spirit of the Dietary Guidelines. These groups encourage people to modify their eating behavior in ways that are both healthful and pleasurable.

**The Dietary Guidelines and You** When using the Dietary Guidelines, you should consider your state of health. Make specific changes and see whether they are effective. Results are sometimes disappointing, even when you are following a diet change very closely. Some people can eat a lot of saturated fat and still keep blood cholesterol under control. Other people, unfortunately, have high blood cholesterol even if they eat a diet low in saturated fat. Differences in genetic background are a key reason for these different responses, as you will learn in Chapter 3. Thus, we have different individual nutritional needs and risks of developing certain diseases. One's diet should be planned with this individuality in mind, taking into account when

Dietary Guidelines
for Americans
2005

**CRITICAL THINKING**

Shannon has grown up eating the typical American diet. Having recently read and heard many media reports about the relationship between nutrition and health, she is beginning to look critically at her diet and is considering making changes. However, she doesn't know where to begin. What advice would you give her?

## ADEQUATE NUTRIENTS WITHIN ENERGY NEEDS

- Consume a variety of nutrient-dense foods and beverages within and among the basic food groups while choosing foods that limit the intake of saturated and *trans* fats, cholesterol, added sugars, salt, and alcohol.

- Meet recommended intakes within energy needs by adopting a balanced eating pattern, such as MyPyramid or the DASH diet (see chapter 14).

### Key Recommendations for Specific Population Groups

- *People over age 50.* Consume vitamin B-12 in its crystalline form (i.e., fortified foods or supplements).

- *Women of childbearing age who may become pregnant.* Eat foods high in iron from animal products and/or consume iron-rich plant foods or iron-fortified foods with an enhancer of iron absorption, such as vitamin C–rich foods.

- *Women of childbearing age who may become pregnant and those in the first few months of pregnancy.* Consume adequate amount of the synthetic form of the B vitamin folate (i.e., folic acid) daily (from fortified foods or supplements) in addition to food forms of folate found in a varied diet.

- *Older adults, people with dark skin, and people exposed to insufficient ultraviolet band radiation (i.e., sunlight).* Consume extra vitamin D from vitamin D–fortified foods and/or supplements.

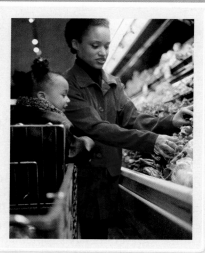

## WEIGHT MANAGEMENT

- To maintain body weight in a healthy range, balance calorie intake from foods and beverages with energy expended.

- To prevent gradual weight gain over time, make small decreases in calorie intake from food and beverages and increase physical activity.

### Key Recommendations for Specific Population Groups

- *Those who need to lose weight.* Aim for a slow, steady weight loss by decreasing calorie intake while maintaining an adequate nutrient intake and increasing physical activity.

- *Overweight children.* Reduce the rate of body weight gain while allowing for growth and development. Consult a health-care provider before placing a child on a weight-reduction diet.

- *Pregnant women.* Ensure appropriate weight gain as specified by a health-care provider.

- *Breastfeeding women.* Moderate weight reduction is safe and does not compromise weight gain of the breastfeeding infant.

- *Overweight adults and overweight children with chronic diseases and/or on medication.* Consult a health-care provider about weight-loss strategies prior to starting a weight-reduction program to ensure appropriate management of other health conditions.

## FOOD GROUPS TO ENCOURAGE

- Consume a sufficient amount of fruits and vegetables while staying within calorie needs. Two cups of fruit and 2½ cups of vegetables per day are recommended for a reference 2000-kcal intake, with higher or lower amounts depending on one's calorie needs.

- Choose a variety of fruits and vegetables each day. In particular, select from all 5 vegetable subgroups (dark green vegetables, orange vegetables, legumes, starchy vegetables, and other vegetables) several times a week.

- Consume 3 or more ounce-equivalents of whole-grain products per day, with the rest of the recommended grains coming from enriched or whole-grain products. In general, at least half the grains should come from whole grains.

- Consume 3 cups per day of fat-free or low-fat milk or equivalent milk products.

### Key Recommendations for Specific Population Groups

- *Children and adolescents.* Consume whole-grain products often; at least half the grains should be whole grains. Children 2 to 8 years should consume 2 cups per day of fat-free or low-fat milk or equivalent milk products. Children 9 years of age and older should consume 3 cups per day of fat-free or low-fat milk or equivalent milk products.

**FIGURE 2-8 ▶** Key Recommendations within each general topic from the latest Dietary Guidelines for Americans.

## PHYSICAL ACTIVITY

- Engage in regular physical activity and reduce sedentary activities to promote health, psychological well-being, and a healthy body weight.

- To reduce the risk for chronic disease in adulthood: engage in at least 30 minutes of moderate-intensity physical activity, above usual activity, at work or home on most days of the week.

- For most people, greater health benefits can be obtained by engaging in physical activity of more vigorous intensity or longer duration.

- To help manage body weight and prevent gradual, unhealthy body weight gain in adulthood: engage in approximately 60 minutes of moderate- to vigorous-intensity activity on most days of the week while not exceeding energy intake needs.

- To sustain weight loss in adulthood: participate in at least 60 to 90 minutes of daily moderate-intensity physical activity while not exceeding calorie needs. Some people (men over 40 years of age and women over 50 years of age) may need to consult with a health-care provider before participating in this level of activity.

- Achieve physical fitness by including cardiovascular conditioning, stretching exercises for flexibility, and resistance exercises or calisthenics for muscle strength and endurance.

### Key Recommendations for Specific Population Groups

- *Children and adolescents.* Engage in at least 60 minutes of physical activity on most, preferably all, days of the week.

- *Pregnant women.* In the absence of medical complications, incorporate 30 minutes or more of moderate-intensity physical activity on most, if not all, days of the week. Avoid activities with a high risk of falling or abdominal trauma.

- *Breastfeeding women.* Be aware that neither acute nor regular exercise adversely affects the mother's ability to breastfeed successfully.

- *Older adults.* Participate in regular physical activity to reduce functional declines associated with aging and to achieve the other benefits of physical activity identified for all adults.

## SODIUM AND POTASSIUM

- Consume less than 2300 mg of sodium per day (approximately 1 tsp of salt).

- Choose and prepare foods with little salt. At the same time, consume potassium-rich foods, such as fruits and vegetables.

### Key Recommendations for Specific Population Groups

- *Individuals with hypertension, blacks, and middle-aged and older adults.* Aim to consume no more than 1500 mg of sodium per day, and meet the potassium recommendation (4700 mg per day) with food.

## ALCOHOLIC BEVERAGES

- Those who choose to drink alcoholic beverages should do so sensibly and in moderation—defined as the consumption of up to 1 drink per day for women and up to 2 drinks per day for men (12 oz of a regular beer, 5 oz of wine, or 1½ oz of 80–proof distilled spirits count as 1 drink).

- Alcoholic beverages should not be consumed by some individuals, including those who cannot restrict their alcohol intake, women of childbearing age who may become pregnant, pregnant and lactating women, children and adolescents, individuals taking medications that can interact with alcohol, and those with specific medical conditions.

- Alcoholic beverages should be avoided by individuals engaging in activities that require attention, skill, or coordination, such as driving or operating machinery.

**FIGURE 2-8** ▶ *Continued.*

## FATS

- Consume less than 10% of calories from saturated fatty acids and less than 300 mg per day of cholesterol, and keep *trans* fatty acid consumption as low as possible.

- Keep total fat intake between 20 and 35% of calorie intake, with most fats coming from sources of polyunsaturated and monounsaturated fatty acids, such as fish, nuts, and vegetable oils.

- When selecting and preparing meat, poultry, dry beans, and milk or milk products, make choices that are lean, low-fat, or fat-free.

- Limit intake of fats and oils high in saturated and/or *trans* fatty acids, and choose products low in such fats and oils.

### Key Recommendations for Specific Population Groups

- *Children and adolescents.* Keep total fat intake between 30 and 35% of calorie intake for children 2 to 3 years of age and between 25 and 35% of calorie intake for children and adolescents 4 to 18 years of age, with most fats coming from sources of polyunsaturated and monounsaturated fatty acids, such as fish, nuts, and vegetable oils.

## FOOD SAFETY

To Avoid Microbial Foodborne Illness

- Clean hands, food contact surfaces, and fruits and vegetables. Meat and poultry should *not* be washed or rinsed to avoid spreading bacteria to other foods.

- Separate raw, cooked, and ready-to-eat foods while shopping, preparing, and storing foods.

- Cook foods to a safe temperature to kill microorganisms.

- Chill (refrigerate) perishable food promptly and defrost foods safely.

- Avoid raw (unpasteurized) milk or any products made from unpasteurized milk, raw or partially cooked eggs or foods containing raw eggs, and raw or undercooked meat and poultry, unpasteurized juices, and raw sprouts.

### Key Recommendations for Specific Population Groups

- *Infants and young children, pregnant women, older adults, and those who are immunocompromised.* Do not eat or drink raw (unpasteurized) milk or any products made from unpasteurized milk, raw or partially cooked eggs or foods containing raw eggs, raw or undercooked meat and poultry, raw or undercooked fish or shellfish, unpasteurized juices, and raw sprouts.

- *Pregnant women, older adults, and those who are immunocompromised.* Eat only certain deli meats and frankfurters that have been reheated to steaming hot.

## CARBOHYDRATES

- Choose fiber-rich fruits, vegetables, and whole grains often.

- Choose and prepare foods and beverages with little added sugars or caloric sweeteners, such as amounts suggested by MyPyramid.

- Reduce the incidence of dental caries by practicing good oral hygiene and consuming sugar- and starch-containing foods and beverages less frequently.

**FIGURE 2-8** ▶ *Continued.*

**TABLE 2-7** Recommended Diet Changes Based on the Dietary Guidelines

| If You Usually Eat This, | Try This Instead | Benefit |
|---|---|---|
| White bread | Whole-wheat bread | • Higher nutrient density, due to less processing<br>• More fiber |
| Sugary breakfast cereal | Low-sugar, high-fiber cereal with fresh fruit | • Higher nutrient density<br>• More fiber<br>• More phytochemicals |
| Cheeseburger with French fries | Hamburger and baked beans | • Less saturated fat and *trans* fat<br>• Less cholesterol<br>• More fiber<br>• More phytochemicals |
| Potato salad | Three-bean salad | • More fiber<br>• More phytochemicals |
| Doughnuts | Bran muffin/bagel with light cream cheese | • More fiber<br>• Less fat |
| Regular soft drinks | Diet soft drinks | • Fewer calories |
| Boiled vegetables | Steamed vegetables | • Higher nutrient density, due to reduced loss of water-soluble vitamins |
| Canned vegetables | Fresh or frozen vegetables | • Higher nutrient density, due to reduced loss of heat-sensitive vitamins<br>• Lower in sodium |
| Fried meats | Broiled meats | • Less saturated fat |
| Fatty meats, such as ribs or bacon | Lean meats, such as ground round, chicken, or fish | • Less saturated fat |
| Whole milk | Low-fat or fat-free milk | • Less saturated fat<br>• Fewer calories<br>• More calcium |
| Ice cream | Sherbet or frozen yogurt | • Less saturated fat<br>• Fewer calories |
| Mayonnaise or sour cream salad dressing | Oil and vinegar dressings or light creamy dressings | • Less saturated fat<br>• Less cholesterol<br>• Fewer calories |
| Cookies | Popcorn (air popped with minimal margarine or butter) | • Fewer calories and *trans* fat |
| Heavily salted foods | Foods flavored primarily with herbs, spices, lemon juice | • Lower in sodium |
| Chips | Pretzels | • Less fat |

▲ Choose low-sugar, high-fiber cereal with fresh fruit instead of sugary breakfast cereal.

▲ Choose popcorn, pretzels, or nuts instead of cookies and chips.

possible, one's current health status and family history for specific diseases. However, tailoring a unique nutrition program for every North American citizen is currently unrealistic. MyPyramid and the 2005 Dietary Guidelines provide typical adults with simple advice, which can be actively practiced by anyone willing to take a step toward good health.

**T**he *2008 Physical Activity Guidelines for Americans* were recently published by the U.S. Department of Health and Human Services. These guidelines were established in response to information indicating that inactivity remains high among American children, adolescents, and adults, and that little progress has been made in increasing levels of physical activity among Americans. The current inactivity puts Americans at unnecessary risk. The Guidelines provide science-based guidance to help Americans aged six and older improve their health through appropriate physical activity. The Guidelines will be used by health professionals and policymakers to help Americans:

- Learn about the health benefits of physical activity
- Understand how to do physical activity in a manner that meets the Guidelines
- Understand how to reduce the risks of activity-related injury
- Assist others in participating regularly in physical activity

*Be Active, Healthy, and Happy!*

*www.health.gov/paguidelines*

▲ http://www.health.gov/PAGuidelines/.

**Dietary Reference Intakes (DRIs)** Term used to encompass nutrient recommendations made by the Food and Nutrition Board of the National Academy of Sciences. These include RDAs, EARs, AIs, EERs, and ULs.

**Recommended Dietary Allowance (RDA)** Nutrient intake amount sufficient to meet the needs of 97% to 98% of the individuals in a specific life stage.

There is no "optimal" diet. Instead, there are numerous healthful diets. For additional information, visit the website of the International Food Information Council (www.ific.org). This site is a great resource for current nutrition information.

## 2.5 Specific Nutrient Standards and Recommendations

The overarching goal of any healthy diet plan is to meet nutrient needs. To begin, we must determine what amount of each essential nutrient is needed to maintain health. The standards that have been developed for such nutrient needs are abbreviated DRI, RDA, AI, EER, and UL and can often seem like an alphabet soup of abbreviations. However, you can more easily sift through these nutrient standards if you have a knowledge base about their development and use (Table 2-8).

▲ Does everyone in this photo have the same nutrient needs?

Most of the terms that describe nutrient needs fall under one umbrella term—**Dietary Reference Intakes (DRIs).** The development of DRIs is an ongoing, collaborative effort between the Food and Nutrition Board of the Institute of Medicine in the United States and Health Canada. Included under the DRI umbrella are **Recommended Dietary Allowances (RDAs), Adequate Intakes (AIs), Estimated Energy Requirements (EERs),** and **Tolerable Upper Intake Levels (Upper Levels or ULs).**

### Recommended Dietary Allowance

A Recommended Dietary Allowance (RDA) is the recommended amount of a nutrient based on meeting the needs of nearly all individuals (about 97%) in a particular age and gender group. A person can compare his or her individual intake of specific nutrients to the RDA. Although an intake slightly above or below the RDA for a particular nutrient is no reason for concern, a significant deviation below (about 70%) or above (about three times or more for some nutrients) the RDA for an extended time can eventually result in a deficiency or toxicity of that nutrient, respectively.

**TABLE 2-8** Recommendations within the Dietary Reference Intakes

| RDA | Recommended Dietary Allowance. Use to evaluate your current intake for a specific nutrient. The further you stray above or below this value, the greater your chances of developing nutritional problems. |
|---|---|
| AI | Adequate Intake. Use to evaluate your current intake of nutrients, but realize that an AI designation implies that further research is required before scientists can establish a more definitive recommendation. |
| EER | Estimated Energy Requirement. Use to estimate calorie needs of the average person within a specific height, weight, gender, age, and physical activity pattern. |
| UL | Upper Level. Use to evaluate the highest amount of daily nutrient intake unlikely to cause adverse health effects in the long run in almost all people (97% to 98%) in a population. This number applies to chronic use and is set to protect even very susceptible people in the healthy general population. As intake increases above the Upper Level, the potential for adverse effects generally increases. |
| DV | Daily Value. Use as a rough guide for comparing the nutrient content of a food to approximate human needs. Typically, the Daily Value used on food labels refers to ages 4 years through adulthood. It is based on a 2000 kcal diet. Some Daily Values also increase slightly with higher calorie intakes (see Fig. 2-12 in the following section on food labeling). |

Although nutrition recommendations are often made for the entire healthy population, each of us have individual needs based on our particular health status and genetic background. It would be more appropriate, but also more expensive, if recommendations were made on an individual basis once a person's health status is known.

**Adequate Intake (AI)** Nutrient intake amount set for any nutrient for which insufficient research is available to establish an RDA. AIs are based on estimates of intakes that appear to maintain a defined nutritional state in a specific life stage.

**Estimated Energy Requirement (EER)** Estimate of the energy (kcal) intake needed to match the energy use of an average person in a specific life stage.

**Tolerable Upper Intake Level (UL)** Maximum chronic daily intake level of a nutrient that is unlikely to cause adverse health effects in almost all people in a specific life stage.

## Adequate Intake

An RDA can be set for a nutrient only if there is sufficient information on the human needs for that particular nutrient. Today, there is not enough information on some nutrients, such as calcium, to set such a precise standard as an RDA. For this and other nutrients, the DRIs include a category called an Adequate Intake (AI). This standard is based on the dietary intakes of people that appear to be maintaining nutritional health. That amount of intake is assumed to be adequate, as no evidence of a nutritional deficiency is apparent.

## Estimated Energy Requirement

For calorie needs, we use the Estimated Energy Requirement (EER) instead of an RDA or AI. As described, the RDAs are set somewhat higher than the average needs for nutrients. This is fine for nutrients rather than calories because a slight excess of vitamins and minerals is not harmful. However, a long-term excess of calories will lead to weight gain. Therefore, the calculation of EER needs to be more specific, taking into account age, gender, height, weight, and physical activity (e.g., sedentary or moderately active). In some cases, the additional calorie needs for growth and lactation are also included (see Chapters 7, 14, and 15 for the specific formulas used). The EER also is based on the "average" person. Thus it can only serve as a starting point for estimating calorie needs.

## Tolerable Upper Intake Level

A Tolerable Upper Intake Level (Upper Level or UL) has been set for some vitamins and minerals (see the inside cover). The UL is the highest amount of a nutrient unlikely to cause adverse health effects in the long run. As intake exceeds the UL, the risk of ill effects increases. These amounts generally should not be exceeded day after day, as toxicity could develop. For people eating a varied diet and/or using a balanced multivitamin and mineral supplement, exceeding the UL is unusual. Problems are more likely to arise with diets that promote excessive intakes of a limited variety of foods or with the use of many fortified foods or excessive doses of individual vitamins or minerals.

▲ With a little bit of study, you can master the alphabet soup of nutrition recommendations.

## Daily Value

A nutrition standard more relevant to everyday life is the Daily Value (DV). This is a generic standard used on food labels. It is applicable to both genders from 4 years of age through adulthood, and is based on consuming a 2000 kcal diet. DVs are mostly set at or close to the highest RDA value or related nutrient standard seen in the various age and gender categories for a specific nutrient (see Appendix B). DVs have been set for vitamins, minerals, protein, and other dietary components. DVs allow consumers to compare their intake from a specific food to desirable (or maximum) intakes.

### MAKING DECISIONS

#### Using Nutrient Recommendations

As nutrient intake increases, the Recommended Dietary Allowance (RDA) for the nutrient, if set, is eventually met and a deficient state is no longer present. An individual's needs most likely will be met since RDAs are set high to include almost all people. Related to the RDA concept of meeting an individual's needs are the standards of Adequate Intake (AI) and the Estimated Energy Requirement (EER). These can be used to estimate an individual's needs for some nutrients and calories, respectively. Still, keep in mind that these standards do not share the same degree of accuracy as the RDA. For example, EER may have to be adjusted upward if the individual is very physically active. Finally, as nutrient intake increases above the Upper Level (UL), poor nutritional health is again likely. However, this poor health is due now to the toxic effects of a nutrient, rather than those of a deficiency.

### CONCEPT CHECK

Dietary Guidelines for Americans have been set by government organizations. These guidelines are designed to reduce the risk of developing obesity, hypertension, type 2 diabetes, cardiovascular disease, alcoholism, and foodborne illness. In general, they recommend eating a variety of foods, fostered by following MyPyramid. They also recommend performing regular physical activity, aiming for a healthy weight, and moderating total fat, saturated fat, *trans* fat, salt, sugar, and alcohol intake, while focusing more on fruits, vegetables, and whole-grain products in daily menu planning. Safe food preparation and storage are also highlighted. All of the specific dietary standards are included in the broad category of Dietary Reference Intakes (DRIs). The Recommended Dietary Allowances (RDAs) are the amounts of each nutrient that will meet the needs of healthy individuals within specific gender and age categories. If not enough information is available to set an RDA, an Adequate Intake (AI) value is used. Tolerable Upper Intake Levels (ULs) are the highest amounts of a nutrient unlikely to cause adverse health effects. ULs have been set for some vitamins and minerals.

### How Should these Nutrient Standards Be Used?

To sum up the acronyms described so far, the type of standard set for nutrients depends on the quality of available evidence. A nutrient recommendation backed by lots of experimental research will have an RDA. For a nutrient that still requires more research, only an AI is presented. We use the EER as a starting point for determining calorie needs. Some nutrients also have a UL if information on toxicity or adverse health effects is available. Periodically, new DRIs become available as expert committees review and interpret the available research.

RDAs and related standards are intended mainly for diet planning. Specifically, a diet plan should aim to meet the RDA or AI as appropriate and not to exceed the UL over the long term (Fig. 2-9). Specific RDA, AI, EER, and UL standards are printed on the inside cover of this book. To learn more about these nutrient standards, visit the link for Food and Nutrition on the Institute of Medicine's web page (www.iom.edu).

## 2.6 Using the Scientific Method to Determine Nutrient Needs

How do we know what we know about nutrient needs? In a word, research. Like other sciences, the research that sets the foundation for nutrition knowledge has developed through the use of the *scientific method,* a testing procedure designed to detect and eliminate error.

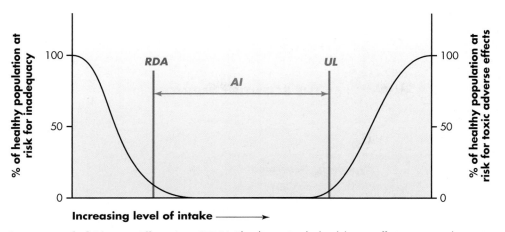

**FIGURE 2-9 ▶** This figure shows the relationship of the Dietary Reference Intakes (DRIs) to each other and the percent of the population covered by each. At intakes between the RDA and the UL, the risk of either an inadequate diet or adverse effects from the nutrient in question is close to 0. The UL is then the highest level of nutrient intake likely to pose no risks of adverse health effects to almost all individuals in the general population. At intakes above the UL, the margin of safety to protect against adverse effects is reduced. The AI is set for some nutrients instead of an RDA. The Food and Nutrition Board states that there is no established benefit for healthy individuals if they consume nutrient intakes above the RDA or AI.

*Recommended Dietary Allowance (RDA):* The dietary intake level that is sufficient to meet the nutrient requirement of nearly all (97% to 98%) healthy individuals in a particular life stage and gender group. When set for a nutrient, aim for this intake.

*Adequate Intake (AI):* A recommended intake value based on observed or experimentally determined approximations or estimates of nutrient intake by a group (or groups) of healthy people that is assumed to be adequate — used when an RDA cannot be determined. When set for a nutrient, aim for this intake.

*Tolerable Upper Intake Level (Upper Level or UL):* The highest level of nutrient intake that is likely to pose no risk of adverse health effects for almost all individuals in the general population. As intake increases above the Upper Level, the risk of adverse effects increases.

The first step of the scientific method is the observation of a natural phenomenon. Scientists then suggest possible explanations, called **hypotheses,** about its cause. At times, historical events can provide clues to important relationships in nutrition science, such as the link between vitamin C and **scurvy** (see Chapter 8). In a related approach, scientists may study the dietary and disease patterns among various populations, a research method called **epidemiology.**

Historical and epidemiological findings can *suggest* hypotheses about the role of diet in various health problems. *Proving* the role of particular dietary components, however, requires controlled experiments. The data gathered from experiments may either support or refute each hypothesis. If the results of many experiments support a hypothesis, the hypothesis becomes generally accepted by scientists and can be called a **theory** (such as the theory of gravity). Often, the results from one experiment suggest a new set of questions (Fig. 2-10).

The most rigorous type of controlled experiment follows a randomized, double-blind, placebo-controlled study design. In this type of study, a group of participants—the experimental group—follows a specific protocol (e.g., consuming a certain food or nutrient), and participants in a corresponding **control group** follow their normal habits or consume a **placebo.** People are randomly assigned to each group, such as by the flip of a coin. Scientists then observe the experimental group over time to see if there is any effect not found in the control group.

Human experiments provide the most convincing evidence about relationships between nutrients and health, but they are often not practical or ethical. Thus, much of what we know about human nutritional needs and functions has been generated from animal experiments. The use of animal experiments to study the role of nutrition in certain human diseases depends on the availability of an **animal model**—a disease in laboratory animals that closely mimics a particular human disease. Often, however, if no animal model is available and human experiments are ruled out, scientific knowledge cannot advance beyond what can be learned from epidemiological studies.

**hypotheses** Tentative explanations by a scientist to explain a phenomenon.

**scurvy** The deficiency disease that results after a few weeks to months of consuming a diet that lacks vitamin C; pinpoint sites of bleeding on the skin are an early sign.

**epidemiology** The study of how disease rates vary among different population groups.

**theory** An explanation for a phenomenon that has numerous lines of evidence to support it.

**control group** Participants in an experiment who are not given the treatment being tested.

**placebo** Generally a fake medicine or treatment used to disguise the treatments given to the participants in an experiment.

**animal model** Use of animals to study disease to understand more about human disease.

**case-control study** A study in which individuals who have a disease or condition, such as lung cancer, are compared with individuals who do not have the condition.

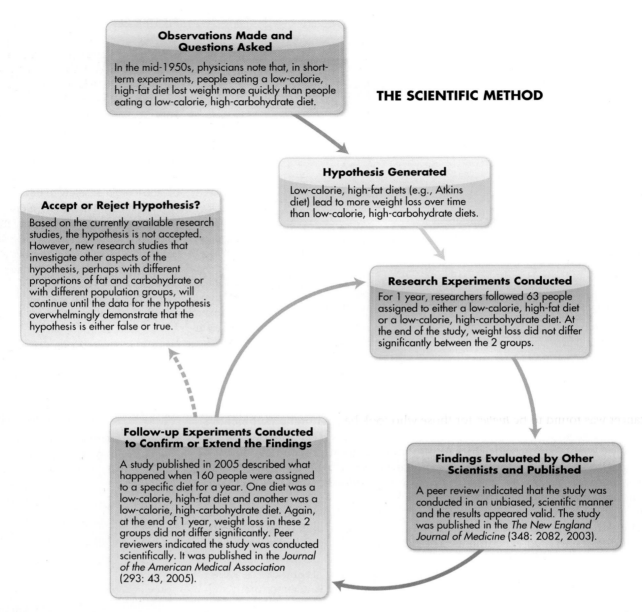

**THE SCIENTIFIC METHOD**

**Observations Made and Questions Asked**

In the mid-1950s, physicians note that, in short-term experiments, people eating a low-calorie, high-fat diet lost weight more quickly than people eating a low-calorie, high-carbohydrate diet.

**Hypothesis Generated**

Low-calorie, high-fat diets (e.g., Atkins diet) lead to more weight loss over time than low-calorie, high-carbohydrate diets.

**Accept or Reject Hypothesis?**

Based on the currently available research studies, the hypothesis is not accepted. However, new research studies that investigate other aspects of the hypothesis, perhaps with different proportions of fat and carbohydrate or with different population groups, will continue until the data for the hypothesis overwhelmingly demonstrate that the hypothesis is either false or true.

**Research Experiments Conducted**

For 1 year, researchers followed 63 people assigned to either a low-calorie, high-fat diet or a low-calorie, high-carbohydrate diet. At the end of the study, weight loss did not differ significantly between the 2 groups.

**Follow-up Experiments Conducted to Confirm or Extend the Findings**

A study published in 2005 described what happened when 160 people were assigned to a specific diet for a year. One diet was a low-calorie, high-fat diet and another was a low-calorie, high-carbohydrate diet. Again, at the end of 1 year, weight loss in these 2 groups did not differ significantly. Peer reviewers indicated the study was conducted scientifically. It was published in the *Journal of the American Medical Association* (293: 43, 2005).

**Findings Evaluated by Other Scientists and Published**

A peer review indicated that the study was conducted in an unbiased, scientific manner and the results appeared valid. The study was published in the *The New England Journal of Medicine* (348: 2082, 2003).

**FIGURE 2-10** ▶ This example shows how the scientific method was used to test a hypothesis about the effects of low-calorie, high-fat diets on weight loss. Scientists consistently follow these steps when testing all types of hypotheses. Scientists do not accept a nutrition or another scientific hypothesis until it has been thoroughly tested using the scientific method.

Once an experiment is complete, scientists summarize the findings and seek to publish the results in scientific journals. Generally, before articles are published in scientific journals, they are critically reviewed by other scientists familiar with the subject, which helps to ensure that only high-quality, objective research findings are published.

Keep in mind, one experiment is never enough to prove a particular hypothesis or provide a basis for nutritional recommendations. Rather, through follow-up studies, the results obtained in one laboratory must be confirmed by experiments conducted in other laboratories, and possibly under varying circumstances. Only then can we really trust and use the results. The more lines of evidence available to support an idea, the more likely it is to be true (Fig. 2-11).

## MAKING DECISIONS

### Research on Stomach Ulcers

Overall, the scientific method requires a skeptical attitude. A recent example of this need for skepticism involves stomach **ulcers.** Not so many years ago, everyone "knew" that stomach ulcers were caused by a stressful lifestyle and a poor diet. Then, in 1983, an Australian physician, Dr. Barry Marshall, reported in a respected medical journal that ulcers are usually caused by a common **microorganism** called *Helicobacter pylori*. Furthermore, he stated that a cure is possible using antibiotics. At first, other physicians were skeptical about this finding and continued to prescribe medications such as antacids that reduce stomach acid. But, as more studies were published demonstrating that patients using antibiotics were cured of ulcers, the medical profession eventually accepted the findings. Today, ulcers are managed for the most part by medications that destroy the microorganism. (We will discuss the treatment of stomach ulcers in more detail in Chapter 3.) Sound scientific discoveries will always be subject to challenge and change.

▲ Careful research contributes to scientifically valid nutrition knowledge.

Epidemiological studies may suggest hypotheses, but controlled experiments are needed to rigorously test hypotheses before nutrition recommendations can be made. For example, epidemiologists found that smokers who regularly consumed fruits and vegetables had a lower risk for lung cancer than smokers who ate few fruits and vegetables. Some scientists proposed that beta-carotene, a pigment present in many fruits and vegetables, may be responsible for reducing the damage that tobacco smoke creates in the lungs. However, in **double-blind studies** involving heavy smokers, the risk of lung cancer was found to be *higher* for those who took beta-carotene supplements than for those who did not (this is not true for the small amount of beta-carotene found naturally in foods). Soon after these results were reported, the U.S. federal agency supporting two other large ongoing studies that employed beta-carotene supplements called a halt to the research, stating that these supplements are ineffective in preventing both lung cancer and cardiovascular disease.

**ulcer** Erosion of the tissue lining, usually in the stomach (gastric ulcer) or the upper small intestine (duodenal ulcer). As a group these are generally referred to as peptic ulcers.

**microorganism** Bacteria, virus, or other organism invisible to the naked eye, some of which cause diseases. Also called *microbes*.

**double-blind study** An experimental design in which neither the participants nor the researchers are aware of each participant's assignment (test or placebo) or the outcome of the study until it is completed. An independent third party holds the code and the data until the study has been completed.

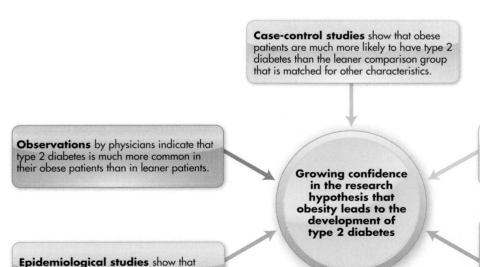

**FIGURE 2-11 ▶** Data from a variety of sources can come together to support a research hypothesis. This diagram shows how various types of research data support the hypothesis that obesity leads to the development of type 2 diabetes (see Chapter 4).

## 2.7 Food Labels and Diet Planning

Today, nearly all foods sold in stores must be in a package that has a label containing the following information: the product name, name and address of the manufacturer, amount of product in the package, and ingredients listed in descending order by weight. This food and beverage labeling is monitored in North America by government agencies such as the Food and Drug Administration (FDA) in the United States. The listing of certain food constituents also is required—specifically, on a Nutrition Facts panel (Fig. 2-12). Use the information in the Nutrition Facts panel to learn more about what you eat. The following components must be listed: total calories (kcal), calories from fat, total fat, saturated fat, *trans* fat, cholesterol, sodium, total carbohydrate, fiber, sugars, protein, vitamin A, vitamin C, calcium, and iron. In addition to these required components, manufacturers can choose to list polyunsaturated and monounsaturated fat, potassium, and others. Listing these components becomes *required* if the food is fortified with that nutrient or if a claim is made about the health benefits of the specific nutrient (see the upcoming section in Chapter 2 entitled "Health Claims on Food Labels").

Remember that the Daily Value is a generic standard used on the food label. The percentage of the Daily Value (% Daily Value or % DV) is usually given for each nutrient per serving. These percentages are based on a 2000 kcal diet. In other words, they are not as applicable to people who require considerably more or less than 2000 kcal per day with respect to fat and carbohydrate intake. DVs are mostly set at or close to the highest RDA value or related nutrient standard seen in the various age and gender categories for a specific nutrient.

Serving sizes on the Nutrition Facts panel must be consistent among similar foods. This means that all brands of ice cream, for example, must use the same serving size on their label. (These serving sizes may differ from those of MyPyramid because those on food labels are based on typical serving sizes.) In addition, food claims made on packages must follow legal definitions (Table 2-9). For example, if a product claims to be "low sodium," it must have 140 milligrams of sodium or less per serving.

Many manufacturers list the Daily Values set for dietary components such as fat, cholesterol, and carbohydrate on the Nutrition Facts panel. This can be useful as a reference point. As noted, they are based on 2000 kcal; if the label is large enough, amounts based on 2500 kcal are listed as well for total fat, saturated fat, carbohydrate, and other components. As mentioned, DVs allow consumers to compare their intake from a specific food to desirable (or maximum) intakes.

### Exceptions to Food Labeling

Foods such as fresh fruits and vegetables, fish, meats, and poultry currently are not required to have Nutrition Facts labels. However, many grocers and some meat packers have voluntarily chosen to provide their customers with information about these products. Nutrition Facts labels on meat products will likely be required in the coming years. The next time you are at the grocery store, ask where you might find information on the fresh products that do not have a Nutrition Facts panel. You will likely find a poster or pamphlet near the product; often, these pamphlets contain recipes that use your favorite fruit, vegetable, or cut of meat. They may even assist you in your endeavor to improve your diet.

Protein deficiency is not a public health concern in the United States, so declaration of the % Daily Value for protein is not mandatory on foods for people over 4 years of age. If the % Daily Value for protein is given on a label, FDA requires that the product be analyzed for protein quality. This procedure is expensive

**T**he nutrition label uses the term calorie to express energy content in some cases, but kilocalorie (kcal) values are actually listed.

**N**utrient and herbal supplement labels have a different layout with a "Supplement Facts" heading. The Nutrition and Your Health section at the end of this chapter and Chapter 8 show examples of these labels.

▼ Use the Nutrition Facts label to learn more about the nutrient content of the foods you eat. Nutrient content is expressed as a percent of Daily Value. Canadian food laws and related food labels have a slightly different format (review Appendix C).

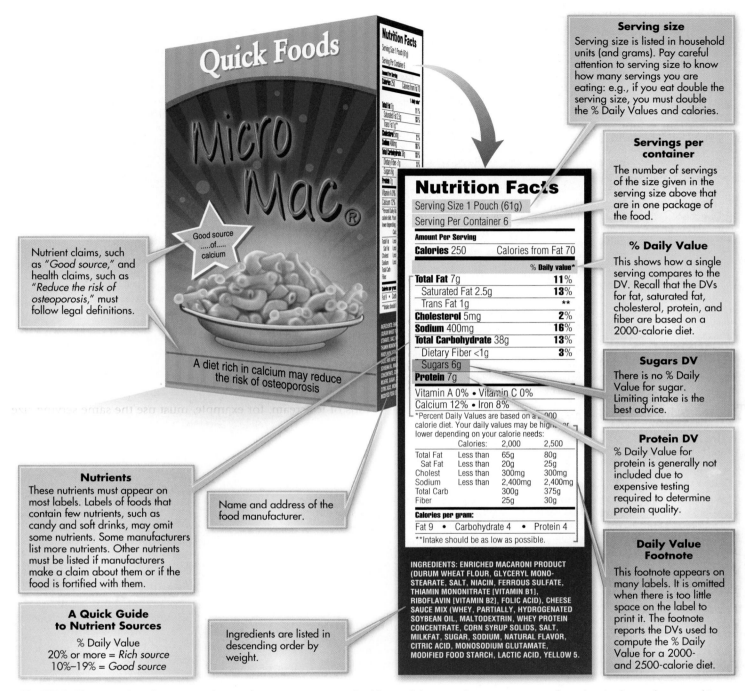

**Serving size**

Serving size is listed in household units (and grams). Pay careful attention to serving size to know how many servings you are eating: e.g., if you eat double the serving size, you must double the % Daily Values and calories.

**Servings per container**

The number of servings of the size given in the serving size above that are in one package of the food.

**% Daily Value**

This shows how a single serving compares to the DV. Recall that the DVs for fat, saturated fat, cholesterol, protein, and fiber are based on a 2000-calorie diet.

**Sugars DV**

There is no % Daily Value for sugar. Limiting intake is the best advice.

**Protein DV**

% Daily Value for protein is generally not included due to expensive testing required to determine protein quality.

**Daily Value Footnote**

This footnote appears on many labels. It is omitted when there is too little space on the label to print it. The footnote reports the DVs used to compute the % Daily Value for a 2000- and 2500-calorie diet.

Nutrient claims, such as "Good source," and health claims, such as "Reduce the risk of osteoporosis," must follow legal definitions.

**Nutrients**

These nutrients must appear on most labels. Labels of foods that contain few nutrients, such as candy and soft drinks, may omit some nutrients. Some manufacturers list more nutrients. Other nutrients must be listed if manufacturers make a claim about them or if the food is fortified with them.

**A Quick Guide to Nutrient Sources**

% Daily Value
20% or more = Rich source
10%–19% = Good source

Name and address of the food manufacturer.

Ingredients are listed in descending order by weight.

**Nutrition Facts**

Serving Size 1 Pouch (61g)

Serving Per Container 6

**Amount Per Serving**

**Calories** 250          Calories from Fat 70

|  | % Daily value* |
|---|---|
| **Total Fat** 7g | **11**% |
| Saturated Fat 2.5g | **13**% |
| Trans Fat 1g | ** |
| **Cholesterol** 5mg | **2**% |
| **Sodium** 400mg | **16**% |
| **Total Carbohydrate** 38g | **13**% |
| Dietary Fiber <1g | **3**% |
| Sugars 6g | |
| **Protein** 7g | |

Vitamin A 0% • Vitamin C 0%

Calcium 12% • Iron 8%

*Percent Daily Values are based on a 2,000 calorie diet. Your daily values may be higher or lower depending on your calorie needs:

| | Calories: | 2,000 | 2,500 |
|---|---|---|---|
| Total Fat | Less than | 65g | 80g |
| Sat Fat | Less than | 20g | 25g |
| Cholest | Less than | 300mg | 300mg |
| Sodium | Less than | 2,400mg | 2,400mg |
| Total Carb | | 300g | 375g |
| Fiber | | 25g | 30g |

**Calories per gram:**

Fat 9    •    Carbohydrate 4    •    Protein 4

**Intake should be as low as possible.

INGREDIENTS: ENRICHED MACARONI PRODUCT (DURUM WHEAT FLOUR, GLYCERYL MONO-STEARATE, SALT, NIACIN, FERROUS SULFATE, THIAMIN MONONITRATE [VITAMIN B1], RIBOFLAVIN [VITAMIN B2], FOLIC ACID), CHEESE SAUCE MIX (WHEY, PARTIALLY, HYDROGENATED SOYBEAN OIL, MALTODEXTRIN, WHEY PROTEIN CONCENTRATE, CORN SYRUP SOLIDS, SALT, MILKFAT, SUGAR, SODIUM, NATURAL FLAVOR, CITRIC ACID, MONOSODIUM GLUTAMATE, MODIFIED FOOD STARCH, LACTIC ACID, YELLOW 5.

**FIGURE 2-12** ▶ Food packages must list product name, name and address of the manufacturer, amount of product in the package, and ingredients. The Nutrition Facts panel is required on virtually all packaged food products. The % Daily Value listed on the label is the percent of the amount of a nutrient needed daily that is provided by a single serving of the product.

and timeconsuming, so many companies opt not to list a % Daily Value for protein. However, labels on food for infants and children under 4 years of age must include the % Daily Value for protein, as must the labels on any food carrying a claim about protein content (see Chapter 15).

**TABLE 2-9** Definitions for Nutrient Claims Allowed on Food Labels

### Sugar

- **Sugar free:** less than 0.5 grams (g) per serving.
- **No added sugar; without added sugar; no sugar added:**
  - No sugars were added during processing or packing, including ingredients that contain sugars (for example, fruit juices, applesauce, or jam).
  - Processing does not increase the sugar content above the amount naturally present in the ingredients. (A functionally insignificant increase in sugars is acceptable for processes used for purposes other than increasing sugar content.)
  - The food that it resembles and for which it substitutes normally contains added sugars.
  - If the food doesn't meet the requirements for a low- or reduced-calorie food, the product bears a statement that the food is not low calorie or calorie reduced and directs consumers' attention to the Nutrition Facts panel for further information on sugars and calorie content.
- **Reduced sugar:** at least 25% less sugar per serving than reference food

### Calories

- **Calorie free:** fewer than 5 kcal per serving
- **Low calorie:** 40 kcal or less per serving and, if the serving is 30 g or less or 2 tablespoons or less, per 50 g of the food
- **Reduced or fewer calories:** at least 25% fewer kcal per serving than reference food

### Fiber

- **High fiber:** 5 g or more per serving. (Foods making high-fiber claims must meet the definition for low fat, or the level of total fat must appear next to the high-fiber claim.)
- **Good source of fiber:** 2.5 to 4.9 g per serving
- **More or added fiber:** at least 2.5 g more per serving than reference food

### Fat

- **Fat free:** less than 0.5 g of fat per serving
- **Saturated fat free:** less than 0.5 g per serving, and the level of *trans* fatty acids does not exceed 0.5 g per serving

- **Low fat:** 3 g or less per serving and, if the serving is 30 g or less or 2 tablespoons or less, per 50 g of the food. 2% milk can no longer be labeled low fat, as it exceeds 3 g per serving. *Reduced fat* will be the term used instead.
- **Low saturated fat:** 1 g or less per serving and not more than 15% of kcal from saturated fatty acids
- **Reduced or less fat:** at least 25% less per serving than reference food
- **Reduced or less saturated fat:** at least 25% less per serving than reference food

### Cholesterol

- **Cholesterol free:** less than 2 milligrams (mg) of cholesterol and 2 g or less of saturated fat per serving
- **Low cholesterol:** 20 mg or less cholesterol and 2 g or less of saturated fat per serving and, if the serving is 30 g or less or 2 tablespoons or less, per 50 g of the food
- **Reduced or less cholesterol:** at least 25% less cholesterol and 2 g or less of saturated fat per serving than reference food

### Sodium

- **Sodium free:** less than 5 mg per serving
- **Very low sodium:** 35 mg or less per serving and, if the serving is 30 g or less or 2 tablespoons or less, per 50 g of the food
- **Low sodium:** 140 mg or less per serving and, if the serving is 30 g or less or 2 tablespoons or less, per 50 g of the food
- **Light in sodium:** at least 50% less per serving than reference food
- **Reduced or less sodium:** at least 25% less per serving than reference food

### Other Terms

- **Fortified or enriched:** Vitamins and/or minerals have been added to the product in amounts in excess of at least 10% of that normally present in the usual product. Enriched generally refers to replacing nutrients lost in processing, whereas fortified refers to adding nutrients not originally present in the specific food.
- **Healthy:** An individual food that is low fat and low saturated fat and has no more than 360 to 480 mg of sodium or 60 mg of cholesterol per serving can be labeled "healthy" if it provides at least 10% of the Daily Value for vitamin A, vitamin C, protein, calcium, iron, or fiber.

- **Light or lite:** The descriptor *light* or *lite* can mean two things: first, that a nutritionally altered product contains one-third fewer kcal or half the fat of reference food (if the food derives 50% or more of its kcal from fat, the reduction must be 50% of the fat) and, second, that the sodium content of a low-calorie, low-fat food has been reduced by 50%. In addition, "light in sodium" may be used for foods in which the sodium content has been reduced by at least 50%. The term *light* may still be used to describe such properties as texture and color, as long as the label explains the intent—for example, "light brown sugar" and "light and fluffy."

**Diet:** A food may be labeled with terms such as *diet, dietetic, artificially sweetened,* or *sweetened with nonnutritive sweetener* only if the claim is not false or misleading. The food can also be labeled *low calorie* or *reduced calorie.*

**Good source:** *Good source* means that a serving of the food contains 10% to 19% of the Daily Value for a particular nutrient. If 5% or less it is a *low source.*

**High:** *High* means that a serving of the food contains 20% or more of the Daily Value for a particular nutrient.

**Organic:** Federal standards for organic foods allow claims when much of the ingredients do not use chemical fertilizers or pesticides, genetic engineering, sewage sludge, antibiotics, or irradiation in their production. At least 95% of ingredients (by weight) must meet these guidelines to be labeled "organic" on the front of the package. If the front label instead says "made with organic ingredients," only 70% of the ingredients must be organic. For animal products, the animals must graze outdoors, be fed organic feed, and cannot be exposed to large amounts of antibiotics or growth hormones.

**Natural:** The food must be free of food colors, synthetic flavors, or any other synthetic substance.

### The following terms apply only to meat and poultry products regulated by USDA.

**Extra lean:** less than 5 g of fat, 2 g of saturated fat, and 95 mg of cholesterol per serving (or 100 g of an individual food)

**Lean:** less than 10 g of fat, 4.5 g of saturated fat, and 95 mg of cholesterol per serving (or 100 g of an individual food)

Many definitions are from FDA's *Dictionary of Terms,* as established in conjunction with the 1990 Nutrition Education and Labeling Act (NELA).
g = grams; mg = milligrams

## Health Claims on Food Labels

As a marketing tool directed toward the health-conscious consumer, food manufacturers like to claim that their products have all sorts of health benefits. The FDA has legal oversight over most food products and permits some health claims with certain restrictions.

Overall, claims on foods fall into one of four categories:

- Health claims—closely regulated by FDA
- Preliminary health claims—regulated by FDA but evidence may be scant for the claim
- Nutrient claims—closely regulated by FDA (review Table 2-9)
- Structure/function claims—as discussed in the Nutrition and Your Health section at the end of this chapter, these are not FDA approved or necessarily valid

Table 2-9 lists the definitions for nutrient claims on food labels. Currently, FDA limits the use of health messages to specific instances in which there is significant scientific agreement that a relationship exists between a nutrient, food, or food constituent and the disease. The claims allowed at this time may show a link between the following:

- A diet with enough calcium and a reduced risk of osteoporosis
- A diet low in total fat and a reduced risk of some cancers
- A diet low in saturated fat and cholesterol and a reduced risk of cardiovascular disease (typically referred to as heart disease on the label)
- A diet rich in fiber—containing grain products, fruits, and vegetables—and a reduced risk of some cancers
- A diet low in sodium and high in potassium and a reduced risk of hypertension and stroke
- A diet rich in fruits and vegetables and a reduced risk of some cancers
- A diet adequate in the synthetic form of the vitamin folate (called folic acid) and a reduced risk of neural tube defects (a type of birth defect) (see Chapter 8)
- Use of sugarless gum and a reduced risk of tooth decay, especially when compared with foods high in sugars and starches
- A diet rich in fruits, vegetables, and grain products that contain fiber and a reduced risk of cardiovascular disease. Oats (oatmeal, oat bran, and oat flour) and psyllium are two fiber-rich ingredients that can be singled out in reducing the risk of cardiovascular disease, as long as the statement also says the diet should also be low in saturated fat and cholesterol.
- A diet rich in whole-grain foods and other plant foods, as well as low in total fat, saturated fat, and cholesterol, and a reduced risk of cardiovascular disease and certain cancers
- A diet low in saturated fat and cholesterol that also includes 25 grams of soy protein and a reduced risk of cardiovascular disease. The statement "one serving of the (name of food) provides _____ grams of soy protein" must also appear as part of the health claim.
- Fatty acids from oils present in fish and a reduced risk of cardiovascular disease
- Margarines containing plant stanols and sterols and a reduced risk of cardiovascular disease (see Chapter 5 for more details on plant stanols and sterols)

A "may" or "might" qualifier must be used in the statement.

**Health Claims Report Card**

| A | **High** Significant scientific agreement | 1 |
| B | **Moderate** Evidence is not conclusive | 2 |
| C | **Low** Evidence is limited and not conclusive | 3 |
| D | **Extremely Low** Little scientific evidence supporting this claim | 4 |

▲ In 2003, FDA unveiled a new process, including the Health Claims Report card, to provide more science-based, FDA-regulated health information on food product labels. This new process is used to rank the claim based on the amount of scientific evidence and agreement. Only the first three classes are allowed.

▲ The nutrition information on the Nutrition Facts panels on these products can be combined to determine the nutrient intake for a peanut butter and jelly sandwich.

▲ Specific health claims can be made on food labels for whole-grain cereals.

In addition, before a health claim can be made for a food product, it must meet two general requirements. First, the food must be a "good source" (before any fortification) of fiber, protein, vitamin A, vitamin C, calcium, or iron. The legal definition of "good source" appears in Table 2-9. Second, a single serving of the food product cannot contain more than 13 grams of fat, 4 grams of saturated fat, 60 milligrams of cholesterol, or 480 milligrams of sodium. If a food exceeds any one of these requirements, no health claim can be made for it, despite its other nutritional qualities. For example, even though whole milk is high in calcium, its label can't make the health claim about calcium and osteoporosis because whole milk contains 5 grams of saturated fat per serving. In another example, a health claim regarding fat and cancer can be made only if the product contains 3 grams or less of fat per serving, the standard for low-fat foods.

## MAKING DECISIONS

### Health Claims

FDA allows the three preliminary classes of health claims shown on page 69 as long as the label qualifies the food with a disclaimer such as "this evidence is not conclusive." These preliminary health claims haven't shown up on many foods at this time (nuts, such as walnuts, and fish have been some of the first examples). These claims also cannot be used on foods considered unhealthy (review Table 2-9 for the definition of healthy with regard to a food).

## CONCEPT CHECK

The Nutrition Facts panel on a food label provides key information for helping track one's food intake. Nutrient quantities are compared with the Daily Values and expressed on a percentage basis (% Daily Value). This information can be used to either increase or reduce intake of specific nutrients. Health and nutrient claims on food labels are closely regulated by FDA. Fruits, vegetables, whole-grain breads and cereals, soy, and good sources of calcium are prominent among the foods that can make specific health claims.

**C**anadian food labels use a slightly different group of health claims and label descriptors (see Appendix C).

**T**he **Exchange System** is a final menu-planning tool. This tool organizes foods based on calorie, protein, carbohydrate, and fat content. The result is a manageable framework for designing diets, especially for treatment of diabetes. For more information on the Exchange System see Appendix D.

## 2.8 Epilogue

The tools discussed in Chapter 2 greatly aid in menu planning. Menu planning can start with MyPyramid. The totality of choices made within the groups can then be evaluated using the Dietary Guidelines. Individual foods that make up a diet can be examined more closely using the Daily Values listed on the Nutrition Facts panel of the product. For the most part, these Daily Values are in line with the Recommended Dietary Allowances and related nutrient standards. The Nutrition Facts panel is especially useful in identifying nutrient-dense foods—foods high in a specific nutrient, such as the vitamin folate, but low in the relative amount of calories provided—and the energy-dense foods—foods that fill you up without providing a lot of calories. Generally speaking, the more you learn about and use these tools, the more they will benefit your diet.

# Evaluating Nutrition Claims and Dietary Supplements

The following suggestions should help you make healthful and logical nutrition decisions:

1. Apply the basic principles of nutrition as outlined in this chapter (along with the 2005 Dietary Guidelines for Americans and related resources in Chapter 2) to any nutrition claim including those on websites. Do you note any inconsistencies? Do reliable references support the claims? Beware of the following:
   - Testimonials about personal experience
   - Disreputable publication sources
   - Promises of dramatic results (rarely true)
   - Lack of evidence from other scientific studies

2. Examine the background and scientific credentials of the individual, organizations, or publication making the nutritional claim. Usually, a reputable author is one whose educational background or present affiliation is with a nationally recognized university or medical center that offers programs or courses in the field of nutrition, medicine, or a closely allied specialty.

3. Be wary if the answer is "Yes" to any of the following questions about a health-related nutrition claim:
   - Are only advantages discussed and possible disadvantages ignored?
   - Are claims made about "curing" disease? Do they sound too good to be true?
   - Is extreme bias against the medical community or traditional medical treatments evident? Physicians as a group strive to cure diseases in their patients, using what proven techniques are available. They do not ignore reliable cures.
   - Is the claim touted as a new or secret scientific breakthrough?

4. Note the size and duration of any study cited in support of a nutrition claim. The larger it is and the longer it went on, the more dependable its findings. Also consider the type of study: epidemiology versus case-control versus double-blind. Check out the group studied; a study of men or women in Sweden may be less relevant than one of men or women of Southern European, African, or Hispanic descent, for example. Keep in mind that "contributes to," "is linked to," or "is associated with" does not mean "causes."

5. Beware of press conferences and other hype regarding the latest findings. Much of this will not survive more detailed scientific evaluation.

6. When you meet with a nutrition professional, you should expect that he or she will do the following:
   - Ask questions about your medical history, lifestyle, and current eating habits.
   - Formulate a diet plan tailored to your needs, as opposed to simply tearing a form from a tablet that could apply to almost anyone.
   - Schedule follow-up visits to track your progress, answer any questions, and help keep you motivated.
   - Involve family members in the diet plan, when appropriate.
   - Consult directly with your physician and readily refer you back to your physician for those health problems a nutrition professional is not trained to treat.

7. Avoid practitioners who prescribe **megadoses** of vitamin and mineral supplements for everyone.

8. Examine product labels carefully. Be skeptical of any promotional information about a product that is not clearly stated on the label. A product is not likely to do something not specifically claimed on its label or package insert (legally part of the label).

**megadose** Large intake of a nutrient beyond estimates of needs or what would be found in a balanced diet; 2 to 10 times human needs is a starting point.

## Dietary Supplements

A cautious approach to nutrition-related advice and products is even more important today because of broad changes in U.S. federal law passed in 1994.

The Dietary Supplement Health and Education Act (DSHEA) of 1994 classified vitamins, minerals, amino acids, and herbal remedies as "foods," which restrains the U.S. Food and Drug Administration (FDA) from regulating them as tightly as drugs and food additives. According to this act, rather than the manufacturer having to prove a dietary supplement is safe, FDA must prove it is unsafe before preventing its sale. In contrast, the safety of food additives and drugs must be demonstrated to FDA's satisfaction before they are marketed.

► Recently major nutrition organizations put together 10 red flags that they consider signals for poor nutrition advice:

1. Recommendations that promise a quick fix
2. Dire warnings of dangers from a single product or regimen
3. Claims that sound too good to be true
4. Simplistic conclusions drawn from a complex study
5. Recommendations based on a single study
6. Dramatic statements refuted by reputable scientific organizations
7. Lists of "good" and "bad" foods
8. Recommendations made to help sell a product
9. Recommendations based on studies published without peer review
10. Recommendations from studies that ignore differences among individuals or groups

► FDA can act if evidence accumulates showing that a product is harmful. This has been true for some herbal remedies marketed as dietary supplements, such as ephedra.

Currently, a dietary supplement (or herbal product) can be marketed in the United States without FDA approval if (1) there is a history of its use or other evidence that it is expected to be reasonably safe when used under the conditions recommended or suggested in its labeling, and (2) the product is labeled as a dietary supplement. The "Supplement Facts" panel resembles the Nutrition Facts panel on foods and is required on all dietary supplements. It is permissible for the labels on such products to claim a benefit related to a classic nutrient-deficiency disease, describe how a nutrient affects human body structure or function (called structure/function claims), and claim that general well-being results from consumption of the ingredient(s). Examples could be "maintains bone health" or "improves blood circulation." However, the label of products bearing such claims also must prominently display in boldface type the following disclaimer: "This statement has not been evaluated by the Food and Drug Administration. This product is not intended to diagnose, treat, cure, or prevent disease" (Fig. 2-13). Despite this warning, when consumers find these products on the shelves of supermarkets,

health-food stores, and pharmacies, they may mistakenly assume FDA has carefully evaluated the products.

Many of us are willing to try untested nutrition products and believe in their miraculous actions. Popular products claim to increase muscle growth, enhance sexuality, boost energy, reduce body fat, increase strength, supply missing nutrients, increase longevity, and even improve brain function. Clearly, many nutritional products commonly found in stores are not strictly regulated in terms of effectiveness and safety. The amount and potency of dietary supplmements have also been in question. In June 2007, FDA issued long-awaited standards that will require supplement manufacturers to test the purity, strength, and composition of all their products. Large companies will be the first to comply (by June 2008), whereas small companies have until 2010. Until then, national brands are more reliable. The usefulness of supplements is discussed further in the Nutrition and Your Health section in Chapter 8, "Dietary Supplements—Who Needs Them?"

If you embark on a self-cure by means of such products, you will probably waste money and possibly risk ill health. A better approach is to consult a physician or **registered dietitian** first. You can find a registered dietitian in North America by consulting the Yellow Pages in the telephone directory, contacting the local dietetic association, calling the dietary department of a local hospital, or visiting www.eatright.org/ or www.dietitians.ca. Make sure the person has the credentials "R.D." after his/her name ("R.D.N." is also used in Canada). This indicates the person has completed rigorous classroom and clinical training in nutrition and participates in continuing education. Appendix H also lists many reputable sources of nutrition advice for your use. Finally, the

**registered dietitian (R.D.)** A person who has completed a baccalaureate degree program approved by the American Dietetic Association, performed at least 900 hours of supervised professional practice, and passed a registration examination.

# Supplement Facts

Serving Size 1 Softgel — Suggested serving size

**Each Softgel Contains**     % DV *
Ginseng Extract (Panax ginseng) (root) 100 mg — Product and amount
  (Standardized to 4% Ginsenosides)

*Daily Value (DV) not established.

**INGREDIENTS:** Gelatin, Soybean Oil, Panax Ginseng Extract, Vegetable Oil, Lecithin, Palm Oil, Glycerin, Sorbitol, Yellow Beeswax, Hydrogenated Coconut Oil, Titanium Dioxide, Yellow 5, Blue 1, Red 40, Green 3, Chlorophyll.

**DIST. BY NUTRA ASSOC., INC.**
**4411 WHITE POINT RD., SPRING CITY, IL 12345** — Name and address of manufacturer

**Suggested use:** Adults- 1 to 2 capsules daily taken with a full glass of water, or as a tea, add one to two capsules to a cup of hot water. — Suggested use

When you need to perform your best, take ginseng. — Structure/function claim

This statement has not been evaluated by the Food and Drug Administration. This product is not intended to diagnose, treat, cure, or prevent disease. — Standard FDA disclaimer

**FIGURE 2-13** ► Supplement Facts label on an herbal product. Note the structure/function claim and the FDA disclaimer. Any nutrients or other food constituents would also be listed if contained in the product.

following websites can help you evaluate ongoing nutrition and health claims:

http://www.acsh.org/
American Council on Science and Health

http://www.quackwatch.org/
Quackwatch: Your Guide to Quackery, Health Fraud, and Intelligent Decisions

http://www.ncahf.org/
National Council Against Health Fraud

http://dietary-supplements.info.nih.gov/
National Institutes of Health, Office of Dietary Supplements

http://www.fda.gov/
U.S. Food and Drug Administration

Overall, nutrition is a rapidly advancing field and there are always new findings.

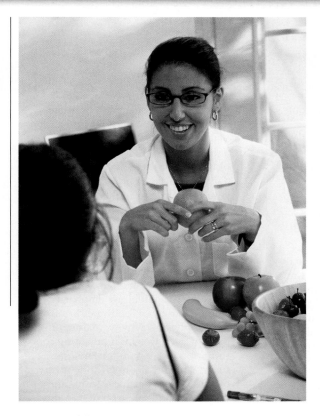

◄ Registered dietitians are a reliable source of nutrition advice.

## Case Study Dietary Supplements

While Whitney was driving to campus last week, she heard an advertisement for a supplement containing a plant substance recently imported from China. It supposedly gives people more energy and helps one cope with the stress of daily life. This advertisement caught Whitney's attention because she has been feeling run down lately. She is taking a full-course load and has been working 30 hours a week at a local restaurant to try to make ends meet. Whitney doesn't have a lot of extra money. Still, she likes to try new things and this recent breakthrough from China sounded almost too good to be true. After searching for more information about this supplement on the Internet, she discovered that the recommended dose would cost $60 per month. Because Whitney is looking for some help with her low energy level, she decides to order a 1-month supply.

Answer the following questions, and check your response in Appendix A.

1. Is the advertised supplement regulated by the FDA or other government agency?

2. What type of label claim is the phrase "increases energy," and does it require government approval?

3. Can Whitney feel confident that the supplement is safe and effective?

4. Is the amount of active ingredients in supplements tightly controlled?

5. Does it make sense for Whitney to spend the extra $60 per month for this supplement?

6. What advice would you give Whitney about the fact that she has been feeling run down lately?

▲ Do you agree with Whitney's decision to try this supplement?

## Summary

1. A healthy eating plan is based on consuming a *variety* of foods *balanced* by a moderate intake of each food and will minimize the risk of developing nutrition-related diseases.

   Nutrient density reflects the nutrient content of a food in relation to its calorie content. Nutrient-dense foods are relatively rich in nutrients, in comparison with calorie content.

   Energy density of a food is determined by comparing calorie content with the weight of food. A food rich in calories but weighing relatively very little, such as nuts, cookies, fried foods in general, and most snack foods (including fat-free brands), is considered energy dense. Foods with low energy density include fruits, vegetables, and any food that incorporates lots of water during cooking, such as oatmeal.

2. A person's nutritional state can be categorized as *desirable nutrition,* in which the body has adequate stores for times of increased needs; *undernutrition,* which may be present with or without clinical symptoms; and *over-nutrition,* which can lead to vitamin and mineral toxicities and various chronic diseases.

   Evaluation of nutritional state involves analyzing background factors, as well as anthropometric, biochemical, clinical, dietary, and environmental assessments. It is not always possible to detect nutritional inadequacies via nutrition assessment because symptoms of deficiencies are often nonspecific and may not appear for many years.

3. MyPyramid is designed to translate nutrient recommendations into a food plan that exhibits variety, balance, and moderation. The best results are obtained by using low-fat or fat-free dairy products; incorporating some vegetable proteins in the diet in addition to animal-protein foods; including citrus fruits and dark green vegetables; and emphasizing whole-grain breads and cereals.

4. Dietary Guidelines for Americans have been issued to help reduce chronic diseases. The guidelines emphasize eating a variety of foods; performing regular physical activity; maintaining or improving weight; moderating consumption of fat, *trans* fat, cholesterol, sugar, salt, and alcohol; eating plenty of whole-grain products, fruits, and vegetables; and safely preparing and storing foods, especially perishable foods.

5. Recommended Dietary Allowances (RDAs) are set for many nutrients. These amounts yield enough of each nutrient to meet the needs of healthy individuals within specific gender and age categories. Adequate Intake (AI) is the standard used when not enough information is available to set a more specific RDA. Estimated Energy Requirements (EERs) set calorie needs for both genders at various ages and physical activity patterns. Tolerable Upper Intake Levels (Upper Levels or ULs) for nutrient intake have been set for some vitamins and minerals.

All of the many dietary standards fall under the term *Dietary Reference Intakes (DRIs).* Daily Values are used as a basis for expressing the nutrient content of foods on the Nutrition Facts panel and are based for the most part on the RDAs.

6. The scientific method is the procedure for testing the validity of possible explanations of a phenomenon, called hypotheses. Experiments are conducted to either support or refute a specific hypothesis. Once we have enough experimental information to support a specific hypothesis, it then can be called a theory. All of us need to be skeptical of new ideas in the nutrition field, waiting until many lines of experimental evidence support a concept before adopting any suggested dietary practice.

7. Food labels, especially the Nutrition Facts panels, are a useful tool to track your nutrient intake and learn more about the nutritional characteristics of the foods you eat. Any health claims listed must follow criteria set by FDA.

8. Apply the basic principles of nutrition to evaluate any nutrition claim Dietary supplements can be marketed in the United States without FDA approval. Certain health claims can be made on supplement labels, although few have been thoroughly evaluated by reputable scientists.

## Study Questions

1. Relate the importance of variety in a diet, especially with regard to fruit and vegetable choices, to the discovery of various phytochemicals in foods.

2. How would you explain the concepts of nutrient density and energy density to a fourth grade class?

3. Trace the progression, in terms of physical results, of a person who went from an overnourished to an undernourished state.

4. How could the nutritional state of the person at each state in question 3 be evaluated?

5. Describe the philosophy underlying the creation of MyPyramid. What dietary changes would you need to make to meet the pyramid guidelines on a regular basis?

6. Describe the intent of the Dietary Guidelines for Americans. Point out

one criticism for its general application to all North American adults.

7. Based on the discussion of the Dietary Guidelines for Americans, suggest two key dietary changes the typical North American adult should consider making.

8. How do RDAs and AIs differ from Daily Values in intention and application?

9. Nutritionists encourage all people to read labels on food packages to learn more about what they eat. What four nutrients could easily be tracked

in your diet if you read the Nutrition Facts panels regularly on food products?

10. Explain why consumers can have confidence in FDA-approved health claims on food packages.

## Check Your Knowledge

Answers to the following multiple choice questions are below

1. Anthropometric measurements include
   a. height, weight, skinfolds, and body circumferences.
   b. blood concentrations of nutrients.
   c. a diet history of the previous days' intake.
   d. blood levels of enzyme activities.

2. Foods with *high* nutrient density offer the _____ nutrients for the _____ calories.
   a. least, lowest
   b. least, most
   c. most, lowest
   d. most, most

3. The steps on the side of the MyPyramid remind us to be physically active at least _____ minutes per day.
   a. 5           c. 20
   b. 10          d. 30

4. The Dietary Guidelines for Americans were recently revised in
   a. 2000        c. 2003
   b. 2001        d. 2005

5. The term Daily Value is used on
   a. restaurant menus.
   b. food labels.
   c. medical charts.
   d. None of the above.

6. The Tolerable Upper Intake Level, or UL, is to
   a. estimate calorie needs of the average person.
   b. evaluate the highest amount of daily nutrient intake unlikely to cause adverse health effects.
   c. evaluate your current intake for a specific nutrient.
   d. compare the nutrient content of a food to approximate human needs.

7. The current food label must list
   a. a picture of the product.

   b. a uniform and realistic serving size.
   c. the RDA for each age group.
   d. ingredients alphabetically.

8. Dietary supplements are tightly regulated by the
   a. FDA.
   b. USDA.
   c. FTC.
   d. None of the above.

9. The scientific method begins with
   a. a hypothesis.
   b. research experiments.
   c. publication of research findings.
   d. observations made and questions asked.

10. The most common type of malnutrition in industrialized nations, such as the United States, is
   a. anorexia.
   b. protein deficiency.
   c. obesity.
   d. iron deficiency.

Answer Key: 1. a, 2. c, 3. d, 4. d, 5. b, 6. b, 7. b, 8. d, 9. d, 10. d

## Further Readings

1. ADA Reports: Position of the American Dietetic Association: Food and nutrition misinformation. *Journal of the American Dietetic Association* 106:601, 2006.

   *Much food and nutrition misinformation pervades North American society. Individuals should carefully consider the training of those who give such advice and be assured that registered dietitians are a reliable source.*

2. Barr SI: Introduction to dietary reference intakes. *Applied Physiology, Nutrition, and Metabolism* 31:61, 2006.

   *The development of the dietary reference intakes (DRIs) was a joint initiative by the United States and Canada to update and replace the former Recommended Nutrient Intakes for Canadians and the Recommended Dietary*

*Allowances for Americans. The new DRIs are described.*

3. Birt DF: Phytochemicals and cancer prevention: From epidemiology to mechanism of action. *Journal of the American Dietetic Association* 106:20, 2006.

   *Studies in laboratory animals and cell cultures indicate a role for many components of fruits and vegetables in cancer prevention. Numerous human case-control studies have suggested that vegetable intake reduces the risk of a variety of cancers. These results have not been demonstrated for fruits. In addition, prospective studies have not supported a relationship between fruit and vegetable intake and cancer prevention. Although the relationship between fruit and vegetable intake and cancer risk is still unclear, a diet rich in fruits and vegetables is*

*still one of the best recommendations to improve health and reduce overall chronic disease.*

4. Borra S: Consumer perspectives on food labels. *American Journal of Clinical Nutrition* 83:1235S, 2006.

   *An important goal of the nutrition and ingredient information on food labels is to help consumers make nutritious dietary choices. This article summarizes the results of recent quantitative and qualitative research on consumers' use and understanding of the food label information.*

5. He FJ and others: Fruit and vegetable consumption and stroke: Meta-analysis of cohort studies. *Lancet* 367:320, 2006.

   *Increased fruit and vegetable intake was associated with a reduced risk of both ischemic and* hemorrhagic stroke. *Compared to individuals who had less than 3 servings of fruit and vegetables per day, the risk was reduced for those with 3 to 5 servings per day and even more reduced for those with more than 5 servings per day.*

6. Johnston CS: Uncle Sam's diet sensation: MyPyramid—an overview and commentary. *Medscape General Medicine* 7:78, 2005.

   *This overview of the Internet-based MyPyramid points out several strengths of the new educational tool. These include the focus on reducing calories and increasing physical activity in an effort to address the obesity crisis. In addition, areas that the federal government still needs to address, such as access to this information by the underprivileged, are discussed.*

7. Kennedy ET: Evidence for nutritional benefits in prolonging wellness. *American Journal of Clinical Nutrition* 83:410S, 2006.

   *The interaction between genes; the environment; and lifestyle factors, especially diet and physical activity, are involved in healthy aging. The need to consider all the lifestyle and environmental factors contributing to suboptimal eating and lifestyle patterns is discussed.*

8. Kretser AJ: The new Dietary Reference Intakes in food labeling: The food industry's perspective. *American Journal of Clinical Nutrition* 83:1231S, 2006.

   *The food industry is prepared to update food labels using new nutrient recommendations. The Grocery Manufacturers Association welcomes the opportunity to coordinate nutrition information across the Dietary Guidelines for Americans 2005, MyPyramid, and the food label.*

9. Meyer TE and others: Long-term caloric restriction ameliorates the decline in diastolic function in humans. *Journal of the American College of Cardiology* 47:398, 2006.

   *Cardiovascular aging is associated with an increased likelihood of developing cardiovascular diseases, such as myocardial infarction (heart attack), stroke, and congestive heart failure. Calorie restriction (1671 kcal vs. 2445 kcal) affected heart functions that typically decline with age. Eating the nutrient-rich diet of less than 2000 kcal slowed the decline in diastolic function, a well-recognized marker of cardiovascular aging in humans. The results suggest that cutting calories will lead to a longer life.*

10. Pavia M and others: Association between fruit and vegetable consumption and oral cancer: A meta-analysis of observational studies. *American Journal of Clinical Nutrition* 83:1126, 2006.

    *Results showed that for each portion of fruit and vegetable consumed per day, the risk of oral cancer was reduced by 49% to 50%. The lower risk of oral cancer associated with fruit consumption was influenced by the type of fruit consumed.*

11. Reedy J and Krebs-Smith SM: A comparison of food-based recommendations and nutrient values of three food guides: USDA's MyPyramid, NHLBI's dietary approaches to stop hypertension eating plan, and Harvard's healthy eating pyramid. *Journal of the American Dietetic Association* 108: 522, 2008.

    *The three food guides share consistent messages to eat more fruits, vegetables, legumes, and whole grains; eat less added sugar and saturated fat; and emphasize plant oils.*

12. Rolls B: *The volumetric eating plan: Techniques and recipes for feeling full on fewer calories.* Harper, New York, 2005.

    *Studies by Dr. Rolls have shown that the amount of calories in a given volume of food makes a big difference in how many calories people consume at a given meal, and throughout the day. The greater the energy density (more calories packed into a given weight or volume of food) the easier it is to overeat. The eating plan includes techniques and recipes such as increasing the fruits and vegetables in dishes so they are higher in fiber and water which will help people lower their calories without feeling deprived.*

13. Seal CJ: Whole grains and CVD risk. *Proceedings of the Nutrition Society* 65:24, 2006.

    *Evidence from population and epidemiological studies suggest a strong inverse relationship between the consumption of whole-grain foods and the risk of cardiovascular diseases (CVD). This evidence has resulted in recommendations to consume at least 3 servings of whole-grains per day. The mechanisms by which whole-grain foods have this effect on CVD, however, are poorly understood. Intervention studies are needed to support the health claims and promote whole-grain consumption.*

14. Sheth A and others: Potential liver damage associated with over-the-counter vitamin supplements. *Journal of the American Dietetic Association* 108: 1536, 2008.

    *This is a case report of a patient that developed liver cirrhosis after long-term (2 years) daily ingestion of over-the-counter dietary supplements containing 13,000 micrograms of vitamin A. This case provides is an example of the potential for liver damage that may be associated with long-term intakes of OTC vitamin supplements. These adverse effects indicate the need for medical supervision of these types of products.*

15. Sofi F and others: Adherence to Mediterranean diet and health status: meta-analysis. *British Medical Journal* 337:a1344, 2008.

    *A systematic review of all prospective cohort studies that have analyzed the relationship between adherence to a Mediterranean diet, mortality, and incidence of chronic diseases found that greater adherence to a Mediterranean diet is associated with a significant improvement in health status. A significant reduction in overall mortality (9%), mortality from cardiovascular diseases (9%), incidence of or mortality from cancer (6%), and incidence of Parkinson's disease and Alzheimer's disease (13%) was found. These results indicate that a Mediterranean-like dietary pattern should be encouraged for primary prevention of major chronic diseases.*

16. Taylor CL and Wilkening VL: How the nutrition food label was developed, part 1: The nutrition facts panel. Part 2: The purpose and promise of nutrition claims. *The Journal of the American Dietetic Association* 108: 437, 618, 2008.

    *These articles offer insight into the development of the nutrition label and discuss its role in improving the diet and health of Americans. The issues discussed highlight the fact that the nutrition label is a "work in progress."*

17. U.S. Department of Health and Human Services. *2008 Physical Activity Guidelines for Americans.* 2008. http://www.health. gov/PAGuidelines/.

    *Inactivity remains high among American children, adolescents, and adults, putting Americans at unnecessary risk of disease. The Guidelines provide science-based guidance to help Americans aged six and older improve their health through appropriate physical activity.*

18. United States Department of Agriculture: Diet Quality of Americans in 1994–96 and 2001–02 as measured by the Healthy Eating Index-2005. *Nutrition Insight* 37, December 2007.

    *This report provides Healthy Eating Index-2005 (HEI-2005) scores for the total U.S. population estimated from national surveys conducted in 1994–96 and in 2001–02 and reflects the quality of the American diet prior to the implementation of the 2005 Dietary Guideline. The survey found that the HEI-2005 scores were low for the "food groups to encourage" identified in the Dietary Guidelines for Americans 2005 and concludes that the diet quality of Americans needs to be improved.*

19. Woolf SH: Weighing the evidence to formulate dietary guidelines. *Journal of the American College of Nutrition* 25:277S, 2006.

    *The steps involved in dietary guideline development are discussed. These include some combination of (1) specification of the topic and the guideline development methodology; (2) systematic review of the evidence; (3) consideration of expert opinion; (4) public policy analysis; (5) drafting of the document; and (6) peer review.*

20. Yeager D: Got organic? *Today's Dietitian*, p. 60, October 2008.

    *Regulation of the organic milk industry is discussed. The United States Department of Agriculture now regulates the organic industry. The National Organic Program certifies that food is produced using organic practices. Most milk companies follow the regulations stringently when it comes producing organic milk.*

# RATE YOUR PLATE

## I. Does your Diet Meet MyPyramid Recommendations?

Using your food-intake record from Chapter 1, place each food item in the appropriate group of the accompanying MyPyramid chart. That is, for each food item, indicate how many servings it contributes to each group based on the amount you ate (see Food Composition Table Supplement for serving sizes). Many of your food choices may contribute to more than one group. For example, toast with soft margarine contributes to two categories: (1) the grains group; and (2) the oils group. After entering all the values, add the number of servings consumed in each group. Finally, compare your total in each food group with the recommended number of servings shown in Table 2-4 or obtained from the www.MyPyramid.gov website. Enter a minus sign (−) if your total falls below the recommendation or a plus sign (+) if it equals or exceeds the recommendation.

Indicate the number of servings from MyPyramid that each food yields:

| Food or Beverage | Amount Eaten | Milk | Meat & Beans | Fruits | Vegetables | Grains | Oils |
|---|---|---|---|---|---|---|---|
|  |  |  |  |  |  |  |  |
|  |  |  |  |  |  |  |  |
|  |  |  |  |  |  |  |  |
|  |  |  |  |  |  |  |  |
|  |  |  |  |  |  |  |  |
|  |  |  |  |  |  |  |  |
|  |  |  |  |  |  |  |  |
|  |  |  |  |  |  |  |  |
|  |  |  |  |  |  |  |  |
|  |  |  |  |  |  |  |  |
|  |  |  |  |  |  |  |  |
|  |  |  |  |  |  |  |  |
|  |  |  |  |  |  |  |  |
|  |  |  |  |  |  |  |  |
|  |  |  |  |  |  |  |  |
|  |  |  |  |  |  |  |  |
| Group totals |  |  |  |  |  |  |  |
| Recommended servings |  |  |  |  |  |  |  |
| Shortages in numbers of servings |  |  |  |  |  |  |  |

## II. Are You Putting the Dietary Guidelines into Practice?

As noted in this chapter, the advice provided by the 2005 Dietary Guidelines for Americans can be summarized into three main points and a number of related activities. Fill out the following inventory to see to what extent you are following the basic intent of the Guidelines.

### Food Intake

Do you:

[ Y ]  [ N ]  Consume a variety of nutrient-dense foods and beverages within and among the basic food groups of MyPryamid?

Choose foods that limit the intake of:

[ Y ]  [ N ]  Saturated fat

[ Y ]  [ N ]  *Trans* fat

[ Y ]  [ N ]  Cholesterol

[ Y ]  [ N ]  Added sugars

[ Y ]  [ N ]  Salt

[ Y ]  [ N ]  Alcohol (if used)

Emphasize in your food choices:

[ Y ]  [ N ]  Vegetables

[ Y ]  [ N ]  Fruits

[ Y ]  [ N ]  Legumes (beans)

[ Y ]  [ N ]  Whole-grain breads and cereals

[ Y ]  [ N ]  Fat-free or low-fat milk or equivalent milk products

### Body Weight

[ Y ]  [ N ]  Maintain body weight in a healthy range by balancing energy intake from foods and beverages with energy expended?

[ Y ]  [ N ]  Engage in at least 30 minutes of moderate-intensity physical activity, above usual activity, at work or home on most days of the week?

### Safe Food Handling

[ Y ]  [ N ]  Clean hands, food contact surfaces, and fruits and vegetables before preparation?

[ Y ]  [ N ]  Cook foods to a safe temperature to kill microorganisms?

Figure 2-8 points to other health practices that are part of the 2005 Dietary Guidelines for Americans, but this abbreviated list includes the major points to consider.

## III. Applying the Nutrition Facts Label to Your Daily Food Choices

Imagine that you are at the supermarket looking for a quick meal before a busy evening. In the frozen food section, you find two brands of frozen cheese manicotti (see labels a and b). Which of the two brands would you choose? What information on the Nutrition Facts label in the figure contributed to this decision?

_____

_____

_____

_____

(a)                                    (b)

# CHAPTER 3 The Human Body: A Nutrition Perspective

## Student Learning Outcomes After studying Chapter 3 you will be able to:

1. Identify the functions of the common cellular components.

2. Define tissue, organ, and organ system.

3. List some basic characteristics of the 12 organ systems and outline a role for each related to nutrition.

4. Outline the overall processes of digestion and absorption in the mouth, stomach, small intestine, and large intestine, as well as the roles played by the liver, gallbladder, and pancreas.

5. Understand the role of genetic background in the development of nutrition-related diseases.

6. Identify the major nutrition-related gastro-intestinal health problems and approaches to treatment.

## Chapter Outline

Student Learning Outcomes

Refresh Your Memory

3.1 Human Physiology

3.2 The Cell: Structure, Function, and Metabolism

3.3 Organization of the Body

3.4 Cardiovascular System and Lymphatic System

3.5 Nervous System

3.6 Endocrine System

3.7 Immune System

3.8 Digestive System

3.9 Urinary System

3.10 Storage Capabilities

3.11 A Closer Look at *Genetics and Nutrition*

Nutrition and Your Health: *Common Problems with Digestion*

Case Study: Gastroesophageal Reflux Disease

Summary/Study Questions/Check Your Knowledge/Further Readings

Rate Your Plate

MERELY EATING FOOD WON'T NOURISH YOU. You must first digest the food—break it down into usable forms of the essential nutrients that can be absorbed into the bloodstream. Once nutrients are taken up by the bloodstream, they can be distributed to and used by body cells.

We rarely think about, let alone control, digesting and absorbing foods. Except for a few voluntary responses—such as deciding what and when to eat, how well to chew food, and when to eliminate the remains—most digestion and absorption processes control themselves. As suggested in the comic in this chapter, we don't consciously decide when the pancreas will secrete digestive substances into the small intestine or how quickly foodstuffs will be propelled down the intestinal tract. Various hormones and the nervous system mostly control these functions. Your only awareness of these involuntary responses may be a hunger pang right before lunch or a "full" feeling after eating that last slice of pizza.

Let's examine digestion and absorption as well as other aspects of human physiology that support nutritional health. In the process you will become acquainted with the basic anatomy (structure) and physiology (function) of the circulatory system, nervous system, endocrine system, immune system, digestive system, urinary system, and storage capabilities of the human body.

**Refresh Your Memory**

As you begin your study of human physiology in Chapter 3, you may want to review:

- Cell structure and function from previous coursework in university-level biology courses
- Each of the body's organ systems from any previous biology training

## 3.1 Human Physiology

The human body is composed of trillions of cells. Each cell is a self-contained, living entity. Cells of the same type normally join together, using intercellular substances to form **tissues,** such as muscle tissue. One, two, or more tissues then combine in a particular way to form more complex structures, called **organs.** All organs contribute to nutritional health, and a person's overall nutritional state determines how well each organ functions. At a still higher level of coordination, several organs can cooperate for a common purpose to form an **organ system,** such as the digestive system. Overall, the human body is a coordinated unit of many highly structured organ systems (Fig. 3-1).

Chemical processes (reactions) occur constantly in every living cell: The production of new substances is balanced by the breaking down of older ones. An example is the constant formation and degradation of bone. For this turnover of substances to occur, cells require a continuous supply of energy in the form of dietary carbohydrate, protein, and/or fat. Cells also need water; building supplies, especially protein and minerals; and chemical regulators, such as the vitamins. Almost all cells also need a steady supply of oxygen. These substances enable the tissues, made from individual cells, to function properly.

Getting an adequate supply of all nutrients to the body's cells begins with a healthy diet. To assure optimal use of nutrients, the body's cells, tissues, organs, and organ systems also must work efficiently.

**tissues** Collections of cells adapted to perform a specific function.

**organ** A group of tissues designed to perform a specific function—for example, the heart, which contains muscle tissue, nerve tissue, and so on.

**organ system** A collection of organs that work together to perform an overall function.

**FRANK & ERNEST®** by Bob Thaves

Some popular (fad) diets suggest not combining meat and potatoes to improve digestion and that fruit should only be eaten before noon. These diets might also purport that foods get stuck in the body and in turn putrefy and create toxins. Are there any scientific reasons to suggest that the timing of our food intake should optimize digestion? Do certain food practices improve digestion and subsequent absorption? This chapter provides some answers.

FRANK AND ERNEST reprinted by permission of Newspaper Enterprise Association, Inc.

**1 Chemical level.** Atoms combine to form molecules.

**2 Cell level.** Molecules form organelles, such as the nucleus and mitochondria, which make up cells.

**3 Tissue level.** Similar cells and surrounding materials make up tissues.

**4 Organ level.** Different tissues combine to form organs, such as the stomach.

**5 Organ system level.** Organs such as the stomach and intestines make up an organ system.

**6 Organism level.** Organ systems make up an organism.

**FIGURE 3-1** ▶ The levels of organization of the human body are chemical, cell, tissue, organ, organ system, and organism. Each level is more complex than the previous level. The organ system shown is the digestive system.

Chapter 3 covers the anatomy and physiology of the cell and major organ systems, especially as they relate to human nutrition. The information you are about to study is limited to the components of the various organ systems specifically influenced by the more than 45 essential nutrients discussed in this text.

## 3.2 The Cell: Structure, Function and Metabolism

The cell is the basic structural and functional component of life. Living organisms are made of many different kinds of cells specialized to perform particular functions, and all cells are derived from preexisting cells. In the human body, all cells have certain common features. These cells have compartments and specialized structures that perform particular functions; these components are called **organelles** (Fig. 3-2). There are at least 15 different organelles. Eight of the most important organelles will be discussed. The numbers following the names of the cell structures correspond to the structures illustrated in Figure 3-2. Metabolism, the chemical processes that take place in body cells, will also be discussed.

**organelles** Compartments, particles, or filaments that perform specialized functions within a cell.

### Cell (Plasma) Membrane 1

There is an outside and inside to every cell, as defined by the cell (plasma) membrane. This membrane holds the cellular contents together and regulates the direction and flow of substances into and out of the cell. Cell-to-cell communication also occurs by way of this membrane.

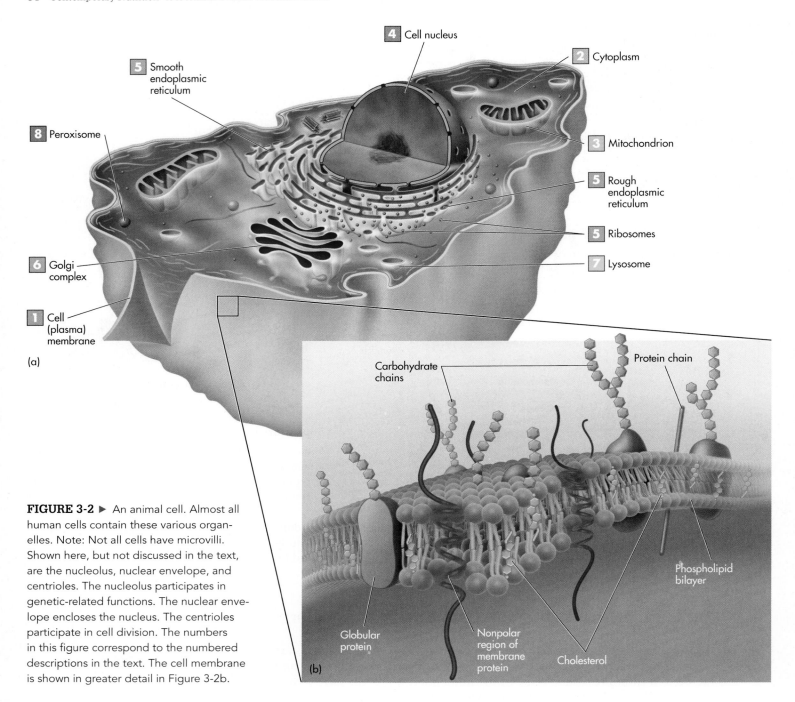

(a)

**FIGURE 3-2** ▶ An animal cell. Almost all human cells contain these various organelles. Note: Not all cells have microvilli. Shown here, but not discussed in the text, are the nucleolus, nuclear envelope, and centrioles. The nucleolus participates in genetic-related functions. The nuclear envelope encloses the nucleus. The centrioles participate in cell division. The numbers in this figure correspond to the numbered descriptions in the text. The cell membrane is shown in greater detail in Figure 3-2b.

(b)

**phospholipid** Any of a class of fat-related substances that contain phosphorus, fatty acids, and a nitrogen-containing component. Phospholipids are an essential part of every cell.

**enzyme** A compound that speeds the rate of a chemical process but is not altered by that process. Almost all enzymes are proteins.

The cell membrane, illustrated in Figure 3-2(b), is a lipid bilayer (or double membrane) of **phospholipids** with their water-soluble heads facing both the interior of the cell and the exterior of the cell. Their water-insoluble tails are tucked into the center portion of the cell membrane.

Cholesterol is one component of the cell membrane. It is fat soluble, so it is embedded within the bilayer. This cholesterol provides rigidity and thus stability to the membrane.

There are also various proteins embedded in the cell membrane. Proteins provide structural support, act as transport vehicles, and function as **enzymes** that affect chemical processes within the membrane (see the later section on digestion for more about enzymes). Some proteins form open channels that allow water-soluble substances to pass into and out of the cell. Proteins on the outside surface of the membrane act as receptors, snagging essential substances that the cell needs and drawing them into the cell. Other proteins act as gates, opening and closing to control the flow of various particles into and out of the cell.

In addition to the lipid and protein, the membrane also contains carbohydrates that mark the exterior of the cell. These carbohydrates are combined either with protein or fat and provide a delivery service for sending messages to the cell's organelles. These carbohydrate structures also act as identification markers for the cell. In addition, they detect invaders and initiate defensive actions. In sum, these carbohydrates provide tags that are important to cellular identity and interaction.

## Cytoplasm 2

The **cytoplasm** is the combination of fluid material and organelles within the cell, not including the nucleus. A small amount of energy for use by the cell can be produced by chemical processes that occur in the cytoplasm. This contributes to the survival of all cells and is the sole source of energy production in red blood cells. This energy production is called **anaerobic** metabolism because it doesn't require oxygen.

**Organelles.** Included within the cytoplasm are organelles. As described in the next two pages, they carry out vital roles in cell functions.

## Mitochondria 3

**Mitochondria** are sometimes called the "power plants," or the powerhouse of the cell. These organelles are capable of converting the energy in energy-yielding nutrients from food (carbohydrate, protein, and fat) to a form of energy that cells can use. This is an **aerobic** process that uses the oxygen we inhale, as well as water, enzymes, and other compounds (see Chapter 10 for details). With the exception of red blood cells, all cells contain mitochondria; only the size, shape, and quantity vary.

## Cell Nucleus 4

With the exception of the red blood cell, all cells have one or more nuclei. The **cell nucleus** is bounded by its own double membrane. The nucleus contains the genetic material responsible for controlling actions that occur in the cell. The genetic material consists of **genes** on **chromosomes** made up of **deoxyribonucleic acid (DNA).** DNA is the "code book" that contains directions for making substances, specifically proteins, the cell needs. This code book remains in the nucleus of the cell, but sends its information to other cell organelles by way of a similar "messenger" molecule called **ribonucleic acid (RNA).** The information on the DNA is copied onto the RNA through the process of **transcription** and then moves out to the cytoplasm through pores in the nuclear membrane. The RNA carries the transcribed DNA code to protein-synthesizing sites called **ribosomes.** There, the RNA code is used in the process of **translation** to make a specific protein (see Chapter 6 for details on protein synthesis). This process is also known as **gene expression.**

All of the DNA in a cell is copied during cell replication. DNA is a double-stranded molecule, and when the cell begins to divide, each strand is separated and an identical copy of each is made. Thus, each new DNA contains one new strand of DNA and one strand from the original DNA. In this way, the genetic code is preserved from one cell generation to the next. (The mitochondria contain their own DNA, so they reproduce themselves within a cell independent of action in the cell's nucleus.)

**cytoplasm** The fluid and organelles (except the nucleus) in a cell.

**anaerobic** Not requiring oxygen.

**mitochondria** The main sites of energy production in a cell. They also contain the pathway for oxidizing fat for fuel, among other metabolic pathways.

**aerobic** Requiring oxygen.

**cell nucleus** An organelle bound by its own double membrane and containing chromosomes, the genetic information for cell protein synthesis and cell replication.

**gene** A specific segment on a chromosome. Genes provide the blueprint for the production of cell proteins.

**chromosome** A single, large DNA molecule and its associated proteins; contains many genes to store and transmit genetic information.

**deoxyribonucleic acid (DNA)** The site of hereditary information in cells; DNA directs the synthesis of cell proteins.

**ribonucleic acid (RNA)** The single-stranded nucleic acid involved in the transcription of genetic information and translation of that information into protein structure.

**transcription** Information on DNA needed to make a protein is copied onto RNA.

**ribosomes** Cytoplasmic particles that mediate the linking together of amino acids to form proteins; may exist freely in the cytoplasm or attached to endoplasmic reticulum.

**translation** The information contained in RNA is used to determine the amino acids in a protein.

**gene expression** Use of DNA information on a gene to produce a protein. Thought to be a major determination of cell development.

▲ Genes are present on DNA—a double helix. The cell nucleus contains most of the DNA in the body.

**endoplasmic reticulum (ER)** An organelle in the cytoplasm composed of a network of canals running through the cytoplasm. Part of the endoplasmic reticulum contains ribosomes.

**Golgi complex** The cell organelle near the nucleus that processes newly synthesized protein for secretion or distribution to other organelles.

**secretory vesicles** Membrane-bound vesicles produced by the Golgi apparatus; contains protein and other compounds to be secreted by the cell.

**lysosome** A cellular organelle that contains digestive enzymes for use inside the cell for turnover of cell parts.

**peroxisome** A cell organelle that destroys toxic products within the cell.

**adenosine triphosphate (ATP)** The main energy currency for cells. ATP energy is used to promote ion pumping, enzyme activity, and muscular contraction.

## Endoplasmic Reticulum (ER) 5

The outer membrane of the cell nucleus is continuous with a network of tubes called the **endoplasmic reticulum (ER).** Part of the endoplasmic reticulum (termed the rough [as opposed to smooth] endoplasmic reticulum) contains the ribosomes, where the RNA code is translated into proteins during protein synthesis. Many of these proteins play a central role in human nutrition. Parts of the endoplasmic reticulum also are involved in lipid synthesis, detoxification of toxic substances, and calcium storage and release in the cell.

## Golgi Complex 6

The **Golgi complex** is a packaging site for proteins used in the cytoplasm or exported from the cell. It consists of sacs within the cytoplasm in which proteins are "packaged" as **secretory vesicles** for secretion by the cell.

## Lysosomes 7

**Lysosomes** are the cell's digestive system. They are sacs that contain enzymes for the digestion of foreign material. Sometimes known as "suicide bags," they are responsible for digesting worn-out or damaged cell components. Certain cells associated with immune functions contain many lysosomes (see the later section on the immune system).

## Peroxisomes 8

**Peroxisomes** contain enzymes that detoxify harmful chemicals. Peroxisomes get their name from the fact that hydrogen peroxide ($H_2O_2$) is formed as a result of such enzyme action. Peroxisomes also contain a protective enzyme called *catalase*, which prevents excessive accumulation of hydrogen peroxide in the cell, which would be very damaging. Peroxisomes also play a minor role in metabolizing one possible source of energy for cells—alcohol.

## Cell Metabolism

Metabolism refers to the entire network of chemical processes involved in maintaining life. It encompasses all the sequences of chemical reactions that occur in the body's cells. These biochemical reactions take place in the cell cytoplasm and organelles that we have just discussed. They enable us to release and use energy from foods, synthesize one substance from another, and prepare waste products for excretion.

The reactions of metabolism that take place within your body can be categorized into one of two types. One type of reaction, anabolic, puts different molecules together and, therefore, requires energy. The other type of reaction, catabolic, takes molecules apart and, therefore, releases energy. The metabolism of the nutrients, carbohydrates, proteins, and fats are interrelated and yield energy. The other nutrients, vitamins and minerals, contribute to the enzyme activity that supports metabolic reactions in the cell.

As we discussed earlier, the metabolism of energy production begins in the cytoplasm with the initial anaerobic breakdown of glucose. The remaining aerobic steps of energy production take place in the mitochondria. Ultimately, the cells of the body use these interconnected processes to convert the energy found in food to energy stored in the high-energy compound, **adenosine triphosphate (ATP).** You will learn more about the metabolism of energy sources in Chapter 10.

## CONCEPT CHECK

In Chapter 1, you learned that fat (lipids), protein, and carbohydrate function as fuels. Now you recognize that these organic nutrients also serve as structural materials in the cell membrane. This is typical of many nutrients; they can carry out multiple functions. The cell receives nutrients and other substances through the cell membrane by using various transport systems.

The basic structural unit in the body is the cell. Within the cell are a variety of organelles with unique functions to perform. Although there is no typical cell, virtually all cells have the same organelles, each performing the same essential task.

## 3.3 Organization of the Body

As noted earlier, when groups of similar cells work together to accomplish a specialized task, the arrangement is referred to as a tissue. Humans are composed of four primary types of tissue: **epithelial, connective, muscle,** and **nervous.** Epithelial tissue is composed of cells that cover surfaces both inside and outside the body. For example, the lining of the respiratory tract is made up of epithelial cells. These cells of epithelial tissue secrete important substances, absorb nutrients, and excrete waste. Connective tissue supports and protects the body, stores fat, and produces blood cells. Muscle tissue is designed for movement. Nervous tissue found in the brain and spinal cord is designed for communication. These four types of tissues then go on to form various organs, and ultimately, organ systems (Table 3-1).

We will be particularly concerned in Chapter 3 with the digestive system. The nutrients we consume in food are unavailable until such time as they have been processed by the digestive system. This employs chemical and mechanical means to alter food so that the nutrients can be released and absorbed into the body for distribution to body tissues.

Sometimes organs within a system can serve another system. For example, the basic function of the digestive system is to convert the food we eat into absorbable nutrients. At the same time, the digestive system serves the immune system by preventing dangerous pathogens from invading the body and causing illness. As you study nutrition, you will note the multiple roles played by many organs (Fig. 3-3).

The overriding theme of human nutrition is to understand the actions of nutrients as they affect different cells, tissues, organs, and organ systems. Each type of organ system is impacted by nutrient intake and simultaneously determines how each nutrient is used.

Our task now is to explore the key systems in the body as they specifically relate to the study of human nutrition: circulatory (cardiovascular and lymphatic), nervous, endocrine, immune, digestive, and urinary systems. This part of Chapter 3 will set the stage for a more detailed look at these and other organ systems in later chapters covering various aspects of human nutrition.

Also in this chapter, we will introduce the emerging area of genetics and nutrition. Throughout this book, discussions will point out how you can personalize nutrition advice based on your genetic background. In this way, you can identify and avoid the "controllable" risk factors that would contribute to development of genetically linked diseases present in your family.

**epithelial tissue** The surface cells that line the outside of the body and all external passages within it.

**connective tissue** Protein tissue that holds different structures in the body together. Some structures are made up of connective tissue—notably, tendons and cartilage. Connective tissue also forms part of bone and the nonmuscular structures of arteries and veins.

**muscle tissue** A type of tissue adapted to contract to cause movement.

**nervous tissue** Tissue composed of highly branched, elongated cells, which transport nerve impulses from one part of the body to another.

**urea** Nitrogenous waste product of protein metabolism; major source of nitrogen in the urine.

**cardiovascular system** The body system consisting of the heart, blood vessels, and blood. This system transports nutrients, waste products, gases, and hormones throughout the body and plays an important role in immune responses and regulation of body temperature.

**lymphatic system** A system of vessels and lymph that accepts fluid surrounding cells and large particles, such as products of fat absorption. Lymph eventually passes into the bloodstream from the lymphatic system.

## 3.4 Cardiovascular System and Lymphatic System

The body has two separate organ systems that circulate fluids in the body: the **cardiovascular system** and the **lymphatic system.** The cardiovascular system consists of the heart and blood vessels. The lymphatic system consists of lymphatic vessels and

**TABLE 3-1** Organ Systems of the Body

| System | Major Components | Functions Related to Nutrition |
|---|---|---|
| Cardiovascular | Heart, blood vessels, and blood | Transports nutrients, waste products, gases, and hormones throughout the body and plays a role in the immune response and the regulation of body temperature |
| Lymphatic | Lymph vessels, lymph nodes, and other lymph organs | Removes foreign substances from the blood and lymph, combats disease, maintains tissue fluid balance, and aids in fat absorption |
| Nervous | Brain, spinal cord, nerves, and sensory receptors | A major regulatory system: detects sensation, controls movements, and controls physiological and intellectual functions |
| Endocrine | Endocrine glands, such as the pituitary, thyroid, and adrenal glands | A major regulatory system: participates in the regulation of metabolism, reproduction, and many other functions through the action of hormones |
| Immune | White blood cells, lymph vessels and nodes, spleen, thymus gland, and other lymph tissues | Provides defense against foreign invaders; formation of white blood cells |
| Digestive | Mouth, esophagus, stomach, intestines, and accessory structures (liver, gallbladder, and pancreas) | Performs the mechanical and chemical processes of digestion, absorption of nutrients, and elimination of wastes |
| Urinary | Kidneys, urinary bladder, and the ducts that carry urine | Removes waste products from the circulatory system and regulates the acidity, chemical composition, and water content of the blood |
| Integumentary | Skin, hair, nails, and sweat glands | Protects the body, regulates temperature, prevents water loss, and produces a substance that converts to vitamin D upon sun exposure |
| Skeletal | Bones, associated cartilage, and joints | Supports the body, and allows for body movement, produces blood cells, and stores minerals |
| Muscular | Smooth, cardiac, and skeletal muscle | Produces body movement, maintains posture, and produces body heat |
| Respiratory | Lungs and respiratory passages | Exchanges gases (oxygen and carbon dioxide) between the blood and the atmosphere and regulates blood acid-base (pH) balance |
| Reproductive | Gonads, accessory structures, and genitals of males and females | Performs the processes of reproduction and influences sexual functions and behaviors |

**lymph** A clear fluid that flows through lymph vessels; carries most forms of fat after their absorption by the small intestine.

**plasma** The fluid, extracellular portion of the circulating blood. This includes the blood serum plus all blood-clotting factors. In contrast, serum is the fluid that remains after clotting factors have been removed from plasma.

a number of lymph tissues. Blood flows through the cardiovascular system, while **lymph** flows through the lymphatic system.

## Cardiovascular System

The heart is a muscular pump that normally contracts and relaxes 50 to 90 times per minute when the body is at rest. This continual pumping, measured by taking your pulse, keeps blood moving through the blood vessels. The blood that flows through the cardiovascular system is composed of **plasma,** red blood cells, white blood cells, platelets, and many other substances. It travels two basic routes. In the first route, blood circulates from the right side of the heart, through the lungs, and then back to the heart. In the lungs, blood picks up oxygen and releases carbon dioxide. After this exchange of gases has taken place, blood is said to be *oxygenated* and returns to the left side of your heart. In the second route, the oxygenated blood circulates from the left side of the heart to all other body cells, eventually returning back to the right side of the heart (Fig. 3-4). After blood has circulated throughout the body, it is *deoxygenated.* (As you review the cardiovascular system, recall from your previous studies of biology that *left* and *right* designations of the heart refer to the left and right sides of your body, not of the page in your textbook.)

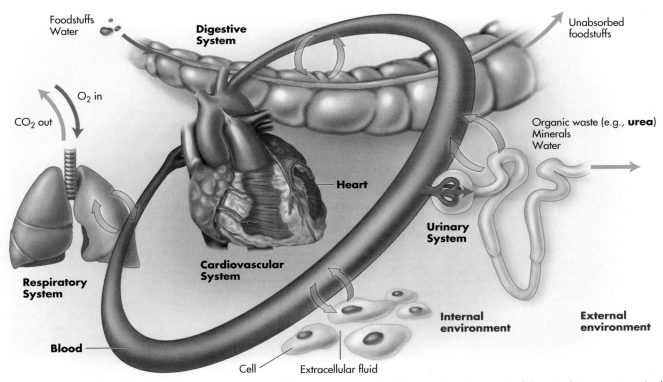

Foodstuffs
Water

**Digestive System**

Unabsorbed foodstuffs

$O_2$ in

$CO_2$ out

Organic waste (e.g., **urea**)
Minerals
Water

— **Heart**

**Urinary System**

**Cardiovascular System**

**Respiratory System**

Internal environment

External environment

**Blood** —

Cell    Extracellular fluid

**FIGURE 3-3** ▶ Exchanges of nutrients occur between our external environment and the internal environment of the circulatory system via the digestive, respiratory, and urinary systems. Overall, the human body is a combination of 12 systems working together to support cell needs.

In the cardiovascular system, blood leaves the heart via **arteries**, which branch into **capillaries**, a network of tiny blood vessels. Exchange of nutrients, oxygen, and waste products between the blood and cells occurs through the minute, web-like pores of the capillaries (Fig. 3-5). Capillaries service every region of the body via individual capillary beds only one cell layer thick. The blood then returns to the heart via the **veins.**

The cardiovascular system distributes nutrients absorbed from food and oxygen from the air to all body cells (review Fig. 3-3). Other functions include delivery of hormones to their target cells, maintenance of a constant body temperature, and distribution of white blood cells throughout the body to protect against pathogens as part of the immune system (see the later section, "Immune System").

**Portal Circulation in the Gastrointestinal Tract.** Water and nutrients are transferred to the circulatory system through capillary beds. Once absorbed through the stomach or intestinal wall, nutrients reach one of two destinations. Some nutrients are taken up by cells in the intestines and portions of the stomach to nourish those organs. Most of the nutrients from recently eaten foods, however, are transferred into **portal circulation.** To enter portal circulation, the nutrients pass from the intestinal capillaries into veins that eventually merge into a very large vein called a **portal vein.** Unlike most veins in the body—which carry blood back to the heart—this portal vein leads directly to the liver. This enables the liver to process absorbed nutrients before they enter the general circulation of the bloodstream. Overall, portal circulation represents a special form of circulation in the cardiovascular system.

## Lymphatic System

The **lymphatic system** is also a circulatory system. It consists of a network of lymphatic vessels and the fluid (lymph) that moves through them. Lymph is similar to

▲ The body is made up of numerous organ systems including the endocrine, nervous, and circulatory systems shown here.

**artery** A blood vessel that carries blood away from the heart.

**capillary** A microscopic blood vessel that connects the smallest arteries and veins; site of nutrient, oxygen, and waste exchange between body cells and the blood.

**vein** A blood vessel that carries blood to the heart.

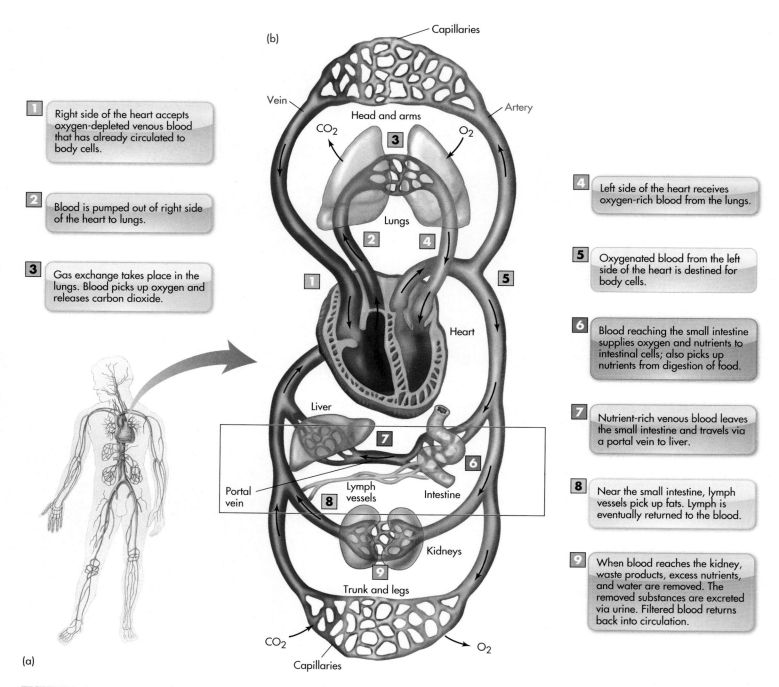

(b)

**1** Right side of the heart accepts oxygen-depleted venous blood that has already circulated to body cells.

**2** Blood is pumped out of right side of the heart to lungs.

**3** Gas exchange takes place in the lungs. Blood picks up oxygen and releases carbon dioxide.

**4** Left side of the heart receives oxygen-rich blood from the lungs.

**5** Oxygenated blood from the left side of the heart is destined for body cells.

**6** Blood reaching the small intestine supplies oxygen and nutrients to intestinal cells; also picks up nutrients from digestion of food.

**7** Nutrient-rich venous blood leaves the small intestine and travels via a portal vein to liver.

**8** Near the small intestine, lymph vessels pick up fats. Lymph is eventually returned to the blood.

**9** When blood reaches the kidney, waste products, excess nutrients, and water are removed. The removed substances are excreted via urine. Filtered blood returns back into circulation.

Capillaries
Vein
Head and arms
$CO_2$
$O_2$
Artery
Lungs
Heart
Liver
Portal vein
Lymph vessels
Intestine
Kidneys
Trunk and legs
$CO_2$
$O_2$
Capillaries

(a)

**FIGURE 3-4** ▶ Blood circulation through the body. Figure (a) shows the heart and some examples of the major arteries and veins of the cardiovascular system. Figure (b) shows the paths that blood takes from the heart to the lungs (**1**–**3**), back to the heart (**4**), and through the rest of the body (**5**–**9**). The red color indicates blood richer in oxygen; blue is for blood carrying more carbon dioxide. Keep in mind that arteries and veins go to all parts of the body.

**portal circulation** The portion of the circulatory system that uses a large vein (portal vein) to carry nutrient-rich blood from capillaries in the intestines and portions of the stomach to the liver.

blood, consisting largely of blood plasma that has found its way out of capillaries and into the spaces between cells. It contains a full array of the various white blood cells that play an important role in the immune system. However, neither red blood cells nor platelets are present. Lymph is collected in tiny lymph vessels all over the body and moves through even larger vessels until it eventually enters the cardiovascular system through major veins near the heart. This flow is driven by muscle contractions arising from normal body movements.

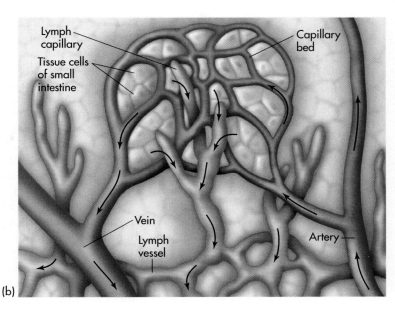

**FIGURE 3-5** ▶ Capillary and lymph vessels. (a) Exchange of oxygen ($O_2$) and nutrients for carbon dioxide ($CO_2$) and waste products occurs between the capillaries and the surrounding tissue cells. (b) Lymph vessels are also present in capillary beds, such as in the small intestine. Lymph vessels in the small intestine are also called lacteals. The lymph vessels have closed ends.

**Lymphatic Circulation in the Gastrointestinal Tract.** Besides contributing to the defense of the body against invading pathogens, lymphatic vessels that serve the small intestine play an important role in nutrition. These vessels pick up and transport the majority of products of fat digestion and fat absorption. These fat-related products are too large to enter the bloodstream directly and therefore are generally emptied into the bloodstream only after passing through the lymphatic system. The lymph vessels also take up excess fluid that collects between cells and returns it to the bloodstream.

**portal vein** Large vein leaving from the intestine and stomach and connecting to the liver.

**nervous system** The body system consisting of the brain, spinal cord, nerves, and sensory receptors. This system detects sensations, directs movements, and controls physiological and intellectual functions.

### CONCEPT CHECK

Blood is transported from the right side of the heart to the capillaries in the lungs. Carbon dioxide is removed and oxygen is taken up by red blood cells. The oxygenated blood returns to the left side of the heart. Here it is pumped into general circulation. In the capillaries, oxygen is released from the red blood cells and delivered through pores in the capillaries to the surrounding cells. Nutrients also are distributed from the bloodstream to body cells via the capillaries. Carbon dioxide released from cells travels through the capillary pores to the blood.

The lymph system serves several purposes: the transport of absorbed dietary fats, the uptake and return to the bloodstream of excess fluid that collects between cells, and the defense of the body against invading pathogens.

## 3.5 Nervous System

The **nervous system** is a regulatory system that centrally controls most body functions. The nervous system can detect changes occurring in various organs and the external environment and initiate corrective action when needed to maintain a constant internal environment. The nervous system also regulates activities that change almost instantly, such as muscle contractions and perception of danger. The body has many receptors that receive information about what is happening within the body and in the outside environment. For the most part these receptors are found in our

**neuron** The structural and functional unit of the nervous system. Consists of a cell body, dendrites, and an axon.

**synapse** The space between one neuron and another neuron (or cell).

**neurotransmitter** A compound made by a nerve cell that allows for communication between it and other cells.

eyes, ears, skin, nose, and stomach. We act on information from these receptors via the nervous system.

The basic structural and functional unit of the nervous system is the **neuron.** These are elongated, highly branched cells. The body contains about 100 billion neurons. Neurons respond to electrical and chemical signals, conduct electrical impulses, and release chemical regulators. Overall, neurons allow us to perceive what is occurring in our environment, engage in learning, store vital information in memory, and control the body's voluntary (and involuntary) actions.

The brain stores information, reacts to incoming information, solves problems, and generates thoughts. In addition, the brain plans a course of action based on the other sensory inputs. Responses to the stimuli are carried out mostly through the rest of the nervous system.

Simply put, the nervous system receives information through stimulation of various receptors, processes this information, and sends out signals through its various branches for an action that needs to be taken. Actual transmission of the signal occurs through a change in the sodium and potassium concentration in the neuron. There is an influx of sodium into the neuron and a loss of potassium as the message is sent. Concentrations of these minerals are then restored to normal amounts in the neuron after the signal passes, making it ready to conduct another message.

When the signal must bridge a gap **(synapse)** between the branches of different neurons, the message is generally converted to a chemical signal called a **neurotransmitter.** The neurotransmitter is then released into the gap, and its target may be another neuron or another type of cell, such as a muscle cell (Fig. 3-6). If the signal

**FIGURE 3-6 ▶** Transmission of a message from one neuron to another neuron or to another type of cell that relies on neurotransmitters. Vesicles containing neurotransmitters, formed within the neuron, fuse with the membrane of the neuron and the neurotransmitter is released into the synapse. The neurotransmitter then binds to the receptors on the nearby neuron (or cell). In this way, the message is transmitted from one neuron to another or to the cell that ultimately performs the action directed by the message.

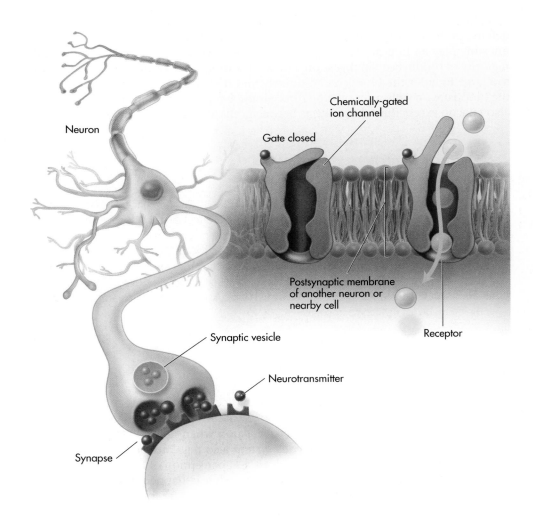

is sent to another neuron, this allows it to continue on to its final destination. The neurotransmitters used in this process are often made from common nutrients found in foods, such as amino acids. The amino acid tryptophan is converted to the neurotransmitter serotonin, and the amino acid tyrosine is converted to the neurotransmitters **norepinephrine** and **epinephrine** (also called adrenaline).

Other nutrients also play a role in the nervous system. Calcium is needed for the release of neurotransmitters from neurons. Vitamin B-12 plays a role in the formation of the **myelin sheath,** which provides insulation around specific parts of most neurons. Finally, a regular supply of carbohydrate in the form of glucose is important for supplying fuel for the brain. The brain can use other calorie sources, but generally relies on glucose.

## 3.6 Endocrine System

The **endocrine system** plays a major role in the regulation of metabolism, reproduction, water balance, and many other functions by producing hormones in the **endocrine glands** of the body and subsequently releasing them into the blood (Fig. 3-7). The term *hormone* comes from the Greek word for "to stir or excite." A true hormone is a regulatory compound that has a specific site of synthesis from which it then enters the bloodstream to reach target cells. Hormones are the messengers of the body. They can be permissive (turn on), antagonistic (turn off), or synergistic (work

**norepinephrine** A neurotransmitter from nerve endings and a hormone from the adrenal gland. It is released in times of stress and is involved in hunger regulation, blood glucose regulation, and other body processes.

**epinephrine** A hormone also known as *adrenaline;* it is released by the adrenal glands (located on each kidney) at times of stress. It acts to increase glycogen breakdown in the liver, among other functions.

**myelin sheath** A lipid and protein combination (lipoprotein) that covers nerve fibers.

**endocrine system** The body system consisting of the various glands and the hormones these glands secrete. This system has major regulatory functions in the body, such as reproduction and cell metabolism.

**endocrine gland** A hormone-producing gland.

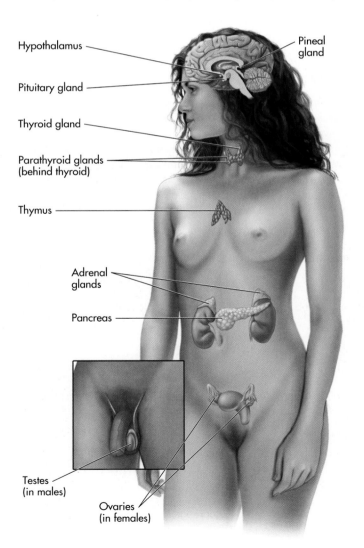

Hypothalamus

Pineal gland

Pituitary gland

Thyroid gland

Parathyroid glands (behind thyroid)

Thymus

Adrenal glands

Pancreas

Testes (in males)

Ovaries (in females)

**FIGURE 3-7** ▶ The endocrine system is made up of several glands that act in the regulation of metabolism, reproduction, water balance, and many other functions.

in cooperation with another hormone) in performing a task. Some compounds must undergo chemical changes before they can function as hormones. For example, vitamin D, synthesized in the skin or obtained from food, is converted into an active hormone by chemical changes made in the liver and kidneys.

The hormone **insulin,** synthesized in and released from the pancreas, helps control the amount of glucose in the blood. Insulin is mostly produced when glucose in the blood rises to a certain level, usually after a meal. At this point, insulin is released and it travels to the muscle, adipose, and liver cells of the body. Among its many functions, insulin allows for the movement of glucose from the blood into muscle and adipose cells. In the liver cells, insulin causes an increase in stored glycogen by stimulating the synthesis of glycogen from glucose. Once a sufficient amount of glucose has been cleared from the blood, the production of insulin lessens. The hormones epinephrine, norepinephrine, glucagon, and growth hormone have just the opposite effect on blood glucose. They all cause an increase in blood glucose through a variety of actions (Table 3-2). **Thyroid hormones,** synthesized in and released from the thyroid gland (Fig. 3-7), help to control the body's rate of metabolism. Other hormones are especially important in regulating digestive processes (see the later section, "Digestive System").

Hormones are not available to all cells in the body, but only those with the correct **receptor** protein. These binding sites are highly specific for a certain hormone. They are generally found on the cell membrane. The hormone attaches to its receptor on the cell membrane. This binding activates additional compounds called second messengers within the cell to carry out the assigned task. This is true of insulin. A few hormones can penetrate the cell membrane and eventually bind to receptors on the DNA in the nucleus (e.g., thyroid hormone and estrogen).

**thyroid hormones** Hormones produced by the thyroid gland that among their functions increase the rate of overall metabolism in the body.

**receptor** A site in a cell at which compounds (such as hormones) bind. Cells that contain receptors for a specific compound are partially controlled by that compound.

## CONCEPT CHECK

The functional unit of the nervous system is the neuron. Communication between neurons themselves, and other types of cells, is via neurotransmitters released into the synapse between the cells.

In the endocrine system, hormones are produced by glands in response to a change in the internal or external environment of the body. The gland secretes the hormone into the blood, and the blood delivers it to target cells. The hormone either attaches to receptors in the cell membrane and, through the action of second messengers, causes changes within the cell, or enters the cell and binds to the DNA in the cell to cause changes within the cell.

**TABLE 3-2** Some Hormones of the Endocrine System with Nutritional Significance

| Hormone | Gland/Organ | Target | Effect | Role in Nutrition |
|---------|-------------|--------|--------|-------------------|
| Insulin | Pancreas | Adipose (fat) and muscle cells | Decreased blood glucose | Uptake and storage of glucose, fat, and amino acids by cells |
| Glucagon | Pancreas | Liver | Increased blood glucose | Release of glucose from liver stores, release of fat from adipose tissue |
| Epinephrine, Norepinephrine | Adrenal glands | Heart, blood vessels, brain, lungs | Increased body metabolism and blood glucose | Release of glucose and fat into the blood |
| Growth hormone | Pituitary gland | Most cells | Promotion of amino acid uptake by cells, increased blood glucose | Promotion of protein synthesis and growth, increased fat use for energy |
| Thyroid hormones | Thyroid gland | Most organs | Increased oxygen consumption, overall growth, brain development of the nervous system | Protein synthesis, increased body metabolism |

# 3.7 Immune System

Many types of body cells and body components work in cooperation as part of the **immune system** to maintain a defense against infection (Fig. 3-8). The components that work as part of the immune system include the skin, intestinal cells, and white blood cells. Several nutrients, including protein; minerals iron, copper, and zinc; and vitamins A, B-6, B-12, C, and folate have important roles in the immune system. These nutrients are key factors in the synthesis, growth, development, and activity of immune cells and additional factors that kill pathogens. It is easy to demonstrate the importance of nutritional health for immune function. Early humans were plagued by famine and thus, malnutrition; this contributed to infections, often leading to death. Today, largely because of better nutrition, most of the world avoids that cycle.

We are born with most aspects of immune function; these are termed **non-specific** (or innate) because the targets are a variety of microorganisms. In contrast, white blood cells produce **immunoglobulins**, also called **antibodies**, that target specific organisms or foreign proteins called **antigens**. These immunoglobulins constitute **specific** (or adaptive) immune function. Once exposed, a memory is created such that a second exposure to the substance will produce a more vigorous and rapid attack.

## Skin

The skin is a large component of the immune system, forming an almost continuous barrier surrounding the body. Invading microorganisms have difficulty penetrating the skin. However, if the skin is split by lesions, bacteria can easily penetrate this barrier. Skin health is poor during deficiencies of such nutrients as essential fatty acids, vitamin A, niacin, and zinc. Vitamin A deficiency also decreases gland secretions in the skin that contain the enzyme **lysozyme,** capable of killing bacteria. Bacterial eye infections are common in developing countries, often as a result of a vitamin A deficiency.

## Intestinal Cells

The cells of the intestines form an important barrier to invading microorganisms. The cells are packed closely together, producing a physical barrier to microorganisms. In addition, specialized cells that produce immune factors—such as immunoglobulins—are scattered throughout the intestinal tract. These immune factors bind to the invading microorganisms, preventing them from entering the bloodstream. These factors are part of the mucosal membrane aspect of immunity.

Nutrient deficiencies can cause the intestinal cells to break down weakening the mucosal membrane so that microorganisms more easily enter the body and cause infections. Thus, two common results of undernutrition related to an impaired immune system are diarrhea and bacterial infections of the bloodstream. To protect the health of the intestinal tract, an adequate nutrient intake is necessary—especially of protein, vitamin A, vitamin B-6, vitamin B-12, vitamin C, folate, and zinc.

## MAKING DECISIONS

### Immune Status

Although many studies show that a healthy nutritional state is associated with good immune status, other studies show that an overabundance of certain nutrients can harm the immune system. For example, taking too much zinc may decrease immune function (see Chapter 9).

**FIGURE 3-8 ▶** Just as the roof and other external structures of a house protect the inside environment from outside elements, host protective factors (shown on the bricks) of the immune system "shelter" humans from threats such as diseases and toxins (shown in the rain).

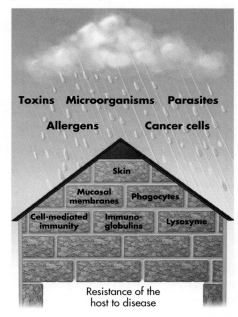

**immune system** The body system consisting of white blood cells, lymph glands and vessels, and various other body tissues. The immune system provides defense against foreign invaders, primarily due to the action of various types of white blood cells.

**non-specific immunity** Defenses that stop the invasion of pathogens; requires no previous encounter with a pathogen.

**immunoglobulins** Proteins found in the blood that bind to specific antigens; also called antibodies. The five major classes of immunoglobulins play different roles in antibody-mediated immunity.

**antigen** Any substance that induces a state of sensitivity and/or resistance to microorganisms or toxic substances after a lag period; foreign substance that stimulates a specific aspect of the immune system.

**antibody** Blood protein (immunoglobulin) that binds foreign proteins found in the body. This helps to prevent and control infections.

**specific immunity** Function of lymphocytes directed at specific antigens.

**lysozyme** An enzyme produced by a variety of cells; it can destroy bacteria by rupturing their cell membranes.

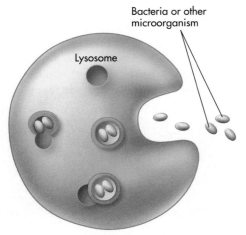

Phagocyte

**FIGURE 3-9** ▶ One class of white blood cell, phagocytes, can ingest bacteria, fungi, viruses, and other foreign particles in the process of phagocytosis. An indentation is formed and the particle is engulfed by the cell. The foreign material is eventually digested by lysosomes in the cell.

**white blood cells** One of the formed elements of the circulating blood system; also called *leukocytes*. White blood cells are able to squeeze through intracellular spaces and migrate. They phagocytize bacteria, fungi, and viruses, as well as detoxify proteins that may result from allergic reactions, cellular injury, and other immune system cells.

**phagocytes** Cells that engulf substances; include neutrophils and macrophages.

**phagocytosis** Process in which a cell forms an indentation, and particles or fluids enter the indentation and are engulfed by the cell.

**cell-mediated immunity** A process in which certain white blood cells come in contact with the invading cells to destroy them.

**digestive system** System consisting of the gastrointestinal tract and accessory structures (liver, gallbladder, and pancreas). This system performs the mechanical and chemical processes of digestion, absorption of nutrients, and elimination of wastes.

**digestion** Process by which large ingested molecules are mechanically and chemically broken down to produce basic nutrients that can be absorbed across the wall of the GI tract.

**absorption** The process by which substances are taken up from the GI tract and enter the bloodstream or the lymph.

## White Blood Cells

Once a microorganism enters the bloodstream, **white blood cells** move in to attack it. A variety of types of white blood cells participate in this response and function in unique ways. For example, a class called **phagocytes** circulates throughout the circulatory system and ingests and sometimes digests microorganisms and foreign particles (via lysosomes present in the cells) in a process called **phagocytosis** (Fig. 3-9). Other white blood cells participate in **cell-mediated immunity,** achieved when certain immune cells recognize foreign cells or proteins and directly attack and destroy them. Immunoglobulins in their role as antibodies elicit an antibody-antigen response that binds microorganisms and proteins that are foreign to the body and destroys them, and then creates a template (memory) that allows future recognition of the microorganism or foreign protein. Recognition allows more rapid attacks in the future.

Some white blood cells live only a few days. Their constant resynthesis requires steady nutrient intake. The immune system needs (1) iron to produce an important killing factor; (2) copper for the synthesis of a specific type of white blood cell; and (3) adequate amounts of protein, vitamin B-6, vitamin B-12, vitamin C, and folate for general cell synthesis and, later, cell activity. Zinc and vitamin A are also needed for the overall growth and development of immune cells.

### CONCEPT CHECK

Many types of body cells and body components work in cooperation as part of the immune system to maintain a defense against infection. The skin forms an almost continuous barrier surrounding the body. Cell secretions contain the enzyme lysozyme. Specialized cells in the intestines and certain white blood cells secrete antibodies (immunoglobulins). Phagocytes roam throughout the circulatory system and ingest and sometimes digest microorganisms and foreign particles. Other white blood cells participate in cell-mediated immunity. This occurs when certain immune cells recognize foreign cells and directly attack them. Many nutrients, including protein, iron, copper, zinc, vitamin B-6, B-12, C, and folate, are needed for the overall growth and development of immune cells.

## 3.8 Digestive System

The foods and beverages we consume, for the most part, must undergo extensive alteration by the **digestive system** to provide us with usable nutrients. The processes of **digestion** and **absorption** take place in a long tube that is open at both ends and extends from the mouth to the anus. This tube is called the **gastrointestinal (GI) tract** (Fig. 3-10). Nutrients from the food we eat must pass through the walls of the GI tract—from the inside to the outside—to be absorbed into the bloodstream. The organs that make up the GI tract, as well as some additional accessory organs located nearby, are collectively known as the digestive system.

In the digestive system, food is broken down mechanically and chemically. Mechanical digestion takes place as soon as you begin chewing your food and continues as muscular contractions simultaneously mix and move food through the length of the GI tract (as part of a process known as **motility**). Chemical digestion refers to the chemical breakdown of foods by substances secreted into the GI tract. Finally, the digestive system eliminates wastes. In addition to nutrients that arise from digestion of food, the bacteria that live in the large intestine produce vitamin K and the vitamin biotin, some of which we can absorb and use.

Most of the processes of digestion and absorption are under autonomic control; that is, they are involuntary. Almost all of the functions involved in digestion and absorption are controlled by signals from the nervous system, hormones from the

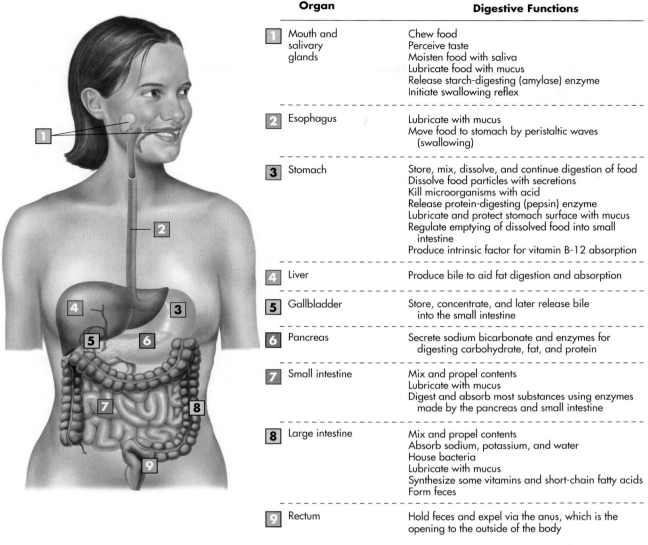

| Organ | Digestive Functions |
|---|---|
| **1** Mouth and salivary glands | Chew food<br>Perceive taste<br>Moisten food with saliva<br>Lubricate food with mucus<br>Release starch-digesting (amylase) enzyme<br>Initiate swallowing reflex |
| **2** Esophagus | Lubricate with mucus<br>Move food to stomach by peristaltic waves (swallowing) |
| **3** Stomach | Store, mix, dissolve, and continue digestion of food<br>Dissolve food particles with secretions<br>Kill microorganisms with acid<br>Release protein-digesting (pepsin) enzyme<br>Lubricate and protect stomach surface with mucus<br>Regulate emptying of dissolved food into small intestine<br>Produce intrinsic factor for vitamin B-12 absorption |
| **4** Liver | Produce bile to aid fat digestion and absorption |
| **5** Gallbladder | Store, concentrate, and later release bile into the small intestine |
| **6** Pancreas | Secrete sodium bicarbonate and enzymes for digesting carbohydrate, fat, and protein |
| **7** Small intestine | Mix and propel contents<br>Lubricate with mucus<br>Digest and absorb most substances using enzymes made by the pancreas and small intestine |
| **8** Large intestine | Mix and propel contents<br>Absorb sodium, potassium, and water<br>House bacteria<br>Lubricate with mucus<br>Synthesize some vitamins and short-chain fatty acids<br>Form feces |
| **9** Rectum | Hold feces and expel via the anus, which is the opening to the outside of the body |

**FIGURE 3-10 ▶** Physiology of the GI tract. Many organs cooperate in a regulated fashion to allow the digestion and absorption of nutrients in foods.

endocrine system, and hormone-like compounds. Many common ailments arise from problems with the digestive system. Several of these digestive problems are discussed in the "Nutrition and Your Health" section at the end of this chapter.

The digestive system is composed of six separate organs; each organ performs one, or more, specific job(s). Let's look briefly at the role of each organ. These organs are listed in the flow chart on this page. More detailed descriptions of digestive processes will be explained in later chapters as each nutrient is introduced.

## Mouth

The mouth performs many functions in the digestion of food. Besides chewing food to reduce it to smaller particles, the mouth also senses the taste of the foods we consume. The tongue, through the use of its taste buds, identifies foods on the basis of their specific flavor(s). Sweet, sour, salty, bitter, and **umami** comprise the primary taste sensations we experience. Surprisingly, the nose and our sense of smell greatly contribute to our ability to sense the taste of food. When we chew a food, chemicals are released that stimulate the nasal passages. Thus, it makes perfect sense that when

**gastrointestinal (GI) tract** The main sites in the body used for digestion and absorption of nutrients. It consists of the mouth, esophagus, stomach, small intestine, large intestine, rectum, and anus. Also called the *digestive tract*.

**motility** Generally, the ability to move spontaneously. It also refers to movement of food through the GI tract.

**umami** A brothy, meaty, savory flavor in some foods. Monosodium glutamate enhances this flavor when added to foods.

### GI Tract Components and Flow

Mouth
↓
Esophagus (10 inches long)
↓
Stomach—4-cup (1-liter) capacity. Food remains about 2 to 3 hours, or longer for large meals.
↓
Small intestine—duodenum (10 in long), jejunum (4 ft long), ileum (5 ft long)— about 10 ft (3.1 meters) in total length. Food remains about 3 to 10 hours.
↓
Large intestine (colon)—cecum, ascending colon, transverse colon, descending colon, sigmoid colon—3½ ft (1.1 meters) in total length. Food can remain up to 72 hours.
↓
Rectum
↓
Anus

**saliva** Watery fluid, produced by the salivary glands in the mouth, that contains lubricants, enzymes, and other substances.

**salivary amylase** A starch-digesting enzyme produced by salivary glands.

we have a cold and our noses are stuffed up and congested, even our most favorite foods will not taste as good as they normally do.

The taste of food, or the anticipation of it, signals the rest of the GI tract to prepare for the digestion of food. Once in the mouth, mechanical and chemical digestion begins. Salivary glands produce **saliva,** which functions as a solvent so that food particles can be further separated and tasted. In addition, saliva contains a starch-digesting enzyme, **salivary amylase** (see Chapter 4 for more on starch-digesting enzymes).

Enzymes are a key part of digestion. Each enzyme is specific to one type of chemical process. For example, enzymes that recognize and digest table sugar (sucrose) ignore milk sugar (lactose). Besides working on only specific types of chemicals, enzymes are sensitive to acidic and alkaline conditions, temperature, and the types of vitamins and minerals they require. Digestive enzymes that work in the acidic environment of the stomach do not work well in the alkaline environment of the small intestine. Overall, enzymes work to hasten certain events that take place in the body (Fig. 3-11).

The pancreas and the small intestine produce most of the digestive enzymes; however, the mouth and the stomach also contribute their own enzymes to digestion. **Mucus,** another component of saliva, makes it easy to swallow a mouthful of food. The food then travels to the esophagus. The important secretions and products of digestion are listed in Table 3-3.

## MAKING DECISIONS

### Enzymes and Digestion

The authors of some popular (fad) diet books contend that eating certain combinations of foods, such as meats and fruits together, hinders the digestive process. However, does this make sense in light of our newly gained knowledge about GI tract physiology? The body is able to increase the production of certain digestive enzymes in response to the type of diet consumed. The GI tract can respond to the nutritional makeup and amount of food consumed because of this fine-tuning. Once consumed, foods are attacked by multiple enzymes to release nutrients and other compounds for absorption.

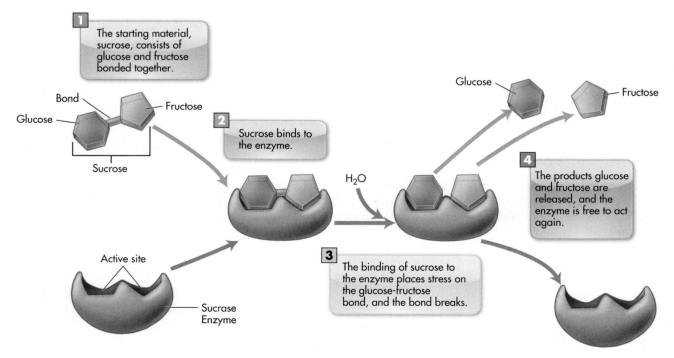

**FIGURE 3-11** ► A model of enzyme action. The enzyme sucrase splits the sugar sucrose into two simpler sugars; glucose and fructose. [Note that sometimes energy input is needed to make reactions occur.]

**TABLE 3-3** Important Secretions and Products of the Digestive Tract

| Secretion | Site of Production | Purpose |
|---|---|---|
| Saliva | Mouth | Partial starch digestion using **salivary amylase,** lubrication of food for swallowing |
| **Mucus** | Mouth, stomach, small intestine, large intestine | Protects GI tract cells, lubricates food as it travels through the GI tract |
| Enzymes | Mouth, stomach, small intestine, pancreas | Promote digestion of carbohydrates, fats, and proteins into forms small enough for absorption (Examples: **amylases, lipases, proteases**) |
| Acid | Stomach | Promotes digestion of protein among other functions |
| Bile | Liver (stored in gallbladder) | Aids fat digestion in the small intestine by suspending fat in water using **bile acids, cholesterol,** and **lecithin** |
| Bicarbonate | Pancreas, small intestine | Neutralizes stomach acid when it reaches the small intestine |
| Hormones | Stomach, small intestine, pancreas | Stimulate production and/or release of acid, enzymes, bile, and bicarbonate; help regulate peristalsis and overall GI tract flow (Examples: gastrin, secretin, insulin, cholecystokinin, glucagon) |

▲ The body digests the foods as they are presented—the order in which foods are eaten plays no role in digestion.

## Esophagus

The **esophagus** is a long tube that connects the **pharynx** with the stomach. Near the pharynx is a flap of tissue (called the **epiglottis**) that prevents the **bolus** of swallowed food from entering the trachea (wind pipe) (Fig. 3-12). During swallowing, food lands on the epiglottis, folding it down to cover the opening of the trachea. Breathing also stops automatically. These responses ensure that swallowed food will only travel down the esophagus. If food instead travels down the trachea, choking may occur (the victim will not be able to speak or breathe). A group of techniques to treat such a person are called the Heimlich maneuver (see www.heimlichinstitute.org for details).

At the top of the esophagus, nerve fibers release signals to tell the GI tract that food has been consumed. This results in an increase in gastrointestinal muscle action, called **peristalsis.** Continual waves of muscle contractions, followed by muscle relaxation, force the food down the digestive tract from the esophagus onward (Fig. 3-13).

At the end of the esophagus is the **lower esophageal sphincter,** a muscle that constricts (closes) after food enters the stomach (Fig. 3-14). The main function of sphincters is to prevent the backflow of GI tract contents. Sphincters respond to various stimuli, such as signals from the nervous system, hormones, acidic versus alkaline conditions, and pressure that builds up around the sphincter. The primary function of the lower esophageal sphincter is to prevent the acidic contents of the stomach from flowing back up into the esophagus—which can cause some of the health problems we will discuss in the "Nutrition and Your Health" section at the end of Chapter 3.

## Stomach

The stomach is a large sac that can hold up to 4 cups (or 1 quart) of food for several hours until all of the food is able to enter the small intestine. Stomach size varies individually and can be reduced surgically as a radical treatment for obesity (more on this in Chapter 7). While in the stomach, the food is mixed with gastric juice,

**mucus** A thick fluid secreted by many cells throughout the body. It contains a compound that has both carbohydrate and protein parts. It acts as a lubricant and means of protection for cells.

**amylase** Starch-digesting enzyme produced by the salivary glands and pancreas.

**lipase** Fat-digesting enzyme produced by the salivary glands, stomach, and pancreas.

**protease** Protein-digesting enzyme produced by the stomach, small intestine, and pancreas.

**esophagus** A tube in the GI tract that connects the pharynx with the stomach.

**pharynx** The organ of the digestive tract and respiratory tract located at the back of the oral and nasal cavities, commonly known as the throat.

**epiglottis** The flap that folds down over the trachea during swallowing.

**bolus** A moistened mass of food swallowed from the oral cavity into the pharynx.

**peristalsis** A coordinated muscular contraction used to propel food down the gastrointestinal tract.

**lower esophageal sphincter** A circular muscle that constricts the opening of the esophagus to the stomach. Also called the *gastroesophageal sphincter.*

**FIGURE 3-12** ▶ The process of swallowing. (a) During swallowing, food does not normally enter the trachea because the epiglottis closes over the larynx. (b) The closed epiglottis allows food to proceed down the esophagus. When a person chokes, food becomes lodged in the trachea, blocking air flow to the lungs. (c) The food should move down the esophagus.

Bolus of food
Tongue
Epiglottis
Larnyx
Trachea
(a)

Esophagus
(b)

(c)

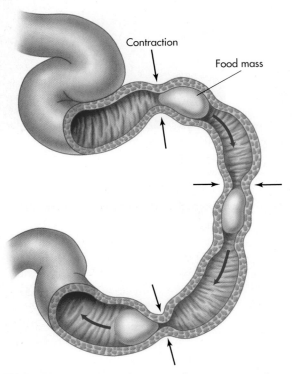

Contraction
Food mass

**FIGURE 3-13** ▶ Peristalsis. Peristalsis is a progressive type of movement, propelling material from point to point along the GI tract. To begin this, a ring of contraction occurs where the GI wall is stretched, passing the food mass forward. The moving food mass triggers a ring of contraction in the next region, which pushes the food mass even farther along. The result is a ring of contraction that moves like a wave along the GI tract, pushing the food mass down the tract.

**chyme** A mixture of stomach secretions and partially digested food.

**pyloric sphincter** Ring of smooth muscle between stomach and small intestine.

**villi** (singular, **villus**) The fingerlike protrusions into the small intestine that participate in digestion and absorption of food.

**absorptive cells** Intestinal cells that line the villi; and participate in nutrient absorption.

which contains water, a very strong acid, and enzymes. (Gastric is a term pertaining to the stomach.) The acid in the gastric juice maintains the acidity of the stomach contents and, thereby destroys the biological activity of proteins, converts inactive digestive enzymes to their active form, partially digests food protein, and makes dietary minerals soluble so that they can be absorbed. The mixing that takes place in the stomach produces a watery food mixture, called **chyme,** which slowly leaves the stomach a teaspoon (5 milliliters) at a time and enters the small intestine. Following a meal, the stomach contents are emptied into the small intestine over the course of 1 to 4 hours. The **pyloric sphincter,** located at the base of the stomach, controls the rate at which the chyme is released into the small intestine (review Fig. 3-14). There is very little absorption of nutrients from the stomach, except for some alcohol.

You might wonder how the stomach prevents itself from being digested by the acid and enzymes it produces. First, the stomach has a thick layer of mucus that lines and protects it. The production of acid and enzymes also requires the release of a specific hormone (gastrin). This release happens primarily when we are eating or thinking about eating. Last, as the concentration of acid in the stomach increases, hormonal control causes acid production to taper off.

One other important function of the stomach is the production of a substance called **intrinsic factor.** This vital material is essential for the absorption of vitamin B-12.

## Small Intestine

The small intestine is about 10 feet (3 meters) long, beginning at the stomach on the "north" and ending at the large intestine (colon) on the "south (Fig. 3-15)." The small intestine is considered "small" because of its narrow (1 inch [2.5 centimeters]) diameter. Most of the digestion and absorption of food occurs in the small intestine. The chyme secreted from the stomach is moved through the small intestine by peristaltic contractions so that it can be well mixed with the digestive juices of the small intestine (review Fig. 3-13). These juices contain many enzymes that function in the breakdown of carbohydrates, protein, and fat, as well as in the preparation of vitamins and minerals for absorption.

The physical structure of the small intestine is very important to the body's ability to digest and absorb the nutrients it needs. The lining of the small intestine is called the mucosa and is folded many times; within these folds are fingerlike projections called **villi.** These "fingers" are constantly moving, which helps them trap food to enhance absorption. Each individual villus (singular) is made up of many **absorptive cells,** and each of these cells has a highly folded cap. The combined folds, villi, and caps in the small intestine increase its surface area 600 times beyond that of a simple tube (Fig. 3-16).

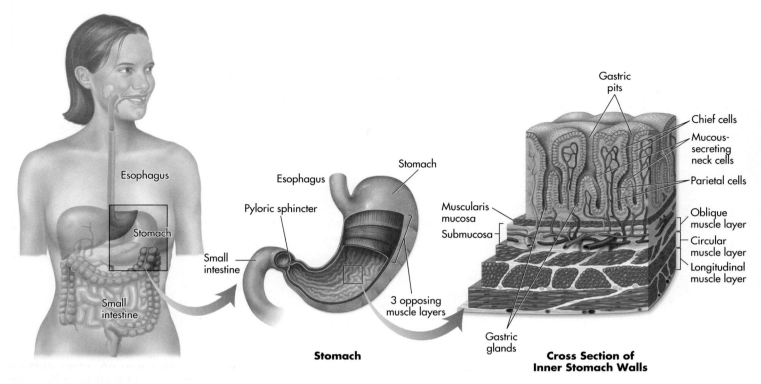

**FIGURE 3-14** ▶ Physiology of the stomach. Surface mucous cells produce mucus for protection from stomach acid and enzymes. Parietal cells produce the hydrochloric acid (HCL), and chief cells produce the enzymes. Mucous neck cells, scattered among the cells in the gastric pits, also produce mucus.

**FIGURE 3-15** ▶ The small intestine and beginning of the large intestine. The three parts of the small intestine are the duodenum, jejunum, and ileum. Notice the smaller diameter of the small intestine, compared with the large intestine.

The absorptive cells have a short life. New intestinal absorptive cells are constantly produced in the crypts of the small intestine (Fig. 3-16) and appear daily along the surface of each villus "finger." This is probably because absorptive cells are subjected to a harsh environment, so renewal of the intestinal cell lining is necessary. This rapid cell turnover leads to high nutrient needs for the small intestine. Fortunately, many of

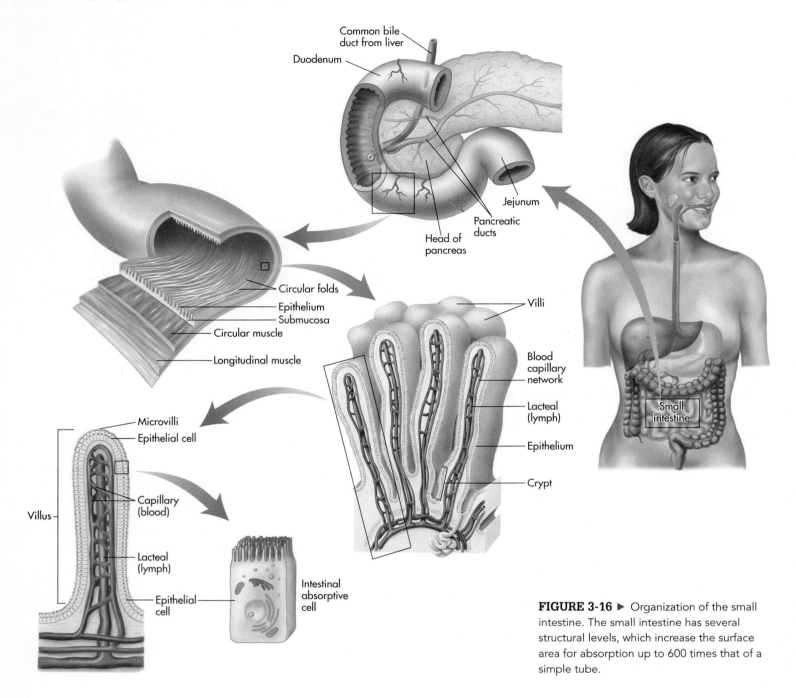

**FIGURE 3-16** ▶ Organization of the small intestine. The small intestine has several structural levels, which increase the surface area for absorption up to 600 times that of a simple tube.

the old cells can be broken down and have their component parts reused. The health of the cells is further enhanced by various hormones and other substances that participate in or are produced as part of the digestive process.

The small intestine absorbs nutrients through the intestinal wall through various means and processes, as illustrated in Figure 3-17:

- **Passive diffusion:** When the nutrient concentration is higher in the cavity (lumen) of the small intestine than in the absorptive cells, the difference in nutrient concentration drives the nutrient into the absorptive cells by diffusion. Fats, water, and some minerals are absorbed by passive diffusion.
- **Facilitated diffusion:** Some compounds require a carrier protein to drive them into absorptive cells. This type of absorption is called faciliated diffusion. Fructose

Intestinal lumen

energy used

Interior of absorptive cell

**FIGURE 3-17** ▶ Nutrient absorption relies on four major absorptive processes. **1** Passive diffusion (in green) is diffusion of nutrients across the absorptive cell membranes. **2** Facilitated diffusion (in blue) uses a carrier protein to move nutrients down a concentration gradient. **3** Active absorption (in red) involves a carrier protein as well as energy to move nutrients (against a concentration gradient) into absorptive cells. **4** Phagocytosis and pinocytosis (in green and brown) are forms of active transport in which the absorptive cell membrane forms an indentation that engulfs a nutrient to bring it into the cell.

is one example of a compound that makes use of such a carrier to allow for facilitated diffusion.

- **Active absorption:** In addition to the need for a carrier protein, some nutrients also require energy input to move from the lumen of the small intestine into the absorptive cells. This mechanism makes it possible for cells to take up nutrients even when they are consumed in low concentrations. Some sugars, such as glucose, are actively absorbed, as are amino acids.
- **Phagocytosis** and **pinocytosis:** In a further means of active absorption, absorptive cells literally engulf compounds (phagocytosis) or liquids (pinocytosis). As described earlier, a cell membrane can form an indentation of itself so that when particles or fluids move into the indentation, the cell membrane surrounds and engulfs them. This process is used when an infant absorbs immune substances from human milk (see Chapter 14).

Once absorbed, water-soluble compounds such as glucose and amino acids go to the capillaries and then on to the portal vein. Recall that the liver is the end of this process. Most fats eventually go into the lymph vessels. In doing so, they can eventually enter the bloodstream (see the earlier section on the circulatory system for details; and review Figs. 3-4 and 3-5).

Undigested food cannot be absorbed into cells of the small intestine. Any undigested food that reaches the end of the small intestine must pass through the **ileocecal sphincter** on the way to the large intestine (Fig. 3-18). This sphincter prevents the contents of the large intestine from reentering the small intestine.

**ileocecal sphincter** The ring of smooth muscle between the end of the small intestine and the large intestine.

## Large Intestine

When the contents of the small intestine enter the large intestine, the material left bears little resemblance to the food originally eaten. Under normal circumstances, only a minor amount (5%) of carbohydrate, protein, and fat escape absorption to reach the large intestine (Fig. 3-19).

Physiologically, the large intestine differs from the small intestine in that there are no villi or digestive enzymes. The absence of villi means that little absorption takes place in the large intestine in comparison to the small intestine. Nutrients absorbed

**FIGURE 3-18** ▶ The parts of the colon: cecum ascending colon, transverse colon, descending colon, and sigmoid colon.

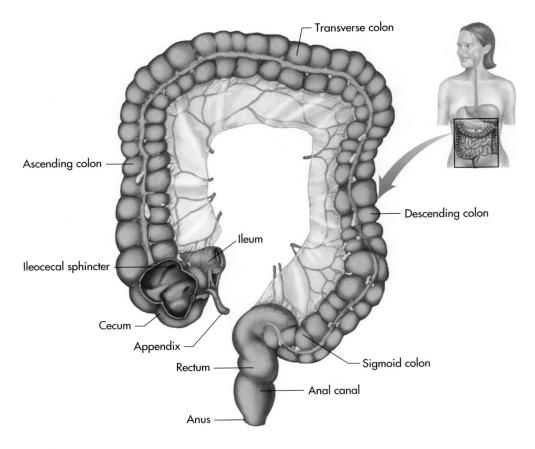

from the large intestine include water, some vitamins, some fatty acids, and the minerals sodium and potassium. Unlike the small intestine, the large intestine has a number of mucus-producing cells. The mucus secreted by these cells functions to hold the feces together and to protect the large intestine from the bacterial activity within it. The large intestine is home to a large population of bacteria (over 500 different species). Whereas the stomach and small intestine have some bacterial activity, the large intestine is the organ most heavily colonized with bacteria. Starting at infancy, the diet plays a major part in determining the type of bacteria in our digestive tracts. The number and type of bacteria in the human colon recently has become of great interest. Research has shown that intestinal bacteria play a significant role in the maintenance of health, especially health of the colon. It is speculated that higher levels of beneficial organisms can reduce the activity of disease-causing bacteria. This is another illustration of the intestinal tract working as an important immune organ. The strains *bifidobacteria* and *lactobacilli* are typically associated with health, whereas *clostridia* are considered problematic. These bacteria are able to break down some of the remaining food products that enter the large intestine, such as the milk sugar lactose (in lactose intolerant people), and some components of fiber. The products of bacterial metabolism in the large intestine, which include various acids, can then be absorbed.

Foods containing certain microorganisms such as lactobacilli are getting a lot of attention. The term **probiotic** is used for these microorganisms because once consumed, they take up residence in the large intestine and lead to some health benefits, such as improving intestinal tract health. You can find these probiotic microorganisms in certain forms of fluid milk, fermented milk, and yogurt. They can even be found in pill form. A related term is **prebiotic.** These are substances that increase growth of probiotic microorganisms. One example is fructooligosaccharides (see Table 1-5 in

**prebiotic** Substance that stimulates bacterial growth in the large intestines.

**probiotic** Product that contains specific types of bacteria. Use is intended to colonize the large intestine with the specific bacteria in the product. An example is yogurt.

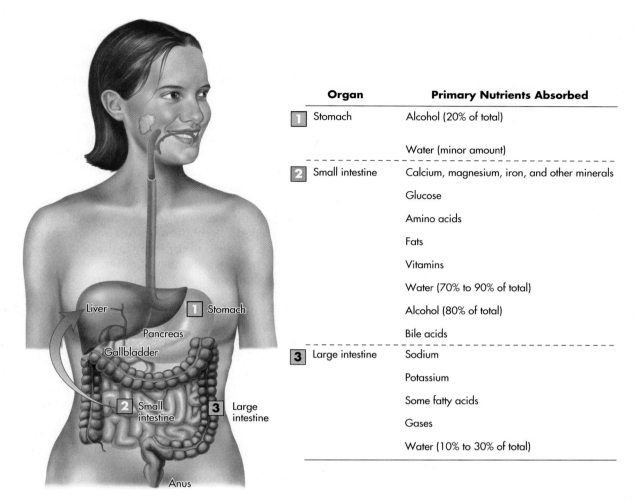

| Organ | Primary Nutrients Absorbed |
|---|---|
| 1 Stomach | Alcohol (20% of total) |
| | Water (minor amount) |
| 2 Small intestine | Calcium, magnesium, iron, and other minerals |
| | Glucose |
| | Amino acids |
| | Fats |
| | Vitamins |
| | Water (70% to 90% of total) |
| | Alcohol (80% of total) |
| | Bile acids |
| 3 Large intestine | Sodium |
| | Potassium |
| | Some fatty acids |
| | Gases |
| | Water (10% to 30% of total) |

**FIGURE 3-19** ▶ Major sites of absorption along the GI tract. Some absorption of vitamin K and biotin takes place in the large intestine. With the exception of fat soluble nutrients, most nutrients travel through the portal vein to the liver after their absorption.

Chapter 1 for dietary sources). The beneficial organisms of the large intestine will be discussed further in Chapter 4 when we explore their use as probiotics.

The small intestine absorbs only 70% to 90% of the fluid it receives, which includes large amounts of GI-tract secretions produced during digestion. Therefore, some water remains in the material that enters the large intestine. The remnants of a meal also contain some minerals and some fiber. Because water is removed from the large intestine, its contents become semisolid by the time they have passed through the first two-thirds of it. What remains in the **feces,** besides water and undigested fiber, is tough connective tissues (from animal foods); bacteria from the large intestine; and some body wastes, such as parts of dead intestinal cells.

## Rectum

The feces or stool remains in the last portion of the large intestine, the **rectum,** until muscular movements push it into the **anus** to be eliminated. The presence of feces in the rectum stimulates elimination. The anus contains two **anal sphincters** (internal and external), one of which is under voluntary control (external sphincter). Relaxation of this sphincter allows for elimination.

**rectum** Terminal portion of the large intestine.

**anus** Last portion of the GI tract; serves as an outlet for that organ.

**anal sphincters** A group of two sphincters (inner and outer) that help control expulsion of feces from the body.

**gallbladder** An organ attached to the underside of the liver; site of bile storage, concentration, and eventual secretion.

**bile** A liver secretion stored in the gallbladder and released through the common bile duct into the first segment of the small intestine. It is essential for the digestion and absorption of fat.

 See *Nutrition and Your Health: Common Problems with Digestion* at the end of Chapter 3.

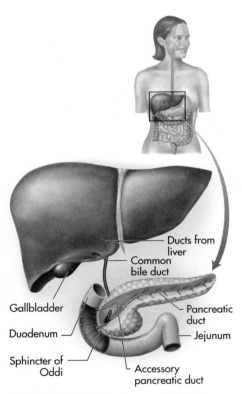

Ducts from liver
Common bile duct
Gallbladder
Duodenum
Sphincter of Oddi
Pancreatic duct
Jejunum
Accessory pancreatic duct

**FIGURE 3-20 ▶** The liver, gallbladder, and pancreas are accessory organs that work with the GI tract. The liver produces bile, stored in the gallbladder and released into the duodenum portion of the small intestine, via the common bile duct, to help digest fat. The pancreas secretes pancreatic juice containing water, bicarbonate, and digestive enzymes into the duodenum via the common bile duct. The common bile duct from the liver and gallbladder and the pancreatic duct join together at the sphincter of Oddi to deliver bile, pancreatic enzymes, and bicarbonate to the duodenum.

## Accessory Organs

The liver, **gallbladder,** and pancreas work with the GI tract and are considered accessory organs to the process of digestion (review Fig. 3-10). These accessory organs are not part of the GI tract through which food passes, but they play necessary roles in the process of digestion. These organs secrete digestive fluids into the GI tract and enable the process of converting food into absorbable nutrients.

The liver produces a substance called **bile.** The bile is stored and concentrated in the gallbladder until the gallbladder receives a hormonal signal to release the bile. This signal is induced by the presence of fat in the small intestine. Bile is released and delivered to the small intestine via a tube called the bile duct (Fig. 3-20).

In action, bile is like soap. Components of the bile enable large portions of fat to break into smaller bits so that they can be suspended in water (Chapter 5 will cover this process in detail). Interestingly, some of the bile constituents can be "recycled" in a process known as **enterohepatic circulation.** These components of bile are reabsorbed from the small intestine, returned to the liver via the portal vein, and reused.

In addition to bile, the liver releases a number of other unwanted substances that travel with the bile to the gallbladder and end up in the small intestine and eventually in the large intestine for excretion. The liver functions in this manner to remove unwanted substances from the blood. (Other byproducts are excreted via the urine; see the next section, "Urinary System.")

The pancreas manufactures hormones and pancreatic juice. The hormones include glucagon and insulin, which as noted earlier function in glucose regulation. Pancreatic juice contains water, bicarbonate, and a variety of digestive enzymes capable of breaking apart carbohydrates, proteins, and fats into small fragments. Bicarbonate is a base that neutralizes the acidity of chyme as it moves from the stomach into the small intestine. Recall that the stomach produces a thick layer of mucus to protect itself from the acid of gastric secretions. The small intestine, however, does not have a protective layer of mucus, because mucus would impede nutrient absorption. Instead, the neutralizing capacity of bicarbonate from the pancreas protects the walls of the small intestine from erosion by acid, which would otherwise lead to formation of an ulcer (see the "Nutrition and Your Health" section at the end of Chapter 3).

### CONCEPT CHECK

Digestion is a mechanical and chemical process mediated by enzymes and coordinated by hormones and nerves. Whereas swallowing and ultimate elimination of feces from the anus are voluntary, the majority of the digestive processes are involuntary. The stomach initiates the process of digestion by mixing food with gastric juice and converting this partially digested food into chyme. The products of digestion are molecules of the original food or beverage small enough to be absorbed into the villi of the small intestine and transferred to the blood or lymph. For the most part, nutrients are absorbed in the small intestine; only a few are absorbed in the large intestine. Any dietary component that escapes digestion by human or bacterial enzymes exits the body as feces.

## 3.9 Urinary System

The **urinary system** is composed of two kidneys, one on each side of the spinal column. Each kidney is connected to the bladder by a **ureter.** The bladder is emptied by way of the **urethra** (Fig. 3-21). The main function of the kidneys is to remove waste from the body. The kidneys are constantly filtering blood to control its composition. This results in the formation of urine, mostly water, along with dissolved waste products such as urea, and excess and unneeded water-soluble vitamins and various minerals.

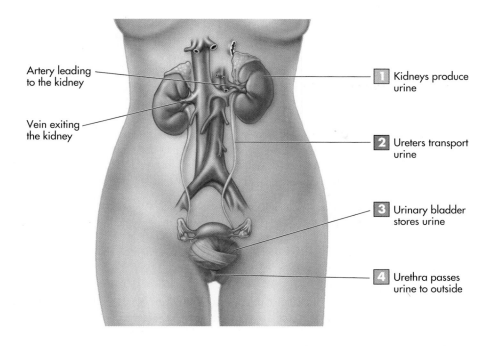

Artery leading to the kidney

Vein exiting the kidney

**1** Kidneys produce urine

**2** Ureters transport urine

**3** Urinary bladder stores urine

**4** Urethra passes urine to outside

**FIGURE 3-21** ▶ Organs of the urinary system. The kidneys **1** bean-shaped organs located on either side of the spinal column, filter waste from the blood and form urine, which is transported to the bladder by the ureters **2** and stored in the bladder **3** as urine. The urethra **4** transports the urine to outside the body. The urinary system of the female is shown. The male's urinary system is the same, except that the urethra extends through the penis.

**enterohepatic circulation** A continual recycling of compounds between the small intestine and the liver; bile acids are one example of a recycled compound.

**urinary system** The body system consisting of the kidneys, urinary bladder, and the ducts that carry urine. This system removes waste products from the circulatory system and regulates blood acid-base balance, overall chemical balance, and water balance in the body.

**ureter** Tube that transports urine from the kidney to the urinary bladder.

**urethra** Tube that transports urine from the urinary bladder to the outside of the body.

**pH** A measure of relative acidity or alkalinity of a solution. The pH scale is 0 to 14. A pH below 7 is acidic; a pH above 7 is alkaline.

**erythropoietin** A hormone secreted mostly by the kidneys that enhances red blood cell synthesis and stimulates red blood cell release from bone marrow.

Together with the lungs, the kidneys also maintain the acid-base balance **(pH)** of the blood. The kidneys also convert a form of vitamin D into its active hormone form and produce a hormone that stimulates red blood cell synthesis (**erythropoietin;** see Chapter 10 for information on misuse of this hormone by some athletes). During times of fasting, the kidneys even produce glucose from certain amino acids. Thus, the kidneys perform many important functions and are a vital component of the body.

The proper function of the kidneys is closely tied to the strength of the cardiovascular system, particularly its ability to maintain adequate blood pressure, and the consumption of sufficient fluid. Uncontrolled diabetes, hypertension, and drug abuse are harmful to the kidneys.

## 3.10 Storage Capabilities

The human body must maintain reserves of nutrients, otherwise we would need to eat continuously. Storage capacity varies for each different nutrient. Most fat is stored in adipose tissue, made up of cells designed specifically for this. Short-term storage of carbohydrate occurs in muscle and liver in the form of glycogen. The blood maintains a small reserve of glucose and amino acids. Many vitamins and minerals are stored in the liver, while other nutrient stores are found in other sites in the body.

When people do not meet certain nutrient needs, these nutrients are obtained by breaking down a tissue that contains high concentrations of the nutrient. For example, calcium is taken from bone and protein is taken from muscle. In cases of long-term deficiency, these nutrient losses weaken and harm these tissues.

Many people believe that if too much of a nutrient is obtained—for example, from a vitamin or mineral supplement—only what is needed is stored and the rest is excreted by the body. Though true for some nutrients, such as vitamin C, the large dosages of other nutrients frequently found in supplements, such as vitamin A and iron, can cause harmful side effects because they are not readily excreted. This is one reason why obtaining your nutrients primarily (or exclusively) from a balanced diet is the safest means to acquire the building blocks you need to maintain the good health of all organ systems.

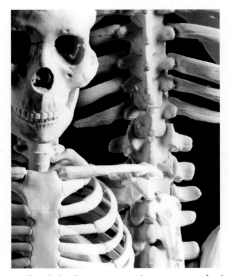

▲ The skeletal system provides a reserve of calcium for day-to-day needs when dietary intake is inadequate. Long-term use of this reserve, however, reduces bone strength.

## CONCEPT CHECK

The urinary system removes the wastes produced by the body and many nutrients ingested in excess of storage capacity and need. The kidneys maintain the chemical composition and acidity of the blood. In addition, the kidneys help convert vitamin D to its active form and produce a hormone needed for red blood cell synthesis.

In well-nourished individuals, nutrients are constantly present in the blood for immediate use and are stored in the body tissues for later use when sufficient amounts are not consumed from food. However, when the body suffers a nutrient deficiency after an inadequate diet is consumed over a long period, vital tissues will be broken down for their nutrients, which can lead to ill health. Additionally, too much of any nutrient can be detrimental. It's best to focus primarily (or exclusively) on obtaining all essential nutrients from a balanced diet rather than mostly from dietary supplements.

## 3.11 A Closer Look at Genetics and Nutrition

Once nutrients and other dietary components are taken up by cells, they may interact with our genes and have an effect on gene expression. The growth, development, and maintenance of cells, and ultimately of the entire organism, are directed by genes present in the cells. Each gene essentially represents a recipe, noting the ingredients (amino acids) and how those ingredients should be put together (to make proteins). The products (proteins) of all the recipes in the cookbook (the human genome) would then make up the human organism. The genome and the epigenome, the way the genome is marked and packaged inside a cell's nucleus, control the expression of individual traits, such as height, eye color, and susceptibility to many diseases. Epigenetics refers to inherited changes in gene expression caused by mechanisms other than changes in the underlying DNA sequence. While our genome contains the code for the proteins that can be made by our bodies, our epigenome is an extra layer of instructions that influences gene activity. In many cases it is the epigenome that can be repaired by treatments, or affected by diet, rather than the genetics.

The causes of chronic diseases are complex and include a significant genetic component. Fortunately, the science of genetics is moving swiftly such that medical breakthroughs are beginning to touch our lives. Genetic discoveries are leading to new drugs that disrupt disease processes at the molecular level and to tests that predict our risk for disease. In 2008, scientists discovered more than 100 genetic variations associated with many medical conditions associated with aging, including type 2 diabetes, Alzheimer's disease, osteoporosis, high blood pressure, and heart disease.

**A** genetic variation can directly affect the proteins encoded by our genes and result in different:

- nutrient requirements among individuals.
- susceptibilities to diseases.
- effects of environmental factors (such as our diet) on our genes and their proteins.

**nutrigenomics** Study of how food impacts health through its interaction with our genes and its subsequent effect on gene expression.

### The Emerging Field of Nutrigenomics

In the near future, genetic information will enhance the ability of health professionals to help individuals manage diseases and optimize health. Nutritional genomics or **nutrigenomics** is the study of how food impacts health through its interaction with our genes and its subsequent effect on gene expression. Nutrigenomics includes the study of how genes determine our nutritional requirements. Research in this area highlights the fallacy of a "one-size-fits-all" approach to nutrition interventions for disease prevention and management. It is becoming clear that the general nutrient requirements do not apply to certain genetic subgroups. Research is very active in identifying these subgroups and classifying the human genetic variation that may affect nutrient utilization and physiological function and therefore their unique nutrient requirements.

In addition to the direct effect of genes on disease risk, in many cases, genes influence the effect of diet and nutrition on disease development and progression. In some cases, a food component can cause a gene to be turned on or off, thus manipulating the production of proteins that can affect—positively or negatively—development or progression of diseases. With a better understanding of the interactions between genes and our diet, it will not be long before dietary recommendations may be personalized to help those with various genetically-linked diseases.

## Nutritional Diseases with a Genetic Link

Studies of families, including those with twins and adopted children, provide strong support for the effects of genetics in various disorders. In fact, family history is considered to be an important risk factor in the development of many nutrition-related diseases.

▲ Studies of twins have provided strong evidence for the interaction between genes and diet and their combined effects on disease risk.

**Cardiovascular Disease.** There is strong evidence that cardiovascular disease is the result of gene-environment interactions. About 1 of every 500 people in North America has a defective gene that greatly delays cholesterol removal from the bloodstream. As you saw in Chapter 1, elevated blood cholesterol is one major risk factor for development of cardiovascular disease. The gene-diet interactions being discovered for cardiovascular disease, particularly the cases of high blood lipid levels, will likely be the first to lead to nutrition plans personalized to decrease cardiovascular disease risk. Another type of genetic variation can cause a person to have abnormally high levels of an amino acid called homocysteine, which increases cardiovascular disease risk. Diet changes can help these people, but medications and even surgery are needed to address these problems.

**Obesity.** Most obese North Americans have at least one obese parent. This strongly suggests a genetic link. Findings from many human studies suggest that a variety of genes (likely 60 or more) are involved in the regulation of body weight. Little is known, however, about the specific nature of these genes in humans or how the actual changes in body metabolism (such as lower calorie-burning in general or fat use in particular) are produced.

Still, although some individuals may be genetically predisposed to store body fat, whether they do so depends on how many calories they consume relative to their needs. A common concept in nutrition is that *nurture*—how people live and the environmental factors that influence them—allows *nature*—each person's genetic potential—to be expressed. Although not every person with a genetic tendency toward obesity becomes obese, those genetically predisposed to weight gain have a higher lifetime risk than individuals without a genetic predisposition to obesity.

**Diabetes.** Both of the two common types of diabetes—type 1 and type 2—have genetic links. Evidence for these genetic links comes from studies of families and twins and from the high incidence of diabetes among certain population groups (e.g., South Asians or Pima Indians). Diabetes, in fact, is a complex disease with more than 200 genes identified as possible causes. Only sensitive and expensive testing can determine who is at risk. Type 2 diabetes is the most common form of diabetes (90% of all cases), and also has a strong link to obesity. Typically a genetic tendency for type 2 diabetes is expressed once a person becomes obese but often not before, again illustrating that nurture affects nature.

**Cancer.** A few types of cancer (e.g., some forms of colon [*colon* is another name for large intestine] and breast cancer) have a strong genetic link, and genetics may play a role in others, such as **prostate cancer**. Because obesity increases the risk of several forms of cancer, a long-standing excess calorie intake is also a risk factor. Although genes are an important determinant in the development of cancer, environmental

## CRITICAL THINKING

Wesley notices that at family gatherings his parents, uncles, aunts, and older siblings typically drink excessive amounts of alcohol. His father has been arrested for driving while intoxicated, as has one of his aunts. Two of his uncles died before the age of 60 from alcohol abuse. As Wesley approaches the age of legal drinking, he wonders if he is destined to fall into the pattern of alcohol abuse. What advice would you give to Wesley concerning his future use of alcohol?

▲ Genetic testing for disease susceptibility will be more common in the future as the genes that increase the risk of developing various diseases are isolated and decoded.

The following weblinks will help you gather more information about genetic conditions and testing:

http://nutrigenomics.ucdavis.edu/
Center for Excellence for Nutritional Genomics. Website dedicated to promoting the new science of nutritional genomics

www.geneticalliance.org
Alliance of Genetic Support Groups

www.kumc.edu/gec/support
Information on genetic and rare conditions

www.cancer.gov/cancertopics/
prevention-genetics-causes
Genetics information from the National Cancer Institute

http://www.genome.gov/
National Human Genome Research Institute (at the National Institutes of Health) website. Describes the latest research finding, discusses some ethical issues, and provides a talking glossary.

http://history.nih.gov/exhibits/genetics/
Revolution in Progress: Human Genetics and Medical Research

and lifestyle factors, such as excessive sun exposure and a poor diet, also contribute significantly to the risk profile.

## MAKING DECISIONS

Research is opening the way for "personalized nutrition" that uses the results of genetic testing to determine which diet will work most effectively with the person's genetic makeup. There are genetic tests available for at least 1,500 diseases and conditions, but mechanisms are not in place to ensure that the tests are based on adequate evidence or that marketing claims are truthful. Many companies are already tailoring genetic testing services and products for certain genetic profiles even though there are insufficient data on which to base genotype-specific recommendations. Most of these offers are online. As we discussed in chapter 2, caution is always needed when evaluating nutrition information and claims. Genetic testing is no exception. Some DNA testing companies are responsible organizations, and some are not. Some are offering DNA tests to determine the best weight-loss diets or the best supplements. These marketing schemes belittle the science of genetics to consumers. Use the principles outlined in Chapter 2 to evaluate any genetic testing services or products.

## Your Genetic Profile

From this discussion, you can see that your genes can greatly influence your risk of developing certain diseases. By recognizing your potential for developing a particular disease, you can avoid behavior that further raises your risk. How can you figure out your genetic profile? Genetic testing can be valuable if it confirms that you carry a gene for a disease that you can do something about in terms of protecting against it. Testing is also of interest when you do not know your family medical history or there are gaps in your family tree. About 1,000 genetic tests have become available in recent years. It typically costs about $1,000 to have your DNA read to reveal the diseases to which you are most susceptible. Many tests are covered by health insurance plans. The Genetic Information Nondiscrimination Act (GINA) became a law in May 2008, and prohibits health insurers from raising premiums or denying coverage based on genetic information and applies to people who have genes that carry the risk of disease. DNA testing includes providing a saliva sample from which your DNA will be separated. Certain areas of the genome are then read and measured in the process known as genotyping. After this one- to two-month process, you receive your DNA profile, which will supplement what you already know about your family history. You can also compare your DNA profile to future findings from DNA research.

Many of the genes involved in common diseases, such as diabetes, are still unknown. Although there are genetic tests available for some diseases, your family history of certain diseases is still a much better indicator of your genetic profile and risk of disease. Put together a family tree of illnesses and deaths by compiling a few key facts on your primary relatives: siblings, parents, aunts and uncles, and grandparents, as suggested in the "Rate Your Plate" section. In general, the greater number of your relatives who had a genetically transmitted disease and the closer they are related to you, the greater your risk. If there is a significant family history of a certain disease, lifestyle changes may be appropriate. For example, women with a family history of breast cancer should avoid becoming obese, should minimize alcohol use, and should obtain mammograms regularly.

Figure 3-22 shows an example of a family tree (also called a *genogram*). High-risk conditions include two or more first-degree relatives in a family with a specific disease (first-degree relatives include one's parents, siblings, and offspring). Another sign of risk of inherited disease is development of the disease in a first-degree relative before

50 to 60 years. In the family depicted in Figure 3-22, prostate cancer killed the man's father. Knowing this, the man should be tested regularly for prostate cancer. His sisters should consider frequent mammograms and other preventive practices because their mother died of breast cancer. Because heart attack and stroke are also common in the family, all the children should adopt a lifestyle that minimizes the risk of developing these conditions, such as avoiding excessive animal fat and salt intake. Colon cancer is also evident in the family, so careful screening throughout life is important.

Information about our genetic makeup will increasingly influence our dietary and lifestyle choices. Throughout this book we will discuss "controllable" risk factors that could contribute to development of genetically linked diseases present in your family. This information will help you personalize nutrition advice based on your genetic background and identify and avoid the risk factors that could lead to the diseases present in your family.

This review of human anatomy, physiology, and genetics from a nutrition perspective sets the stage for developing a more detailed understanding of the nutrients. Chapters 4, 5, and 6 will build on this information.

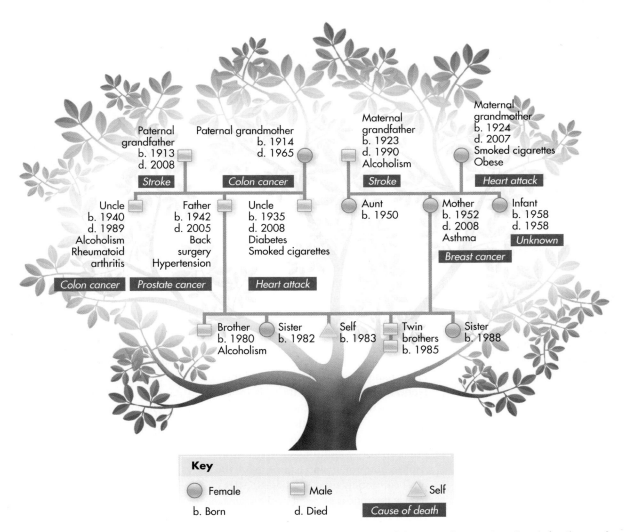

**FIGURE 3-22** ▶ Example of a family tree for Justin, designated as "Self" at the trunk of the tree. The gender of each family member is identified by color (blue squares for males, orange circles for females). Dates of birth (b) and death (d) are listed below each family member. If deceased, the cause of death is highlighted using white text against a red background. In addition to causes of death, medical conditions the family members experienced are noted beneath each name. Create your own family tree of frequent diseases using this figure as a guide. Then show your family tree to your physician to get a more complete picture of what the information means for your health.

# Common Problems with Digestion

The fine-tuned organ system we call the digestive system can develop problems. Knowing about these common problems can help you avoid or lessen them. Two common GI tract-related problems are diverticulosis and lactose maldigestion and intolerance. These disorders will be discussed in Chapter 4 after you learn more about carbohydrates.

## Ulcers

A peptic **ulcer** can occur when the lining of the esophagus, stomach, or small intestine is eroded by the acid secreted by the stomach cells (Fig. 3-23). As the stomach lining deteriorates in ulcer development, it loses its protective mucus layer, and the acid further erodes the stomach tissue. Acid can also erode the lining of the esophagus and the first part of the small intestine, the duodenum. In young people, most ulcers occur in the small intestine, wheras in older people they occur primarily in the stomach.

Millions of North Americans develop ulcers during their lifetimes. As a result, billions of healthcare dollars are spent annually on the treatment of peptic ulcers and their complications. Fortunately, our understanding of ulcer formation has increased, resulting in a variety of improved treatment options. The typical symptom of an ulcer is pain about 2 hours after eating. Stomach acid acting on a meal irritates the ulcer after most of the meal has moved from the site of the ulcer.

Not long ago, the major cause of ulcer disease was thought to be excess acid. Therefore, neutralizing and curtailing the secretion of stomach acid were the logical treatment choices. Although acid is still a significant player in ulcer formation, the principal causes of ulcer disease are currently thought to be infection of the stomach by the acid-resistant bacteria, *Helicobacter pylori (H. pylori)*; heavy use of nonsteroidal anti-inflammatory drugs **(NSAIDS),** such as aspirin; and disorders that cause excessive acid production in the stomach. Stress is regarded as a predisposing factor for ulcers, especially if the person is infected with *H. pylori* or has certain anxiety disorders. Cigarette smoking is also known to cause ulcers, increase ulcer complications such as bleeding, and lead to ulcer treatment failure.

The *H. pylori* bacteria is common but results in ulcer disease in only 10% to 15% of those infected. The bacteria is found in more than 80% of patients with stomach and duodenal ulcers. Although the mechanism of how *H. pylori* causes ulcers is not well understood, treatment of the infection with antibiotics heals the ulcers and prevents their recurrence. Two Australian physicians were awarded the Nobel Prize in 2005 "for their discovery of the bacterium *Helicobacter pylori* and its role in gastritis and peptic ulcer disease."

NSAIDs are medications for painful inflammatory conditions such as arthritis. Aspirin, ibuprofen, and naproxen are the most commonly used NSAIDs. NSAIDs reduce the mucus secreted by the stomach. Newer medications, called "Cox-2 inhibitors" (e.g., celecoxib [Celebrex]), have been used as a replacement for NSAIDs because they are less likely to cause stomach ulcers. They do offer some advantages over NSAIDs, but they may not be totally safe for some people, especially those with a history of cardiovascular disease or strokes.

The primary risk associated with an ulcer is the possibility that it will erode entirely through the stomach or intestinal wall. The GI contents could then spill into the body cavities, causing a massive infection. In addition, an ulcer may erode a blood vessel, leading to substantial blood loss. For these reasons, it is important not to ignore the early warning signs of ulcer development, including a persistent gnawing or burning near the stomach that may occur immediately following a meal or awaken you at night. In addition to the pain that may improve with food, other signs and symptoms of ulcers are weight loss, nausea, vomiting, loss of appetite, and abdominal bloating.

In the past, milk and cream therapy was used to help cure ulcers. Clinicians now know that milk and cream are two of the worst foods for an ulcer. The calcium in these foods stimulates stomach acid secretion and actually inhibits ulcer healing.

Today, a combination of approaches is used for ulcer therapy. People infected with *H. pylori* are given antibiotics as well as stomach acid-blocking medications

**ulcer** Erosion of the tissue lining, usually in the stomach or the upper small intestine. As a group these are generally referred to as *peptic ulcers.*

**NSAIDs** Nonsteroidal anti-inflammatory drugs; includes aspirin, ibuprofen (Advil®), and naproxen (Aleve®).

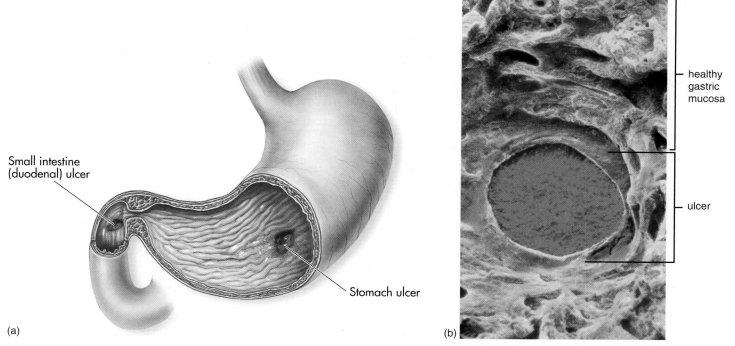

(a)

(b)

**FIGURE 3-23** ▶ (a) A peptic ulcer in the stomach or small intestine. *H. pylori* bacteria and NSAIDs (e.g., aspirin) cause ulcers by impairing mucosal defense, especially in the stomach. In the same way, smoking, genetics, and stress can impair mucosal defense, as well as cause an increase in the release of pepsin and stomach acid. All of these factors can contribute to ulcers. (b) Close-up of a stomach ulcer. This needs to be treated or eventual perforation of the stomach is possible.

▶ When suffering from persistent heartburn or GERD, see a doctor if you have

- Difficulty swallowing or pain when swallowing
- Heartburn that has persisted for more than 10 years
- Initial onset of heartburn after age 50
- Heartburn that resists treatment with medications
- Sudden, unexplained weight loss
- Chest pain
- Blood loss or anemia
- Blood in stool or vomit

called **proton pump inhibitors** (e.g., omeprazole [Prilosec], esomeprazole [Nexium], and lansoprazole [Prevacid]) and possibly bismuth. (Proton is another name for the hydrogen ion that creates acidity.) In many cases, there is a 90% cure rate for *H. pylori* infections in the first week of this treatment. Recurrence is unlikely if the infection is cured, but an incomplete cure almost certainly leads to repeated ulcer formation.

Antacid medications may also be part of ulcer care, as is a class of medicines called **H$_2$ blockers.** These include cimetidine (Tagamet), ranitidine (Zantac), nizatidine (Axid), and famotidine (Pepcid), all of which prevent **histamine**-related acid secretion in the stomach. Medications that coat the ulcer, such as sucralfate (Carafate), are also commonly used.

People with ulcers should refrain from smoking and minimize the use of aspirin and related NSAIDs. These practices reduce the mucus secreted by the stomach. Overall, a combination of lifestyle therapy and medical

treatment has so revolutionized ulcer therapy that dietary changes are of minor importance today. Current diet-therapy approaches recommend avoiding foods that increase ulcer symptoms (Table 3-4).

**proton pump inhibitor** A medication that inhibits the ability of gastric cells to secrete hydrogen ions. Low doses of this class of medications are also available without prescription (e.g., omeprazole [Prilosec]).

**H$_2$ blocker** Medication, such as cimetidine (Tagamet®), that blocks the increase of stomach acid production caused by histamine.

**histamine** A breakdown product of the amino acid histidine that stimulates acid secretion by the stomach and has other effects on the body, such as contraction of smooth muscles, increased nasal secretions, relaxation of blood vessels, and changes in relaxation of airways.

**TABLE 3-4** Recommendations to Prevent Ulcers and Heartburn from Occurring or Recurring

| Ulcers |
|---|
| 1.Stop smoking if you are now a smoker. |
| 2. Avoid large doses of aspirin, ibuprofen, and other NSAID compounds unless a physician advises otherwise. For people who must use these medications, FDA has approved an NSAID combined with a medication to reduce gastric damage. The medication reduces gastric acid production and enhances mucus secretion. |
| 3. Limit consumption of coffee, tea, and alcohol (especially wine), if this helps. |
| 4. Limit consumption of pepper, chili powder, and other strong spices, if this helps. |
| 5. Eat nutritious meals on a regular schedule; include enough fiber (see Chapter 4 for sources of fiber). |
| 6. Chew foods well. |
| 7. Lose weight if you are currently overweight. |

| Heartburn |
|---|
| 1. Follow ulcer prevention recommendations. |
| 2. Wait about 2 hours after a meal before lying down. |
| 3. Don't overeat. Eat smaller meals that are low in fat. |
| 4. Elevate the head of the bed at least 6 inches. |

## Heartburn

About half of North American adults experience occasional heartburn, also known as acid reflux (Fig. 3-24). This gnawing pain in the upper chest is caused by the movement of acid from the stomach into the esophagus. The recurrent and therefore more serious form of the problem is called **gastroesophageal reflux disease (GERD).** Unlike the stomach, the esophagus has very little mucus lining to protect it, so acid quickly erodes the lining of the esophagus, causing pain. Symptoms may also include nausea, gagging, cough, or hoarseness. GERD is characterized by the occurrence of such symptoms of acid reflux two or more times per week. People who have GERD experience occasional relaxation of the gastroesophageal sphincter. Typically it should be relaxed only during swallowing, but in individuals with GERD it is relaxed at other times as well.

The majority of heartburn sufferers say it significantly affects their quality of life, particularly their enjoyment of many favorite foods. On a more serious note, however, if left untreated, heartburn can, over time, damage the lining of the esophagus, leading to chronic esophageal inflammation and an increased risk of esophageal cancer. Heartburn sufferers should follow the general recommendations given in Table 3-4 . For occasional heartburn, quick relief can be found with over-the-counter (OTC) antacids. Taking antacids will reduce the acid in the stomach but will not stop the acid reflux. For more persistent (few days a week or everyday) heartburn or GERD, the H$_2$ blockers or PPIs, discussed in the previous section on ulcers, may be needed. PPIs provide long-lasting relief by reducing stomach acid production and must be taken at the right time. PPIs should be taken before the first meal of the day because they take longer to work. If the proper medications

**gastroesophageal reflux disease (GERD)** Disease that results from stomach acid backing up into the esophagus. The acid irritates the lining of the esophagus, causing pain.

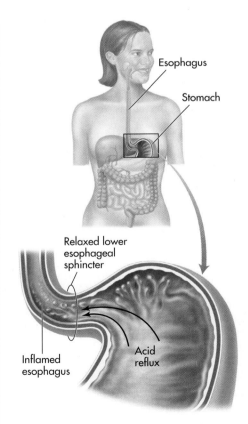

**FIGURE 3-24** ▶ Heartburn results from stomach acid refluxing into the esophagus.

Esophagus

Stomach

Relaxed lower esophageal sphincter

Inflamed esophagus

Acid reflux

▲ Dried fruits are a natural source of fiber and can help prevent constipation when consumed with an adequate amount of fluid.

are not effective at controlling GERD, surgery may be needed to strengthen the weakened esophageal sphincter. A popular theory is that relaxation of the lower esophageal sphincter allows acid and stomach contents to flow back into the esophagus. This situation will be more of a problem when lying down.

Both pregnancy and obesity can lead to heartburn because these conditions result in increased production of estrogen and progesterone. These hormones relax the lower esophageal sphincter, making heartburn more likely. In the case of obesity, adipose tissue turns certain circulating hormones into estrogen; thus, the more adipose tissue one has, the more estrogen produced.

## Constipation and Laxatives

**Constipation,** difficult or infrequent evacuation of the bowels, is commonly reported by adults. Slow movement of fecal material through the large intestine causes constipation. As fluid is increasingly absorbed during the extended time the feces stay in the large intestine, they become dry and hard.

Constipation can result when people regularly inhibit their normal bowel reflexes for long periods. People may ignore normal urges when it is inconvenient to interrupt occupational or social activities. Muscle spasms of an irritated large intestine can also slow the movement of feces and contribute to constipation. Calcium, iron supplements, and medications such as antacids can also cause constipation.

Eating foods with plenty of fiber, such as whole-grain breads and cereals, along with drinking adequate fluid to avoid dehydration, is the best method for treating mild cases of constipation. Fiber stimulates peristalsis by drawing water into the large intestine and helping form a bulky, soft fecal output. Dried fruits are a good source of fiber and therefore can also help stimulate the bowel. Additional fluid should be consumed to facilitate fiber's action in the large intestine. In addition, people with constipation may need to develop more regular bowel habits; allowing the

same time each day for a bowel movement can help train the large intestine to respond routinely. Finally, relaxation facilitates regular bowel movements, as does regular physical activity.

**Laxatives,** as well as various other medications, can also lessen constipation. Some laxatives work by irritating the intestinal nerve junctions to stimulate the peristaltic muscles, while others that contain fiber draw water into the intestine to enlarge fecal output. The larger output stretches the peristaltic muscles, making them rebound and then constrict. Regular use of laxatives, however, should be supervised by a physician. Overall the bulk-forming fiber laxatives are the safest to use.

## Hemorrhoids

**Hemorrhoids,** also called *piles,* are swollen veins of the rectum and anus. The blood vessels in this area are subject to intense pressure, especially during bowel movements. Added stress to the vessels from pregnancy, obesity, prolonged sitting, violent coughing or sneezing, or straining during bowel movements, particularly with constipation, can lead to a hemorrhoid. Hemorrhoids can develop unnoticed until a strained bowel movement precipitates symptoms, which may include pain, itching, and bleeding.

Itching, caused by moisture in the anal canal, swelling, or other irritation, is perhaps the most common symptom. Pain, if present, is usually aching and steady. Bleeding may result from a hemorrhoid and appear in the toilet as a bright red streak in the feces. The sensation of a mass in the anal canal after a bowel movement is symptomatic of an internal hemorrhoid that protrudes through the anus.

Anyone can develop a hemorrhoid, and about half of adults over age 50 do. Pressure from prolonged sitting or

**constipation** A condition characterized by infrequent bowel movements.

**laxative** A medication or other substance that stimulates evacuation of the intestinal tract.

exertion is often enough to bring on symptoms, although diet, lifestyle, and possibly heredity play a role. For example, a low-fiber diet can lead to hemorrhoids as a result of straining during bowel movements. If you think you have a hemorrhoid, you should consult your physician. Rectal bleeding, although usually caused by hemorrhoids, may also indicate other problems, such as cancer.

A physician may suggest a variety of self-care measures for hemorrhoids. Pain can be lessened by applying warm, soft compresses or sitting in a tub of warm water for 15 to 20 minutes. Dietary recommendations are the same as those for treating constipation, emphasizing the need to consume adequate fiber and fluid. Over-the-counter remedies, such as Preparation H, can also offer relief of symptoms.

## Irritable Bowel Syndrome

Many adults (25 million or more in the United States alone) have irritable bowel syndrome, noted as a combination of cramps, gassiness, bloating, and irregular bowel function (diarrhea, constipation, or alternating episodes of both). It is more common in younger women than in younger men. In older adults the ratio is closer to 50:50. The disease leads to about 3.5 million visits to physicians in the United States each year.

Symptoms associated with irritable bowel syndrome include visible abdominal distention, pain relief after a bowel movement, increased stool frequency, loose stools with pain onset, mucus in stool, and a feeling of incomplete elimination even after a bowel movement.

The cause is thought to be altered intestinal peristalsis coupled with a decreased pain threshold for abdominal distension—in other words, a minor amount of abdominal bloating causes pain that the average person would not sense. It is also noteworthy that up to 50% of sufferers report a history of verbal or sexual abuse.

Therapy is individualized and can include a trial of high-fiber foods (soluble fiber is more effective than insoluble fiber) or elimination diets that focus on avoiding dairy products and gas-forming foods, such as legumes, certain vegetables (cabbage, beans, and broccoli), and some fruits (grapes, raisins, cherries, and cantaloupe). Herbal formulations, certain probiotics, and cognitive behavioral therapy have been shown to decrease symptoms of irritable bowel syndrome and improve overall quality of life. The patient should have only moderate caffeine intake or eliminate caffeine-containing foods/beverages altogether. Low-fat and more frequent, small meals may help the patient because large meals can trigger contractions of the large intestine. Other strategies include a reduction in stress, psychological counseling, and certain antidepressant and other medications. Hypnosis has been shown to relieve symptoms in severe cases.

Referral to a registered dietitian can be beneficial, as many patients experience improvement with the elimination of specific problem foods. A good patient/physician relationship is also necessary for the treatment of irritable bowel syndrome; however, before any single treatment is applauded, note that response to placebos alone has been as high as 70% in this population. Although irritable bowel syndrome can be uncomfortable and upsetting, it is harmless as it carries no risk for cancer or other serious digestive problems. The website www.ibsgroup.org provides further information.

## Diarrhea

Diarrhea, a GI tract disease that generally lasts only a few days, is defined as increased fluidity, frequency, or amount of bowel movements compared to a person's usual pattern. Most cases of diarrhea result from infections in the intestines, with bacteria and viruses the usual offending agents. They produce substances that cause the intestinal cells to secrete fluid rather than absorb fluid. Another form of diarrhea can be caused by consumption of substances not readily absorbed, such as the sugar alcohol sorbitol found in sugarless gum (see Chapter 4) or large amounts of a high-fiber source such as bran. When consumed in large amounts, the unabsorbed substance draws much water into the intestines, in turn leading to diarrhea. Treatment of diarrhea generally requires drinking lots of fluid during the affected stage; reduced intake of the poorly absorbed substance also is important if that is a cause. Prompt treatment—within 24 to 48 hours—is especially important for infants and older people, as they are more susceptible to the effects of dehydration associated with diarrhea (see Chapters 15 and 16). Diarrhea that lasts more than 7 days in adults should be investigated by a physician as it can be a symptom of more serious intestinal disease, especially if there is also blood in the stool.

## Gallstones

Gallstones are a major cause of illness and surgery, affecting 10% to 20% of U.S. adults. Gallstones are pieces of solid material that develop in the gallbladder when substances in the bile—primarily cholesterol (80% of gallstones)—form crystal-like particles. They may be as small as a grain of sand or as large as a golf ball. These stones are caused by a combination of factors, with excess weight being the primary modifiable factor, especially in women 20 to 60 years old. Other factors include genetic background (e.g., Native Americans), advanced age (> 60 years for both women and men), reduced activity of the gallbladder (contracts less than normal), altered bile composition (e.g., too much cholesterol or not enough bile salts), diabetes, and diet (e.g., low-fiber diets). In addition, gallstones may develop during rapid weight loss or prolonged fasting (as the liver metabolizes more fat, it secretes more cholesterol into the bile).

Attacks due to gallstones include intermittent pain in the upper right abdomen, gas and bloating, nausea or vomiting, or other health problems. Surgical removal of the gallbladder is the most common method for treating gallstones (500,000 surgeries per year in the United States).

Prevention of gallstones revolves around avoiding becoming overweight, especially for women. Avoiding rapid weight loss (> 3 lbs. per week), limiting animal protein and focusing more on plant protein intake (especially some nut intake), and following a high-fiber diet can help as well. Regular physical activity is also recommended, as is moderate to no caffeine and alcohol intake.

**Less Common Digestive Disorders**

In **cystic fibrosis**—an inherited disease of infants, children, and sometimes adults—the pancreas often develops thick mucus that blocks its ducts, and active cells then die. As a result, the pancreas is not able to effectively deliver its digestive enzymes into the small intestine. Digestion of carbohydrate, protein, and—most notably—fat then is impaired. Often the missing enzymes must be ingested in capsule form with meals to aid in digestion. Another intestinal problem gaining attention is **celiac disease.** People with this disease experience an allergic reaction to the protein gluten in certain cereals, such as wheat and rye. This reaction damages the absorptive cells, resulting in a much-reduced surface area due to flattening of the villi. Elimination of wheat, rye, and certain other grains from the diet typically cures the problem.

## Summary

Overall, typical medical disorders of the GI tract arise from differences in anatomical features and lifestyle habits among individuals. Because of the importance of various nutrition and lifestyle habits, such as adequate fiber and fluid intake, as well as not smoking or abusing NSAID medications, nutrition and lifestyle therapy is often effective in helping treat GI tract disorders.

**cystic fibrosis** Inherited disease that can cause overproduction of mucus. Mucus can block the pancreatic duct, decreasing enzyme output.

**celiac disease** Immunological or allergic reaction to the protein gluten in certain grains, such as wheat and rye. The effect is to destroy the intestinal enterocytes, resulting in a much reduced surface area due to flattening of the villi. Elimination of wheat, rye, and certain other grains from the diet restores the intestinal surface.

▲ Gallbladder and gallstones seen after surgical removal from the body. Size and composition of the stones vary from one case to another.

## Case Study Gastroesophageal Reflux Disease

Caitlin is a 20-year-old college sophomore. Over the last few months, she has been experiencing regular bouts of heartburn. This usually happens after a large lunch or dinner. Occasionally she has even bent down after dinner to pick up something and had some stomach contents travel back up her esophagus and into her mouth. This especially frightened Caitlin, so she visited the University Health Center.

The nurse practitioner at the Center told Caitlin it was good that she came in for a checkup because she suspects Caitlin has a disease called gastroesophageal reflux disease (GERD). She tells Caitlin that this can lead to serious problems, such as a rare form of cancer if not controlled. She provides Caitlin with a pamphlet describing GERD and schedules an appointment with a physician for further evaluation.

Answer the following questions, and check your response in Appendix A.

1. What dietary and lifestyle habits likely contribute to Caitlin's symptoms of GERD?
2. What is the dietary and lifestyle management advice that will help Caitlin cope with this health problem?
3. What types of medications have been especially useful for treating this problem?
4. Overall, how will Caitlin cope with this health problem, and will it ever go away?
5. Why is management of GERD so important?

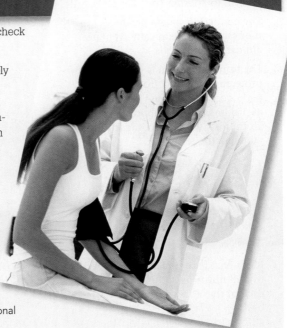

▶ Caitlin was wise to see a health professional about her persistent heartburn.

# Summary

1. The basic structural unit of the human body is the cell. Although almost all cells contain the same collection of organelles (nucleus, mitochondria, endoplasmic reticulum, lysosomes, peroxisomes, and cytoplasm), cell structure varies according to the type of job they must perform.

2. Cells join together to make up tissues, tissues unite to form organs, and organs work together as an organ system.

3. Blood is pumped from the heart to the lungs, picking up oxygen. Then, the blood delivers essential nutrients, oxygen, and water to all body cells. Nutrients and wastes are exchanged between the blood and cells across the cell membrane. This exchange occurs in the capillaries. Water-soluble compounds absorbed by the small intestine cells enter the portal vein and travel to the liver. Fat-soluble compounds enter the lymphatic system, which eventually connects to the bloodstream.

   The nervous system's neurons are the body's communication network. They control and manage all other organ systems of the body. Neurotransmitters are used to carry the message from one neuron to another (or to another cell).

   The endocrine system produces hormones, which chemically regulate almost all other cells.

   The immune system is responsible for protecting the body from invading pathogens. We activate immunity, such as production of antibodies (immunoglobulins), when we come in contact with a pathogen.

   The urinary system, including the kidneys, is responsible for filtering the blood, removing body wastes, and maintaining the chemical composition of the blood.

   Limited stores of nutrients are present in the blood for immediate use and stored to a greater or lesser extent in body tissues for later use when sufficient food is unavailable. When the body suffers a nutrient deficiency caused by a poor diet, it breaks down vital tissues for their nutrients, which can lead to ill health. Additionally, too much of any nutrient can be detrimental.

4. The gastrointestinal (GI) tract consists of the mouth, esophagus, stomach, small intestine, large intestine (colon), rectum, and anus.

   Spaced along the GI tract are ring-like valves (sphincters) that regulate the flow of foodstuffs. Muscular contractions, called *peristalsis*, move the foodstuffs down the GI tract. A variety of nerves, hormones, and other substances control the activity of sphincters and peristaltic muscles.

   Digestive enzymes are secreted by the mouth, stomach, wall of the small intestine, and pancreas. The presence of food in the small intestine stimulates the release of pancreatic enzymes.

   The major absorptive sites consist of fingerlike projections called *villi*, located in the small intestine. Absorptive cells cover the villi. This intestinal lining is continually renewed. Absorptive cells can perform various

   forms of passive diffusion and active absorption.

   Little digestion and absorption occur in the stomach or large intestine, but some protein is digested in the stomach. Some constituents of fiber and undigested starch are broken down by bacteria in the large intestine and some of the products are absorbed; any undigested fiber that remains is eliminated in the feces.

   Final water and mineral absorption takes place in the large intestine. Products from bacterial breakdown of some fibers and other substances are also absorbed here. The presence of feces in the rectum provides the impetus for elimination.

   The liver, gallbladder, and pancreas participate in digestion and absorption. Products from these organs, such as enzymes and bile, enter the small intestine and play important roles in digesting protein, fat, and carbohydrate.

5. Genetic background influences the risk for many health-related diseases. Examining one's family tree provides clues for an individual to such risks. Preventative measures are then important to implement, especially with respect to diet.

6. Common GI-tract diseases, such as heartburn, constipation, and irritable bowel syndrome, can be treated with diet changes. These can include increasing fiber intake and avoiding large meals high in fat. Medications are also very helpful in many cases.

# Study Questions

1. Identify at least one contribution to overall nutrition status provided by each of the 12 organ systems of the body.

2. Draw and label parts of the cell, and explain the function of each organelle

   discussed in the text as it relates to human nutrition.

3. Trace the flow of blood from the right side of the heart around the body and back to the same site. How is blood routed through the small intestine?

   Which class of nutrients enters the body via the blood? Via the lymph?

4. Explain why the small intestine is better suited than the other GI tract organs to carry out the absorptive process.

5. Identify the four basic tastes. Give an example of one food that exemplifies each of these basic taste sensations. Why can't you taste food when you have a cold? What is umami?

6. What is one role of acid in the process of digestion? Where is it secreted?

7. Contrast the processes of active absorption and passive diffusion of nutrients.

8. Identify the two accessory organs that empty their contents into the small intestine. How do the digestive substances secreted by these organs contribute to the digestion of food?

9. In which organ systems would the following substances be found?

   chyme
   plasma
   lymph
   urine

10. What is the difference between nature and nurture? Relate these terms to the attempt to prevent three common chronic diseases.

---

## Check Your Knowledge

Answers to the following multiple choice questions are below:

1. The stomach is protected from digesting itself by producing
   a. bicarbonate only when food is in the stomach.
   b. a thick layer of mucus to coat the lining of the stomach.
   c. hydroxyl ions to neutralize the acid.
   d. antipepsin that destroys digestive substances.

2. The lower esophageal sphincter is located between the
   a. stomach and esophagus.
   b. stomach and duodenum.
   c. ileum and the cecum.
   d. sigmoid colon and the anus.

3. A coordinated muscular contraction that propels food down the GI tract is called
   a. a sphincter.
   b. enterohepatic circulation.

   c. gravitational pull.
   d. peristalsis.

4. Bicarbonate ions ($HCO_3-$) from the pancreas
   a. neutralize the acid when it is in the stomach.
   b. are synthesized in the pyloric sphincter.
   c. neutralize the bile in the duodenum.
   d. neutralize the acid contents in the duodenum.

5. Most of the digestive processes occur in the
   a. mouth.
   b. stomach.
   c. small intestine.
   d. large intestine.
   e. colon.

6. Bile is formed in the _____ and stored in the _____.
   a. stomach, pancreas
   b. duodenum, kidney
   c. liver, gallbladder
   d. gallbladder, liver

7. Much of the digestion that occurs in the large intestine is caused by
   a. lipase.          c. saliva.
   b. pepsin.          d. bacteria.

8. Nexium ("the purple pill") is a popular drug that acts as a(n)
   a. $H_2$ blocker.
   b. laxative.
   c. analgesic.
   d. proton pump inhibitor.

9. The study of how food impacts health through its interaction with our genes is called
   a. nutrigenomics.
   b. epidemiology.
   c. immunology.
   d. genetics.

10. Energy production that takes place in the cytoplasm is called anaerobic metabolism because it does not require
   a. water.
   b. oxygen.
   c. anabolic steroids.
   d. anaerobic bacteria.

Answers: 1. b, 2. a, 3. d, 4. d, 5. c, 6. c, 7. d, 8. d, 9. a, 10. b

---

## Further Readings

1. Broekaert IJ, Walker WA: Probiotics and chronic disease. *Journal of Clinical Gastroenterology* 40:270, 2006.
   *Probiotic research has suggested several ways that they can be beneficial for the human body. Clinical research has demonstrated its preventive and curative potential in several intestinal diseases. The potential role of probiotics in the prevention and treatment of a wide variety of chronic diseases is reviewed.*

2. Camilleri M: Probiotics and irritable bowel syndrome: Rationale, putative mechanisms, and evidence of clinical efficacy. *Journal of Clinical Gastroenterology* 40:264, 2006.
   *The evidence that Bifidobacteria or Lactobacilli species alone or in the specific probiotic combination of VSL#3 are beneficial for treatment of symptoms in IBS is discussed.*

3. Gosden RG, Feinberg AP, Genetics and epigenetics, Nature's pen-and-pencil set.

*New England Journal of Medicine* 356:731; 2007.
   *Epigenetics refers to inherited changes in gene expression caused by mechanisms other than changes in the underlying DNA sequence. The epigenetic information is more like a code written in pencil in the margins around the DNA, which is written in indelible ink. In many cases it is the epigenome that can be repaired by treatments, or affected by diet, rather than the genetics.*

4. Gropper SS and others: *Advanced nutrition and human metabolism.* 4th ed. Belmont CA: Thomson Wadsworth, 2005.

   *Chapter 2 of this textbook provides a detailed description of the digestive processes of the human body. Students seeking more details about digestion and absorption will find this chapter helpful.*

5. Heartburn. How to relieve the discomfort. *Mayo Clinic Health Letter* 24: 1, 2006.

   *Steps to soothe the fire of heartburn are offered, including foods to limit, medications to take properly, and raising your bed.*

6. Institute of Medicine: *Nutrigenomics and beyond: Informing the future.* Washington, DC: The National Academy Press, 2007.

   *This report summarizes the results of a workshop convened by the Institute of Medicine to review the state of the nutritional genomics research and policy. It includes guidance for further development and translation of this knowledge into nutrition practice and policy.*

7. Jacobson BC and others: Body-mass index and symptoms of gastroesophageal reflux in women. *New England Journal of Medicine* 354:2340, 2006.

   *BMI was associated with symptoms of gastroesophageal reflux disease in 10,545 participants in the Nurses' Health Study. Even moderate weight gain was found to cause or exacerbate symptoms of reflux.*

8. Katsanis SH and others: A case study of personalized medicine. *Science* 320: 53, 2008.

   *Personalized medicine promises to revolutionize health care by tailoring treatments based on individual genetic information. The need for regulating personalized genomic medicine in a manner beneficial to public health is discussed. Currently, in most states companies are not required to demonstrate clinical validity before offering new genetic tests to health care providers and the public.*

9. Layke JC, Lopez PP: Esophageal cancer. A review and update. *American Family Physician* 73:2187, 2006.

   *Esophageal cancer is aggressive and is commonly diagnosed at an advanced stage with a poor prognosis. The associations between the development of esophageal cancer and Helicobacter pylori infection and gastroesophageal reflux disease are discussed along with other factors. Despite the increased use of proton pump inhibitors and the eradication of H. pylori, the number of new cases of esophageal cancer continues to grow.*

10. Lynch A, Webb C: What are the most effective nonpharmacologic therapies for irritable bowel syndrome? *Journal of Family Practice* 57:57, 2008.

    *This article provides insight into recommendations that have been shown to be helpful in the treatment of irritable bowel syndrome. Herbal formulations, certain probiotics, elimination diets based on immunoglobulin G antibodies, cognitive behavioral therapy, and self-help books are discussed because they have been shown to decrease global symptoms of irritable bowel syndrome (IBS) and improve overall quality of life. Hypnosis has been shown to relieve symptoms for patients with severe refractory IBS. Soluble fiber is more effective than insoluble fiber at improving IBS symptoms.*

11. Muller-Lisser and others: Myths and misconceptions about constipation. *American Journal of Gastroenterology* 100:232, 2005.

    *Increasing fiber intake and avoiding dehydration often helps in mild cases of constipation. More difficult cases require a careful physician evaluation and likely the use of laxatives and other medications. Often very helpful, the latter are reviewed in the article.*

12. Niewinski MM: Advances in celiac disease and gluten-free diet. *Journal of the American Dietetic Association* 108:661, 2008.

    *The recognition of celiac disease as a disorder, especially in adults, is increasing. This review focuses on the gluten-free diet and emphasizes the importance for all patients with celiac disease to receive expert dietary counseling. Recent advances in the gluten-free diet are discussed.*

13. Omoruyi O, Holten KB. How should we manage GERD?: The Journal of Family Practice 55:410, 2006.

    *Guidelines for the use of proton pump inhibitors, histamine type 2 receptor antagonists (H$_2$ blockers), and surgery for the treatment of GERD are presented.*

14. Santosa S and others: Probiotics and their potential health claims. *Nutrition Reviews* 64:265, 2006.

    *This paper reviews evidence of the ability of different probiotic strains to prevent and treat diarrhea, treat irritable bowel syndrome, treat inflammatory bowel disease, and prevent colon cancer. The strongest evidence is related to prevention and treatment of diarrhea and some forms of irritable bowel syndrome.*

15. Schardt D: Not everybody must get stones. *Nutrition and Action Healthletter,* p. 89, November 2004.

    *Excess body weight is the primary modifiable risk factor for developing gallbladder stones. Low-fiber diets are also implicated.*

16. Seeley RR and others: *Anatomy and physiology.* 7th ed. Boston: McGraw-Hill, 2006.

    *This text provides comprehensive coverage of the anatomy and physiology of the gastrointestinal tract, as well as other related body systems.*

17. Shanta-Retelny V: Living bacteria: The body's natural defense. *Today's Dietitian,* p. 44, May, 2005.

    *Evidence that bacteria play an important role in health maintenance is discussed. Many interesting "gut flora" facts are presented. In addition, the idea that probiotics can play a therapeutic role in gut health is introduced. It is speculated that new, well-characterized, scientifically proven probiotic strains with specific health benefits will be developed in the future.*

18. Stover PJ: Influence of human genetic variation on nutritional requirements. *American Journal of Clinical Nutrition* 83:436S, 2006.

    *The complexity of the interaction between genes and diet is discussed as well as the opportunities to reevaluate the criteria used to determine RDAs relative to the contribution of genetic variation to optimal nutrition for individuals.*

19. Stover PJ, Caudill MA: Genetic and epigenetic contributions to human nutrition and health: Managing genome-diet interactions. *Journal of the American Dietetic Association* 108:1480, 2008.

    *Nutritional genomics promises to revolutionize clinical and public health nutrition practice. This article discusses ways that nutritional genomics will facilitate the establishment of genome-informed nutrient and food-based dietary guidelines for disease prevention and healthful aging, individualized medical nutrition therapy for disease management, and better targeted public health nutrition interventions that maximize benefits and minimize adverse outcomes within genetically diverse human populations.*

20. The low-down on hemorrhoids. *UC Berkeley Wellness Letter,* p. 4, July, 2004.

    *Hemorrhoids are commonly experienced by many adults. Measures to reduce such risk and as well treat the problem are discussed, such as an adequate fluid and fiber intake. Fortunately hemorrhoids rarely lead to serious health problems.*

## I. Are You Taking Care of Your Digestive Tract?

People need to think about the health of their digestive tracts. There are symptoms we need to notice, as well as habits we need to practice to protect it. The following assessment is designed to help you examine your habits and symptoms associated with the health of your digestive tract. Put a *Y* in the blank to the left of the question to indicate yes and an *N* to indicate no.

_____  1. Are you currently experiencing greater than normal stress and tension?

_____  2. Do you have a family history of digestive tract problems (e.g., ulcers, hemorrhoids, recurrent heartburn, constipation)?

_____  3. Do you experience pain in your stomach region about 2 hours after you eat?

_____  4. Do you smoke cigarettes?

_____  5. Do you take aspirin frequently?

_____  6. Do you have heartburn at least once per week?

_____  7. Do you commonly lie down after eating a large meal?

_____  8. Do you drink alcoholic beverages more than two or three times per day?

_____  9. Do you experience abdominal pain, bloating, or gas 1½ to 2 hours after consuming milk products?

_____  10. Do you often have to strain while having a bowel movement?

_____  11. Do you consume less than 9 (women) or 13 (men) cups of a combination of water and other fluids per day?

_____  12. Do you perform physical activity for less than 60 minutes or more on most or all days of the week (e.g., jog, swim, walk briskly, row, stair climb)?

_____  13. Do you eat a diet relatively low in fiber (recall that significant fiber is found in whole fruits, vegetables, legumes, nuts and seeds, whole-grain breads, and whole-grain cereals)?

_____  14. Do you frequently have diarrhea?

_____  15. Do you frequently use laxatives or antacids?

Add up the number of yes answers and record the total. If your score is from 8 to 15, your habits and symptoms put you at risk for experiencing future digestive tract problems. Take particular note of the habits to which you answered yes. Consider trying to cooperate more with your digestive tract.

## II. Create Your Family Tree for Health-Related Concerns

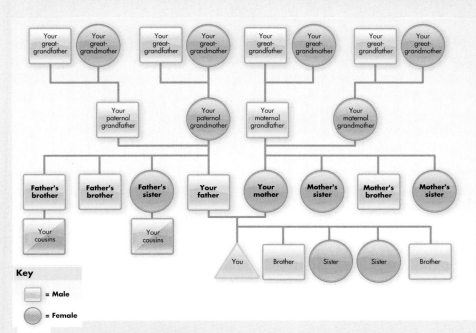

Adapt this diagram to your family tree. Under each heading, list year born, year died (if applicable), major diseases that developed during the person's lifetime, and cause of death (if applicable). Figure 3-22 provides one such example.

You are likely to be at risk for any diseases listed. Creating a plan for preventing such diseases when possible, especially those that developed in your family members before age 50 to 60 years, is advised. Speak with your physician about any concerns arising from this exercise.

# CHAPTER 4 Carbohydrates

## Student Learning Outcomes  After studying Chapter 4 you will be able to:

1. Identify the basic structures and food sources of the major carbohydrates—monosaccharides, disaccharides, polysaccharides (e.g., starches), and fiber.

2. Describe food sources of carbohydrate and list some alternative sweeteners.

3. Explain how carbohydrates are digested and absorbed, including the consequences of lactose maldigestion (and lactose intolerance).

4. List the functions of carbohydrate in the body and the problems that result from not eating enough carbohydrate.

5. Describe the regulation of blood glucose and discuss how other nutrients can be converted to blood glucose.

6. Outline the beneficial effects of fiber on the body.

7. State the RDA for carbohydrate and various guidelines for carbohydrate intake.

8. Identify the consequences of diabetes, and explain appropriate dietary measures that will reduce the adverse effects of this health problem.

## Chapter Outline

Student Learning Outcomes

Refresh Your Memory

4.1 Carbohydrates—An Introduction

4.2 Simple Carbohydrates

4.3 Complex Carbohydrates

4.4 Fiber

4.5 Carbohydrates in Foods

4.6 Making Carbohydrates Available for Body Use

4.7 Putting Simple Carbohydrates to Work in the Body

4.8 Putting Fiber to Work

4.9 Carbohydrate Needs

4.10 Health Concerns Related to Carbohydrate Intake

Nutrition and Your Health: Diabetes—When Blood Glucose Regulation Fails

Case Study: Problems with Milk Intake

Summary/Study Questions/Check Your Knowledge/Further Readings

Rate Your Plate

**WHAT DID YOU EAT TO OBTAIN THE ENERGY YOU ARE USING RIGHT NOW?** Chapters 4, 5, and 6 will examine this question by focusing on the main nutrients the human body uses for fuel. These nutrients are carbohydrates (on average, 4 kcal per gram) and fats and oils (on average, 9 kcal per gram). Although protein (on average, 4 kcal per gram) *can* be used for energy needs, the body typically reserves this nutrient for other processes. Most people know that potatoes are rich in carbohydrates and steak contains mostly fat and protein, but many people do not know how to use this information.

It is likely that you have recently consumed fruits, vegetables, dairy products, cereal, breads, and pasta. These foods supply carbohydrates. Although some carbohydrate sources are more beneficial than others (for example, whole grain bread compared to white bread, as suggested in the Ziggy comic in this chapter), carbohydrates should be a major part of our diets. Many people think carbohydrate-rich foods are fattening but they are not any more so than fat or protein. In fact, pound for pound, carbohydrates are much less fattening than fats and oils. Furthermore, high-carbohydrate foods, especially fiber-rich foods such as fruits, vegetables, whole-grain breads and cereals, and legumes, provide many important health benefits in addition to the calories they contain. Some people think sugars cause hyperactivity in children—not so, according to well-designed scientific investigations. Almost all carbohydrate-rich foods, except pure sugars, provide several essential nutrients and should generally constitute 45% to 65% of our daily calorie intake. Let's take a closer look at carbohydrates, including why the recent craze of carbohydrate-bashing was misguided.

 **Refresh Your Memory**

As you begin your study of carbohydrates in Chapter 4, you may want to review:

- The concept of energy density and the health claims for various carbohydrates in Chapter 2
- The processes of digestion and absorption in Chapter 3
- The hormones that regulate blood glucose in Chapter 3

## 4.1 Carbohydrates—An Introduction

Carbohydrates are a main fuel source for some cells, especially those in the brain, nervous system, and red blood cells. Muscles also rely on a dependable supply of carbohydrate to fuel intense physical activity. Carbohydrates provide on average 4 kcal per gram and are a readily available fuel for all cells, both in the form of blood glucose and **glycogen** stored in the liver and muscles. The glycogen stored in the liver can be used to maintain blood glucose concentrations in times when you have not eaten for several hours or the diet does not supply enough carbohydrate. Regular intake of carbohydrate is important, because liver glycogen stores are depleted in about 18 hours if no carbohydrate is consumed. After that point, the body is forced to produce carbohydrate, largely from breakdown of proteins in the body. This eventually leads to health problems including the loss of muscle tissue. To obtain adequate energy, the Food and Nutrition Board recommends that 45% to 65% of the calories we consume each day be from carbohydrates. (See the Acceptable Macronutrient Distribution Range table in the DRI charts in the back pages of this book.)

**glycogen** A carbohydrate made of multiple units of glucose with a highly branched structure. It is the storage form of glucose in humans and is synthesized (and stored) in the liver and muscles.

The class of carbohydrate that has gained the most attention recently is fiber. Why is this so? As Ziggy is reminded, White bread is a poor source of fiber. Which health problems typically result from a limited intake of fiber? Which foods are good sources of fiber? How much fiber is enough? Too much? Chapter 4 provides some answers.

Humans have sensors on our tongues that recognize the sweetness of carbohydrates. Researchers speculate that this sweetness indicated a safe energy source to early humans, and so it became an important energy source.

Despite their important role as a calorie source, some forms of carbohydrate promote health more than others. As you will see in this chapter, whole-grain breads and cereals have greater health benefits than refined and processed forms of carbohydrate. Choosing the healthiest carbohydrate sources most often, while moderating intake of less healthful sources, contributes to a healthy diet. It is difficult to eat so little carbohydrate that body fuel needs are not met, but it is easy to overconsume the simple carbohydrates that can contribute to health problems. Let's explore this concept further as we look at carbohydrates in detail.

Green plants create the carbohydrates in our foods. Leaves capture the sun's solar energy in their cells and transform it to chemical energy. This energy is then stored in the chemical bonds of the carbohydrate glucose as it is produced from carbon dioxide from the air and water from the soil. This complex process is called **photosynthesis** (Fig. 4-1).

$$\text{6 carbon dioxide} + \text{6 water (solar energy)} \rightarrow \text{glucose} + \text{6 oxygen}$$
$$(CO_2) \qquad\qquad (H_2O) \qquad\quad (C_2H_{12}O_6) \quad (O_2)$$

Translated into English, this reads: 6 molecules of carbon dioxide combine with 6 molecules of water to form one molecule of **glucose**. Converting solar energy into chemical bonds in the sugar is a key part of the process. Six molecules of oxygen are then released into the air.

## 4.2 Simple Carbohydrates

As the name suggests, most carbohydrate molecules are composed of carbon, hydrogen, and oxygen atoms. Simple forms of carbohydrates are called **sugars**. Larger, more complex forms are primarily called either **starches** or **fibers**, depending on their digestibility by human GI tract enzymes. Starches are the digestible form. The Concept Map on pg. 127 summarizes the forms and characteristics of carbohydrates.

Monosaccharides and disaccharides are often referred to as *simple sugars* because they contain only one or two sugar units. Food labels lump all of these sugars under one category, listing them as "sugars."

▲ Fruits such as oranges and pears are an excellent source of carbohydrate, including sugar, starch, and fiber.

**photosynthesis** Process by which plants use energy from the sun to synthesize energy-yielding compounds, such as glucose.

**glucose** A six-carbon monosaccharide that usually exists in a ring form; found as such in blood, and in table sugar bonded to fructose; also known as *dextrose*.

**sugar** A simple carbohydrate with the chemical composition $(CH_2O)_n$. The basic unit of all sugars is glucose, a six-carbon ring structure. The primary sugar in the diet is sucrose, which is made up of glucose and fructose.

**starch** A carbohydrate made of multiple units of glucose attached together in a form the body can digest; also known as *complex carbohydrate*.

**fiber** Substances in plant foods not digested by the processes that take place in the stomach or small intestine. These add bulk to feces. Fibers naturally found in foods are also called dietary fiber.

**6 carbon dioxide (CO$_2$) + 6 water (H$_2$O)**

Sun

**Energy** →

**Glucose (C$_6$H$_{12}$O$_6$) + 6 oxygen (O$_2$)**

**FIGURE 4-1** ▶ A summary of photosynthesis. Plants use carbon dioxide, water, and energy to produce glucose. Glucose is then stored in the leaf but can also undergo further metabolism to form starch and fiber in the plant. With the addition of nitrogen from soil or air, glucose also can be transformed into protein.

**FIGURE 4-2** ▶ Chemical forms of the important monosaccharides.

**Monosaccharides**

Glucose            Fructose            Galactose

## Monosaccharides—Glucose, Fructose, and Galactose

**Monosaccharides** are the simple sugar units (*mono* means one) that serve as the basic unit of all carbohydrate structures. The most common monosaccharides in foods are glucose, fructose, and galactose (Fig. 4-2).

Glucose is the major monosaccharide found in the body. Glucose is also known as *dextrose,* and glucose in the bloodstream may be called blood sugar. Glucose is an important source of energy for human cells, although foods contain very little carbohydrate as this single sugar. Most glucose comes from the digestion of starches and **sucrose** (common table sugar) from our food. The latter is made up of the monosaccharides glucose and fructose. For the most part, sugars and other carbohydrates in foods are eventually converted to glucose in the liver. This glucose then goes on to serve as a source of fuel for cells.

**Fructose,** also called *fruit sugar,* is another common monosaccharide. After it is consumed, fructose is absorbed by the small intestine and then transported to the liver, where it is quickly metabolized. Much is converted to glucose, but the rest goes on to form other compounds, such as fat, if fructose is consumed in very high amounts. Most of the free fructose in our diets comes from the use of **high-fructose corn syrup** in soft drinks, candies, jams, jellies, and many other fruit products and desserts (see the later discussion on nutritive sweeteners). Fructose also is found naturally in fruits and forms half of each sucrose molecule, as previously noted.

The sugar **galactose** has nearly the same structure as glucose. Large quantities of pure galactose do not exist in nature. Instead, galactose is usually found bonded to glucose in **lactose,** a sugar found in milk and other milk products. After lactose is digested and absorbed, galactose arrives in the liver. There it is either transformed into glucose or further metabolized into glycogen.

**sucrose**  Fructose bonded to glucose; table sugar.

**fructose**  A six-carbon monosaccharide that usually exists in a ring form; found in fruits and honey; also known as *fruit sugar.*

**galactose**  A six-carbon monosaccharide that usually exists in a ring form; closely related to glucose.

**lactose**  Glucose bonded to galactose; also known as *milk sugar.*

**maltose**  Glucose bonded to glucose.

---

### MAKING DECISIONS

#### Nutrient Metabolism

Now is a good time to begin emphasizing a key concept in nutrition: the difference between *intake* of a substance and the body's *use* of that substance. The body often does not use all nutrients in their original states. Some of these substances are broken down and later reassembled into the same or a different substance when and where they are needed. For example, much of the galactose in the diet is metabolized to glucose. When later required for the production of milk in the mammary gland of a lactating female, galactose is resynthesized from glucose to help form the milk sugar lactose. Knowing this, do you think it is necessary for a lactating women to drink milk to make milk?

---

## Disaccharides—Sucrose, Lactose, and Maltose

**Disaccharides** are formed when two monosaccharides combine (*di* means two). The disaccharides in food are sucrose, lactose, and **maltose**. All contain glucose.

## Disaccharides

Sucrose:  glucose + fructose
Lactose:  glucose + galactose
Maltose:  glucose + glucose

CH$_2$OH

Sucrose

**FIGURE 4-3** ▶ Chemical form of the disaccharide sucrose.

Sucrose forms when the two sugars glucose and fructose bond together (Fig. 4-3). Sucrose is found naturally in sugarcane, sugar beets, honey, and maple sugar. These products are processed to varying degrees to make brown, white, and powdered sugars. Animals do not produce sucrose or much of any carbohydrate except glycogen.

Lactose forms when glucose bonds with galactose during the synthesis of milk. Again, our major food source for lactose is milk products. A later section on lactose maldigestion and lactose intolerance discusses the problems that result when a person can't readily digest lactose.

◀ This Concept Map summarizes the various forms and characteristics of the simple and complex carbohydrates.

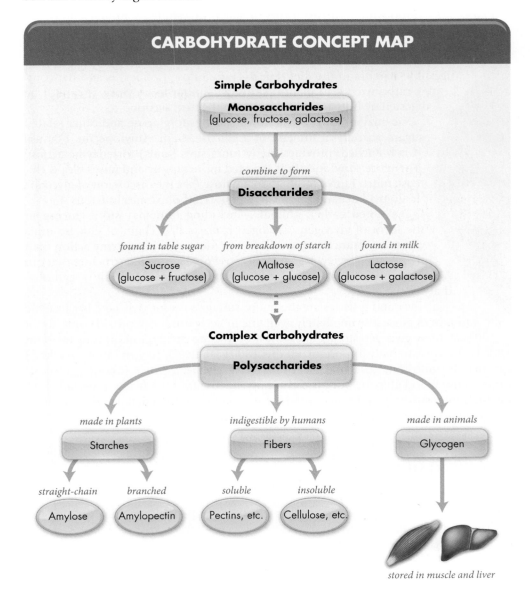

## CARBOHYDRATE CONCEPT MAP

**Simple Carbohydrates**

**Monosaccharides**
(glucose, fructose, galactose)

*combine to form*

**Disaccharides**

*found in table sugar*
Sucrose
(glucose + fructose)

*from breakdown of starch*
Maltose
(glucose + glucose)

*found in milk*
Lactose
(glucose + galactose)

**Complex Carbohydrates**

**Polysaccharides**

*made in plants*
Starches

*indigestible by humans*
Fibers

*made in animals*
Glycogen

*straight-chain*
Amylose

*branched*
Amylopectin

*soluble*
Pectins, etc.

*insoluble*
Cellulose, etc.

*stored in muscle and liver*

Maltose results when starch is broken down to just two glucose molecules bonded together. Maltose plays an important role in the beer and liquor industry. In the production of alcoholic beverages, starches in various cereal grains are first converted to simpler carbohydrates by enzymes present in the grains. The products of this step—maltose, glucose, and other sugars—are then mixed with yeast cells in the absence of oxygen. The yeast cells convert most of the sugars to alcohol (ethanol) and carbon dioxide, a process called **fermentation**. Little maltose remains in the final product. Few other food products or beverages contain maltose. In fact, most maltose that we ultimately digest in the small intestine is produced during our own digestion of starch.

**fermentation** The conversion of carbohydrates to alcohols, acids, and carbon dioxide without the use of oxygen.

**polysaccharides** Carbohydrates containing many glucose units, from 10 to 1000 or more.

**amylose** A digestible straight-chain type of starch composed of glucose units.

**amylopectin** A digestible branched-chain type of starch composed of glucose units.

## 4.3 Complex Carbohydrates

In many foods, single-sugar units are bonded together to form a chain, known as a polysaccharide (*poly* means many). **Polysaccharides**, also called *complex carbohydrates* or *starch*, may contain 1000 or more glucose units and are found chiefly in grains, vegetables, and fruits. When food labels list "Other Carbohydrates," this primarily refers to starch content.

Plants store carbohydrate in two forms of starch digestible by humans: **amylose** and **amylopectin**. Amylose, a long, straight chain of glucose units, comprises about 20% of the digestible starch found in vegetables, beans, breads, pasta, and rice. Amylopectin is a highly branched chain and makes up the remaining 80% of digestible starches in the diet (Fig. 4-4). Cellulose (a fiber) is another complex carbohydrate in plants. Although similar to amylose, it cannot be digested by humans, as discussed in the next section.

The enzymes that break down starches to glucose and other related sugars act only at the end of a glucose chain. Amylopectin, because it is branched, provides many more sites (ends) for enzyme action. Therefore, amylopectin is digested more rapidly and raises blood glucose much more readily than amylose (see the discussion of glycemic load in a later section of Chapter 4, "Carbohydrates in Foods").

As noted earlier, animals—including humans—store glucose in the form of glycogen. Glycogen consists of a chain of glucose units with many branches, providing even more sites for enzyme action than amylopectin (review Fig. 4-4). Because of its branched structure that can be broken down quickly, glycogen is an ideal storage form of carbohydrate in the body.

The liver and muscles are the major storage sites for glycogen. Because the amount of glucose immediately available in body fluids can provide only about 120 kcal, these glycogen storage sites for carbohydrate energy—amounting to about 1800 kcal—are extremely important. Of this 1800 kcal, liver glycogen (about 400 kcal) can readily contribute to blood glucose. Muscle glycogen stores (about 1400 kcal) cannot raise blood glucose, but instead supply glucose for muscle use, especially during high-intensity and endurance exercise (see Chapter 10 for a detailed discussion of carbohydrate use in exercise).

▲ Root vegetables such as potato, yams and tapioca are high in amylopectin starch.

### MAKING DECISIONS

#### Animal Sources of Carbohydrates

If animals store glycogen in their muscles, are meats, fish, and poultry a good source of carbohydrates? No—animal products are not good food sources of this (or any other) carbohydrate because glycogen stores quickly degrade after the animal dies.

**FIGURE 4-4 ►** Some common starches and glycogen. We consume essentially no glycogen. All glycogen found in the body is made by our cells, primarily in the liver and muscles.

## 4.4 Fiber

Fiber as a class is mostly made up of polysaccharides, but they differ from starches insofar as the chemical links that join the individual sugar units cannot be digested by human enzymes in the GI tract. This prevents the small intestine from absorbing the sugars that make up the various fibers. Fiber is not a single substance but a group of substances with similar characteristics (Table 4-1). The group is comprised of the carbohydrates **cellulose**, **hemicelluloses**, **pectins**, **gums**, and **mucilages**, as well as the noncarbohydrate, **lignin**. In total, these constitute all the nonstarch polysaccharides in foods. Nutrition Facts labels generally do not list these individual forms of fiber, but instead lump them together under the term **dietary fiber**.

Cellulose, hemicelluloses, and lignin form the structural parts of plants. Bran fiber is rich in hemicelluloses and lignin. (The woody fibers in broccoli are partly lignin.) Bran layers form the outer covering of all grains, so **whole grains** (i.e., unrefined) are good sources of bran fiber (Fig. 4-5). Because the majority of these fibers neither readily dissolve in water nor are easily metabolized by intestinal bacteria, they are called **nonfermentable** or insoluble fibers.

Pectins, gums, and mucilages are contained around and inside plant cells. These fibers either dissolve or swell when put into water and are therefore called **viscous** or soluble fibers. They also are readily fermented by bacteria in the large intestine. These fibers are found in salad dressings, some frozen desserts, jams, and jellies as gum arabic, guar gum, locust bean gum, and various pectin forms. Some forms of hemicelluloses also fall into the soluble category.

Most foods contain mixtures of soluble and insoluble fibers. Food labels do not generally distinguish between the two types, but, manufacturers have the option to do so. Often, if food is listed as a good source of one type of fiber, it usually contains some

**cellulose** An undigestible nonfermentable straight-chain polysaccharide made of glucose molecules.

**hemicellulose** A nonfermentable fiber containing xylose, galactose, glucose, and other monosaccharides bonded together.

**pectin** A viscous fiber containing chains of galacturonic acid and other monosaccharides; characteristically found between plant cell walls.

**mucilages** A viscous fiber consisting of chains of galactose, mannose, and other monosaccharides; characteristically found in seaweed.

**lignins** A nonfermentable fiber made up of a multiringed alcohol (noncarbohydrate) structure.

**dietary fiber** Fiber found in food.

**whole grains** Grains containing the entire seed of the plant, including the bran, germ, and endosperm (starchy interior). Examples are whole-wheat and brown rice.

**nonfermentable fiber** A fiber that is not easily metabolized by intestinal bacteria.

**TABLE 4-1** Classification of Fibers

| Type | Component(s) | Physiological Effects | Major Food Sources |
|---|---|---|---|
| **Nonfermentable or Insoluble** | | | |
| Noncarbohydrate form | Lignin | Increases fecal bulk | Whole grains, wheat bran |
| Carbohydrate form | Cellulose, hemicelluloses | Increases fecal bulk Decreases intestinal transit time | All plants, wheat products Wheat, rye, rice, vegetables |
| **Viscous or Soluble** | | | |
| Carbohydrate form | Pectins, gums, mucilages, some hemicelluloses | Delays stomach emptying; slows glucose absorption; can lower blood cholesterol | Citrus fruits, apples, bananas, oat products, carrots, barley, beans, thickeners added to foods |

**FIGURE 4-5** ▶ Viscous and nonfermentable fiber. (a) The skin of an apple consists of the nonfermentable fiber cellulose, which provides structure for the fruit. The viscous fiber pectin "glues" the fruit cells together. (b) The outside layer of a wheat kernel is made of layers of bran—primarily hemicellulose, a nonfermentable fiber—making this whole grain a good source of fiber. Overall, fruits, vegetables, whole-grain breads and cereals, and beans are rich in fiber.

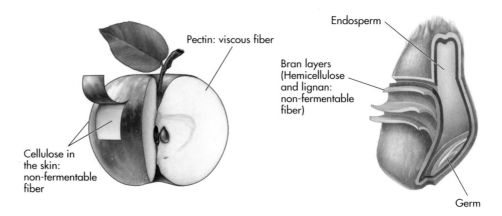

**viscous fiber** A fiber that is readily fermented by bacteria in the large intestine.

**functional fiber** Fiber added to foods that has been shown to provide health benefits.

**total fiber** Combination of dietary fiber and functional fiber in a food. Also just called *fiber*.

of the other type of fiber as well. The definition of fiber has recently been expanded to include both the dietary fiber found naturally in foods and additional fiber that is added to foods. This second category is called **functional fiber;** a fiber of this type must show beneficial effects in humans to be included in the category. **Total fiber** (or just the term *fiber*) is then the combination of dietary fiber and functional fiber in the food product. Currently the Nutrition Facts label only includes the category dietary fiber; the label has yet to be updated to reflect the latest definition of fiber.

A newly studied category of functional fiber are the prebiotics. Prebiotics include a group of short-chain carbohydrates or oligosaccharides, resistant to digestion, but fermented by bacteria in the colon. They are thought to stimulate the growth or activity of beneficial bacteria in the large intestine and therefore promote the host's health.

### CONCEPT CHECK

Important monosaccharides in nutrition are glucose, fructose, and galactose. Glucose is a primary energy source for body cells. Disaccharides form when two monosaccharides bond together. Important disaccharides in nutrition are sucrose (glucose + fructose), maltose (glucose + glucose), and lactose (glucose + galactose). Once digested into monosaccharides and absorbed, most carbohydrates are transformed into glucose by the liver.

Amylose, amylopectin, and glycogen are all polysaccharides, which function as storage forms of glucose. Amylose and amylopectin are the major digestible plant polysaccharides and contain multiple glucose units bonded together. Glycogen is a storage form of glucose in our liver and muscle cells.

Fiber is essentially the portion of plant food that remains undigested as it enters the large intestine. There are two general classes of fiber: nonfermentable and viscous. Nonfermentable (insoluble) fibers are mostly made up of cellulose, hemicelluloses, and lignins. Viscous (soluble) fibers are made up mostly of pectins, gums, and mucilages. Both nonfermentable and viscous fibers are resistant to human digestive enzymes, but bacteria in the large intestine can break down viscous fibers.

## 4.5 Carbohydrates in Foods

The food components that yield the highest percentage of calories from carbohydrates are table sugar, honey, jam, jelly, fruit, and plain baked potatoes (Fig. 4-6). Corn flakes, rice, bread, and noodles all contain at least 75% of calories as carbohydrates. Foods with moderate amounts of carbohydrate calories are peas, broccoli, oatmeal, dry beans and other legumes, cream pies, French fries, and fat-free milk. In these foods, the carbohydrate content is diluted either by protein, as in the case of fat-free milk, or by fat, as in the case of a cream pie. Foods with essentially no carbohydrates include beef, eggs, chicken, fish, vegetable oils, butter, and margarine.

## Food Sources of Carbohydrate

| Food Item | Carbohydrate (grams) | % RDA |
|---|---|---|
| **RDA** | 130 | 100% |
| Baked potato, 1 each | 51 | 39% |
| Cola drink, 12 fluid oz | 39 | 30% |
| Plain M&M's, ½ oz | 30 | 23% |
| Banana, 1 each | 28 | 22% |
| Cooked rice, ½ cup | 22 | 17% |
| Cooked corn, ½ cup | 21 | 16% |
| Light yogurt, 1 cup | 19 | 15% |
| Kidney beans, ½ cup | 19 | 15% |
| Spaghetti noodles, ½ cup | 19 | 15% |
| Orange, 1 each | 16 | 12% |
| Seven grain bread, 1 slice | 12 | 9% |
| Fat-free milk, 1 cup | 12 | 9% |
| Pineapple chunks, ½ cup | 10 | 8% |
| Cooked carrots, ½ cup | 8 | 6% |
| Peanuts, 1 ounce | 6 | 5% |

**Key:**
- Grains
- Vegetables
- Fruits
- Oils
- Milk
- Meat & Beans
- Discretionary calories

**FIGURE 4-6** ▶ Food sources of carbohydrates compared to the RDA of 130 grams for carbohydrate.

The percentage of calories from carbohydrate is more important than the total amount of carbohydrate in a food when planning a healthy high-carbohydrate diet. Figure 4-7 shows that the grain, vegetable, fruit, and milk groups contain the most nutrient-dense sources of carbohydrate. In planning a high-carbohydrate diet, you need to emphasize grains, pasta, fruits, and vegetables. On the other hand, you can't create a diet high in carbohydrate calories from chocolate, potato chips, and French fries because these foods contain too much fat. Currently, the top five carbohydrate sources for U.S. adults are white bread, soft drinks, cookies and cakes (including doughnuts), sugars/syrups/jams, and potatoes. Clearly, many North Americans (teenagers included) should take a closer look at their main carbohydrate sources and strive to improve them from a nutritional standpoint by including more whole grains, fruits, and vegetables.

## Starch

Starches contribute much of the carbohydrate in our diets. Recall that plants store glucose as polysaccharides in the form of starches. Thus, plant-based foods, such as legumes, tubers, and the grains (wheat, rye, corn, oats, barley, and rice) used to make breads, cereals, and pasta, are the best sources of starch. A diet rich in these starches provides ample carbohydrate, as well as many micronutrients.

## Fiber

Fiber can be found in many of the same foods as starch, so a diet rich in grains, legumes, and tubers also can provide significant amounts of dietary fiber (especially insoluble cellulose, hemicellulose, and lignins). Because much of the fiber in whole

▲ Breads are a rich source of carbohydrate, especially starch and fiber.

## MyPyramid: Sources of Carbohydrates

| Food Group | Grains | Vegetables | Fruits | Oils | Milk | Meat & Beans | |
|---|---|---|---|---|---|---|---|
| **Sources of Carbohydrate** | • All varieties | • All varieties | • All varieties | • None | • Milk<br>• Yogurt | • Beans | • Nuts |
| **Grams per Serving** | 15 | 5 | 18 | 0 | 12 | 10 | 4 |

**FIGURE 4-7 ▶** Sources of carbohydrates from MyPyramid. The height of the background color (none, 1/3, 2/3, or completely covered) within each group in the pyramid indicates the average nutrient density for carbohydrate in that group. Overall, the grain group, vegetable group, fruit group, and milk group contain many foods that are nutrient-dense sources of carbohydrate. With regard to physical activity, carbohydrates are a key fuel in most endeavors.

grains is found in the outer layers, which are removed in processing, highly processed grains are low in fiber. Soluble fibers (pectin, gums, mucilages) are found in the skins and flesh of many fruits and berries; as thickeners and stabilizers in jams, yogurts, sauces, and fillings; and in products that contain psyllium and seaweed.

For individuals who have difficulties consuming adequate dietary fiber, fiber is available as a supplement or as an additive to certain foods (functional fiber). In this way, individuals with relatively low dietary fiber intakes can still obtain the health benefits of fiber.

### Nutritive Sweeteners

The various substances that impart sweetness to foods fall into two broad classes: nutritive sweeteners, which can provide calories for the body; and alternative sweeteners, which for the most part provide no calories. As shown in Table 4-2, the alternative sweeteners are much sweeter on a per-gram basis than the nutritive sweeteners. The taste and sweetness of sucrose make it the benchmark against which all other sweeteners are measured. Sucrose is obtained from sugar cane and sugar beet plants. Both sugars and sugar alcohols provide calories along with sweetness. Sugars are found in many different food products, whereas sugar alcohols have rather limited uses.

**Sugars.** All of the monosaccharides (glucose, fructose, and galactose) and disaccharides (sucrose, lactose, and maltose) discussed earlier are designated *nutritive sweeteners*

**TABLE 4-2** The Sweetness of Sugars (Nutritive) and Alternative Sweeteners

| Type of Sweetener | Relative Sweetness*<br>(Sucrose = 1) | Typical Sources |
|---|---|---|
| **Sugars** | | |
| Lactose | 0.2 | Dairy products |
| Maltose | 0.4 | Sprouted seeds |
| Glucose | 0.7 | Corn syrup |
| Sucrose | 1.0 | Table sugar, most sweets |
| Invert sugar[†] | 1.3 | Some candies, honey |
| Fructose | 1.2–1.8 | Fruit, honey, some soft drinks |
| **Sugar Alcohols** | | |
| Sorbitol | 0.6 | Dietetic candies, sugarless gum |
| Mannitol | 0.7 | Dietetic candies |
| Xylitol | 0.9 | Sugarless gum |
| Maltitol | 0.9 | Baked goods, chocolate, candies |
| **Alternative Sweeteners** | | |
| Tagatose Naturlose® | 0.9 | Ready-to-eat breakfast cereals, diet soft drinks, meal replacement bars, frozen desserts, candy, frosting |
| Cyclamate[‡] | 30 | Tabletop sweetener, medicines |
| Aspartame (Equal®) | 180 | Diet soft drinks, diet fruit drinks, sugarless gum, powdered diet sweetener |
| Acesulfame-K (Sunette®) | 200 | Sugarless gum, diet drink mixes, powdered diet sweeteners, puddings, gelatin desserts |
| Saccharin (sodium salt) (Sweet'N Low®) | 300 | Diet soft drinks, powdered diet sweetener |
| Sucralose (Splenda®) | 600 | Diet soft drinks, powdered diet sweetener, sugarless gums, jams, frozen desserts |
| Neotame | 7000 to 13,000 | Powdered diet sweetener, baked goods, frozen desserts, jams |

*On a per gram basis.

[†]Sucrose broken down into glucose and fructose.

[‡]Not available in the United States, but available in Canada.

From the American Dietetic Association, 2004, and other sources.

▲ Soft drinks are typical sources of either sugars or alternative sweeteners, depending on the type of soft drink chosen.

(Table 4-3). Many forms of sugar are used in food products and result in an intake of about 82 grams or 16 teaspoons of sugar per day.

High-fructose corn syrup, generally 55% fructose, is used extensively in the food industry. High-fructose corn syrup is made by treating cornstarch with acid and enzymes. This treatment breaks down much of the starch into glucose. Then some of the glucose is converted by enzymes into fructose. The final syrup is usually as sweet as sucrose. Its major advantage is that it is cheaper than sucrose. Also, it doesn't form crystals and it has better freezing properties. High-fructose corn syrups are used in soft drinks, candies, jam, jelly, other fruit products, and desserts (e.g., packaged cookies).

In addition to sucrose and high-fructose corn syrup, brown sugar, turbinado sugar (sold as raw sugar), honey, maple syrup, and other sugars are also added to foods.

▲ There are many forms of sugar on the market. Used in many foods, together they contribute to our daily intake of approximately 82 grams (16 teaspoons) of sugars in our diets.

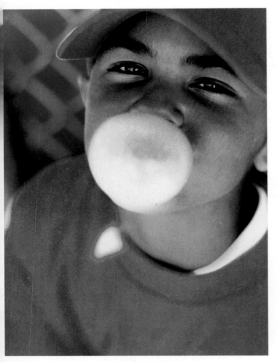

▲ Sugarless gum is typically sweetened with sugar alcohols.

**sorbitol** Alcohol derivative of glucose that yields about 3 kcal/g but is slowly absorbed from the small intestine; used in some sugarless gums and dietetic foods.

**xylitol** Alcohol derivative of the 5-carbon monosaccharide xylose.

**TABLE 4-3** Names of Sugars Used in Foods

| | | | |
|---|---|---|---|
| Sugar | Invert sugar | Honey | Maple syrup |
| Sucrose | Glucose | Corn syrup or sweeteners | Dextrose |
| Brown sugar | Sorbitol | | Fructose |
| Confectioner's sugar (powdered sugar) | Levulose | High-fructose corn syrup | Maltodextrins |
| | Polydextrose | Molasses | Caramel |
| Turbinado sugar | Lactose | Date sugar | Fruit sugar |

Brown sugar is essentially sucrose containing some molasses; either the molasses is not totally removed from the sucrose during processing or it is added to the sucrose crystals. Turbinado sugar, a partially refined version of raw sucrose, has a slight molasses flavor.

Maple syrup is made by boiling down and concentrating the sap that runs during the late winter in sugar maple trees. Most pancake syrup sold in supermarkets is not pure maple syrup, which is expensive. Instead, it is primarily corn syrup and high-fructose corn syrup with maple flavor added.

Honey is a product of plant nectar that has been altered by bee enzymes. The enzymes break down much of the nectar's sucrose into fructose and glucose. Honey offers essentially the same nutritional value as other simple sugars—a source of energy and little else. However, honey is not safe to feed to infants because it can contain spores of the bacterium *Clostridium botulinum*. These spores can become the bacteria that cause fatal food-borne illness. Honey does not pose the same threat to adults because the acidic environment of an adult's stomach inhibits the growth of the bacteria. An infant's stomach, however, does not produce much acid, making infants susceptible to the threat that this bacterium poses.

**Sugar Alcohols** Food manufacturers and consumers have numerous options for obtaining sweetness while consuming less sugar and calories. Overall, sugar alcohols and alternative sweeteners enable people with diabetes to enjoy the flavor of sweetness while controlling sugars in their diets; they also provide noncaloric or very-low-calorie sugar substitutes for persons trying to lose (or control) body weight.

Sugar alcohols such as **sorbitol** and **xylitol** are used as nutritive sweeteners. Sugar alcohols contribute fewer calories (about 2.6 kcal per gram) than sugars. They also are absorbed and metabolized to glucose more slowly than are simple sugars. Because of this, they remain in the intestinal tract for a longer time and in large quantities can cause diarrhea. In fact, any products that may be consumed in amounts that may result in a daily ingestion of 50 grams of sugar alcohols, must bear this labeling statement: "Excess consumption may have a laxative effect."

Sugar alcohols are used in sugarless gum, breath mints, and candy. Unlike sucrose, sugar alcohols are not readily metabolized by bacteria to acids in the mouth and thus do not promote tooth decay (see the later section on problems linked to carbohydrate intake).

Sugar alcohols must be listed on labels. If only one sugar alcohol is used in a product, its name must be listed. However, if two or more are used in one product, they are grouped together under the heading "sugar alcohols." The caloric value of each sugar alcohol used in a food product is calculated so that when one reads the total amount of calories a product provides, it includes the sugar alcohols in the overall amount.

## Alternative Sweeteners

Often called artificial sweeteners, alternative sweeteners include **saccharin**, cyclamate, **aspartame**, **sucralose**, **neotame**, and **acesulfame-K**. Unlike sugar alcohols, alternative sweeteners yield little or no calories when consumed in amounts typically used in food products. Six are currently available in the United States: saccharin, aspartame, sucralose, neotame, acesulfame-K, and tagatose. Cyclamate was banned for use in the United States in 1970, although it has never been conclusively proven to cause health problems when used appropriately. Cyclamate is used in Canada as a sweetener in medicines and as a tabletop sweetener.

The safety of sweeteners is determined by the FDA and is indicated by an **Acceptable Daily Intake (ADI)** guideline. The ADI is the amount of alternative sweetener considered safe for daily use over one's lifetime. ADIs are based on studies in laboratory animals and are set at a level 100 times less than the level at which no harmful effects were noted in animal studies. Alternative sweeteners can be used safely by adults and children. Although general use is considered safe during pregnancy, pregnant women may want to discuss this issue with their health-care providers.

**Saccharin.** The oldest alternative sweetener, saccharin, was first produced in 1879 and is currently approved for use in more than 90 countries. It represents about half of the alternative sweetener market in North America (typically packaged in pink packets, including Sweet 'N Low®). Based on laboratory animal studies, saccharin was once thought to increase the risk of bladder cancer but it is no longer listed as a potential cause of cancer.

**Aspartame.** Aspartame is in widespread use throughout the world (typically packaged in blue packets, including Equal®). It has been approved for use by more than 90 countries, and its use has been endorsed by the World Health Organization, the American Medical Association, the American Diabetes Association, and other groups.

The components of aspartame are the amino acids phenylalanine and aspartic acid, along with methanol. Recall that amino acids are the building blocks of proteins, so aspartame is more of a protein than a carbohydrate. Aspartame yields about 4 kcal per gram, but it is about 200 times sweeter than sucrose. Thus, only a small amount of aspartame is needed to obtain the desired sweetness, and the amount of calories added is insignificant unless the product is consumed in unusually high amounts. Aspartame is used in beverages, gelatin desserts, chewing gum, toppings and fillings in precooked bakery goods, and cookies. Aspartame does not cause tooth decay. Like other proteins, however, aspartame is damaged when heated for a long time and thus would lose its sweetness if used in products requiring cooking.

Some complaints have been filed with FDA by people claiming to have had adverse reactions to aspartame: headaches, dizziness, seizures, nausea, and other side effects. It is important for people who are sensitive to aspartame to avoid it, but the percentage of sensitive people is likely to be extremely small.

The acceptable daily intake of aspartame set by FDA is 50 milligrams per kilogram of body weight. This is equivalent to the aspartame in about 14 cans of diet soft drink for an adult or about 80 packets of Equal®. Aspartame appears to be safe for pregnant women and children, but some scientists suggest cautious use by these groups, especially young children, who need ample calories to grow.

**Sucralose.** Sucralose (Splenda®) is 600 times sweeter than sucrose. It is made by adding three chlorines to sucrose. Sucralose is approved for use as an additive to foods such as soft drinks, gum, baked goods, syrups, gelatins, frozen dairy desserts such as ice cream, jams, processed fruits and fruit juices, and for tabletop use. Sucralose doesn't break down under high heat conditions and can be used in cooking and baking. It is also excreted as such in the feces. The small amount absorbed is excreted in the urine.

---

**S**ugar alcohols as a class are also called polyols.

**saccharin** Alternative sweetener that yields no energy to the body; 300 times sweeter than sucrose.

**aspartame** Alternative sweetener made of 2 amino acids and methanol; about 200 times sweeter than sucrose.

**sucralose** Alternative sweetener that has chlorines in place of 3 hydroxyl (—OH) groups on sucrose; 600 times sweeter than sucrose.

**neotame** General-purpose, non-nutritive sweetener that is approximately 7000 to 13,000 times sweeter than table sugar. It has a chemical structure similar to aspartame's. Neotame is heat stable and can be used as a tabletop sweetener, as well as in cooking applications. It is not broken down to its amino acid components in the body after consumption.

**P**ersons with an uncommon disease called **phenylketonuria (PKU),** which interferes with the metabolism of phenylalanine, should avoid aspartame because of its high phenylalanine content. A warning label is required on products containing aspartame, alerting people with PKU that a product with aspartame contains phenylalanine.

INGREDIENTS: SORBITOL, GUM BASE, MANNITOL, GLYCEROL, HYDROGENATED GLUCOSE SYRUP, XYLITOL, ARTIFICIAL AND NATURAL FLAVORS, ASPARTAME, RED 40, YELLOW 6 AND BHT (TO MAINTAIN FRESHNESS). PHENYLKETONURICS: CONTAINS PHENYLALANINE.

*Sugarless Gum*

▲ Sugar alcohols and the alternative sweetener aspartame are used to sweeten this product. Note the warning for people with phenylketonuria PKU that this product is made with aspartame and, thus, contains phenylalanine.

**acesulfame K** Alternative sweetener that yields no energy to the body; 200 times sweeter than sucrose.

**Acceptable Daily Intake (ADI)** Estimate of the amount of a sweetener that an individual can safely consume daily over a lifetime. ADIs are given as mg per kg of body weight per day.

**phenylketonuria (PKU)** Disease caused by a defect in the liver's ability to metabolize the amino acid phenylalanine into the amino acid tyrosine; untreated, toxic by-products of phenylalanine build up in the body and lead to mental retardation.

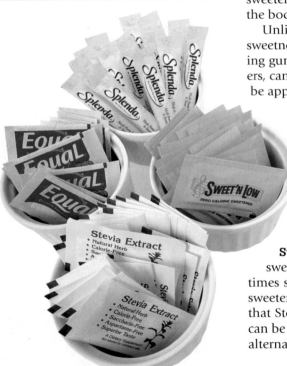

▲ A variety of alternative sweeteners are available.

**Neotame.** Neotame was recently approved by FDA for use as a general-purpose sweetener in a wide variety of food products, other than meat and poultry. Neotame is a nonnutritive, high-intensity sweetener that, depending on its food application, is approximately 7000 to 13,000 times sweeter than table sugar. It has a chemical structure similar to aspartame. Neotame is heat stable and can be used as a tabletop sweetener as well as in cooking applications. Examples of uses for which it has been approved include baked goods, nonalcoholic beverages (including soft drinks), chewing gum, confections and frostings, frozen desserts, gelatins and puddings, jams and jellies, processed fruits and fruit juices, toppings, and syrups. Neotame is safe for use by the general population, including children, pregnant and lactating women, and people with diabetes. In addition, no special labeling for people with phenylketonuria is needed because neotame is not broken down in the body to its amino acid components.

**Acesulfame-K.** The alternative sweetener acesulfame-K (the *K* stands for potassium; Sunette®) was approved by the FDA in July 1988. It is approved for use in more than 40 countries and has been in use in Europe since 1983. Acesulfame-K is 200 times sweeter than sucrose. It contributes no calories to the diet because it is not digested by the body, and it does not cause dental caries.

Unlike aspartame, acesulfame-K can be used in baking because it does not lose its sweetness when heated. In the United States, it is currently approved for use in chewing gum, powdered drink mixes, gelatins, puddings, baked goods, tabletop sweeteners, candy, throat lozenges, yogurt, and nondairy creamers; additional uses may soon be approved. One recent trend is to combine it with aspartame in soft drinks.

**Tagatose.** Tagatose, sold as Naturlose,® is a slightly altered form of the simple sugar fructose. It is approved for use in ready-to-eat breakfast cereals, diet soft drinks, meal replacement bars, frozen desserts, candy, frosting, and chewing gum. Tagatose is poorly absorbed, so it yields only 1.5 kcal per gram to the body. Use also does not raise the risk for dental caries, nor does it increase blood glucose. Eventual fermentation in the large intestine may even lead to a beneficial effect on that organ (i.e., a prebiotic effect, covered in Chapter 3).

**Stevia.** Stevia, sold as the dietary supplement Sweet Leaf®, is an alternative sweetener derived from a South American shrub. Stevia extracts are 100 to 300 times sweeter than sucrose but provide no energy. It has been used in teas and as a sweetener in Japan since the 1970s, and the FDA recently (December 2008) stated that Stevia is considered generally recognized as safe (GRAS) for use in foods. Stevia can be purchased as a dietary supplement in natural and health food stores and as an alternative sweetener in grocery stores.

---

### CONCEPT CHECK

Table sugar, honey, jam, fruit, and plain baked potatoes contain the highest percentage of calories from carbohydrates. Foods such as cream pies, potato chips, whole milk, and oatmeal contain moderate amounts of carbohydrate. Common nutritive sweeteners added to foods include sucrose, maple sugar, honey, brown sugar, and high-fructose corn syrup. For people who want to limit calories from sugar intake, other sweeteners are available and include the sugar alcohols, saccharin, aspartame, sucralose, neotame, acesulfame-K, and tagatose. Of these, aspartame is the most common alternative sweetener in use.

## 4.6 Making Carbohydrates Available for Body Use

As discussed in Chapter 3, simply eating a food does not supply nutrients to body cells. Digestion and absorption must occur first.

## Digestion

Food preparation can be viewed as the start of carbohydrate digestion because cooking softens tough connective structures in the fibrous parts of plants, such as broccoli stalks. When starches are heated, the starch granules swell as they soak up water, making them much easier to digest. All of these effects of cooking generally make carbohydrate-containing foods easier to chew, swallow, and break down during digestion.

The enzymatic digestion of starch begins in the mouth, when the saliva, which contains an enzyme called salivary **amylase**, mixes with the starchy products during the chewing of the food. This amylase breaks down starch into many smaller units, primarily disaccharides, such as maltose (Fig. 4-8). You can taste this conversion while chewing a saltine cracker. Prolonged chewing of the cracker causes it to taste sweeter as some starch breaks down into the sweeter disaccharides, such as maltose. Still, food is in the mouth for such a short amount of time that this phase of digestion is negligible. In addition, once the food moves down the esophagus and reaches the stomach, the acidic environment inactivates salivary amylase.

> **amylase**  Starch-digesting enzyme from the salivary glands or pancreas.

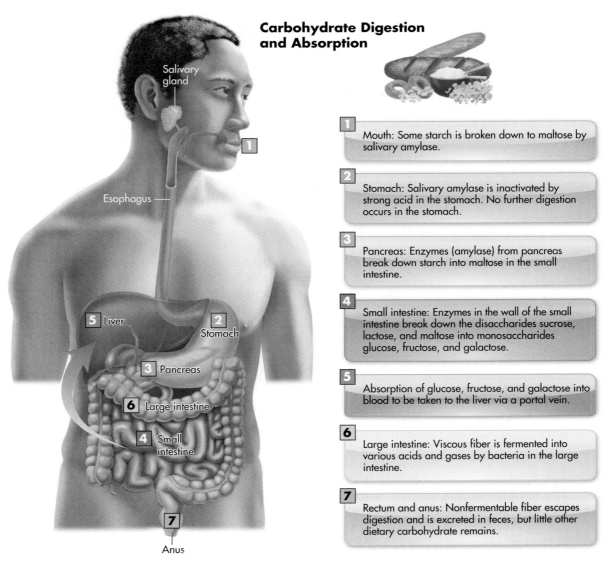

**Carbohydrate Digestion and Absorption**

**1** Mouth: Some starch is broken down to maltose by salivary amylase.

**2** Stomach: Salivary amylase is inactivated by strong acid in the stomach. No further digestion occurs in the stomach.

**3** Pancreas: Enzymes (amylase) from pancreas break down starch into maltose in the small intestine.

**4** Small intestine: Enzymes in the wall of the small intestine break down the disaccharides sucrose, lactose, and maltose into monosaccharides glucose, fructose, and galactose.

**5** Absorption of glucose, fructose, and galactose into blood to be taken to the liver via a portal vein.

**6** Large intestine: Viscous fiber is fermented into various acids and gases by bacteria in the large intestine.

**7** Rectum and anus: Nonfermentable fiber escapes digestion and is excreted in feces, but little other dietary carbohydrate remains.

**FIGURE 4-8** ▶ Carbohydrate digestion and absorption. Enzymes made by the mouth, pancreas, and small intestine participate in the process of digestion. Most carbohydrate digestion and absorption takes place in the small intestine. Chapter 3 covered the physiology of digestion and absorption in detail.

When the carbohydrates reach the small intestine, the more alkaline environment of the intestine is better suited for further carbohydrate digestion. The pancreas releases enzymes, such as pancreatic amylase, to aid the last stage of starch digestion. After amylase action, the original carbohydrates in a food are now present in the small intestine as the monosaccharides glucose and fructose, originally present as such in food, and disaccharides (maltose from starch breakdown, lactose mainly from dairy products, and sucrose from food and that added at the table).

The disaccharides are digested to their monosaccharide units once they reach the wall of the small intestine, where the specialized enzymes on the absorptive cells digest each disaccharide into monosaccharides. The enzyme **maltase** acts on maltose to produce two glucose molecules. **sucrase** acts on sucrose to produce glucose and fructose. **Lactase** acts on lactose to produce glucose and galactose.

**Lactose Maldigestion and Lactose Intolerance. Lactose maldigestion** is a normal pattern of physiology that often begins to develop after early childhood, at about ages 3 to 5 years. It can lead to symptoms of abdominal pain, gas, and diarrhea after consuming lactose, generally when eaten in large amounts. This *primary* form of lactose maldigestion is estimated to be present in about 75% of the world's population, although not all of these individuals experience symptoms. (When significant symptoms develop after lactose intake it is then called **lactose intolerance**.) Another form of the problem, *secondary* lactose maldigestion, is a temporary condition in which lactase production is decreased in response to another condition, such as intestinal diarrhea. The symptoms of lactose intolerance include gas, abdominal bloating, cramps, and diarrhea. The bloating and gas are caused by bacterial fermentation of lactose in the large intestine. The diarrhea is caused by undigested lactose in the large intestine as it draws water from the circulatory system into the large intestine.

In North America, approximately 25% of adults show signs of decreased lactose digestion in the small intestine. Many lactose maldigesters are Asian Americans, African Americans, and Latino/Hispanic Americans, and the occurrence increases as people age. It is hypothesized that approximately 3000 to 5000 years ago, a genetic mutation occurred in regions that relied on milk and dairy foods as a main food source, allowing those individuals (mostly in northern Europe, pastoral tribes in Africa, and the Middle East) to retain the ability to maintain high lactase output for their entire lifetime.

Still, many of these individuals can consume moderate amounts of lactose with minimal or no gastrointestinal discomfort because of eventual lactose breakdown by bacteria in the large intestine. Thus, it is unnecessary for these people to greatly restrict their intake of lactose-containing foods, such as milk and milk products. These calcium-rich food products are important for maintaining bone health. Obtaining enough calcium and vitamin D from the diet is much easier if milk and milk products are included in a diet.

Studies have shown that nearly all individuals with decreased lactase production can tolerate ½ to 1 cup of milk with meals, and that most individuals adapt to intestinal gas production resulting from the fermentation of lactose by bacteria in the large intestine. Combining lactose-containing foods with other foods also helps because certain properties of foods can have positive effects on rates of digestion. For example, fat in a meal slows digestion, leaving more time for lactase action. Hard cheese and yogurt also are more easily tolerated than milk. Much of the lactose is lost in the production of cheese, and the active bacteria cultures in yogurt digest the lactose when these bacteria are broken apart in the small intestine and release their lactase. In addition, an array of products, such as low-lactose milk and lactase pills, are available to assist lactose maldigesters when needed.

## Absorption

Monosaccharides found naturally in foods and those formed as by-products of starch and disaccharide digestion in the mouth and small intestine generally follow an active

**maltase** An enzyme made by absorptive cells of the small intestine; this enzyme digests maltose to two glucoses.

**sucrase** An enzyme made by absorptive cells of the small intestine; this enzyme digests sucrose to glucose and fructose.

**lactase** An enzyme made by absorptive cells of the small intestine; this enzyme digests lactose to glucose and galactose.

**lactose maldigestion (primary and secondary)** Primary lactose maldigestion occurs when production of the enzyme lactase declines for no apparent reason. Secondary lactose maldigestion occurs when a specific cause, such as long-standing diarrhea, results in a decline in lactase production. When significant symptoms develop after lactose intake, it is then called lactose intolerance.

**lactose intolerance** A condition in which symptoms such as abdominal gas and bloating appear as a result of severe lactose maldigestion.

absorption process. Recall from Chapter 3 that this is a process that requires a specific carrier and energy input for the substance to be taken up by the absorptive cells in the small intestine. Glucose and its close relative, galactose, undergo active absorption. They are pumped into the absorptive cells along with sodium.

Fructose is taken up by the absorptive cells via facilitated diffusion. In this case, a carrier is used, but no energy input is needed. This absorptive process is thus slower than that seen with glucose or galactose. So, large doses of fructose are not readily absorbed and can contribute to diarrhea as the monosaccharide remains in the small intestine and attracts water.

Once glucose, galactose, and fructose enter the absorptive cells, some fructose is metabolized into glucose. The single sugars in the absorptive cells are then transferred to the portal vein that goes directly to the liver. The liver then metabolizes those sugars by transforming the monosaccharides galactose and fructose into glucose and:

- Releasing it directly into the bloodstream for transport to organs such as the brain, muscles, kidneys, and adipose tissues
- Producing glycogen for storage of carbohydrate
- Producing fat (minor amount, if any)

Of these three options, producing fat is the least likely, except when carbohydrates are consumed in high amounts and overall calorie needs are exceeded.

Unless an individual has a disease that causes malabsorption, or an intolerance to a carbohydrate such as lactose (or fructose), only a minor amount of some sugars (about 10%) escapes digestion. Any undigested carbohydrate travels to the large intestine and is fermented there by bacteria. The acids and gases produced by bacterial metabolism of the undigested carbohydrate are absorbed into the bloodstream. Scientists suspect that some of these products of bacterial metabolism promote the health of the large intestine by providing it with a source of calories.

▲ Use of yogurt helps lactose maldigesters meet calcium needs.

## MAKING DECISIONS

### Fermentable Fiber

Bacteria in the large intestine ferment soluble fibers into such products as acids and gases. The acids, once absorbed, also provide calories for the body. In this way, soluble fibers provide about 1.5 to 2.5 kcal per gram. Although the intestinal gas (flatulence) produced by this bacterial fermentation is not harmful, it can be painful and sometimes embarrassing. Over time, however, the body tends to adapt to a high-fiber intake, eventually producing less gas.

    Name some potentially gas-forming foods. Are these foods good sources of soluble fiber?

## CONCEPT CHECK

Carbohydrate digestion is the process of breaking down larger carbohydrates into smaller units, and eventually to monosaccharide forms. The enzymatic digestion of starches in the body begins in the mouth with salivary amylase. Enzymes made by the pancreas and small intestine complete the digestion of carbohydrates to single sugars in the small intestine. Lactose maldigestion is a condition that results when cells of the intestine do not make sufficient lactase, the enzyme necessary to digest lactose, resulting in symptoms such as abdominal gas, pain, and diarrhea. Most people with lactose maldigestion can tolerate cheeses and yogurt, as well as moderate amounts of milk. When significant symptoms develop after lactose intake, it is called lactose intolerance. Following primarily an active absorption process, glucose and galactose, (resulting from the digestive process or present in the meal), are taken up by absorptive cells in the intestine. Fructose undergoes facilitated absorption. All of the monosaccharides then enter the portal vein that goes directly to the liver. The liver finally exercises its metabolic options, producing glucose, glycogen, and even fat if carbohydrates are consumed in great excess and overall calorie needs are exceeded.

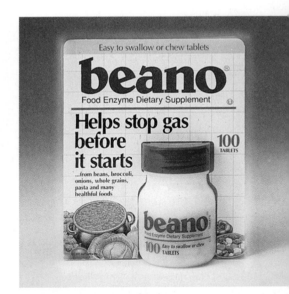

▲ Beano® is a dietary supplement that contains natural digestive enzymes. Such products can be used to reduce intestinal gas produced by bacterial metabolism of undigested sugars in beans and some vegetables in the large intestine.

# 4.7 Putting Simple Carbohydrates to Work In The Body

As just discussed, all of the digestible carbohydrate that we eat is eventually converted to glucose. Glucose then is the form of carbohydrate that goes on to function in body metabolism. The other sugars can generally be converted to glucose and the starches are broken down to yield glucose, so the functions described here apply to most carbohydrates. The functions of glucose in the body start with supplying calories to fuel the body.

## Yielding Energy

The main function of glucose is to supply calories for use by the body. Certain tissues in the body, such as red blood cells, can use only glucose and other simple carbohydrate forms for fuel. Most parts of the brain and central nervous system also derive energy only from glucose, unless the diet contains almost none. In that case, much of the brain can use partial breakdown products of fat—called **ketone bodies**—for energy needs. Other body cells, including muscle cells, can use simple carbohydrates as fuel but many of these cells can also use fat or protein for energy needs.

## Sparing Protein from Use as an Energy Source and Preventing Ketosis

A diet that supplies enough digestible carbohydrates to prevent breakdown of proteins for energy needs is considered *protein sparing*. Under normal circumstances, digestible carbohydrates in the diet mostly end up as blood glucose, and protein is reserved for functions such as building and maintaining muscles and vital organs. However, if you don't eat enough carbohydrates, your body is forced to make glucose from body proteins, draining the pool of amino acids available in cells for other critical functions. During long-term starvation, the continuous withdrawal of proteins from the muscles, heart, liver, kidneys, and other vital organs can result in weakness, poor function, and even failure of body systems.

In addition to the loss of protein, when you don't eat enough carbohydrates, the metabolism of fats is inefficient. In the absence of adequate carbohydrate, fats don't break down completely in metabolism and instead form ketone bodies. This condition, known as **ketosis**, should be avoided because it disturbs the body's normal acid-base balance and leads to other health problems. This is a good reason to question the long-term safety of the low-carbohydrate diets that have been popular.

**ketone bodies** Partial breakdown products of fat that contain three or four carbons.

**ketosis** The condition of having a high concentration of ketone bodies and related breakdown products in the bloodstream and tissues.

### MAKING DECISIONS

#### Carbohydrates and Protein Sparing

The wasting of protein that occurs during long-term fasting can be life threatening. This has prompted companies that make formulas for rapid weight loss to include sufficient carbohydrate in the products to decrease protein breakdown and thereby protect vital tissues and organs, including the heart. Most of these very low-calorie products are powders that can be mixed with different types of fluids and are consumed five or six times per day. When considering any weight-loss products, be sure that your total diet provides at least the RDA for carbohydrate.

## Regulating Glucose

Under normal circumstances, a person's blood glucose concentration is regulated within a narrow range. Recall from Chapter 3 that when carbohydrates are digested

▲ When following a weight-loss diet, be sure that your diet provides at least the RDA for carbohydrate and taken up by the absorptive cells of the small intestine, the resulting monosaccharides are transported directly to the liver. One of the liver's roles, then, is to guard against excess glucose entering the bloodstream after a meal. The liver works in concert with the pancreas to regulate blood glucose.

When the concentration of glucose in the blood is high, such as during and immediately after a meal, the pancreas releases the hormone **insulin** into the bloodstream. Insulin delivers two different messages to various body cells to cause the level of glucose in the blood to fall. First, insulin directs the liver to store the glucose as glycogen. Second, insulin directs muscle, adipose, and other cells to remove glucose from the bloodstream by taking it into those cells. By triggering both glycogen synthesis in the liver and glucose movement out of the bloodstream into certain cells, insulin keeps the concentration of glucose from rising too high in the blood (Fig. 4-9).

On the other hand, when a person has not eaten for a few hours and blood glucose begins to fall, the pancreas releases the hormone **glucagon**. This hormone has the opposite effect of insulin. It prompts the breakdown of liver glycogen into glucose, which is then released into the bloodstream. In this way, glucagon keeps blood glucose from falling too low.

A different mechanism increases blood glucose during times of stress. **Epinephrine** (adrenaline) is the hormone responsible for the "flight or fight" reaction. Epinephrine and a related compound are released in large amounts from the adrenal glands (located on each kidney) and various nerve endings in response to a perceived threat, such as a car approaching head-on. These hormones cause glycogen in the liver to be quickly broken down into glucose. The resulting rapid flood of glucose from the liver into the bloodstream helps promote quick mental and physical reactions.

In essence, the actions of insulin on blood glucose are balanced by the actions of glucagon, epinephrine, and other hormones. If hormonal balance is not maintained, such as during over- or underproduction of insulin or glucagon, major changes in blood glucose concentrations occur. The disease, type 1 diabetes, is an example of the under-production of insulin. To maintain blood glucose within an acceptable range, the body relies on a complex regulatory system. This provides a safeguard against extremely high blood glucose (**hyperglycemia**) or low blood glucose (**hypoglycemia**). The failure of blood glucose regulation will be discussed in the "Nutrition and Your Health" section at the end of this chapter.

**insulin**  A hormone produced by the pancreas. Among other processes, insulin increases the synthesis of glycogen in the liver and the movement of glucose from the bloodstream into body cells.

**glucagon**  A hormone made by the pancreas that stimulates the breakdown of glycogen in the liver into glucose; this ends up increasing blood glucose. Glucagon also performs other functions.

**epinephrine**  A hormone also known as *adrenaline*; it is released by the adrenal glands (located on each kidney) and various nerve endings in the body. It acts to increase glycogen breakdown in the liver, among other functions.

**hyperglycemia**  High blood glucose, above 125 milligrams per 100 milliliters of blood.

**hypoglycemia**  Low blood glucose, below 40 to 50 milligrams per 100 milliliters of blood.

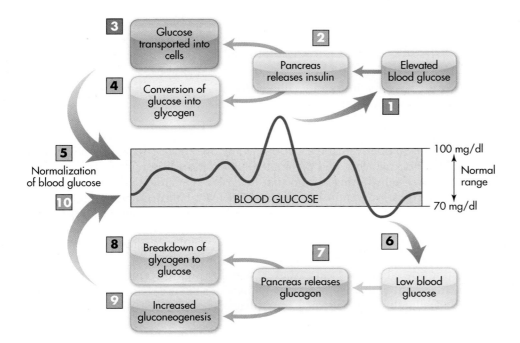

**FIGURE 4-9** ▶ Regulation of blood glucose. Insulin and glucagon are key factors in controlling blood glucose. When blood glucose rises above the normal range of 70 to 90 milligrams per deciliter (mg/dL) **1**, insulin is released **2** to lower it **3** and **4**. Blood glucose then falls back into the normal range **5**. When blood glucose falls below the normal range **6**, glucagon is released **7**, which has the opposite effect of insulin **8** and **9**. This then restores blood glucose to the normal range **10**. Other hormones, such as epinephrine, norepinephrine, cortisol, and growth hormone, also contribute to blood glucose regulation.

See *Nutrition and Your Health: Diabetes-When Blood Glucose Regulation Fails* at the end of Chapter 4.

**A** term you might see on food labels is *net carbs*. Although this term is not FDA-approved, sometimes it is used to describe the carbohydrates that increase blood glucose. Fiber and sugar alcohol content are subtracted from the total carbohydrate content to yield net carbs because they have a negligible effect on blood glucose.

**glycemic index (GI)** The blood glucose response of a given food, compared to a standard (typically, glucose or white bread). Glycemic index is influenced by starch structure; fiber content; food processing; physical structure; and macronutrients in the meal, such as fat.

**glycemic load (GL)** The amount of carbohydrate in a serving of food multiplied by the glycemic index of that carbohydrate. The result is then divided by 100.

▲ Carrots, criticized in the popular press for having a high glycemic index (which isn't even true), actually contribute a low glycemic load to a diet.

## The Glycemic Index and Glycemic Load of Carbohydrate Sources

Our bodies react uniquely to different sources of carbohydrates, such that a serving of a high-fiber food, such as baked beans, results in lower blood glucose levels compared to the same size serving of mashed potatoes. Why are we concerned with the effects of various foods on blood glucose? Foods that result in a high blood glucose elicit a large release of insulin from the pancreas. Chronically high insulin output leads to many deleterious effects on the body: high blood triglycerides, increased fat deposition in the adipose tissue, increased tendency for blood to clot, increased fat synthesis in the liver, and a more rapid return of hunger after a meal (insulin rapidly lowers the macronutrients in the blood as it stimulates their storage, signaling hunger). Over time, this increase in insulin output may cause the muscles to become resistant to the action of insulin, and eventually lead to type 2 diabetes in some people. Two food measurements have been developed that are useful in predicting the blood sugar response to various foods and for planning a diet to avoid hyperglycemia (high blood glucose).

The first of these tools is **glycemic index (GI)**. Glycemic index is a ratio of the blood glucose response to a given food compared to a standard (typically, glucose or white bread) (Table 4-4). Glycemic index is influenced by starch structure, fiber content, food processing, physical structure, and other macronutrients in the meal, such as fat. Foods with particularly high glycemic index values are potatoes, especially baking potatoes (due to higher amylopectin content compared to red potatoes), mashed potatoes (due to greater surface area exposed), short grain white rice, honey, and jelly beans. A major shortcoming of glycemic index is that the measurement is based on a serving of food that would provide 50 grams of carbohydrate. As you can imagine, this amount of food may not reflect the amount typically consumed.

Another way of describing how different foods affect blood glucose (and insulin) levels is **glycemic load (GL)**. The glycemic load is more useful because it takes into account the glycemic index and the amount of carbohydrate consumed. Glycemic load, therefore, better reflects a food's effect on one's blood glucose than either number alone. To calculate the glycemic load of a food, the amount (in grams) of carbohydrate in a serving of the food is multiplied by the glycemic index of that food, and then divided by 100 (because glycemic index is a percentage). For example, vanilla wafers have a glycemic index of 77, and a small serving contains 15 grams of carbohydrate:

$$(\text{Glycemic Index} \times \text{Grams of Carbohydrate}) \div 100 = \text{Glycemic Load}$$
$$(77 \times 15) \div 100 = 12$$

Even though the glycemic index of vanilla wafers (77) is considered high, the glycemic load calculation shows that the impact of this food on blood glucose levels is fairly low (review Table 4-4)

There are many ways to address this problem of high glycemic load foods. The most important is to not overeat these foods at any one meal. This greatly minimizes their effects on blood glucose and the related increased insulin release. At least once per meal, consider substituting a food that has a low glycemic load for one with a higher value, such as long grain rice or spaghetti for a baked potato. Combining a low glycemic load food, such as an apple, kidney beans, milk, or salad with dressing, with a high glycemic load food also reduces the effect on blood glucose. In addition, maintaining a healthy body weight and performing regular physical activity further reduces the effects of a high glycemic load diet.

Substituting low glycemic load carbohydrates for high glycemic load foods can help in the treatment of diabetes; Chapter 10 discusses the use of foods with different glycemic load values in planning diets for athletes.

**TABLE 4-4**  Glycemic Index (GI) and Glycemic Load (GL) of Common Foods

Reference food glucose = 100
Low GI foods—below 55                          Low GL foods—below 15
Intermediate GI foods—between 55 and 70        Intermediate GL foods—between 15 and 20
High GI foods—more than 70                     High GL foods—more than 20

| | Serving Size (grams) | Glycemic Index (GI) | Carbohydrate (grams) | Glycemic Load (GL) |
|---|---|---|---|---|
| **Pastas/Grains** | | | | |
| White, long grain | 1 cup | 56 | 45 | 25 |
| White, short grain | 1 cup | 72 | 53 | 38 |
| Spaghetti | 1 cup | 41 | 40 | 16 |
| **Vegetables** | | | | |
| Carrots, boiled | 1 cup | 49 | 16 | 8 |
| Sweet corn | 1 cup | 55 | 39 | 21 |
| Potato, baked | 1 cup | 85 | 57 | 48 |
| **Dairy Foods** | | | | |
| Milk, skim | 1 cup | 32 | 12 | 4 |
| Yogurt, low-fat | 1 cup | 33 | 17 | 6 |
| Ice cream | 1 cup | 61 | 31 | 19 |
| **Legumes** | | | | |
| Baked beans | 1 cup | 48 | 54 | 26 |
| Kidney beans | 1 cup | 27 | 38 | 10 |
| Navy beans | 1 cup | 38 | 54 | 21 |
| **Sugars** | | | | |
| Honey | 1 tsp | 73 | 6 | 4 |
| Sucrose | 1 tsp | 65 | 5 | 3 |
| Fructose | 1 tsp | 23 | 5 | 1 |
| **Breads and Muffins** | | | | |
| Bagel | 1 small | 72 | 30 | 22 |
| Whole-wheat bread | 1 slice | 69 | 13 | 9 |
| White bread | 1 slice | 70 | 10 | 7 |
| **Fruits** | | | | |
| Apple | 1 medium | 38 | 22 | 8 |
| Banana | 1 medium | 55 | 29 | 16 |
| Orange | 1 medium | 44 | 15 | 7 |
| **Beverages** | | | | |
| Orange juice | 1 cup | 46 | 26 | 13 |
| Gatorade | 1 cup | 78 | 15 | 12 |
| Coca-Cola | 1 cup | 63 | 26 | 16 |
| **Snack Foods** | | | | |
| Potato chips | 1 oz | 54 | 15 | 8 |
| Vanilla wafers | 5 cookies | 77 | 15 | 12 |
| Jelly beans | 1 oz | 80 | 26 | 21 |

Source: Foster-Powell K and others: International table of glycemic index and glycemic load. *American Journal of Clinical Nutrition* 76:5, 2002.

▲ A food such as potato chips, with a low glycemic index, can still have a high glycemic load if eaten in large portions.

**Y**ou might wonder why the glycemic index and glycemic load of white bread and whole wheat are similar. This is because whole-wheat flour is typically so finely ground that it is quickly digested. Thus the effect of fiber in slowing digestion and related absorption of glucose is no longer present. Some experts suggest we focus more on minimally processed (e.g., coarsely ground, steel cut, or rolled) grains, such as with whole-wheat flour and oatmeal, to get the full benefits of these fiber sources in reducing blood glucose levels.

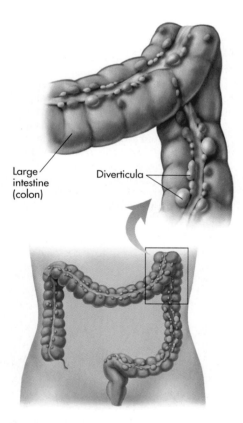

**R**ecall from Chapter 2 that FDA has approved the following claim: "Diets rich in whole-grain foods and other plant foods and low in total fat, saturated fat, and cholesterol may decrease the risk for cardiovascular (heart) disease and certain cancers."

**diverticula** Pouches that protrude through the exterior wall of the large intestine.

**hemorrhoid** A pronounced swelling of a large vein, particularly veins found in the anal region.

**diverticulosis** The condition of having many diverticula in the large intestine.

**diverticulitis** An inflammation of the diverticula caused by acids produced by bacterial metabolism inside the diverticula.

**FIGURE 4-10** ▶ Diverticula in the large intestine. A low-fiber diet increases the risk of developing diverticula. About one-third of people over age 45 have diverticulosis, while two-thirds of people over 85 do.

## CONCEPT CHECK

Carbohydrates provide glucose for the energy needs of red blood cells and parts of the brain and nervous system. Eating too little carbohydrates forces the body to make glucose using primarily amino acids from proteins found in muscles and other vital organs. A low glucose supply in cells also inhibits efficient metabolism of fats. Ketosis can then result.

Blood glucose concentration is maintained within a narrow range. When blood glucose rises after a meal, the hormone insulin is released in great amounts from the pancreas. Insulin acts to lower blood glucose by increasing glucose storage in the liver and glucose up-take by other body cells. If blood glucose falls during fasting, glucagon and other hormones increase the liver's release of glucose into the bloodstream to restore normal blood glucose concentrations. In a similar way, the hormone epinephrine can make more glucose available in response to stress. This balance in hormone activity helps maintain blood glucose within a healthy range.

## 4.8 Putting Fiber to Work

### Promoting Bowel Health

Fiber supplies mass to the feces, making elimination much easier. This is especially true for insoluble fibers. When enough fiber is consumed, the stool is large and soft because many types of plant fibers attract water. The larger size stimulates the intestinal muscles to contract, which aids elimination. Consequently, less pressure is necessary to expel the stool.

When too little fiber is eaten, the opposite can occur: very little water is present in the feces, making it small and hard. Constipation may result, which forces one to exert excessive pressure in the large intestine during defecation. This high pressure can force parts of the large intestine (colon) wall out from between the surrounding bands of muscle, forming many small pouches called **diverticula** (Fig. 4-10). **Hemorrhoids** may also result from excessive straining during defecation (review Chapter 3).

Diverticula are asymptomatic in about 80% of affected people; that is, they are not noticeable. The asymptomatic form of this disease is called **diverticulosis**. If the diverticula become filled with food particles, such as hulls and seeds, they may eventually become inflamed and painful, a condition known as **diverticulitis**. Surprisingly, intake of fiber then should be reduced to limit further bacterial activity. Once the inflammation subsides, a high-fiber diet is resumed to ease stool elimination and reduce the risk of a future attack.

Over the past 30 years, many population studies have shown a link between increased fiber intake and a decrease in colon cancer development. Most of the research on diet and colon cancer is focusing on the potential preventive effects of fruits, vegetables, whole-grain breads and cereals, and beans (rather than just fiber). Smoking, obesity in men, excessive alcohol use, starch- and sugar-rich foods, and processed meat intake are under study as potential causes of colon cancer. Overall, the health benefits to the colon that stem from a high-fiber diet are partially due to the nutrients that are commonly present in most high-fiber foods, such as vitamins, minerals, phytochemicals, and in some cases essential fatty acids. Thus it is more advisable to increase fiber intake using fiber-rich foods, rather than mostly relying on fiber supplements.

### Reducing Obesity Risk

Aside from its role in maintaining bowel regularity, the consumption of fiber has many additional health benefits. A diet high in fiber likely controls weight and reduces the risk of developing obesity. The bulky nature of high-fiber foods requires more time to chew and fills us up without yielding many calories. Increasing intake of foods rich in fiber is one strategy for feeling satisfied or full after a meal (review the discussion of energy density in Chapter 2). This is still another reason to question the low-carbohydrate diets—where is the whole-grain fiber going to come from?

### Enhancing Blood Glucose Control

Consuming large amounts of viscous fibers, such as oat fiber, slow glucose absorption from the small intestine, and so contribute to better blood glucose regulation. This effect can be helpful in the treatment of diabetes. In fact, adults whose main carbohydrate source is low-fiber foods are much more likely to develop diabetes than those who have high-fiber diets.

### Reducing Cholesterol Absorption

Recall that good sources of viscous fiber are apples, bananas, oranges, carrots, barley, oats, and kidney beans. A high intake of viscous fiber also inhibits absorption of cholesterol and cholesterol-rich bile acids from the small intestine, thereby reducing blood cholesterol and possibly reducing the risk of cardiovascular disease and gallstones. The beneficial bacteria in the large intestine degrade soluble fiber and produce certain fatty acids that probably also reduce cholesterol synthesis in the liver. In addition, the slower glucose absorption that occurs with diets high in viscous fiber is linked to a decrease in insulin release. One of the effects of insulin is to stimulate cholesterol synthesis in the liver, so this reduction in insulin may contribute to the ability of viscous fiber to lower blood cholesterol. Overall, a fiber-rich diet containing fruits, vegetables, beans, and whole-grain breads and cereals (including whole-grain breakfast cereals) is advocated as part of a strategy to reduce cardiovascular disease (coronary heart disease and stroke) risk. And again, this is something that a low-carbohydrate diet can't promise.

▲ Oatmeal is a rich source of viscous fiber. FDA allows a health claim for the benefits of oatmeal to lower blood cholesterol that arise from the effects of this viscous fiber.

### CONCEPT CHECK

Fiber forms a vital part of the diet by adding mass to the stool, which eases elimination. Fiber-rich foods also help in weight control and reduce the risk of developing obesity and cardiovascular disease, and possibly colon cancer. Soluble fiber can also be useful for controlling blood glucose in patients with diabetes and in lowering blood cholesterol. Whole-grain breads and cereals, vegetables, beans, and fruits are excellent sources of fiber.

## 4.9 Carbohydrate Needs

Currently, recommendations for carbohydrate intake vary widely in the scientific literature and popular press. The RDA for carbohydrates is 130 grams per day for adults. This is based on the amount needed to supply adequate glucose for the brain and nervous system, without having to rely on ketone bodies from incomplete fat breakdown as a calorie source. Somewhat exceeding this amount is fine; the Food and Nutrition Board recommends that carbohydrate intake should range from 45% to 65% of total calorie intake. The Nutrition Facts panel on food labels uses 60% of calorie intake as the standard for recommended carbohydrate intake. This would be 300 grams of carbohydrate when consuming a 2000-calorie diet.

North American adults consume about 180 to 330 grams of carbohydrates per day, which supply about 50% of calorie intake. Worldwide, however, carbohydrates account for about 70% of all calories consumed, and in some countries, up to 80% of the calories consumed. One recommendation on which almost all experts agree is that one's carbohydrate intake should be based primarily on fruits, vegetables, whole-grain breads and cereals, and beans, rather than on refined grains, potatoes, and sugar.

▲ The 2005 Dietary Guidelines define whole grain as the entire grain seed or kernel made of three components: bran, germ, and endosperm.

The 2005 Dietary Guidelines for Americans recommend that we choose fiber-rich fruits, vegetables, and whole grains often. More specifically, three or more ounces of grains, roughly one-half of one's grains, should be whole. Remember that the 2005 Dietary Guidelines define whole grain as the entire grain seed or kernel made of three components: the bran, germ, and endosperm, which must be in nearly the same relative proportions as the original grain if cracked, crushed, or flaked.

### How Much Fiber Do We Need?

An Adequate Intake for fiber has been set based on the ability of fiber to reduce risk of cardiovascular disease (and likely many cases of diabetes). The Adequate Intake for fiber for adults is 25 grams per day for women and 38 grams per day for men. The goal is to provide at least 14 grams per 1000 kcal in a diet. After age 50, the Adequate Intake falls to 21 grams per day and 30 grams per day, respectively. The Daily Value used for fiber on food and supplement labels is 25 grams for a 2000 kcal diet. In North America, fiber intake averages 13 grams per day for women and 17 grams per day for men and the average whole-grain intake is less than one serving per day. This low intake is attributed to the lack of knowledge on the benefits of whole grains, and the inability to recognize whole-grain products at the time of purchase. Thus, most of us should increase our fiber intake. At least three servings of whole grains per day is recommended. Eating a high-fiber cereal (at least 3 grams of fiber per serving) for breakfast is one easy way to increase fiber intake (Fig. 4-11).

The "Rate Your Plate" exercise shows a diet containing 25 or 38 grams of fiber within moderate calorie intakes. Diets to meet the fiber recommendations are possible and enjoyable if you incorporate plenty of whole-wheat bread, fruits, vegetables, and beans. Use the "Rate Your Plate" exercise to estimate the fiber content of your diet. What is *your* fiber score?

▲ Look for the term "whole-grain" or "whole-wheat" flour on the label for breads that are an excellent source of fiber.

The 2005 Dietary Guidelines for Americans provide the following advice regarding carbohydrate intake:

- Choose fiber-rich fruits, vegetables, and whole grains often. (In general, at least half of one's intake of grains [3 ounces or more] should come from whole grains.)

- Choose and prepare foods and beverages with little added sugars or caloric sweeteners, such as in amounts suggested by MyPyramid.

- Reduce the incidence of dental caries by practicing good oral hygiene and consuming sugar- and starch-containing foods and beverages less frequently.

### MAKING DECISIONS

#### Whole Grains

When buying bread, if you see the name "wheat bread" on the label, do you think you are buying a whole-wheat product? Most people do. The flour is from the wheat plant, so manufacturers correctly list enriched white (refined) flour as wheat flour on food labels. However, if the label does not list "whole-wheat flour" first, then the product is not primarily a whole-wheat bread and thus does not contain as much fiber as it could. Careful reading of labels is important in the search for more fiber. Look especially for the term whole grains on the food label to ensure that you are getting a good source of natural fiber.

In the final analysis, keep in mind that any nutrient can lead to health problems when consumed in excess. High carbohydrate, high fiber, and low fat does not mean zero calories. Carbohydrates help moderate calorie intake in comparison with fats, but high-carbohydrate foods also contribute to total calorie intake.

## 4.10 Health Concerns Related to Carbohydrate Intake

Aside from the health risks related to ketosis, both excessive fiber and sugar intakes can pose health problems. Too much lactose in the diet is also a problem for some people.

### Problems with High-Fiber Diets

Very high intakes of fiber—for example, 60 grams per day—can pose some health risks and therefore should be followed only under the guidance of a physician. Increased

## Nutrition Facts

Serving Size 1 cup (55g/2.0 oz.)
Servings Per Container 10

| Amount Per Serving | Cereal | Cereal with ½ Cup Vitamins A & D Skim Milk |
|---|---|---|
| **Calories** | 170 | 210 |
| Calories from Fat | 10 | 10 |
| | **% Daily Value\*\*** | |
| **Total Fat** 1.0g\* | **2**% | **2**% |
| Sat. Fat 0g | **0**% | **0**% |
| *Trans* Fat 0g | | \* |
| **Cholesterol** 0mg | **0**% | **0**% |
| **Sodium** 300mg | **13**% | **15**% |
| **Potassium** 340mg | **10**% | **16**% |
| **Total Carbohydrate** 43g | **14**% | **16**% |
| Dietary Fiber 7g | **28**% | **28**% |
| Sugars 16g | | |
| Other Carbohydrate 20g | | |
| **Protein** 4g | | |
| Vitamin A | 15% | 20% |
| Vitamin C | 20% | 22% |
| Calcium | 2% | 15% |
| Iron | 65% | 65% |
| Vitamin D | 10% | 25% |
| Thiamin | 25% | 30% |
| Riboflavin | 25% | 35% |
| Niacin | 25% | 25% |
| Vitamin B$_6$ | 25% | 25% |
| Folic acid | 30% | 30% |
| Vitamin B$_{12}$ | 25% | 35% |
| Phosphorus | 20% | 30% |
| Magnesium | 20% | 25% |
| Zinc | 25% | 25% |
| Copper | 10% | 10% |

\*Amount in cereal. One half cup skim milk contributes an additional 40 calories, 65mg sodium, 6g total carbohydrate (6g sugars), and 4g protein.
\*\*Percent Daily Values are based on a 2,000 calorie diet. Your daily values may be higher or lower depending on your calorie needs:

| | Calories: | 2,000 | 2,500 |
|---|---|---|---|
| Total Fat | Less than | 65g | 80g |
| Sat Fat | Less than | 20g | 25g |
| Cholesterol | Less than | 300mg | 300mg |
| Sodium | Less than | 2,400mg | 2,400mg |
| Potassium | | 3,500mg | 3,500mg |
| Total Carbohydrate | | 300g | 375g |
| Dietary Fiber | | 25g | 30g |

Calories per gram:
Fat 9 • Carbohydrate 4 • Protein 4

\*Intake of *trans* fat should be as low as possible.

**Ingredients:** Wheat bran with other parts of wheat, raisins, sugar, corn syrup, salt, malt flavoring, glycerin, iron, niacinamide, zinc oxide, pyridoxine hydrochloride (vitamin B₆), riboflavin (vitamin B₂), vitamin A palmitate, thiamin hydrochloride (vitamin B₁), folic acid, vitamin B₁₂, and vitamin D.

## Nutrition Facts

Serving Size: ¾ Cup (30g)
Servings Per Package: About 17

| Amount Per Serving | Cereal | Cereal With ¹/₂ Cup Skim Milk |
|---|---|---|
| **Calories** | 170 | 210 |
| Calories from Fat | 0 | 5 |
| | | **%Daily Value\*\*** |
| **Total Fat** 0g\* | **0**% | **1**% |
| Saturated Fat 0g | **0**% | **1**% |
| *Trans* Fat 0g | | \* |
| **Cholesterol** 0mg | **0**% | **1**% |
| **Sodium** 60mg | **2**% | **4**% |
| **Potassium** 80mg | **2**% | **8**% |
| **Total Carbohydrate** 35g | **9**% | **11**% |
| Dietary Fiber 1g | **4**% | **4**% |
| Sugars 20g | | |
| Other Carbohydrate 13g | | |
| **Protein** 3g | | |
| Vitamin A | 25% | 30% |
| Vitamin C | 0% | 2% |
| Calcium | 0% | 15% |
| Iron | 10% | 10% |
| Vitamin D | 10% | 20% |
| Thiamin | 25% | 25% |
| Riboflavin | 25% | 35% |
| Niacin | 25% | 25% |
| Vitamin B$_6$ | 25% | 25% |
| Folic acid | 25% | 25% |
| Vitamin B$_{12}$ | 25% | 30% |
| Phosphorus | 4% | 15% |
| Magnesium | 4% | 8% |
| Zinc | 10% | 10% |
| Copper | 2% | 2% |

\*Amount in Cereal. One-half cup skim milk contributes an additional 65mg sodium, 6g total carbohydrate (6g sugars), and 4g protein.
\*\*Percent Daily Values are based on a 2,000 calorie diet. Your daily values may be higher or lower depending on your calorie needs:

| | Calories: | 2,000 | 2,500 |
|---|---|---|---|
| Total Fat | Less than | 65g | 80g |
| Sat. Fat | Less than | 20g | 25g |
| Cholesterol | Less than | 300mg | 300mg |
| Sodium | Less than | 2,400mg | 2,400mg |
| Potassium | | 3,500mg | 3,500mg |
| Total Carbohydrate | | 300g | 375g |
| Dietary Fiber | | 25g | 30g |

Calories per gram:
Fat 9 • Carbohydrate 4 • Protein 4

\*Intake of *trans* fat should be as low as possible.

**Ingredients:** Wheat, Sugar, Corn Syrup, Honey, Caramel Color, Partially Hydrogenated Soybean Oil, Salt, Ferric Phosphate, Niacinamide (Niacin), Zinc Oxide, Vitamin A (Palmitate), Pyridoxine Hydrochloride (Vitamin B6), Riboflavin, Thiamin Mononitrate, Folic Acid (Folate), Vitamin B12 and Vitamin D.

**FIGURE 4-11** ▶ Reading the Nutrition Facts on food labels helps us choose more nutritious foods. Based on the information from these nutrition labels, which cereal is the better choice for breakfast? Consider the amount of fiber in each cereal. Did the ingredient lists give you any clues? (Note: Ingredients are always listed in descending order by weight on a label.) When choosing a breakfast cereal, it is generally wise to focus on those that are rich sources of fiber. Sugar content can also be used for evaluation. However, sometimes this number does not reflect added sugar but simply the addition of fruits, such as raisins, complicating the evaluation.

▲ Whole-grain foods, such as granola, are excellent sources of fiber.

fluid intake is extremely important with a high-fiber diet. Inadequate fluid intake can leave the stool very hard and painful to eliminate. In more severe cases, the combination of excess fiber and insufficient fluid may contribute to blockages in the intestine, which may require surgery.

Aside from problems with the passage of materials through the GI tract, a high-fiber diet may also decrease the availability of nutrients. Certain components of fiber may bind to essential minerals, keeping them from being absorbed. For example, when fiber is consumed in large amounts, zinc and iron absorption may be hindered. In children, a very high fiber intake may reduce overall calorie intake, because fiber can quickly fill a child's small stomach before food intake meets energy needs.

## Problems with High-Sugar Diets

The main problems with consuming an excess amount of sugar are that it provides empty calories and increases the risk for dental decay.

**Diet Quality Declines When Sugar Intake Is Excessive.**  Overcrowding the diet with sweet treats can leave little room for important, nutrient-dense foods, such as fruits and vegetables. Children and teenagers are at the highest risk for overconsuming empty calories in place of nutrients essential for growth. Many children and teenagers are drinking an excess of sugared soft drinks and other sugar-containing beverages and much less milk than ever before. This exchange of soft drinks for milk can compromise bone health because milk contains calcium and vitamin D, both essential for bone health.

Supersizing sugar-rich beverages is also a growing problem; for example, in the 1950s a typical serving size of a soft drink was a 6½ ounce bottle, and now a 20 ounce plastic bottle is a typical serving. This one change in serving size contributes 170 extra kcal of sugars to the diet. Most convenience stores now offer cups that will hold 64 ounces of soft drinks. Filling up on sugared soft drinks in place of foods is not a healthy practice, but enjoying an occasional soft drink or limiting intake to one 12 ounce serving a day is generally fine. Switching to diet soft drinks would spare the simple sugar calories, but still lacks nutritional value, except for the fluid.

The sugar found in cakes, cookies, and ice cream also supplies many extra calories that promote weight gain, unless an individual is physically active. Today's low-fat and fat-free snack products usually contain lots of added sugar to produce a product with an acceptable taste. The result is to produce a high-calorie food equal to or greater in calorie content than the high-fat food product it was designed to replace.

With regard to sugar intake, an upper limit of 25% of total calorie intake from "added sugars" has been set by the Food and Nutrition Board (sugars added to foods during processing and preparation). Diets that go beyond this upper limit are likely to be deficient in vitamins and minerals. The World Health Organization suggests that added sugars provide no more than 10% of total daily calorie intake.

A moderate intake of about 10% of calorie intake corresponds to a maximum of approximately 50 grams (or 12 tsp) of sugars per day, based on a 2000 kcal diet. Most of the sugars we eat come from foods and beverages to which sugar has been added during processing and/or manufacture. On average, North Americans eat about 82 grams of added sugars daily, amounting to about 16% of calorie intake. Major sources of added sugars include soft drinks; cakes; cookies; fruit punch; and dairy desserts, such as ice cream. Following the recommendation of having no more than 10% of added calories from sugars is easier if sweet desserts such as cakes, cookies, and ice cream (full and reduced fat) are consumed sparingly (Table 4-5).

An excess intake of sugared soft drinks has recently been linked to a risk for both weight gain and type 2 diabetes in adults.

▲ Cookies and cakes are one of the top five carbohydrate sources for U.S. adults.

## MAKING DECISIONS

### Sugar and Hyperactivity

There is a widespread notion that high sugar intake by children causes hyperactivity, typically part of the syndrome called *attention deficit hyperactivity disorder (ADHD)*. However, most researchers find that sucrose may have the opposite effect. A high-carbohydrate meal, if also low in protein and fat, has a calming effect and induces sleep; this effect may be linked to changes in the synthesis of certain neurotransmitters in the brain, such as serotonin. If there is a problem, it is probably the excitement or tension in situations in which high sugar-rich foods are served, such as at birthday parties and on Halloween.

**TABLE 4-5** Suggestions for Reducing Simple-Sugar Intake

Many foods we enjoy are sweet. These should be eaten in moderation.

**At the Supermarket**

- Read ingredient labels. Identify all the added sugars in a product. Select items lower in total sugar when possible.
- Buy fresh fruits or fruits packed in water, juice, or light syrup rather than those packed in heavy syrup.
- Buy fewer foods that are high in sugar, such as prepared baked goods, candies, sugared cereals, sweet desserts, soft drinks, and fruit-flavored punches. Substitute vanilla wafers, graham crackers, bagels, English muffins, diet soft drinks, and other low sugar alternatives.
- Buy reduced-fat microwave popcorn to replace candy for snacks.

**In the Kitchen**

- Reduce the sugar in foods prepared at home. Try new low-sugar recipes or adjust your own. Start by reducing the sugar gradually until you've decreased it by one-third or more.
- Experiment with spices, such as cinnamon, cardamom, coriander, nutmeg, ginger, and mace, to enhance the flavor of foods.
- Use home-prepared items with less sugar instead of commercially prepared ones that are higher in sugar.

**At the Table**

- Reduce your use of white and brown sugars, honey, molasses, syrups, jams, and jellies.
- Choose fewer foods high in sugar, such as prepared baked goods, candies, and sweet desserts.
- Reach for fresh fruit instead of cookies or candy for dessert and between-meal snacks.
- Add less sugar to foods—coffee, tea, cereal, and fruit. Cut back gradually to a quarter or half the amount. Consider using sugar alternatives to substitute for some sugar.
- Reduce the number of sugared soft drinks, punches, and fruit juices you drink. Substitute water, diet soft drinks, and whole fruits.

▲ Many foods we enjoy are sweet. These should be eaten in moderation.

## Dental Caries

Sugars in the diet (and starches readily fermented in the mouth, such as crackers and white bread) also increase the risk of developing **dental caries**. Recall that caries, also known as cavities, are formed when sugars and other carbohydrates are metabolized into acids by bacteria that live in the mouth (Fig. 4-12). These acids dissolve the tooth enamel and underlying structure. Bacteria also use the sugars to make plaque, a sticky substance that both adheres acid-producing bacteria to teeth and diminishes the acid-neutralizing effect of saliva.

The worst offenders in terms of promoting dental caries are sticky and gummy foods high in sugars, such as caramel, because they stick to the teeth and supply the bacteria with a long-lived carbohydrate source. Frequent consumption of liquid sugar sources (e.g., fruit juices) can also cause dental caries. Snacking regularly on sugary foods is also likely to cause caries because it gives the bacteria on the teeth a steady source of carbohydrate from which to continually make acid. Sugared gum chewed between meals is a prime example of a poor dental habit. Still, sugar-containing foods are not the only foods that promote acid production by bacteria in the mouth. As mentioned, if starch-containing foods (e.g., crackers and bread) are held in the mouth for a long time, the starch will be broken down to sugars by enzymes in the mouth; bacteria can then produce acid from these sugars. Overall, the sugar and starch content of a food and its ability to remain in the mouth largely determine its potential to cause caries.

**dental caries** Erosions in the surface of a tooth caused by acids made by bacteria as they metabolize sugars.

**FIGURE 4-12** ▶ Dental caries. Bacteria can collect in various areas on a tooth. Using simple sugars such as sucrose, bacteria then create acids that can dissolve tooth enamel, leading to caries. If the caries process progresses and enters the pulp cavity, damage to the nerve and resulting pain are likely. The bacteria also produce plaque whereby they adhere to the tooth surface.

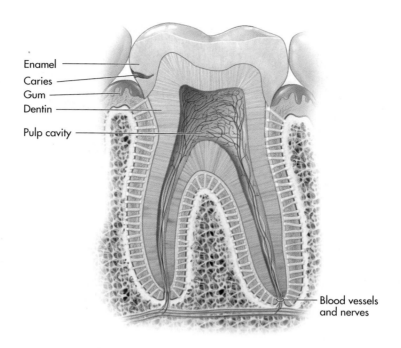

Enamel
Caries
Gum
Dentin
Pulp cavity
Blood vessels and nerves

## CRITICAL THINKING

John and Mike are identical twins who like the same games, sports, and foods. However, John likes to chew sugar-free gum and Mike doesn't. At their last dental visit, John had no cavities, but Mike had two. Mike wants to know why John, who chews gum after eating, doesn't have cavities and he does. How would you explain this to him?

Fluoridated water and toothpaste have contributed to fewer dental caries in North American children over the past 20 years due to fluoride's tooth-strengthening effect (see Chapter 9). Research has also indicated that certain foods—such as cheese, peanuts, and sugar-free chewing gum—can help reduce the amount of acid on teeth. In addition, rinsing the mouth after meals and snacks reduces the acidity in the mouth. Certainly, good nutrition, habits that do not present an overwhelming challenge to oral health (e.g., chewing sugar-free gum), and routine visits to the dentist all contribute to improved dental health.

## CONCEPT CHECK

The RDA for carbohydrate is 130 grams per day. The typical North American diet provides 180 to 330 grams per day. A reasonable goal is to have about half of our calorie intake coming from starch and our total carbohydrate intake making up about 60% of our calorie intake, with a range of 45% to 65%. This should allow for the recommended intake of 25 to 38 grams of fiber per day for women and men, respectively. High-fiber diets must be accompanied by adequate fluid intakes to avoid constipation and should be followed only under a physician's guidance.

North Americans eat about 82 grams of sugars added to foods each day. Most of these sugars are added to foods and beverages in processing. To reduce consumption of sugars, one must reduce consumption of items with added sugars, such as some baked goods, sweetened beverages, and presweetened ready-to-eat breakfast cereals. This is one practice that can help reduce the development of dental caries and likely improve diet quality and various aspects of health.

# Diabetes—When Blood Glucose Regulation Fails

Improper regulation of blood glucose results in either hyperglycemia (high blood glucose) or hypoglycemia (low blood glucose) as noted in this chapter. High blood glucose is most commonly associated with diabetes (technically, *diabetes mellitus*), a disease that affects 6.5% of the North American population. Of these, it is estimated one-third to one-half of these people do not know that they have the disease. Diabetes leads to about 200,000 deaths each year in North America. Diabetes is currently increasing in epidemic proportions in North America. New recommendations promote testing fasting blood glucose in adults over age 45 every 3 years to help diagnose the problem. Diabetes is diagnosed when one's fasting blood glucose is 126 milligrams per 100 milliliters of blood or greater. In contrast, low blood glucose is a much rarer condition.

## Diabetes

There are two major forms of diabetes: **type 1** (formerly called insulin-dependent or juvenile-onset diabetes), and **type 2 diabetes** (formerly called non–insulin-dependent or adult-onset diabetes) (Table 4-6). The change in names to type 1 and type 2 diabetes stems from the fact that many type 2 diabetics eventually must also rely on insulin injections as a part of their treatment. In addition, many children today have type 2 diabetes. A third form, called gestational diabetes, occurs in some pregnant women (see Chapter 14). It is usually treated with an insulin regimen and diet and resolves after delivery of the baby. However, women who have gestational diabetes during pregnancy are at high risk for developing type 2 diabetes later in life.

Traditional symptoms of diabetes are excessive urination, excessive thirst, and excessive hunger. No one symptom is diagnostic of diabetes, and other

**TABLE 4-6** Comparison of Type 1 and Type 2 Diabetes

|  | Type 1 Diabetes | Type 2 Diabetes |
|---|---|---|
| **Occurrence** | 5–10% of cases of diabetes | 90% of cases of diabetes |
| **Cause** | Autoimmune attack on the pancreas | Insulin resistance |
| **Risk Factors** | Moderate genetic predisposition | Strong genetic predisposition<br>Obesity and physical inactivity<br>Ethnicity<br>Metabolic Syndrome<br>Pre-diabetes |
| **Characteristics** | Distinct symptoms (frequent thirst, hunger, and urination)<br>Ketosis<br>Weight loss | Mild symptoms, especially in early phases of the disease (fatigue and nighttime urination)<br>Ketosis does not generally occur. |
| **Treatment** | Insulin<br>Diet<br>Exercise | Diet<br>Exercise<br>Oral medications to lower blood glucose<br>Insulin (in advanced cases) |
| **Complications** | Cardiovascular disease<br>Kidney disease<br>Nerve disease<br>Blindness<br>Infections | Cardiovascular disease<br>Kidney disease<br>Nerve damage<br>Blindness<br>Infections |
| **Monitoring** | Blood glucose<br>Urine ketones<br>HbA1c* | Blood glucose<br>HbA1c |

*Hemoglobin A1c

**type 1 diabetes** A form of diabetes prone to ketosis and that requires insulin therapy.

**type 2 diabetes** A form of diabetes characterized by insulin resistance and often associated with obesity. Insulin therapy can be used but is often not required.

symptoms—such as unexplained weight loss, exhaustion, blurred vision, tingling in hands and feet, frequent infections, poor wound healing, and impotence—often accompany traditional symptoms.

## Type 1 Diabetes

Type 1 diabetes often begins in late childhood, around the age of 8 to 12 years, but can occur at any age. The disease runs in certain families, indicating a clear genetic link. Children usually are admitted to the hospital with abnormally high blood glucose after eating, as well as evidence of ketosis.

The onset of type 1 diabetes is generally associated with decreased release of insulin from the pancreas. As insulin in the blood declines, blood glucose increases, especially after eating. Figure 4-13 shows a typical glucose tolerance curve observed in a patient with this form of diabetes after consuming about 75 grams of glucose. When blood glucose levels are high, the kidneys let excess glucose spill into the urine, resulting in frequent urination of urine high in sugar.

A common clinical method to determine a person's success in controlling blood glucose is to measure glycated (also termed glycosylated) hemoglobin (hemoglobin A1c). Over time, blood glucose attaches to (glycates) hemoglobin in red blood cells and more so when blood glucose remains elevated. A hemoglobin A1c value of over 7% indicates poor blood glucose control. An acceptable value is 6% or less. Maintaining near-normal hemoglobin A1c levels greatly reduces the risk of death and developing other diseases in people with diabetes. Elevated blood glucose also leads to glycation of other proteins and fats in the body, forming what are called advanced glycation endproducts (AGEs). These have been shown to be toxic to cells, especially those of the immune system and kidneys.

Most cases of type 1 diabetes begin with an immune system disorder, which causes destruction of the insulin-producing cells in the pancreas. Most likely, a virus or protein foreign to the body sets off the destruction. In response to their damage, the affected pancreatic cells release other proteins, which stimulate a more furious

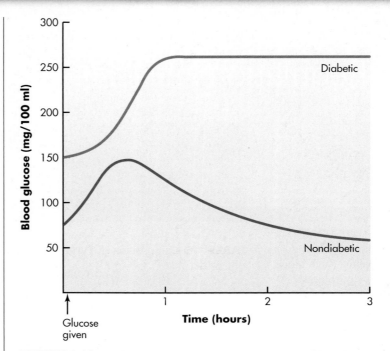

**FIGURE 4-13** ▶ Glucose tolerance test. A comparison of blood glucose concentrations in untreated diabetic and healthy nondiabetic persons after consuming a 75-g test load of glucose.

attack. Eventually, the pancreas loses its ability to synthesize insulin, and the clinical stage of the disease begins. Consequently, early treatment to stop the immune-linked destruction in children may be important. Research into this area is ongoing.

Type 1 diabetes is treated primarily by insulin therapy, either with injections two to six times per day or with an insulin pump. The pump dispenses insulin at a steady rate into the body, with greater amounts delivered after each meal. Inhaled forms of insulin also are available. Dietary therapy includes three regular meals and one or more snacks (including one at bedtime) and having a regulated ratio of carbohydrate:protein:fat to maximize insulin action and minimize swings in blood glucose. If one does not eat often enough, the injected insulin can cause a severe drop in blood glucose or hypoglycemia, because it acts on whatever glucose is available. The diet should be moderate in simple carbohydrates, include ample fiber and polyunsaturated fat, but be low in both animal and *trans* fats, supply an amount of calories in balance with needs, and include fish twice a week. Meeting magnesium needs is also helpful, as well as a moderate intake of coffee.

▶ **Symptoms of Diabetes**

The symptoms of diabetes may occur suddenly, and include one or more of the following:

- Extreme thirst
- Frequent urination
- Drowsiness, lethargy
- Sudden vision changes
- Increased appetite
- Sudden weight loss
- Sugar in urine
- Fruity, sweet, or winelike odor on breath
- Heavy, labored breathing
- Stupor, unconsciousness

▲ Regularly checking blood glucose is part of diabetes therapy.

If a high carbohydrate intake raises triglycerides and cholesterol in the blood beyond desired ranges, carbohydrate intake can be reduced and replaced with unsaturated fat. Surprisingly, this change tends to reduce blood triglycerides and cholesterol. Chapter 5 discusses how to implement such a diet (as well as when certain related medications may be beneficial). Some consumption of sugars with meals is fine, as long as blood glucose regulation is preserved and the sugars replace other carbohydrates in the meal, so that undesirable weight gain does not take place.

The latest evidence suggests that diabetes essentially guarantees development of cardiovascular disease. Because people with diabetes (type 1, as well as type 2) are at a high risk for cardiovascular disease and related heart attacks, they should take an aspirin each day (generally 80 to 160 milligrams per day) if their physicians find no reason not to do so. Blood cholesterol lowering medications also may be prescribed. As discussed in Chapter 5, these practices reduce the risk of heart attack.

The hormone imbalances that occur in people with untreated type 1 diabetes—chiefly, not enough insulin—lead to mobilization of body fat, taken up by liver cells. Ketosis is the result because the fat is partially broken down to ketone bodies. Ketone bodies can rise excessively in the blood, eventually forcing ketone bodies into the urine. These pull sodium and potassium ions and water with them into the urine. This series of events also causes frequent urination and can contribute to a chain reaction that eventually leads to dehydration; ion imbalance; coma; and even death, especially in patients with poorly controlled type 1 diabetes. Treatment includes provision of insulin, fluids, and minerals such as sodium and potassium.

In addition to cardiovascular disease, other degenerative complications that result from poor blood glucose regulation, specifically long-term hyperglycemia, include blindness, kidney disease, and deterioration of nerves. The high blood sugar concentration physically deteriorates small blood vessels (capillaries) and nerves. When improper nerve stimulation occurs in the intestinal tract, intermittent diarrhea and constipation result. Because

of nerve deterioration in the extremities, many people with diabetes lose the sensation of pain associated with injuries or infections. They do not have as much pain, so they often delay treatment of hand or foot problems. This delay, combined with a rich environment for bacterial growth (bacteria thrive on glucose) sets the stage for damage and death of tissues in the extremities, sometimes leading to the need for amputation of feet and legs. Current research has shown that the development of blood vessel and nerve complications of diabetes can be slowed with aggressive treatment directed at keeping blood glucose within the normal range. The therapy poses some risks of its own, such as hypoglycemia, so it must be implemented under the close supervision of a physician.

A person with diabetes generally must work closely with a physician and registered dietitian to make the correct alterations in diet and medications and to perform physical activity safely. Physical activity enhances glucose uptake by muscles independent of insulin action, which in turn can lower blood glucose. This outcome is beneficial, but people with type 1 diabetes need to be aware of their blood glucose response to physical activity and compensate appropriately.

## Type 2 Diabetes

Type 2 diabetes usually begins after age 40. This is the most common type of diabetes, accounting for about 90% of the cases diagnosed in North America. Minority populations such as Latino/Hispanic Americans, African Americans, Asian Americans, Native Americans, and those from Pacific Islands are at particular risk. As noted in the introduction, the overall number of people affected also is on the rise, primarily because of widespread inactivity and obesity in our population. There has been a substantial increase in type 2 diabetes in children, due mostly to an increase in over-weight in this population (coupled with limited physical activity). Type 2 diabetes is also genetically linked, so family history is an important risk factor. However, the initial problem is not with the insulin-secreting cells of the pancreas. Instead, type 2 diabetes arises when the insulin receptors on the cell surfaces of certain body tissues, especially muscle tissue, become insulin resistant. In this case, blood glucose is not readily transferred into cells, so the person develops high blood glucose as a result of the glucose remaining in the bloodstream. The pancreas attempts to increase insulin output to compensate, but there is a limit to its ability to do this. Thus, rather than insufficient insulin production, there is an abundance of insulin, particularly during the onset of the disease. As the disease develops, pancreatic function can fail, leading to reduced insulin output. Because of the genetic link for type 2 diabetes, those who have a family history should schedule regular blood glucose tests and be careful to avoid risk factors such as obesity, inactivity, a diet rich in animal and *trans* fats, and simple carbohydrates.

Many cases of type 2 diabetes (about 80%) are associated with obesity (especially with fat located in the abdominal region), but high blood glucose is not directly caused by the obesity. In fact, some lean people also develop this type of diabetes. Obesity associated with oversized adipose cells increases the risk for insulin resistance by the body as more fat is added to these cells during weight gain.

Type 2 diabetes linked to obesity often disappears if the obesity is corrected. Achieving a healthy weight therefore should be a primary goal of treatment, but even limited weight loss can lead to better blood glucose regulation. Although many cases of type 2 diabetes can be relieved by reducing excess adipose tissue stores, many people are not able to lose weight. They remain affected with diabetes and may experience the degenerative complications seen in the type 1 form of the disease. Ketosis, however, is not usually seen in type 2 diabetes. Certain oral medications can also help control blood glucose. Adequate chromium intake is also important for blood glucose regulation (see Chapter 9). Patients with type 2 diabetes may experience decreased effectiveness of their treatments over time resulting in spikes in blood glucose after meals and weight gain. New classes of drugs that mimic gut hormones are helping diabetic patients overcome the chronic

▲ Regular exercise is a key part of a plan to prevent (and control) type 2 diabetes.

problems that conventional treatments alone have been unable to control.

Sometimes it may be necessary to provide insulin injections in type 2 diabetes because nothing else is able to control the disease. (This eventually becomes true in about half of all cases of type 2 diabetes.) Regular physical activity also helps the muscles take up more glucose. And regular meal patterns, with an emphasis on control of calorie intake and consumption of mostly fiber-rich carbohydrates, as well as regular fish intake, is important therapy. Nuts help fulfill the goal of increased fiber consumption. (An almost daily intake of nuts was even shown to reduce the risk of developing type 2 diabetes in one study.) Some sugar consumption is fine with meals, but again these must be substituted for other carbohydrates, not simply added to the meal plan. Distributing carbohydrates throughout the day is also important, as this helps minimize the high and low swings in blood glucose concentrations. Moderate alcohol use is acceptable (1 serving per day) and has been shown to substantially reduce heart attack risk in people with type 2 diabetes. Still, the person must be warned that alcohol can lead to hypoglycemia and that regular testing for this possibility is necessary. And, as mentioned

before, meeting magnesium needs and moderate coffee intake are also helpful.

People with type 2 diabetes who have high blood triglycerides should moderate their carbohydrate intake and increase their intake of unsaturated fat and fiber, as noted earlier for people with type 1 diabetes.

## Hypoglycemia

As noted earlier, people with diabetes who are taking insulin sometimes have hypoglycemia if they don't eat frequently enough. Hypoglycemia can also develop in nondiabetic individuals. The two common forms of nondiabetic hypoglycemia are termed *reactive* and *fasting*.

**Reactive hypoglycemia** occurs 2 to 4 hours after eating a meal, especially a meal high in simple sugars. It results

▶ For more information on diabetes, consult the following websites: **www.diabetes.org** and **ndep.nih.gov**.

**reactive hypoglycemia** Low blood glucose that follows a meal high in simple sugars, with corresponding symptoms of irritability, headache, nervousness, sweating, and confusion; also called *postprandial hypoglycemia*.

in irritability, nervousness, headache, sweating, and confusion. The cause of reactive hypoglycemia is unclear, but it may be overproduction of insulin by the pancreas in response to rising blood glucose. In **fasting hypoglycemia**, blood glucose falls to low concentrations after fasting for about 8 hours to 1 day. It usually is caused by pancreatic cancer, which may lead to excessive insulin secretion. This form of hypoglycemia is rare.

The diagnosis of hypoglycemia requires the simultaneous presence of low blood glucose and the typical hypoglycemic

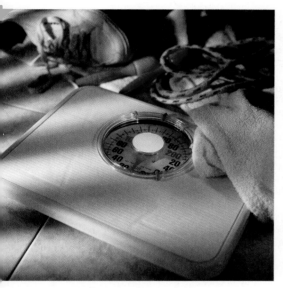

▲ Decreasing body weight and increasing physical activity are interventions to help prevent the metabolic syndrome.

**reactive hypoglycemia** Low blood glucose that follows a meal high in simple sugars, with corresponding symptoms of irritability, headache, nervousness, sweating, and confusion; also called *postprandial hypoglycemia*.

**fasting hypoglycemia** Low blood glucose that follows about a day of fasting.

**metabolic syndrome** A condition in which a person has poor blood glucose regulation, hypertension, increased blood triglycerides, and other health problems. This condition is usually accompanied by obesity, lack of physical activity, and a diet high in refined carbohydrates. Also called Syndrome X.

symptoms. Blood glucose of 40 to 50 milligrams per 100 milliliters is suggestive, but just having low blood glucose after eating is not enough evidence to make the diagnosis of hypoglycemia. Although many people think they have hypoglycemia, few actually do.

It is normal for healthy people to have some hypoglycemic symptoms, such as irritability, headache, and shakiness, if they have not eaten for a prolonged period. If you sometimes have symptoms of hypoglycemia, you need to eat regular meals, make sure you have some protein and fat in each meal, and eat complex carbohydrates with ample soluble fiber. Avoid meals or snacks that contain little more than simple carbohydrates. This standard nutrition therapy is one we all could follow. If symptoms continue, try small protein-containing snacks or fruits and juice between meals. Fat, protein, and viscous fiber in the diet tend to moderate swings in blood glucose. Last, moderate caffeine and alcohol intake.

## Metabolic Syndrome

**Metabolic syndrome**, also known as Syndrome X, is characterized by the occurrence of several risk factors for diabetes and cardiovascular disease. The precise definition and criteria for diagnosis have recently been debated by health scholars. A person with metabolic syndrome has several or all of the following conditions: abdominal obesity (accumulation of fat around and within the midsection), high blood triglycerides, low HDL or "good" cholesterol, hypertension, high fasting blood glucose, increased blood clotting, and increased inflammation (Fig. 4-14). Each aspect of metabolic syndrome is a unique health problem with its own treatment. In metabolic syndrome, however, these risk factors are clustered together, making a person twice as likely to develop cardiovascular disease and five times more likely to develop diabetes.

It is generally accepted that one key element unifies all the aspects of metabolic syndrome: *insulin resistance*. As you learned in this chapter, insulin is a hormone that directs tissues to pull glucose out of the blood and into cells for storage or fuel.

With insulin resistance, the pancreas produces plenty of insulin, but the cells of the body do not respond to it effectively. Instead, excess glucose stays in the bloodstream. For a while the pancreas may be able to compensate for the resistance of cells to insulin by over-producing insulin. Over time, however, the pancreas is unable to keep up the accelerated insulin production and blood glucose levels remain elevated. With metabolic syndrome, blood glucose is not high enough to be classified as diabetes ($\geq$ 126 milligrams per deciliter), but without intervention, it is likely to get worse and eventually lead to diabetes.

Genetics and aging contribute to the development of insulin resistance and the other elements of metabolic syndrome, but environmental factors such as diet and activity play an important role. Obesity, particularly abdominal obesity, is highly related to insulin resistance. More than half of adults in the United States are over-weight, 30% are obese, and these numbers continue to climb year after year. Increases in body weight among children and adolescents are of great concern because it places them at high risk for these health problems. This increase in body weight has precipitated a dramatic surge in cardiovascular disease and diabetes risk—an estimated 50 million Americans now have metabolic syndrome.

There is controversy among health professionals, over whether to treat each risk factor uniquely or to attempt to integrate therapies to treat all the risk factors simultaneously. For example, the chief culprits contributing to the high blood triglycerides of metabolic syndrome are excessively large meals full of foods rich in simple sugars and refined starches and low in fiber, coupled with little physical activity. Nutrition and lifestyle changes are key strategies in addressing all of the unhealthy conditions of metabolic syndrome as a whole. Suggested interventions include:

- Decrease body weight. Even small improvements (e.g., 5% weight loss) for overweight and obese individuals can lessen disease risk. The most successful weight loss and weight maintenance programs include moderate dietary

## Metabolic Syndrome Risk Indicators

- **High blood pressure**
  130/85 mmHg or higher

- **Low HDL cholesterol**
  - Men with HDL level less than 40 mg/dl
  - Women with HDL level less than 50 mg/dL

- **Elevated glucose**
  Fasting level of 100 mg/dL or higher

- **Elevated triglycerides (blood fat)**
  150 mg/dL or higher

- **Abdominal obesity**
  - Men with waist circumference greater than 42 inches
  - Women with waist circumference greater than 35 inches

## Medical Conditions Related to Metabolic Syndrome

**1 Type 2 diabetes**
Over time, insulin resistance can increase blood glucose levels, which can lead to type 2 diabetes.

**2 Coronary artery disease**
Elevated blood pressure and cholesterol levels can cause plaque to build up inside coronary arteries, which may eventually lead to a heart attack.

**3 Stroke**
Plaque build-up in arteries can lead to blood clots that prevent blood flow to the brain, causing damage to brain tissue.

**FIGURE 4-14** ▶ For a patient to be diagnosed with metabolic syndrome, he or she must have three of the five risk factors listed above.

restriction combined with physical activity.
- Increase physical activity. To alleviate risks for chronic diseases, the Dietary Guidelines for Americans include a recommendation for at least 30 minutes of moderate-intensity physical activity on most days of the week.
- Choose healthy fats. Limiting intakes of total fat, saturated fat, and *trans* fat are generally recommended for improving blood lipids. Including omega-3 fats, such as those found in fish and nuts, is another way to combat chronic disease.
- For those with particularly high risk for cardiovascular disease, medications may be warranted.

## Case Study Problems with Milk Intake

Myeshia is a 19-year-old African-American female who recently read about the health benefits of calcium and decided to increase her intake of dairy products. To start, she drank a cup of 1% milk at lunch. Not long afterward, she experienced bloating, cramping, and increased gas production. She suspected that the culprit of this pain was the milk she consumed, especially because her parents and her sister complain of the same problem. She wanted to determine if other milk products were, in fact, the cause of her discomfort so the next day she substituted a cup of yogurt for the glass of milk at lunch. Subsequently, she did not have any pain.

Answer the following questions, and check your response in Appendix A.

1. Why did Myeshia believe that she was sensitive to milk?
2. What component of milk is likely causing the problems that Myeshia experiences after drinking milk?
3. Why does this component cause intestinal discomfort in some individuals?
4. What is the name of this condition?
5. What groups of people are most likely to experience this condition?
6. Why did consuming yogurt not cause the same effects for Myeshia?
7. Are there any other products on the market that can replace regular milk or otherwise alleviate symptoms for individuals with this problem?
8. Can people with this condition ever drink regular milk?
9. What nutrients may be inadequate in the diet if dairy products are not consumed?
10. Why do some individuals have trouble tolerating milk products during or immediately after an intestinal viral infection?

## Summary

1. The common monosaccharides in food are glucose, fructose, and galactose. Once these are absorbed from the small intestine and delivered to the liver, much of the fructose and galactose is converted to glucose.

   The major disaccharides are sucrose (glucose + fructose), maltose (glucose + glucose), and lactose (glucose + galactose). When digested, these yield their component monosaccharides.

   One major group of polysaccharides consists of storage forms of glucose: starches in plants and glycogen in humans. These can be broken down by human digestive enzymes, releasing the glucose units. The main plant starches—straight-chain amylose and branched-chain amylopectin—are digested by enzymes in the mouth and small intestine. In humans, glycogen is synthesized in the liver and muscle tissue from glucose. Under the influence of hormones, liver glycogen is readily broken down to glucose, which can enter the bloodstream.

   Fiber is composed primarily of the polysaccharides cellulose, hemicellulose, pectin, gum, and mucilage, as well as the noncarbohydrate lignins. These substances are not broken down by human digestive enzymes. However, soluble (also called viscous) fiber is fermented by bacteria in the large intestine.

2. Table sugar, honey, jelly, fruit, and plain baked potatoes are some of the most concentrated sources of carbohydrates. Other high-carbohydrate foods, such as pie and fat-free milk, are diluted by either fat or protein. Nutritive sweeteners in food include sucrose, high-fructose corn syrup, brown sugar, and maple syrup. Several alternative sweeteners are approved for use by FDA: saccharin, aspartame, sucralose, neotame, acesulfame-K, and tagatose.

3. Some starch digestion occurs in the mouth. Carbohydrate digestion is completed in the small intestine. Some plant fibers are digested by the bacteria present in the large intestine; undigested plant fibers become part

of the feces. Monosaccharides in the intestinal contents mostly follow an active absorption process. They are then transported via the portal vein that leads directly to the liver.

The ability to digest large amounts of lactose often diminishes with age. People in some ethnic groups are especially affected. This condition often develops early in childhood and is referred to as *lactose maldigestion.* Undigested lactose travels to the large intestine, resulting in such symptoms as abdominal gas, pain, and diarrhea. Most people with lactose maldigestion can tolerate cheese, yogurt, and moderate amounts of milk.

4. Carbohydrates provide calories (on average, 4 kcal per gram), protect against wasteful breakdown of food and body protein, and prevent ketosis. The RDA for carbohydrate is 130 grams per day. If carbohydrate intake is inadequate for the body's needs, protein is metabolized to provide glucose for energy needs. However, the price is loss of body protein, ketosis, and eventually a general body weakening. For this reason, low-carbohydrate diets are not recommended for extended periods.

5. Blood glucose concentration is regulated within a narrow range of 70 to 99 mg/dL. Insulin and glucagon are hormones that control blood glucose concentration. When we eat a meal, insulin promotes glucose uptake by cells. When fasting, glucagon promotes glucose release from glycogen stores in the liver.

6. Insoluble (also called nonfermentable) fiber provides mass to the feces, thus easing elimination. In high doses, soluble fiber can help control blood glucose in diabetic people and lower blood cholesterol.

7. Diets high in complex carbohydrates are encouraged as a replacement for high-fat diets. A goal of about half of calories as complex carbohydrates is a good one, with about 45% to 65% of total calories coming from carbohydrates in general. Foods to consume are whole-grain cereal products, pasta, legumes, fruits, and vegetables. Many of these foods are rich in fiber.

Moderating sugar intake, especially between meals, reduces the risk of dental caries. Alternative sweeteners, such as aspartame, aid in reducing intake of sugars.

8. Diabetes is characterized by a persistent high blood glucose concentration. A healthy diet and regular physical activity are helpful in treating both type 1 and type 2 diabetes. Insulin is the main medication employed—it is required in type 1 diabetes and may be used in type 2 diabetes.

## Study Questions

1. Outline the basic steps in blood glucose regulation, including the roles of insulin and glucagon.

2. What are the three major monosaccharides and the three major disaccharides? Describe how each plays a part in the human diet.

3. Why are some foods that are high in carbohydrates, such as cookies and fat-free milk, not considered to be concentrated sources of carbohydrates?

4. Describe the digestion of the various types of carbohydrates in the body.

5. Describe the reason why some people are unable to tolerate high intakes of milk.

6. What are the important roles that fiber plays in the diet?

7. What, if any, are the proven ill effects of sugar in the diet?

8. Why do we need carbohydrates in the diet?

9. Summarize current carbohydrate intake recommendations.

10. List three alternatives to simple sugars for adding sweetness to the diet.

## Check Your Knowledge

Answers to the following multiple choice questions are below.

1. Dietary fiber
   a. raises blood cholesterol levels.
   b. speeds up transit time for food through the digestive tract.
   c. causes diverticulosis.
   d. causes constipation.

2. When the pancreas detects excess glucose, it releases the
   a. enzyme amylase.
   b. monosaccharide glucose.
   c. hormone insulin.
   d. hormone glucagon.

3. Cellulose is a(n)
   a. indigestible fiber.
   b. simple carbohydrate.
   c. energy-yielding nutrient.
   d. animal polysaccharide.

4. Digested white sugar is broken into _____ and _____.
   a. glucose, lactose
   b. glucose, fructose
   c. sucrose, maltose
   d. fructose, sucrose

5. Starch is a
   a. complex carbohydrate.
   b. fiber.
   c. simple carbohydrate.
   d. gluten.

6. Fiber content of the diet can be increased by adding
   a. fresh fruits.
   b. fish and poultry.
   c. eggs.
   d. whole grains and cereals.
   e. Both a and d.

7. Which form of diabetes is most common?
   a. type 1
   b. type 2
   c. type 3
   d. gestational

8. The recommended daily intake for fiber is approximately _____ grams.
   a. 5           c. 100
   b. 30          d. 450

9. Glucose, galactose, and fructose are
   a. disaccharides.
   b. sugar alcohols.
   c. monosaccharides.
   d. polysaccharides.

10. One of the components of metabolic syndrome is
   a. obesity.
   b. diabetes.
   c. low blood sugar.
   d. low blood pressure.

Answers: 1. b, 2. c, 3. a, 4. b, 5. a, 6. e, 7. b, 8. b, 9. c, 10. b

# Further Readings

1. ADA Reports: Position of the American Dietetic Association: Use of nutritive and nonnutritive sweeteners. *Journal of the American Dietetic Association* 104:225, 2004.

   *When currently recommended diet practices are met, such as the Dietary Guidelines for Americans, use of some nutritive and nonnutritive sweeteners is acceptable. The text of the article explores in detail both classes of sweeteners, in turn supporting this overall conclusion.*

2. American Diabetes Association: Nutrition recommendations and interventions for diabetes: A position statement of the American Diabetes Association. *Diabetes Care* 31 (suppl 1): S61, 2008.

   *This article provides a comprehensive look at the treatment of diabetes. Goals for therapy and medical tools to help reach those goals are highlighted.*

3. American Diabetes Association and American Dietetic Association: *Choose your foods: Exchange lists for diabetes.* 2008.

   *This update of a booklet that has been in existence for more than 50 years is used as the basis for nutrition education for diabetes meal planning. Foods are grouped into general categories (or lists) that, per serving size, are similar in macronutrients and calories. Changes have been made so they are easier to use and foods within the lists have been updated.*

4. Artificial Sweeteners: No calories. . .Sweet! *FDA Consumer* 40(4):406, 2006.

   *This article is an update on the artificial sweeteners approved by the FDA. To date, five artificial sweeteners are approved by the FDA: aspartame, saccharin, acesulfame-K, neotame, and sucralose. The typical amount of each of these sweeteners used by U.S. consumers is well within designated levels that can be consumed safely every day over a lifetime. The article provides a detailed look at each of the sweeteners.*

5. Cowie CC and others: Prevalence of diabetes and impaired fasting glucose in adults in the U.S. population. *Diabetes Care* 29:1263, 2006.

   *The results of this study of the National Health And Nutrition Examination Survey (NHANES) suggest that 73 million Americans have diabetes or are at risk based on higher-than-normal blood glucose levels. The prevalence of diagnosed diabetes increased significantly over the last decade, and minority groups remain disproportionately affected. The overall prevalence of total diabetes in 1999–2002 was 9.3% (19.3 million), consisting of 6.5% diagnosed and 2.8% undiagnosed. The prevalence of diagnosed diabetes rose from 5.1% in 1988–1994 to 6.5% in 1999–2002. The prevalence of total diabetes was much greater (21.6%) in older individuals aged ≥ 65 years. Diagnosed diabetes was twice as prevalent in non-Hispanic blacks and Mexican-Americans compared with non-Hispanic whites.*

6. Ebbeling CB and others: Effects of decreasing sugar-sweetened beverage consumption on body weight in adolescents: A randomized, controlled pilot study. *Pediatrics* 117:673, 2006.

   *The consumption of sugar-sweetened drinks by children has increased dramatically over the past 20 years right along with the rise in childhood obesity. A new intervention aimed at limiting consumption of sugary drinks had a beneficial effect on weight loss in teens. The intervention was the home delivery of noncaloric beverages (water and artificially sweetened drinks) to displace sugar-sweetened beverages. The teens were also instructed on how to choose noncaloric drinks outside the home. The intervention decreased consumption of sugary drinks by 82%. The heavier the teen, the greater was the effect on body weight. The authors calculate that a single 12-ounce sugar-sweetened beverage per day results in about 1 pound of weight gain over 3 to 4 weeks.*

7. Food and Nutrition Board: *Dietary reference intakes for energy, carbohydrate, fiber, fat, fatty acids, cholesterol, protein, and amino acids.* Washington, DC: National Academy Press, 2005.

   *This report provides the latest guidance for macronutrient intakes. With regard to carbohydrate, the RDA has been set at 130 grams per day. Carbohydrate intake should range from 45% to 65% of calorie intake. Sugars added to foods should constitute no more than 25% of calorie intake.*

8. Grundy SM: Does a diagnosis of metabolic syndrome have a value in clinical practice? *American Journal of Clinical Nutrition* 83:1248, 2006.

   *The metabolic syndrome concept has led to the development of clinical guidelines by the World Health Organization and the National Cholesterol Education Program. These guidelines have been well accepted by medical professionals. This article reviews the new diagnosis of metabolic syndrome and discusses why organizations including the American Diabetes Association and many diabetes specialists have not embraced the clustering of its risk factors.*

9. Hayes C, Kriska A: Role of physical activity in diabetes management and prevention. *Journal of the American Dietetic Association* 108: S19, 2008.

   *Evidence supporting the important role of physical activity in the prevention and treatment of diabetes has accumulated. Despite the benefits of physical activity, many people are physically inactive. As the prevalence of overweight and obesity, prediabetes, and type 2 diabetes rises, physical inactivity has become an urgent public health concern. This article reviews research about physical activity/exercise in diabetes and summarizes the current exercise recommendations. This information can be used by health professionals to make safe and effective recommendations for integrating physical activity/ exercise into plans for individuals with or at risk of developing diabetes.*

10. McMillan-Price J and others: Comparison of 4 diets of varying glycemic load on weight loss and cardiovascular risk reduction in overweight and obese young adults. *Archives of Internal Medicine* 166:1466, 2006.

    *In this study of 128 overweight or obese young adults, both high-protein and low-glycemic index diets increased body fat loss. Cardiovascular disease risk was decreased best with a high-carbohydrate, low-glycemic index diet.*

11. Park Y and others: Dietary fiber intake and risk of colorectal cancer. *Journal of the American Medical Association* 294:2849, 2005.

    *In this large analysis of pooled data from 13 prospective studies, dietary fiber was inversely associated with risk of colorectal cancer when data were adjusted for age. However, when other dietary risk factors (red meat, total milk, and alcohol intake) were accounted for, high-dietary fiber intake was not associated with a decreased risk of colorectal cancer. The authors conclude that a diet high in dietary fiber from whole plant foods can still be advised because this has been related to lower risks of other chronic conditions, including heart disease and diabetes.*

12. Pastors JG: Metabolic syndrome—is obesity the culprit? *Today's Dietitian* 8(3):12, 2006.

    *Metabolic syndrome, especially its link to obesity, has become better understood in recent years. This article reviews the role of obesity, the dilemmas of diagnosis, new diet and activity guidelines, and the need for a combination of therapeutic approaches for metabolic syndrome.*

13. Savaiano DA and others: Lactose intolerance symptoms assessed by meta-analysis: A grain of truth that leads to exaggeration. *Journal of Nutrition* 136: 1107, 2006.

    *An analysis of the results of 21 studies of lactose intolerance revealed that lactose is not a major cause of symptoms for lactose maldigesters after a moderate intake of dairy foods equaling about 1 cup.*

14. Slavin J and others: How fiber affects weight regulation. *Food Technology*, p. 34, February 2008.

    *High-fiber diets are linked to lower body weight. This article discusses the effect of different fibers on satiety and food intake. Dietary fiber has intrinsic, hormonal, and intestinal effects that decrease food intake by promoting satiety. Examples of these effects include decreased gastric emptying and/or slowed energy and nutrient absorption.*

15. Swann L: Educate your brain about whole grain. *Today's Dietitian* 8(6):36, 2006.

    *The 2005 Dietary Guidelines recommend 3 or more ounces of whole-grain products per day. This equals about one-half of one's intake from the grain group. Recent surveys, however, have found that only 5% of American adults eat*

*one-half of their grains as whole grains. This article discusses the need to better educate consumers about whole grain including better definitions and ways of measuring these foods.*

16. Sweeteners can sour your health. *Consumer Reports on Health* p. 8, January 2005.

    *Limiting simple sugars in a diet is important to lessen the risk of developing obesity, diabetes, and dental caries, as well as increasing diet quality. Moderate use of the alternative sweeteners listed in the article helps one meet that goal.*

17. The whole grain story. *Tufts University Health & Nutrition Letter* p. 4, July 2005.

    *Regular whole-grain consumption may help prevent cardiovascular disease, unnecessary weight gain, and the metabolic syndrome. This is easier to do today because many whole-grain products are available.*

18. Wang Y and others: Comparison of abdominal adiposity and overall obesity in predicting risk of type 2 diabetes in men. *American Journal of Clinical Nutrition* 81:555, 2005.

    *Obesity and excess upper body fat stores are both risk factors for developing type 2 diabetes. Avoiding both conditions is important, especially excess upper body fat distribution.*

19. Warshaw HS: FAQs about polyols. *Today's Dietitian* p. 37, April 2004.

    *Polyols (i.e., sugar alcohols) yield from 0.2–3.0 kcal per gram, so still need to be considered when calculating the calorie content of a diet. A major attribute of these products is that they do not increase the risk for dental caries.*

# RATE YOUR PLATE

## I. Estimate Your Fiber Intake

Review the sample menus shown in Table 4-7. The first menu contains 1600 kcal and 25 grams of fiber (AI for women); the second menu contains 2100 kcal and 38 grams of fiber (AI for men).

**TABLE 4-7** Sample Menus Containing 1600 kcal with 25 g of Fiber and 2000 kcal with 38 g of Fiber*

| Menu | 25 g Fiber | | | 38 g Fiber | | |
|---|---|---|---|---|---|---|
| | Serving Size | Carbohydrate Content (g) | Fiber Content (g) | Serving Size | Carbohydrate Content (g) | Fiber Content (g) |
| **Breakfast** | | | | | | |
| Muesli cereal | 1 cup | 60 | 6 | 1 cup | 60 | 6 |
| Raspberries | ½ cup | 11 | 2 | ½ cup | 11 | 2 |
| Whole-wheat toast | 1 slice | 13 | 2 | 2 slices | 26 | 4 |
| Margarine | 1 tsp | 0 | 0 | 1 tsp | 0 | 0 |
| Orange juice | 1 cup | 28 | 0 | 1 cup | 28 | 0 |
| 1% milk | 1 cup | 24 | 0 | 1 cup | 24 | 0 |
| Coffee | 1 cup | 0 | 0 | 1 cup | 0 | 0 |
| **Lunch** | | | | | | |
| Bean and vegetable burrito | 2 small | 50 | 4.5 | 3 small | 75 | 7 |
| Guacamole | ¼ cup | 5 | 4 | ¼ cup | 5 | 4 |
| Monterey Jack cheese | 1 oz | 0 | 0 | 1 oz | 0 | 0 |
| Pear (with skin) | 1 | 25 | 4 | 1 | 25 | 4 |
| Carrot sticks | — | — | — | ¾ cup | 6 | 3 |
| Sparkling water | 2 cups | 0 | 0 | 2 cups | 0 | 0 |
| **Dinner** | | | | | | |
| Grilled chicken (no skin) | 3 oz | 0 | 0 | 3 oz | 0 | 0 |
| Salad | ½ cup red cabbage ½ cup romaine ¼ cup peach slices | 7 | 3 | ½ cup red cabbage ½ cup romaine 1 cup peach slices | 19 | 6 |
| Toasted almonds | — | — | — | ½ oz | 3 | 2 |
| Fat-free salad dressing | 2 tbsp. | 0 | 0 | 2 tbsp. | 0 | 0 |
| 1% milk | 1 cup | 24 | 0 | 1 cup | 24 | 0 |
| Total | | 247 | 25 | | 306 | 38 |

*The overall diet is based on MyPyramid Breakdown of approximate energy content: carbohydrate 58%; protein 12%; fat 30%.

To roughly estimate your daily fiber consumption, determine the number of servings that you ate yesterday from each food category listed here. If you are not meeting your needs, how could you do so? Multiply the serving amount by the value listed and then add up the total amount of fiber.

| Food | Servings | Grams |
|---|---|---|
| **Vegetables** <br> (serving size: 1 cup raw leafy greens or 1/2 cup other vegetables) | _____ ×2 | _____ |
| **Fruits** <br> (serving size: 1 whole fruit; 1/2 grapefruit; 1/2 cup berries or cubed fruit; <br> 1/4 cup dried fruit) | _____ ×2.5 | _____ |
| **Beans, lentils, split peas** <br> (serving size: 1/2 cup cooked) | _____ ×7 | _____ |
| **Nuts, seeds** <br> (serving size: 1/4 cup; 2 tbsp peanut butter) | _____ ×2.5 | _____ |
| **Whole grains** <br> (serving size: 1 slice whole-wheat bread; 1/2 cup whole-wheat pasta, brown rice, or other whole grain; 1/2 each bran or whole-grain muffin) | _____ ×2.5 | _____ |
| **Refined grains** <br> (serving size: 1 slice bread, 1/2 cup pasta, rice, or other processed grains; and 1/2 each refined bagels or muffins) | _____ ×1 | _____ |
| **Breakfast cereals** <br> (serving size: check package for serving size and amount of fiber per serving) | _____ × grams of fiber per serving | _____ |
| **Total Grams of Fiber =** | | _____ |

Adapted from Fiber: Strands of protection. *Consumer Reports on Health*, p. 1, August 1999.

How does your total fiber intake for yesterday compare with the general recommendation of 25 to 38 g of fiber per day for women and men, respectively? If you are not meeting your needs, how could you do so?

## II. Can You Choose the Sandwich with the Most Fiber?

Assume the sandwiches on this blackboard are available at your local deli and sandwich shop. All of the sandwiches provide about 350 kcal. The fiber content ranges from about 1 gram to about 7.5 grams. Rank the sandwiches from highest amount of fiber to lowest amount; then check your answers at the bottom of the page.

### Deli Specials

**Turkey & Swiss on Rye**
Served with tomato slices, sliced cucumbers, romaine lettuce, and mustard

**Ham & Swiss on Sourdough**
Extra-lean ham served with mayonnaise

**Tuna Salad on Whole Wheat**
Our tuna salad contains tuna, grated carrots, onions, and mayonnaise, and is served with alfalfa sprouts, romaine lettuce, and cucumber slices

**Hot Dog**
Served on a white bun with relish, mustard, and catsup

**Soyburger**
Served on a whole-wheat English muffin with tomato and pickle slices, romaine lettuce, and mayonnaise

**PB & J**
Soft white bread with strawberry jelly and smooth peanut butter

**Answer Key:**
1. Soyburger: 7.5 grams
2. Tuna Salad on Whole Wheat: 7 grams
3. Turkey & Swiss on Rye: 4 grams
4. PB & J: 3 grams
5. Ham & Swiss on Sourdough: 1.5 grams
6. Hot Dog: 1 gram

# CHAPTER 5 Lipids

## Student Learning Outcomes  After studying Chapter 5 you will be able to:

1. List four classes of lipids (fats) and the role of each in nutritional health.

2. Distinguish between fatty acids and triglycerides.

3. Differentiate among saturated, monounsaturated, and polyunsaturated fatty acids in terms of structure and food sources.

4. Explain how lipids are digested and absorbed.

5. Name the classes of lipoproteins and classify them according to their functions.

6. List the function of lipids, including the two essential fatty acids.

7. Discuss the implications of various fats, including omega-3 fatty acids, with respect to cardiovascular disease.

8. Characterize the symptoms of cardiovascular disease and highlight some known risk factors.

## Chapter Outline

Student Learning Outcomes

Refresh Your Memory

5.1 Lipids: Common Properties

5.2 Lipids: Main Types

5.3 Fats and Oils in Foods

5.4 Making Lipids Available for Body Use

5.5 Carrying Lipids in the Bloodstream

5.6 Essential Functions of Fatty Acids

5.7 Broader Roles for Fatty Acids and Triglycerides in the Body

5.8 Phospholipids in the Body

5.9 Cholesterol in the Body

5.10 Recommendations for Fat Intake

Nutrition and Your Health: Lipids and Cardiovascular Disease

Case Study: Planning a Heart Healthy Diet

Summary/Study Questions/Check Your Knowledge/Further Readings

Rate Your Plate

YOUR BILL FROM A MEDICAL LABORATORY READS "BLOOD LIPID PROFILE—$95." Your doctor informs you that your "triglycerides are too high." A health-food advertisement suggests using Benecol margarine to lower blood cholesterol. Advertisers plug foods "lowest in saturated fat." All of these substances—triglycerides, cholesterol, and saturated fat—are lipids, a collective term referring to fats and oils.

Lipids contain more than twice the calories per gram (on average, 9 kcal) as proteins and carbohydrates (on average, 4 kcal each). Consumption of common saturated fatty acids also contributes to the risk of cardiovascular disease. As the comic in this chapter suggests, for these reasons, some concern about certain lipids is warranted, but lipids also play vital roles both in the body and in foods. Their presence in the diet is essential to good health, and in general, lipids such as those found in vegetable oils should comprise 20% to 35% of an adult's total calorie intake.

Let's look at lipids in detail—their forms, functions, metabolism, and food sources. Chapter 5 will also look at the link between various lipids and the major "killer" disease in North America: cardiovascular disease, which involves the heart, including the coronary arteries (coronary heart disease), as well as other arteries in the body.

### Refresh Your Memory

As you begin your study of lipids in Chapter 5, you may want to review:

- Legal definitions for various label descriptors, such as low-fat and fat-free in Chapter 2
- The concept of energy density in Chapter 2
- The processes of digestion and absorption in Chapter 3
- The metabolic syndrome in Chapter 4

## 5.1 Lipids: Common Properties

Humans need very little fat in their diet to maintain health. In fact, the body's need for the essential fatty acids can be met by daily consumption of about 2 to 4 tablespoons of plant oil incorporated into foods and consumption of fatty fish such as salmon or tuna at least twice weekly. If fish is not consumed, the essential fatty acids in canola oil, soybean oil, and walnuts contribute much of the same health benefits as those found in fish. Thus, one could follow a purely vegetarian diet containing about 10% of calories from fat and still maintain health. However, as long as saturated fat, cholesterol, and partially-hydrogenated fat (which contains *trans* fat) is minimized, fat intake can safely be higher than that 10% allotment. The Food and Nutrition Board suggests that fat intake can be as high as 35% of calories consumed for an adult (the Acceptable Macronutrient Distribution Range for fat is 20%–35% of calories consumed for adults). Some experts suggest that an intake as high as 40% of calories is appropriate. After learning more about lipids—fats, oils, and related compounds—in Chapter 5, you can decide for yourself how much fat you want to consume, as well as how to track your daily intake.

Lipids are a diverse group of chemical compounds. They share one main characteristic: They do not readily dissolve in water. Think of an oil and vinegar salad dressing. The oil is not soluble in the water-based vinegar; on standing, the two separate into distinct layers, with oil on top and vinegar on the bottom.

High fat, low fat, no fat—which is best? And why is there such a debate? Would it be easier just to avoid fat altogether? Doesn't a high-fat diet lead to obesity? To cardiovascular disease? Overall, which are the "best" fats, and why are French fries, doughnuts, stick margarine, and crackers getting such a bad rap? Chapter 5 provides some answers.

# 5.2 Lipids: Main Types

The chemical structure of lipids is diverse. **Triglycerides** are the most common type of lipid found in the body and in foods. Each triglyceride molecule consists of three fatty acids bonded to **glycerol. Phospholipids** and **sterols,** including **cholesterol,** are also classified as lipids, although their structures can be quite different from the structure of triglycerides. All of these lipid compounds are described in Chapter 5.

Food experts, such as chefs, call lipids that are solid at room temperature *fats,* and lipids that are liquid *oils.* Most people use the word *fat* to refer to all lipids because they don't realize there is a difference. However, *lipid* is a generic term that includes triglycerides and many other substances. To simplify our discussion, Chapter 5 primarily uses the term *fat.* When necessary for clarity, the name of a specific lipid, such as cholesterol, will be used. This word use is consistent with the way many people use these terms.

## Fatty Acids: The Simplest Form of Lipids

In the body and in foods, fatty acids are found in the main form of lipids, triglycerides. A fatty acid is basically a long chain of carbons bonded together and flanked by hydrogens. At one end of the molecule (the alpha end), is an **acid group.** At the other end (the omega end), is a **methyl group** (Fig. 5-1).

Fats in foods are not composed of a single type of fatty acid. Rather, each dietary fat, or triglyceride, is a complex mixture of many different fatty acids, the combination of which provides each food its unique taste and smell.

Recall from Chapter 1 that fatty acids can be saturated or unsaturated. Chemically speaking, a carbon atom can form four bonds. Within the carbon chain of a fatty acid, the carbons bond to other carbons and to hydrogens. The carbons that make up the chain of a **saturated fatty acid** are all connected to each other by single bonds. This allows for the maximum number of hydrogens to be bound. Just as a sponge can be saturated (full) with water, a saturated fatty acid such as stearic acid is saturated with hydrogen (Fig. 5-1a).

As noted earlier, most fats high in saturated fatty acids, such as animal fats, remain solid at room temperature. A good example is the solid fat surrounding a piece of uncooked steak. Chicken fat, semisolid at room temperature, contains less saturated fat than beef fat. However, in some foods, saturated fats are suspended in liquid, such as the butterfat in whole milk, so the solid nature of these fats at room temperature is less apparent.

If the carbon chain of a fatty acid contains a double bond, those carbons in the chain have fewer bonds to share with hydrogen, and the chain is said to be *unsaturated.* A fatty acid with only one double bond is **monounsaturated** (Fig. 5-1b). Canola and olive oils contain a high percentage of monounsaturated fatty acids. Likewise, if two or more of the bonds between the carbons are double bonds, the fatty acid is even less saturated with hydrogens, and so it is **polyunsaturated** (Fig. 5-1c, d). Corn, soybean, sunflower, and safflower oils are rich in polyunsaturated fatty acids.

Unsaturated fatty acids can exist in two different structural forms, the *cis* and *trans* forms. The form of fatty acids known as *trans* fatty acids was briefly described in Chapter 1. In their natural form, monounsaturated and polyunsaturated fatty acids usually are in the *cis* form (Fig. 5-2). By definition, the resulting ***cis* fatty acid** has the hydrogens on the same side of the carbon-carbon double bond. During certain types of food processing (discussed later in this chapter), some hydrogens are transferred to opposite sides of the carbon-carbon double bond, creating the *trans* form, or a ***trans* fatty acid.** As seen in Figure 5-2, the *cis* bond causes the fatty acid backbone to bend, whereas the *trans* bond allows the backbone to remain straighter. This makes it similar to the shape of a saturated fatty acid. The Food and Nutrition Board suggests limiting intake of *trans* fatty acids in processed foods (also referred to as *trans* fats) as much as possible. Later you will see why.

**triglyceride** The major form of lipid in the body and in food. It is composed of three fatty acids bonded to glycerol, an alcohol.

**glycerol** A three-carbon alcohol used to form triglycerides.

**phospholipid** Any of a class of fat-related substances that contain phosphorus, fatty acids, and a nitrogen-containing base. The phospholipids are an essential part of every cell.

**sterol** A compound containing a multi-ring (steroid) structure and a hydroxyl group (–OH). Cholesterol is a typical example.

**cholesterol** A waxy lipid found in all body cells. It has a structure containing multiple chemical rings that is found only in foods that contain animal products.

**saturated fatty acid** A fatty acid containing no carbon-carbon double bonds.

**monounsaturated fatty acid** A fatty acid containing one carbon-carbon double bond.

**polyunsaturated fatty acid** A fatty acid containing two or more carbon-carbon double bonds.

acid group     $-\overset{\displaystyle O}{\underset{\displaystyle |}{\overset{\displaystyle \|}{C}}}-OH$

methyl group   $-CH_3$

▲ Saturated fats, such as butter, are solid at room temperature, whereas unsaturated fats, such as olive and corn oil, are liquid at room temperature.

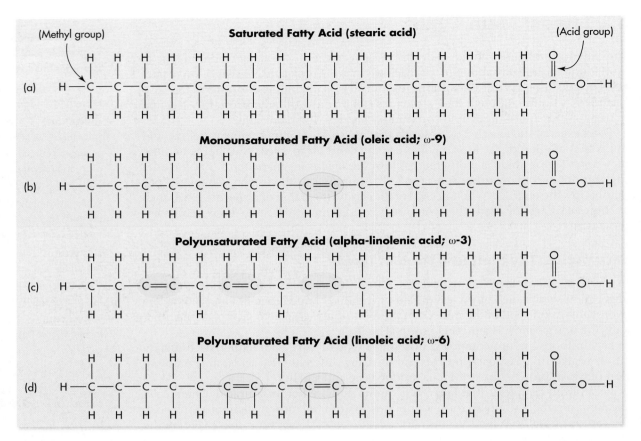

**FIGURE 5-1** ▶ Chemical forms of saturated, monounsaturated, and polyunsaturated fatty acids. Each of the depicted fatty acids contains 18 carbons, but they differ from each other in the number and location of double bonds. The double bonds are shaded. The linear shape of saturated fatty acids, as shown in (a), allows them to pack tightly together and so form a solid at room temperature. In contrast, unsaturated fatty acids have "kinks" where double bonds interrupt the carbon chain (see Figure 5-2). Thus, unsaturated fatty acids pack together only loosely, and are usually liquid at room temperature.

*cis* **fatty acid** A form of an unsaturated fatty acid that has the hydrogens lying on the same side of the carbon-carbon double bond.

*trans* **fatty acid** A form of an unsaturated fatty acid, usually a monounsaturated one when found in food, in which the hydrogens on both carbons forming the double bond lie on opposite sides of that bond.

**long-chain fatty acid** A fatty acid that contains 12 or more carbons.

**omega-3 (ω-3) fatty acid** An unsaturated fatty acid with the first double bond on the third carbon from the methyl end (—CH$_3$).

You may be surprised to learn that some *trans* fatty acids, known as conjugated linoleic acid (CLA), occur naturally. CLA is a family of derivatives of the fatty acid linoleic acid. The bacteria that live in the rumens of some animals (cows, sheep, and goats, for example) produce *trans* fatty acids that eventually appear in foods such as beef, milk, and butter. These naturally occurring *trans* fats are currently under study for possible health benefits, including prevention of cancer, decreasing body fat, and improvement in insulin levels in diabetics. About 20% of *trans* fatty acids in our diets come from this source. Dietary supplements of CLA are available but are highly variable in their quality.

Overall, a fat or an oil is classified as saturated, monounsaturated, or polyunsaturated based on the type of fatty acids present in the greatest concentration (Fig. 5-3). Fats in foods that contain primarily saturated fatty acids are solid at room temperature, especially if the fatty acids have long carbon chains (i.e., a **long-chain fatty acid**), as opposed to shorter versions. In contrast, fats containing primarily polyunsaturated or monounsaturated fatty acids (long chain or shorter) are usually liquid at room temperature. Almost all fatty acids in the body and in foods are long-chain varieties.

An important characteristic of unsaturated fatty acids is the location of the double bonds. If the first double bond starts three carbons from the methyl (omega) end of

*Cis* form
(Causes backbone of molecule to bend)

*Trans* form

**Oleic acid**

**Elaidic acid**

**FIGURE 5-2** ▶ *Cis* and *trans* fatty acids. In the *cis* form at carbon-carbon double bonds in a fatty acid, the hydrogens (in blue) lie on the same side of the double bond. This causes a "kink" at that point in the fatty acid, typical of unsaturated fatty acids in foods. In contrast, in the *trans* form at carbon-carbon double bonds in a fatty acid, the hydrogens lie across from each other at the double bond. This causes the fatty acid to exist in a linear form, like a saturated fatty acid. *Cis* fatty acids are much more common in foods than *trans* fatty acids. The latter are primarily found in foods containing partially-hydrogenated fats, notably stick margarine, shortening, and deep-fat fried foods.

**omega-6 (ω-6) fatty acid** An unsaturated fatty acid with the first double bond on the sixth carbon from the methyl end (—CH₃).

**alpha-linolenic acid** An essential omega-3 fatty acid with 18 carbons and three double bonds.

**linoleic acid** An essential omega-6 fatty acid with 18 carbons and two double bonds.

**essential fatty acids** Fatty acids that must be supplied by the diet to maintain health. Currently, only linoleic acid and alpha-linolenic acid are classified as essential.

**oleic acid** An omega-9 fatty acid with 18 carbons and one double bond.

**diglyceride** A breakdown product of a triglyceride consisting of two fatty acids bonded to a glycerol backbone.

**monoglyceride** A breakdown product of a triglyceride consisting of one fatty acid attached to a glycerol backbone.

the fatty acid, it is an **omega-3 (ω-3) fatty acid** (review Fig. 5-1c). If the first double bond is located six carbons from the omega end, it is an **omega-6 (ω-6) fatty acid** (review Fig. 5-1d). Following this scheme, an omega-9 fatty acid has its first double bond starting at the ninth carbon from the methyl end (review Fig. 5-1b). In foods, **alpha-linolenic acid** is the major omega-3 fatty acid; **linoleic acid** is the major omega-6 fatty acid. These are also the **essential fatty acids** we need to consume (more on this in the later section about putting lipids to work in the body). **Oleic acid** is the major omega-9 fatty acid.

## Triglycerides

Fats and oils in foods are mostly in the form of triglycerides. The same is true for fats found in body structures. Although some fatty acids are transported in the bloodstream attached to proteins, most fatty acids are formed into triglycerides by cells in the body.

As noted before, triglycerides contain a simple three-carbon alcohol, glycerol, which serves as a backbone for the three attached fatty acids (Fig. 5-4a). Removing one fatty acid from a triglyceride forms a **diglyceride.** Removing two fatty acids from a triglyceride forms a **monoglyceride.** Later you will see that before most dietary fats are absorbed in the small intestine, the two outer fatty acids are typically removed from the triglyceride. This produces a mixture of fatty acids and monoglycerides, absorbed into the intestinal cells. After absorption, the fatty acids and monoglycerides are mostly re-formed into triglycerides.

▲ Plant oils vary in their content of specific fatty acids. Oils similar in appearance may vary significantly in fatty acid composition. Olive and canola oils are rich in monounsaturated fat; olive oil has been awarded much attention in recent years. Canola oil, however, is a much less expensive choice of monounsaturated fat. Safflower oil is rich in polyunsaturated fat.

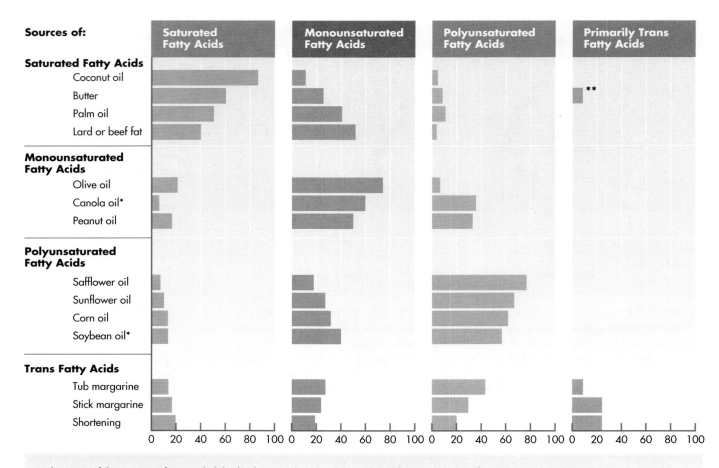

*Rich source of the omega-3 fatty acid alpha-linolenic acid (7% and 12% of total fatty acid content for soybean oil and canola oil, respectively).

**The natural *trans* fatty acids in butter are not harmful and may even have health-promoting properties, such as preventing certain forms of cancer.

**FIGURE 5-3** ▶ Saturated, monounsaturated, polyunsaturated, and *trans* fatty acid composition of common fats and oils (expressed as % of all fatty acids in the product).

## Phospholipids

Phospholipids are another class of lipid. Like triglycerides, they are built on a backbone of glycerol. However, at least one fatty acid is replaced with a compound containing phosphorus (and often other elements, such as nitrogen) (Fig. 5-4b). Many types of phospholipids exist in the body, especially in the brain. They form important parts of cell membranes. **Lecithin** is a common example of a phospholipid. Various forms are found in body cells and they participate in fat digestion, absorption, and transport. The body is able to produce all the phospholipids it needs. Even though lecithin is sold as a dietary supplement and is present as an additive in many foods, phospholipids such as this one are not essential components of the diet.

**lecithin** A group of compounds that are major components of cell membranes.

## Sterols

Sterols are the last class of lipids Chapter 5 covers. Their characteristic multi-ringed structure makes them different from the other lipids already discussed (Fig. 5-4c). The most common example of a sterol is cholesterol. This waxy substance doesn't look like a triglyceride—it doesn't have a glycerol backbone or any fatty acids. Still, because it doesn't readily dissolve in water, it is a lipid. Among other functions, cholesterol is used to form certain hormones and bile acids and is incorporated into cell structures. The body can make all the cholesterol it needs.

**FIGURE 5-4** ▶ Chemical forms of common lipids: (a) triglyceride, (b) phospholipid (in this case, lecithin), and (c) sterol (in this case, cholesterol).

## CONCEPT CHECK

Lipids are a group of compounds that do not dissolve readily in water. Included in this group are fatty acids, triglycerides, phospholipids, and sterols. Fatty acids can be distinguished from one another by the length of the carbon skeleton and the number and position of double bonds along that skeleton. Saturated fatty acids contain no double bonds within their carbon skeleton; that is, they are fully saturated with hydrogens. Monounsaturated fatty acids contain one carbon-carbon double bond, and polyunsaturated fatty acids contain two or more of these bonds. Certain omega-3 and omega-6 fatty acids are essential in the human diet.

Triglycerides are the major form of fat in the body and in foods. These consist of three fatty acids bonded to a glycerol backbone. Phospholipids are similar to triglycerides in structure, but at least one fatty acid is replaced by another compound containing phosphorus. Phospholipids play an important structural role in cell membranes. Sterols, another class of lipids, do not resemble either triglycerides or phospholipids, but instead have a multi-ringed structure. Cholesterol, one example of a sterol, forms parts of cells, some hormones, and bile acids. Whereas certain essential fatty acids (as components of triglycerides) are needed in the diet, the body produces all the triglycerides, phospholipids, and cholesterol it needs. Next we will discuss the sources of fat in foods (Fig. 5-5).

# MyPyramid: Sources of Fats

| Food Group | Grains | Vegetables | Fruits | Oils | Milk | Meat & Beans |
|---|---|---|---|---|---|---|
| Sources of Fat | • Crackers<br>• Pasta dishes with added fat | • French fried potatoes | • Fruit pies<br>• Avocados | • All | • Whole milk<br>• Some yogurts<br>• Many cheeses<br>• Premium ice cream | • Marbled meat<br>• Bacon<br>• Poultry (skin)<br>• Deep-fat fried meat<br>• Nuts |
| Grams per Serving | 0–18 | 0–27 | 0–11 | 12–14 | 0–10 | 7–17 |

**FIGURE 5-5** ▶ Sources of fats from MyPyramid. The height of the background color (none, 1/3, 2/3, or completely covered) within each group in the pyramid indicates the average nutrient density for fat in that group. The fruit group and vegetable groups are generally low in fat. In the other groups, both high-fat and low-fat choices are available. Careful reading of food labels can help you choose lower-fat versions of some foods. In general, any type of frying adds significant amounts of fat to a product, as with French fries and fried chicken. With regard to physical activity, fats are a key fuel in prolonged events, such as long-distance cycling, long-distance running, and prolonged slow to brisk walking.

## 5.3 Fats and Oils in Foods

▲ The North American diet contains many high-fat foods—including typical pastry choices. Portion control with these foods is thus important, especially if one is trying to control calorie intake.

Lipids in the form of triglycerides are abundant in the North American diet. The foods highest in fat (and therefore energy dense) include salad oils and spreads such as butter, margarine, and mayonnaise. All of these foods contain close to 100% of calories as fat. In reduced-fat margarines, water replaces some of the fat. Whereas regular margarines are 80% fat by weight (11 grams per tablespoon), some reduced-fat margarines are as low as 30% fat by weight (4 grams per tablespoon). When used in recipes, the extra water added to these margarines can cause texture and volume changes in the finished product. Cookbooks can provide guidance for appropriate use of these products by suggesting alterations in recipes to compensate for the increased water content.

Still considering the overall fat content, whole foods highest in fat include nuts, bologna, avocados, and bacon, which have about 80% of calories as fat. Next, peanut butter and cheddar cheese have about 75%. Marbled steak and hamburgers (ground chuck) have about 60%, and chocolate bars, ice cream, doughnuts, and whole milk have about 50% of calories as fat. Eggs, pumpkin pie, and cupcakes have 35%, as do lean cuts of meat, such as top round (and ground round) and sirloin. Bread contains about 15%. Finally, foods such as cornflakes, sugar, and fat-free milk have essentially no fat. Careful label reading is necessary to determine the true fat content of food—these are only rough guidelines (Fig. 5-6).

The type of fat in food is important to consider along with the total amount of fat. Animal fats are the chief contributors of saturated fatty acids to the North American diet. About 40% to 60% of total fat in dairy and meat products is in the form of saturated fatty acids. In contrast, plant oils contain mostly unsaturated fatty acids, ranging from 73% to 94% of total fat. A moderate to high proportion of total fat (49% to 77%) is supplied by monounsaturated fatty acids in canola oil, olive oil, and peanut oil. Some animal fats are also good sources of monounsaturated fatty acids (30% to 47%) (review Fig. 5-3). Corn, cottonseed, sunflower, soybean, and safflower oils contain mostly polyunsaturated fatty acids (54% to 77%). These plant oils supply the majority of the linoleic and alpha-linolenic acid in the North American food supply.

Wheat germ, peanuts, egg yolk, soy beans, and organ meats are rich sources of phospholipids. Phospholipids such as lecithin, a component of egg yolks, are often added to salad dressing. Lecithin is used as an **emulsifier** in these and other products because of its ability to keep mixtures of lipids and water from separating (see Fig. 5-7). Emulsifiers are added to salad dressings to keep the vegetable oil suspended in water. Eggs added to cake batters likewise emulsify the fat with the milk.

Cholesterol is found only in animal foods (Table 5-1). An egg yolk contains about 210 milligrams of cholesterol. Eggs are our main dietary source of cholesterol, along

▲ Peanuts are a source of lecithins, as are wheat germ and egg yolks.

**emulsifier** A compound that can suspend fat in water by isolating individual fat droplets, using a shell of water molecules or other substances to prevent the fat from coalescing.

**FIGURE 5-6** ▶ Food sources of fat compared to the American Heart Association (AHA) recommendation of 70 grams per day, or 30% of calories from fat for a 2100 kcal diet.

## Food Sources of Fat

| Food Item | Fat (grams) | Calories from Fat % | % AHA Recommendation |
|---|---|---|---|
| **AHA Recommendation** | 70 | 30% | 100% |
| T-bone steak, 3 ounces | 17 | 66% | 24% |
| Mixed nuts, 1 ounce | 16 | 78% | 23% |
| Canola oil, 1 tablespoon | 14 | 100% | 20% |
| Hamburger with bun, 1 each | 12 | 39% | 17% |
| Margarine, 1 tablespoon | 12 | 100% | 17% |
| Avocado, 1/2 cup | 11 | 86% | 16% |
| Cheddar cheese, 1 ounce | 10 | 74% | 14% |
| Whole milk, 1 cup | 8 | 49% | 11% |
| Chicken breast with skin, 3 ounces | 7 | 36% | 10% |
| Whole milk yogurt, 8 ounces | 7 | 28% | 10% |
| Snack crackers, 1 ounce | 7 | 45% | 10% |
| Baked beans, 1/2 cup | 7 | 31% | 10% |
| M&M chocolate candies, 1 ounce | 6 | 39% | 9% |
| Flax seeds, 1 tablespoon | 3 | 62% | 4% |
| Fig Newton cookies, 2 each | 3 | 23% | 4% |

Key:
■ Grains
■ Vegetables
■ Fruits
□ Oil
■ Milk
■ Meat & Beans
□ Discretionary calories

**FIGURE 5-7 ▶** Emulsifiers in action. Emulsifiers prevent many brands of salad dressings and other condiments from separating into layers of water and fat. Emulsifiers attract fatty acids inside and have a water-attracting group on the outside. Add them to salad dressing, shake well, and they hold the oil in the dressing away from the water. Emulsification is important in both food production and fat digestion/absorption.

**Emulsifiers and Agitation in Salad Dressing**

Oil

Water

Water

Emulsified fat

Oil droplet attracted to fatty acid core

Water attracted to shell

Phospholipid acting as an emulsifier

**TABLE 5-1** Cholesterol Content of Foods

| | |
|---|---|
| 3 oz beef brains | 2635 mg |
| 3 oz beef liver | 337 mg |
| 1 large egg yolk* | 209 mg |
| 3 oz shrimp | 166 mg |
| 3 oz beef* | 75 mg |
| 3 oz pork | 75 mg |
| 3 oz chicken or turkey (white meat)* | 75 mg |
| 1 cup ice cream | 63 mg |
| 3 oz trout | 60 mg |
| 3 oz tuna | 45 mg |
| 3 oz hot dog | 38 mg |
| 1 oz cheddar cheese* | 30 mg |
| 1 cup whole milk* | 24 mg |
| 1 cup 1% milk | 12 mg |
| 1 cup fat-free milk | 5 mg |
| 1 large egg white | 0 mg |

*Leading dietary sources of cholesterol in American diets.

with meats and whole milk. Manufacturers who advertise their brand of peanut butter, vegetable shortening, margarines, and vegetable oils as "cholesterol-free" are taking advantage of uninformed consumers—all of these products are naturally cholesterol-free. Some plants contain other sterols similar to cholesterol, but they do not pose the heart health risks associated with cholesterol. In fact, some plant sterols have blood cholesterol-lowering properties (see the later section on medical interventions to lower blood lipids).

## Fat Is Hidden in Some Foods

Some fat discussed so far is obvious: butter on bread, mayonnaise in potato salad, and marbling in raw meat. Fat is harder to detect in other foods that also contribute significant amounts of fat to our diets. Foods that contain hidden fat include whole milk, pastries, cookies, cake, cheese, hot dogs, crackers, French fries, and ice cream. When we try to cut down on fat intake, hidden fats need to be considered, along with the more obvious sources.

A place to begin searching for hidden fat is on the Nutrition Facts labels of foods you buy. Some signals from the ingredient list that can alert you to the presence of fat are animal fats, such as bacon, beef, ham, lamb, pork, chicken, and turkey fats; lard; vegetable oils; nuts; dairy fats, such as butter and cream; egg and egg-yolk solids; and partially-hydrogenated shortening or vegetable oil. Conveniently, the label lists ingredients by order of weight in the product. If fat is one of the first ingredients listed, you are probably looking at a high-fat product. Use food labels to learn more about the fat content of the foods you eat (Fig. 5-8).

The definitions for various fat descriptors on food labels, such as "low-fat," "fat-free," and "reduced-fat," were listed in Table 2-9 in Chapter 2 and are reprinted in the margin here. Recall that "low-fat" indicates, in most cases, that a product contains no more than 3 grams of fat per serving. Products marketed as "fat-free" must have less than one-half of a gram of fat per serving. A claim of "reduced-fat" means the product has at least 25% less fat than is usually found in that type of food. When there is no Nutrition Facts label to inspect, controlling portion size is a good way to control fat intake.

When many North Americans think of a low-fat diet, they include reduced-fat versions of pastries, cookies, and cakes. When health professionals refer to a low-fat diet,

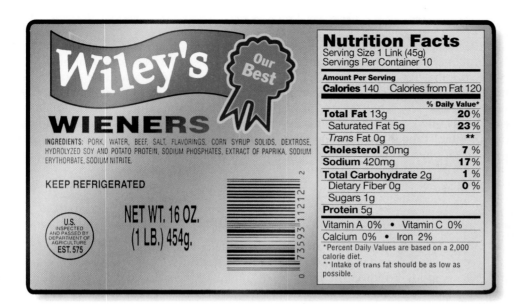

**FIGURE 5-8** ▶ Reading labels helps locate hidden fat. Who would think that wieners (hot dogs) can contain about 85% of food calories as fat? Looking at the hot dog does not suggest that almost all of its food calories comes from fat, but the label shows otherwise. Let's do the math: 13 grams total fat × 9 kcal per gram of fat = 120 kcal from fat; 120 kcal/140 kcal per link = 0.86 or 86% kcal from fat.

they often have a different plan in mind: focusing primarily on fruits, vegetables, and whole-grain breads and cereals. Whether to choose a fat-rich food should depend on how much fat you have eaten or will eat during that particular day. So, if you plan to eat high-fat foods at your evening meal, you could reduce your fat intake at a previous meal to balance overall fat intake for the day.

## Fat in Food Provides Some Satiety, Flavor, and Texture

Fat in foods has generally been considered to be the most satiating of all the macronutrients. However, studies show that protein and carbohydrate probably lead to the most satiety (gram for gram). High-fat meals do provide satiety, but primarily because one consumes a lot of calories in the process. A high-fat meal is likely to be a high-calorie meal.

Various fats play important roles in foods, so much ingenuity must go into the production of reduced-fat products to preserve flavor and texture. In some cases, "fat-free" also means tasteless. Fat components in foods provide important textures and carry flavors. If you've ever eaten a high-fat yellow cheese or cream cheese, you probably agree that fat melting on the tongue feels good. The fat in reduced-fat and whole milk also gives body, which fat-free milk lacks. The most tender cuts of meat are high in fat, visible as the marbling of meat. In addition, many flavorings dissolve in fat. Heating spices in oil intensifies the flavors of an Indian curry or a Mexican dish, carried to the sensory cells that discriminate taste and smell in the mouth.

### MAKING DECISIONS

#### Low-Fat Diets

A person who has been following a typical North American diet will probably need some time to adjust to the taste of a lower-fat diet. Emphasizing flavorful fruits, vegetables, and whole grains will help one to adapt to a low-fat diet. Interestingly, after an adjustment period, higher-fat foods may not be as palatable or may lead to gastrointestinal discomfort. For example, after switching from whole to 1% low-fat milk for a few weeks, whole milk begins to taste more like cream than milk. It is certainly possible to make the change from a higher-fat diet to a lower-fat diet. The benefits of weight control and reduced risk for several chronic diseases make the adjustment worth the effort.

▶ **Definitions for Nutrient Claims About Fat and Cholesterol on Food Labels**

**Fat**

- **Fat free:** less than 0.5 g of fat per serving
- **Saturated fat free:** less than 0.5 g per serving, and the level of *trans* fatty acids does not exceed 0.5 g per serving
- **Low fat:** 3 g or less per serving and, if the serving is 30 g or less or 2 tablespoons or less, per 50 g of the food. 2% milk can no longer be labeled low fat, as it exceeds 3 g per serving. *Reduced fat* will be the term used instead.
- **Low saturated fat:** 1 g or less per serving and not more than 15% of kcal from saturated fatty acids
- **Reduced or less fat:** at least 25% less per serving than reference food
- **Reduced or less saturated fat:** at least 25% less per serving than reference food

**Cholesterol**

- **Cholesterol free:** less than 2 milligrams (mg) of cholesterol and 2 g or less of saturated fat per serving
- **Low cholesterol:** 20 mg or less cholesterol and 2 g or less of saturated fat per serving and, if the serving is 30 g or less or 2 tablespoons or less, per 50 g of the food
- **Reduced or less cholesterol:** at least 25% less cholesterol and 2 g or less of saturated fat per serving than reference food

▲ Dairy products are a primary contributor of saturated fat to our diets.

## Wise Use of Reduced-Fat Foods Is Important

Manufacturers have introduced reduced-fat versions of numerous food products. The fat content of these alternatives ranges from 0% in fat-free Fig Newtons to about 75% of the original fat content in other products. However, the total calorie content of most fat-reduced products is not substantially lower than that of their conventional versions. Generally, when fat is removed from a product, something must be added—commonly, sugars—in its place. It is difficult to reduce both the fat and sugar contents of a product at the same time and maintain flavor and texture. For this reason, many reduced-fat products (e.g., cakes and cookies) are still energy dense. Use the Nutrition Facts label to choose the portion size with the desired calories.

## Fat Replacement Strategies for Foods

To help consumers trim their fat intake and still enjoy the mouthfeel sensations fat provides, food companies offer low-fat versions of many foods. To lower the fat in foods, manufacturers may replace some of the fat with water, protein (Dairy-Lo®), or forms of carbohydrates such as starch derivatives (Z-trim®), fiber (Maltrin®, Stellar™, Oatrim), and gums. Manufacturers also may use engineered fats, such as olestra (Olean®) and salatrim (Benefat®), that are made with fat and sucrose (table sugar) but that provide few or no calories because they cannot be digested and/or absorbed well.

So far, fat replacements have had little impact on our diets, partly because the currently approved forms are either not very versatile or not used extensively by manufacturers. In addition, fat replacements are not practical for use in the foods that provide the most fat in our diets—beef, cheese, whole milk, and pastries.

## CONCEPT CHECK

Fat-dense foods—those with more than 60% of total calories as fat—include plant oils, butter, margarine, mayonnaise, nuts, bacon, avocados, peanut butter, cheddar cheese, steak, and hamburger. Of the foods we typically eat, cholesterol is found naturally only in those of animal origin, with eggs being a primary source. Emulsifiers, such as the phospholipids, lecithins, are added to salad dressings and other fat-rich products to keep the vegetable oils and other fats suspended in the water. Hidden fat exists in foods such as whole milk, pastries, cookies, cake, cheese, hot dogs, crackers, French fries, and ice cream. Fat has a variety of roles in foods, including that of contributing to flavor and texture. Fat also provides the pleasurable mouth feel of many of our favorite foods, intensifies the taste of many spices, and tenderizes many popular cuts of meat. Fat free doesn't mean calorie free; moderation in the use of reduced-fat products is still important.

## CRITICAL THINKING

Allison has decided to start eating a low-fat diet. Allison has mentioned to you that all she needs to do is add less butter, oil, or margarine to her foods and she will dramatically lower her fat intake. How can you explain to Allison that she needs to be aware of the hidden fats in her diet as well?

## Fat Rancidity Limits Shelf Life of Foods

Decomposing oils emit a disagreeable odor and taste sour and stale. Stale potato chips are a good example. The double bonds in unsaturated fatty acids break down, producing rancid by-products. Ultraviolet light, oxygen, and certain procedures can break double bonds and, in turn, destroy the structure of polyunsaturated fatty acids. Saturated fats and *trans* fats can much more readily resist these effects because they contain fewer carbon-carbon double bonds.

Rancidity is not a major problem for consumers because the odor and taste generally discourage us from eating enough to become sick. However, rancidity is a problem for manufacturers because it reduces a product's shelf life. To increase shelf life, manufacturers often add partially-hydrogenated plant oils to products. Foods most likely to become rancid are deep-fried foods and foods with a large amount of exposed surface. The fat in fish is also susceptible to rancidity because it is highly polyunsaturated.

Antioxidants such as vitamin E help protect foods against rancidity by guarding against fat breakdown. The vitamin E naturally occurring in plant oils reduces the breakdown of double bonds in fatty acids. When food manufacturers want to prevent rancidity in polyunsaturated fats, they often add the synthetic antioxidants **BHA** and **BHT** or vitamin C to products that contain fat such as salad dressings and cake mixes. Manufacturers also tightly seal products and use other methods to reduce oxygen levels inside packages.

## Hydrogenation of Fatty Acids in Food Production Increases *Trans* Fatty Acid Content

As mentioned previously, most fats with long-chain saturated fatty acids are solid at room temperature, and those with unsaturated fatty acids are liquid at room temperature. In some kinds of food production, solid fats work better than liquid oils. In pie crust, for example, solid fats yield a flaky product, whereas crusts made with liquid oils tend to be greasy and more crumbly. If oils with unsaturated fatty acids are used to replace solid fats, they often must be made more saturated (with hydrogen), as this solidifies the vegetable oils into shortenings and margarines. Hydrogen is added by bubbling hydrogen gas under pressure into liquid vegetable oils in a process called **hydrogenation** (Fig. 5-9). The fatty acids aren't fully hydrogenated to the saturated fatty acid form, as this would make the product too hard and brittle. Partial hydrogenation—leaving some monounsaturated fatty acids—creates a semisolid product.

The process of hydrogenation produces *trans* fatty acids as was described earlier in this chapter. Most natural monounsaturated and polyunsaturated fatty acids exist in the *cis* form, causing a bend in the carbon chain, whereas the straighter carbon forms of *trans* fat more closely resemble saturated fatty acids. This may be the mechanism

▲ Fat replacements such as gum fiber are typically seen in soft serve ice cream.

**C**anada has not approved the use of olestra in food products; the United States is the sole country that permits the use of this fat substitute in foods.

**BHA, BHT** Butylated hydroxyanisole and butylated hydroxytoluene—two common synthetic antioxidants added to foods.

**hydrogenation** The addition of hydrogen to a carbon-carbon double bond, producing a single carbon-carbon bond with two hydrogens attached to each carbon. Hydrogenation of unsaturated fatty acids in a vegetable oil increases its hardness, so this process is used to convert liquid oils into more solid fats, used in making margarine and shortening. *Trans* fatty acids are a by-product of hydrogenation of vegetable oils.

← Hydrogen source

Unsaturated vegetable oil (liquid)

(a)

Adding hydrogen under pressure

(b)

Partially hydrogenated fat (semisolid)

(c)

**FIGURE 5-9** ▶ How liquid oils become solid fats. (a) Unsaturated fatty acids are present in liquid form. (b) Hydrogens are added (hydrogenation), changing some carbon-carbon double bonds to single bonds and producing some *trans* fatty acids. (c) The partially-hydrogenated product is likely to be used in margarine, shortening, or for deep-fat frying.

▲ The American Heart Association's national public health campaign called "Face the Fats" emphasizes that "some are bad, some are better". The Bad Fats Brothers, Trans and Sat, urge us to cut down on *trans* and saturated fat. The Better Fats Sisters, Poly named for polyunsaturated fat, and Mon, short for monounsaturated fat encourage us "to replace bad fats with foods that will be better choices." (check out this program at www.american.heart.org/FaceTheFats)

whereby *trans* fat increases the risk for heart disease. Studies also indicate that *trans* fats increase overall inflammation in the body, which is not healthful. Thus, people should limit intake of partially-hydrogenated fat and thus *trans* fat. This may not be such a concern for the average person, as long as *trans* fat intake is not excessive and the diet is adequate in polyunsaturated fat. However, because *trans* fatty acids serve no particular role in maintaining body health, the latest Dietary Guidelines for Americans, the American Heart Association, and the Food and Nutrition Board each recommend minimal *trans* fat intake.

Not so long ago, public pressure persuaded manufacturers to eliminate the tropical oils rich in saturated fat (palm, palm olein, and coconut) from food processing. Partially-hydrogenated soybean oil—rich in *trans* fat—became the major replacement. Currently, *trans* fat intake in North America is estimated to contribute about 3% to 4% of total calories, amounting to 10 grams per day, on average. Table 5-2 lists typical sources.

FDA is now requiring the *trans* fat content of foods on food labels (review Fig. 5-8). The food labels in Canada also must list *trans* fat content. FDA hopes to make consumers more aware of the amounts of *trans* fat in foods as well as the negative health consequences associated with their excessive consumption. North American companies are already responding to this issue by creating products free of *trans* fat. For example, Promise, Smart Beat, and some Fleischmann's margarines are lower in or free of *trans* fat (less than 0.5 grams per serving) compared to typical margarines.

This addition of the *trans* fat listing on labels helps consumers at the supermarket, but when dining out, consumers are "left in the dark" as to which foods contain *trans* fat. Knowing which foods are low in *trans* fat when ordering at a restaurant is difficult because information about preparation methods and precise

**TABLE 5-2** Main Sources of Fatty acids and Their State at Room Temperature

| Type and Health Effects | Main Sources | State at Room Temperature |
|---|---|---|
| **Saturated Fatty Acids** Increase blood levels of cholesterol | | |
| Long Chain | Lard; fat in beef, pork, and lamb | Solid |
| Medium and Short Chain | Milk fat (butter), coconut oil, palm oil, palm kernel oil | Soft or liquid |
| **Monounsaturated Fatty Acids** Decrease blood levels of cholesterol | Olive oil, canola oil, peanut oil | Liquid |
| **Polyunsaturated Fatty Acids** Decrease blood levels of cholesterol | Sunflower oil, corn oil, safflower oil, fish oil | Liquid |
| **Essential Fatty Acids** Omega 3: alpha—linolenic acid Reduces inflammation responses, blood clotting, and plasma triglycerides | Cold-water fish (salmon, tuna, sardines, mackerel), walnuts, flaxseed, hemp oil, canola oil, soybean oil | Liquid |
| Omega 6: Linoleic Acid Regulates blood pressure and increases blood clotting | Beef, poultry, safflower oil, sunflower oil, corn oil | Solid to liquid |
| **Trans Fatty Acids** Increase blood cholesterol more than saturated fat | Margarine (squeeze, tub, stick), shortening | Soft to very solid |

fat composition is rarely available. To minimize *trans* fat intake, a general guideline is to limit consumption of fried (especially deep-fat fried) food items, any pastries or flaky bread products (such as pie crusts, crackers, croissants, and biscuits), and cookies.

Until all foods are labeled with *trans* fat content, consumers can also make educated guesses on the *trans* fat content of foods by examining the list of ingredients on the food label. If partially-hydrogenated vegetable oil is one of the first three ingredients on the label, you can assume there is a significant amount of *trans* fat in the product.

Limiting *trans* fat at home is a much easier task. Most importantly, use little or no stick margarine or shortening. Instead, substitute vegetable oils and softer tub margarines (whose labels list vegetable oil or water as the first ingredient). Avoid deep-fat frying any food in shortening. Substitute baking, panfrying, broiling, steaming, grilling, or deep-fat frying in unhydrogenated vegetable oils. Replace nondairy creamers with reduced-fat or fat-free milk, since most nondairy creamers are rich in partially-hydrogenated vegetable oils. Finally, read the ingredients on food labels, using the previous tips to estimate *trans* fat content.

▲ Fried foods are a rich source of fat and *trans* fats. Reducing the intake of these foods can help lower blood lipid levels.

## CONCEPT CHECK

Hydrogenation of unsaturated fatty acids is the process of adding hydrogen to carbon-carbon double bonds to produce single bonds. This results in the creation of some *trans* fatty acids. Hydrogenation changes vegetable oil to solid fat. It is wise to monitor *trans* fat intake, as this form of fat increases the risk for heart disease.

The carbon-carbon double bonds in polyunsaturated fatty acids are easily broken, yielding products responsible for rancidity. The presence of antioxidants, such as vitamin E in oils, naturally protects unsaturated fatty acids against oxidative destruction. Manufacturers can use hydrogenated fats and add natural or synthetic antioxidants to reduce the likelihood of rancidity.

# 5.4 Making Lipids Available for Body Use

It's no secret that fats and oils make foods more appealing. Their presence in foods adds flavor, lubrication, and texture. What happens to lipids once they are eaten? Let's take a closer look at the digestion, absorption, and physiological roles of lipids in the body.

## Digestion

In the first phase of fat digestion, the stomach (and salivary glands to some extent) secretes **lipase.** This enzyme acts primarily on triglycerides that have fatty acids with short chain lengths, such as those found in butterfat. The action of salivary and stomach lipase, however, is usually dwarfed by that of the lipase enzyme released from the pancreas and active in the small intestine. Triglycerides and other lipids found in common vegetable oils and meats have longer chain lengths and are generally not digested until they reach the small intestine (Fig. 5-10).

In the small intestine, triglycerides are broken down by lipase into smaller products, namely monoglycerides (glycerol backbones with a single fatty acid attached) and fatty acids. Under the right circumstances, digestion is rapid and thorough. The "right" circumstances include the presence of bile from the gallbladder. Bile acids present in the bile act as emulsifiers on the digestive products of lipase action, suspending the monoglycerides and fatty acids in the watery digestive juices. This emulsification improves digestion and absorption because as large fat globules are broken down into smaller ones, the total surface area for lipase action increases (Fig. 5-11).

**lipase** Fat-digesting enzyme produced by the salivary glands, stomach, and pancreas.

**FIGURE 5-10** ▶ A summary of fat digestion and absorption. Chapter 3 covered general aspects of this process.

## Fat Digestion and Absorption

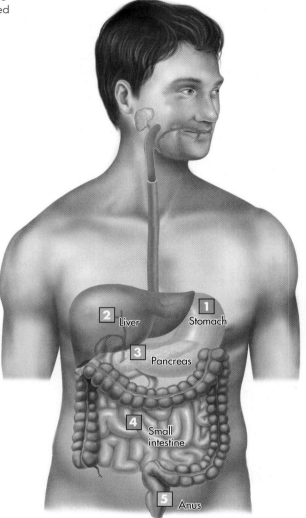

**1** Stomach: Only minor digestion of fat takes place in the stomach through the action of lipase enzymes.

**2** Liver: The liver produces bile, stored in the gallbladder and released through the bile duct into the small intestine. Bile aids in fat digestion and absorption by emulsifying lipids in the digestive juices.

**3** Pancreas: The pancreas secretes a mixture of enzymes, including lipase, into the small intestine.

**4** Small intestine: The small intestine is the primary site for digestion and absorption of lipids. Once absorbed, long-chain fatty acids are packaged for transport through the lymph and bloodstream. (Shorter-chain fatty acids are absorbed directly into portal circulation.)

**5** Large intestine: Less than 5% of ingested fat is normally excreted in the feces.

**I**f the gallbladder is surgically removed (e.g., in cases of gallstone formation), bile will enter the small intestine directly from the liver.

With regard to phospholipid digestion, certain enzymes from the pancreas and cells in the wall of the small intestine digest phospholipids. The eventual products are glycerol, fatty acids, and remaining parts. With regard to cholesterol digestion, any cholesterol with a fatty acid attached is broken down to free cholesterol and fatty acids by certain enzymes released from the pancreas.

## MAKING DECISIONS

### Bile Acids

During meals, bile acids circulate in a path that begins in the liver, goes on to the gallbladder, and then moves to the small intestine. After participating in fat digestion, most bile acids are absorbed and end up back at the liver. Approximately 98% of the bile acids are recycled. Only 1% to 2% ends up in the large intestine to be eliminated in the feces. Using medicines that block some of this reabsorption of bile acids is one way to treat high blood cholesterol. The liver takes cholesterol from the bloodstream to form replacement bile acids. Viscous fiber in the diet can also bind to bile acids to produce the same effect (see a later section on medical interventions related to cardiovascular disease for details).

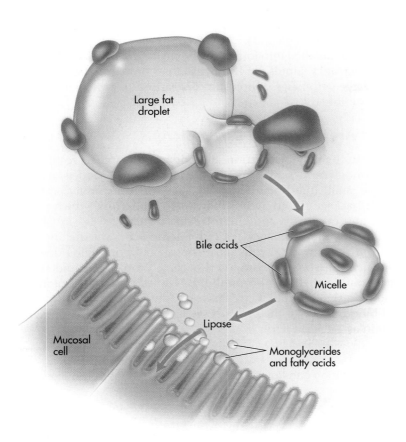

**FIGURE 5-11** ▶ Bile acids mix with fats to form small droplets called micelles that facilitate the absorption of monoglycerides and fatty acids into the mucosal cells of the small intestine.

## Absorption

The products of fat digestion in the small intestine are fatty acids and monoglycerides. These products diffuse into the absorptive cells of the small intestine. About 95% of dietary fat is absorbed in this way. The chain length of fatty acids affects the ultimate fate of fatty acids and monoglycerides after absorption. If the chain length of a fatty acid is less than 12 carbon atoms, it is water soluble and will therefore probably travel as such through the portal vein that connects directly to the liver. If the fatty acid is a more typical long-chain variety, it must be reformed into a triglyceride in the intestinal absorptive cell and eventually enter circulation via the lymphatic system (review Chapter 3 for an overview of this process).

### CONCEPT CHECK

In the small intestine, a lipase enzyme released from the pancreas digests dietary triglycerides into monoglycerides (glycerol backbones with single fatty acids attached) and fatty acids. These breakdown products then diffuse into the absorptive cells of the small intestine. Long-chain fatty acids are transported through the lymphatic system, whereas fatty acids with shorter carbon chains are absorbed directly into the portal vein that connects directly to the liver. Other lipids are prepared for absorption by different enzymes.

## 5.5 Carrying Lipids in the Bloodstream

As noted earlier, fat and water don't mix easily. This incompatibility presents a challenge for the transport of fats through the watery media of the blood and lymph.

**lipoprotein** A compound found in the bloodstream containing a core of lipids with a shell composed of protein, phospholipid, and cholesterol.

**chylomicron** Lipoprotein made of dietary fats surrounded by a shell of cholesterol, phospholipids, and protein. Chylomicrons are formed in the absorptive cells of the small intestine after fat absorption and travel through the lymphatic system to the bloodstream.

**Lipoproteins** serve as vehicles for transport of lipids from the small intestine and liver to the body tissues (Table 5-3).

Lipoproteins are classified into four groups—chylomicrons, VLDL, LDL, and HDL—based on their densities. Lipids are less dense than proteins. Therefore, lipoproteins that contain a large percentage of lipids in comparison to protein are less dense than those depleted of lipids.

## Dietary Fats Are Carried by Chylomicrons

As you learned in the previous section, digestion of dietary fats results in a mixture of glycerol, monoglycerides, and fatty acids. Once these products are absorbed by the cells of the small intestine, they are reassembled into triglycerides. Then, the intestinal cells package the triglycerides into **chylomicrons,** which enter the lymphatic system and eventually the bloodstream (review Fig. 3-5 in Chapter 3 for a depiction of lymphatic circulation). Chylomicrons contain dietary fat and originate only from the intestinal cells. Like the other lipoproteins described in the next section, chylomicrons are composed of large droplets of lipid surrounded by a thin, water-soluble shell of phospholipids, cholesterol, and protein (Fig. 5-12). The water-soluble shell around a chylomicron allows the lipid to float freely in the water-based blood. Some of the proteins present may also help other cells identify the lipoprotein as a chylomicron.

**TABLE 5-3** Composition and Roles of the Major Lipoproteins in the Blood

| Lipoprotein | Primary Component | Key Role |
|---|---|---|
| Chylomicron | Triglyceride | Carries dietary fat from the small intestine to cells |
| VLDL | Triglyceride | Carries lipids made and taken up by the liver to cells |
| LDL | Cholesterol | Carries cholesterol made by the liver and from other sources to cells |
| HDL | Protein | Contributes to cholesterol removal from cells and, in turn, excretion of it from the body |

**FIGURE 5-12** ▶ The structure of a lipoprotein, in this case an LDL. This structure allows fats to circulate in the water-based bloodstream. Various lipoproteins are found in the bloodstream. The primary component of LDL is cholesterol.

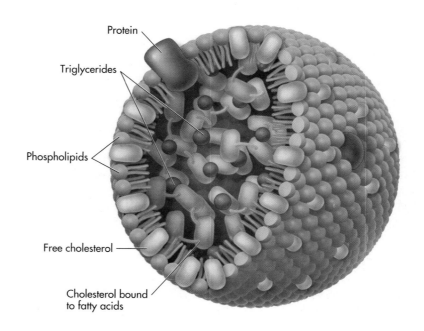

Protein

Triglycerides

Phospholipids

Free cholesterol

Cholesterol bound to fatty acids

Once a chylomicron enters the bloodstream, the triglycerides in its core are broken down into fatty acids and glycerol by an enzyme called **lipoprotein lipase,** attached to the inside walls of the blood vessels (Fig. 5-13). As soon as the fatty acids are released to the bloodstream, they are absorbed by cells in the vicinity, while much of the glycerol circulates back to the liver. Muscle cells can immediately use the absorbed fatty acids for fuel. Adipose cells, on the other hand, tend to re-form the fatty acids into triglycerides for storage. After triglycerides have been removed, a chylomicron remnant remains. Chylomicron remnants are removed from circulation by the liver and their components are recycled to make other lipoproteins and bile acids.

**lipoprotein lipase** An enzyme attached to the cells that form the inner lining of blood vessels; it breaks down triglycerides into free fatty acids and glycerol.

## Other Lipoproteins Transport Lipids from the Liver to the Body Cells

The liver takes up various lipids from the blood. The liver also is the manufacturing site for lipids and cholesterol. The raw materials for lipid and cholesterol synthesis include free fatty acids taken up from the bloodstream, as well as carbon and hydrogen derived from carbohydrates, protein, and alcohol. The liver then must package these synthesized lipids as lipoproteins for transport in the blood to body tissues.

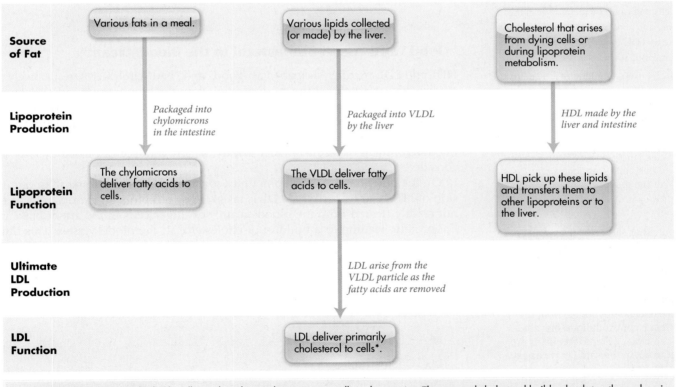

**FIGURE 5-13** ▶ Lipoprotein production and function. Chylomicrons carry absorbed fat to body cells. VLDL carries fat taken up from the bloodstream by the liver, as well as any fat made by the liver, to body cells. LDL arises from VLDL and carries mostly cholesterol to cells. HDL arises mostly from the liver and intestine. HDL carries cholesterol from cells to other lipoproteins and to the liver for excretion.

**very-low-density lipoprotein (VLDL)** The lipoprotein created in the liver that carries cholesterol and lipids that have been taken up or newly synthesized by the liver.

**low-density lipoprotein (LDL)** The lipoprotein in the blood containing primarily cholesterol; elevated LDL is strongly linked to cardiovascular disease risk.

**high-density lipoprotein (HDL)** The lipoprotein in the blood that picks up cholesterol from dying cells and other sources and transfers it to the other lipoproteins in the bloodstream, as well as directly to the liver; low HDL increases the risk for cardiovascular disease.

**menopause** The cessation of the menstrual cycle in women, usually beginning at about 50 years of age.

**scavenger cells** Specific form of white blood cells that can bury themselves in the artery wall and accumulate LDL. As these cells take up LDL, they contribute to the development of atherosclerosis.

**atherosclerosis** A buildup of fatty material (plaque) in the arteries, including those surrounding the heart.

See *Nutrition and Your Health: Lipids and Cardiovascular Disease* at the end of Chapter 5.

It appears that saturated fatty acids promote an increase in the amount of free cholesterol (not attached to fatty acids) in the liver, whereas unsaturated fatty acids do the opposite. As free cholesterol in the liver increases, it causes the liver to reduce cholesterol uptake from the bloodstream, contributing to elevated LDL in the blood. (*Trans* fatty acids are thought to act in the same ways as saturated fatty acids.)

First in our discussion of lipoproteins made by the liver are **very-low-density lipoproteins (VLDL).** These particles are composed of cholesterol and triglycerides surrounded by a water-soluble shell. VLDLs are rich in triglycerides and thus are very low in density. Once in the bloodstream, lipoprotein lipase on the inner surface of the blood vessels breaks down the triglyceride in the VLDL into fatty acids and glycerol. Fatty acids and glycerol are released into the bloodstream and taken up by the body cells.

As its triglycerides are released, the VLDL becomes proportionately denser. Much of what eventually remains of the VLDL fraction is then called **low-density lipoprotein (LDL);** this is composed primarily of the remaining cholesterol. The primary function of LDL is to transport cholesterol to tissues. LDL particles are taken up from the bloodstream by specific receptors on cells, especially liver cells, and are then broken down. The cholesterol and protein components of LDL provide some of the building blocks necessary for cell growth and development, such as synthesis of cell membranes and hormones.

The final group of lipoproteins, **high-density lipoproteins (HDL),** is a critical and beneficial participant in this process of lipid transport. Its high proportion of protein makes it the densest lipoprotein. The liver and intestine produce most of the HDL in the blood. It roams the bloodstream, picking up cholesterol from dying cells and other sources. HDL donates the cholesterol primarily to other lipoproteins for transport back to the liver to be excreted. Some HDL travels directly back to the liver.

## "Good" and "Bad" Cholesterol in the Bloodstream

HDL and LDL are often described as "good" and "bad" cholesterol, respectively. Many studies demonstrate that the amount of HDL in the bloodstream can closely predict the risk for cardiovascular disease. Risk increases with low HDL because little cholesterol is transported back to the liver and excreted. Women tend to have high amounts of HDL, especially before **menopause,** compared to men. High amounts of HDL slow the development of cardiovascular disease, so any cholesterol carried by HDL can be considered "good" cholesterol.

On the other hand, LDL is sometimes considered "bad" cholesterol. In our discussion of LDL, you learned that LDL is taken up by receptors on various cells. If LDL is not readily cleared from the bloodstream, **scavenger cells** in the arteries take up the lipoprotein, leading to a buildup of cholesterol in the blood vessels. This buildup, known as **atherosclerosis,** greatly increases the risk for cardiovascular disease (see the following "Nutrition and Your Health" section). LDL is only a problem when it is too high in the bloodstream because low amounts are needed as part of routine body functions.

## MAKING DECISIONS

### LDL Cholesterol

The cholesterol in foods is not designated as "good" or "bad." It is only after cholesterol has been made or processed by the liver that it shows up in the bloodstream as LDL or HDL. Dietary patterns can affect the metabolism of cholesterol, however. Diets low in saturated fat, *trans* fat, and cholesterol encourage the uptake of LDL by the liver, thereby removing LDL from the bloodstream and decreasing the ability of scavenger cells to form atherosclerotic plaques in the blood vessels. Likewise, diets high in saturated fat, *trans* fat, and cholesterol reduce the uptake of LDL by the liver, increasing cholesterol in the blood and the risk for cardiovascular disease. What foods in your diet are high in saturated fat, *trans* fat, or cholesterol?

## 5.6 Essential Functions of Fatty Acids

The various classes of lipids have diverse functions in the body. All are necessary for health, but, as mentioned earlier, many can be made by the body and therefore are not needed in our diet. Of all the classes of lipids, only certain polyunsaturated fatty acids are essential parts of a diet.

### The Essential Fatty Acids

We must obtain linoleic acid (an omega-6 fatty acid) and alpha-linolenic acid (an omega-3 fatty acid) from foods to maintain health, so they are called *essential* fatty acids (Fig. 5-14). These omega-6 and omega-3 fatty acids form parts of vital body structures, perform important roles in immune system function and vision, help form cell membranes, and produce hormone-like compounds. Omega-6 and omega-3 fatty acids must be obtained through the diet because human cells lack the enzymes needed to produce these fatty acids. Other fatty acids, such as omega-9 fatty acids, can be synthesized in the body, and therefore are not essential components of the diet.

**Omega-3 Fatty Acids in Fish (grams per 3 ounce serving)**

| | |
|---|---|
| Atlantic salmon | 1.8 |
| Anchovy | 1.7 |
| Sardines | 1.4 |
| Rainbow trout | 1.0 |
| Coho salmon | 0.9 |
| Bluefish | 0.8 |
| Striped bass | 0.8 |
| Tuna, white, canned | 0.7 |
| Halibut | 0.4 |
| Catfish, channel | 0.2 |

Recommended omega-3 fatty acid (alpha-linolenic acid) intake per day:
| | |
|---|---|
| Men | 1.6 grams |
| Women | 1.1 grams |

**FIGURE 5-14** ▶ The essential fatty acid (EFA) family. Linoleic acid and alpha-linolenic acid are available from dietary sources; and must be consumed as body synthesis does not take place. These are the essential fatty acids. The other fatty acids in this figure can be synthesized from the essential fatty acids.

**eicosapentaenoic acid (EPA)** An omega-3 fatty acid with 20 carbons and five carbon-carbon double bonds. It is present in large amounts in fatty fish and is slowly synthesized in the body from alpha-linolenic acid.

**docosahexaenoic acid (DHA)** An omega-3 fatty acid with 22 carbons and six carbon-carbon double bonds. It is present in large amounts in fatty fish and is slowly synthesized in the body from alpha-linolenic acid. DHA is especially present in the retina and brain.

**arachidonic acid** An omega-6 fatty acid made from linoleic acid with 20 carbon atoms and 4 carbon-carbon double bonds.

**hemorrhagic stroke** Damage to part of the brain resulting from rupture of a blood vessel and subsequent bleeding within or over the internal surface of the brain.

▲ The American Heart Association recommends eating fatty fish such as salmon at least twice a week. As a source of omega-3 fatty acids, fish is a heart-healthy alternative to other animal sources of protein, which can be high in saturated fat and cholesterol.

See *Nutrition and Your Health: Lipids and Cardiovascular Disease* at the end of Chapter 5.

Still, we need to consume only about 5% of our total calories per day from essential fatty acids. That corresponds to about 2 to 4 tablespoons of plant oil each day. We can easily get that much—from mayonnaise, salad dressings, and other foods—without much effort. Regular consumption of vegetables and whole-grain breads and cereals also helps to supply enough essential fatty acids.

Research also suggests that we include a regular intake of the omega-3 fatty acids, **eicosapentaenoic acid (EPA)** and **docosahexaenoic acid (DHA),** which can be made from alpha-linolenic acid. EPA and DHA are naturally high in fatty fish such as salmon, tuna, sardines, anchovies, striped bass, catfish, herring, mackerel, trout, or halibut. Consumption of one or more of these fish at least twice a week is recommended to obtain EPA and DHA. Additional sources of omega-3 fatty acids include canola and soybean oils, walnuts, flax seeds, mussels, crab, and shrimp.

## MAKING DECISIONS

### Mercury in Fish

Consumption of fatty fish at least twice a week is recommended as a good source of the omega-3 fatty acids. Some fish can be a source of mercury, toxic in high amounts, especially swordfish, shark, king mackerel, and tile fish (see Chapter 13). Albacore tuna also is a potential source, while other forms of tuna are much lower in mercury. Those fish low in mercury are salmon, sardines, bluefish, and herring. Shrimp is also low in mercury. For others, varying your choices rather than always eating the same species of fish and limiting overall intake to 12 ounces per week (on average 2 to 3 meals of fish or shellfish per week) is recommended to reduce mercury exposure, especially for pregnant women and children. Existing research indicates that the benefits of fish intake, especially in reducing the risk of cardiovascular disease, outweigh the possible risks of mercury contamination.

The recommendation to consume omega-3 fatty acids stems from the observation that compounds made from omega-3 fatty acids tend to decrease blood clotting and inflammatory processes in the body. The omega-6 fatty acids, notably **arachidonic acid** made from linoleic acid, generally increase clotting and inflammation, and saturated fatty acids also increase blood clotting.

Some studies show that people who eat fish at least twice a week (total weekly intake: 8 ounces [240 grams]) run lower risks for heart attack than do people who rarely eat fish. In these cases, the omega-3 fatty acids in fish oil are probably acting to reduce blood clotting. As will be covered in detail in the "Nutrition and Your Health" section, blood clots are part of the heart attack process. In addition, these omega-3 fatty acids have a favorable effect on heart rhythm. Consequently, the risk of heart attack decreases with the consumption of omega-3 fatty acids from fish, especially for people already at high risk.

We need to remember, however, that blood clotting is a normal body process. Certain groups of people, such as Eskimos in Greenland, eat so much seafood that their normal blood-clotting ability can be impaired. An excess of omega-3 fatty acid intake can allow uncontrolled bleeding and may cause **hemorrhagic stroke.** However, no increase in risk of stroke has been observed in studies using moderate amounts of omega-3 fatty acids.

Studies also have shown that large amounts of omega-3 fatty acids from fish (2 to 4 grams per day) can lower blood triglycerides in people with high triglyceride concentrations. In addition, these omega-3 fatty acids are suspected to be helpful in managing the pain of inflammation associated with rheumatoid arthritis by suppressing immune system responses. This may also help with certain behavioral disorders and cases of mild depression.

In some instances, fish oil capsules can be safely substituted for fish consumption if a person does not like fish. Generally, about 1 gram of omega-3 fatty acids (about three capsules) from fish oil per day is recommended, especially for people with evidence of cardiovascular disease. (Freezing fish oil capsules before consumption or using enteric coated capsules will reduce the fishy aftertaste.) The American Heart Association also recently suggested that fish oil supplements (providing 2 to 4 grams of omega-3 fatty acids per day) could be employed to treat elevated blood triglycerides, as previously noted. However, fish oil capsules should be limited for individuals who have bleeding disorders, take anticoagulant medications, or anticipate surgery, because they may increase risk of uncontrollable bleeding and hemorrhagic stroke. Thus for fish oil capsules, as well as other dietary supplements, it is important to follow a physician's recommendations. Remember that fish oil supplements are not regulated by the FDA. The quality of these supplements, therefore, is not standardized, and contaminants naturally present in the fish oil may not have been removed.

In summary, the regular consumption of fatty fish is advised. Consuming whole fish is thought to have greater benefits and be safer than using fish oil supplements. Fish is not only a rich source of omega-3 fatty acids, but is also a valuable source of protein and trace elements that may also provide protective effects for the cardiovascular system. Broiled or baked fish is recommended rather than fried fish because frying may decrease the ratio of omega-3 to omega-6 fatty acids and may produce *trans* fatty acids and oxidized lipid products that may increase cardiovascular disease risk.

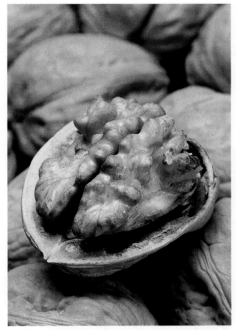

▲ Walnuts are one of the richest plant sources of the omega-3 fatty acid, alpha-linolenic acid, and are also a good source of plant sterols.

## MAKING DECISIONS

### Flax Seeds or Walnuts?

Flax seeds and walnuts are getting attention today because they are rich vegetable sources of the omega-3 alpha-linolenic acid. About 2 tablespoons of flax seed per day is typically recommended if used as an omega-3 fatty acid source. Flax seeds can be purchased in many natural food stores rather inexpensively. These need to be chewed thoroughly or they will pass through the GI tract undigested. Many people find it easier to grind them in a coffee grinder before eating them. Flax seed oil is also available, but it turns **rancid** very quickly, especially if not refrigerated. Compared to other nuts and seeds, walnuts are one of the richest sources of alpha-linolenic acid (2.6 grams per 1-ounce serving or 14 walnut halves). The DRI for alpha-linolenic acid is 1.6 grams/day for men and 1.1 grams/day for women. In addition, walnuts are a rich source of plant sterols known to inhibit intestinal absorption of cholesterol.

## Effects of a Deficiency of Essential Fatty Acids

If humans fail to consume enough essential fatty acids, their skin becomes flaky and itchy, and diarrhea and other symptoms such as infections often are seen. Growth and wound healing may be restricted. These signs of deficiency have been seen in people fed intravenously by **total parenteral nutrition** containing little or no fat for 2 to 3 weeks, as well as in infants receiving formulas low in fat. However, because our bodies need the equivalent of only about 2 to 4 tablespoons of plant oils a day, even a lowfat diet will provide enough essential fatty acids if it follows a balanced plan such as MyPyramid and includes a serving of fatty fish at least twice a week.

## CRITICAL THINKING

Advertisements often claim that fats are bad. Your classmate Mike asks, "If fats are so bad for us, why do we need to have any in our diets?" How would you answer him?

**rancid**  Containing products of decomposed fatty acids that have an unpleasant flavor and odor.

**total parenteral nutrition**  The intravenous feeding of all necessary nutrients, including the most basic forms of protein, carbohydrates, lipids, vitamins, minerals, and electrolytes.

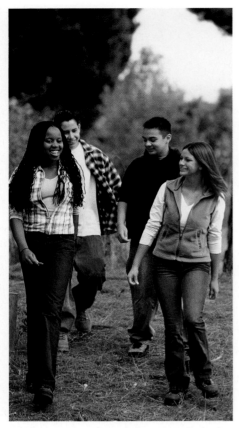

▲ When at rest or during light activity, the body uses mostly fatty acids for fuel.

## 5.7 Broader Roles for Fatty Acids and Triglycerides in the Body

Many key functions of fat in the body require the use of fatty acids in the form of triglycerides. Triglycerides are used for energy storage, insulation, and transportation of fat-soluble vitamins.

### Providing Energy

Triglycerides contained in the diet and stored in adipose tissue provide the fatty acids that are the main fuel for muscles while at rest and during light activity. Muscles use carbohydrate for fuel in addition to fatty acids supplied by triglycerides only in endurance exercise, such as long-distance running and cycling, or in short bursts of intense activity, such as a 200-meter run. Other body tissues also use fatty acids for energy needs. Overall, about half of the energy used by the entire body at rest and during light activity comes from fatty acids. When considering the whole-body, the use of fatty acids by skeletal and heart muscle is balanced by the use of glucose by the nervous system and red blood cells. Recall from Chapter 4 that cells need a supply of carbohydrate to efficiently process fatty acids for fuel. The details about how we burn fat as a fuel will be discussed in Chapter 7.

### Storing Energy for Later Use

We store energy mainly in the form of triglycerides. The body's ability to store fat is essentially limitless. Its fat storage sites, adipose cells, can increase about 50 times in weight. If the amount of fat to be stored exceeds the ability of the existing cells to expand, the body can form new adipose cells.

An important advantage of using triglycerides to store energy in the body is that they are energy dense. Recall that these yield, on average, 9 kcal per gram, whereas proteins and carbohydrates yield only about 4 kcal per gram. In addition, triglycerides are chemically stable, so they are not likely to react with other cell constituents, making them a safe form for storing energy. Finally, when we store triglycerides in adipose cells, we store little else, especially water. Adipose cells contain about 80% lipid and only 20% water and protein. In contrast, imagine if we were to store energy as muscle tissue, which is about 73% water. Body weight linked to energy storage would increase dramatically. The same would be true if we stored energy primarily as glycogen, as about 3 grams of water are stored for every gram of glycogen.

Nucleus

Cell membrane

Fat droplet

**Adipose cell**

## Insulating and Protecting the Body

The insulating layer of fat just beneath the skin is made mostly of triglycerides. Fat tissue also surrounds and protects some organs—kidneys, for example—from injury. We usually don't notice the important insulating function of fat tissue, because we wear clothes and add more as needed. A layer of insulating fat is important in animals living in cold climates. Polar bears, walruses, and whales all build a thick layer of fat tissue around themselves to insulate against cold-weather environments. The extra fat also provides energy storage for times when food is scarce.

## Transporting Fat-Soluble Vitamins

Triglycerides and other fats in food carry fat-soluble vitamins to the small intestine and aid their absorption. People who absorb fat poorly, such as those with the disease cystic fibrosis, are at risk for deficiencies of fat-soluble vitamins, especially vitamin K. A similar risk comes from taking mineral oil as a laxative at mealtimes. The body cannot digest or absorb mineral oil, so the undigested oil carries the fat-soluble vitamins from the meal into the feces, where they are eliminated. Unabsorbed fatty acids can bind minerals, such as calcium and magnesium, and draw them into the stool for elimination. This can harm mineral status (see Chapter 9). Recall that the main problem with the fat replacer, olestra, is that it can bind the fat-soluble vitamins and reduce their absorption.

## 5.8 Phospholipids in the Body

Many types of phospholipids exist in the body, especially in the brain. They form important parts of cell membranes. Phospholipids are found in body cells, and they participate in fat digestion in the intestine. Recall that the various forms of lecithin (discussed earlier) are common examples of phospholipids (review Fig. 5-4b).

Cell membranes are composed primarily of phospholipids. A cell membrane looks much like a sea of phospholipids with protein "islands" (Fig. 5-15). The proteins

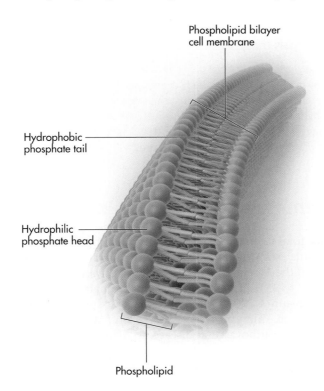

Phospholipid bilayer cell membrane

Hydrophobic phosphate tail

Hydrophilic phosphate head

Phospholipid

**FIGURE 5-15** ▶ Phospholipids are the main components of cell membranes, forming a double or bilayer of lipid.

form receptors for hormones, function as enzymes, and act as transporters for nutrients. The fatty acids on the phospholipids serve as a source of essential fatty acids for the cell. Some cholesterol is also present in the membrane.

In some foods, phospholipids function as emulsifiers (as covered earlier) allowing fat and water to mix. By breaking fat globules into small droplets, emulsifiers enable a fat to be suspended in water. They act as bridges between the oil and water that in turn lead to the formation of tiny oil droplets surrounded by thin shells of water. In an emulsified solution, such as salad dressing or mayonnaise, millions of tiny oil droplets are separated by shells of water (review Fig. 5-7).

The body's main emulsifiers are the lecithins and bile acids, produced by the liver and released into the small intestine via the gallbladder during digestion.

## 5.9  Cholesterol in the Body

Cholesterol plays many vital roles in the body. It forms part of some important hormones, such as estrogen, testosterone, and a form of the active vitamin D hormone. Cholesterol is also the building block of bile acids, needed for fat digestion. Finally, cholesterol is an essential structural component of cells and the outer layer of the lipoprotein particles that transport lipids in the blood. The cholesterol content of the heart, liver, kidney, and brain is high, reflecting its critical role in these organs.

About two-thirds of the cholesterol circulating through your body is made by body cells; the remaining one-third is consumed in the diet. Each day, our cells produce approximately 875 milligrams of cholesterol. Of the 875 milligrams of cholesterol made by the body, about 400 milligrams are used to make new bile acids to replenish those lost in the feces, and about 50 milligrams are used to make hormones. In addition to all the cholesterol cells make, we consume about 180 to 325 milligrams of cholesterol per day from animal-derived food products, with men consuming the higher amount compared to women. Absorption of cholesterol from food ranges from about 40% to 65%. The effect of blood cholesterol, especially LDL cholesterol, on cardiovascular disease risk will be discussed in the "Nutrition and Your Health" section.

See *Nutrition and Your Health: Lipids and Cardiovascular Disease* at the end of Chapter 5.

### CONCEPT CHECK
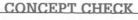

Triglycerides are the major form of fat in the body. They are used for energy and stored in adipose tissue, they insulate and protect body organs, and they transport fat-soluble vitamins. Phospholipids are emulsifiers—compounds that can suspend fat in water. Phospholipids also form parts of cell membranes and various compounds in the body. Cholesterol, a sterol, forms part of cell membranes, hormones, and bile acids. If sufficient amounts are not consumed, the body makes what phospholipids and cholesterol it needs.

▲ Trimming the fat off meats can help reduce saturated fat intake. Limiting intake of meat that is highly marbled with fat (streaks of fat running through the lean) helps, too.

## 5.10  Recommendations for Fat Intake

There is no RDA for total fat intake for adults, although there is an Adequate Intake set for total fat for infants (see Chapter 15). The 2005 Dietary Guidelines for Americans recommendation and the Acceptable Macronutrient Distribution Range is that total fat intake should be 20% to 35% of total calories, which equates to 44 to 78 grams per day for a person who consumes 2000 kcal daily. The most specific recommendations for fat intake come from the American Heart Association (AHA). Many North Americans are at risk for developing cardiovascular disease, so AHA promotes dietary and lifestyle goals aimed at reducing this risk. The AHA diet and lifestyle goals for cardiovascular disease risk reduction for the general public are presented in Table 5-4. These goals include aiming for an overall healthy eating pattern; appropriate body weight; and a desirable

**TABLE 5-4** American Heart Association 2006 Diet and Lifestyle Goals for Cardiovascular Disease Risk Reduction

- Consume an overall healthy diet.

- Aim for a healthy body weight.

- Aim for recommended levels of low-density lipoprotein (LDL) cholesterol, high-density lipoprotein (HDL) cholesterol, and triglycerides.

- Aim for a normal blood pressure.

- Aim for a normal blood glucose level.

- Be physically active.

- Avoid use of and exposure to tobacco products.

From: Lichtenstein AH et al: Diet and lifestyle recommendations revision 2006. A scientific statement from the American Heart Association Nutrition Committee. *Circulation* 114:82, 2006.

**O**ne goal of *Healthy People 2010* is to increase the proportion of persons age 2 years and older who consume less than 10% of calorie intake from saturated fat.

blood cholesterol profile, blood pressure, and blood glucose level. In Table 5-5 , a more detailed list of recommendations is provided for those who currently are at high risk or have cardiovascular disease.

To reduce risk for cardiovascular disease, the AHA recommends that no more than 7% of total calories come from saturated fat and no more than 1% from *trans* fat. These are the primary fatty acids that raise LDL. In addition, cholesterol should amount to a maximum of 300 mg per day. This often happens along with the reduction in saturated fat and *trans* fat intake. Table 5-6 is an example of a diet that adheres to 20% or 30% of calories as fat. Compare these recommendations to the actual dietary intake patterns of these fats by North Americans: 33% of calories from total fat, about 13% of calories from saturated fat, and 180 to 320 milligrams of cholesterol each day.

**TABLE 5-5** American Heart Association 2006 Diet and Lifestyle Recommendations for Cardiovascular Disease Risk Reduction

- Balance calorie intake and physical activity to achieve or maintain a healthy body weight.

- Consume a diet rich in vegetables and fruits.

- Choose whole-grain, high-fiber foods.

- Consume fish, especially oily fish, at least twice a week.

- Limit your intake of saturated fat to less than 7% of energy, *trans* fat to less than 1% of energy, and cholesterol to less than 300 milligrams per day by
  — choosing lean meats and vegetable alternatives;
  — selecting fat-free (skim), 1%-fat, and low-fat dairy products; and
  — minimizing intake of partially hydrogenated fats.

- Minimize your intake of beverages and foods with added sugars.

- Choose and prepare foods with little or no salt.

- If you consume alcohol, do so in moderation.

- When you eat food prepared outside of the home, follow the AHA Diet and Lifestyle Recommendations.

From: Lichtenstein AH and others: Diet and lifestyle recommendations revision 2006. A scientific statement from the American Heart Association Nutrition Committee. *Circulation* 114:82, 2006.

**S**ome advice regarding fat intake from the 2005 Dietary Guidelines:
- Limit intake of fats and oils high in saturated and/or *trans* fatty acids, and choose products low in such fats and oils.
- Consume fats high in polyunsaturated and monounsaturated fatty acids, such as from fish, nuts, and vegetable oils.
- When selecting and preparing meat, poultry, dry beans, and milk or milk products, make choices that are lean, low-fat, or fat-free.

**TABLE 5-6** Daily Menu Examples Containing 2000 kcal and 30% or 20% of Calories as Fat

| | 30% of Calories as Fat | | 20% of Calories as Fat | |
| --- | --- | --- | --- | --- |
| Food | | Fat (grams) | Food | Fat (grams) |
| **Breakfast** | | | | |
| Orange juice, 1 cup | | 0.5 | Same | 0.5 |
| Shredded wheat, ¾ cup | | 0.5 | Shredded wheat, 1 cup | 0.7 |
| Toasted bagel | | 1.1 | Same | 1.1 |
| Tub margarine, 3 teaspoons | | 11.4 | Tub margarine, 2 teaspoons | 7.6 |
| 1% low-fat milk, 1 cup | | 2.5 | Fat-free milk, 1 cup | 0.6 |
| **Lunch** | | | | |
| Whole-wheat bread, 2 slices | | 2.4 | Same | 2.4 |
| Roast beef, 2 ounces | | 4.9 | Light turkey roll, 2 ounces | 0.9 |
| Mayonnaise, 3 teaspoons | | 11.0 | Mayonnaise, 2 teaspoons | 7.3 |
| Lettuce | | — | Same | — |
| Tomato | | — | Same | — |
| Oatmeal cookie, 1 | | 3.3 | Oatmeal cookie, 2 | 6.6 |
| **Snack** | | | | |
| Apple | | — | Same | — |
| **Dinner** | | | | |
| Chicken tenders frozen meal | | 18.0 | Fat-free chicken tenders | — |
| Carrots, ½ cup | | — | Same | — |
| Dinner roll, 1 | | 2.0 | Same | 2.0 |
| Margarine, 1 teaspoon | | 3.8 | Same | 3.8 |
| Banana | | 0.6 | Same | 0.6 |
| 1% low-fat milk, 1 cup | | 2.5 | Fat-free milk, 1 cup | 0.6 |
| **Snack** | | | | |
| Raisins, 2 teaspoons | | — | Raisins, ½ cup | — |
| Air-popped popcorn, 3 cups | | 1.0 | Air-popped popcorn, 6 cups | 2.0 |
| Margarine, 2 teaspoons | | 7.6 | Same | 7.6 |
| **Totals** | | **73.1** | | **44.3** |

▲ **Whole grains** (shredded wheat, whole-wheat bread, oatmeal cookies, popcorn), **fruits** (orange juice, apple, banana, raisins), **vegetables** (carrots, lettuce, tomato), **lean meats** (roast beef, turkey, chicken), and **fat-free milk** are the primary components of the low-fat menus in Table 5-6.

**T**he advice to consume 20% to 35% of calories as fat does not apply to infants and toddlers below the age of 2 years. These youngsters are forming new tissue that requires fat, especially in the brain, so their intake of fat and cholesterol should not be greatly restricted.

Both the National Cholesterol Education Program (NCEP) and the Food and Nutrition Board are in agreement with the advice of the AHA. One exception in the latest guidelines from the NCEP is that fat intake could be as high as 35% of total calories as long as intakes of saturated fat, cholesterol, and *trans* fat are minimized. The Food and Nutrition Board combines the AHA and NCEP recommendations, suggesting that fat provide a range of 20% to 35% of calories. The 2005 Dietary Guidelines also support this advice. In addition to fat intake, controlling total calorie intake is also significant, as weight control is a vital component of cardiovascular disease prevention.

Regarding essential fatty acids, the Food and Nutrition Board has issued recommendations for both omega-6 and omega-3 fatty acids. The amounts listed in Table 5-7 work out to about 5% of calorie in-take for the total of both essential fatty acids. Infants and children have lower needs (again, see Chapter 15). Consumption of fish at least twice a week is one step toward meeting requirements for essential fatty acids.

The typical North American diet derives about 7% of calories from polyunsaturated fatty acids, and thus meets essential fatty acid needs. An upper limit of 10% of calorie intake as polyunsaturated fatty acids is often recommended, in part because the breakdown (oxidation) of those present in lipoproteins is linked to increased cholesterol deposition in the arteries (see the "Nutrition and Your Health" section in

**TABLE 5-7** Food and Nutrition Board Recommendations for Omega-6 and Omega-3 Fatty Acids per Day

|  | Men (grams per day) | Women (grams per day) |
|---|---|---|
| Linoleic acid (omega-6) | 17 | 12 |
| Alpha-linolenic acid (omega-3) | 1.6 | 1.1 |

this chapter). Depression of immune function is also suspected to be caused by an excessive intake of polyunsaturated fatty acids.

In recent years, the Mediterranean diet has attracted a lot of attention as a result of lower rates of chronic diseases seen in people following such a diet plan. The major sources of fat in the Mediterranean diet include liberal amounts of olive oil compared to a small amount of animal fat (from animal flesh and dairy products). In contrast, major sources of fat in the typical North American diet include animal flesh, whole milk, pastries, cheese, margarine, and mayonnaise. While dietary fat sources definitely play a role in prevention of chronic disease, it is important to remember that other aspects of one's lifestyle also contribute to disease risk. People who follow a Mediterranean diet also tend to consume moderate alcohol (usually in the form of red wine, which contains many antioxidants), eat plenty of whole grains and few refined carbohydrates, and are also more physically active than typical North Americans.

An alternative plan for reduction of cardiovascular disease is Dr. Dean Ornish's purely vegetarian (**vegan**) diet plan. This diet is very low in fat, including only a scant quantity of vegetable oil used in cooking and the small amount of oils present in plant foods. Individuals restricting fat intake to 20% of calories should be monitored by a physician, as the resulting increase in carbohydrate intake can increase blood triglycerides in some people, which is not a healthful change. Over time, however, the initial problem of high blood triglycerides on a low-fat diet may self-correct. Among people following the Ornish plan, blood triglycerides initially increased, but within a year, fell to normal values as long as they emphasized high-fiber carbohydrate sources, controlled (or improved) body weight, and followed a regular exercise program.

In summary, the general consensus among nutrition experts suggests that limitation of saturated fat, cholesterol, and *trans* fat intake should be the primary focus, and that the diet needs to contain some omega-3 and omega-6 fatty acids (Table 5-8). Furthermore, if fat intake exceeds 30% of total calories, the extra fat should come from monounsaturated fat.

▲ If you are looking to decrease the amount of saturated and *trans* fats in your diet, it is a good idea to opt for lower-fat substitutes for some of your current high-fat food choices. How do you think this meal compares with the fried meal on p. 179.

**vegan** A person who eats only plant foods.

## CONCEPT CHECK

There is no RDA for fat. We need about 5% of total calorie intake from plant oils to obtain the needed essential fatty acids. Eating fatty fish at least twice a week is also advised to supply omega-3 fatty acids. Many health-related agencies recommend a diet containing no more than 35% of calorie intake as fat, with no more than 7% to 10% of calorie intake as a combination of saturated fat and *trans* fat for the general public. Cholesterol intake should be limited to 200 to 300 milligrams per day. These practices help maintain a normal LDL value in the blood. The North American diet contains about 33% of calories as fat, with about 13% of calories as saturated fat and about 3% as *trans* fatty acids. Cholesterol intake varies from about 200 to 400 milligrams per day.

**TABLE 5-8** Tips for Avoiding Too Much Fat, Saturated Fat, Cholesterol, and *Trans* Fat

| | Eat Less of These Foods | Eat More of These Foods |
|---|---|---|
| Grains | • Pasta dishes with cheese or cream sauces<br>• Croissants<br>• Pastries<br>• Doughnuts<br>• Pie crust | • Whole-grain breads<br>• Whole-grain pasta<br>• Brown rice<br>• Angel food cake<br>• Animal or graham crackers<br>• Air-popped popcorn |
| Vegetables | • French fries<br>• Potato chips<br>• Vegetables cooked in butter, cheese, or cream sauces | • Fresh, frozen, baked, or steamed vegetables |
| Fruit | • Fruit pies | • Fresh, frozen, or canned fruits |
| Milk | • Whole milk<br>• Ice cream<br>• High-fat cheese<br>• Cheesecake | • Fat-free and reduced-fat milk<br>• Low-fat frozen desserts (e.g., yogurt, sherbet, ice milk)<br>• Reduced-fat/part-skim cheese |
| Meat and beans | • Bacon<br>• Sausage<br>• Organ meats (e.g., liver)<br>• Egg yolks | • Fish<br>• Skinless poultry<br>• Lean cuts of meat (with fat trimmed away)<br>• Soy products<br>• Egg whites/egg substitutes |
| Oils | • Butter and stick margarine | • Canola oil or olive oil<br>• Tub or liquid margarine (in small amounts) |

▲ To avoid too much saturated fat and cholesterol, for breakfast eat fewer foods like bacon, sausage, hash browns and whole eggs and more foods like whole-grain waffles and fresh fruit.

# LIPIDS CONCEPT MAP

**LIPIDS-Fats & Oils**

*main form of fat in food and body*

**Triglycerides**
(glycerol+3 fatty acids)

*in lipid bilayer in cell membranes*

**Phospholipids**

Example: lecithin

*released from fat stores broken down to release energy*

**Fatty Acids**

*formed during fat digestion*

Monoglycerides

**Sterols**

**Cholesterol**

*in animal fats & tropical oils*

Saturated

*in plant oils*

**Unsaturated**

*activated in skin by uv radiation*

Vitamin D

**Steroid Hormones**

*aids fat digestion*

Bile

*high in olive oil*

Monounsaturated
(one double bond)

**Polyunsaturated**
(two or more double bonds)

Examples:
estrogen,
testosterone

*high in fish oil*

*high in plant oils*

*Omega*-3 Fatty Acids

*Omega*-6 Fatty Acids

Essential Fatty Acid
alpha-linolenic acid

Essential Fatty Acid
linolenic acid

# Lipids and Cardiovascular Disease

Cardiovascular disease is the major killer of North Americans. Cardiovascular disease typically involves the coronary arteries and, thus, frequently the term coronary heart disease (CHD) or coronary artery disease (CAD) is used. Each year about 500,000 people die of coronary heart disease in the United States, about 60% more than die of cancer. The figure rises to almost 1 million if strokes and other circulatory diseases are included in the global term *cardiovascular disease*. About 1.5 million people in the United States each year have a heart attack. The overall male-to-female ratio for cardiovascular disease is about 2:1. Women generally lag about 10 years behind men in developing

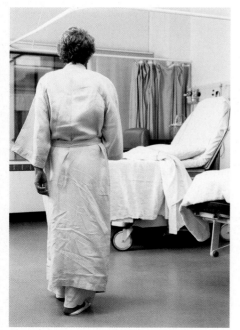

▲ Cardiovascular disease kills more women than any other disease—twice as many as does cancer.

the disease. Still, it eventually kills more women than any other disease—twice as many as does cancer. And, for each person in North America who dies of cardiovascular disease, 20 more (over 13 million people) have symptoms of the disease.

## Development of Cardiovascular Disease

The symptoms of cardiovascular disease develop over many years and often do not become obvious until old age. Nonetheless, autopsies of young adults under 20 years of age have shown that many of them had atherosclerotic **plaque** in their arteries (Fig. 5-16). This finding indicates that plaque buildup can begin in childhood and continue throughout life, although it usually goes undetected for some time.

The typical forms of cardiovascular disease—coronary heart disease and strokes—are associated with inadequate blood circulation in the heart and brain related to buildup of this plaque. Blood supplies the heart muscle, brain, and other body organs with oxygen and nutrients. When blood flow via the coronary arteries surrounding the heart is interrupted, the heart muscle can be damaged. A heart attack, or **myocardial infarction,** may result (review Fig. 5-16). This may cause the heart to beat irregularly or to stop. About 25% of people do not survive their first heart attack. If blood flow to parts of the brain is interrupted long enough, part of the brain dies, causing a **cerebrovascular accident,** or stroke.

A heart attack can strike with the sudden force of a sledgehammer, with pain radiating up the neck or down the arm.

It can sneak up at night, masquerading as indigestion, with slight pain or pressure in the chest. Many times, the symptoms are so subtle in women that death occurs before she or the health professional realizes that a heart attack is taking place. If there is any suspicion at all that a heart attack is taking place, the person should first call 911 and then chew an aspirin (325 milligrams) thoroughly. Aspirin helps reduce the blood clotting that leads to a heart attack.

Continuous formation and breakdown of blood clots in the blood vessels is a normal process. However, in areas where plaques build up, blood clots are more likely to remain intact and then lead to a blockage, cutting off or diminishing the supply of blood to the heart (via the coronary arteries) or brain (via the carotid arteries). More than 95% of heart attacks are caused by such blood clots. Heart attacks generally are caused by total blockage of the coronary arteries due to a blood clot forming in an area of the artery already partially blocked by plaque. Disruption of the plaque may even lead to eventual clot formation.

---

**plaque** A cholesterol-rich substance deposited in the blood vessels; it contains various white blood cells, smooth muscle cells, various proteins, cholesterol and other lipids, and eventually calcium.

**myocardial infarction** Death of part of the heart muscle. Also termed a *heart attack.*

**cerebrovascular accident (CVA)** Death of part of the brain tissue due typically to a blood clot. Also termed a *stroke.*

> Typical warning signs of a heart attack are:

- Intense, prolonged chest pain or pressure, sometimes radiating to other parts of the upper body (men and women)
- Shortness of breath (men and women)
- Sweating (men and women)
- Nausea and vomiting (especially women)
- Dizziness (especially women)
- Weakness (men and women)
- Jaw, neck, and shoulder pain (especially women)
- Irregular heartbeat (men and women)

▲ At the first sign of a possible heart attack, the person should first call 911 and then thoroughly chew an aspirin.

> *Healthy People 2010* has set a goal of reducing death from coronary heart disease by 30%, compared with today's incidence.

**FIGURE 5-16** ▶ The road to a heart attack. Injury to an artery wall begins the process. This is followed by a progressive buildup of plaque in the artery walls. The heart attack represents the terminal phase of the process. Blockage of the left coronary artery by a blood clot is evident. The heart muscle served by the portion of the coronary artery beyond the point of blockage lacks oxygen and nutrients and is damaged and may die. This damage can lead to a significant drop in heart function and often total heart failure.

Atherosclerosis probably first develops to repair damage in a vessel lining. The damage that starts this process can be caused by smoking, diabetes, hypertension, LDL, and viral and bacterial infection. Ongoing inflammation in the blood vessel is also suspected to cause blood vessel damage. (A laboratory test for c-reactive protein in the blood is used to assess if inflammation is present.) Atherosclerosis can be seen in arteries throughout the body. The damage develops especially at points where an artery branches into two smaller vessels. A great deal of stress is placed on the vessel walls at these points due to changes in blood flow.

Once blood vessel damage has occurred, the next step in the development of atherosclerosis is the progression phase. This step is characterized by deposition of plaque at the site of initial damage. The rate of plaque buildup during the progression phase is directly related to the amount of LDL in the blood. The form of LDL that contributes to atherosclerosis is **oxidized** LDL. This form is preferentially

**oxidize** In the most basic sense, the loss of an electron or gain of an oxygen by a chemical substance. This change typically alters the shape and/or function of the substance.

taken up by scavenger cells in the arterial wall. Nutrients and phytochemicals that have **antioxidant** properties may reduce LDL oxidation. Fruits and vegetables are particularly rich in these compounds. Eating fruits and vegetables regularly is one positive step we can make to reduce plaque buildup and slow the progression of cardiovascular disease. Some fruits and vegetables particularly helpful in this regard include legumes (beans), nuts, dried plums (prunes), raisins, berries, plums, apples, cherries, oranges, grapes, spinach, broccoli, red bell peppers, potatoes, and onions. Tea and coffee are also sources of antioxidants.

As plaque accumulates, arteries harden, narrow, and lose their elasticity. Affected arteries become further damaged as blood pumps through them and pressure increases. Finally, in the terminal phase, a clot or spasm in a plaque-clogged artery leads to a heart attack.

Factors that typically bring on a heart attack in a person already at risk include dehydration; acute emotional stress (such as firing an employee); strenuous physical activity when not otherwise physically fit (shoveling snow, for example); waking during the night or getting up in the morning (linked to an abrupt increase in stress); and consuming large, high-fat meals (increases blood clotting).

## Risk Factors for Cardiovascular Disease

Many of us are free of the risk factors that contribute to rapid development of atherosclerosis. If so, the advice of health experts is to consume a balanced diet, perform regular physical activity, have a complete fasting lipoprotein analysis performed at age 20 or beyond, and reevaluate risk factors every 5 years.

For most people, however, the most likely risk factors are:

- **Total blood cholesterol over 200 milligrams per 100 milliliters of blood** (mg/dl; dl is short for deciliter or 100 milliliters). Risk is especially high when total cholesterol is at or over 240 mg/dl and LDL-cholesterol readings are over 130 to 160 mg/dl. (The terms LDL-cholesterol and HDL-cholesterol are used when expressing the blood concentration because it is the cholesterol content of these lipoproteins that is measured.)

- **Smoking.** Smoking is the main cause of about 20% of cardiovascular disease deaths and generally negates the female advantage of later occurrence of the disease. A combination of smoking and oral contraceptive use increases the risk of cardiovascular disease in women even more. Smoking greatly increases the expression of a person's genetically linked risk for cardiovascular disease, even if one's blood lipids are low. Smoking also makes blood more likely to clot. Even secondhand smoke has been implicated as a risk factor.

- **Hypertension. Systolic blood pressure** over 139 (millimeters of mercury) and **diastolic blood pressure** over 89 indicate hypertension. Healthy blood pressure values are less than 120 and 80, respectively. (Treatment of hypertension is reviewed in Chapter 9.)

- **Diabetes.** Diabetes virtually guarantees development of cardiovascular disease, and so puts a person with diabetes in the high-risk group. Insulin increases cholesterol synthesis in the liver, in turn increasing LDL in the bloodstream. This disease negates any female advantage.

▲ Smoking is one of the four major risk factors for developing cardiovascular disease.

**antioxidant** Generally a compound that stops the damaging effects of reactive substances seeking an electron (i.e., oxidizing agents). This prevents breakdown (oxidizing) of substances in foods or the body, particularly lipids.

**systolic blood pressure** The pressure in the arterial blood vessels associated with the pumping of blood from the heart.

**diastolic blood pressure** The pressure in the arterial blood vessels when the heart is between beats.

### MAKING DECISIONS

#### Antioxidant Supplements and Cardiovascular Disease

Are large doses of antioxidant vitamin supplements a reliable way to reduce LDL oxidation, and thereby prevent cardiovascular disease? Controversy about such dietary supplementation exists among the experts, as will be detailed in Chapter 8. The American Heart Association does not support use of antioxidant supplements (such as vitamin E) to reduce cardiovascular disease risk. This is because large-scale studies have shown no decrease in cardiovascular disease risk with use of antioxidant supplements. One study even showed a modest increase for heart failure in people with diabetes or otherwise at high risk for cardiovascular disease after taking antioxidant supplements. However, further trials of antioxidant supplementation (e.g., 600 IU of vitamin E every other day) for prevention of heart disease in men are ongoing. With regard to women, 600 IU of natural-source vitamin E taken every other day provided no overall benefit for major cardiovascular events (or cancer). More research is warranted, however, as a decrease in sudden cardiac death was seen in a subset of older women in this study. Some experts suggest daily vitamin E supplementation (100 IU to 400 IU) may be helpful for *preventing* cardiovascular disease, while other experts recommend against the practice. One thing is certain: any supplementation of vitamin E should be taken only under the guidance of a physician, because of interactions with vitamin K and anticlotting medications (and possibly high-dose aspirin use).

▶ For more information on cardiovascular disease, see the website of the American Heart Association at www.americanheart.org or the heart disease section of Healthfinder at www.healthfinder.gov/tours/heart.htm. This is a site created by the U.S. government for consumers. In addition, visit the website www.nhlbi.nih.gov/.

▶ *Healthy People 2010* has set a goal of reducing total blood cholesterol among adults from the average of 206 mg/dl to 199 mg/dl, as well as reducing the percentage of adults with high blood cholesterol from 21% to 17%.

▶ **Cardiovascular Disease Risk Factors**

- Total blood cholesterol > 200 mg/dl
- Smoking
- Hypertension
- Diabetes
- HDL cholesterol < 40 mg/dl
- Age: Men > 45 yr; Women > 55 yr
- Family history of cardiovascular disease
- Blood triglycerides > 200 mg/dl
- Obesity
- Inactivity

▶ Two approaches have been shown to cause reversal of atherosclerosis in the body. One employs a vegan diet and other lifestyle changes that are part of the Dr. Dean Ornish program. The other employs aggressive LDL lowering with medications.

▶ As noted earlier, aspirin in small doses reduces blood clotting. It is often used under a physician's guidance to treat people at risk for heart attack or stroke, especially if one has already occurred. About 80 to 160 milligrams per day is needed for such benefits. Individuals who may especially benefit from aspirin therapy are men over 40, smokers, postmenopausal women, and people with diabetes, hypertension, or a family history of cardiovascular disease.

Together, the previous four risk factors explain most cases of cardiovascular disease.

Other risk factors to consider:

- HDL-cholesterol under 40 mg/dl, especially when the ratio of total cholesterol to HDL-cholesterol is greater than 4:1 (3.5:1 or less is optimal). Women often have high values for HDL-cholesterol, and therefore it is important for this to be measured in women to establish cardiovascular disease risk. A value of 60 mg/dl or more is especially protective. Exercising for at least 45 minutes four times a week can increase HDL by about 5 mg/dl. Losing excess weight (especially around the waist) and avoiding smoking and overeating also help maintain or raise HDL, as does moderate alcohol consumption.
- Age. Men over 45 years and women over 55 years.
- Family history of cardiovascular disease, especially before age 50.
- Blood triglycerides 200 mg/dl or greater in the fasting state (less than 100 mg/dl is optimal).
- Obesity (especially fat accumulation in the waist). Typical weight gain seen in adults is a chief contributor to the increase in LDL seen with aging. Obesity also typically leads to insulin resistance, creating a diabetes-like state, and ultimately the disease itself. It also increases overall inflamation throughout the body.
- Inactivity. Exercise conditions the arteries to adapt to physical stress. Regular exercise also improves insulin action in the body. The corresponding reduction in insulin output leads to a reduction in lipoprotein synthesis in the liver. Both regular aerobic exercise and resistance exercise are recommended. A person with existing cardiovascular disease should seek physician approval before starting such a program, as should older adults.

Researchers are trying to unravel and quantify numerous other factors that may be linked to premature cardiovascular disease, such as the connection between inadequate intake of vitamin B-6, folate, and vitamin B-12, which can lead to increased

homocysteine in the blood. As noted, homocysteine may damage the cells lining the blood vessels, in turn promoting atherosclerosis. Studies show that supplementation with folic acid and B vitamins does not reduce risk of recurrent cardiovascular disease in patients that had previous heart attacks or had existing vascular diseases.

The term *risk factor* is not equivalent to cause of disease; nevertheless, the more of these risk factors one has, the greater the chances of ultimately developing cardiovascular disease. A good example is the **metabolic syndrome** (also called *Syndrome X*) discussed in Chapter 4. A person with the metabolic syndrome would have abdominal obesity, high blood triglycerides, low HDL-cholesterol, hypertension, poor blood glucose regulation (i.e., high fasting blood glucose), and increased blood clotting. This profile raises the risk for cardiovascular disease considerably. On a positive note, cardiovascular disease is rare in populations who have low LDL-cholesterol, normal blood pressure, and do not smoke or have diabetes. By minimizing these risk factors, as well as following the dietary recommendations of the American Heart Association on page 193 and staying physically active, one will most likely reduce many of the other controllable risk factors listed. In other words, develop and follow a total lifestyle plan. Medications may also be added to lower blood lipids, as discussed next. Finally, if a person has a family history of cardiovascular disease but the usual risk factors aren't present, a rarer defect might be the cause. In this case, having a detailed physical examination for other potential causes is advised.

## Medical Interventions to Lower Blood Lipids

Some people need even more aggressive therapy added to their regimen of a diet and lifestyle overhaul to treat elevated blood lipids. The clearest indication for this more aggressive approach is in people who already have had a heart attack or have cardiovascular disease symptoms or diabetes.

Medications are the cornerstone of this more aggressive therapy. The National

Cholesterol Education Program in the United States has developed a formula based on age, total blood cholesterol, HDL-cholesterol, smoking history, and blood pressure to determine who needs such medications. Check out this formula at http://hp2010.nhlbihin.net/atpiii/calculator.asp?usertype=pub. This formula provides an estimate for having a heart attack in the next 10 years.

Medications work to lower LDL in one of two ways. Some reduce cholesterol synthesis in the liver. Such medicines are known as "statins" (e.g., atorvistatin [Lipitor]). The cost of treatment with one of these drugs can be from $1,600 or more per year, depending on the dose needed. These medications lead to problems in some people, and so require physician monitoring, especially of liver function. Another group of medications binds bile acids or the cholesterol that is part of bile secreted into the small intestine. This binding leads to their elimination in the feces and so requires the liver to synthesize new bile acids and/or cholesterol. The liver removes LDL from the blood to do this. Some of these medications taste gritty and therefore are not popular.

The current therapeutic goal for people with (or at high risk for) cardiovascular disease (Table 5-9) is to drive LDL down to less than 70 mg/dl.

The statin drug simvastatin (Zocor) has been combined with another drug (ezetimibe) and is marketed as Vytorin, a drug that will treat the two sources of cholesterol, "food and family." While the statin reduces the cholesterol made by the liver, the ezetimibe helps block the absorption of cholesterol from food.

A third group of drugs can be used to lower blood triglycerides by decreasing the triglyceride production of the liver. These include gemfibrozil (Lopid) and megadoses of the vitamin nicotinic acid. The use of nicotinic acid does result in pesky side effects, however, but these are typically manageable.

## Other Possible Medical Therapies for Cardiovascular Disease

FDA has approved two margarines that have positive effects on blood cholesterol levels—Benecol and Take Control. These margarines contain plant stanols/sterols.

The plant stanols/sterols, also called phytosterols, work by reducing cholesterol absorption in the small intestine and lowering its return to the liver. The liver responds by taking up more cholesterol from the blood so it can continue to make bile acids. The studies done on the cholesterol-lowering effect of these margarines have found that 2 to 5 grams of plant stanols/sterols per day reduces total blood cholesterol by 8% to 10% and LDL-cholesterol by 9% to 14% (similar to what is seen with some cholesterol-lowering drugs).

Benecol is made from plant stanols extracted from wood pulp. This product is sold as margarine and has been added to salad dressings. Take Control is made from plant sterols isolated from soybeans. The recommended amount for both is about 2 to 3 grams per day as part of at least two meals; this works out to about 1 tablespoon of Benecol or 2 tablespoons of Take Control per day. Use would cost about $1.00 per day, as these margarines are more expensive than regular margarines.

In people who have borderline high total blood cholesterol (between 200 and 239 mg/dl), these margarines can be helpful in avoiding future drug therapy. Plant stanols/sterols have been made available in pill form as well. Remember that plant sterols are naturally present in nuts in high concentrations. Wheat germ, sesame seeds, pistachios, and sunflower seeds are some of the richest sources.

The two most common surgical treatments for coronary artery blockage are percutaneous transluminal coronary angioplasty (PTCA) and coronary artery bypass graft (CABG). PTCA involves the insertion of a balloon catheter into an artery. Once it is advanced to the area of the lesion, the balloon is expanded to crush the lesion. This method works best when only one vessel is blocked, and it may be held open with metal mesh, called a stent. CABG involves the removal and use of a saphenous vein, a large vein in the leg, or use of a mammary artery. The relocated vein is sewn to the main heart vessel (aorta) and then used to bypass the blocked artery. The procedure can be performed on one or more blockages.

▲ Benecol and Take Control are margarines that are examples of "functional foods" because they contain added cholesterol-lowering plant stanols/sterols.

**TABLE 5-9** Sorting Out One's Goals for Cardiovascular Disease Prevention/Treatment

| Risk Class | This Is You If . . . | Your LDL (mg/dl) Goal |
|---|---|---|
| Very high | You have cardiovascular disease and other risk factors such as diabetes, obesity, smoking | Below 70 |
| High | You have cardiovascular disease or diabetes or two or more risk factors for cardiovascular disease (e.g., smoking, hypertension) | Below 100 |
| Moderately high | You have cardiovascular disease risks and an increased 10-year risk of developing a heart attack | 100–130 |
| Moderate | You have 2 or more risk factors and a marginal chance of developing cardiovascular disease in the next 10 years. | Below 130 |
| Low | You have few or no cardiovascular disease risk factors | Below 160 |

## Case Study **Planning a Heart Healthy Diet**

Jackie is a 21-year-old health-conscious individual majoring in business. She recently learned that a diet high in saturated fat can contribute to high blood cholesterol and that exercise is beneficial for the heart. Jackie now takes a brisk 30-minute walk each morning before going to class, and she has started to cut as much fat out of her diet as she can, replacing it mostly with carbohydrates. A typical day for Jackie now begins with a bowl of Fruity Pebbles with 1 cup of skim milk and ½ cup of apple juice. For lunch, she might pack a turkey sandwich on white bread with lettuce, tomato, and mustard; a small package of fat-free pretzels; and a handful of reduced-fat vanilla wafers. Dinner could be a large portion of pasta with some olive oil and garlic mixed in, and a small iceberg lettuce salad with lemon juice squeezed over it. Her snacks are usually baked chips, low-fat cookies, fat-free frozen yogurt, or fat-free pretzels. She drinks diet soft drinks throughout the day as her main beverage.

Answer the following questions, and check your response in Appendix A.

1. Has Jackie made the best diet changes with regard to lowering blood cholesterol and maintaining heart health?
2. Is there much fat left in Jackie's new diet plan? Is it necessary for her to drastically lower her fat intake?
3. What types of fat should Jackie try to consume? Why are these types of fat the most desirable?
4. What types of foods has Jackie used to replace the fat in her diet?
5. What food groups are missing from her new diet plan? How many servings should she be including from these food groups?
6. Is Jackie's new exercise routine appropriate?

▲ Are there important food groups missing from Jackie's new diet plan?

## Summary

1. Lipids are a group of compounds that do not dissolve in water. Fatty acids are the simplest form of lipid. There are three fatty acids on every triglyceride, the most common type of lipid found in the body and foods. Phospholipids and sterols are two other classes of lipids in food and our bodies.

2. Saturated fatty acids contain no carbon-carbon double bonds, mono-unsaturated fatty acids contain one carbon-carbon double bond, and polyunsaturated fatty acids contain two or more carbon-carbon double bonds in the carbon chain. In omega-3 polyunsaturated fatty acids, the first of the carbon-carbon double bonds is located three carbons from the methyl end of the carbon chain. In omega-6 polyunsaturated fatty acids, the first carbon-carbon double bond counting from the methyl end occurs at the sixth carbon. Both omega-3 and omega-6 fatty acids are essential fatty acids; these must be included in the diet to maintain health.

3. Triglycerides are formed from a glycerol backbone with three fatty acids. Triglycerides rich in long-chain saturated fatty acids tend to be solid at room temperature, whereas those rich in mono-unsaturated and polyunsaturated fatty acids are liquid at room temperature. Triglyceride is the major form of fat in both food and the body. It allows for efficient energy storage, protects certain organs, transports fat-soluble vitamins, and helps insulate the body.

4. Phospholipids are derivatives of triglycerides in which one or two of the fatty acids are replaced by phosphorus-containing compounds. Phospholipids are important parts of cell membranes, and some act as efficient emulsifiers.

5. Cholesterol forms vital biological compounds, such as hormones, components of cell membranes, and bile acids. Cells in the body make cholesterol whether we eat it or not. It is not a necessary part of an adult's diet.

6. Foods rich in fat include salad oils, butter, margarine, and mayonnaise. Nuts, bologna, avocados, and bacon are also high in fat, as are peanut butter and cheddar cheese. Steak and hamburger are moderate in fat content, as is whole milk. Many grain products, and fruits and vegetables in general, are low in fat.

7. Fats and oils have several functions as components of foods. Fats add flavor and texture to foods and provide some satiety after meals. Some phospholipids are used in foods as emulsifiers, which suspend fat in water. When fatty acids break down, food becomes rancid, resulting in a foul odor and unpleasant flavor.

8. Hydrogenation is the process of converting carbon-carbon double bonds into single bonds by adding hydrogen

at the point of unsaturation. The partial-hydrogenation of fatty acids in vegetable oils changes the oils to semisolid fats and helps in food formulation and reduces rancidity. Hydrogenation also increases *trans* fatty acid content. High amounts of *trans* fat in the diet are discouraged, as these increase LDL and reduce HDL.

9. Fat digestion takes place primarily in the small intestine. Lipase enzyme released from the pancreas digests long-chain triglycerides into smaller breakdown products—namely, monoglycerides (glycerol backbones with single fatty acids attached) and fatty acids. The breakdown products are then taken up by the absorptive cells of the small intestine. These products are mostly remade into triglycerides and eventually enter the lymphatic system, in turn passing into the bloodstream.

10. Lipids are carried in the bloodstream by various lipoproteins, which consist of a central triglyceride core encased in a shell of protein, cholesterol, and

phospholipid. Chylomicrons are released from intestinal cells and carry lipids arising from dietary intake. Very-low-density lipoprotein (VLDL) and low-density lipoprotein (LDL) carry lipids both taken up by and synthesized in the liver. High-density lipoprotein (HDL) picks up cholesterol from cells and facilitates its transport back to the liver.

11. The essential fatty acids are linoleic acid (an omega-6 fatty acid) and alpha-linolenic acid (on omega-3 fatty acid). Body cells can synthesize hormone-like compounds from both omega-3 and omega-6 fatty acids. The compounds produced from omega-3 fatty acids tend to reduce blood clotting, blood pressure, and inflammatory responses in the body. Those produced from omega-6 fatty acids tend to increase blood clotting.

12. There is currently no RDA for fat for adults. Plant oils should contribute about 5% of total calories to achieve the Adequate Intakes proposed for

essential fatty acids (linoleic acid and alpha-linolenic acid). Fatty fish are a rich source of omega-3 fatty acids and should be consumed at least twice a week.

13. Many health agencies and scientific groups suggest a fat intake of no more than 30% to 35% of total calories. Some health experts advocate an even further reduction to 20% of calorie intake for some people to maintain a normal LDL value, but such a diet requires professional guidance. Medications such as "statins" may be added also to lower LDL. If fat intake exceeds 30% of total calories, the diet should emphasize monounsaturated fat. The typical North American diet contains about 33% of total calories as fat.

14. In the blood, elevated amounts of LDL and low amounts of HDL are strong predictors of the risk for cardiovascular disease. Additional risk factors for the disease are smoking, hypertension, diabetes, obesity, and inactivity.

## Study Questions

1. Describe the chemical structures of saturated and polyunsaturated fatty acids and their different effects in both food and the human body.

2. Relate the need for omega-3 fatty acids in the diet to the recommendation to consume fatty fish at least twice a week.

3. Describe the structures, origins, and roles of the four major blood lipoproteins.

4. What are the recommendations from various health-care organizations

regarding fat intake? What does this mean in terms of food choices?

5. What are two important attributes of fat in food? How are these different from the general functions of lipids in the human body?

6. Describe the significance of and possible uses for reduced-fat foods.

7. Does the total cholesterol concentration in the bloodstream tell the whole story with respect to cardiovascular disease risk?

8. List the four main risk factors for the development of cardiovascular disease.

9. What three lifestyle factors decrease the risk of cardiovascular disease development?

10. When are medications most needed in cardiovascular disease therapy, and how in general do the various classes of medications operate to reduce risk?

## Check Your Knowledge

Answers to the following multiple choice questions are below the questions.

1. Margarine usually is made by a process called _____, in which hydrogen atoms are added to carbon-carbon

double bonds in the polyunsaturated fatty acids found in vegetable oils.
  a. saturation
  b. esterification
  c. isomerization
  d. hydrogenation

2. Essential fatty acids that cause a decrease in blood clotting are
  a. omega-3.      c. omega-9.
  b. omega-6.      d. prostacyclins.

3. Cholesterol is
   a. a dietary essential; the human body cannot synthesize it.
   b. found in foods of plant origin.
   c. an important part of human cell membranes and necessary to make some hormones.
   d. All of the above.

4. Which of the following groups of foods would be important sources of saturated fatty acids?
   a. olive oil, peanut oil, canola oil
   b. palm oil, palm kernel oil, coconut oil
   c. safflower oil, corn oil, soybean oil
   d. All of the above.

5. Lipoproteins are important for
   a. transport of fats in the blood and lymphatic system.
   b. synthesis of triglycerides.
   c. synthesis of adipose tissue.
   d. enzyme production.

6. Which of the following foods is the best source of omega-3 fatty acids?
   a. fatty fish
   b. peanut butter and jelly
   c. lard and shortenings
   d. beef and other red meats

7. Immediately after a meal, newly digested and absorbed dietary fats appear in the lymph, and then blood, as part of which of the following?
   a. LDL
   b. HDL
   c. chylomicrons
   d. cholesterol

8. High blood concentrations of _____ decrease the risk for cardiovascular disease.
   a. low-density lipoproteins
   b. chylomicrons
   c. high-density lipoproteins
   d. cholesterol

9. Phospholipids such as lecithin are used extensively in food preparation because they
   a. provide the agreeable feel of fat melting on the tongue.
   b. are excellent emulsifiers.
   c. provide important textural features.
   d. impart delicate flavors.

10. The main form of lipid found in the food we eat is
    a. cholesterol.
    b. phospholipids.
    c. triglycerides.
    d. plant sterols

Answers: 1. d, 2. a, 3. c, 4. b, 5. a, 6. a, 7. c, 8. c, 9. b, 10. c

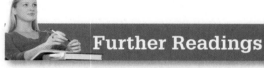

## Further Readings

1. ADA Reports: Position of the American Dietetic Association: Fat replacers. *Journal of the American Dietetic Association* 105:266, 2005.

   *The majority of fat replacers, when used in moderation by adults, can be safe and useful adjuncts to lowering the fat content of foods and may play a role in decreasing total calorie and fat intake. Still, consumers should not be led to believe that fat and calorie-reduced products can be consumed in unlimited amounts*

2. Fisler JS, Warden CH: Dietary fat and genotype: Toward individualized prescriptions for lifestyle changes. *American Journal of Clinical Nutrition* 81:1255, 2005.

   *There is great variation in the effect of dietary fat on blood lipids. At least part of that variation is due to genetics. This article discusses the challenges involved in identifying the interactive effects of nutrients and genes in the area of lipids, cholesterol, and coronary artery disease.*

3. Getz L: A burger and fries (hold the trans fats). *Today's Dietitian* 11(2):35, 2009.

   *Several cities across the U.S., including New York, Philadelphia, and Boston, have banned* trans *fat use in restaurants. Most eating establishments have willingly responded to the demand for healthier oils. It is important to remember that choosing* trans *fat-free foods does not necessarily make it a healthy choice.*

4. Grundy SM and others: Diagnosis and management of the metabolic syndrome. *Circulation* 112: 1350, 2005.

   *The constellation of metabolic risk factors known as metabolic syndrome consists of many factors, including elevated blood triglycerides, low HDL cholesterol concentrations, elevated blood pressure, elevated blood glucose, increased blood clotting, and an inflammatory state in the body. The most important of these underlying risk factors are abdominal obesity and insulin resistance. Other associated conditions include physical inactivity, aging, hormonal imbalance, and genetic or ethnic predisposition.*

5. Hansson GK: Inflammation, atherosclerosis, and coronary artery disease. *The New England Journal of Medicine* 352:1685, 2005.

   *Excellent review of the role of inflammation in causing cardiovascular disease. Identifying atherosclerosis as an inflammatory disease offers new opportunities for the prevention and treatment of coronary artery disease.*

6. He KA, Daviglus ML: A few more thoughts about fish and fish oil. *Journal of the American Dietetic Association* 105:428, 2005.

   *Fish consumption has been shown to have beneficial effects on cardiovascular disease. Consuming whole fish is thought to have greater benefits and be safer than using fish oil supplements. Fish is not only a rich source of omega-3 fatty acids, but is also a valuable source of protein and trace elements that may also provide protective effects for the cardiovascular system. Broiled or baked fish is recommended rather than fried fish because frying may decrease the ratio of omega-3 to omega-6 fatty acids and may produce* trans *fatty acids and oxidized*

   *lipid products that may increase cardiovascular disease risk.*

7. Kris-Etherton PM, Hill AM: n-3 fatty acids: Food or supplements? *Journal of the American Dietetic Association* 108: 1125, 2008.

   *A food-based approach is recommended for all fatty acids including the n-3 fatty acids. If an individual does not eat fish, the richest source of n-3 fatty acids, other options such as "designer" foods high in n-3 fatty acids, foods fortified with these fatty acids, or even supplements can be used. For vegans, algal supplements are an alternative source of DHA instead of fish or fish oil.*

8. Kuller LH: Nutrition, lipids, and cardiovascular disease. *Nutrition Reviews* 64:S15, 2006.

   *The development of coronary heart disease is discussed as an epidemic due to increased consumption of saturated fat and cholesterol, low intakes of polyunsaturated fat, and obesity. The risk of the disease is increased by hypertension, smoking, and diabetes. The careful monitoring and prevention of this disease beginning in young adults is important but expensive.*

9. Lau VWY and others: Plant sterols are efficacious in lowering plasma LDL and non-HDL cholesterol in hypercholesterolemic type 2 diabetic and nondiabetic persons. *American Journal of Clinical Nutrition* 81:1351, 2005.

   *Incorporation of plant sterols into a low-saturated-fat and low-cholesterol diet for persons at increased risk of CVD mortality could* have a positive effect on reducing the mortality rate, including in those people with type 2 diabetes.

10. Lee I and others: Vitamin E in the primary prevention of cardiovascular disease and cancer: The women's health study: A randomized controlled trial. *Journal of the American Medical Association* 294:56, 2005.

The data from this large trial indicated that 600 IU of natural-source vitamin E taken every other day provided no overall benefit for major cardiovascular events or cancer. These data do not support recommending vitamin E supplementation for cardiovascular disease or cancer prevention among healthy women, but more research is warranted, as a decrease in sudden cardiac death was seen in a subset of older women in this study.

11. Lewis NM and others: The walnut: A nutritional nut case. *Today's Dietitian* 6(8):36, 2004.

Compared to other nuts and seeds, walnuts are one of the richest sources of alpha-linolenic acid (2.6 grams per 1-ounce serving or 14 walnut halves). The DRI for alpha-linolenic acid is 1.6 grams/day for men and 1.1 grams/day for women. In addition, walnuts are a rich source of plant sterols known to inhibit intestinal absorption of cholesterol.

12. Lichtenstein AH and others: Diet and lifestyle recommendations revision 2006. A scientific statement from the American Heart Association Nutrition Committee. *Circulation* 114:82, 2006.

The American Heart Association presents recommendations designed to reduce the risk of cardiovascular disease in the general population. Specific goals are presented and include consuming an overall healthy diet; to aim for a healthy body weight, recommended levels of low-density lipoprotein cholesterol, high-density lipoprotein cholesterol, and triglycerides; normal blood pressure; normal blood glucose level; being physically active; and avoiding the use of and exposure to tobacco products.

13. Lonn E and others: Effects of long-term vitamin E supplementation on cardiovascular events and cancer: A randomized controlled trial. *Journal of the American Medical Association* 293:1338, 2005.

No significant differences were noted between the vitamin E supplementation group and the control group in the incidence of cancer or deaths related to cancer. There also were no differences in the main composite of cardiovascular outcomes including death or rehospitalization.

A significant increased risk in heart failure and related complications occurred in the vitamin E group.

14. Meisinger C and others: Plasma oxidized low-density lipoprotein, a strong predictor for acute coronary heart disease events in apparently healthy, middle-aged men from the general population. *Circulation* 112:651, 2005.

Elevated concentrations of oxidized low-density lipoprotein are predictive of future coronary heart disease events in apparently healthy men. Thus, oxidized LDL may represent a promising risk marker for clinical coronary heart disease complications and should be evaluated in further studies.

15. Micallef MA, Garg ML: The lipid-lowering effects of phytosterols and (n-3) polyunsaturated fatty acids are synergistic and complementary in hyperlipidemic men and women. *Journal of Nutrition* 138: 1086, 2008.

Phytosterols are plant compounds with structures similar to cholesterol. Some margarines and other products are enriched with phytosterols. Consuming phytosterols can reduce the intestinal absorption of cholesterol by 30% to 40%. Fish oils are rich in omega-3 polyunsaturated fatty acids (PUFA) and can reduce blood triglycerides and raise HDL-cholesterol. The combined effect of phytosterols and omega-3 PUFA on blood lipid profiles was studied in individuals with high blood lipids. The combined supplementation with phytosterols and omega-3 PUFA had synergistic and complementary lipid-lowering effects in men and women with high blood lipids, resulting in a reduction in plasma total and LDL-cholesterol concentrations, an increase in HDL-cholesterol concentration, and a decrease in plasma triglyceride concentration.

16. Ohr LM: The (heart) beat goes on. *Food Technology* 60(6):87, 2006.

Research and ingredient innovations in the food industry related to the heart-health field are described. Ingredients that have the advantage of a heart-health claim include omega-3 fatty acids and plant sterols. Also discussed are dietary fiber and grains, soy, antioxidants, and nuts.

17. Phillips KM and others: Phytosterol composition of nuts and seeds commonly consumed in the United States. *Journal of Agriculture and Food Chemistry* 53:9436, 2005.

This study set out to find the nuts and seeds that could provide the most heart-protective

benefits. Of the 27 nuts and seeds analyzed, wheat germ and sesame seeds had the greatest concentration of phytosterols and Brazil nuts and walnuts ranked the lowest. Pistachio and sunflower seeds were the richest sources of phytosterols for products typically consumed as snack foods.

18. Reese MATB: Beyond the headlines: The lowdown on low-fat diets. *Today's Dietitian* 8(6):32, 2006.

Results of the 8-year Women's Health Initiative study showed that a reduction in dietary fat had almost no effect on the incidence of heart attacks and strokes or breast and colon cancer. This article explains some of the study characteristics that most likely contributed to the unexpected results. Most important to consider is that the subjects were all postmenopausal women who had all been on a high-fat diet. The results suggest that starting a low-fat diet at 50 to 79 years may be too late to see extraordinary benefits.

19. Shai I and others: Weight loss with a low-carbohydrate, Mediterranean, or low-fat diet. *New England Journal of Medicine* 359:229, 2008.

Moderately obese adults (mean age, 52 years) were assigned to one of three diets: low-fat, restricted-calorie; Mediterranean, restricted-calorie; or low-carbohydrate, non-restricted-calorie, and studied for two years. The diet was monitored for various components, including amount and type of carbohydrates, fat, protein, and cholesterol. The mean weight loss among the 272 participants who remained on their diets was 3.3 kg for the low-fat group, 4.6 kg for the Mediterranean-diet group, and 5.5 kg for the low-carbohydrate group. The results indicate that Mediterranean and low-carbohydrate diets may be effective alternatives to low-fat diets. The more favorable effects on lipids (with the low-carbohydrate diet) and on glycemic control (with the Mediterranean diet) suggest that personal preferences and metabolic considerations might inform individualized tailoring of dietary interventions.

20. Wang C and others: n-3 fatty acids from fish or fish-oil supplements, but not alpha-linolenic acid, benefit cardiovascular disease outcomes in primary- and secondary-prevention studies: A systematic review. *American Journal of Clinical Nutrition* 84:5, 2006.

This review of previous studies found that consumption of omega-3 fatty acids from fish or fish oil but not alpha-linolenic acid, significantly reduced all-cause mortality, myocardial infarction, cardiac and sudden death, or stroke.

## I. Is Your Diet High in Saturated and *Trans* Fat?

Instructions: In each row of the following list, circle your typical food selection from column A or B.

| Column A | or | Column B |
|---|---|---|
| Bacon and eggs | or | Ready-to-eat whole-grain breakfast cereal |
| Doughnut or sweet roll | or | Whole-wheat roll, bagel, or bread |
| Breakfast sausage | or | Fruit |
| Whole milk | or | Reduced-fat, low-fat, or fat-free milk |
| Cheeseburger | or | Turkey sandwich, no cheese |
| French fries | or | Plain baked potato with salsa |
| Ground chuck | or | Ground round |
| Soup with cream base | or | Soup with broth base |
| Macaroni and cheese | or | Macaroni with marinara sauce |
| Cream/fruit pie | or | Graham crackers |
| Cream-filled cookies | or | Granola bar |
| Ice cream | or | Frozen yogurt, sherbet, or reduced-fat ice cream |
| Butter or stick margarine | or | Vegetable oils or soft margarine in a tub |

### Interpretation

The foods listed in column A tend to be high in saturated fat, *trans* fatty acids, cholesterol, and total fat. Those in column B generally are low in these dietary components. If you want to help reduce your risk of cardiovascular disease, choose more foods from column B and fewer from column A.

# II. Applying the Nutrition Facts Label to Your Daily Food Choices

Imagine that you are at the supermarket looking for a quick snack to help you keep your energy up during afternoons. In the snack section, you settle on two choices (see labels a and b). Evaluate the products using the table on the left.

| Compare the nutrients in each product by completing this list. For each serving, which product is lower in each of the following? | | | |
|---|---|---|---|
| Calories | (a) | (b) | no difference |
| Calories from Fat | (a) | (b) | no difference |
| Total Fat | (a) | (b) | no difference |
| Saturated Fat | (a) | (b) | no difference |
| Trans Fat | (a) | (b) | no difference |
| Cholesterol | (a) | (b) | no difference |
| Sodium | (a) | (b) | no difference |
| Total Carbohydrates | (a) | (b) | no difference |
| Dietary Fiber | (a) | (b) | no difference |
| Sugars | (a) | (b) | no difference |
| Protein | (a) | (b) | no difference |
| Iron | (a) | (b) | no difference |
| Which package has more servings per container? (a) (b) no difference | | | |
| Which of the two brands would you choose? (a) (b) no difference | | | |
| What information on the Nutrition Facts labels contributed to your decision? | | | |

## (a)

### Nutrition Facts

Serving Size: 2 bars (42g)
Servings Per Container: 6

| Amount Per Serving | 2 bars | |
|---|---|---|
| **Calories** 180 | Calories from Fat 50 | |
| | | **% Daily Value*** |
| **Total Fat** 6g | | **9**% |
| Saturated Fat 0.5g | | **3**% |
| Trans fat 0g | | ** |
| **Cholesterol** 0mg | | **0**% |
| **Sodium** 160mg | | **7**% |
| **Total Carbohydrates** 29g | | **10**% |
| Dietary Fiber 2g | | **8**% |
| Sugars 11g | | |
| **Protein** 4g | | |
| Iron | 6% | |

Not a significant source of Vitamin A, Vitamin C, and calcium.

** Intake of trans fat should be as low as possible.

* Daily values are based on a 2,000 calorie diet. Your daily values may be higher or lower depending on your calorie needs:

| ** Intake should be as low as possible. | Calories | 2,000 | 2,500 |
|---|---|---|---|
| **Total Fat** | Less than | 65g | 80g |
| Saturated Fat | Less than | 20g | 25g |
| **Cholesterol** | Less than | 300mg | 300mg |
| **Sodium** | Less than | 2,400mg | 2,400mg |
| **Total Carbohydrates** | | 300g | 375g |
| Dietary Fiber | | 25g | 30g |

**INGREDIENTS:** WHOLE GRAIN ROLLED OATS, SUGAR, CANOLA OIL, CRISP RICE WITH SOY PROTEIN (RICE FLOUR, SOY PROTEIN CONCENTRATE, SUGAR, MALT, SALT), HONEY, BROWN SUGAR SYRUP, HIGH FRUCTOSE CORN SYRUP, SALT, SOY LECITHIN, BAKING SODA, NATURAL FLAVOR, PEANUT FLOUR, ALMOND FLOUR, HAZELNUT FLOUR, WALNUT FLOUR, PECAN FLOUR.

## (b)

### Nutrition Facts

Serving Size: 2 cookies (38g)
Servings Per Container: about 12

| Amount Per Serving | | |
|---|---|---|
| **Calories** 180 | | Calories from Fat 70 |
| | | **% Daily Value*** |
| **Total Fat** 7g | | **11**% |
| Saturated Fat 2g | | **10**% |
| Trans fat 2g | | ** |
| **Cholesterol** 0mg | | **0**% |
| **Sodium** 100mg | | **4**% |
| **Total Carbohydrate** 26g | | **9**% |
| Dietary Fiber 1g | | **4**% |
| Sugars 12g | | |
| **Protein** 2g | | |

| Vitamin A 0% | • | Vitamin C 0% |
|---|---|---|
| Calcium 0% | • | Iron 2% |

** Intake of trans fat should be as low as possible.

* Daily values are based on a 2,000 calorie diet. Your daily values may be higher or lower depending on your calorie needs:

| ** Intake should be as low as possible. | Calories | 2,000 | 2,500 |
|---|---|---|---|
| **Total Fat** | Less than | 65g | 80g |
| Saturated Fat | Less than | 20g | 25g |
| **Cholesterol** | Less than | 300mg | 300mg |
| **Sodium** | Less than | 2,400mg | 2,400mg |
| **Total Carbohydrates** | | 300g | 375g |
| Dietary Fiber | | 25g | 30g |

Calories per gram: • Fat 9 • Carbohydrate 4
• Protein 4

**INGREDIENTS:** ENRICHED FLOUR (WHEAT FLOUR, NIACIN, REDUCED IRON, THIAMINE MONONITRATE, RIBOFLAVIN, FOLIC ACID), SUGAR, VEGETABLE OIL SHORTENING (PARTIALLY HYDROGENATED SOYBEAN, COCONUT, COTTONSEED, CORN AND/OR SAFFLOWER AND/OR CANOLA OIL), CORN SYRUP, HIGH FRUCTOSE CORN SYRUP, WHEY (A MILK INGREDIENT), CORN STARCH, SALT, SKIM MILK, LEAVENING (BAKING SODA, AMMONIUM BICARBONATE), ARTIFICIAL FLAVOR, SOYBEAN LECITHIN, COLOR (CONTAINING FD&C YELLOW #5 LAKE).

# CHAPTER 6 Proteins

## Student Learning Outcomes  After studying Chapter 6 you will be able to:

1. Describe how amino acids form proteins.

2. Distinguish between essential and non-essential amino acids and explain why adequate amounts of each of the essential amino acids are required for protein synthesis.

3. Distinguish between high-quality and low-quality proteins, identify examples of each,

and describe the concept of complementary proteins.

4. Describe how protein is digested and absorbed in the body.

5. List the primary functions of protein in the body.

6. Calculate the RDA for protein for an adult when a healthy weight is given.

7. Describe what is meant by positive protein balance, negative protein balance, and protein equilibrium.

8. Describe how protein-calorie malnutrition eventually can lead to disease in the body.

9. Develop vegetarian diet plans that meet the body's nutritional needs.

## Chapter Outline

Student Learning Outcomes

Refresh Your Memory

6.1 Protein—An Introduction

6.2 Proteins—Amino Acids Bonded Together

6.3 Protein in Foods

6.4 Protein Digestion and Absorption

6.5 Putting Proteins to Work in the Body

6.6 Protein Needs

6.7 Does Eating a High-Protein Diet Harm You?

6.8 Protein-Calorie Malnutrition

Nutrition and Your Health: Vegetarian and Plant-Based Diets

Case Study: Planning a Vegetarian Diet

Summary/Study Questions/Check Your Knowledge/Further Readings

Rate Your Plate

CONSUMING ENOUGH PROTEIN IS VITAL FOR MAINTAINING HEALTH. Proteins form important structures in the body, make up a key part of the blood, help regulate many body functions, and can fuel body cells.

North Americans generally eat more protein than is needed to maintain health. Our daily protein intake comes mostly from animal sources such as meat, poultry, fish, eggs, milk, and cheese. In contrast, in the developing world, diets can be deficient in protein. High-protein diets have come and gone over the past 30 years. Recently, these have become popular as weight-loss diets, with some containing about 35% of calories as protein. This figure falls within the latest advice for protein intake from the Food and Nutrition Board (10% to 35% of calorie intake), so in general these diets are appropriate if otherwise nutritionally sound (e.g., they follow MyPyramid).

Diets that are mostly vegetarian still predominate in much of Asia and areas of Africa, and, as suggested in the comic on the next page, some North Americans are currently adopting the practice. Plant sources of protein are worthy of more attention from North Americans. In the early 1900s, plant sources of proteins—nuts, seeds, and legumes—were consumed just as often as animal proteins. Over the years, though, plant proteins have been sidelined by meats. During this time, nuts have been viewed as high-fat foods, and beans have gotten the inferior reputation of "the poor man's meat." Contrary to these popular misconceptions, sources of plant proteins offer a wealth of nutritional benefits—from lowering blood cholesterol to preventing certain forms of cancer.

We could benefit from eating more plant sources of proteins. As shown in the comic in this chapter, it takes some knowledge to do so. It is possible—and desirable—to enjoy the benefits of animal and plant protein as we work toward the goal of meeting protein needs. This chapter takes a close look at protein, including the benefits of plant proteins in a diet. It will also examine vegetarian diets: their benefits and their risks, if not properly planned. Let's see why a detailed study of protein is worth your attention.

### Refresh Your Memory

As you begin your study of proteins in Chapter 6, you may want to review:

- Organization of the cell in Chapter 3
- The processes of digestion and absorption in Chapter 3
- The nervous system and immune system in Chapter 3
- The role of carbohydrates in preventing ketosis in Chapter 4

## 6.1 Protein—An Introduction

Diets in the developed parts of the world, such as the United States and Canada, are typically rich in protein, and therefore a specific focus on eating enough protein is generally not needed. In the developing world, however, it is important to focus on protein in diet planning because diets in those areas of the world can be deficient in protein.

**FRANK & ERNEST® by Bob Thaves**

Can a vegetarian diet provide enough protein? What is prompting the growing interest in various forms of vegetarian diets? Why are plant protein sources, especially soy and nuts, gaining more attention? Should meat-eaters abandon that dietary practice? Chapter 6 provides some answers.

FRANK & ERNEST © United Features Syndicate. Reprinted by Permission.

High-protein diets have been popular as weight-loss diets over the years. The latest advice from the Food and Nutrition Board allows for up to 35% of total calorie intake to be supplied by protein, so in general these diets are appropriate if otherwise nutritionally sound, especially with regard to being moderate in fat and having enough fiber. Still, as discussed in Chapter 7, these types of diets are hardly a magic wand for weight loss.

Thousands of substances in the body are made of proteins. Aside from water, proteins form the major part of lean body tissue, totaling about 17% of body weight. Amino acids—the building blocks for proteins—are unique in that they contain nitrogen bonded to carbon. Plants combine nitrogen from the soil with carbon and other elements to form amino acids. They then link these amino acids together to make proteins. We get the nitrogen we need by consuming dietary proteins. Proteins are thus an essential part of a diet because they supply nitrogen in a form we can readily use—namely, amino acids. Using simpler forms of nitrogen is, for the most part, impossible for humans.

Proteins are crucial to the regulation and maintenance of the body. Body functions such as blood clotting, fluid balance, hormone and enzyme production, visual processes, transport of many substances in the bloodstream, and cell repair require specific proteins. The body makes proteins in many configurations and sizes so that they can serve these greatly varied functions. Formation of these body proteins begins with amino acids from both the protein-containing foods we eat and those synthesized from other compounds within the body. Proteins can also be broken down to supply energy for the body—on average, 4 kcal per gram.

If you fail to consume an adequate amount of protein for weeks at a time, many metabolic processes slow down. This is because the body does not have enough amino acids available to build the proteins it needs. For example, the immune system no longer functions efficiently when it lacks key proteins, thereby increasing the risk of infections, disease, and death.

## Amino Acids

Amino acids—the building blocks of proteins—are formed mostly of carbon, hydrogen, oxygen, and nitrogen. The following diagram shows the structure of a generic amino acid and also what one of the specific amino acids, glutamic acid, looks like. The amino acids have different chemical makeups, but all are slight variations of the generic amino acid pictured (see Appendix F). Each amino acid has an "acid" group; an "amino" group; and a "side" or R group specific to the amino acid.

The R group on some amino acids has a branched shape, like a tree. These so-called **branched-chain amino acids** are leucine, isoleucine, and valine (see Appendix F for the chemical structures of the amino acids). The branched-chain amino acids are the primary amino acids used by muscles for energy needs. This is one reason why proteins from milk (e.g., whey proteins) are popular with strength-training athletes (see Chapter 10 for details).

**branched-chain amino acids** Amino acids with a branching carbon backbone; these are leucine, isoleucine, and valine. All are essential amino acids.

Acid group - - - - - - - -

Side group - - - - - - - -

Amino group - - - - - - - -

"Generic" amino acid. The R signifies another chemical group that would be present.

One example of an R group

Part of generic amino acid foundation

Glutamic acid

**nonessential amino acids** Amino acids that can be synthesized by a healthy body in sufficient amounts; there are 11 nonessential amino acids. These are also called *dispensable amino acids.*

**essential amino acids** The amino acids that cannot be synthesized by humans in sufficient amounts or at all and therefore must be included in the diet; there are nine essential amino acids. These are also called *indispensable amino acids.*

**limiting amino acid** The essential amino acid in lowest concentration in a food or diet relative to body needs.

**TABLE 6-1** Classification of Amino Acids

| Essential Amino Acids | Nonessential Amino Acids |
|---|---|
| Histidine | Alanine |
| Isoleucine* | Arginine |
| Leucine* | Asparagine |
| Lysine | Aspartic acid |
| Methionine | Cysteine |
| Phenylalanine | Glutamic acid |
| Threonine | Glutamine |
| Tryptophan | Glycine |
| Valine* | Proline |
| | Serine |
| | Tyrosine |

*A branched-chain amino acid

Your body needs to use 20 different amino acids to function (Table 6-1). Although all these commonly found amino acids are important, 11 are considered **nonessential** (also called *dispensable*) with respect to our diets. Human cells can produce these certain amino acids as long as the right ingredients are present—the key factor being nitrogen that is already part of another amino acid. Therefore it is not essential that these amino acids be in our diet.

The nine amino acids the body cannot make in sufficient amounts or at all are known as **essential** (also called *indispensable*)—they must be obtained from foods. This is because body cells either cannot make the needed carbon-based foundation of the amino acid, cannot put a nitrogen group on the needed carbon-based foundation, or just cannot do the whole process fast enough to meet body needs.

Eating a balanced diet can supply us with both the essential and nonessential amino-acid building blocks needed to maintain good health. Both nonessential and essential amino acids are present in foods that contain protein. If you don't eat enough essential amino acids, your body first struggles to conserve what essential amino acids it can. However, eventually your body progressively slows production of new proteins until at some point you will break protein down faster than you can make it. When that happens, health deteriorates.

The essential amino acid in smallest supply in a food or diet in relation to body needs becomes the limiting factor (called the **limiting amino acid**) because it limits the amount of protein the body can synthesize. For example, assume the letters of the alphabet represent the 20 or so different amino acids we consume. If *A* represents an essential amino acid, we need three of these letters to spell the hypothetical protein *BANANA*. If the body had a *B*, two *N*s, but only two *A*s, the "synthesis" of *BANANA* would not be possible. *A* would then be seen as the limiting amino acid.

Adults need only about 11% of their total protein requirement to be supplied by essential amino acids. Typical diets supply an average of 50% of protein as essential amino acids.

The estimated needs for essential amino acids for infants and preschool children are 40% of total protein intake; however, in later childhood the need drops to 20%.

▲ When combined with vegetables, high-protein foods such as meats also help balance the amino acid content of the diet.

## MAKING DECISIONS

### Phenylketonuria

Some of the nonessential amino acids are also classed as conditionally essential. This means they must be made from essential amino acids if insufficient amounts are eaten. When that occurs, the body's supply of certain essential amino acids is depleted. Tyrosine is an example of a conditionally essential amino acid that can be made from the essential amino acid phenylalanine.

The disease phenylketonuria (PKU) illustrates the importance of phenylalanine to make tyrosine. Recall from Chapter 4 that a person with PKU has a limited ability to metabolize the essential amino acid phenylalanine. Normally, the body uses an enzyme to convert much of our dietary phenylalanine intake into tyrosine.

In PKU-diagnosed persons, the activity of the enzyme used in processing phenylalanine to tyrosine is insufficient. When the enzyme cannot synthesize enough tyrosine, both amino acids must be derived from foods. The point is that phenylalanine and tyrosine become *essential* in terms of dietary needs because the body can't produce enough tyrosine from phenylalanine. Phenylalanine levels in the blood increase because it is not converted to tyrosine. PKU is treated by limiting the consumption of phenylalanine with a special diet so that phenylalanine and its by-products do not rise to toxic concentrations in the body and cause the severe mental retardation seen in untreated PKU cases.

Rina is 7 months pregnant and has read about various tests that her baby will undergo when he or she is born. How can you explain to Rina the purpose and significance of one of those tests, the one that screens for PKU?

▲ Within the first few days of life all newborns are tested for phenylketonuria.

Diets designed for infants and young children need to take this into account to make sure enough proteins are present to yield a high-quality protein intake. Including some animal products in the diet, such as human milk or formula for infants, or cow's milk for children, helps ensure this. Otherwise, complementary amino acids from plant proteins should be consumed in each meal or within two subsequent meals. A major health risk for infants and children occurs in famine situations in which only one type of cereal grain is available, increasing the probability that one or more of the nine essential amino acids is lacking in the total diet. This is discussed further in a later section on protein-calorie malnutrition.

### CONCEPT CHECK

The human body uses 20 different amino acids from protein-containing foods. A healthy body can synthesize 11 of the amino acids, so it is not necessary to obtain all amino acids from foods—only nine of these must come from the diet and are therefore termed *essential (indispensable) amino acids.* The essential amino acid in smallest supply in a food in relation to body needs is called the limiting amino acid because it limits the amount of protein the body can synthesize.

## 6.2 Proteins—Amino Acids Bonded Together

Amino acids are linked together by chemical bonds—technically called **peptide bonds**—to form proteins. Although these bonds are difficult to break, acids, enzymes, and other agents are able to do so—for example, during digestion.

The body can synthesize many different proteins by linking together the 20 common types of amino acids with peptide bonds.

**peptide bond** A chemical bond formed between amino acids in a protein.

**polypeptide** A group of amino acids bonded together, from 50 to 2000 or more.

▲ Genes are present on DNA—a double-stranded helix. The cell nucleus contains most of the DNA in the body.

## Protein Synthesis

Our discussion of protein synthesis, begins with DNA. DNA is present in the nucleus of the cell and contains coded instructions for protein synthesis (i.e., which specific amino acids are to be placed in a protein and in which order). Recall from Chapter 3 that DNA is a double-stranded molecule.

Protein synthesis in a cell, however, takes place in the cytoplasm, not in the nucleus. Thus, the DNA code used for synthesis of a specific protein must be transferred from the nucleus to the cytoplasm to allow for protein synthesis. This transfer is the job of messenger RNA (mRNA). Enzymes in the nucleus read the code on one segment (a gene) of one strand of the DNA and *transcribe* that information into a single-stranded mRNA molecule (Fig. 6-1). This mRNA undergoes processing and then it is ready to leave the nucleus.

Once in the cytoplasm, mRNA travels to the ribosomes. The ribosomes read the mRNA code and *translate* those instructions to produce a specific protein. Amino acids are added one at a time to the growing **polypeptide** chain according to the instructions on the mRNA. Another key participant in protein synthesis, transfer RNA (tRNA), is responsible for bringing the specific amino acids to the ribosomes as needed during protein synthesis (review Fig. 6-1). Energy input is required to add each amino acid to the chain, making protein synthesis "costly" in terms of calorie use.

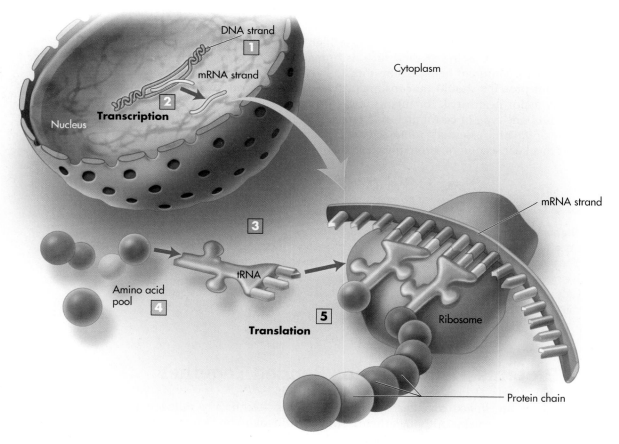

**1** DNA contains the information necessary to produce proteins.

**2** Transcription or copying of a segment of DNA results in mRNA, a copy of the information in DNA needed to make a protein.

**3** The mRNA leaves the nucleus and goes to a ribosome.

**4** Amino acids, the building blocks of proteins, are carried to the ribosome by tRNAs containing the code that matches that on the mRNA.

**5** In the process of translation, the information contained in mRNA is used to determine the number, types, and arrangement of amino acids in the protein.

DNA strand

**1**

mRNA strand

**2**

**Transcription**

Nucleus

Cytoplasm

mRNA strand

**3**

tRNA

Amino acid pool

**4**

**5**

**Translation**

Ribosome

Protein chain

**FIGURE 6-1** ▶ Protein synthesis (simplified). Once the mRNA is fully read, the amino acids have been connected into the polypeptide which is released into the cytoplasm. It generally is then processed further to become a cell protein.

Once synthesis of a polypeptide is complete, it twists and folds into the appropriate three-dimensional structure of the intended protein. These structural changes occur based on specific interactions between the amino acids that make up the polypeptide chain (see the next section on protein organization for details). Some polypeptides, such as the hormone insulin, also undergo further changes in the cell before they are functional.

The important message in this discussion is the relationship between DNA and the proteins eventually produced by a cell. If the DNA code contains errors, an incorrect mRNA will be produced. The ribosomes will then read this incorrect message and an incorrect amino acid will be added and an incorrect polypeptide chain will be produced. As discussed in Chapter 3, genetic engineering may ultimately be able to correct many gene defects in humans, by placing the correct DNA code in the nucleus, so that the correct protein can be made by the ribosomes.

**FIGURE 6-2** ▶ Protein organization. Proteins often form a coiled shape, as shown by this drawing of the blood protein hemoglobin. This shape is dictated by the order of the amino acids in the protein chain. To get an idea of its size, consider that each teaspoon (5 milliliters) of blood contains about $10^{18}$ hemoglobin molecules. One billion is $10^9$.

## Protein Organization

As noted before, by bonding together various combinations of the 20 common types of amino acids, the body synthesizes thousands of different proteins. The sequential order of the amino acids then ultimately determines the protein's shape. The main point is that only correctly positioned amino acids can interact and fold properly to form the intended shape for the protein. The resulting unique, three-dimensional form goes on to dictate the function of each particular protein (Fig. 6-2). If it lacks the proper structure, a protein cannot function.

**Sickle cell disease** (also called **sickle cell anemia**) is one example of what happens when amino acids are out of order on a protein. North Americans of African descent are especially prone to this genetic disease. It occurs because of defects in the structure of the protein chains of hemoglobin, a protein that carries oxygen in red blood cells. In two of its four protein chains, an error in the amino-acid order occurs. This error produces a profound change in hemoglobin structure. It can no longer form the shape needed to carry oxygen efficiently inside the red blood cell. Instead of forming normal circular disks, the red blood cells collapse into crescent (or sickle) shapes (Fig. 6-3). Health deteriorates, and eventually episodes of severe pain in the bones and joints, abdominal pain, headaches, convulsions, and paralysis may occur.

These life-threatening symptoms are caused by a minute, but critical, error in the hemoglobin amino-acid order. Why does this error happen? It results from a defect in a person's genetic blueprint, DNA, inherited through one's parents. A defect in the DNA can dictate that a wrong amino acid will be built into the sequence of the body proteins. Many diseases, including cancer, stem from errors in the DNA code.

**sickle cell disease (sickle cell anemia)** An illness that results from a malformation of the red blood cell because of an incorrect structure in part of its hemoglobin protein chains. The disease can lead to episodes of severe bone and joint pain, abdominal pain, headache, convulsions, paralysis, and even death.

**denaturation** Alteration of a protein's three-dimensional structure, usually because of treatment by heat, enzymes, acid or alkaline solutions, or agitation.

## Denaturation of Proteins

Exposure to acid or alkaline substances, heat, or agitation can alter a protein's structure, leaving it uncoiled or otherwise deformed. This process of altering the three-dimensional structure of a protein is called **denaturation** (see Fig. 6-7 on p. 222). Changing a protein's shape often destroys its ability to function normally, such that it loses its biological activity.

Denaturation of proteins is useful for some body processes, especially digestion. The heat produced during cooking denatures some proteins. After food is ingested, the secretion of stomach acid denatures some bacterial proteins, plant hormones, many active enzymes, and other forms of proteins in foods, making it safer to eat. Digestion is also enhanced by denaturation because the unraveling increases exposure of the polypeptide chain to digestive enzymes. Denaturing proteins in some foods can also reduce their tendencies to cause allergic reactions.

**FIGURE 6-3** ▶ An example of the consequences of errors in DNA coding of proteins. (*a*) Normal red blood cell; (*b*) red blood cell from a person with sickle-cell anemia—note its abnormal crescent (sickle-like) shape.

Recall that we need the essential amino acids that the proteins in the diet supply—not the proteins themselves. We dismantle ingested dietary proteins and use the amino acid building blocks to assemble the proteins we need.

### CONCEPT CHECK

Amino acids are bonded together in specific sequences to form distinct proteins. DNA provides the directions for synthesizing these new proteins. Specifically, DNA directs the order of the amino acids on the protein. The amino acid order within a protein determines its ultimate shape and function. Destroying the shape of a protein denatures it. Stomach acid, heat, and other factors can denature proteins, causing them to lose their biological activity. Proteins must be denatured during digestion so that amino acids are available for absorption.

## 6.3 Protein in Foods

Of the typical foods we eat, about 70% of our protein comes from animal sources (Fig. 6-4). The most nutrient-dense source of protein is water-packed tuna, which has 87% of calories as protein (Fig. 6-5). The top five contributors of protein to the North American diet are beef, poultry, milk, white bread, and cheese. In North America, meat and poultry consumption amounts to about 150 pounds per person per year. Worldwide, 35% of protein comes from animal sources. In Africa and East Asia, only about 20% of the protein eaten comes from animal sources.

### Protein Quality of Foods

Animal and plant proteins can differ greatly in their proportions of essential and non-essential amino acids. Animal proteins contain ample amounts of all nine essential amino acids. (Gelatin—made from the animal protein collagen—is an exception because it loses one essential amino acid during processing and is low in other essential amino acids.) With the exception of soy protein, plant proteins don't match our need for essential amino acids as precisely as animal proteins. Many plant proteins, especially those found in grains, are low in one or more of the nine essential amino acids.

As you might expect, human tissue composition resembles animal tissue more than it does plant tissue. The similarities enable us to use proteins from any single animal source more efficiently to support human growth and maintenance than we do those from any single plant source. For this reason, animal proteins, except gelatin, are considered **high-quality** (also called **complete**) **proteins,** which contain the nine essential amino acids we need in sufficient amounts. Individual plant sources of proteins, except for soy beans, are considered **lower-quality** (also called **incomplete**) **proteins** because their amino-acid patterns can be quite different from ours. Thus, a single plant protein source, such as corn alone, cannot easily support body growth and maintenance. To obtain a sufficient amount of essential amino acids, a variety of plant proteins need to be consumed because each plant protein lacks adequate amounts of one or more essential amino acids.

When only lower-quality protein foods are consumed, enough of the essential amino acids needed for protein synthesis may not be obtained. Therefore, when compared to high-quality proteins, a greater amount of lower-quality protein is needed to meet the needs of protein synthesis. Moreover, once any of the nine essential amino acids in the plant protein we have eaten is used up, further protein synthesis becomes impossible. Because the depletion of just one of the essential amino acids prevents protein synthesis, the process illustrates the *all-or-none principle:* Either all essential

▲ Small amounts of animal protein in a meal easily add up to meet daily protein needs.

**high-quality (complete) proteins**
Dietary proteins that contain ample amounts of all nine essential amino acids.

**lower-quality (incomplete) proteins**
Dietary proteins that are low in or lack one or more essential amino acids.

## MyPyramid: Food Sources of Protein

| Food Group | Grains | Vegetables | Fruits | Oils | Milk | Meat & Beans |
|---|---|---|---|---|---|---|
| **Sources of Protein** | • Bread<br>• Breakfast cereals<br>• Rice<br>• Noodles | • Carrots<br>• Corn<br>• Broccoli | • Apples<br>• Oranges<br>• Bananas | • None | • Milk<br>• Yogurt<br>• Cheese | • Meat<br>• Eggs<br>• Fish<br>• Dry beans<br>• Nuts |
| **Grams per Serving** | 2–3 | 2–3 | <1 | <1 | 8–10 | 7 |

**FIGURE 6-4 ▶** Sources of protein from MyPyramid. The height of the background color (none, 1/3, 2/3, or completely covered) within each group in the pyramid indicates the average nutrient density for protein in that group. Overall, the milk group and the meat & beans group contain many foods that are nutrient-dense sources of protein. Based on serving sizes listed for MyPyramid, the fruits group and oils group provide little or no protein (less than 1 gram per serving). Food choices from the vegetables group and grains group provide moderate amounts of protein (2 to 3 grams per serving). The milk group provides much protein (8 to 10 grams per serving), as does the meat & beans group (7 grams per serving). With regard to physical activity, proteins are a minor source of fuel for most endeavors, but can become somewhat important during endurance activities.

amino acids are available or none can be used. The remaining amino acids would then be used for energy needs, or converted to carbohydrate or fat.

When two or more proteins combine to compensate for deficiencies in essential amino acid content in each protein, the proteins are called **complementary proteins.** Mixed diets generally provide high-quality protein because a complementary protein pattern results. Therefore, healthy adults should have little concern about balancing foods to yield the proteins needed to obtain enough of all nine essential amino acids. Even on plant-based diets, complementary proteins need not be consumed at the same meal by adults. Meeting amino-acid needs over the course of a day is a reasonable goal because there is a ready supply of amino acids from those present in body cells and in the blood (see Fig. 6-10 on page 226).

In general, plant sources of protein deserve more attention and use than they currently receive from many North Americans. Plant foods contribute fewer calories to the diet than most animal products and they supply an ample amount of protein, plus magnesium, plenty of fiber, and several other nutritional benefits (Fig. 6-6). The vegetable proteins we eat are a heart-healthy alternative to animal proteins because they contain no cholesterol and little saturated fat, aside from that added during processing or cooking. Legumes and nut sources of protein especially have received a lot of recent attention.

**complementary proteins** Two food protein sources that make up for each other's inadequate supply of specific essential amino acids; together they yield a sufficient amount of all nine and, so provide high-quality (complete) protein for the diet.

## CRITICAL THINKING

Evan, a vegetarian, has heard of the "all-or-none principle" of protein synthesis but doesn't understand how this principle applies to protein synthesis in the body. He asks you, "How important is this nutritional concept for diet planning?" How would you answer his question?

**FIGURE 6-5** ▶ Food sources of protein compared to the RDA of 56 grams for a 70 kg man.

## Food Sources of Protein

| Food Item and Amount | Protein (grams) | % RDA |
|---|---|---|
| **RDA** | 56* | 100% |
| Canned tuna, 3 ounces | 21.6 | 38.6% |
| Broiled chicken, 3 ounces | 21.3 | 38% |
| Beef chuck, 3 ounces | 15.3 | 27% |
| Yogurt, 1 cup | 10.6 | 19% |
| Kidney beans, 1/2 cup | 8.1 | 14.5% |
| 1% low-fat milk, 1 cup | 8.0 | 14% |
| Peanuts, 1 ounce | 7.3 | 13% |
| Cheddar cheese, 1 ounce | 7.0 | 12.5% |
| Egg, 1 | 5.5 | 10% |
| Cooked corn, 1/2 cup | 2.7 | 5% |
| Seven grain bread, 1 slice | 2.6 | 4.6% |
| White rice, 1/2 cup | 2.1 | 4% |
| Pasta, 1 ounce | 1.2 | 2% |
| Banana, 1 | 1.2 | 2% |

\* for 70 kg man

**Key:**
- Grains
- Vegetables
- Fruits
- Oils
- Milk
- Meat & Beans

yogurt

**FIGURE 6-6** ▶ Legumes are rich sources of protein. One-half cup meets about 10% of protein needs, but contributes only about 5% of energy needs.

## A Closer Look at Plant Sources of Proteins

In proportion to the amount of calories they supply, plant foods provide not only protein, but also magnesium, fiber, folate, vitamin E, iron (absorption is increased by the vitamin C also present), zinc, and some calcium. In addition, phytochemicals from these foods are implicated in prevention of a wide variety of chronic diseases.

Nuts have a hard shell surrounding an edible kernel. Almonds, pistachios, walnuts, and pecans are some common examples. The defining characteristic of a nut is that it grows on a tree. (Peanuts, because they grow underground, are legumes.) Seeds (such as pumpkin, sesame, and sunflower seeds) differ from nuts in that seeds grow on vegetable or flowering plants, but they are similar to nuts in nutrient composition. In general, nuts and seeds supply 160 to 190 kcal, 6 to 10 grams of protein, and 14 to 19 grams of fat per 1 ounce serving. Although they are a dense source of calories, nuts and seeds make a powerful contribution to health when consumed in moderation.

Legumes are a plant family with pods that contain a single row of seeds. Besides peanuts, examples include garden and black-eyed peas, kidney beans, great northern beans, lentils, and soy beans. Dried varieties of the mature legume seeds—what we know as beans—also make an impressive contribution to the protein, vitamin, mineral, and fiber content of a meal. A one-half cup serving of legumes provides 100 to 150 kcal, 5 to 10 grams of protein, less than one gram of fat, and about 5 grams of fiber. Recall from Chapter 4 that consumption of beans can lead to intestinal gas because our bodies lack the enzymes to break down certain carbohydrates that beans contain. An over-the counter preparation called Beano® can greatly lessen symptoms if taken right before the meal. It is also helpful to soak dry beans in water, which leaches the indigestible carbohydrates into the water so they can be disposed. However, intestinal gas is not harmful. In fact, fermentation products of ingestible carbohydrates promote the health of your colon (review Chapter 3 for more information on probiotics and prebiotics).

The impact of plant proteins on health will be discussed in the "Nutrition and Your Health" section at the end of this chapter.

---

### MAKING DECISIONS

#### Soy and Nut Allergies

For some of us, food allergies from soy, peanuts and tree nuts (e.g., almonds and walnuts), and wheat are a concern. Overall, food allergies occur in up to 8% of children 4 years of age or younger and in up to 2% of adults. Eight foods account for 90% of food-related allergies; soy, peanuts, tree nuts, and wheat are four of these foods. (The other foods are milk, egg, fish, and shellfish.) The allergic reactions can range from a mild intolerance to fatal allergic reactions (see Chapter 15 for details). Current guidelines regarding plant sources of allergens advise that infants not be fed wheat products before 6 months of age. Children less than 3 years of age should not eat peanuts or tree nuts. In addition, any of the plant sources of allergens need to be avoided in children and adults who continue to experience such allergies.

---

In sum, plant proteins are a nutritious alternative to animal proteins. They are inexpensive, versatile, tasty, add color to your plate, and benefit health beyond their contribution of protein to the diet. Simply adding these foods to your diet can lead to weight gain, but learning to substitute plant proteins in place of other less healthy foods is one way to reduce your risk for many diseases. Watch for news about additional research progress into this area.

## 6.4 Protein Digestion and Absorption

As with carbohydrate digestion, protein digestion begins with the cooking of food. Cooking unfolds (denatures) proteins (Fig. 6-7) and softens tough connective tissue in meat. Cooking also makes many protein-rich foods easier to chew and swallow, and facilitates their breakdown during later digestion and absorption. As you will see in Chapter 13, cooking also makes many protein-rich foods, such as meats, eggs, fish, and poultry, much safer to eat.

### Digestion

The enzymatic digestion of protein begins in the stomach (Fig. 6-8). Proteins are first denatured by stomach acid. **Pepsin,** a major stomach enzyme for digesting proteins, then goes to work on the unraveled polypeptide chains. Pepsin breaks the polypeptide into shorter chains of amino acids because it can break only a few of the many peptide bonds found in these large molecules. The release of pepsin is controlled by the hormone gastrin. Thinking about food or chewing food stimulates gastrin release in the stomach. Gastrin also strongly stimulates the stomach to produce acid.

The partially-digested proteins move from the stomach into the small intestine along with the rest of the nutrients and other substances in a meal (chyme). Once in the small intestine, the partially-digested proteins (and any fats accompanying them) trigger the release of the hormone cholecystokinin (CCK) from the walls of the small intestine. CCK, in turn, travels through the bloodstream to the pancreas where it causes the pancreas to release protein-splitting enzymes, such as **trypsin.** These digestive enzymes further divide the chains of amino acids into segments of two to three amino acids and some individual amino acids. Eventually, this mixture is digested

See *Nutrition and Your Health: Vegetarian and Plant-Based Diets* at the end of Chapter 6.

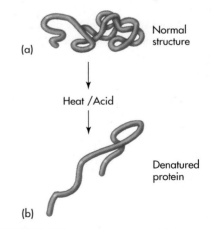

(a)   Normal structure

Heat /Acid

(b)   Denatured protein

**FIGURE 6-7** ▶ Denaturation. (a) Protein showing typical coiled state. (b) Protein is now partly uncoiled. This uncoiling can reduce biological activity and allow digestive enzymes to act on peptide bonds.

**pepsin** A protein-digesting enzyme produced by the stomach.

**trypsin** A protein-digesting enzyme secreted by the pancreas to act in the small intestine.

into amino acids, using other enzymes from the lining of the small intestine and enzymes present in the absorptive cells themselves.

## Absorption

The short chains of amino acids and any individual amino acids in the small intestine are taken up by active transport into the absorptive cells lining the small intestine. Any remaining peptide bonds are broken down to yield individual amino acids inside the intestinal cells. They are water-soluble, so the amino acids travel to the liver via the portal vein, which drains absorbed nutrients from the intestinal tract. In the liver, individual amino acids can undergo several modifications, depending on the needs of the body. Individual amino acids may be combined into the proteins needed by the body; broken down for energy needs; released into the bloodstream; or converted to nonessential amino acids, glucose, or fat. With excess protein intake, amino acids are converted to fat as a last resort.

Except during infancy, it is uncommon for intact proteins to be absorbed from the digestive tract. In infants up to 4 to 5 months of age, the gastrointestinal tract is somewhat permeable to small proteins, so some whole proteins can be absorbed. Because proteins from some foods (e.g., cow's milk and egg whites) may predispose an infant to food allergies, pediatricians and registered dietitians recommend waiting until an infant is at least 6 to 12 months of age before introducing commonly allergenic foods (see Chapter 15 for details).

**FIGURE 6-8** ▶ A summary of protein digestion and absorption. Enzymatic protein digestion begins in the stomach and ends in the absorptive cells of the small intestine, where any remaining short groupings of amino acids are broken down into single amino acids. Stomach acid and enzymes contribute to protein digestion. Absorption from the intestinal lumen into the absorptive cells requires energy input.

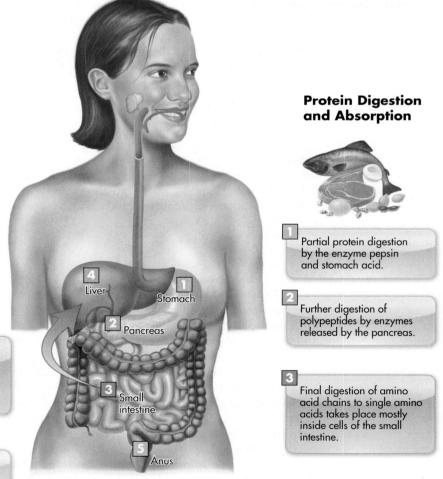

**Protein Digestion and Absorption**

**1** Partial protein digestion by the enzyme pepsin and stomach acid.

**2** Further digestion of polypeptides by enzymes released by the pancreas.

**3** Final digestion of amino acid chains to single amino acids takes place mostly inside cells of the small intestine.

**4** Amino acids absorbed into the portal vein and transported to the liver. From there they enter the general bloodstream.

**5** Little dietary protein is present in feces.

Liver — Stomach — Pancreas — Small intestine — Anus

## CONCEPT CHECK

Protein digestion begins with cooking, as proteins are denatured by heat. Once protein reaches the stomach, enzymes cleave proteins into smaller segments of amino acids. As food travels through the small intestine, protein breakdown products formed in the stomach are broken down further to individual amino acids or short segments of amino acids and taken up into the absorptive cells of the small intestine where final breakdown into amino acids occurs. The amino acids then travel to the liver via the portal vein.

# 6.5 Putting Proteins to Work in the Body

Proteins function in many crucial ways in human metabolism and in the formation of body structures. We rely on foods to supply the amino acids needed to form these proteins. However, only when we also eat enough carbohydrate and fat can food proteins be used most efficiently. If we don't consume enough calories to meet needs, some amino acids from proteins are broken down to produce energy, rendering them unavailable to build body proteins.

## Producing Vital Body Structures

Every cell contains protein. Muscles, connective tissue, mucus, blood-clotting factors, transport proteins in the bloodstream, lipoproteins, enzymes, immune antibodies, some hormones, visual pigments, and the support structure inside bones are primarily made of protein. Excess protein in the diet doesn't enhance the synthesis of these body components, but eating too little protein can prevent it.

Most vital body proteins are in a constant state of breakdown, rebuilding, and repair. For example, the intestinal tract lining is constantly sloughed off. The digestive tract treats sloughed cells just like food particles, digesting them and absorbing their amino acids. In fact, most of the amino acids released throughout the body can be recycled to become part of the pool of amino acids available for synthesis of future proteins. Overall, **protein turnover** is a process by which a cell can respond to its changing environment by producing proteins that are needed and disassembling proteins that are not needed.

During any day, an adult makes and degrades about 250 grams of protein, recycling many of the amino acids. Relative to the 65 to 100 grams of protein typically consumed by adults in North America, recycled amino acids make an important contribution to total protein metabolism.

If a person's diet is low in protein for a long period, the processes of rebuilding and repairing body proteins will slow down. Over time, skeletal muscles; blood proteins; and vital organs, such as the heart and liver, will decrease in size or volume. Only the brain resists protein breakdown.

## Maintaining Fluid Balance

Blood proteins help maintain body fluid balance. Normal blood pressure in the arteries forces blood into capillary beds. The blood fluid then moves from the **capillary beds** into the spaces between nearby cells **(extracellular spaces)** to provide nutrients to those cells (Fig. 6-9). Proteins in the bloodstream are too large however, to move out of the capillary beds into the tissues. The presence of these proteins in the capillary beds attracts the proper amount of fluid back to the blood, partially counteracting the force of blood pressure.

With an inadequate consumption of protein, the concentration of proteins in the bloodstream drops below normal. Excessive fluid then builds up in the surrounding tissues because the counteracting force produced by the smaller amount of blood proteins is too weak to pull enough of the fluid back from the tissues into the bloodstream. As

▲ Protein contributes to the structure and function of muscle.

**protein turnover** The process by which cells break down old proteins and resynthesize new proteins. In this way the cell will have the proteins it needs to function at that time.

**capillary bed** Network of one-cell thick vessels that create a junction between arterial and venous circulation. It is here that gas and nutrient exchange occurs between body cells and the blood.

**extracellular space** The space outside cells; represents one-third of body fluid.

**FIGURE 6-9** ▶ Blood proteins in relation to fluid balance. (a) Blood proteins are important for maintaining the body's fluid balance. (b) Without sufficient protein in the bloodstream, edema develops.

**Arterial end of a capillary bed**

Fluid forced into tissue spaces by blood pressure generated by pumping action of heart

Blood cells

(a)

**Venous end of a capillary bed**

Proteins

Fluid drawn into bloodstream by the proteins as blood pressure declines in the capillary bed

**Normal tissue**

Blood pressure balanced by counteracting force of protein

**Swollen tissue (edema)**

Blood pressure exceeds counteracting force of protein, and so fluid remains in the tissues

(b)

**edema** The buildup of excess fluid in extracellular spaces.

**buffers** Compounds that cause a solution to resist changes in acid-base conditions.

fluids accumulate in the tissues, the tissues swell, causing **edema**. Edema may be a symptom of a variety of medical problems, so its cause must be identified. An important step in diagnosing the cause is to measure the concentration of blood proteins.

## Contributing to Acid-Base Balance

Proteins help regulate acid-base balance in the blood. Proteins located in cell membranes pump chemical ions in and out of cells. The ion concentration that results from the pumping action, among other factors, keeps the blood slightly alkaline. In addition, some blood proteins are especially good **buffers** for the body. Buffers are compounds that maintain acid-base conditions within a narrow range.

## Forming Hormones and Enzymes

Amino acids are required for the synthesis of many hormones—our internal body messengers. Some hormones, such as the thyroid hormones, are made from only one type of amino acid, tyrosine. Insulin, on the other hand, is a hormone composed of 51 total amino acids. Almost all enzymes are proteins or have a protein component.

**N**eurotransmitters, released by nerve endings, are often derivatives of amino acids. This is true for dopamine and norepinephrine (both synthesized from the amino acid tyrosine), and serotonin (synthesized from the amino acid tryptophan).

## Contributing to Immune Function

Proteins are a key component of the cells within the immune system. An example is the antibodies, proteins produced by one type of white blood cell. These antibodies can bind to foreign proteins in the body, an important step in removing invaders from the body. Without sufficient dietary protein, the immune system lacks the materials needed to function properly. For example, a low protein status can turn measles into a fatal disease for a malnourished child.

**T**he vitamin niacin can be made from the amino acid tryptophan, illustrating another role of proteins.

## Forming Glucose

In Chapter 4 you learned that the body must maintain a fairly constant concentration of blood glucose to supply energy for the brain, red blood cells, and nervous tissue. At rest, the brain uses about 19% of the body's energy requirements, and it gets most

## PROTEIN CONCEPT MAP

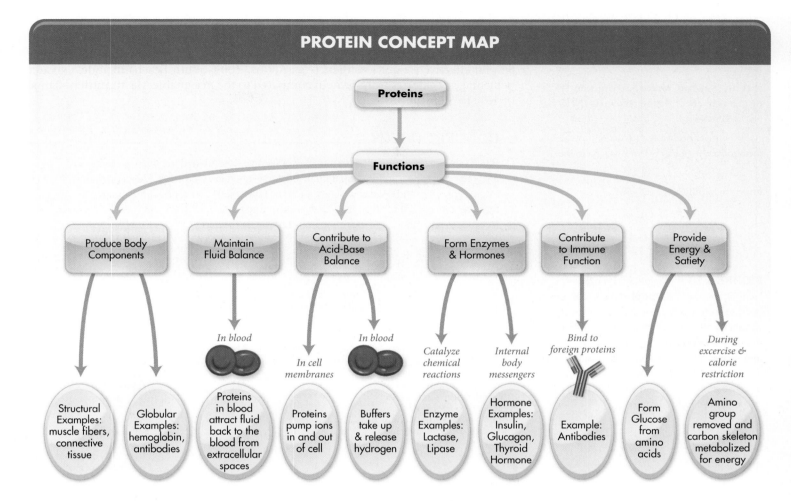

of that energy from glucose. If you don't consume enough carbohydrate to supply the glucose, your liver (and kidneys, to a lesser extent) will be forced to make glucose from amino acids present in body tissues (Fig. 6-10).

Making some glucose from amino acids is normal. For example, when you skip breakfast and haven't eaten since 7 P.M. the preceding evening, glucose must be manufactured. In an extreme situation, however, such as in starvation, amino acids from muscle tissue are converted into glucose, which wastes muscle tissue and can produce edema.

### Providing Energy

Proteins supply little energy for a weight-stable person. Two situations in which a person does use protein to meet energy needs are during prolonged exercise (see Chapter 10 for information about the use of amino acids for energy needs during exercise) and during calorie restriction, as with a weight-loss diet. In these cases, the amino group ($-NH_2$) from the amino acid is removed and the remaining carbon skeleton is metabolized for energy needs (Fig. 6-10). Still, under most conditions, cells primarily use fats and carbohydrates for energy needs. Although proteins contain the same amount of calories (on average, 4 kcal per gram) as carbohydrates, proteins are a costly source of calories, considering the amount of processing the liver and kidneys must perform to use this calorie source.

### Contributing to Satiety

Compared to the other macronutrients, proteins provide the highest feeling of **satiety** after a meal. Thus, including some protein with each meal helps control overall

**satiety** A state in which there is no longer a desire to eat; a feeling of satisfaction.

food intake. Many experts warn against skimping on protein when trying to reduce energy intake to lose weight. Meeting protein needs is still important and exceeding needs somewhat may provide an additional benefit when dieting to lose weight. Several effective weight loss diets (e.g., Atkins, Zone, South Beach) include a greater percentage of calories from protein compared to the Acceptable Macronutrient Range of 10% to 35% for protein.

## CONCEPT CHECK

Vital body constituents—such as muscle, connective tissue, blood transport proteins, enzymes, hormones, buffers, and immune factors—are mainly proteins. The degradation of existing proteins and synthesis of new proteins takes place constantly, amounting to a turnover rate of about 250 grams a day for the entire human body. Proteins can also be used for glucose and other fuel production and contributes to satiety.

**pool** The amount of a nutrient stored within the body that can be mobilized when needed.

**carbon skeleton** Amino acid structure that remains after the amino group ($-NH_2$) has been removed.

**urea** Nitrogenous waste product of protein metabolism; major source of nitrogen in the urine, chemically $NH_2-\underset{\underset{O}{\|}}{C}-NH_2$.

**FIGURE 6-10** ▶ Amino acid metabolism. The amino acid **pool** in a cell can be used to form body proteins, as well as a variety of other possible products. When the **carbon skeletons** of amino acids are metabolized to produce glucose or fat, ammonia ($NH_3$) is a resulting waste product. The ammonia is converted to **urea** and excreted in the urine.

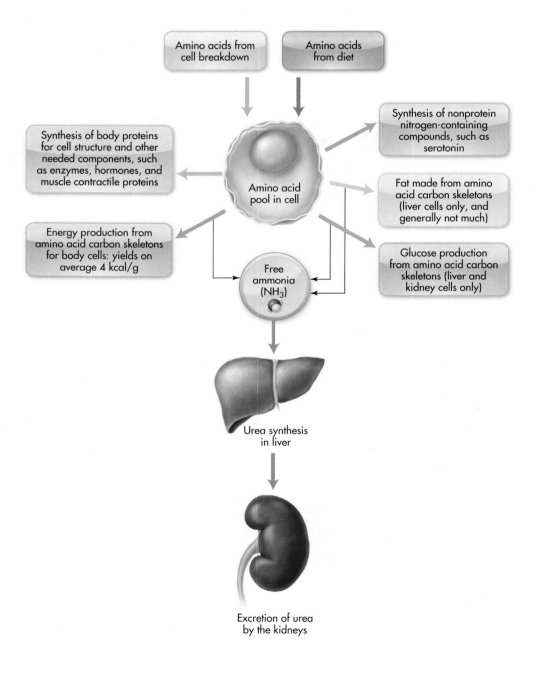

# 6.6 Protein Needs

How much protein (actually, amino acids) do we need to eat each day? People who aren't growing need to eat only enough protein to match whatever they lose daily from protein breakdown. The amount of breakdown can be determined by measuring the amount of urea and other nitrogen-containing compounds in the urine, as well as losses of protein from feces, skin, hair, nails, and so on. In short, people need to balance protein intake with such losses to maintain a state of **protein equilibrium,** also called *protein balance* (Fig. 6-11).

When a body is growing or recovering from an illness or injury, it needs a **positive protein balance** to supply the raw materials required to build new tissues. To achieve this, a person must eat more protein daily than he or she loses. In addition, the hormones insulin, growth hormone, and testosterone all stimulate positive protein balance. Resistance exercise (weight training) also enhances positive protein balance. Consuming less protein than needed leads to **negative protein balance,** such as when acute illness reduces the desire to eat and so one loses more protein than consumed.

For healthy people, the amount of dietary protein needed to maintain protein equilibrium (wherein intake equals losses) can be determined by increasing protein intake until it equals losses of protein and its related breakdown products (e.g., urea). Calorie needs must also be met so that amino acids are not diverted for such use.

Today, the best estimate for the amount of protein required for nearly all adults to maintain protein equilibrium is 0.8 grams of protein per kilogram of healthy

**protein equilibrium** A state in which protein intake is equal to related protein losses; the person is said to be in protein balance.

**positive protein balance** A state in which protein intake exceeds related protein losses, as is needed during times of growth.

**negative protein balance** A state in which protein intake is less than related protein losses, as is often seen during acute illness.

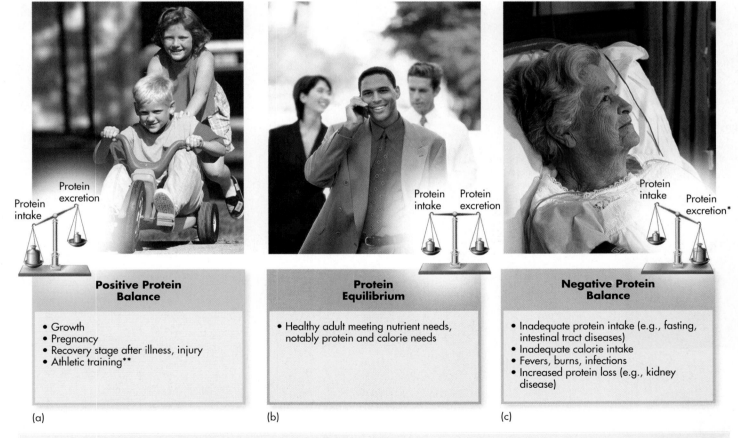

Protein intake / Protein excretion

**Positive Protein Balance**

- Growth
- Pregnancy
- Recovery stage after illness, injury
- Athletic training**

Protein intake / Protein excretion

**Protein Equilibrium**

- Healthy adult meeting nutrient needs, notably protein and calorie needs

Protein intake / Protein excretion*

**Negative Protein Balance**

- Inadequate protein intake (e.g., fasting, intestinal tract diseases)
- Inadequate calorie intake
- Fevers, burns, infections
- Increased protein loss (e.g., kidney disease)

(a)                                                    (b)                                                    (c)

*Based on losses of urea and other nitrogen-containing compounds in the urine, as well as protein lost from feces, skin, hair, nails, and other minor routes.
**Only when additional lean body mass is being gained. Nevertheless, the athlete is probably already eating enough protein to support this extra protein synthesis; protein supplements are not needed.

**FIGURE 6-11** ▶ Protein balance in practical terms: (a) positive protein balance; (b) protein equilibrium; (c) negative protein balance.

body weight. This is the RDA for protein. Requirements are higher during periods of growth, such as pregnancy and infancy (see Chapters 14 and 15 for specific values for pregnant women, infants, and children). Healthy weight is used as a reference in the determination of protein needs because excess fat storage doesn't contribute much to protein needs (see Chapter 7 for insight into the concept of healthy weight). Calculations using this RDA are shown in the margin and estimate a requirement of about 56 grams of protein daily for a typical 70-kilogram (154-pound) man and about 46 grams of protein daily for a typical 57-kilogram (125-pound) woman.

The RDA for protein translates into about 10% of total calories. Many experts recommend up to 15% of total calories to provide more flexibility in diet planning, in turn allowing for the variety of protein-rich foods North Americans typically consume. As noted earlier, the Food and Nutrition Board has set an upper range for protein intake at 35% of calories consumed. It is easy to meet currently suggested daily protein needs (Table 6-2). On a daily basis, typical North American protein intakes are about 100 grams of protein for men and 65 grams for women. Thus, most of us consume much more protein than the RDA recommends because we like many high-protein

**TABLE 6-2** Protein Content of Sample Menus Containing 1600 kcal and 2000 kcal

| Menu | | 1600 kcal | | 2000 kcal | |
|---|---|---|---|---|---|
| | | Serving Size | Protein (g) | Serving Size | Protein (g) |
| **Breakfast** | | | | | |
| | Low-fat granola | ⅔ cup | 5 | ⅔ cup | 5 |
| | Blueberries | 1 cup | 1 | 1 cup | 1 |
| | Fat-free (skim) milk | 1 cup | 8.5 | 1 cup | 8.5 |
| | Coffee | 1 cup | 0 | 1 cup | 0 |
| **Lunch** | | | | | |
| | Broiled chicken breast | 3 oz | 25 | 4 oz | 33 |
| | Salad greens | 3 cups | 5 | 3 cups | 5 |
| | Baked taco shell strips | ½ cup | 2 | ½ cup | 2 |
| | Low-fat salad dressing | 2 tbsp | 0 | 2 tbsp | 0 |
| | Fat-free (skim) milk | 1 cup | 8.5 | 1 cup | 8.5 |
| **Dinner** | | | | | |
| | Yellow rice | 1¼ cups | 5 | 2½ cups | 10 |
| | Shrimp | 4 large | 5 | 6 large | 7 |
| | Mussels | 4 medium | 8 | 6 medium | 12 |
| | Clams | 5 small | 12 | 10 small | 24 |
| | Peas | ¼ cup | 4 | ½ cup | 4 |
| | Sweet red pepper | ¼ cup | 0 | ½ cup | 0 |
| **Snack** | | | | | |
| | Muffin | 1 small | 4 | 1 small | 4 |
| | Swiss cheese | 1 oz | 7.5 | 1 oz | 7.5 |
| | Banana | ½ small | 0.5 | ½ small | 0.5 |
| | Total | | 101 | | 132 |

foods and can afford to buy them. Our bodies cannot store excess protein once it is consumed, so the excess amino acids are converted to carbon skeletons that are turned into glucose or fat and then stored as fat or metabolized for energy needs (review Fig. 6-10).

Mental stress, physical labor, and recreational weekend sports activities do not require an increase in the protein RDA. For some highly trained athletes, such as those participating in endurance or strength training, protein consumption may need to exceed the RDA. This is an area of debate in sports nutrition: the Food and Nutrition Board does not support an increased need, but some experts suggest an increase to about 1.7 grams per kilogram. Many North Americans already consume that much protein, especially men.

| Convert weight from pounds to kilograms: | $\dfrac{154 \text{ pounds}}{2.2 \text{ pounds/kilogram}}$ = 70 kilograms |
|---|---|
| | $\dfrac{125 \text{ pounds}}{2.2 \text{ pounds/kilogram}}$ = 57 kilograms |

**Calculate protein RDA:**

$$70 \text{ kilograms} \times \frac{0.8 \text{ grams protein}}{\text{kilogram body weight}} = 56 \text{ grams}$$

$$57 \text{ kilograms} \times \frac{0.8 \text{ grams protein}}{\text{kilogram body weight}} = 46 \text{ grams}$$

## 6.7  Does Eating a High-Protein Diet Harm You?

People frequently ask about the potential harm of protein intakes in excess of the RDA. Problems with diets that are high in protein foods primarily stem from the fact that they typically rely on animal sources of protein. Diets rich in animal products will most likely be simultaneously low in the beneficial substances found in plant sources, including fiber, some vitamins (e.g., folate), some minerals (e.g., magnesium), as well as phytochemicals, and high in substances such as saturated fat and cholesterol. A high animal-protein diet, therefore, is unlikely to follow the recommendations of the Dietary Guidelines for Americans or the Food and Nutrition Board in terms of reducing risk for cardiovascular disease.

Some, but not all, studies show that high-protein diets can increase calcium losses in urine. For people with adequate calcium intakes, little concern about this relationship is warranted, but keep in mind that calcium is commonly deficient in North American diets.

Meat is one of the richest sources of protein. Excessive intake of red meat, however, especially processed forms, is linked to colon cancer in population studies. There are several possible explanations for this connection. The curing agents used to process meats such as ham and salami may cause cancer. Substances that form during cooking of red meat at high temperatures may also cause cancer. The excessive fat or low-fiber contents of diets rich in red meat may also be a contributing factor. Because of these concerns, some nutrition experts suggest we focus more on poultry, fish, nuts, legumes, and seeds to meet protein needs. In addition, any red or other type of meat should be trimmed of all visible fat before grilling.

Some researchers have expressed concern that a high-protein intake may overburden the kidneys by forcing them to excrete the extra nitrogen as urea. Additionally, animal proteins may contribute to kidney stone formation in certain individuals. There is some support for limiting protein intake for people in the early stages of kidney disease, because low-protein diets somewhat slow the decline in kidney function. Laboratory animal studies show that moderate protein intakes that just meet nutritional needs preserve kidney function over time better than high-protein diets. Preserving kidney function is especially important for those who have diabetes, early signs of kidney disease, or only one functioning kidney, so a high-protein diet is not recommended for these people. High-protein diets increase urine output, in turn posing a risk for dehydration. This is a special concern for athletes (see Chapter 10).

▲ Animal protein foods are typically our main sources of protein in the North American diet.

## MAKING DECISIONS

### Amino Acid Supplements

Protein and amino acid supplements are used primarily by athletes and dieters. Athletes use them hoping they will help build muscle. The branched-chain amino acids described earlier are especially popular with athletes looking to enhance their performance. Dieters have turned to these supplements hoping they will increase their weight loss. Although the right amount of protein in the diet will aid athletic performance and help in weight control, consuming this protein in the form of amino acid supplements cannot be considered safe.

Earlier in this chapter, you learned that the body is designed to handle whole proteins as a dietary source of amino acids. When individual amino acid supplements are taken, they can overwhelm the absorptive mechanisms in the small intestine, triggering amino acid imbalances in the body. Imbalances occur because groups of chemically similar amino acids compete for absorption sites in the absorptive cells. For example, lysine and arginine are absorbed by the same transporter, so an excess of lysine can impair absorption of arginine. The amino acids most likely to cause toxicity when consumed in large amounts are methionine, cysteine, and histidine. Due to the potential for imbalances and toxicities of individual amino acids, the best advice to ensure adequacy is to stick to whole foods rather than supplements as sources of amino acids. Amino acids as such also have a disagreeable odor and flavor and are also much more expensive than food protein. In Canada the sale of individual amino acids to consumers is banned.

### CONCEPT CHECK

The Recommended Dietary Allowance (RDA) for adults is 0.8 grams of protein per kilogram of healthy body weight. This is approximately 56 grams of protein daily for a 70-kilogram (156-pound) person. The average North American man consumes about 100 grams of protein daily, and a woman consumes about 65 grams. Thus, typically we eat more than enough protein to meet our needs. This even includes well-balanced vegetarian diets. Diets high in protein can compromise kidney health in people with diabetes and those with kidney disease, and animal protein sources likely increase cardiovascular disease and kidney stone risk when consumed in high amounts.

## 6.8 Protein-Calorie Malnutrition

**protein-calorie malnutrition (PCM)** A condition resulting from regularly consuming insufficient amounts of calories and protein. The deficiency eventually results in body wasting, primarily of lean tissue, and an increased susceptibility to infections.

**kwashiorkor** A disease occurring primarily in young children who have an existing disease and consume a marginal amount of calories and insufficient protein in relation to needs. The child generally suffers from infections and exhibits edema, poor growth, weakness, and an increased susceptibility to further illness.

**marasmus** A disease resulting from consuming a grossly insufficient amount of protein and calories; one of the diseases classed as protein-calorie malnutrition. Victims have little or no fat stores, little muscle mass, and poor strength. Death from infections is common.

Protein deficiency is rarely an isolated condition and usually accompanies a deficiency of calories and other nutrients resulting from insufficient food intake. In the developed world, alcoholism can lead to cases of protein deficiency because of the low protein content of alcoholic beverages. Protein and calorie malnutrition is a significant problem in hospitals worldwide, affecting patients of all ages from infants to geriatric patients. Malnutrition can be caused by the illnesses or injuries for which the patients are admitted to the hospital and by the hospitalization itself. In developing areas of the world, people often have diets low in calories and also in protein. This state of undernutrition stunts the growth of children and makes them more susceptible to disease throughout life. (Undernutrition is a main focus of Chapter 12.) People who consume too little protein calories can eventually develop **protein-calorie malnutrition (PCM)**, also referred to as *protein-energy malnutrition (PEM)*. In its milder form, it is difficult to tell if a person with PCM is consuming too little calories or protein, or both. When an inadequate intake of nutrients, including protein, is combined with an already existing disease, especially an infection, a form of malnutrition called **kwashiorkor** can develop. But if the nutrient deficiency—especially for calories—becomes severe, a deficiency disease called **marasmus** can result. Both conditions are seen primarily in children, but also may develop in adults, even in those hospitalized in North America. These two conditions form the tip of the iceberg with respect to states of undernutrition, and symptoms of these two conditions can even be present in the same person (Fig. 6-12).

**FIGURE 6-12 ▶** Classification of under-nutrition in children.

*Severe protein (with moderate energy) deficit; often accompanied by infections or other diseases*

**Protein Energy Malnutrition**

*Severe energy and protein deficit*

**Characteristics of Kwashiorkor**

- Edema
- Mild to moderate weight loss
- Maintenance of some muscle and subcutaneous fat
- Growth impairment (60%–80% of normal weight for age)
- Rapid onset
- Fatty liver

**Characteristics of Marasmus**

- Severe weight loss
- Wasting of muscle and body fat (skin and bones appearance)
- Severe growth impairment (less than 60% of normal weight for age)
- Develops gradually

## Kwashiorkor

*Kwashiorkor* is a word from Ghana that means "the disease that the first child gets when the new child comes." From birth, an infant in developing areas of the world is usually breastfed. Often by the time the child reaches 1 to 1.5 years of age, the mother is pregnant or has already given birth again, and the new child gets preference for breastfeeding. The older child's diet then abruptly changes from nutritious human milk to starchy roots and **gruels.** These foods have low-protein densities, compared with total energy. Additionally, the foods are usually full of plant fibers, often bulky, making it difficult for the child to consume enough to meet calorie needs. The child generally also has infections, which acutely raise calorie and protein needs. For these reasons, calorie needs of these children are met just barely, at best, and their protein consumption is grossly inadequate, especially in view of the increased amount needed to combat infections. Many vitamin and mineral needs are also far from being fulfilled. Famine victims face similar problems.

The major symptoms of kwashiorkor are apathy, diarrhea, listlessness, failure to grow and gain weight, and withdrawal from the environment. These symptoms complicate other diseases present. For example, a condition such as measles, a disease that normally makes a healthy child ill for only a week or so, can become severely debilitating and even fatal. Further symptoms of kwashiorkor are changes in hair color, potassium deficiency, flaky skin, fatty liver, reduced muscle mass, and massive edema in the abdomen and legs. The presence of edema in a child who has some subcutaneous fat (i.e., directly under the skin) is the hallmark of kwashiorkor (review Fig. 6-12). In addition, these children seldom move. If you pick them up, they don't cry. When you hold them, you feel the plumpness of edema, not muscle and fat tissue.

Many symptoms of kwashiorkor can be explained based on what we know about proteins. Proteins play important roles in fluid balance, lipoprotein transport, immune function, and production of tissues, such as skin, cells lining the GI tract, and hair. Children with an insufficient protein intake do not grow and mature normally.

If children with kwashiorkor are helped in time—if infections are treated and a diet ample in protein, calories, and other essential nutrients is provided—the disease

**gruels** A thin mixture of grains or legumes in milk or water.

**T**oxic products in moldy grains may also contribute to kwashiorkor.

▲ Unsafe water supplies in developing countries contribute to the incidence of marasmus, particularly in bottle-fed infants.

**preterm** An infant born before 37 weeks of gestation; also referred to as premature.

process reverses. They begin to grow again and may even show no signs of their previous condition, except perhaps shortness of stature. Unfortunately, by the time many of these children reach a hospital or care center, they already have severe infections. Despite the best care, they still die. Or, if they survive, they return home only to become ill again.

## Marasmus

Marasmus typically occurs as an infant slowly starves to death. It is caused by diets containing minimal amounts of calories, as well as too little protein and other nutrients. As previously noted, the condition is also commonly referred to as *protein-calorie malnutrition*, especially when experienced by older children and adults. The word *marasmus* means "to waste away," in Greek. Victims have a "skin-and-bones" appearance, with little or no subcutaneous fat (review Fig. 6-12).

Marasmus commonly develops in infants who either are not breastfed or have stopped breastfeeding in the early months. Often the weaning formula used is improperly prepared because of unsafe water and because the parents cannot afford sufficient infant formula for the child's needs. The latter problem may lead the parents to dilute the formula to provide more feedings, not realizing that this provides only more water for the infant.

Marasmus in infants commonly occurs in the large cities of poverty-stricken countries. When people are poor and sanitation is lacking, bottle feeding often leads to marasmus. In the cities, bottle feeding is often necessary because the infant must be cared for by others when the mother is working or away from home. An infant with marasmus requires large amounts of calories and protein—like a **preterm** infant—and, unless the child receives them, full recovery from the disease may never occur. The majority of brain growth occurs between conception and the child's first birthday. In fact, the brain is growing at its highest rate after birth. If the diet does not support brain growth during the first months of life, the brain may not grow to its full adult size. This reduced or retarded brain growth may lead to diminished intellectual function. Both kwashiorkor and marasmus plague infants and children; mortality rates in developing countries are often 10 to 20 times higher than in North America.

### CONCEPT CHECK

Most undernutrition consists of mild deficits in calories, protein, and often other nutrients. If a person needs more nutrients because of disease and infection but does not consume enough calories and protein, a condition known as kwashiorkor can develop. The person suffers from edema and weakness. Children around age 2 are especially susceptible to kwashiorkor, particularly if they already have other diseases. Famine situations in which only starchy root products are available to eat contribute to this problem. Marasmus is a condition wherein people—infants, especially—starve to death. Symptoms include muscle wasting, absence of fat stores, and weakness. Both an adequate diet and the treatment of concurrent diseases must be promoted to regain and then maintain nutritional health.

# Vegetarian and Plant-Based Diets

Vegetarianism has evolved over the centuries from a necessity into an option. Historically, vegetarianism was linked with specific philosophies and religions or with science. Today, about 1 in 40 adults in the United States (and about 1 in 25 in Canada) is a vegetarian. Vegetarian diets have evolved to include such new products as soy-based sloppy joes, chili, tacos, burgers, and more. In addition, cookbooks that feature the use of a variety of fruits, vegetables, and seasonings are enhancing food selection for vegetarians of all degrees.

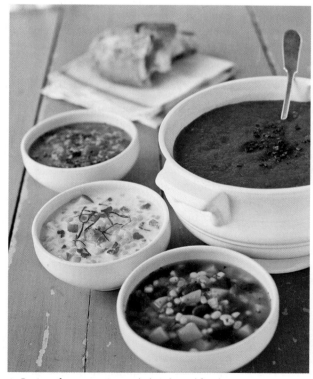

▲ Recipes for vegetarian and plant-based foods are widely available today.

Vegetarianism is popular among college students. Fifteen percent of college students in one survey said they select vegetarian options at lunch or dinner on any given day. In response, dining services offer vegetarian options at every meal, such as pastas with meatless sauce and pizza. Many teenagers are also turning to vegetarianism. In addition, a survey by the National Restaurant Association found that 20% of its customers want a vegetarian option when they eat out. Many customers cite health and taste as reasons for choosing vegetarian meals.

As nutrition science has grown, new information has enabled the design of nutritionally adequate vegetarian diets. It is important for vegetarians to take advantage of this information because a diet of only plant-based foods has the potential to promote various nutrient deficiencies and substantial growth retardation in infants and children. People who choose a vegetarian diet can meet their nutritional needs by following a few basic rules and knowledgeably planning their diets.

Studies show that death rates from some chronic diseases, such as certain forms of cardiovascular disease, hypertention, many forms of cancer, type 2 diabetes, and obesity, are lower for vegetarians than for non-vegetarians. Vegetarians often live longer, as shown in religious groups that practice

vegetarianism. Other aspects of healthful lifestyles, such as not smoking, abstaining from alcohol and drugs, and regular physical activity often go along with vegetarianism and probably partially account for the lower risks of chronic disease and longer lives seen in this population.

As you learned in Chapter 2, MyPyramid and the 2005 Dietary Guidelines for Americans emphasize a plant-based diet of whole-grain breads and cereals, fruits, and vegetables. In addition, the American Institute for Cancer Research promotes "The New American Plate," which includes plant-based foods covering two-thirds (or more) of the plate and meat, fish, poultry, or lowfat dairy covering only one-third (or less) of the plate. Although these recommendations do allow the inclusion of animal products, they are definitely more "vegetarian-like" than typical North American diets.

## Why Do People Become Vegetarians?

People choose vegetarianism for a variety of reasons including ethics, religion, economics, and health. Some believe that killing animals for food is unethical. Hindus and Trappist monks eat vegetarian meals as a practice of their religion. In North America, many Seventh Day Adventists base their practice of vegetarianism on biblical texts and believe it is a more healthful way to live.

Some advocates of vegetarianism base their food preference upon the inefficient use of animals as a source of protein. Forty percent of the world's

# The New American Plate

The New American Plate

2/3 (or more) vegetables, fruits, whole grains and beans

1/3 (or less) animal protein

American Institute for Cancer Research

▶ American Institute for Cancer Research Diet and Health Guidelines for Cancer Prevention

1. Choose a diet rich in a variety of plant-based foods.

2. Eat plenty of vegetables and fruit.

3. Maintain a healthy weight and be physically active

4. Drink alcohol only in moderation, if at all.

5. Select foods low in fat and salt.

6. Prepare and store food safely.

*And always remember. . .*

Do not use tobacco in any form.

grain production is used to raise meat-producing animals. Although animals that humans eat sometimes eat grasses that humans cannot digest, many also eat grains that humans can eat.

People might also practice vegetarianism because it limits saturated fat and cholesterol intake, while encouraging a high intake of complex carbohydrates, vitamins A, E, and C, carotenoids, magnesium, and fiber.

## Good for Your Heart

Plant sources of proteins can positively impact heart health in several ways. First, the plant foods we eat contain no cholesterol nor *trans* fat and little saturated fat. The major type of fats in plant foods are monounsaturated and polyunsaturated fats. Nuts in particular are high in monounsaturated fat, which helps to keep blood cholesterol low.

Beans and nuts contain soluble fiber, which binds to cholesterol in the small intestine and prevents it from being absorbed by the body. Also, due to the activity of some phytochemicals, foods

made from soybeans can lower production of cholesterol by the body. The effect is modest (about a 2% to 6% drop). In 1999, the Food and Drug Administration allowed health claims for the cholesterol-lowering properties of soy foods, and in 2000, the American Heart Association recommended inclusion of some soy protein in the diets of people with high blood cholesterol. As noted in Chapter 2, to list a health claim for soy on the label, a food product must have at least 6.25 grams of soy protein and less than 3 grams of fat, 1 gram of saturated fat, and 20 milligrams of cholesterol per serving.

There are several other compounds in plant foods under study for their heart-protective roles. Some of the phytochemicals may help to prevent blood clots and relax the blood vessels. Nuts are an especially good source of nutrients implicated in heart health, including vitamin E, folate, magnesium, and copper. Frequent consumption of nuts (about 1 ounce of nuts five times per week) is associated with a decreased risk of cardiovascular disease. Recall from Chapter 2 that FDA also allows a provisional health claim to

link nuts with a reduced risk of developing cardiovascular disease. As noted in Chapter 5, a vegan diet coupled with regular exercise and other lifestyle changes can lead to a reversal of atherosclerotic plaque in various arteries in the body.

## Cancer-Fighting Agents

The numerous phytochemicals in plant foods are thought to aid in preventing cancers of the breast, prostate, and colon. Many of the proposed anti-cancer effects of foods containing plant protein are through antioxidant mechanisms.

Consumption of plant sources of proteins can aid in prevention of cardiovascular disease and cancer, but there are also other areas for future study. Some studies show that replacing animal proteins with plant proteins is beneficial for kidney health. However, because plant foods such as soy are high in oxalates, people with a history of kidney stones should probably limit intake of soy (see Chapter 9 for more about oxalates). Plants may be particularly good sources of protein for people with diabetes or impaired glucose tolerance because the high fiber content of plant foods leads to a slower increase in blood glucose (review Chapter 4 for a discussion of glycemic load). Frequent nut consumption may even reduce the risk of developing gallstones; a reduced risk for obesity and type 2 diabetes is also likely. Much of the excitement surrounding the ability of soy to combat a host of medical problems has waned. Several studies have shown little benefit of soy in preventing many forms of cancer, in lowering blood cholesterol, contributing to bone maintenance in women after menopause, and in treating menopausal symptoms in women. A recent review of eighteen studies, however, concluded that soy consumption was associated with a 14% reduction in breast cancer risk.

## Increasing Plant Proteins in Your Diet

Now that you've seen how much you can benefit from including plant proteins in your diet, here are some suggestions for putting the theory onto your plate:

- At your next cookout, try a veggie burger instead of a hamburger. These are usually made from beans and are available in the frozen foods section of the grocery store and come in a variety of delicious flavors. Many restaurants have added veggie burgers to their menus.
- Sprinkle sunflower seeds or chopped almonds on top of your salad to add taste and texture.
- Mix chopped walnuts into the batter of your banana bread to boost your intake of monounsaturated fats.
- Eat soy nuts (oil-roasted soybeans) as a great snack.
- Spread some peanut butter on your bagel instead of butter or cream cheese.
- Instead of having beef or chicken tacos for dinner, heat up a can of great northern beans in your skillet with one half of a packet of taco seasoning and chopped tomatoes. Use this as a filling in a tortilla shell.
- Consider using soy milk, especially if you have lactose malabsorption or lactose intolerance. Look for varieties fortified with calcium.

## Food Planning for Vegetarians

There are a variety of vegetarian diet styles. **Vegans,** or "total vegetarians," eat only plant foods (and do not use animal products for other purposes, such as leather shoes or feather pillows). **Fruitarians** primarily eat fruits, nuts, honey, and vegetable oils. This plan is not recommended because it can lead to nutrient deficiencies in people of all ages. **Lactovegetarians** modify vegetarianism a bit—they include dairy products in their plant-based diet. **Lactoovovegetarians** modify the diet even further and eat dairy products and eggs, as well as plant foods. Including these animal products makes food planning easier because they are rich in some nutrients that are missing or minimal in plants, such as vitamin B-12 and calcium. The more variety in the diet, the easier it is to meet nutritional needs. Thus, the practice of eating no animal sources of food significantly separates the vegans and fruitarians from all other semivegetarian styles.

Most people who call themselves vegetarians consume at least some dairy products, if not all dairy products and eggs. A food-group plan has been developed for lactovegetarians and vegans (Table 6-3). This plan includes servings of nuts, grains, legumes, and seeds to help meet protein needs. There is also a vegetable group, a fruit group, and a milk group.

## Vegan Diet Planning

Planning a vegan diet requires knowledge and creativity to yield high-quality protein and other key nutrients without animal products. Earlier in this chapter, you learned about complementing proteins, whereby the essential amino acids deficient in one protein source are supplied by those of another consumed at the same meal or the next (Fig. 6-13). Many legumes are deficient in the essential amino acid methionine, while cereals are limited in lysine. Eating a combination of legumes and cereals, such as beans and rice, will supply the body with adequate amounts of all essential amino acids (Fig. 6-13). As for any diet, variety is an especially important characteristic of a nutritious vegan diet.

▲ Plant proteins, like those in walnuts, can be incorporated into one's diet in numerous ways, such as adding them to banana bread.

▲ A salad containing numerous types of vegetables and legumes is a healthy vegetarian choice.

**vegan** A person who eats only plant foods.

**fruitarian** A person who primarily eats fruits, nuts, honey, and vegetable oils.

**lactovegetarian** A person who consumes plant products and dairy products.

**lactoovovegetarian** A person who consumes plant products, dairy products, and eggs.

**TABLE 6-3** Food Plan for Vegetarians Based on MyPyramid

| Food Group | MyPyramid Servings | | Key Nutrients Supplied[c] |
| | Lactovegetarian[a] | Vegan[b] | |
| --- | --- | --- | --- |
| Grains | 6–11 | 8–11 | Protein, thiamin, niacin, folate, vitamin E, zinc, magnesium, iron, and fiber |
| Beans and other legumes | 2–3 | 3 | Protein, vitamin B-6, zinc, magnesium, and fiber |
| Nuts, seeds | 2–3 | 3 | Protein, vitamin E, and magnesium |
| Vegetables | 3–5 (include 1 dark green or leafy variety daily) | 4–6 (include 1 dark green or leafy variety daily) | Vitamin A, vitamin C, folate, vitamin K, potassium, and magnesium |
| Fruits | 2–4 | 4 | Vitamin A, vitamin C, and folate |
| Milk | 3 | _____ | Protein, riboflavin, vitamin D, vitamin B-12, and calcium |
| Fortified soy milk | _____ | 3 | Protein, riboflavin, vitamin D, vitamin B-12, and calcium |

[a]This plan contains about 75 grams of protein in 1650 kcal.

[b]This plan contains about 79 grams of protein in 1800 kcal.

[c]One serving of vitamin- and mineral-enriched ready-to-eat breakfast cereal is recommended to meet possible nutrient gaps. Alternatively, a balanced multivitamin and mineral supplement can be used. Vegans also may benefit from the use of fortified soy milk to provide calcium, vitamin D, and vitamin B-12.

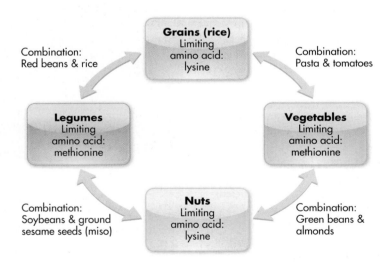

**FIGURE 6-13** ▶ Plant group combinations in which the proteins complement each other in a meal based on their limiting amino acids.

Combination: Red beans & rice

**Grains (rice)**
Limiting amino acid: lysine

Combination: Pasta & tomatoes

**Legumes**
Limiting amino acid: methionine

**Vegetables**
Limiting amino acid: methionine

Combination: Soybeans & ground sesame seeds (miso)

**Nuts**
Limiting amino acid: lysine

Combination: Green beans & almonds

Aside from amino acids, low intakes of certain micronutrients can be a problem for the vegan. At the forefront of nutritional concerns are riboflavin, vitamins D and B-12, iron, zinc, iodide, and calcium. The following dietary advice should be implemented. In addition, use of a balanced multivitamin and mineral supplement can help as well.

Riboflavin can be obtained from green leafy vegetables, whole grains, yeast, and legumes—components of most vegan diets. Alternate sources of vitamin D include fortified foods (e.g., margarine), as well as regular sun exposure (see Chapter 8).

Vitamin B-12 only occurs naturally in animal foods. Plants can contain soil or microbial contaminants that provide trace amounts of vitamin B-12, but these are negligible sources of the vitamin. Because the body can store vitamin B-12 for about 4 years, it may take a long time after removal of animal foods from the diet for a vitamin B-12 deficiency to surface. If dietary B-12 inadequacy persists, deficiency can lead to a form of anemia, nerve damage, and mental dysfunction. These deficiency consequences have been noted in the infants of vegetarian mothers whose breast milk was low in vitamin B-12. Vegans can prevent a vitamin B-12 deficiency by finding a reliable source of vitamin B-12, such as fortified soybean milk,

▲ Keep in mind that amino acids in vegetables are best used when a combination of sources is consumed.

ready-to-eat breakfast cereals, and special yeast grown on media rich in vitamin B-12.

For iron, the vegan can consume whole grains (especially ready-to-eat breakfast cereals), dried fruits and nuts, and legumes. The iron in these foods is not absorbed as well as iron in animal foods. A good source of vitamin C helps with the absorption of iron so it is recommended that vitamin C be consumed with every meal that contains iron-rich plant foods. Cooking in iron pots and skillets can also add iron to the diet (see Chapter 9).

The vegan can find zinc in whole grains (especially ready-to-eat breakfast cereals), nuts, and legumes, but phytic acid and other substances in these foods limit zinc absorption. Breads are a good source of zinc because the leavening process (rising of the bread dough) reduces the influence of phytic acid. Iodized salt is a reliable source of iodide. It should be used instead of plain salt, both of which are found in U.S. supermarkets.

Of all nutrients, calcium is the most difficult to consume in sufficient quantities for vegans. Fortified foods including fortified soy milk, fortified orange juice, calcium-rich tofu (check the label), as well as certain ready-to-eat breakfast cereals and snacks are the vegan's best option for obtaining calcium. Green leafy vegetables and nuts also contain calcium, but the mineral is either not well absorbed or not very plentiful from these sources. Calcium supplements are another option (see Chapter 9). Special diet planning is always required, because even a multivitamin and mineral supplement will not supply enough calcium to meet the needs of the body.

Consuming adequate quantities of omega-3 fatty acids is yet another nutritional concern for vegetarians, especially vegans. Fish and fish oils, abundant

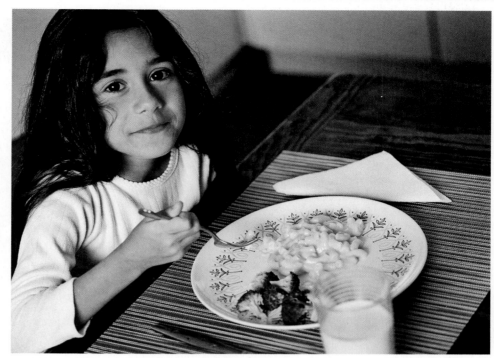

▲ Children can safely enjoy vegetarian and vegan diets as long as certain adjustments are made to meet their age-specific nutritional needs.

sources of these heart-healthy fats, are omitted from many types of vegetarian diets. Alternative plant sources of omega-3 fatty acids include canola oil, soybean oil, seaweed, microalgae, flax seeds, and walnuts.

## Special Concerns for Infants and Children

Infants and children, notoriously picky eaters in the first place, are at highest risk for nutrient deficiencies as a result of improperly planned vegetarian and vegan diets. With the use of complementary proteins and good sources of problem nutrients just discussed, the calorie, protein, vitamin, and mineral needs of vegetarian and vegan infants and children can be met. The most common nutritional concerns for infants and children following vegetarian and vegan diets are deficiencies of iron, vitamin B-12, vitamin D, and calcium.

Vegetarian and vegan diets tend to be high in bulky, high-fiber, low-calorie foods that cause a feeling of fullness. While this is a welcome advantage for adults, children have small stomach volume and relatively high nutrient needs compared to their size, and therefore may feel full before their calorie needs are met. For this reason, the fiber content of a child's diet may need to be decreased by replacing high-fiber sources with some refined grain products, fruit juices, and peeled fruit. Other concentrated sources of calories for vegetarian and vegan children include fortified soy milk, nuts, dried fruits, avocados, and cookies made with vegetable oils or tub margarine.

## Case Study Planning a Vegetarian Diet

Jordan is a freshman in college. He lives in a campus residence hall and teaches martial arts in the afternoon. He eats two or three meals a day at the residence hall cafeteria and snacks between meals. Jordan and his roommate both decided to become vegetarians because they recently read a magazine article describing the health benefits of a vegetarian diet. Yesterday Jordan's vegetarian diet consisted of a Danish pastry for breakfast and a tomato-rice dish (no meat) with pretzels and a diet soft drink for lunch. In the afternoon, after his martial arts class, he had a milk shake and two cookies. At dinnertime he had a vegetarian sub sandwich consisting of lettuce, sprouts, tomatoes, cucumbers, and cheese, with two glasses of fruit punch. In the evening, he had a bowl of popcorn.

Answer the following questions, and check your response in Appendix A.

1. What type of health benefits can Jordan expect from following a well-planned vegetarian diet?
2. What is missing from Jordan's current diet plan in terms of foods that should be emphasized in a vegetarian diet?
3. Which nutrients are missing in this current diet plan?
4. Are there any food components in the current diet plan that should be minimized or avoided?
5. How could he improve his new diet at each meal and snack to meet his nutritional needs and avoid undesirable food components?

▲ Has Jordan planned a healthy and nutritious vegetarian diet?

## Summary

1. Amino acids, the building blocks of proteins, contain a very usable form of nitrogen for humans. Of the 20 common types of amino acids found in food, nine must be consumed in food (essential) and the rest can be synthesized by the body (nonessential).

2. Individual amino acids are bonded together to form proteins. The sequential order of amino acids determines the protein's ultimate shape and function. This order is directed by DNA in the cell nucleus. Diseases such as sickle cell anemia can occur if the amino acids are incorrect on a polypeptide chain. When the three-dimensional shape of a protein is unfolded—denatured—by treatment with heat, acid or alkaline solutions, or other processes, the protein also loses its biological activity.

3. Almost all animal products are nutrient-dense sources of protein. The high quality of these proteins means that they can be easily converted into body proteins. Rich plant sources of protein, such as beans, are also available.

High-quality (complete) protein foods contain ample amounts of all nine essential amino acids. Furthermore, foods derived from animal sources provide high biological value protein. Lower-quality (incomplete) protein foods lack sufficient amounts of one or more essential amino acids. This is typical of plant foods, especially cereal grains. Different types of plant foods eaten together often complement each other's amino-acid deficits, thereby providing high-quality protein in the diet.

4. Protein digestion begins in the stomach, dividing the proteins into breakdown products containing shorter polypeptide chains of amino acids. In the small intestine, these polypeptide chains eventually separate into amino acids in the absorptive cells. The free amino acids then travel via the portal vein that connects to the liver. Some then enter the bloodstream.

5. Important body components—such as muscles, connective tissue, transport proteins in the bloodstream, visual pigments, enzymes, some hormones, and immune cells—are made of proteins. These proteins are in a state of constant turnover. The carbon chains of proteins may be used to produce glucose (or fat) when necessary.

6. The protein RDA for adults is 0.8 grams per kilogram of healthy body weight. For a typical 70-kilogram (154-pound) person, this corresponds to 56 grams of protein daily; for a 57-kilogram (125-pound) person, this corresponds to 46 grams per day. The North American diet generally supplies plenty of protein. Men typically consume about 100 grams of protein daily, and women consume closer to 65 grams. These usual protein intakes are also of sufficient quality to support body functions. This is even true for well-balanced vegetarian diets.

7. People need to balance protein intake with such losses to maintain a state of

protein equilibrium, also called *protein balance.*

When a body is growing or recovering from an illness or injury, it needs a positive protein balance to supply the raw materials required to build new tissues. To achieve this, a person must eat more protein daily than he or she loses. Consuming less protein than needed leads to negative protein balance, such as when acute illness reduces the desire to eat and so one loses more protein than consumed.

8. Undernutrition can lead to protein-calorie malnutrition in the form of kwashiorkor or marasmus. Kwashiorkor results primarily from an inadequate calorie and protein intake in comparison with body needs, which often increase with concurrent disease and infection. Kwashiorkor often occurs when a child is weaned from human milk and fed mostly starchy gruels. Marasmus results from extreme starvation—a negligible intake of both protein and calories. Marasmus commonly occurs during famine, especially in infants.

9. Consumption of vegetarian and other plant-based diets provides many health benefits, including lower risks of chronic diseases including cardiovascular disease, diabetes, and certain cancers. The benefits associated with the plant-based diets appear to stem from the lower content of saturated fat and cholesterol and the higher amount of fiber, vitamins, minerals, and phytochemicals.

## Study Questions

1. Discuss the relative importance of essential and nonessential amino acids in the diet. Why is it important for essential amino acids lost from the body to be replaced in the diet?

2. Describe the concept of complementary proteins.

3. What is a limiting amino acid? Explain why this concept is a concern in a vegetarian diet. How can a vegetarian compensate for limiting amino acids in specific foods?

4. Briefly describe the organization of proteins. How can this organization be altered or damaged? What might be a result of damaged protein organization?

5. Describe four functions of proteins. Provide an example of how the structure of a protein relates to its function.

6. How are DNA and protein synthesis related?

7. What would be one health benefit of reducing high-protein intake(s) to RDA amounts for some people?

8. What characteristics of vegetable proteins could improve the North American diet? What foods would you include to provide a diet that has ample protein from both plant and animal sources but is moderate in fat?

9. Outline the major differences between kwashiorkor and marasmus.

10. What are the possible long-term effects of an inadequate intake of dietary protein among children between the ages of 6 months and 4 years?

## Check Your Knowledge

Answers to the following multiple choice questions are below the questions.

1. The "instructions" for making proteins are located in the
   a. cell membrane.
   b. DNA and RNA genetic material.
   c. stomach.
   d. small intestine.

2. A nutrient that could easily be deficient in the diet of a vegan would be
   a. vitamin C.
   b. folic acid.
   c. calcium.
   d. All of the above.

3. If an essential amino acid is unavailable for protein synthesis, the
   a. cell will make the amino acid.
   b. synthesis of the protein will stop.

   c. cell will continue to attach amino acids to the protein.
   d. partially completed protein will be stored for later completion.

4. An example of protein complementation used in vegetarian diet planning would be the combination of
   a. cereal and milk.
   b. bacon and eggs.
   c. rice and beans.
   d. macaroni and cheese.

5. An individual who eats only plant food is referred to as a
   a. planetarium.
   b. vegan.
   c. lactovegetarian.
   d. ovovegetarian.

6. Which of the following groups accounts for the differences among amino acids?
   a. amine group
   b. side chain
   c. acid group
   d. keto group

7. Absorption of amino acids takes place in the
   a. stomach.
   b. liver.
   c. small intestine.
   d. large intestine.

8. Jack is not an athlete and weighs 176 pounds (80 kilograms). His RDA for protein would be _____ grams.
   a. 32          c. 64
   b. 40          d. 80

9. Which of the following is true about protein intake of people in the United States?
   a. Most do not consume enough protein.
   b. Most consume approximately the amount needed to balance losses.
   c. Athletes generally do not get enough protein without supplementation.
   d. Most consume more than is needed.

10. The basic building block of a protein is called a(n)
    a. fatty acid.
    b. monosaccharide.
    c. amino acid.
    d. gene.

Answers Key: 1. b, 2. c, 3. b, 4. c, 5. b, 6. b, 7. c, 8. c, 9. d, 10. c

## Further Readings

1. ADA Reports: Position of the American Dietetic Association and Dietitians of Canada: vegetarian diets. *Journal of the American Dietetic Association* 103:748, 2003.

   *It is the position of the American Dietetic Association and Dietitians of Canada that appropriately planned vegetarian diets are healthful, nutritionally adequate, and provide health benefits in the prevention and treatment of certain diseases. In some cases, however, use of fortified foods or a multivitamin and mineral supplement may be needed to meet recommendations for individual nutrients.*

2. Aronson D: Vegetarian nutrition. *Today's Dietitian* p. 3, March 2005.

   *This article summarizes the possible nutrient deficiencies that can result from a vegetarian diet. Plant food sources to counteract these risks are reviewed, such as rich sources of calcium.*

3. Barnard ND and others: A low-fat vegan diet improves glycemic control and cardiovascular risk factors in a randomized clinical trial in individuals with type 2 diabetes. *Diabetes Care* 29:1777, 2006.

   *Improvements in glycemic (decreased hemoglobin A1C) and lipid (decreased LDL cholesterol) control were greater in type 2 diabetic patients that followed a low-fat vegan diet compared to a diet based on American Diabetes Association guidelines. In the vegan group, 43% of the subjects reduced their diabetes medications compared to 26% of the subjects on the ADA diet.*

4. Berkow SE, Barnard ND: Blood pressure regulation and vegetarian diets. *Nutrition Reviews* 63:1, 2005.

   *Vegetarian diets are associated with lower blood pressure. It is likely that the fruit, vegetables, legumes, and nuts in such a diet lead to this health benefit.*

5. Chao A and others: Meat consumption and colorectal cancer. *Journal of the American Medical Association* 293:172, 2005.

   *Diets rich in red meat, especially processed meat, increase the risk of colon cancer. Protein from poultry and fish, in contrast, does not pose the same risk.*

6. Fessler TA: Malnutrition: A serious concern for hospitalized patients. *Today's Dietitian* 10 (7): 44, 2008.

   *Malnutrition continues to be a significant problem in hospitals worldwide, affecting patients of all ages from infants to geriatric patients. Malnutrition can be caused by the illnesses or injuries for which the patients are admitted to the hospital and by the hospitalization itself. This article outlines the need for prompt identification, treatment, and monitoring of malnourished patients among healthcare professionals.*

7. Food and Nutrition Board: *Dietary reference intakes for energy, carbohydrate, fiber, fat, fatty acids, cholesterol, protein, and amino acids.* Washington DC: The National Academy Press, 2002.

   *This report provides the latest guidance for macronutrient intakes. With regard to protein intake, the RDA has been set at 0.8 grams per kilogram per day. Protein intake can range from 10% to 35% of calorie intake. The 10% allotment approximates the RDA, based on typical calorie intakes.*

8. Garlick PJ: The nature of human hazards associated with excessive intakes of amino acids. *Journal of Nutrition* 134:1633S, 2004.

   *The most toxic amino acids are methionine, cysteine, and histidine. Possible health risks from excessive intakes of other amino acids are also reviewed. These risks are seen with amino acid supplements, not whole food sources.*

9. Gardner CD and others: The effect of a plant-based diet on plasma lipids in hypercholesterolemic adults. *Annals of Internal Medicine* 142:725, 2005.

   *Adding plant proteins to a diet already low in saturated fat and cholesterol provides additional benefits regarding lowering blood cholesterol. The authors emphasize the importance of including fruits, vegetables, legumes, and whole grains in a diet.*

10. Key TJ and others: Health effects of vegetarian and vegan diets. *Proceedings of the Nutrition Society* 65:35, 2006.

    *This study reviewed recent findings from large studies and summarizes the latest understanding of the health effects of vegetarian and vegan diets. Results indicated that vegetarians have a lower BMI and lower obesity rates than comparable nonvegetarians; total plasma cholesterol is lower in vegetarians that nonvegetarians; between vegetarians and nonvegetarians there is no significant differences in blood pressure; studies of vegetarians indicate a moderate reduction in mortality from ischemic heart disease; and studies showed no differences between vegetarians and nonvegetarians for colorectal cancer, breast cancer, prostate cancer, or total mortality.*

11. Lejeune MP and others: Additional protein intake limits weight regain after weight loss in humans. *British Journal of Nutrition* 93: 281, 2005.

    *Adding 30 grams of protein per day to their usual diets helped people in this study limit weight regain after weight loss. The diet ended up 18% of calorie intake as protein, compared to 15% in the control group. This protein intake in the experimental group would not be considered excessive given an upper limit of 35% of calorie intake set by the Food and Nutrition Board.*

12. Mangels R: Weight control the vegan way. *Vegetarian Journal* XXV (1), 2006.

    *This article provides suggestions for vegans, or people interested in following a vegan diet, who want to lose weight. Two eating plans are included that were developed for people who are moderately active, spending 30-60 minutes daily in moderate physical activity. The first eating plan has approximately 1500 calories and is designed for women who want to lose 1-2 pounds per week. The second has about 1900 calories and is designed for men who want to lose 1-2 pounds per week. Protein foods include kidney beans, chickpeas, and other beans; tofu; lite or plain soymilk; nuts and nut butters; seitan (say-than, wheat meat); and meat analogs. Recipes are also included.*

13. Newby PK: Risk of overweight and obesity among semivegetarian, lactovegetarian, and

vegan women. *American Journal of Clinical Nutrition* 81:1267, 2005.

*Semivegetarian women in this study were less likely to be overweight and obese compared to omnivorous women. Consuming more plant foods and less animal products may help individuals control their weight.*

14. Sabate J: The contribution of vegetarian diets to human health. *Forum of Nutrition* 56:218, 2005.

*Components of a healthy vegetarian diet include a variety of vegetables, fruits, whole-grain breads and cereals, legumes, and nuts. Such a diet contributes to overall health and increased longevity when these foods are emphasized.*

15. Sacks FM and others: Soy protein, iso-flavones, and cardiovascular health. An American Heart Association Science Advisory for Professionals From the Nutrition Committee. *Circulation* 113:1034, 2006.

*This scientific advisory evaluates recent work published on soy protein and its component isoflavones and their potential role in improving risk factors for cardiovascular disease. In the majority of studies, soy protein with isoflavones, as compared with milk or other proteins, decreased LDL cholesterol concentrations; the average effect was ~ 3% and no significant effects on HDL cholesterol, triglycerides, lipoprotein(a), or blood pressure were evident.*

*The authors conclude that soy products should be beneficial to cardiovascular and overall health because of their high content of polyunsaturated fats, fiber, vitamins, and minerals and low content of saturated fat.*

16. Taylor SL: Estimating prevalence of soy protein allergy. *The Soy Connection* 14 (2):1, 2006.

*This article discusses the issue of soy protein allergy. Although soy protein has been designated one of the major allergens by the U.S. Food and Drug Administration, rigorous prevalence data for this allergy are not available, and indirect evidence suggests it occurs less frequently than other common allergens including shellfish, peanuts, tree nuts, and fish.*

17. Trock BJ and others: Meta-analysis of soy intake and breast cancer risk. *Journal of the National Cancer Institute*, 98 (7):459, 2006.

*This study analyzed data from 18 previously published studies and concludes that consumption of soy foods among healthy women was associated with a significant reduction (14%) in breast cancer risk.*

18. WebWatch: Healthy Vegetarian Resources and Recipes. *Obesity Management* August, 2008.

*This summary of websites that provide vegetarian resources includes reviews of American*

*Dietetic Association Alliance Sites, sites that focus on Vegetarian Cooking and Recipes, and other sites with resources and directories, including one that specializes on the vegetarian teen.*

19. Who's the veggie-friendliest of them all? *Vegetarian Journal* XXVII, p. 14, 2008.

*The Vegetarian Resource Group evaluated the menus of the 400 largest restaurant chains in the United States. This article highlights the establishments that appeared to make the best effort at serving vegetarians of diverse needs. You can find more than 2,000 veggie-friendly restaurants at their website www.vrg.org.*

20. Xiao CW: Health effects of soy protein and isoflavones in humans. *Journal of Nutrition* 138: 1244S, 2008.

*The results of epidemiological and clinical studies have suggested that soy consumption may be associated with a lower incidence of certain chronic diseases and a reduction in the risk factors for cardiovascular disease. These results led to an FDA-approved food-labeling health claim for soy proteins in the prevention of coronary heart disease. This article reviews the evidence for health claims on the effects of soy protein and isoflavones in humans and concludes that the existing data are inconsistent or inadequate to support most of the suggested health benefits of consuming soy protein or ISF.*

## I. Protein and the Vegetarian

Alana is excited about all the health benefits that might accompany a vegetarian diet. However, she is concerned that she will not consume enough protein to meet her needs. She is also concerned about possible vitamin and mineral deficiencies. Use Nutrition-Calc Plus or a food composition table to calculate her protein intake and see if her concerns are valid.

|  | Protein (g) |
|---|---|
| **Breakfast**<br>Calcium fortified orange juice, 1 cup<br>Soy milk, 1 cup<br>Fortified bran flakes, 1 cup<br>Banana, medium |  |
| **Snack**<br>Calcium-enriched granola bar |  |
| **Lunch**<br>GardenBurger, 4 oz<br>Whole-wheat bun<br>Mustard, 1 tbsp<br>Soy cheese, 1 oz<br>Apple, medium<br>Green leaf lettuce, 1 ½ cups<br>Peanuts, 1 oz<br>Sunflower seeds, 1/4 cup<br>Tomato slices, 2<br>Mushrooms, 3<br>Vinaigrette salad dressing, 2 tbsp<br>Iced tea |  |
| **Dinner**<br>Kidney beans, ½ cup<br>Brown rice, 3/4 cup<br>Fortified margarine, 2 tbsp<br>Mixed vegetables, 1/4 cup<br>Hot tea |  |
| **Dessert**<br>Strawberries, ½ cup<br>Angel food cake, 1 small slice<br>Soy milk, ½ cup |  |
|  | TOTAL PROTEIN (grams) _____ |

Alana's diet contained 2150 kcal, with _____ grams (you fill in) of protein (Is this plenty for her?), 360 grams of carbohydrate, 57 grams of total dietary fat (only 9 grams of which came from saturated fat), and 50 grams of fiber. Her vitamin and mineral intake with respect to those of concern to vegetarians—vitamin B-12, vitamin D, calcium, iron, and zinc—met her needs.

## II. Meeting Protein Needs When Dieting to Lose Weight

Your father has been steadily gaining weight for the last 30 years and now has developed hypertension and type 2 diabetes as a result. His physician recommends that he lose some weight by following an 1800 kcal diet. You know that it will be important for your father to meet protein needs as he tries to lose weight. Design a 1-day diet for him that contains about 20% of calorie intake as protein. Table 6-2 will provide some help. Will this diet meet his protein RDA? Does the diet look like a plan you could also follow?

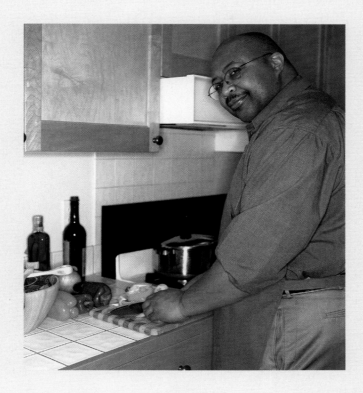

# CHAPTER 7 Energy Balance and Weight Control

## Student Learning Outcomes Chapter 7 is designed to allow you to:

1. Describe energy balance and the uses of energy by the body.

2. Compare methods to determine energy use by the body.

3. Discuss methods for assessing body composition and determining whether body weight and composition are healthy.

4. Outline the risks to health posed by overweight and obesity.

5. List and discuss characteristics of a sound weight-loss program

6. Describe why and how reduced calorie intake, behavior modification, and increased physical activity fit into a weight-loss plan.

7. Outline the benefits and hazards of various weight-loss methods for severe obesity.

8. Discuss the causes and treatment of underweight.

9. Evaluate popular weight-reduction diets and determine which are unsafe, doomed to fail, or both.

## Chapter Outline

Student Learning Outcomes

Refresh Your Memory

7.1 Energy Balance

7.2 Determination of Energy Use by the Body

7.3 Estimation of a Healthy Weight

7.4 Energy Imbalance

7.5 Why Some People Are Obese—Nature Versus Nurture

7.6 Treatment of Overweight and Obesity

7.7 Control of Calorie Intake—The Main Key to Weight Loss and Weight Maintenance

7.8 Regular Physical Activity—A Second Key to Weight Loss and Especially Important for Later Weight Maintenance

7.9 Behavior Modification—A Third Strategy for Weight Loss and Management

7.10 Professional Help for Weight Loss

7.11 Treatment of Underweight

Nutrition and Your Health: *Popular Diets—Cause for Concern*

Case Study: Choosing a Weight-Loss Program

Summary/Study Questions/Check Your Knowledge/Further Readings

Rate Your Plate

IN THE LAST 20 YEARS (THE YEARS SINCE MOST COLLEGE STUDENTS WERE BORN), THERE HAS BEEN A DRAMATIC INCREASE IN THE PERCENTAGE OF INDIVIDUALS WHO ARE OVERWEIGHT OR OBESE. The ranks of the obese are growing in North America and worldwide. Recall from Chapter 1 that an estimated 1 billion people in the world are overweight. This problem is increasing not only in the United States but also globally among affluent peoples and in developing countries where westernized diets (high-fat, high-calorie) are increasing in popularity. Excess weight increases the likelihood of many health problems, such as cardiovascular disease, cancer, hypertension, strokes, certain bone and joint disorders, and type 2 diabetes, especially if a person performs minimal physical activity.

Currently, most weight-reduction efforts fizzle before bodies fall into a healthy weight range. As suggested in this chapter's comic, typical popular ("fad") diets are generally monotonous, ineffective, and confusing. They may even endanger some populations, such as children, teenagers, pregnant women, and people with various health disorders. A more logical approach to weight loss is straightforward: (1) eat less; (2) increase physical activity; and (3) change problematic eating behaviors.

A national commitment has begun from a variety of groups, including government agencies, the food industry, health professionals, and communities, to address the growing weight problem in North America. It has become obvious that, without this national effort to promote weight maintenance and effective new approaches to making our social environment more favorable to maintaining healthy weight, the current trends will not be reversed (Fig. 7-1). Chapter 7 discusses these recommendations to help you understand obesity's causes, consequences, and potential treatments.

 **Refresh Your Memory**

As you begin your study of weight control in Chapter 7, you may want to review:

- Biological and social dimensions of food intake in Chapter 1
- The concept of energy density and appropriate serving sizes for foods in Chapter 2
- The role of fiber in weight regulation in Chapter 4
- The fat content of various foods in Chapter 5
- The long-term risks of high-protein diets in Chapter 6

What components make up a successful diet plan? What constitutes a "fad" diet? Why is overweight and obesity a growing problem worldwide? What might be the future consequences of this trend? Chapter 7 provides some answers.

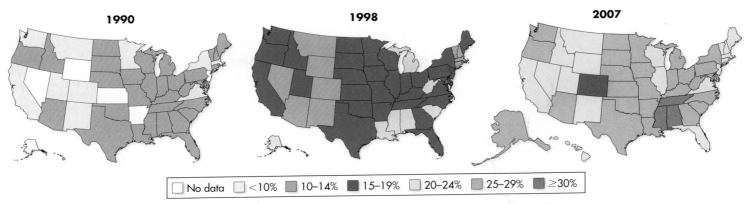

**1990**   **1998**   **2007**

| | | | | | | |
|---|---|---|---|---|---|---|
| ☐ No data | ☐ <10% | ◼ 10–14% | ◼ 15–19% | ☐ 20–24% | ◼ 25–29% | ◼ ≥30% |

**FIGURE 7-1** ▶ Obesity trends among U.S. adults: 1990, 1998, 2007 (BMI ≥ 30, or about 30 lb overweight for 5'4" person).

*Source: CDC Behavioral Risk Factor Surveillance System.*

## 7.1 Energy Balance

We begin this chapter with some good news and some bad news. The good news is that if you stay at a healthy body weight, you increase your chances of living a long and healthy life. The bad news is that currently 65% of all North American adults are overweight, significantly more than in the 1980s. Of those, about 45% (30% of the total population) are obese. There is a good chance that any of us could become part of those statistics if we do not pay attention to the prevention of significant weight gain in adulthood. Gaining more than 10 pounds or 2 inches in waist circumference are signals that a re-evaluation of diet and lifestyle is in order.

*There is no quick cure for overweight, despite what the advertisements claim. Successful weight loss comes from hard work and commitment.* A combination of decreased calorie intake, increased physical activity, and behavior modification is considered to be the most reliable treatment for the overweight condition. And without a doubt, the prevention of the overweight condition in the first place is the most successful approach.

**The Growing Overweight/ Obesity Problem**

Adults 20 to 74 who are overweight or obese:

| | |
|---|---|
| 1960–1962 | **45%** |
| 1971–1974 | **47%** |
| 1976–1980 | **47%** |
| 1988–1994 | **56%** |
| 1999–today | **64.5%** |

### Positive and Negative Energy Balance

A healthy weight can result from paying more attention to the important concept of **energy balance.** Think of energy balance as an equation:

Energy Input    Energy Output
(calories from food intake)   =   (metabolism; digestion, absorption, and transport of nutrients; physical activity)

The balance of calories (measured in kcals) on the two sides of this equation can influence energy stores, especially the amount of triglyceride stored in adipose tissue (Fig. 7-2). Fat tissue contains about 3500 calories per pound. Therefore to lose one pound of fat per week, calorie intake must be decreased by about 500 calories per day. When energy input is greater than energy output, the result is **positive energy balance.** The excess calories consumed are stored, which results in weight gain. There are some situations in which positive energy balance is normal and healthy. During pregnancy, a surplus of calories supports the developing fetus. Infants and children require a positive energy balance for growth and development. In adults, however, even a small positive energy balance is usually in the form of fat storage rather than muscle and bone and, over time, can cause body weight to climb.

**energy balance** The state in which energy intake, in the form of food and beverages, matches the energy expended, primarily through basal metabolism and physical activity.

**positive energy balance** The state in which energy intake is greater than energy expended, generally resulting in weight gain.

**FIGURE 7-2** ▶ A model for energy balance—input vs. output. This figure depicts energy balance in practical terms.

| Intake | Output | Weight Change | Energy Balance |
|---|---|---|---|
| | | | **Energy balance (equilibriuim)** |
| 3000 kcal | 3000 kcal | No change | Calories in — Calories out |
| | | | **Positive energy balance** |
| 4000 kcal | 2000 kcal | Increase | Calories in — Calories out |
| | | | **Negative energy balance** |
| 2000 kcal | 3000 kcal | Decrease | Calories in — Calories out |

## CRITICAL THINKING

A 26-year-old classmate of yours has been thinking about the process of aging. One of the things she fears most as she gets older is gaining weight. How would you explain energy balance to her?

**negative energy balance** The state in which energy intake is less than energy expended, resulting in weight loss.

On the other hand, if energy input is less than energy output, there is a calorie deficit and **negative energy balance** results. A negative energy balance is necessary for successful weight loss. It is important to realize that during negative energy balance, weight loss involves a reduction in both lean and adipose tissue, not just "fat."

The maintenance of energy balance substantially contributes to health and well-being in adults by minimizing the risk of developing many common health problems. Adulthood is often a time of subtle increases in weight gain, which eventually turns into obesity if left unchecked. The process of aging does not cause weight gain; rather the problem stems from a pattern of excess food intake coupled with limited physical activity and slower metabolism. Let's look in detail at the factors that affect the energy balance equation.

# Energy Intake

Energy needs are met by food intake, represented by the number of calories eaten each day. Determining the appropriate amount and type of food to match our energy needs is a challenge for many of us. Our desire to consume food and the ability of our bodies to use it efficiently are survival mechanisms that have evolved with humans. However, because of current North American food supplies and accessibility, many of us are now too successful in obtaining food energy. The abundant food supply has essentially replaced the need to store body fat. Given the wide availability of food in vending machines, drive-up windows, social gatherings, and fast-food restaurants—combined with *super-sized* portions—it is no wonder that the average adult is 8 pounds heavier than just 10 years ago. In response to this cultural trend of food being widely available, "defensive eating" (i.e., making careful and conscious food choices, especially in regard to portion size) on a continual basis is important for many of us.

The number of calories in a food is determined with an instrument called a **bomb calorimeter.** This calorie determination is described in Figure 7-3. The bomb calorimeter measures the amount of calories coming from carbohydrate, fat, protein, and alcohol. Recall that carbohydrates yield about 4 kcal per gram, proteins yield about 4 kcal per gram, fats yield about 9 kcal per gram, and alcohol yields 7 kcal per gram. These energy figures have been adjusted for (1) our ability to digest the food and (2) substances in food, such as fibrous plant parts that burn in the bomb calorimeter but do not provide calories to the human body. The figures are then rounded to whole numbers. However, today it is also possible and more common to determine the calorie content of a food by quantifying its carbohydrate, protein, and fat (and possibly alcohol) content. Then the kcal per gram factors listed previously are used to calculate the total kcals. (Recall that Chapter 1 showed how to do this calculation.)

# Energy Output

So far, some factors concerning energy intake have been discussed. Now let's look at the other side of the equation—energy output.

The body uses energy for three general purposes: basal metabolism; physical activity; and digestion, absorption, and processing of ingested nutrients. A fourth minor form of energy output, known as thermogenesis, refers to energy expended during fidgeting or shivering in response to cold (Fig. 7-4).

▲ The cultural trend of serving large quantities can easily lead to positive energy balance. Sharing your meal with another person is a good way to avoid overeating when served large portions.

**FIGURE 7-3** ▶ Bomb calorimeters measure calorie content by igniting and burning a dried portion of food. The burning food raises the temperature of the water surrounding the chamber holding the food. The increase in water temperature indicates the number of kilocalories in the food because 1 kilocalorie equals the amount of heat needed to raise the temperature of 1 kg of water by 1°C.

**FIGURE 7-4** ▶ The components of energy intake and expenditure. This figure incorporates the major variables that influence energy balance. *Remember that alcohol is an additional source of energy for some of us.* The size of each component shows the relative contribution of that component to energy balance.

**basal metabolism** The minimal amount of calories the body uses to support itself in a fasting state when resting (e.g., 12 hours for both) and awake in a warm, quiet environment. It amounts to roughly 1 kcal per kilogram per hour for men and 0.9 kcal per kilogram per hour for women; these values are often referred to as *basal metabolic rate (BMR)*.

**resting metabolism** The amount of calories the body uses when the person has not eaten in 4 hours and is resting (e.g., 15 to 30 minutes) and awake in a warm, quiet environment. It is roughly 6% higher than basal metabolism due to the less strict criteria for the test; often referred to as *resting metabolic rate (RMR)*.

**lean body mass** Body weight minus fat storage weight equals lean body mass. This includes organs such as the brain, muscles, and liver, as well as bone and blood and other body fluids.

**W**hile a person is resting, the percentage of total energy use and corresponding energy use by various organs is approximately as follows:

| | | |
|---|---|---|
| Brain | 19% | 265 kcal/day |
| Skeletal muscle | 18% | 250 kcal/day |
| Liver | 27% | 380 kcal/day |
| Kidney | 10% | 140 kcal/day |
| Heart | 7% | 100 kcal/day |
| Other | 19% | 265 kcal/day |

**Basal Metabolism.** **Basal metabolism** is expressed as basal metabolic rate (BMR) and represents the minimal amount of calories expended in a fasting state (for 12 hours or more) to keep a resting, awake body alive in a warm, quiet environment. For a sedentary person, basal metabolism accounts for about 60% to 70% of total energy use by the body. Some of the processes involved include the beating of the heart, respiration by the lungs, and the activity of other organs such as the liver, brain, and kidney. It does not include energy used for physical activity or digestion, absorption, and processing of recently consumed nutrients. If the person is not fasting or completely rested, the term **resting metabolism** is used and expressed as resting metabolic rate (RMR). An individual's RMR is typically 6% higher than his or her BMR.

To see how basal metabolism contributes to energy needs, consider a 130-pound woman. First, knowing that there are 2.2 pounds for every kilogram, convert her weight into metric units:

$$130 \text{ lbs} \div 2.2 \text{ lbs/kilograms} = 59 \text{ kilograms}$$

Then, using a rough estimate of basal metabolic rate of 0.9 kcal per kilogram per hour for an average female (1.0 kcal per kilogram per hour is used for an average male), calculate her basal metabolic rate:

$$59 \text{ kg} \times 0.9 \text{ kcal/kg} = 53 \text{ kcal per hour}$$

Finally, use this hourly basal metabolic rate to find her basal metabolic rate for an entire day:

$$53 \text{ kcal/hr} \times 24 \text{ hrs} = 1272 \text{ kcal}$$

These calculations give only an estimate of basal metabolism, as it can vary 25% to 30% among individuals. Factors that increase basal metabolism include:

- Greater **lean body mass**
- Larger body surface area per body volume
- Male gender (caused by greater lean body mass)
- Body temperature (fever or cold environmental conditions)
- Thyroid hormones
- Aspects of nervous system activity (release of norepinephrine)
- Pregnancy
- Caffeine and tobacco use. (Using the practice of smoking to control body weight is not recommended as too many health risks are increased.)

Of those factors, the amount of lean body mass a person has is the most important one.

In contrast to factors that increase basal metabolism, a low calorie intake, such as that during an extreme diet regime, decreases basal metabolism by about 10% to 20% (about 150 to 300 kcal per day) as the body shifts into a conservation mode. This is a barrier to sustained weight loss during dieting that involves extremely low calorie diets. In addition, the effects of aging make weight maintenance a challenge. As lean body mass slowly and steadily decreases, basal metabolism declines 1% to 2% for each decade past the age of 30. However, because physical activity aids in maintenance of lean body mass, remaining active as one ages helps to preserve a high basal metabolism and, in turn, aids in weight control.

**Energy for Physical Activity.** Physical activity increases energy expenditure above and beyond basal energy needs by as much as 25% to 40%. In choosing to be active or inactive, we determine much of our total calorie expenditure for a day. Calorie expenditure from physical activity varies widely among people. For example, climbing stairs rather than riding the elevator, walking rather than driving to the store, and standing in a bus rather than sitting increase physical activity and, hence, energy use. The alarming incidence of and recent increase in obesity in North America are partially the result of our inactivity. Jobs demand less physical activity, and leisure time is often spent in front of a television or computer.

**Thermic Effect of Food (TEF).** In addition to basal metabolism and physical activity, the body uses energy to digest food, and absorb and further process the nutrients recently consumed. Energy used for these tasks is referred to as the **thermic effect of food (TEF).** TEF is similar to a sales tax—it is like being charged about 5% to 10% for the total amount of calories you eat to cover the cost of processing that food eaten. We may even recognize this increase in metabolism as a warming of the body during and right after a meal. Because of this "tax," you must eat between 105 and 110 kcal (5-10 kcal extra) for every 100 kcal needed for basal metabolism and physical activity. If your daily calorie intake was 3000 kcal, TEF would account for 150 to 300 kcal. As with other components of energy output, the total amount can vary somewhat among individuals.

Food composition influences TEF. For example, the TEF value for a protein-rich meal is 20% to 30% of the calories consumed and is higher than that of a carbohydrate-rich (5% to 10%) or fat-rich (0% to 3%) meal. This is because it takes more energy to metabolize amino acids into fat than to convert glucose into glycogen or transfer absorbed fat into adipose stores. In addition, large meals result in higher TEF values than the same amount of food eaten over many hours.

**Thermogenesis.** **Thermogenesis** represents the increase in nonvoluntary physical activity triggered by cold conditions or overeating. Some examples of nonvoluntary activities include shivering when cold, fidgeting, maintenance of muscle tone, and maintaining body posture when not lying down. Studies have shown that some people are able to resist weight gain from overfeeding by inducing thermogenesis, while others are not able to do so to a great extent.

The contribution of thermogenesis to overall calorie output is fairly small. The combination of basal metabolism and TEF accounts for 70% to 80% of energy used by a sedentary person. The remaining 20% to 30% is used mostly for physical activity, with a small amount used for thermogenesis.

**Brown adipose tissue** is a specialized form of adipose tissue that participates in thermogenesis. It is found in small amounts in infants. The brown appearance results from its rich blood flow. Brown adipose tissue contributes to thermogenesis by releasing some of the energy from energy-yielding nutrients into the environment as heat. In infants, brown adipose tissue contributes as much as 5% of body weight and is thought to be important for heat regulation. Hibernating animals also use brown adipose tissue to generate heat to withstand a long winter. Adults have very little brown adipose tissue, and its role in adulthood is unknown.

▲ Classwork leads to mental stress but puts little physical stress on the body. Hence, energy needs are only about 1.5 kcal per minute.

**T**he TEF value for alcohol is 20%.

**thermic effect of food (TEF)** The increase in metabolism that occurs during the digestion, absorption, and metabolism of energy-yielding nutrients. This represents 5% to 10% of calories consumed.

**thermogenesis** This term encompasses the ability of humans to regulate body temperature within narrow limits (thermoregulation). Two visible examples of thermogenesis are fidgeting and shivering when cold.

**brown adipose tissue** A specialized form of adipose tissue that produces large amounts of heat by metabolizing energy-yielding nutrients without synthesizing much useful energy for the body. The unused energy is released as heat.

## CONCEPT CHECK

Energy balance involves matching energy intake with energy output. Energy content of food is expressed in kcals and can be determined using a bomb calorimeter. This analysis yields the 4-9-4-7 estimates for the kcals in a gram of carbohydrate, fat, protein, and alcohol, respectively.

The body uses energy for four main purposes:

1.  Basal metabolism (60% to 70% of total energy output) represents the minimal amount of calories needed to maintain the body at rest. Primary determinants of basal metabolic rate include quantity of lean body mass, amount of body surface, and thyroid hormone concentrations in the bloodstream.
2.  Physical activity calorie expenditure (20% to 30% of total energy output) represents calorie use for total body cell metabolism above what is needed during rest.
3.  Thermic effect of food (5% to 10% of total energy output) represents the calories needed to digest food and absorb and process nutrients recently consumed.
4.  Thermogenesis (small, variable percentage of total energy output) includes nonvoluntary, heat-producing activities, such as fidgeting, as well as shivering when cold.

**FIGURE 7-5** ▶ Indirect calorimetry measures oxygen intake and carbon dioxide output to determine energy expended during daily activities.

**direct calorimetry** A method of determining a body's energy use by measuring heat released from the body. An insulated chamber is usually used.

**indirect calorimetry** A method to measure energy use by the body by measuring oxygen uptake. Formulas are then used to convert this gas exchange value into energy use.

# 7.2 Determination of Energy Use by the Body

The amount of energy a body uses can be measured by both direct and indirect calorimetry or can be estimated based on height, weight, degree of physical activity, and age.

## Direct and Indirect Calorimetry

**Direct calorimetry** measures the amount of body heat released by a person. The subject is put into an insulated chamber, often the size of a small bedroom, and body heat released raises the temperature of a layer of water surrounding the chamber. A kcal, as you recall, is related to the amount of heat required to raise the temperature of water. By measuring the water temperature in the direct calorimeter before and after the body releases heat, scientists can determine the energy expended.

Direct calorimetry works because almost all the energy used by the body eventually leaves as heat. However, few studies use direct calorimetry, mostly because of its expense and complexity.

The most commonly used method of **indirect calorimetry** measures the amount of oxygen a person consumes instead of measuring heat output (Fig. 7-5). A predictable relationship exists between the body's use of energy and oxygen. For example, when metabolizing a typical mixed diet of the energy-yielding nutrients, carbohydrate, fat, and protein, the human body uses 1 liter of oxygen to yield about 4.85 kcal of energy.

Instruments to measure oxygen consumption for indirect calorimetry are widely used. They can be mounted on carts and rolled up to a hospital bed or carried in backpacks while a person plays tennis or jogs. There are even newly developed hand-held instruments (Body Gem). Tables showing energy costs of various forms of exercises rely on information gained from indirect calorimetry studies.

## Estimates of Energy Needs

As covered in Chapter 2, the Food and Nutrition Board has published a number of formulas to estimate energy needs, called Estimated Energy Requirements (EER). Those for adults are shown here (remember to do multiplication and division before addition and subtraction). (Formulas for pregnant women, lactating women, children, and teenagers, are listed in Chapters 14 and 15.) The calories used for basal metabolism are already factored into these formulas.

*Estimated Energy Requirement Calculation for Men 19 years and older*

$$\text{EER} = 662 - (9.53 \times \text{AGE}) + \text{PA} \times (15.91 \times \text{WT} + 539.6 \times \text{HT})$$

*Estimated Energy Requirement Calculation for Women 19 years and older*

$$\text{EER} = 354 - (6.91 \times \text{AGE}) + \text{PA} \times (9.36 \times \text{WT} + 726 \times \text{HT})$$

The variables in the formulas correspond to the following:

$$\text{EER} = \text{Estimated Energy Requirement}$$
$$\text{AGE} = \text{age in years}$$
$$\text{PA} = \text{Physical Activity Estimate (see following table)}$$
$$\text{WT} = \text{weight in kilograms (pounds} \div 2.2)$$
$$\text{HT} = \text{height in meters (inches} \div 39.4)$$

Physical Activity (PA) Estimates

| Activity Level | PA (Men) | PA (Women) |
|---|---|---|
| Sedentary (e.g., no exercise) | 1.00 | 1.00 |
| Low activity (e.g., walks the equivalent of 2 miles per day at 3 to 4 mph) | 1.11 | 1.12 |
| Active (e.g., walks the equivalent of 7 miles per day at 3 to 4 mph) | 1.25 | 1.27 |
| Very active (e.g., walks the equivalent of 17 miles per day at 3 to 4 mph) | 1.48 | 1.45 |

The following is a sample calculation for a man who is 25 years old, 5 feet, 9 inches (1.75 meters), 154 pounds (70 kilograms), and has an active lifestyle. His EER is:

$$EER = 662 - (9.53 \times 25) + 1.25 \times (15.91 \times 70 + 539.6 \times 1.75) = 2997 \text{ kcal}$$

The next equation is a sample calculation for a woman who is 25 years old, 5 feet, 4 inches (1.62 meters), 120 pounds (54.5 kilograms), and has an active lifestyle. Her EER is:

$$EER = 354 - (6.91 \times 25) + 1.27 \times (9.36 \times 54.5 + 726 \times 1.62) = 2323 \text{ kcal}$$

You have determined the man's EER to be about 3000 kcal and the woman's EER to be about 2300 kcal per day. Remember that this is only an estimate; many other factors, such as genetics and hormones, can affect actual energy needs.

A simple method of tracking your energy expenditure, and thus your energy needs, is to use the forms in Appendix E. Begin by taking an entire 24-hour period and listing all activities performed, including sleep. Record the number of minutes spent in each activity; the total should equal 1440 minutes (24 hours). Next record the energy cost for each activity in kcal per minute following the directions in Appendix E. Multiply the energy cost by the minutes. This gives the energy expended for each activity. Total all the kcal values. This gives your estimated energy expenditure for the day.

The MyPyramid.gov website provides one of the easiest tools to estimate your calorie needs. Figure 7-6 shows the low and high ends of the range of activity levels and their calorie recommendations for the various age and gender groups.

| MyPyramid Calorie Guidelines | | |
|---|---|---|
| **Children** | **Sedentary** ⟶ | **Active** |
| 2–3 years | 1000 ⟶ | 1400 |
| **Females** | **Sedentary** ⟶ | **Active** |
| 4–8 years | 1200 ⟶ | 1800 |
| 9–13 | 1600 ⟶ | 2200 |
| 14–18 | 1800 ⟶ | 2400 |
| 19–30 | 2000 ⟶ | 2400 |
| 31–50 | 1800 ⟶ | 2200 |
| 51+ | 1600 ⟶ | 2200 |
| **Males** | **Sedentary** ⟶ | **Active** |
| 4–8 years | 1200 ⟶ | 2000 |
| 9–13 | 1800 ⟶ | 2600 |
| 14–18 | 2200 ⟶ | 3200 |
| 19–30 | 2400 ⟶ | 3000 |
| 31–50 | 2200 ⟶ | 3000 |
| 51+ | 2000 ⟶ | 2800 |

**FIGURE 7-6** ▶ MyPyramid Calorie Guidelines for age and gender groups.

## CONCEPT CHECK

Energy use by the body can be measured as heat given off by direct calorimetry or as oxygen used by indirect calorimetry. A person's Estimated Energy Requirement can be calculated based on the following factors: gender, height, weight, age, and amount of physical activity.

# 7.3 Estimation of a Healthy Weight

Numerous methods are used to establish what body weight should be, typically called *healthy weight*. Healthy weight is currently the preferred term to use for weight recommendations. Older terms, such as *ideal weight* and *desirable weight*, are subjective and are no longer used in medical literature. Several tables exist, generally based on weight-for-height. These tables arise from studies of large population groups. When applied to a population, they provide good estimates of weight associated with health and longevity. However, they do not necessarily indicate the healthiest body weight

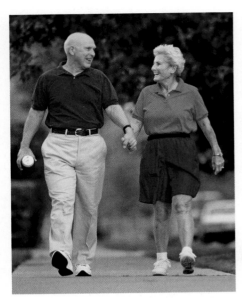

▲ Physical activity, such as walking, is an important component of our energy expenditure.

**O**ne BMI unit = 6–7 pounds

**body mass index (BMI)** Weight (in kilograms) divided by height (in meters) squared; a value of 25 and above indicates overweight and a value of 30 and above indicates obesity.

for each individual. For example, *athletes with large, lean body mass but low-fat content will have greater healthy weights than sedentary individuals.*

Overall, the individual, under a physician's guidance, should establish a "personal" healthy weight (or need for weight reduction) based on weight history, fat distribution patterns, family history of weight-related disease, and current health status. Evidence of the following weight-related conditions is important:

- Hypertension
- Elevated LDL-cholesterol
- Family history of obesity, cardiovascular disease, or certain forms of cancer (e.g., uterus, colon)
- Pattern of fat distribution in the body
- Elevated blood glucose

This assessment points out how well the person is tolerating any existing excess weight. Thus, current height/weight standards are only a rough guide. On a more practical note, other questions can be pertinent: What is the least one has weighed as an adult for at least a year? What is the largest size clothing one would be happy with? What weight has one been able to maintain during previous diets without feeling constantly hungry? Furthermore, a healthy lifestyle may make a more important contribution to a person's health status than the number on the scale. Fit and overweight are not necessarily mutually exclusive (although not often seen together), and neither is thin synonymous with healthy if the person is not also physically active.

### Body Mass Index (BMI)

For the past 50 years, weight-for-height tables issued by the Metropolitan Life Insurance Company have been the typical way healthy weight was established. These tables are organized by gender and frame size, predicting the weight range at a specific height that was associated with the greatest longevity. The latest table (issued in 1983) and methods for determining frame size can be found in Appendix G.

Currently **body mass index (BMI)** is the preferred weight-for-height standard because it is the clinical measurement most closely related to body fat content (Fig. 7-7).

Body mass index is calculated as

$$\frac{body\ weight\ (in\ kilograms)}{height^2\ (in\ meters)}$$

An alternate method for calculating BMI is

$$\frac{weight\ (pounds) \times 703}{height^2\ (inches)}$$

Figure 7-8 lists the BMI for various heights and weights. A healthy weight-for-height is a BMI between 18.5 to 24.9. Health risks from excess weight may begin when the body mass index is 25 or more. What is your BMI? How much would your weight need to change to yield a BMI of 25? 30? These are general cut-off values for the presence of overweight and obesity, respectively. BMI offers another way to define obesity (Fig. 7-8).

| 30–39.9 | Obese | Increased health risk |
| 40 or greater | Severely obese | Major health risk. The number of North Americans falling into this category is increasing rapidly. |

The concept of body mass index is convenient to use because the values apply to both men and women (i.e., gender neutral). However, any weight-for-height standard is a crude measure. Keep in mind, also, that a BMI of 25 to 29.9 is a marker of *overweight* (compared to a standard population) and not necessarily a marker of *overfat*. Many men (especially athletes) have a BMI greater than 25 because of extra muscle tissue. Also, very short adults (under 5 feet tall) may have high BMIs that may not reflect overweight or fatness. For this reason, BMI should be used only as a screening test for overweight or obesity. Even agreed upon weight standards for BMI are not for everyone. Adult BMIs should not be applied to children, still growing adolescents, frail older people, pregnant and lactating women, and highly muscular individuals. Pregnant women and children have unique BMI standards (see Chapters 14 and 15).

Still, overfat and overweight conditions generally appear together. The focus is on BMI in clinical settings mainly because this is easier to measure than total body fat.

## Putting Healthy Weight into Perspective

Listening to the body for hunger cues, regularly eating a healthy diet, and remaining physically active (not to be overlooked) eventually helps one maintain an appropriate height/weight value. This concept will be further addressed in the upcoming discussion on treatment for obesity. Another school of thought is to let nature take its course with regard to body weight. Support for this proposal is that after weight is lost during dieting, people often regain their original weight plus more. The clearest idea regarding a healthy weight is that it is personal. Weight has to be considered in terms of health, not a mathematical calculation.

**FIGURE 7-7** ▶ Estimates of body shapes at different BMI values.

### Weight in pounds

| Height | 120 | 130 | 140 | 150 | 160 | 170 | 180 | 190 | 200 | 210 | 220 | 230 | 240 | 250 |
|---|---|---|---|---|---|---|---|---|---|---|---|---|---|---|
| 4'6" | 29 | 31 | 34 | 36 | 39 | 41 | 43 | 46 | 48 | 51 | 53 | 56 | 58 | 60 |
| 4'8" | 27 | 29 | 31 | 34 | 36 | 38 | 40 | 43 | 45 | 47 | 49 | 52 | 51 | 56 |
| 4'10" | 25 | 27 | 29 | 31 | 34 | 36 | 38 | 40 | 42 | 44 | 46 | 48 | 50 | 52 |
| 5'0" | 23 | 25 | 27 | 29 | 31 | 33 | 35 | 37 | 39 | 41 | 43 | 45 | 47 | 49 |
| 5'2" | 22 | 24 | 26 | 27 | 29 | 31 | 33 | 35 | 37 | 38 | 40 | 42 | 44 | 46 |
| 5'4" | 21 | 22 | 24 | 26 | 28 | 29 | 31 | 33 | 34 | 36 | 38 | 40 | 41 | 43 |
| 5'6" | 19 | 21 | 23 | 24 | 26 | 27 | 29 | 31 | 32 | 34 | 36 | 37 | 39 | 40 |
| 5'8" | 18 | 20 | 21 | 23 | 24 | 26 | 27 | 29 | 30 | 32 | 34 | 35 | 37 | 38 |
| 5'10" | 17 | 19 | 20 | 22 | 23 | 24 | 26 | 27 | 29 | 30 | 32 | 33 | 35 | 36 |
| 6'0" | 16 | 18 | 19 | 20 | 22 | 23 | 24 | 26 | 27 | 28 | 30 | 31 | 33 | 34 |
| 6'2" | 15 | 17 | 18 | 19 | 21 | 22 | 23 | 24 | 26 | 27 | 28 | 30 | 31 | 32 |
| 6'4" | 15 | 16 | 17 | 18 | 20 | 21 | 22 | 23 | 24 | 26 | 27 | 28 | 29 | 30 |
| 6'6" | 14 | 15 | 16 | 17 | 19 | 20 | 21 | 22 | 23 | 24 | 25 | 27 | 28 | 29 |
| 6'8" | 13 | 14 | 15 | 17 | 18 | 19 | 20 | 21 | 22 | 23 | 24 | 26 | 26 | 28 |

Height in feet and inches

☐ Healthy weight   ☐ Overweight   ☐ Obese

Developed by the National Center for Health Statistics in collaboration with the National Center for Chronic Disease Prevention and Health Promotion

**FIGURE 7-8** ▶ Convenient height/weight table based on BMI. A healthy weight for height generally falls within a BMI range of 18.5–24.9 kilograms/meters$^2$.

▲ A high BMI may not reflect overweight or fatness. Extra muscle tissue can result in a BMI greater than 25.

**T**he total cost attributable to weight-related disease is about $90 billion annually in the United States. Half of this cost is borne by the taxpayers through Medicare and Medicaid.

**underwater weighing** A method of estimating total body fat by weighing the individual on a standard scale and then weighing him or her again submerged in water. The difference between the two weights is used to estimate total body volume.

**air displacement** A method for estimating body composition that makes use of the volume of space taken up by a body inside a small chamber.

**bioelectrical impedance** The method to estimate total body fat that uses a low-energy electrical current. The more fat storage a person has, the more impedance (resistance) to electrical flow will be exhibited.

**CONCEPT CHECK**

Healthy body weight is generally determined in a clinical setting using a body mass index or another weight-for-height standard. The presence of existing weight-related diseases should be factored into the determination of healthy body weight. Total health history and lifestyle should be the major considerations when determining healthy weight.

## 7.4 Energy Imbalance

If calorie intake exceeds output over time, overweight (and often obesity) is a likely result. Often, health problems eventually follow (Table 7-1). As just discussed, BMI values can be used as a convenient clinical tool to estimate overweight (BMI ≥ 25), obesity (BMI ≥ 30), and severe obesity (BMI ≥ 40) in individuals greater than 20 years of age. Medical experts, however, recommend that an individual's diagnosis of obesity should not be based primarily on body weight but, rather, on the total amount of fat in the body, the location of body fat, and the presence or absence of weight-related medical problems.

### Estimating Body Fat Content and Diagnosing Obesity

Body fat varies widely among individuals and can range from 2% to 70% of body weight. Desirable amounts of body fat are about 8% to 24% for men and 21% to 35% for women. Men with over 24% body fat and women with over about 35% body fat are considered obese. The higher range of body fat percentage for women is needed physiologically to maintain reproductive functions, including estrogen production.

To measure body fat content accurately using typical methods, both body weight and body volume of the person must be known. Body weight is easy to measure on a conventional scale. Of the typical methods used to estimate body volume, **underwater weighing** is the most accurate. This technique determines body volume using the difference between conventional body weight and body weight under water, along with the relative densities of fat tissue and lean tissue, and a specific mathematical formula. This procedure requires that an individual be totally submerged in a tank of water, with a trained technician directing the procedure (Fig. 7-9). **Air displacement** is another method of determining body volume. Body volume is quantified by measuring the space a person takes up inside a measurement chamber, such as the BodPod (Fig. 7-10). A less accurate method to measure body volume is to submerge a person in a tank and observe the level of the water before and after submersion. The volume of the displaced water is then calculated.

Once body volume is known, it can be used along with body weight in the following equation to calculate body density. Then using body density, body fat content finally can be determined.

$$\text{Body density} = \frac{\text{body weight}}{\text{body volume}}$$
$$\% \text{ body fat} = (495 \div \text{body density}) - 450$$

For example, assume that the individual in the underwater weighing tank in Figure 7-9 has a body density of 1.06 grams per centimeter$^3$. We can use the second formula to calculate that he has 17% body fat ([495 ÷ 1.06] − 450 = 17).

Skinfold thickness is also a common anthropometric method to estimate total body fat content, although there are some limits to its accuracy. Clinicians use calipers to measure the fat layer directly under the skin at multiple sites and then plug these values into a mathematical formula (Fig. 7-11).

The technique of **bioelectrical impedance** is also used to estimate body fat content. The instrument sends a painless, low-energy electrical current to and from the

**TABLE 7-1** Health Problems Associated with Excess Body Fat

| Health Problem | Partially Attributable To |
| --- | --- |
| Surgical risk | Increased anesthesia needs, as well as greater risk of wound infections (the latter is linked to a decrease in immune function) |
| Pulmonary disease and sleep disorders | Excess weight over lungs and pharynx |
| Type 2 diabetes | Enlarged adipose cells, which poorly bind insulin and poorly respond to the message insulin sends to the cell; less synthesis of factors that aid insulin action, and greater synthesis of factors by adipose cells that lessen insulin action |
| Hypertension | Increased miles of blood vessels found in the adipose tissue, increased blood volume, and increased resistance to blood flow related to hormones made by adipose cells |
| Cardiovascular disease (e.g., coronary heart disease and stroke) | Increases in LDL-cholesterol and triglyceride values, low HDL-cholesterol, decreased physical activity, and increased synthesis of blood clotting and inflamatory factors by enlarged adipose cells. A greater risk for heart failure is also seen, due in part to altered heart rhythm. |
| Bone and joint disorders (including gout) | Excess pressure put on knee, ankle, and hip joints |
| Gallstones | Increased cholesterol content of bile |
| Skin disorders | Trapping of moisture and microorganisms in tissue folds |
| Various cancers, such as in the kidney, gall-bladder, colon and rectum, uterus (women), and prostate gland (men) | Estrogen production by adipose cells; animal studies suggest excess calorie intake encourages tumor development |
| Shorter stature (in some forms of obesity) | Earlier onset of puberty |
| Pregnancy risks | More difficult delivery, increased number of birth defects, and increased needs for anesthesia |
| Reduced physical agility and increased risk of accidents and falls | Excess weight that impairs movement |
| Menstrual irregularities and infertility | Hormones produced by adipose cells, such as estrogen |
| Vision problems | Cataracts and other eye disorders are more often present |
| Premature death | A variety of risk factors for disease listed in this table |
| Infections | Reduced immune system activity |
| Liver damage and eventual failure | Excess fat accumulation in the liver |
| Erectile dysfunction in men | Low-grade inflammation caused by excess fat mass and reduced function of the cells lining the blood vessels associated with being overweight |

The greater the degree of obesity, the more likely and the more serious these health problems generally become. They are much more likely to appear in people who show an upper-body fat distribution pattern and/or are greater than twice healthy body weight.

body via wires and electrode patches to estimate body fat. This estimation is based on the assumption that adipose tissue resists electrical flow more than lean tissue because it has a lower electrolyte and water content than lean tissue. More adipose tissue therefore means proportionately greater electrical resistance. Within a few seconds, bioelectrical impedance analyzers convert body electrical resistance into an approximate estimate of total body fat, as long as body hydration status is normal (Fig. 7-12). Body composition monitors, better known as body fat calculators, that use bioelectric impedence are now available for home use. These machines are similar in shape and use to bathroom scales but their main purpose is to measure body fat. A current passes easily through conductive foot pads and/or handheld electrodes. These in-home devices will hopefully encourage people to be less concerned with what they weigh than whether their weight comes from fat or muscle.

**FIGURE 7-9** ▶ Underwater weighing. In this technique the subject exhales as much air as possible and then holds his or her breath and bends over at the waist. Once the subject is totally submerged, the underwater weight is recorded. Using this value, body volume can be calculated.

**FIGURE 7-10** ▶ BodPod. This device determines body volume based on the volume of displaced air, measured as a person sits in a sealed chamber for a few minutes.

**FIGURE 7-11** ▶ Skinfold measurements. Using proper technique and calibrated equipment, skinfold measurements around the body can be used to predict body fat content in about 10 minutes. Measurements are made at several locations including the triceps (photo and drawing) skinfolds.

Caliper

Triceps brachii muscle

Skin

Bone

Fat

**FIGURE 7-12** ▶ Bioelectrical impedance estimates total body fat in less than 5 minutes and is based on the principle that body fat resists the flow of electricity, since it is low in water and electrolytes. The degree of resistance to electrical flow is used to estimate body fatness.

A more advanced determination of body fat content can be made using **dual energy X-ray absorptiometry (DEXA).** DEXA is considered the most accurate way to determine body fat, but the equipment is expensive and not widely available for this use. This X-ray system allows the clinician to separate body weight into three separate components—fat, fat-free soft tissue, and bone mineral. The usual whole-body scan requires about 5 to 20 minutes and the dose of radiation is less than a chest X ray. An assessment of bone mineral density and the risk of osteoporosis also can be made using this method (Fig. 7-13).

Another method to assess body fat is to measure total-body electrical conductance (TOBEC) when placed in an electromagnetic field. Still another method, convenient and inexpensive, but not very accurate is **near-infrared reactance.** This method exposes the bicep muscle to a beam of near-infrared light and assesses the interactions of the light beam with fat and lean tissues in the upper arm after only 2 seconds.

In summary, although the DEXA is considered most accurate, the underwater weighing and air displacement methods of body fat estimation are also accurate because both body weight and body volume are measured. The adaptation of the bioelectrical impedence technology for in-home use is also a useful tool, providing valuable information about whether weight gain is coming from fat or muscle.

## Using Body Fat Distribution to Further Evaluate Obesity

In addition to the amount of fat we store, the location of that body fat is an important predictor of health risks. Some people store fat in upper-body areas, whereas others store fat lower on the body. Excess fat in either location generally spells trouble, but each storage space also has its unique risks. **Upper-body obesity,** characterized by a large abdomen, is more often related to cardiovascular disease, hypertension, and type 2 diabetes. Whereas other adipose cells empty fat into general blood circulation, the fat released from abdominal adipose cells goes directly to the liver, by way of the portal vein. This process likely interferes with the liver's ability to use insulin and negatively affects lipoprotein metabolism by the liver. These abdominal adipose cells also make substances that increase insulin resistance, blood clotting, blood vessel constriction, and inflammation in the body. These changes can lead to long-term health problems.

High blood testosterone (primarily a male hormone) levels apparently encourage upper-body obesity, as does a diet with a high glycemic load, alcohol intake, and smoking. This characteristic male pattern of fat storage is also called android obesity and is commonly known as the apple shape (large abdomen [pot belly] and small buttocks and thighs). Upper-body obesity is assessed by measuring the waist at the widest point just above the hips when relaxed. A waist circumference more than 40 inches (102 centimeters) in men and more than 35 inches (88 centimeters) in women indicates upper-body obesity (Fig. 7-14). If BMI is also 25 or more, health risks are significantly increased.

Estrogen and progesterone (primarily female hormones) encourage lower-body fat storage and **lower-body (gynecoid or gynoid) obesity**—the typical female pattern. The small abdomen and much larger buttocks and thighs give a pear-like appearance. Fat deposited in the lower body is not mobilized as easily as the other type and often resists being shed. After menopause, blood estrogen falls, encouraging upper-body fat distribution.

**dual energy X-ray absorptiometry (DEXA)** A highly accurate method of measuring body composition and bone mass and density using multiple low-energy X-rays.

**upper-body obesity** The type of obesity in which fat is stored primarily in the abdominal area; defined as a waist circumference more than 40 inches (102 centimeters) in men and more than 35 inches (89 centimeters) in women; closely associated with a high risk for cardiovascular disease, hypertension, and type 2 diabetes. Also known as android obesity.

**lower-body obesity** The type of obesity in which fat storage is primarily located in the buttocks and thigh area. Also known as gynoid or gynecoid obesity.

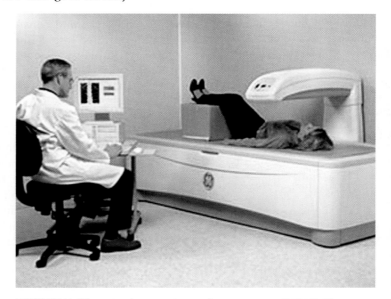

**FIGURE 7-13** ▶ Dual energy X-ray absorptiometry (DEXA). This method measures body fat by passing small doses of radiation through the body. The radiation reacts differently with fat, lean tissue, or bone allowing these components to be quantified. The scanner arm moves from head to toe and in doing so can determine body fat as well as bone density. DEXA is currently considered the most accurate method for determining body fat (as long as the person can fit under the arm of the instrument). The radiation dose is minimal.

44"

32"

Upper-body fat
distribution
(android: apple shape)

Lower-body fat
distribution
(gynoid: pear shape)

**FIGURE 7-14** ▶ Body fat stored primarily in the upper-body (android) form brings higher risks of ill health associated with obesity than does lower-body (gynoid) fat. The woman's waist circumference of 32 inches and the man's waist circumference of 44 inches indicate that the man has upper-body fat distribution but the woman does not, based on a cutoff of 35 inches for women and 40 inches for men.

▲ Waist circumference is an important measure of weight-related health risk.

**identical twins** Two offspring that develop from a single ovum and sperm and, consequently, have the same genetic makeup.

## CONCEPT CHECK

Overweight and obesity typically are associated with excessive body fat storage. The risk of health problems related to being overweight especially increases under the following conditions:

- A man's percentage of body fat exceeds 25%; a woman's exceeds about 35%.
- Excess fat is primarily stored in the upper-body region.
- Body mass index (BMI) is 30 or more (calculated as weight in kilograms divided by height squared in meters).

However, these are merely guidelines. A more individualized approach to assessment is warranted as long as a person is following a healthy lifestyle and has no existing health problems.

Body fat content can be estimated using a variety of methods such as underwater weighing, air displacement, skinfold thickness, bioelectrical impedance, and DEXA. Fat storage distribution further specifies an obese state as either upper-body or lower-body. Obesity leads to an increased risk for cardiovascular disease, some types of cancer, hypertension, type 2 diabetes, certain bone and joint disorders, and some digestive disorders. The risks for some of these diseases are greater with upper-body fat storage.

## 7.5 Why Some People Are Obese—Nature versus Nurture

Both genetic (nature) and environmental (nurture) factors can increase the risk for obesity (Table 7-2). The eventual location of fat storage is strongly influenced by genetics. Consider the possibility that obesity is nurture allowing nature to express itself. Some obese people begin life with a slower basal metabolism; maintain an inactive lifestyle; and consume highly-refined, calorie-dense diets. These people in turn are nurtured into gaining weight, promoting their natural tendency toward obesity.

Still, genes do not fully control destiny. With increased physical activity and decreased food consumption, even those with a genetic tendency toward obesity can attain a healthier body weight.

### How Does Nature Contribute to Obesity?

Studies in pairs of **identical twins** give us some insight into the contribution of nature to obesity. Even when identical twins are raised apart, they tend to show similar weight gain patterns, both in overall weight and body fat distribution. It appears that nurture—eating habits and nutrition, which varies between twins raised apart—has less to do with obesity than nature does. In fact, research suggests that genes account for up to 70% of weight differences between people. A child with no obese parent has only a 10% chance of becoming obese. When a child has one obese parent (common in our society), that risk advances up to 40%, and with two obese parents, it soars to 80%. Our genes help determine metabolic rate, fuel use, and differences in brain chemistry—all of which affect body weight.

We also inherit specific body types. Tall, thin people appear to have an inherently easier time maintaining healthy body weight. This is probably because basal metabolism increases as body surface increases, and therefore taller people use more calories than shorter people, even at rest.

Many of us probably have inherited a thrifty metabolism that enables us to store fat more readily than the typical human, so that we require fewer calories to get through the day. In earlier times, when food supplies were scarce, a thrifty metabolism would have been a built-in safeguard against starvation. Now, with a general abundance of

**TABLE 7-2** What Encourages Excess Body Fat Stores and Obesity?

| Factor | How Fat Storage is Affected |
|---|---|
| Age | Excess body fat is more common in adults and middle-age individuals. |
| Menopause | Increase in abdominal fat deposition is typical. |
| Gender | Females have more fat. |
| Positive energy balance | Over a long period promotes storage of fat. |
| Composition of diet | Excess calorie intake from fat, alcohol, and calorie dense (sugary, fat-rich) foods contributes to obesity. |
| Physical activity | Low physical activity ("couch potato") leads to positive energy balance and body fat storage. |
| Basal metabolism | A low BMR is linked to weight gain. |
| Thermic effect of food | Low for some obesity cases. |
| Increased hunger sensations | Some people have trouble resisting the abundant availability of food, which is likely linked to the activity of various brain chemicals. |
| Ratio of fat to lean tissue | A high ratio of fat mass to lean body mass is correlated with weight gain. |
| Fat uptake by adipose tissue | This is high in some obese individuals and remains high (perhaps even increases) with weight loss. |
| Variety of social and behavioral factors | Obesity is associated with socioeconomic status; familial conditions; network of friends; busy lifestyles that discourage balanced meals; binge eating; easy availability of inexpensive, "super-sized" high-fat food; pattern of leisure activities; television time; smoking cessation; excessive alcohol intake; and number of meals eaten away from home. |
| Undetermined genetic characteristics | These affect components of energy balance, particularly energy expenditure, the deposition of the energy surplus as adipose tissue or as lean tissue, and the relative proportion of fat and carbohydrate used by the body. |
| Race | In some ethnic groups, higher body weight may be more socially acceptable. |
| Certain medications | Food intake increases. |
| Childbearing | Women may not lose all weight gained in pregnancy. |
| National region | Regional differences, such as high-fat diets and sedentary lifestyles in the Midwest and areas of the South, lead to geographically different rates of obesity. |

food, people operating in this low gear require much physical activity and wise food choices to prevent obesity. If you think you are prone to weight gain, you likely have inherited a thrifty metabolism.

**set point** Often refers to the close regulation of body weight. It is not known what cells control this set point or how it functions in weight regulation. There is evidence, however, that mechanisms exist that help regulate weight.

## Does the Body Have a Set Point for Weight?

The **set-point** theory of weight maintenance proposes that humans have a genetically predetermined body weight or body fat content, which the body closely regulates. Some research suggests that the hypothalamus monitors the amount of body fat in humans and tries to keep that amount constant over time. Recall from Chapter 1 that the hormone *leptin* forms a communication link between adipose cells and the brain, which allows for some weight regulation.

Several physiological changes that occur during calorie reduction and weight loss also endorse the set-point theory. For example, when calorie intake is reduced, the blood concentration of thyroid hormones falls, which slows basal metabolism. In addition, as weight is lost, the calorie cost of weight-bearing activity decreases, so that

▶ Does the difference in body fat between the grandfathers and the grandsons arise from nature or nurture, or both?

an activity that burned 100 kcal before weight loss may only burn 80 kcal after weight loss. Furthermore, with weight loss, the body becomes more efficient at storing fat by increasing the activity of the enzyme *lipoprotein lipase,* which takes fat into cells. All of these changes protect the body from losing weight.

If a person overeats, in the short run, basal metabolism tends to increase. This causes some resistance to weight gain. However, in the long run, resistance to weight gain is much less than resistance to weight loss. When a person gains weight and stays at that weight for a while, the body tends to establish a new set point.

Opponents of the set-point theory argue that weight does not remain constant throughout adulthood—the average person gains weight slowly, at least until old age. Also, if an individual is placed in a different social, emotional, or physical environment, weight can be altered and maintained markedly higher or lower. These arguments suggest that humans, rather than having a set point determined by genetics or the number of adipose cells, settle into a particular stable weight based on their circumstances, often regarded as a "settling point."

The size-acceptance nondiet movement, "Health at Every Size," indirectly refers to a set point for weight by defining healthy weight as the natural weight the body adopts, given a healthy diet and meaningful levels of physical activity. Overall, the set point is weaker in preventing weight gain than in preventing weight loss. Even with a set point helping us, the odds are in favor of eventual weight gain unless we devote effort to a healthy lifestyle.

▼ Body weight is influenced by many factors related to both nature and nurture. We resemble our parents because of the genes we have inherited, as well as the lifestyle habits, including diet, that we have learned from them.

## Does Nurture Have a Role?

Some would argue that body weight similarities between family members stem more from learned behaviors rather than genetic similarities. Even couples, who have no genetic link, may behave similarly toward food and eventually assume similar degrees of leanness or fatness. Proponents of nurture pose that environmental factors, such as high-fat diets and inactivity, literally shape us. This seems likely when we consider that our gene pool has not changed much in the past 50 years, whereas according to the U.S. Centers for Disease Control and Prevention the ranks of obese people have grown in epidemic proportions over the last 10 years.

Adult obesity in women is often rooted in childhood obesity. In addition, relative inactivity, periods of stress or boredom, as well as excess weight gain during pregnancy, contribute to female obesity. (Chapter 14 notes that breastfeeding one's infant contributes to loss of some of the excess fat associated with pregnancy.) These patterns suggest both social and genetic links. Male obesity, however, is not strongly linked to childhood obesity and, instead, tends to appear after age 30. This powerful and prevalent pattern suggests a primary role of nurture in obesity, with less genetic influence.

Is poverty associated with obesity? Ironically, the answer is often yes. North Americans of lower socioeconomic status, especially females, are more likely to be obese than those in upper socioeconomic groups. Several social and behavioral factors promote fat storage. These factors include lower socioeconomic status, overweight friends and family, a cultural/ethnic group that prefers higher body weight, a lifestyle that discourages healthy meals and adequate exercise, easy availability of inexpensive high-calorie food, excessive television viewing, smoking cessation, lack of adequate sleep, emotional stress, and frequently eaten meals away from home.

## 7.6 Treatment of Overweight and Obesity

Treatment of overweight and obesity should be long-term, similar to that for any chronic disease. Treatments require long-term lifestyle changes, rather than a quick fix promoted by many popular (also called fad) diet books. We often view a "diet" as something one goes on temporarily, only to resume prior (typically poor) habits once satisfactory results have been achieved. This is a big reason that so many people regain lost weight. Instead, an emphasis on healthy, active living with acceptable dietary modifications will promote weight loss and later weight maintenance.

### What to Look for in a Sound Weight-Loss Plan

A dieter can develop a plan of action by seeking advice from a health professional, such as a registered dietitian, or by using the interactive tools at MyPyramid.gov. Either way, a sound weight-loss program (Fig. 7-15) should especially include these components:

1. Control of calorie intake. One recommendation is to decrease calorie intake by 100 kcal per day (and increase physical activity by 100 kcal per day). This should allow for slow and steady weight loss.
2. Increased physical activity.
3. Acknowledgment that maintenance of a healthy weight requires lifelong changes in habits, not a short-term weight-loss period.

A one-sided approach that focuses only on restricting calories is a difficult plan of action. Instead, adding physical activity and an appropriate psychological component

▲ Student life is often full of physical activity. This is not necessarily true for a person's later working life; hence, weight gain is a strong possibility.

▶ **Weight-Control objectives from *Healthy People 2010***

Increase by 40% the proportion of adults who are at a healthy weight (body mass index between 18.5 and 25).

Reduce by 50% the proportion of adults who are obese (body mass index of 30 or more).

Reduce by 50% the proportion of children and adolescents who are overweight or obese.

**A**s you read brochures, articles, or research reports about specific diet plans, look beyond the weight loss promoted by the diet's advocate to see if the reported weight loss was maintained. If the weight maintenance aspect was missing, then the program was not successful.

### MAKING DECISIONS

#### Losing Body Fat

Rapid weight loss cannot consist primarily of fat loss because a high calorie deficit is needed to lose a large amount of adipose tissue. Adipose tissue, mostly fat, contains about 3500 kcal per pound. Weight loss, however, includes adipose tissue plus lean tissues that support it and represents approximately 3300 kcal per pound (about 7.2 kcal per gram). Therefore, to lose 1 pound of adipose tissue per week, calorie intake must be decreased by approximately 500 kcal per day, or physical activity must be increased by 500 kcal per day. Alternately, a combination of both strategies can be used. Diets that promise 10 to 15 pounds of weight loss per week cannot ensure that the weight loss is from adipose tissue stores alone. How many calories would need to be eliminated from the diet per day to lose 10 pounds per week? Is it possible to subtract enough calories from one's daily intake to lose that amount of adipose tissue? Lean tissue and water, rather than adipose tissue, account for the major part of the weight lost during these dramatic weight-loss programs.

**FIGURE 7-15** ▶ Characteristics of a sound weight-loss diet. Use this checklist to evaluate any new diet plan before putting it into practice.

### RATE OF LOSS

☐ Encourages slow and steady weight loss, rather than rapid weight loss, to promote lasting weight

☐ Sets goal of 1 lb of fat loss per week

☐ Includes a period of weight maintenance for a few months after 10% of body weight is lost

☐ Evaluates need for further dieting before more weight loss begins

### FLEXIBILITY

☐ Supports participation in normal activities (e.g., parties, restaurants)

☐ Adapts to individual habits and tastes

### INTAKE

☐ Meets nutrient needs (except for energy needs)

☐ Includes common foods, with no foods being promoted as magical or special

☐ Recommends a fortified ready-to-eat breakfast cereal or balanced multivitamin/mineral supplement, especially when intake is less than 1600 kcal per day

☐ Uses MyPyramid as a pattern for food choices

### BEHAVIOR MODIFICATION

☐ Focuses on maintenance of healthy lifestyle (and weight) for a lifetime

☐ Promotes reasonable changes that can be maintained

☐ Encourages social support

☐ Includes plans for relapse, so that one does not quit after a setback

☐ Promotes changes that control problem eating behaviors

### OVERALL HEALTH

☐ Requires screening by a physician for people with existing health problems, those over 40 (men) to 50 (women) years of age who plan to increase physical activity substantially, and those who plan to lose weight rapidly

☐ Encourages regular physical activity, sufficient sleep, stress reduction, and other healthy changes in lifestyle

☐ Addresses underlying psychological weight issues, such as depression or marital stress

▲ Making a commitment to a healthier diet and lifestyle can be a challenge for many individuals. A sound weight-loss plan, however, does not require you to completely avoid certain favorite foods. Practical strategies include substituting lower-calorie choices, choosing high-calorie treats less often, and limiting portion sizes.

will contribute to success in weight loss and eventual weight maintenance (Fig. 7-16). From the 2005 Dietary Guidelines for Americans section on weight management, the key recommendations for those who need to lose weight is to aim for a slow, steady weight loss by decreasing calorie intake while maintaining an adequate nutrient intake and increasing physical activity.

## Weight Loss in Perspective

These principles point to the importance of preventing obesity. This concept has wide support because conquering the disorder is so difficult. Public health strategies to address the current obesity problem must speak to all age groups. There is a particular need to focus on children and adolescents because patterns of excess weight and sedentary lifestyle developed during youth may form the basis for a lifetime

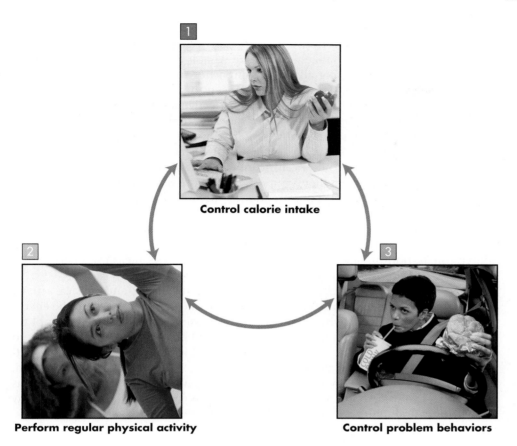

**FIGURE 7-16** ▶ Weight-loss triad. The key to weight loss and maintenance can be thought of as a triad which consists of three parts (1) controlling calorie intake, (2) performing regular physical activity, and (3) controlling problem behaviors. The three parts of the triad support each other in that without one part the triad, weight loss and later maintenance become unlikely.

**1** Control calorie intake

**2** Perform regular physical activity

**3** Control problem behaviors

**F**or more information on weight control, obesity, and nutrition, visit the Weight-Control Information Network (WIN) at **www.niddk.nih.gov/index.htm** or call 800-WIN-8098. Complete guidelines for weight management are available at **www.nhlbi.nih.gov/guidelines/index. htm**. Other websites include **www.caloriecontrol.org**, **www.weight.com**, **www. obesity.org**, and **www.cyberdiet.com**.

### CONCEPT CHECK

Obesity is a chronic disease that necessitates lifelong treatment. Emphasis should be placed especially on preventing obesity, because overcoming this disorder is difficult. Appropriate weight-loss programs have the following characteristics in common: (1) They meet nutritional needs; (2) they can adjust to accommodate habits and tastes; (3) they emphasize readily obtainable foods; (4) they promote changing habits that discourage overeating; (5) they encourage regular physical activity; and (6) they help change obesity-promoting beliefs and rally healthy social support.

of weight-related illness and increased mortality. In the adult population, attention should be directed toward weight maintenance and increased physical activity.

## 7.7 Control of Calorie Intake—The Main Key to Weight Loss and Weight Maintenance

A goal of losing 1 pound or so of stored fat per week may require limiting calorie intake to 1200 kcal per day for women and 1500 kcal for men. The calorie allowance could also be higher for very active people. Keep in mind that, in our sedentary society, decreasing calorie intake is vital because it is difficult to burn much energy without ample physical activity. With regard to consuming fewer calories, some

▲ Slow, steady weight loss is one of the characteristics of a sound weight-loss program.

For interactive dietary and physical activity tools, check out the MyPyramid Tracker and Menu Planner at MyPyramid.gov.

experts suggest consuming less fat (especially saturated fat and *trans* fat), while others suggest consuming less carbohydrate, especially refined (high glycemic load) carbohydrate sources. Protein intakes in excess of what is typically needed by adults are also receiving attention. Using all these approaches simultaneously is fine. At this time the low-fat, high-fiber approaches have been the most successful in long-term studies. There is no long-term evidence of the effectiveness of the other approaches. Finding what works for an individual is a process of trial and error. The notion that any type of diet promotes significantly greater calorie use by the body is unfounded, despite the marketing claims for low-carbohydrate diets.

One way for a dieter to monitor calorie intake at the start of a weight-loss program is by reading labels. Label reading is important, because many foods are more energy dense than people suppose (Fig. 7-17). Another method is to write down food intake for 24 hours (Appendix E) and then calculate calorie intake from the food table in the textbook supplement or by using your diet analysis software. With knowledge of current calorie intake, future food choices can be adjusted as needed. People often underestimate portion size when recording food intake, so measuring cups and a food scale can help.

The MyPyramid Tracker at MyPyramid.gov is an online dietary and physical activity assessment tool that tracks the food calories you eat and compares them to the energy you expend in physical activity. The MyPyramid Menu Planner is an online tool for planning menus based on your personal MyPyramid goals. Table 7-3 shows how to start reducing calorie intake. As you should realize, it is best to consider healthy eating a lifestyle change, rather than a weight-loss plan. Also, liquids deserve attention, because liquid calories do not stimulate satiety mechanisms to the same extent as solid foods. The corresponding advice from experts is to use beverages that have few or no calories and limit sugar-sweetened beverages.

**FIGURE 7-17** ▶ Reading labels helps you choose foods with fewer calories. Which of these frozen desserts is the best choice, per ½ cup serving, for a person on a weight-loss diet? The % Daily Values are based on a 2000 kcal diet.

**TABLE 7-3** Lowering Kcal: Point of Purchase and Consumption Decisions

| Instead of | Try | Number of Kcal Saved |
|---|---|---|
| 3 oz well-marbled meat (prime rib) | 3 oz lean meat (eye of round) | 140 |
| ½ chicken breast, batter-fried | ½ chicken breast, broiled with lemon | 175 |
| ½ cup beef stroganoff | 3 oz lean roast beef (or use a fat-reduced recipe) | 210 |
| ½ cup home-fried potatoes | 1 medium baked potato | 65 |
| ½ cup green bean-mushroom casserole | ½ cup cooked green beans | 50 |
| ½ cup potato salad | 1 cup raw vegetable salad | 140 |
| ½ cup pineapple chunks in heavy syrup | ½ cup pineapple chunks canned in juice | 25 |
| 2 tbsp bottled French dressing | 2 tbsp low-calorie French dressing | 150 |
| ⅛ 9-inch apple pie | 1 baked apple, unsweetened | 308 |
| 3 oatmeal-raisin cookies | 1 oatmeal-raisin cookie | 125 |
| ½ cup ice cream | ½ cup ice milk | 45 |
| 1 danish pastry | ½ English muffin | 150 |
| 1 cup sugar-coated corn flakes | 1 cup plain corn flakes | 60 |
| 1 cup whole milk | 1 cup 1% low-fat milk | 45 |
| 1-oz bag potato chips | 1 cup plain popcorn | 120 |
| $\frac{1}{12}$ 8-inch white layer cake with chocolate frosting | $\frac{1}{12}$ angel food cake, 10-inch tube | 185 |
| 12 fluid ounce cola | 12 fluid ounce diet cola | 150 |

## 7.8 Regular Physical Activity—a Second Key to Weight Loss and Especially Important for Later Weight Maintenance

▲ Physical activity complements any diet plan.

Regular physical activity is important for everyone, especially those trying to lose weight or maintain a lower body weight. Calorie burning is enhanced both during and after physical activity. Therefore, activity greatly complements a reduction in calorie intake for weight loss. Many of us rarely do more than sit, stand, and sleep. More calories are used during physical activity than at rest. Expending only 100 to 300 extra kcal per day above and beyond normal daily activity, while controlling calorie intake, can lead to a steady weight loss. Furthermore, physical activity has so many other benefits, including a boost for overall self-esteem. The latest advice for adults from the 2005 Dietary Guidelines is 60 minutes of physical activity per day to maintain body weight and prevent weight gain and 60 to 90 minutes per day for maintenance of weight loss.

Adding any of the activities in Table 7-4 to one's lifestyle can increase calorie use. Duration and regular performance, rather than intensity, are the keys to success with this approach to weight loss. One should search for activities that can be continued over time. In this regard, walking vigorously 3 miles per day can be as helpful as aerobic dancing or jogging, if it is maintained. Moreover, activities of lighter intensity are less likely to lead to injuries. Some resistance exercises (weight training) also

**TABLE 7-4** Approximate Calorie Costs of Various Activities, and Specific Calorie Costs Projected for a 150-Pound (68 kilogram) Person

| Activity | Kcal per kilogram per Hour | Total Kcal per Hour | Activity | Kcal per kilogram per Hour | Total Kcal per Hour |
|---|---|---|---|---|---|
| Aerobics—heavy | 8.0 | 544 | Horseback riding | 5.1 | 346 |
| Aerobics—medium | 5.0 | 340 | Ice skating (10 MPH) | 5.8 | 394 |
| Aerobics—light | 3.0 | 204 | Jogging—medium | 9.0 | 612 |
| Backpacking | 9.0 | 612 | Jogging—slow | 7.0 | 476 |
| Basketball—vigorous | 10.0 | 680 | Lying—at ease | 1.3 | 89 |
| Bowling | 3.9 | 265 | Racquetball—social | 8.0 | 544 |
| Calisthenics—heavy | 8.0 | 544 | Roller skating | 5.1 | 346 |
| Calisthenics—light | 4.0 | 272 | Running or jogging (10 MPH) | 13.2 | 897 |
| Canoeing (2.5 MPH) | 3.3 | 224 | Skiing downhill (10 MPH) | 8.8 | 598 |
| Cleaning (female) | 3.7 | 253 | Sleeping | 1.2 | 80 |
| Cleaning (male) | 3.5 | 236 | Swimming (.25 MPH) | 4.4 | 299 |
| Cooking | 2.8 | 190 | Tennis | 6.1 | 414 |
| Cycling (13 MPH) | 9.7 | 659 | Volleyball | 5.1 | 346 |
| Cycling (5.5 MPH) | 3.0 | 204 | Walking (3.75 MPH) | 4.4 | 299 |
| Dressing/showering | 1.6 | 106 | Walking (2.5 MPH) | 3.0 | 204 |
| Driving | 1.7 | 117 | Water skiing | 7.0 | 476 |
| Eating (sitting) | 1.4 | 93 | Weight lifting—heavy | 9.0 | 612 |
| Food shopping | 3.6 | 245 | Weight lifting—light | 4.0 | 272 |
| Football—touch | 7.0 | 476 | Window cleaning | 3.5 | 240 |
| Golf (using power cart) | 3.6 | 244 | Writing (sitting) | 1.7 | 118 |

The values in Table 7-4 refer to total energy expenditure, including that needed to perform the physical activity, plus that needed for basal metabolism, the thermic effect of food, and thermogenesis. Use your diet analysis software for your personal estimate.

▲ Fruit is a great low-cal snack—high in nutrient density and low in calories.

should be added to increase lean body mass and, in turn, fat use (see Chapter 10). As lean muscle mass increases, so will one's overall metabolic rate. An added benefit of including exercise in a weight reduction program is maintenance of bone health.

Unfortunately, opportunities to expend calories in our daily lives are diminishing as technology systematically eliminates almost every reason to move our muscles. The easiest way to increase physical activity is to make it an enjoyable part of a daily routine. To start, one might pack a pair of sneakers and walk around the parking lot before coming home after school or work every day. Other ideas are avoiding elevators in favor of stairs and parking the car farther away from the shopping mall.

A pedometer is an inexpensive device that monitors activity as steps. A recommended goal for activity is to take at least 10,000 steps per day—typically we take half that many or less. A pedometer tracks this activity. Calorie counters, such as the Bodybugg, are new devices that track calorie expenditures throughout the day. The counters calculate calories by measuring heart rate, sweat rate, or heat loss and production. Like pedometers, calorie counters can motivate users to do more activity.

# 7.9  Behavior Modification—A Third Strategy for Weight Loss and Management

Controlling calorie intake, so important to weight loss, also means modifying *problem* behaviors. Only the dieter can decide what behaviors keep him or her from reaching for the wrong foods at the wrong times for the wrong reasons.

What events cause us to start (or stop) eating? What factors influence food choices? Psychologists often use terms such as *chain-breaking, stimulus control, cognitive restructuring, contingency management,* and *self-monitoring* when discussing behavior modification (Table 7-5). These factors help place the problem in perspective and organize the intervention strategy into manageable steps.

**Chain-breaking** separates behaviors that tend to occur together—for example, snacking on chips while watching television. Although these activities do not have to occur together, they often do. Dieters may need to break the chain reaction (see "Rate Your Plate" at the end of this chapter for more details).

**Stimulus control** puts us in charge of temptations. Options include pushing tempting food to the back of the refrigerator, removing fat-laden snacks from the kitchen counter, and avoiding the path by the vending machines. Provide a positive stimulus by keeping low-fat snacks available to satisfy hunger/appetite.

**Cognitive restructuring** changes our frame of mind. For example, after a hard day, avoid using alcohol or comfort foods as quick relief for stress. Instead, plan for healthful, relaxing activities for stress reduction. For example, take a walk around the neighborhood or have a satisfying talk with a friend.

Labeling some foods as "off limits" sets up an internal struggle to resist the urge to eat that food. This hopeless battle can keep us feeling deprived. We lose the fight. Managing food choices with the principle of moderation is best. If a favorite food becomes troublesome, place it off limits only temporarily, until it can be enjoyed in moderation.

**Contingency management** prepares one for situations that may trigger overeating (e.g., when snacks are served at a party) or hinder physical activity (e.g., rain).

A **self-monitoring** record can reveal patterns—such as unconscious overeating—that may explain problem eating habits. This record can encourage new habits that will counteract unwanted behaviors. Obesity experts note that this is the key behavioral tool to use in any weight-loss program. See the margin for a list of free online tools available for self-monitoring.

Overall, it's important to address specific problems, such as snacking, compulsive eating, and mealtime overeating. Behavior Modification principles (review Table 7-5) end up as critical components of weight reduction and maintenance. Without behavior modification, it is difficult to make lifelong lifestyle changes needed to meet weight-control goals.

## Relapse Prevention Is Important

Preventing relapse is thought to be the hardest part of weight control—even harder than losing weight. A dieter can tolerate an occasional lapse but needs to plan for lapses. The key is not to overreact, but take charge immediately. Change responses such as "I ate that cookie; I'm a failure" to "I ate that cookie, but I did well to stop after only one!" When dieters lapse from their diet plan, newly learned food habits should steer them back toward the plan. This should enable dieters to avoid the lapse-relapse-collapse trap. Without a strong behavioral program for **relapse prevention** in place, a lapse frequently turns into a relapse. Once a pattern of poor food choices begins, dieters may feel that they have failed and stray farther from the plan. As the relapse lengthens, the diet plan collapses, and dieters fall short of their weight-loss goal. Even with a good behavioral plan, one may fail at a diet. Losing weight is difficult. Overall, maintenance of weight loss is fostered by the "3 *Ms*": motivation, movement, and monitoring.

**T**he motivation to lose weight and keep it off generally comes with a proverbial "flip of the switch," in which the desire to lose weight finally becomes more important than the desire to overeat.

**chain-breaking** Breaking the link between two or more behaviors that encourage overeating, such as snacking while watching television.

**stimulus control** Altering the environment to minimize the stimuli for eating—for example, removing foods from sight and storing them in kitchen cabinets.

**cognitive restructuring** Changing one's frame of mind regarding eating—for example, instead of using a difficult day as an excuse to overeat, substituting other pleasures for rewards, such as a relaxing walk with a friend.

**contingency management** Forming a plan of action to respond to a situation in which overeating is likely, such as when snacks are within arm's reach at a party.

**self-monitoring** Tracking foods eaten and conditions affecting eating; actions are usually recorded in a diary, along with location, time, and state of mind. This is a tool to help people understand more about their eating habits.

**relapse prevention** A series of strategies used to help prevent and cope with weight-control lapses, such as recognizing high-risk situations and deciding beforehand on appropriate responses.

**Food and Activity Tracking**
Here are some websites where you can record your food and physical activity online for free:

www.fitday.com
www.mypyramidtracker.gov
www.nutritiondata.com
www.sparkpeople.com

▲ Large portions of food, such as this steak, provide us with many opportunities to overeat. It takes much perseverance to eat sensibly.

Successful weight losers and maintainers from the National Weight Control Registry:

• Eat a low-fat, high-carbohydrate diet (on average 25% of calorie intake as fat).
• Eat breakfast almost every day.
• Self-monitor by regularly weighing oneself and keeping a food journal.
• Exercise for about 1 hour per day.
• Eat at restaurants only once or twice per week.

Other recent studies support this approach, especially the last four characteristics.

**TABLE 7-5** Behavior Modification Principles for Weight Loss

**Shopping**
1. Shop for food after eating—buy nutritious foods.
2. Shop from a list; limit purchases of irresistible "problem" foods. Shopping for fresh foods around the perimeter of the store first helps.
3. Avoid ready-to-eat foods.
4. Put off food shopping until absolutely necessary.

**Plans**
1. Plan to limit food intake as needed.
2. Substitute periods of physical activity for snacking.
3. Eat meals and snacks at scheduled times; don't skip meals.

**Activities**
1. Store food out of sight, preferably in the freezer, to discourage impulsive eating.
2. Eat all food in a "dining" area.
3. Keep serving dishes off the table, especially dishes of sauces and gravies.
4. Use smaller dishes and utensils.

**Holidays and Parties**
1. Drink fewer alcoholic beverages.
2. Plan eating behavior before parties.
3. Eat a low-calorie snack before parties.
4. Practice polite ways to decline food.
5. Don't get discouraged by an occasional setback.

**Eating Behavior**
1. Put fork down between mouthfuls.
2. Chew thoroughly before taking the next bite.
3. Leave some food on the plate.
4. Pause in the middle of the meal.
5. Do nothing else while eating (for example, reading, watching television).

**Reward**
1. Plan specific rewards for specific behavior (behavioral contracts).
2. Solicit help from family and friends and suggest how they can help you. Encourage family and friends to provide this help in the form of praise and material rewards.
3. Use self-monitoring records as basis for rewards.

**Self-Monitoring**
1. Note the time and place of eating.
2. List the type and amount of food eaten.
3. Record who is present and how you feel.
4. Use the diet diary to identify problem areas.

**Cognitive Restructuring**
1. Avoid setting unreasonable goals.
2. Think about progress, not shortcomings.
3. Avoid imperatives such as *always* and *never*.
4. Counter negative thoughts with positive restatements.

**Portion Control**
1. Make substitutions, such as a regular hamburger instead of a "quarter pounder" or cucumbers instead of croutons in salads.
2. Think small. Order the entrée and share it with another person. Order a cup of soup instead of a bowl or an appetizer in place of an entrée.
3. Use a doggie bag. Ask your server to put half the entrée in a doggie bag before bringing it to the table.

As we said at the start of this chapter, many of us need to become "defensive eaters." Know when to refuse food after satiety registers, and reduce portion sizes.

## Social Support Aids Behavioral Change

Healthy social support is helpful in weight control. Helping others understand how they can be supportive can make weight control easier. Family and friends can provide praise and encouragement. A registered dietitian or other weight-control professional can keep dieters accountable and help them learn from difficult situations. Long-term contact with a professional can be helpful for later weight maintenance. Groups of individuals attempting to lose weight or maintain losses can provide empathetic support.

## Societal Efforts to Reduce Obesity

The incidence of obesity in the United States is now considered an epidemic. Public, private, and nonprofit organizations have begun to work together to address and reverse this public health crisis. For example, the U.S. Food and Drug Administration has brought together leaders from industry, government, academia, and the public health community to seek solutions to the obesity epidemic by making changes in foods eaten outside the home (restaurant and carry-out foods). These groups have collaborated and made recommendations to support the consumer's ability to manage calorie intake. Recommendations include "social marketing" programs that promote healthy eating and active living.

### CONCEPT CHECK

Increasing physical activity in daily life should be part of any weight-loss plan. Daily activity, such as walking and stair climbing, is recommended. Behavior Modification can improve conditions for losing weight. One key step is to break behavior chains that encourage overeating, such as snacking while watching television. Another tactic is to modify the environment to reduce temptation; for example, put foods into cupboards to keep them out of sight. In addition, rethinking attitudes about eating—for example, substituting pleasures other than food as a reward for coping with a stressful day—can be important for altering undesirable behavior. Advanced planning to prevent and deal with lapses is vital, as is rallying healthy social support. Finally, careful observation and recording of eating habits can reveal subtle cues that lead to overeating. Overall, weight loss and maintenance are fostered by controlling calorie intake, performing regular physical activity, and modifying "problem" behaviors.

## 7.10 Professional Help for Weight Loss

The first professional to see for advice about a weight-loss program is one's family physician. Doctors are best equipped to assess overall health and the appropriateness of weight loss. The physician may then recommend a registered dietitian for a specific weight-loss plan and answers to diet-related questions. Registered dietitians are uniquely qualified to help design a weight-loss plan because they understand both food composition and the psychological importance of food. Exercise physiologists can provide advice about programs to increase physical activity. From the 2005 Dietary Guidelines for Americans, the key Recommendations for overweight adults and overweight children with chronic diseases and/or on medication is to consult a healthcare provider about weight loss strategies prior to starting a weight-reduction program to ensure appropriate management of other health conditions. The expense

**CRITICAL THINKING**

With regard to readiness to lose weight, what would you say to a young woman who has just had a baby, needs to find a new job, and recently has gone back to school part-time?

▲ Individuals who successfully maintain their weight loss employ a variety of strategies to cope with the stresses and challenges of changing problem behaviors.

▲ All weight loss programs should begin with a visit to your family physician.

**amphetamine** A group of medications that induce stimulation of the central nervous system and have other effects in the body. Abuse is linked to physical and psychological dependence.

for such professional interventions is tax deductible in the United States in some cases (see a tax advisor) and often covered by health insurance plans if prescribed by a physician.

Many communities have a variety of weight-loss organizations. These include self-help groups, such as Take Off Pounds Sensibly and Weight Watchers. Other programs, such as Jenny Craig and Physicians' Weight Loss Center, are less desirable for the average dieter. Often, the employees are not registered dietitians or other appropriately trained health professionals. These programs also tend to be expensive because of their requirements for intense counseling or mandatory diet foods and supplements. In addition, the Federal Trade Commission has charged these and other commercial diet-program companies with misleading consumers through unsubstantiated weight-loss claims and deceptive testimonials.

North Americans are willing to try almost anything to shed unwanted pounds. Operation Waistline is a program designed by the U.S. Federal Trade Commission to terminate fraudulent claims being made by weight-loss charlatans with regard to diet products. The program hopes to put an end to the $6 billion spent annually in the United States on counterfeit products. The Enforma Natural Products Corporation had to pay $10 million in response to false claims for its "Fat Trapper" product.

## Medications for Weight Loss

Candidates for medications for obesity include those with a BMI of 30 or more, or a BMI of 27 to 29.9 with weight-related health conditions, such as type 2 diabetes, cardiovascular disease, hypertension, or excess waist circumference; those with no contraindications to use the medication; and those ready to undertake lifestyle change. Drug therapy alone has not been found to be successful. Success with medications has been shown only in those who also modify their behavior, decrease calorie intake, and increase physical activity. In addition, if a person has not lost at least 4.4 pounds (2 kilograms) after 4 weeks, it is not likely that the person will benefit from further use of the medication.

Three main classes of medications are used. An **amphetamine**-like medication (phenteramine [Fastin or Ionamin]) prolongs the activity of epinephrine and norepinephrine in the brain. This therapy is effective for some people in the short run but has not yet been proven effective in the long run. Most state medical boards limit use of this drug to 12 weeks unless the person is participating in a medical study using the product. The medication should not be used in pregnant or nursing women or those under 18 years of age.

Sibutramine (Meridia) is a second class of medication that has been approved by FDA for weight loss. It enhances both norepinephrine and serotonin activity in the brain by reducing reuptake of these neurotransmitters by nerve cells. The neurotransmitters then remain active in the brain for a longer time and so prolong a sense of reduced hunger. The most common side effects are constipation, dry mouth, insomnia, and a mild increase in blood pressure in some people. Thus, sibutramine should be used with caution in people with a history of hypertension (or cardiovascular disease). Studies have shown that it is effective in helping some people who already eat healthy diets, but just eat too much. The main effect is to moderately reduce appetite so that people eat less. Sibutramine is safe and effective only when combined with a comprehensive weight-control program and when supervised by a physician.

The third class of medication approved by FDA for weight loss is orlistat (Xenical). This medication reduces fat digestion by about 30% by inhibiting lipase enzyme action in the small intestine (Fig. 7-18). This cuts absorption of dietary fat by one-third for about 2 hours when taken along with a meal containing fat. This malabsorbed fat is deposited in the feces. *Fat intake has to be controlled,* however, because large amounts of fat in the feces cause numerous side effects, such as gas, bloating, and oily discharge. Interestingly, orlistat use can remind the person to follow a fat-controlled diet, as the symptoms resulting from consuming a high-fat meal are unpleasant and

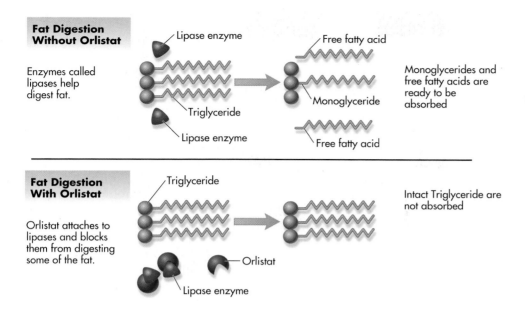

**FIGURE 7-18** ▶ Orlistat is a weight-loss drug that works in the digestive system to block digestion of about one-third of the fat in the food we eat. A low-dose form of this drug (Alli™) is now available without a prescription.

develop quickly. Orlistat is taken with each meal containing fat. The malabsorbed fat also carries fat-soluble vitamins into the feces, so the person taking orlistat must take a multivitamin and mineral supplement at bedtime. In this way, any micronutrients not absorbed during the day can be replaced; fat malabsorption from the dinner meal will not greatly influence micronutrient absorption in the late evening.

The only two weight-loss medications currently approved by FDA for long-term use are sibutramine (Meridia) and orlistat (Xenical). A low-dose form of orlistat (Alli™) is now available over-the-counter without a prescription. Drug companies are working on many other types of medications (e.g., rimonabant) and have high hopes that some of these will prove to be safe and effective for weight loss. In addition, physicians may prescribe medications not approved for weight loss *per se* but can have weight loss as a side effect. Certain antidepressants (e.g., bupropion [Wellbutrin]) are an example. Such an application is termed *off-label*, because the product label does not include weight loss as an FDA-approved use. Consumers need to educate themselves about weight-loss products before trying them. Over-the-counter medications and supplements are widely marketed as miracle cures for obesity, but in some cases, they do more harm than good. One woman developed liver failure after using a so-called weight-loss aid called usnic acid. Her purchase was via the Internet. Today more than ever, let the buyer beware concerning any purported weight-loss aid not prescribed by a physician.

Overall, in skilled hands, prescription medications can aid weight loss in some instances. However, they do not replace the need for reducing calorie intake, modifying "problem" behaviors, and increasing physical activity, both during and after therapy. Often, any weight loss during drug treatment can be attributed mostly to the individual's hard work at balancing calorie intake with calorie output.

## Treatment of Severe Obesity

Severe (morbid) obesity, having a BMI greater than or equal to 40 or weighing at least 100 pounds over healthy body weight (or twice one's healthy body weight), requires professional treatment. Because of the serious health implications of severe obesity, drastic measures may be necessary. Such treatments are recommended only when traditional diets and medications fail. Drastic weight-loss procedures are not without side effects, both physical and psychological, making careful monitoring by a physician a necessity.

**very-low-calorie diet (VLCD)** Known also as *protein-sparing modified fast (PSMF)*, this diet allows a person 400 to 800 kcal per day, often in liquid form. Of this, 120 to 480 kcal is carbohydrate, and the rest is mostly high-quality protein.

**bariatrics** The medical specialty focusing on the treatment of obesity.

**adjustable gastric banding** A restrictive procedure in which the opening from the esophagus to the stomach is reduced by a hollow gastric band.

**gastroplasty** Gastric bypass surgery performed on the stomach to limit its volume to approximately 30 milliliters. Also referred to as stomach stapling.

**Very-Low-Calorie Diets.** If more traditional diet changes have failed, treating severe obesity with a **very-low-calorie diet (VLCD)** is possible, especially if the person has obesity-related diseases that are not well controlled (e.g., hypertension, type 2 diabetes). Some researchers believe that people with body weight greater than 30% above their healthy weight are appropriate candidates. VLCD programs are offered almost exclusively by medical centers or clinics since careful monitoring by a physician is crucial throughout this very restrictive form of weight loss. Major health risks include heart problems and gallstones. Optifast is one such commercial program. In general, the diet allows a person to consume only 400 to 800 kcal per day, often in liquid form. (These diets were previously known as protein-sparing modified fasts.) Of this amount, about 30 to 120 grams (120 to 480 kcal) is carbohydrate. The rest is high-quality protein, in the amount of about 70 to 100 grams per day (280 to 400 kcal). This low carbohydrate intake often causes ketosis, which may decrease hunger. However, the main reasons for weight loss are the minimal energy consumption and the absence of food choice. About 3 to 4 pounds can be lost per week; men tend to lose at a faster rate than women. When physical activity and resistance training augment this diet, a greater loss of adipose tissue occurs.

Weight regain remains a nagging problem, especially without a behavioral and physical activity component. If behavioral therapy and physical activity supplement a long-term support program, maintenance of the weight loss is more likely but still difficult. Any program under consideration should include a maintenance plan. Today, antiobesity medications also may be included in this phase of the program.

**Bariatric Surgery.** **Bariatrics** is the medical specialty focusing on the treatment of obesity. Bariatric surgery is only considered for people with severe obesity and includes operations aimed at promoting weight loss. Two types of bariatric operations are now common and effective. Both procedures can be performed using an open incision (8- to 10-inch) in the middle of the abdomen or a laparoscopic approach in which several smaller incisions (½ - to 2-inch) are used that allow cameras and instruments to enter the abdomen. **Adjustable gastric banding** (also known as the lap-band procedure) is a restrictive procedure in which the opening from the esophagus to the stomach is reduced by a hollow gastric band. This creates a small pouch and a narrow passage into the rest of the stomach and thus decreases the amount of food that can be eaten comfortably. The band can be inflated or deflated via an access port placed just under the skin. Studies have demonstrated that adjustable gastric banding is more effective long term than a very low-calorie diet (500 kcal) for people who are about 50 pounds overweight.

Gastric bypass (also called **gastroplasty** or stomach stapling) is another bariatric surgical procedure used for treating severe obesity. The most common and effective approach (the Roux-en-Y gastric bypass procedure) works by reducing the stomach capacity to about 30 milliliters (the volume of one egg or shot glass) and bypassing a short segment of the upper small intestine (Fig. 7-19). Weight loss is promoted mainly because overeating of solid foods is now less likely due to rapid satiety and discomfort or vomiting after overeating. About 75% of people with severe obesity eventually lose 50% or more of excess body weight with this method. In addition, the surgery's success at long-term maintenance often leads to dramatic health improvements, such as reduced blood pressure and elimination of type 2 diabetes. Risks of the surgery include bleeding, blood clots, hernias, and severe infections. In the long run, nutrient deficiencies can develop if the person is not adequately treated in the years following the surgery. Anemia and bone loss might then be the result. Risk of death from this demanding surgery can be as high as 2% (less risk with experienced surgeons).

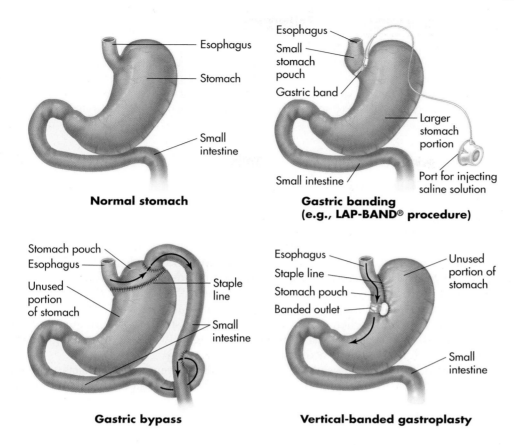

**Normal stomach**

**Gastric banding
(e.g., LAP-BAND® procedure)**

**Gastric bypass**

**Vertical-banded gastroplasty**

**FIGURE 7-19** ▶ The most common forms of gastroplasty for treating severe obesity. The gastric bypass is the most effective method. In banded gastroplasty, the band prevents expansion of the outlet for the stomach pouch.

Patient selection criteria for bariatric surgery include:

- BMI should be greater than 40.
- BMI between 35 and 40 is considered when there are serious obesity-related health concerns.
- Obesity must be present for a minimum of 5 years, with several nonsurgical attempts to lose weight.
- There should be no history of alcoholism or major untreated psychiatric disorders.

The person also must consider that the surgery is costly ($12,000 to $40,000 or more) and may not be covered by medical insurance. In addition, follow-up surgery is often needed after weight loss to correct stretched skin, previously filled with fat. Furthermore, the surgery necessitates major lifestyle changes, such as the need to plan frequent, small meals. Therefore, the dieter who has chosen this drastic approach to weight loss faces months of difficult adjustments.

## MAKING DECISIONS

### Lipectomy

Spot-reducing by using diet and physical activity is not possible. "Problem" local fat deposits can be reduced in size, however, using suction lipectomy. Lipectomy means surgical removal of fat. A pencil-thin tube is inserted into an incision in the skin, and the fat tissue, such as that in the buttocks and thigh area, is suctioned. This procedure carries some risks, such as infection; lasting depressions in the skin; and blood clots, which can lead to kidney failure and sometimes death. The procedure is designed to help a person lose about 4 to 8 pounds per treatment. Cost is about $1600 per site; total costs range as high as $2600 to $9000.

# 7.11 Treatment of Underweight

**underweight** A body mass index below 18.5. The cutoff is less precise than for obesity because this condition has been less studied.

**Underweight** is defined by a BMI less than 18.5 and can be caused by a variety of factors, such as cancer, infectious disease (e.g., tuberculosis), digestive tract disorders (e.g., chronic inflammatory bowel disease), and excessive dieting or physical activity. Genetic background may also lead to a higher resting metabolic rate, a slight body frame, or both. Health problems associated with underweight include the loss of menstrual function, low bone mass, complications with pregnancy and surgery, and slow recovery after illness. Significant underweight is also associated with increased death rates, especially when combined with cigarette smoking. We frequently hear about the risks of obesity, but seldom of underweight. In our culture, being underweight is much more socially acceptable than being obese.

Sometimes being underweight requires medical intervention. A physician should be consulted first to rule out hormonal imbalances; depression; cancer; infectious disease; digestive tract disorders; excessive physical activity; and other hidden disease, such as a serious eating disorder (see Chapter 11 for a detailed discussion of eating disorders).

The causes of underweight are not altogether different from the causes of obesity. Internal and external satiety-signal irregularities, the rate of metabolism, hereditary tendencies, and psychological traits can all contribute to underweight.

In growing children, the high demand for calories to support physical activity and growth can cause underweight. During growth spurts in adolescence, active children may not take the time to consume enough calories to support their needs. Moreover, gaining weight can be a formidable task for an underweight person. An extra 500 kcal per day may be required to gain weight, even at a slow pace, in part because of the increased expenditure of energy in thermogenesis. In contrast to the weight loser, the weight gainer may need to increase portion sizes.

When underweight requires a specific intervention, one approach for treating adults is to gradually increase their consumption of calorie-dense foods, especially those high in vegetable fat. Italian cheeses, nuts, and granola can be good calorie sources with low saturated-fat content. Dried fruit and bananas are good fruit choices. If eaten at the end of a meal, they don't cause early satiety. The same advice applies to salads and soups. Underweight people should replace such foods as diet soft drinks with good calorie sources, such as fruit juices and smoothies.

Encouraging a regular meal and snack schedule also aids in weight gain and maintenance. Sometimes underweight people have experienced stress at work or have been too busy to eat. Making regular meals a priority may not only help them attain an appropriate weight but also help with digestive disorders, such as constipation, sometimes associated with irregular eating times.

Excessively physically active people can reduce activity. If their weight remains low, they can add muscle mass through a resistance training (weight-lifting) program, but they must also increase their calorie intake to support that physical activity. Otherwise, weight gain will be hindered.

If these efforts fail to help a person achieve a healthy weight, they should at least prevent the health problems associated with being underweight. After achieving that, they may have to accept their lean frames.

▲ Underweight is frequently the result of gastrointestinal disorders such as inflammatory bowel disease.

## Nutrition and Your Health

# Popular Diets—Cause for Concern

Many overweight people try to help themselves by using the latest popular (also called fad) diet book. But, as you will see, most of these diets do not help, and some can actually harm those who follow them (Table 7-6). Research has shown that early dieting and other unhealthful weight control practices in adolescents lead to an increased risk of weight gain, overweight, and eating disorders.

Recently, weight-loss experts came together at the request of the USDA to evaluate weight-loss diets. They came to this conclusion: Forget these fads when it comes to dieting. Most of the popular diets are nutritionally inadequate and include certain foods that people would not normally choose to consume in large amounts. The experts stated that eating less of one's favorite foods and becoming more physically active can be much more effective when trying to implement a weight-loss diet. People need a plan they can live with in the long run so that weight control becomes permanent. The goal should be weight control over a lifetime, not immediate weight loss. Every popular diet leads to some immediate weight loss simply because daily in-take is monitored and monotonous food choices are typically part of the plan. A well-known example of the effectiveness of monotony contributing to weight loss is the experience of Jared Fogle. He ate primarily Subway sandwiches for 11 months and lost 245 pounds. He notes however that this is not a miracle diet—it takes a lot of hard work to lead to the success he experienced. There are also many other examples where diet monotony has led to weight loss. Overall, a traditional moderate diet coupled with regular physical activity is adequate for weight loss.

People on diets often fall within a healthy BMI of 18.5 to 25. Rather than worrying about weight loss, these individuals should be focusing on a healthy lifestyle that allows for weight maintenance. Incorporating necessary lifestyle changes and learning to accept one's particular body characteristics should be the overriding goals.

The dieting mania can be viewed as mostly a social problem, stemming from unrealistic weight expectations (especially for women) and lack of appreciation for the natural variety in body shape and weight. Not every woman can look like a fashion model, nor can every man look like a Greek god, but all of us can strive for good health and, if physically possible, an active lifestyle.

The size-acceptance nondiet movement, "Health at Every Size," has attempted to shift the paradigm away from the use of "popular" weight loss diets. The goals of the movement are all independent of body weight and include improvement of self-image, normalization of eating behavior, and increase in physical activity.

## How to Recognize an Unreliable Diet

The criteria for evaluating weight-loss programs with regard to their safety and effectiveness were discussed previously (review Fig. 7-15). In contrast, unreliable diets typically share some common characteristics:

1. They promote quick weight loss. This is the primary temptation that the dieter falls for. As mentioned, this initial weight loss primarily results from water loss and lean muscle mass depletion.

2. They limit food selections and dictate specific rituals, such as eating only fruit for breakfast or cabbage soup every day.

3. They use testimonials from famous people and tie the diet to well-known cities, such as Beverly Hills and South Beach.

4. They bill themselves as cure-alls. These diets claim to work for everyone, whatever the type of obesity or the person's specific strengths and weaknesses.

5. They often recommend expensive supplements.

6. No attempts are made to change eating habits permanently. Dieters follow the diet until the desired weight is reached and then revert to old eating habits—they are told, for example, to eat rice for a month, lose weight, and then return to old habits.

7. They are generally critical of and skeptical about the scientific community. The lack of a quick fix from medical and dietetic professionals has led some of the public to seek advice from those who appear to have the answer.

8. They claim that there is no need to exercise.

Probably the cruelest characteristic of these diets is that they essentially guarantee failure for the dieter. The diets are not designed for permanent weight loss. Habits are not changed, and the food selection is so limited that the person cannot follow the diet in the long run. Although dieters assume they have lost fat, they have lost mostly muscle and other lean tissue mass. As soon as they begin

**TABLE 7-6** Summary of Popular Diet Approaches to Weight Control

| Approach | Examples* | Characteristics | Dietitian's Review |
|---|---|---|---|
| Moderate calorie restriction | • *Dieting for Dummies* (2003)<br>• *Dieting with the Duchess* (2000)<br>• *Dr. Phil's Ultimate Weight Solution* (2003, 2005)<br>• Flat Belly Diet (2008)<br>• Jenny Craig (1980s)<br>• *Picture Perfect Weight Loss* (2003)<br>• Slim-fast (1980s)<br>• *Sonoma Diet* (2005)<br>• *Volumetrics* (2000)<br>• *Wedding Dress Diet* (2000)<br>• Weight Watchers (1960s)<br>• *You on a Diet* (2006) | • Generally 1200 to 1800 kcal per day<br>• Moderate fat intake<br>• Reasonable balance of macronutrients<br>• Encourage exercise<br>• May use behavioral approach | These diets are acceptable if a multivitamin and mineral supplement is used and permission of family physician is granted. |
| Carbohydrate focused | • *Carbohydrate Addicts Diet* (1993, 2001)<br>• *Dr. Atkin's Diet Revolution* (1973, 2002)<br>• *Dr. Gott's No Flour, No Sugar Diet* (2006)<br>• *Eat, Drink & Weigh Less* (2006)<br>• *G.I. (Glycemic Index) Diet* (2003)<br>• *Healthy for Life* (2005)<br>• *New Glucose Revolution* (2002)<br>• Nutrisystem (2003)<br>• *South Beach Diet* (especially initial phases) (2003)<br>• *Sugar Busters Diet* (1998, 2003)<br>• *Zone Diet* (1995) | • Restricted carbohydrate diets generally advise consumption of less than 100 grams of carbohydrate per day<br>• Some plans focus on carbohydrate choices (e.g., choosing low rather than high glycemic index foods) | Selecting high-fiber, whole-grain sources of carbohydrates is an advisable practice for weight control and prevention of several chronic diseases. However, severe carbohydrate restriction may lead to ketosis, reduced exercise capacity (due to poor glycogen stores in the muscles), excessive animal fat intake, constipation, headaches, halitosis (bad breath), and muscle cramps. Severe carbohydrate restriction is not a nutritionally sound, long-term, weight-loss solution. |
| Low fat | • *20/30 Fat and Fiber Diet Plan* (2000)<br>• *Complete Hip and Thigh Diet* (1989, 1999)<br>• *Eat More, Weigh Less* (1993, 2001)<br>• *Fit or Fat* (1977, 2005)<br>• *Foods That Cause You to Lose Weight* (1992, 2003)<br>• *McDougall Program* (1983, 1995)<br>• *Pritikin Diet* (1984, 1995)<br>• *Rice Diet Solution* (2005)<br>• *T-Factor Diet* (1989, 2001)<br>• *Okinawa Program* (2002) | • Generally less than 20% of calories from fat<br>• Limited (or elimination of) animal protein sources; also limited plant oils, nuts, seeds | Low-fat diet plans are not necessarily to be avoided, but certain aspects may be unacceptable. Some potentially negative outcomes include flatulence, poor mineral absorption (from excess fiber intake), and a sense of deprivation (due to limited food choices). |
| Novelty diets | • 3-Hour Diet (2005)<br>• *Beverly Hills Diet* (1981, 1996)<br>• Cabbage-Soup Diet (2004)<br>• *Eat Right 4 Your Type* (1996)<br>• *Fat Smash Diet* (2006)<br>• *Fit for Life* (1987, 2001)<br>• *Metabolic Typing Diet* (2002)<br>• *New Hilton Head Metabolism Diet* (1983, 1996)<br>• *Ultrametabolism* (2006)<br>• *Weigh Down Diet* (2002) | • Promote certain nutrients, foods, or combinations of foods as having unique, magical, or previously undiscovered qualities | Novelty diets are usually not nutritionally balanced, thus malnutrition is a possible result. Also, failure to make long-term changes may lead to relapse, and unrealistic food choices lead to possible bingeing. |

*Dates listed are original release date followed by most recent release date, if applicable.

eating normally again, much of the lost tissue is replaced. In a matter of weeks, most of the lost weight is back. The dieter appears to have failed, when actually the diet has failed. The gain and loss cycle is called weight cycling or "yo-yo" dieting. This whole scenario can add more blame and guilt, challenging the self-worth of the dieter. It can also come with some health costs, such as increased upper-body fat deposition. If someone needs help losing weight, professional help is advised. It is unfortunate that current trends suggest that people are spending more time and money on "quick fixes" rather than on such professional help.

## Types of Popular Diets

### Low- or Restricted-Carbohydrate Approaches

Low-carbohydrate diets have recently been the most popular diets. The low-carbohydrate intake leads to less glycogen synthesis, and therefore less water in the body (about 3 grams of water are stored per gram of glycogen). As discussed in Chapter 4, a very-low-carbohydrate intake also forces the liver to produce needed glucose. The source of carbons for this glucose is mostly proteins from tissues such as muscle resulting in loss of protein tissue, about 72% water. Essential ions, such as potassium are also lost in the urine. With the loss of glycogen stores, lean tissue and water, the dieter loses weight very rapidly. When a normal diet is resumed, the protein tissue is rebuilt and the weight is regained.

Although low-carbohydrate diets work in the short run primarily because they limit total food intake, recent results indicate that low-carbohydrate diets may be effective alternatives to low-fat diets. In a recent 2-year study published in the New England Journal of Medicine, moderately obese adults on a low-carbohydrate diet lost and kept off about 12 pounds, compared to 10 pounds for those following the traditional Mediterranean diet, and 7 pounds for those on a restricted-fat plan.

▲ In time, the very-low-carbohydrate, high-protein diets typically leave a person wanting more variety in meals, and so the diets are abandoned. Dropout rates are high on these diets.

The most popular diet using a low-carbohydrate approach is the Dr. Atkins' New Diet Revolution. More moderate approaches are found in the various Zone diets (40% of calorie intake as carbohydrate), Sugar Busters diet, and the South Beach diet (especially initial phases).

### Carbohydrate-Focused Diets

Several recent diets, including Sugar Busters the Glucose Revolution, and Eat, Drink and Weigh Less, do not restrict carbohydrates, but rather emphasize the "good" carbohydrates in place of the "bad" or "harmful" ones. These diets recommend eating plenty of fruits, vegetables, whole grains, and cutting out simple sugars and processed grains. The carbohydrate-focused diets rely largely on low glycemic index and low glycemic load foods. In theory, these foods will cause a slow, steady rise in blood sugar, which will help control hunger.

### Low-Fat Approaches

The very-low-fat diets contain approximately 5% to 10% of calories as fat and are very high in carbohydrates. The most notable are the Pritikin Diet and the Dr. Dean Ornish "Eat More, Weigh Less" diet plans. This approach is not harmful for healthy adults, but it is difficult to follow. People are quickly bored with this type of diet because they cannot eat many of their favorite foods. These dieters eat primarily grains, fruits, and vegetables, which most people cannot do for very long. Eventually, the person wants some foods higher in fat or protein. These diets are just too different from the typical North American diet for many adults to follow consistently, but may be acceptable for some people.

### Novelty Diets

A variety of diets are built on gimmicks. Some novelty diets emphasize one food or food group and exclude almost all others. A rice diet was designed in the 1940s to lower blood pressure; now it has resurfaced as a weight-loss diet. The first phase consists of eating only rice and fruit. On the Beverly Hills Diet, you eat mostly fruit.

The rationale behind these diets is that you can eat only rice or fruit for just so long before becoming bored and, in theory, reducing your calorie intake. However,

chances are that you will abandon the diet entirely before losing much weight.

The most questionable of the novelty diets propose that "food gets stuck in your body." Fit for Life, the Beverly Hills Diet, and Eat Great, Lose Weight are examples. The supposition is that food gets stuck in the intestine, putrefies, and creates toxins, which invade the blood and cause disease. In response, recommendations are to not consume meat with potatoes or to consume fruits only after noon. These recommendations make no physiological sense.

### Meal Replacements

Meal replacements come in many forms, including beverages or formulas, frozen or shelf-stable entrees, and meal or snack bars. Most meal replacements are fortified with vitamins and minerals and are appropriate to replace one or two regular meals or snacks per day. Although they are not a "magic bullet" for weight loss, they have been shown to help some people lose weight. Advantages of these convenient products are that they provide portion- and calorie-controlled foods that can serve as a visual education on appropriate portion sizes.

### Quackery Is Characteristic of Many Popular Diets

Many popular diets fall under the category of quackery—people taking advantage of others. They usually involve a product or service that costs a considerable amount of money. Often, those offering the product or service don't realize that they are promoting quackery, because they were victims themselves. For example, they tried the product and by pure coincidence it worked for them, so they wish to sell it to all their friends and relatives.

Numerous other gimmicks for weight loss have come and gone and are likely to resurface. If in the future an important aid for weight loss is discovered, you can feel confident that major journals, such as the *Journal of the American Dietetic Association*, the *Journal of the American Medical Association*, or *The New England Journal of Medicine*, will report it. You don't need to rely on paperback books, infomercials, billboards, or newspaper advertisements for information about weight loss.

## Case Study Choosing a Weight-Loss Program

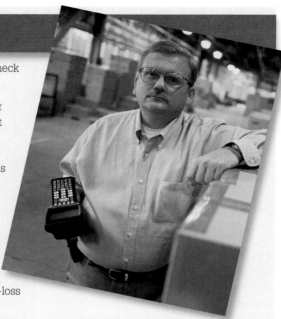

Joe has a hectic schedule. During the day he works full-time at a warehouse distribution center filling orders. At night, three times a week, he attends class at the local community college in pursuit of computer certification. On weekends he likes to watch sports on TV, spend time with family and friends, and study. Joe has little time to think about what he eats—convenience rules. He stops for coffee and a pastry on his way to work, has a burger or pizza for lunch at a quick service restaurant, and for dinner picks up fried chicken or fish at the drive-through on his way to class. Unfortunately, over the past few years Joe's weight has been climbing. Watching a game on television a few nights ago, he saw an infomercial for a product that promises he can eat large portions of tasty foods but not gain weight. A famous actor supports the claim that this product allows one to eat at will and not gain weight. This claim is tempting to Joe.

Answer the following questions, and check your response in Appendix A.

1. Has Joe been experiencing positive or negative energy balance over the past few years?
2. What aspects of Joe's lifestyle (other than diet) are causing this effect on his energy balance? What changes could Joe make in his habits to promote weight loss or maintenance?
3. What changes could Joe make in his diet that would promote weight loss or maintenance?
4. Why should Joe be skeptical of the claims he heard about the weight-loss product in the infomercial?
5. What advice can you offer Joe for evaluation of weight-loss programs?

▲ What changes can Joe make in his daily routine and diet to stop his weight gain?

## Summary

1. Energy balance considers energy intake and energy output. Negative energy balance occurs when energy output surpasses energy intake, resulting in weight loss. Positive energy balance occurs when calorie intake is greater than output, resulting in weight gain.

2. Basal metabolism, the thermic effect of food, physical activity, and thermogenesis account for total energy use by the body. Basal metabolism, which represents the minimum amount of calories required to keep the resting, awake body alive, is primarily affected by lean body mass, surface area, and thyroid hormone concentrations. Physical activity is energy use above that expended at rest. The thermic effect of food describes the increase in metabolism that facilitates digestion, absorption, and processing of the nutrients recently consumed. Thermogenesis is heat production caused by shivering

when cold, fidgeting, and other stimuli. In a sedentary person, about 70% to 80% of energy use is accounted for by basal metabolism and the thermic effect of food.

3. A person of healthy weight shows good health and performs daily activities without weight-related problems. A body mass index (weight in kilograms ÷ height$^2$ in meters) of 18.5 to 25 is one measure of healthy weight, although weight in excess of this value may not lead to ill health. A healthy weight is best determined in conjunction with a thorough health evaluation by a physician. A body mass index of 25 to 29.9 represents overweight. Obesity is defined as a total body fat percentage over 25% (men) or 35% (women) or a body mass index of 30 or more.

4. Fat distribution greatly determines health risks from obesity. Upper-body

fat storage, as measured by a waist circumference greater than 40 inches (102 centimeters) for men or 35 inches (88 centimeters) for women typically results in higher risks of hypertension, cardiovascular disease, and type 2 diabetes than does lower-body fat storage.

5. A sound weight-loss program meets the dieter's nutritional needs by emphasizing a wide variety of low-calorie, bulky foods; adapts to the dieter's habits; consists of readily obtainable foods; strives to change poor eating habits; stresses regular physical activity; and stipulates the supervision by a physician if weight is to be lost rapidly or if the person is over the age of 40 (men) or 50 (women) and plans to perform substantially greater physical activity than usual.

6. A pound of adipose tissue contains about 3500 kcal. Loss or gain of a pound of adipose tissue—the fat itself

plus lean support tissue—represents approximately 3300 kcal. Thus, if energy output exceeds calorie intake by about 500 kcal per day, a pound of adipose tissue can be lost per week.

Physical activity as part of a weight-loss program should be focused on duration rather than intensity. Ideally, vigorous activity for 60 minutes should be part of each day to prevent adult weight gain.

Behavior modification is a vital part of a weight-loss program because the dieter may have many habits that discourage weight maintenance. Specific behavior modification techniques, such as stimulus control and self-monitoring, can be used to help change problem behavior.

7. Medications to blunt appetite, such as phenteramine (Fastin) and sibutramine (Meridia), can aid weight-reduction strategies. Orlistat (Xenical) reduces fat absorption from a meal when taken with the meal. Weight-loss drugs are reserved for those who are obese or have weight-related problems, and they must be administered under close physician supervision.

The treatment of severe obesity may include surgery to reduce stomach volume to approximately 30 milliliters (1 ounce) or very-low-calorie diets containing 400 to 800 kcal per day. Both of these measures should be reserved for people who have failed at more conservative approaches to weight loss. They also require close medical supervision.

8. Underweight can be caused by a variety of factors, such as excessive physical activity and genetic background.

Sometimes being underweight requires medical attention. A physician should be consulted first to rule out underlying disease. The underweight person may need to increase portion sizes and learn to like calorie-dense foods. In addition, encouraging a regular meal and snack schedule aids in weight gain, as well as weight maintenance.

9. Many overweight people try popular diets that most often are not helpful and may actually be harmful. Unreliable diets typically share some common characteristics, including promoting quick weight loss, limiting food selections, using testimonials as proof, and requiring no exercise.

## Study Questions

1. After re-examining the nature and nurture aspects of weight control, propose two hypotheses for the development of obesity.

2. Propose two hypotheses for the development of obesity, based on the four contributors to energy expenditure.

3. Define a healthy weight in a way that makes the most sense to you.

4. Describe a practical method to define obesity in a clinical setting.

5. What are the two most convincing pieces of evidence that both genetic and environmental factors play significant roles in the development of obesity?

6. List three health problems that obese people typically face. Describe a possible reason that each problem arises.

7. When searching for a sound weight-loss program, what three key characteristics would you look for?

8. Why is the claim for quick, effortless weight loss by any method always misleading?

9. Define the term *behavior modification*. Relate it to the terms *stimulus control, self-monitoring, chain-breaking, relapse prevention,* and *cognitive restructuring.* Give examples of each.

10. Why should the treatment of obesity be viewed as a lifelong commitment rather than just a short episode of weight loss?

## Check Your Knowledge

Answers to the following multiple choice questions are below.

1. Decreasing energy intake by about 400 to 500 kcal per day would mean a loss of about one pound of body fat stores in _____ days.
   a. 2          c. 10
   b. 7          d. 14

2. Thermic effect of food represents the energy cost of
   a. chewing food.
   b. peristalsis
   c. basal metabolism.

   d. digesting, absorbing, and packaging nutrients.

3. A well-designed diet should
   a. increase physical activity.
   b. alter problem behaviors.
   c. reduce energy intake.
   d. All of the above.

4. Dr. Atkins' New Diet Revolution, The Zone, and the South Beach Diet are all examples of low- _____ diets.
   a. fat
   b. carbohydrate

   c. protein
   d. fiber

5. The intent of bariatric surgery is to
   a. limit stomach volume.
   b. speed transit time.
   c. surgically remove adipose tissue.
   d. prevent snacking.

6. Basal metabolism
   a. represents about 30% of total energy expenditure.
   b. is energy used to maintain heartbeat, respiration, and other basic functions and daily activities.

c.  represents about 60% to 70% of total calories used by the body during a day.

d.  includes the energy used to digest food.

7.  All of the following factors are associated with a higher basal metabolic rate *except*

a.  stress.          c.  fever.

b.  starvation.      d.  pregnancy.

8.  Probably the most important reason for obesity today in the United States is

a.  watching TV.

b.  snacking practices.

c.  inactivity.

d.  eating French fries.

9.  The major goal for weight reduction in the treatment of obesity is the loss of

a.  weight.          c.  body water.

b.  body fat.        d.  body protein.

10. For most adults, the greatest portion of their energy expenditure is for

a.  physical activity.

b.  sleeping.

c.  basal metabolism.

d.  the thermic effect of food.

Answers: 1. b, 2. d, 3. d, 4. b, 5. a, 6. c, 7. b, 8. c, 9. b, 10. c

# Further Readings (See also the May 2005 Supplement on Obesity in the Journal of the American Dietetic Association)

1. Adams KF and others: Overweight, obesity, and mortality in a large prospective cohort of persons 50 to 71 years old. *The New England Journal of Medicine* 355:763, 2006.

   *Although obesity, defined by a body-mass index (BMI) of 30.0 or more, has been associated with an increased risk of death, the relationship between overweight (a BMI of 25.0 to 29.9) and the risk of death is not clear. BMI was prospectively examined in relation to the risk of death from any cause in 527,265 U.S. men and women 50 to 71 years old. Excess body weight during midlife was associated with an increased risk of death. Risk of death increased by 20% to 40% among overweight persons and by two to three times among obese persons.*

2. Blackburn GL, Corliss J: *Break Through Your Set Point.* New York: Harper Collins, 2007.

   *This book outlines strategies for "breaking through" weight loss plateaus by working with, not against, the body's natural tendency to stay at a fixed weight. The key is slow, gradual weight loss, followed by a six-month period of holding steady at your new weight. Dr. Blackburn suggests that your set point can be lowered by consuming at least 450 calories at each meal, getting plenty of sleep, and being as active as possible.*

3. Foster GD and others: Behavioral treatment of obesity. *American Journal of Clinical Nutrition* 82:230S, 2005.

   *The behavior change process is facilitated through the use of self-monitoring, goal-setting, and problem solving. Behavior therapy can help individuals develop a set of skills (such as eating a low-calorie, low-fat diet) to achieve a healthier weight.*

4. Goldberg J, Bucciarelli A: A century of low-carbohydrate diets. *Nutrition Today* 41(3):99, 2006.

   *Low-carbohydrate diets have come and gone and been promising quick and easy weight loss for more than a century. This article is a review of the history of low-carbohydrate diets, their safety and effectiveness, and how they have performed in clinical trials.*

5. Hollis JF and others: Weight loss during the intensive intervention phase of the weight-loss maintenance trial. *American Journal Preventive Medicine* 35:118, 2008.

   *Participants in this study were overweight or obese and lost an average of 12 pounds in this trial. Keeping a daily record of food and physical activity helped them succeed. This study suggests that the willingness to record your eating habits could lead to a healthier weight.*

6. Jakicic JM, Otto AD: Physical activity considerations for the treatment and prevention of obesity. *American Journal of Clinical Nutrition* 82:226S, 2005.

   *Physical activity is an important component of long-term weight control, and therefore adequate levels of activity should be prescribed to combat the obesity epidemic. Although there is evidence that 30 minutes of moderate-intensity physical activity may improve health outcomes, a growing body of scientific literature suggests that at least 60 minutes of moderate-intensity physical activity may be necessary to maximize weight loss and prevent significant weight regain.*

7. Kruger J and others: Dietary and physical activity behaviors among adults successful at weight loss maintenance. *International Journal of Behavioral Nutrition and Physical Activity* 3:17, 2006.

   *Many individuals who lose weight do not keep the weight off and eventually regain most of the lost weight. In this study, weight-loss strategies among adults who reported successful weight-loss attempts (lost weight and were able to keep it off) were compared to persons whose previous attempts to lose weight were unsuccessful or who could not keep the lost weight off. Strategies practiced more frequently by successful weight losers included self-monitoring strategies such as weighing oneself, planning meals, tracking fat and calories, exercising 30 or more minutes daily, and adding physical activity to their daily routines.*

8. Ledikwe JH and others: Low-energy density diets are associated with high diet quality in adults in the United States. *Journal of the American Dietetic Association* 106:1172, 2006.

   *This study demonstrated the beneficial effects of a low-energy-density diet compared with a high-energy-density diet. Benefits included lower energy intakes, higher food intakes, and higher diet quality. A low-energy-density diet should include a variety of fruits and vegetables; low-fat/reduced-fat, nutrient dense, and/or water-rich grains; dairy products; and meats/meat alternatives.*

9. Li Z and others: Meta-analysis: Pharmacologic treatment of obesity. *Annals of Internal Medicine* 142(7):532, 2005.

   *Sibutramine, orlistat, and phentermine promote weight loss for at least 6 months when given along with recommendations for diet (and other behavioral and exercise interventions). The amount of extra weight loss attributable to these medications is modest, but still may be clinically significant. Use of each of these medications is reviewed in detail.*

10. Madan AT, Orth WD: Vitamin and trace mineral levels after laparoscopic gastric bypass. *Obesity Surgery* 16:603, 2006.

    *Vitamin and mineral deficiencies are thought to be a common long-term outcome of bariatric surgery. In this retrospective study, serum pre- and postoperative levels of vitamins and trace elements were measured in 100 patients who underwent laparoscopic Roux-en-Y gastric bypass. Most vitamin and minerals were slightly lower at 1-year postoperative. Significant decreases were observed only for vitamin D and selenium.*

11. National Center for Chronic Disease Prevention and Health Promotion: *Obesity: Halting the Epidemic by Making Health Easier.* Center for Disease Control and Prevention, Department of Health and Human Services, 2009. http://www.cdc.gov/nccdphp/dnpa.

    *Signs of success in the prevention and control of obesity are emerging. In the U.S., obesity rates among children, adolescents, women, and men did not increase significantly between 2003–2004 and 2005–2006. Increased awareness of* obesity as a national health problem is thought to have contributed to the plateau in obesity rates. Innovative policy and environmental changes in communities, work sites, and schools have also likely led to this leveling of rates. Experts believe that increased exercise and reduced consumption of high-calorie and fatty foods has had an impact.

12. O'Brien PE and others: Treatment of mild to moderate obesity with laparoscopic adjustable gastric banding or an intensive medical program: A randomized trial. *Annals of Internal Medicine* 144:625, 2006.

This was one of the first randomized controlled trials comparing adjustable gastric banding to an intensive very-low-calorie liquid diet. Both groups lost an initial mean 13.8% weight at 6 months. The surgical patients continued to lose weight more rapidly for a mean weight loss of 21.6% at 24 months and also had greater improvement in the metabolic syndrome and quality of life. The results suggest that moderate surgery, such as banding, may pose lower risk than gastric bypass with longer duration of weight-loss results.

13. Ogden CL, Carroll MD, McDowell MA, Flegal KM: Obesity among adults in the United States—no change since 2003–2004. NCHS data brief no 1. Hyattsville, MD: National Center for Health Statistics, 2007.

In the U.S., obesity rates among children, adolescents, women and men did not increase significantly between 2003–2004 and 2005–2006.

14. Robb M, Robb N: Tiny pills, big promises. *Today's Diet & Nutrition* 4(4):58, 2008.

Information is provided about the latest dietary aids/diet pills for weight loss. Diet pills rely on one of three strategies: suppressing appetite, boosting metabolism, or blocking absorption of fats or carbohydrates. Each strategy is reviewed. Aids discussed include Phetermine, Meridia, Hoodia gordonii, and Xenical.

15. See R and others: The association of differing measures of overweight and obesity with prevalent atherosclerosis: the Dallas Heart Study. *Journal of American College of Cardiologists* 50: 752, 2007.

In this study of the associations between different measures of obesity (body mass index, waist circumference, and waist-to-hip ratio) and atherosclerosis from the Dallas Heart Study, the authors discovered that waist-to-hip ratio was more strongly associated with atherosclerosis than either body mass index or waist circumference. These results indicate that apple-shaped people (those who have more fat around their middle) are at greater risk for obesity-related diseases and heart attack than pear-shaped ones (those who have a leaner waistline and carry more of their weight elsewhere).

16. Shai I and others: Weight loss with a low-carbohydrate, Mediterranean, or low-fat diet. *New England Journal of Medicine* 359:229, 2008.

Moderately obese adults (mean age, 52 years) were assigned to one of three diets: low-fat, restricted-calorie; Mediterranean, restricted-calorie; or low-carbohydrate, non–restricted-calorie, and studied for 2 years. Participants on the low-carbohydrate diet lost and kept off about 12 pounds; those following the traditional Mediterranean diet, including a lot of vegetables and a moderate amount of olive oil and nuts achieved and maintained a 10 pound weight loss; and those on the restricted-fat plan kept off 7 pounds. The results indicate that Mediterranean and low-carbohydrate diets may be effective alternatives to low-fat diets.

17. Slavin J and others: How fiber affects weight regulation. *Food Technology*, p.34, February 2008.

High-fiber diets are linked to lower body weight. This article discusses the effect of different fibers on satiety and food intake. Dietary fiber has intrinsic, hormonal, and intestinal effects that decrease food intake by promoting satiety. Examples of these effects include decreased gastric emptying and/or slowed energy and nutrient absorption.

18. Spear BA: Does dieting increase the risk for obesity and eating disorders? *Journal of the American Dietetic Association* 106:523, 2006.

This editorial summarizes the results of recent studies on dieting and other unhealthful weight-control methods in adolescents that appear to predict and be associated with later weight gain, overweight, and eating disorders.

19. Svetkey LP and others: Comparison of strategies for sustaining weight loss: The weight loss maintenance randomized controlled trial. *Journal of the American Medical Association* 299:1139, 2008.

Participants in this study weighed an average of 213 pounds and had high blood pressure and/or high blood cholesterol. They followed the Dietary Approaches to Stop Hypertension (DASH) diet for six months and were encouraged to do 180 minutes of moderate exercise (most chose to walk briskly) a week. Average weight loss was 19 pounds. Some dieters had monthly phone conversations or office visits with a behavioral/nutrition counselor, some had access to an interactive website, and some were left to their own devices. After 2 ½ years, dieters kept more weight off if they reported to a nutrition counselor every month.

20. Wing RR, Phelan S: Long-term weight loss maintenance. *American Journal of Clinical Nutrition* 82:222S, 2005.

National Weight Control Registry members provide evidence that long-term weight loss maintenance is possible and help identify the specific approaches associated with long-term success. The article reviews the habits of these participants, such as regularly eating breakfast, self-monitoring weight, and meeting the goal of 60 minutes of physical activity per day.

## I. A Close Look at Your Weight Status

Determine the following two indices of your body status: body mass index and waist circumference.

### Body Mass Index (BMI)

Record your weight in pounds: _____ lb
Divide your weight in pounds by 2.2 to determine your weight in kilograms: _____ kilograms
Record your height in inches: _____ in
Divide your height in inches by 39.4 to determine your height in meters: _____ meters
Calculate your BMI using the following formula:
BMI = weight (kilograms)/height$^2$ (meters)
BMI = _____ kg/ _____ m$^2$ = _____

### Waist Circumference

Use a tape measure to measure the circumference of your waist (at the umbilicus with stomach muscles relaxed). Circumference of waist (umbilicus) = _____ in

### Interpretation

1. When BMI is greater than 25, health risks from obesity often begin. It is especially advisable to consider weight loss if your BMI exceeds 30. Does yours exceed 25 (or 30)?

   Yes _____ No _____

2. When a person has a BMI greater than 25 and a waist circumference of more than 40 inches (102 centimeters) in men or 35 inches (88 centimeters) in women, there is an increased risk of cardiovascular disease, hypertension, and type 2 diabetes. Does your waist circumference exceed the standard for your gender?

   Yes _____ No _____

3. Do you feel you need to pursue a program of weight loss?

   Yes _____ No _____

### Application

From what you've learned in Chapter 7, what can you do to change your patterns of eating and physical activity to lose weight and help ensure maintenance of any loss?

_____

_____

_____

**FIGURE 7-20** ▶ A model for behavior change. It starts with awareness of the problem and ends with the incorporation of new behaviors intended to address the problem.

## II. An Action Plan to Change or Maintain Weight Status

Now that you have assessed your current weight status, do you feel that you would like to make some changes? Following is a step-by-step guide to behavioral change. This process can be useful even for those satisfied with their current weight, as it can be applied to changing exercise habits, self-esteem, and a variety of other behaviors (Fig. 7-20).

### Becoming Aware of the Problem

By calculating your current weight status, you have already become aware of the problem, if one exists. From here, it is important to find out more information about the cause of the problem and whether it is worth working toward a change.

1. What are the factors that most influence your eating habits? Do you eat due to stress, boredom, or depression? Is volume of food your problem, or do you eat mainly the wrong foods for you? Take some time to assess the root causes of your eating habits.

2. Once you have more information about your specific eating practices, you must decide if it is worth changing these practices. A benefits and costs analysis can be a useful tool in evaluating whether it is worth your effort to make life changes. Use the following example as a guide for listing benefits and costs pertinent to your situation (Fig. 7-21).

### Setting Goals

What can we accomplish, and how long will it take? Setting a realistic, achievable goal and allowing a reasonable amount of time to pursue it increases the likelihood of success.

1. Begin by determining the outcome you would like to achieve. If you are trying to change your eating behaviors to be more healthy, list your reasons for doing so (e.g., overall health, weight loss, self-esteem).

   Overall goal:

   _____

   _____

**FIGURE 7-21 ▶** Benefits and costs analysis applied to increasing physical activity. This process helps put behavior change into the context of total lifestyle.

**Benefits and Costs Analysis**

**1 Benefits of changing eating habits?**

What do you expect to get, now or later, that you want?
What may you avoid that would be unpleasant?

*feel better physically and psychologically*
*look better*

**2 Benefits of not changing eating habits?**

What do you get to do that you enjoy doing?
What do you avoid having to do?

*no need for planning*
*can eat without feeling guilty*

**3 Costs involved in changing eating habits?**

What do you have to do that you don't want to do?
What do you have to stop doing that you would rather continue doing?

*take time to plan meals and shop*
*must give up some food volume*

**4 Costs of not changing eating habits?**

What unpleasant or undesirable effects are you likely to experience now or in the future?
What are you likely to lose?

*creeping weight gain*
*low self-esteem and poor health*

Reasons to pursue goal:

_____

_____

_____

2. Now list several steps that will be necessary to achieve your goal. Keep in mind, however, that it is generally best to change only a few specific behaviors at first—walking briskly for 60 minutes each day, reducing fat intake, using more whole-grain products, and not eating after 7 P.M. Attempting small and perhaps easier dietary changes first reduces the scope of the problem and increases the likelihood of success.

Steps toward achieving goal:

1. _____

2. _____

3. _____

If you are having trouble deciphering the steps needed to achieve your goal, health professionals are an excellent resource for aid in planning.

## Measuring Commitment

Now that you have collected information and know what is required to reach your goal, you must ask yourself, "Can I do this?" Commitment is an essential component in the success of behavioral change. Be honest with yourself. Permanent change is not quick or easy. Once you have decided that you have the commitment required to see this through, continue on to the following sections.

## Making It Official with a Contract

Drawing up a behavioral contract often adds incentive to follow through with a plan. The contract could list goal behaviors and objectives, milestones for measuring progress, and regular rewards for meeting the terms of the contract. After finishing a contract, you should sign it in the presence of some friends. This encourages commitment.

Initially, plans should reward positive behaviors, and then they should focus on positive results. Positive behaviors, such as regular physical activity, eventually lead to positive outcomes, such as increased stamina.

Figure 7-22 is a sample contract for increasing physical activity. Keep in mind that this sample contract is only a suggestion; you can add your ideas as well.

## Psyching Yourself Up

Once your contract is in place, you need to psych yourself up. Discouragement from peers and your temptations to stray from your plan need to be anticipated. Psyching yourself up can enable you to progress toward your goals in spite of others' attitudes and

**FIGURE 7-22** ▶ Alan's behavior contract. Completing such a contract can help generate commitment to behavior change. What would your contract look like?

**Name** *Alan Young*

**Goal**
I agree to *ride my exercise bike*
(specify behavior)

under the following circumstances *for 30 minutes, 4 times per week in the evening*
(specify where, when, how much, etc.)

Substitute behavior and/or reinforcement schedule *I will reinforce myself if I've achieved my goal after a month with a weekend off campus with my roommate.*

**Environmental planning**
In order to help me do this, I am going to (1) arrange my physical and social environment by *buying a new portable CD player*

and (2) control my internal environment (thoughts, images) by *coordinating riding the bike with the first T.V. watching I do in the evening*

**Reinforcements**
Reinforcements provided by me daily or weekly (if contract is kept):
*I will buy myself a new piece of clothing for off campus trip*

Reinforcements provided by others daily or weekly (if contract is kept):
*at the end of a month if I've completed my goal my parents will buy me a fitness club membership for winter.*

**Social support**
Behavior change is more likely to take place when other people support you. During the quarter/semester please meet with the other person at least three times to discuss your progress.
The name of my "significant helper" is: *Mr. and Mrs. Young*

This contract should include:
1. Baseline data (one week)
2. Well-defined goal
3. Simple method for charting progress (diary, counter, charts, etc.)
4. Reinforcements (immediate and long-term)
5. Evaluation method (summary of experiences, success, and/or new learnings about self).

opinions. Almost everyone benefits from some assertiveness training when it comes to changing behaviors. The following are a few suggestions. Can you think of any others?

- No one's feelings should be hurt if you say, "No, thank you," firmly and repeatedly when others try to dissuade you from a plan. Tell them you have new diet behavior and your needs are important.

- You don't have to eat a lot to accommodate anyone—your mother, business clients, or the chef. For example, at a party with friends, you may feel you have to eat a lot to participate, but you don't. Another trap is ordering a lot just because someone else is paying for the meal.

- Learn ways to handle put-downs—inadvertent or conscious. An effective response can be to communicate feelings honestly, without hostility. Tell criticizers that they have annoyed or offended you, that you are working to change your habits and would really like understanding and support from them.

## Practicing the Plan

Once you've set up a plan, the next step is to implement it. Start with a trial of at least 6 to 8 weeks. Thinking of a lifetime commitment can be overwhelming. Aim for a total duration of 6 months of new activities before giving up. We may have to persuade ourselves more than once of the value of continuing the program. The following are some suggestions to help keep a plan on track:

- *Focus on reducing, but not necessarily extinguishing, undesirable behaviors.* For example, it's usually unrealistic to say, "I'll never eat a certain food again." It's better to say, "I won't eat that *problem* food as often as before."

- *Monitor progress.* Note your progress in a diary and reward yourself according to your contract. While conquering some habits and seeing improvement, you may find yourself quite encouraged, even enthusiastic, about your plan of action. That can give you the impetus to move ahead with the program.

- *Control environments.* In the early phases of behavioral change, try to avoid problem situations, such as parties, coffee breaks, and favorite restaurants. Once new habits are firmly established, you can probably more successfully resist the temptations of these environments.

## Re-evaluating and Preventing Relapse

After practicing a program for several weeks to months, it is important to reassess the original plan. In addition, you may now be able to pinpoint other problem areas for which you need to plan appropriately.

1. Begin by taking a close and critical look at your original plan. Does it lead to the goals you set? Are there any new steps toward your goal that you feel capable of adding to your contract? Do you need new reinforcements? It may even be necessary to make a new contract. For permanent change, it is worth this time of reassessment.

2. In practicing your plan over the past weeks or months, you have likely experienced relapses. What triggered these relapses? To prevent a total retreat to your old habits, it is important to set up a plan for such relapses. You can do this by identifying high-risk situations, rehearsing a response, and remembering your goals.

You may have noticed a behavior chain in some of your relapses. That is, the relapse may stem from a series of interconnected habitual activities. The way to break the chain is to first identify the activities, pinpoint the weak links, break those links, and substitute other behaviors. Figure 7-23 illustrates a sample behavior chain and a substitute activities list. Consider compiling a list based on your behavior chains.

## Epilogue

If you have used the activities in this section, you are well on your way to permanent behavioral change. Recall that this exercise can be used for a variety of desired changes, including quitting smoking, increasing physical activity, and improving study habits. It is by no means an easy process, but the results can be well worth the effort. Overall, the keys to success are motivation (keeping the problem in the forefront of your mind), having a plan of action, securing the resources and skills needed for success, and looking for help from family, friends, or a group.

SUBSTITUTE ACTIVITIES

Pleasant activities
1. *Singing/washing hair*
2. *Reading comics/biking*
3. *Sewing/calling a friend*

Necessary activities
1. *Ironing*
2. *Vacuuming*
3. *Straightening apartment*

Situations when used
1. *Wanted ice cream — delayed with bath*
2. *Wanted wheat thins — cleaned up apt.*
3. *Wanted snack — went for walk*
4. *Wanted cookies — did dishes first*
5. *Saw leftovers — went for bike ride*
6. *Tempted by cookies — set timer*
7. *Wanted snack — read comics*

BEHAVIOR CHAIN

Identify the links in your eating response chain on the following diagram. Draw a line through the chain where it was interrupted. Add the link you substituted and the new chain of behavior this substitution started.

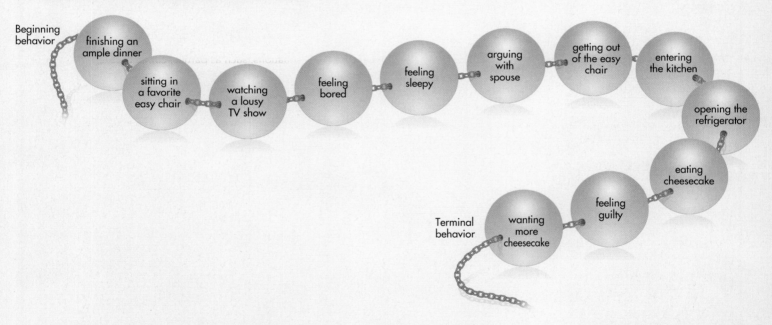

**FIGURE 7-23 ▶** Identifying behavior chains. This is a good tool for understanding more about your habits and pinpointing ways to change unwanted habits. The earlier in the chain you substitute a nonfood link, the easier it is to intervene. Four types of behaviors can be substituted in an ongoing behavior chain.

1. Fun activities (taking a walk, reading a book)
2. Necessary activities (cleaning a room, balancing your checkbook)
3. Incompatible activities (taking a shower)
4. Urge-delaying activities (setting a kitchen timer for 20 minutes before allowing yourself to eat)

Using activities to interrupt behavior patterns that lead to inappropriate eating (or inactivity) can be a powerful means of changing habits.

# CHAPTER 8 Vitamins

## Student Learning Outcomes  After studying Chapter 8, you will be able to:

1. Define the term *vitamin* and list three characteristics of vitamins as a group.

2. Classify the vitamins according to whether they are fat soluble or water soluble.

3. List the major functions and deficiency symptoms for each vitamin.

4. List three important food sources for each vitamin.

5. Describe toxicity symptoms from excess consumption of certain vitamins.

6. Evaluate the use of vitamin supplements with respect to their potential benefits and hazards to the body.

## Chapter Outline

Student Learning Outcomes

8.1 Vitamins: Vital Dietary Components

8.2 The Fat-Soluble Vitamins—A, D, E, and K

8.3 Vitamin A

8.4 Vitamin D

8.5 Vitamin E

8.6 Vitamin K

8.7 The Water-Soluble Vitamins and Choline

8.8 Thiamin

8.9 Riboflavin

8.10 Niacin

8.11 Pantothenic Acid

8.12 Biotin

8.13 Vitamin B-6

8.14 Folate

8.15 Vitamin B-12

8.16 Vitamin C

8.17 Choline

8.18 Vitamin-Like Compounds

Nutrition and Your Health: *Dietary Supplements—Who Needs Them?*

Case Study: Choosing a Dietary Supplement

Summary/Study Questions/Check Your Knowledge/Further Readings

Rate Your Plate

**ALTHOUGH THE VITAMINS ARE ESSENTIAL NUTRIENTS, THE AMOUNT OF VITAMINS WE NEED TO PREVENT DEFICIENCY IS SMALL.** In general, humans require a total of about 1 ounce (28 grams) of vitamins for every 150 pounds (70 kilograms) of food consumed. Some people believe that consuming vitamins far in excess of their needs provides them with extra energy, protection from disease, and prolonged youth. They seem to think that if a little is good, then more must be better. About 40% of adults in the United States take vitamin and/or mineral supplements on a regular basis, some at unsafe levels. They are spending about $17 billion annually on supplements. The health-related value of this practice is hotly debated.

Vitamins are found in plants and animals. Plants synthesize all the vitamins they need and as the chapter comic suggests, are a healthy source of vitamins for animals. Animals vary in their ability to synthesize vitamins. For example, guinea pigs and humans are two of the few organisms unable to make their own supply of vitamin C.

Chapter 8 reviews some general properties of vitamins. These vital nutrients are divided into two groups: the fat-soluble vitamins and the water-soluble vitamins. The chapter focuses on the functions and sources of each vitamin and human needs for them. The current controversy over vitamin and mineral supplement use is also explored.

### ⚡ Refresh Your Memory

As you begin your study of vitamins in Chapter 8, you may want to review:

- Implications of the Dietary Supplement Health and Education Act (DSHEA) in Chapter 2
- The gastrointestinal system for the digestion and absorption of nutrients and the urinary system for vitamin D activation in Chapter 3
- The digestion and absorption of dietary lipids, the formation of lipoproteins, and the definition of antioxidants in Chapter 5
- Amino acid metabolism, protein synthesis, and protein-calorie malnutrition in Chapter 6

## 8.1 Vitamins: Vital Dietary Components

**vitamin** Compound needed in small amounts in the diet to help regulate and support chemical reactions and processes in the body.

**fat-soluble vitamins** Vitamins that dissolve in fat and such substances as ether and benzene but not readily in water. These vitamins are A, D, E, and K.

**water-soluble vitamins** Vitamins that dissolve in water. These vitamins are the B vitamins and vitamin C.

**coenzyme** A compound that combines with an inactive enzyme to form a catalytically active form. In this manner, coenzymes aid in enzyme function.

By definition, **vitamins** are essential organic (carbon-containing) substances needed in small amounts in the diet for normal function, growth, and maintenance of the body. Although vitamins yield no energy to the body, they often participate in energy-yielding reactions. Vitamins A, D, E, and K are **fat soluble,** whereas the B vitamins and vitamin C are **water soluble.** In addition, the B vitamins and vitamin K function as parts of **coenzymes** (compounds that help enzymes function).

Vitamins are generally essential in human diets because they can't be synthesized in the human body or because their synthesis can be decreased by environmental factors. Notable exceptions to having a strict dietary need for a vitamin are vitamin A, which we can synthesize from certain pigments in plants; vitamin D, synthesized in the body if the skin is exposed to adequate sunlight; niacin, synthesized from the

Increasing our intake of fruits and vegetables is one of the recurring Dietary Guidelines. Which vitamins are especially found in fruits and vegetables? What are some other health-related attributes of fruits and vegetables in general? Which chronic diseases are associated with a poor intake of fruits and vegetables? Should we take a daily vitamin supplement if we do not include fruits and vegetables in our diet? Chapter 8 provides some answers.

**ZIGGY**

amino acid tryptophan; and vitamin K and biotin, synthesized to some extent by bacteria in the intestinal tract.

To be classified as a vitamin, a compound must meet the following criteria to be an essential nutrient: (1) the body is unable to synthesize enough of the compound to maintain health; and (2) absence of the compound from the diet for a defined period produces deficiency symptoms that, if caught in time, are quickly cured when the substance is resupplied. A substance does not qualify as a vitamin merely because the body can't make it. Evidence must suggest that health declines when the substance is not consumed.

As scientists began to identify various vitamins, related deficiency diseases such as scurvy, beriberi, pellagra, and rickets were dramatically cured. For the most part, as the vitamins were discovered, they were named alphabetically: A, B, C, D, E, and so on. Later, many substances originally classified as vitamins were found not to be essential for humans and were dropped from the list. Other vitamins, thought at first to be only one chemical turned out to be several chemicals, so the alphabetical names had to be broken down by numbers (B-6, B-12, and so on).

In addition to their use in correcting deficiency diseases, a few vitamins have also proved useful in treating several nondeficiency diseases. These medical applications require administration of pharmacological amounts or **megadoses,** well above typical human needs for the vitamins. For example, megadoses of a form of niacin can be used as part of blood cholesterol–lowering treatment for certain individuals. This chapter will mention others as well. Still, any claimed benefits from use of vitamin supplements, especially intakes in excess of the Upper Level (if set), should be viewed critically because unproven claims are common.

Both plant and animal foods supply vitamins in the human diet. Vitamins isolated from foods or synthesized in the laboratory are the same chemical compounds and generally work equally well in the body. Contrary to claims in the health-food literature, "natural" vitamins isolated from foods are, for the most part, no more healthful than those synthesized in a laboratory, but there are exceptions. Vitamin E is much more potent in its natural form than in its synthetic form. In contrast, synthetic folic acid, the form of the vitamin added to ready-to-eat breakfast cereals and flour, is 1.7 times more potent than the natural vitamin form.

## Have Scientists Found All the Vitamins?

You may wonder whether there are vitamins in foods that have yet to be discovered. After all, the first chemical formula of a vitamin (thiamin) was not determined until 1937, and the last structure was characterized in 1948 (vitamin B-12). Although some optimistic researchers hope to discover that one or more additional compounds (e.g., choline; see p. 332) are vitamins, most scientists are confident that all compounds that meet the criteria for classification as a vitamin have been discovered. Evidence supports this assumption. For example, people have lived well for years when receiving only intravenous administration of solutions that consist of protein, carbohydrate, fat, all the known vitamins, and the essential minerals. With appropriate medical monitoring, these people not only continue to live, but also build new body tissues, heal wounds, fight existing diseases, and even have babies.

## Storage of Vitamins in the Body

Except for vitamin K, the fat-soluble vitamins are not readily excreted from the body. In contrast, excess amounts of the water-soluble vitamins are generally lost from the body rapidly, partly because the water in cells dissolves these vitamins and excretes them out of the body via the kidneys. Water-soluble vitamin B-6 and vitamin B-12 are exceptions; these are stored much more readily than the other water-soluble vitamins.

Because of the limited storage of many vitamins, they should be consumed in the diet daily, although an occasional lapse in the intake of even water-soluble vitamins

**megadose** Intake of a nutrient beyond estimates of needs to prevent a deficiency or what would be found in a balanced diet; 2 to 10 times human needs is a starting point for such a pharmacological dosage.

▲ Vitamins are not likely to be toxic unless taken in large amounts as supplements.

generally causes no harm. Symptoms of a vitamin deficiency occur only when that vitamin is lacking in the diet and body stores are essentially exhausted. For example, an average person must consume no thiamin for 10 days or no vitamin C for 20 to 40 days before developing the first symptoms of deficiency of these vitamins.

## Vitamin Toxicity

Fat-soluble vitamins are not readily excreted, so some can easily accumulate in the body and cause toxic effects. And, although a toxic effect from an excessive intake of any vitamin is theoretically possible, toxicity of the fat-soluble vitamin A is the most frequently observed. Vitamin E and the water-soluble vitamins niacin, vitamin B-6, and vitamin C can also cause toxic effects, but only when consumed in large amounts (15 to 100 times human needs or more). These five vitamins are unlikely to cause toxic effects unless taken in supplement (pill) form. Vitamin A even causes toxicity with long-term intake as little as two times human needs.

A "one-a-day" type of multivitamin and mineral supplement usually contains less than two times the Daily Values of the components, so daily use of these products is unlikely to cause toxic effects in men and nonpregnant women. But consuming many vitamin pills, especially highly potent sources of vitamin A, can cause problems. Today, concentrated vitamin A supplements are widely available in grocery, drug, and health-food stores and pose risks for toxicity when used inappropriately. See the later "Nutrition and Your Health" section to find out more about whether you should take a multivitamin and mineral supplement and, if so, how to do it safely.

See *Nutrition and Your Health: Dietary Supplements—Who Needs Them?* at the end of Chapter 8.

**Community-supported agriculture (CSA)** Farms that are supported by a community of growers and consumers who provide mutual support and share the risks and benefits of food production, usually including a system of weekly delivery or pick-up of vegetables and fruit, sometimes dairy products and meat.

## Preservation of Vitamins in Foods

Substantial amounts of vitamins can be lost from the time a fruit or vegetable is picked until it is eaten. The water-soluble vitamins—particularly thiamin, vitamin C, and folate—can be destroyed with improper storage and excessive cooking. Heat, light, exposure to the air, cooking in water, and alkalinity are all factors that can destroy vitamins. The sooner a food is eaten after harvest, the less chance of nutrient loss. Food cooperatives, **community-supported agriculture (CSA)** and farmers' markets are great sources of freshly harvested fruits and vegetables.

In general, if the food is not eaten within a few days, freezing is the best preservation method to retain nutrients. Fruits and vegetables are often frozen immediately after harvesting, so frozen vegetables and fruits are often as nutrient-rich as freshly picked ones. As part of the freezing process, vegetables are quickly blanched in boiling water. This destroys the enzymes that would otherwise degrade the vitamins. Table 8-1 provides some tips to aid in preserving the vitamins in food.

▲ Frozen fruits and vegetables are often as nutrient-rich as freshly picked ones.

### CONCEPT CHECK

In general, the fat-soluble vitamins—A, D, E, and K—are less readily excreted than the water-soluble B vitamins and vitamin C. Regular consumption of foods rich in both water-soluble and fat-soluble vitamins is important for health. However, the occasional inadequate consumption of any one vitamin is of little health concern, because even water-soluble vitamins persist in the body to some extent. For example, when a person ingests a vitamin-free diet, the first deficiency signs (due to lack of thiamin) will not appear for about 10 days. When taken in supplement form, the fat-soluble vitamin A poses the greatest risk of toxicity. For the most part, there is little risk of toxicity when vitamins are obtained from a variety of foods.

**TABLE 8-1** Tips for Preserving the Vitamin Content of Foods

| What to Do | Why |
|---|---|
| Keep fruits and vegetables cool. | Enzymes in food begin to degrade vitamins once the fruit or vegetable is picked. Chilling reduces this process. Refrigerate fresh produce (except for potatoes, tomatoes, onions, and bananas) until they are consumed. |
| Refrigerate foods in moisture-proof, air-tight containers. | Nutrients keep best at temperatures near freezing, at high humidity, and away from air. |
| Trim, peel, and cut fruits and vegetables minimally—just enough to remove rotten or inedible parts. | Oxygen breaks down vitamins faster when more surface is exposed. Outer leaves of lettuce and other greens have higher values of vitamins and minerals than the inner, tender leaves or stems. Potato skins and apple skins are higher in vitamins and minerals than the inner parts. |
| Microwave, steam, or use a pan or wok with very small amounts of fat and a tight-fitting lid to cook vegetables. | More nutrients are retained when there is less contact with water and shorter cooking time. Whenever possible, cook fruits or vegetables in their skins. |
| Minimize reheating food. | Prolonged reheating reduces vitamin content. |
| Do not add fats to vegetables during cooking if you plan to discard the liquid. | Fat-soluble vitamins will be lost in discarded fat. Add fats to vegetables after they are fully cooked and drained. |
| Do not add baking soda to vegetables to enhance the green color. | Alkalinity destroys much thiamin, and other vitamins. |
| Store canned foods in a cool place. | Canned foods vary in the amount of nutrients lost, largely because of differences in storage time and temperatures. To get maximal nutritive value from canned goods, serve any liquid packed with the food whenever possible. |

▲ Rapid cooking of vegetables in minimal fluids aids in preserving vitamin content. Steaming is one effective method.

## 8.2 The Fat-Soluble Vitamins—A, D, E, and K

Let's look at what we know about the fat-soluble vitamins—vitamins A, D, E, and K.

### Absorption of Fat-Soluble Vitamins

Vitamins A, D, E, and K are absorbed along with dietary fat, because they are fat-soluble. These vitamins then travel with dietary fats through the bloodstream to reach body cells. Special carriers in the bloodstream help distribute some of these vitamins. Fat-soluble vitamins are stored mostly in the liver and fatty tissues.

When fat absorption is efficient, about 40% to 90% of the fat-soluble vitamins are absorbed. Anything that interferes with normal digestion and absorption of fats, however, also interferes with fat-soluble vitamin absorption. For example, people with cystic fibrosis, a disease that often hampers fat absorption, may develop deficiencies of fat-soluble vitamins. Some medications, such as the weight-loss drug orlistat (Xenical), that we discussed in Chapter 7, also interfere with fat absorption. Unabsorbed fat carries these vitamins to the large intestine, where they are excreted in the feces. People with such conditions are especially susceptible to vitamin K deficiency because body stores of vitamin K are lower than those of the other fat-soluble vitamins. Vitamin supplements, taken under a physician's guidance, are part of the treatment for preventing a vitamin deficiency associated with fat malabsorption. Finally, people who use mineral oil as a laxative at mealtimes risk fat-soluble vitamin deficiencies. The intestine does not absorb mineral oil, so fat-soluble vitamins are eliminated with the mineral oil in the feces.

## 8.3 Vitamin A

The amount of vitamin A you consume is important, as both deficiency and toxicity of this vitamin can cause severe problems. In addition, there is a narrow range of optimal intakes between these two states. Vitamin A is found in foods in a variety of forms. **Retinoids,** or preformed vitamin A, are only found in foods of animal origin, such as fish and organ meats. However, plants contain pigments called **carotenoids,** which can be turned into vitamin A in the body as needed. They can be termed **provitamin A.** Only three of the more than 600 carotenoids found in nature are known to serve as provitamin A in humans, but there may be more. Beta-carotene, the orange-yellow pigment in carrots, is the most potent form of provitamin A. The other known provitamin A carotenoids are lutein and zeaxanthin. Together, preformed vitamin A from animal sources and provitamin A carotenoids make up what is generally called vitamin A.

### Functions of Vitamin A and Carotenoids

Vitamin A plays many important roles in the body. The best known and most clearly understood of its roles is in vision. Body changes that occur when vitamin A is lacking provide insight to this and other actions of this fat-soluble nutrient.

**Vision.** Vitamin A performs important functions in light-dark vision, and to a lesser extent, color vision. One form of vitamin A (retinal) allows certain cells in the eye to adjust from bright to dim light (such as after seeing the headlights of an oncoming car). Without sufficient dietary vitamin A, the cells in the eye cannot quickly readjust to dim light. This condition, known as **night blindness,** is an early sign of vitamin A deficiency.

If vitamin A deficiency progresses, the cells that line the cornea of the eye (the clear window of the eye) also lose their ability to produce **mucus.** The eye then becomes dry. Eventually, when dirt particles scratch the dry surface of the eye, bacteria infect it. The infection soon spreads to the entire surface of the eye and leads to blindness. This disease process is called **xerophthalmia,** which means *dry eye* (Fig. 8-1).

Vitamin A deficiency is second only to accidents as a worldwide cause of blindness. North Americans are at little risk because of generally good diets. However, people—especially children—in less-developed nations are susceptible to vitamin A deficiency. Poor vitamin A intakes, low fat intakes that do not allow for sufficient vitamin A absorption, and low stores of vitamin A lessen the ability of the children to meet high needs during rapid childhood growth. Hundreds of thousands of children in developing nations, especially Asia, become blind each year because of vitamin A deficiency and ultimately die from infections. In North America, the leading cause of blindness in adults is diabetes; in children, it is accidents. As covered in more detail in Chapter 12, worldwide attempts to reduce this problem have included giving large doses of vitamin A twice yearly and fortifying sugar, margarine, and monosodium glutamate with vitamin A. These food vehicles are used because they are commonly consumed by the populations of less-developed nations. This effort has proven effective in some countries.

Age-related **macular degeneration** is a leading cause of legal blindness among North American adults over the age of 65 (Fig. 8-2). The disease is associated with changes in the macular area of the eye, which provides the most detailed vision. Age, smoking, and genetics are risk factors. The macula contains the carotenoids lutein and zeaxanthin in high enough concentrations to impart a yellow color. In one study, the higher the total number of carotenoids (beta-carotene, lutein, and zeaxanthin) consumed in the diet, the lower was the risk for age-related macular degeneration. These carotenoids may also decrease the risk of cataracts in the eyes. Consumption of fruits and vegetables high in carotenoids, rather than the intake of these specific carotenoids in supplements, may reduce the risk for these eye disorders. Multivitamin and mineral supplements formulated for older adults (e.g., Centrum Silver™) are being marketed as a source of lutein.

**retinoids** Chemical forms of preformed vitamin A; one source is animal foods.

**carotenoids** Pigment materials in fruits and vegetables that range in color from yellow to orange to red; three of the various carotenoids yield vitamin A. Many are antioxidants.

**provitamin/precursor** A substance that can be made into a vitamin if the body needs it.

**night blindness** A vitamin A deficiency condition in which the retina (in the eye) cannot adjust to low amounts of light.

**mucus** A thick fluid secreted by many cells throughout the body. It contains a compound that has both carbohydrate and protein parts. It acts as a lubricant and means of protection for cells.

**xerophthalmia** Literally "dry eye." This is a cause of blindness that results from a vitamin A deficiency. A lack of mucus production by the eye, which leaves it at a greater risk of damage from surface dirt and bacteria.

**macular degeneration** A painless condition leading to disruption of the central part of the retina (in the eye) and, in turn, blurred vision.

**FIGURE 8-1** ▶ Vitamin A deficiency that eventually led to blindness. Note the severe effects on this eye. This problem is commonly seen today in southeast Asia.

**Health of Other Cells.** Vitamin A also maintains the health of cells that line internal and external surfaces of the lungs, intestines, stomach, vagina, urinary tract, and bladder, as well as those of the eyes and skin. These cells (called **epithelial cells**) serve as important barriers to bacterial infection. As just noted for the eye, some epithelial cells secrete mucus, a needed lubricant. Without vitamin A, mucus-forming cells deteriorate and no longer synthesize mucus. Vitamin A deficiency also causes insufficient mucus production in the intestines and lung cells, and poor health of cells in general. Vitamin A deficiency also reduces the activity of certain immune system cells. Together, these effects leave the vitamin A–deficient person at great risk for infections. For many years, vitamin A has been dubbed the "anti-infection" vitamin.

**Growth, Development, and Reproduction.** Vitamin A participates in the processes of growth, development, and reproduction in several ways. This role has been demonstrated in vitamin A deficient children experiencing growth retardation when vitamin A supplementation increased their growth. At the genetic level, vitamin A (as retinoic acid) binds to receptors on DNA to increase synthesis of a variety of proteins (review Fig. 6-1 regarding the role of DNA in protein synthesis). In doing so, vitamin A is said to be affecting **gene expression.** Some of these proteins are required for growth, such as bone growth. In laboratory animals, another consequence of vitamin A deficiency is an inability to reproduce.

**Cardiovascular Disease Prevention.** Carotenoids may play a role in preventing cardiovascular disease in persons at high risk, possibly linked to carotenoids' antioxidant capability. Until definitive studies are complete, many scientists recommend that we increase our intake of carotenoids and other nutrients and compounds by consuming at least 5 servings of fruits and vegetables per day as part of an effort to reduce the risk of cardiovascular disease.

**Cancer Prevention.** Most forms of cancer arise from cells influenced by vitamin A. Coupled with its ability to aid immune system activity, vitamin A may be a valuable tool in the fight against cancer. This is especially true for skin, lung, bladder, and breast cancers. Still, because of the potential for toxicity, unsupervised use of megadose vitamin A supplements to reduce cancer risk is not advised.

Carotenoids by themselves also may help prevent cancer, acting again as antioxidants. Population studies show that regular consumption of foods rich in carotenoids decreases the risk of lung and oral cancers. Cancer of the **prostate gland** is one of the most common cancers among North American men. The dietary carotenoid found in tomatoes, (the red pigment lycopene) seems to protect against this type of cancer and may also decrease skin cancer risk.

In contrast to the potential benefits of carotenoids in food, recall from Chapter 1 that recent studies from the United States and Finland failed to show a reduction in lung cancer in male smokers and nonsmokers given supplements of the carotenoid beta-carotene for 5 or more years. In fact, beta-carotene use in male smokers increased the number of lung cancer cases compared with the control groups. No comparable studies have been done with women. Although further research continues, most researchers are now convinced that beta-carotene supplementation offers no protection against cancer. Thus, overwhelming advice is to rely on food sources of this or any other carotenoids.

**Vitamin A Analogs for Acne.** The acne medication tretinoin (Retin-A) is made of one **analog** form of vitamin A. It is used as a topical treatment (applied to the skin) for acne. It appears to work by irritating the skin, which leads to opening of pores and a generalized peeling of the skin layer. It also can block the deleterious effects that skin bacteria have on acne lesions. Similar vitamin A derivatives are also used in antiaging creams because they increase cell turnover and interrupt

**FIGURE 8-2 ▶** Age-related macular degeneration causing a blind spot in the center of the visual field. Increased dietary lutein and zeaxanthin are associated with decreased risk of macular degeneration. Further research is needed to better understand the relationship between macular degeneration and carotenoids.

**epithelial cells** The cells that line the outside of the body and the inside of all external passages within it, such as the GI tract.

**gene expression** Use of DNA information on a gene to produce a protein. This is a major determinant of cell development.

**prostate gland** A solid, chestnut-shaped organ surrounding the first part of the urinary tract in the male. The prostate gland secretes substances into the semen.

**analog** A chemical compound that differs slightly from another, usually natural, compound. Analogs generally contain extra or altered chemical groups and may have similar or opposite metabolic effects compared with the native compound. Also spelled *analogue.*

▼ Many vegetables are rich in provitamin A carotenoids.

the pathways of UV skin damage. Another derivative of vitamin A, isotretinoin (Accutane), is an oral drug used to treat serious acne. It acts in part to regulate development of cells in the skin (the gene expression role discussed earlier). Taking high doses of vitamin A itself would not be safe. The use of isotretinoin (Accutane) is strictly monitored by the U.S. Food and Drug Administration (FDA) in order to prevent the use of the drug during pregnancy due to the high risk of birth defects. iPLEDGE is a mandatory distribution program required since March 2006 by the FDA. In order for women to receive this medication, they must have two negative pregnancy tests; sign a patient information/consent form; agree to use two effective forms of birth control; register, along with their doctors and pharmacists, with iPLEDGE by phone or on the Internet, and agree to follow all instructions in the iPLEDGE program.

## Vitamin A Sources and Needs

Preformed vitamin A is found in liver, fish, fish oils, fortified milk and yogurt, and eggs (Fig. 8-3). Although liver is a rich food source of vitamin A and other nutrients that are stored in the liver. Focusing on liver to meet nutrient needs is not a good idea because it also provides a high concentration of cholesterol and other fats. Margarine is also fortified with vitamin A. The provitamin A carotenoids mentioned before are mainly found in dark green and yellow-orange vegetables and some fruits. Carrots, spinach and other greens, winter squash, sweet potatoes, broccoli, mangoes, cantaloupe, peaches, and apricots are examples of such sources. About 65% of the vitamin A in the typical

### Food Sources of Vitamin A

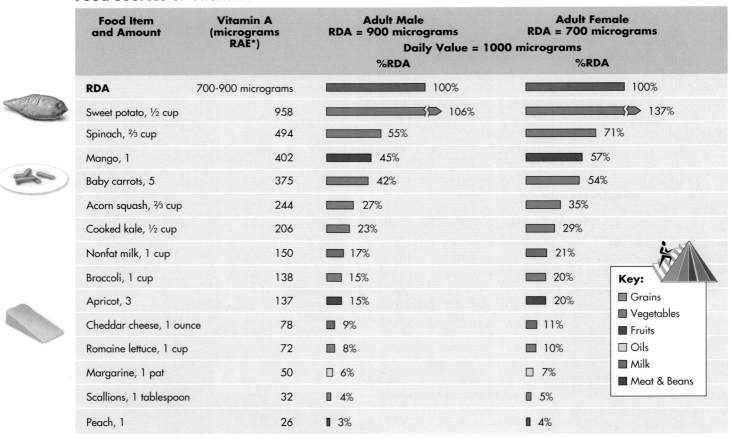

| Food Item and Amount | Vitamin A (micrograms RAE*) | Adult Male RDA = 900 micrograms %RDA | Adult Female RDA = 700 micrograms %RDA |
|---|---|---|---|
| **RDA** | 700-900 micrograms | 100% | 100% |
| Sweet potato, ½ cup | 958 | 106% | 137% |
| Spinach, ⅔ cup | 494 | 55% | 71% |
| Mango, 1 | 402 | 45% | 57% |
| Baby carrots, 5 | 375 | 42% | 54% |
| Acorn squash, ⅔ cup | 244 | 27% | 35% |
| Cooked kale, ½ cup | 206 | 23% | 29% |
| Nonfat milk, 1 cup | 150 | 17% | 21% |
| Broccoli, 1 cup | 138 | 15% | 20% |
| Apricot, 3 | 137 | 15% | 20% |
| Cheddar cheese, 1 ounce | 78 | 9% | 11% |
| Romaine lettuce, 1 cup | 72 | 8% | 10% |
| Margarine, 1 pat | 50 | 6% | 7% |
| Scallions, 1 tablespoon | 32 | 4% | 5% |
| Peach, 1 | 26 | 3% | 4% |

Daily Value = 1000 micrograms

**Key:**
- Grains
- Vegetables
- Fruits
- Oils
- Milk
- Meat & Beans

\* Retinol activity equivalents

**FIGURE 8-3** ▶ Food sources of vitamin A compared to the RDA for adult males and females.

## MyPyramid: Sources of Vitamin A

| Grains | Vegetables | Fruits | Oils | Milk | Meat & Beans |
|---|---|---|---|---|---|
| • Fortified break-fast cereals<br>• Fortified meal replacement bars | • Carrots<br>• Broccoli<br>• Spinach<br>• Squash<br>• Sweet potatoes | • Peaches<br>• Apricots<br>• Cantaloupes<br>• Mangoes<br>• Papayas | • Some forms of palm oil | • Fortified milk<br>• Fortified yogurt<br>• Cheese | • Liver<br>• Eggs |

**FIGURE 8-4** ▶ Sources of vitamin A from MyPyramid. The height of the background color (none, 1/3, 2/3, or completely covered) within each group in the pyramid indicates the average nutrient density for vitamin A in that group. Overall, the vegetables group, fruits group, and certain choices in the meat & beans group provide the richest sources. The grains group contains some foods that are nutrient-dense sources of vitamin A because they are fortified with the vitamin. With regard to physical activity, vitamin A plays no specific role *per se* in such endeavors.

North American diet comes from preformed vitamin A sources, whereas provitamin A dominates in the diet among poor people in other parts of the world.

Among common foods, those especially rich in vitamin A are carrots, spinach and other greens, sweet potatoes, winter squash, romaine lettuce, broccoli, apricots, and fat-free and low-fat milk. Many of the vegetables listed in Figs. 8-3 and 8-4 are good sources of beta-carotene and the other two provitamin A carotenoids. Marine oils are rich in vitamin A, and consumption of large amounts of such oils can lead to symptoms of vitamin A toxicity.

Beta-carotene accounts for some of the orange color of carrots. In vegetables such as broccoli, this yellow-orange color is masked by dark-green chlorophyll pigments. Still, green vegetables contain provitamin A. Green, leafy vegetables, such as spinach and kale, have a high concentration of lutein and zeaxanthin. Tomato juice and other tomato products, such as pizza sauce, contain significant amounts of lycopene.

The RDA for vitamin A is 700 to 900 micrograms of retinol activity equivalents (RAEs). These RAE units take into account the activity of both preformed vitamin A and the three carotenoids that also are known to yield vitamin A in humans. The total RAE value for a food is calculated by adding the concentration of preformed vitamin A to the amount of provitamin A carotenoids in the food that will be converted to vitamin A. The retinol equivalent (RE) is an older unit for vitamin A. This RE is similar to the RAE but assumed that there was a greater contribution to vitamin A needs from carotenoids than we assume today. Food composition tables and nutrient databases still contain some values based on this older RE standard. It will take some time to update these resources. The Daily Value used on food and supplement labels is 1000 micrograms (5000 IU).

▲ Provitamin A carotenoids are the safest way to meet vitamin A needs.

**international unit (IU)** A crude measure of vitamin activity, often based on the growth rate of animals in response to the vitamin. Today IUs have largely been replaced by more precise milligram or microgram measures.

**fetus** The developing human life form from 8 weeks after conception until birth.

## MAKING DECISIONS

### Expressing Vitamin A Content

In the past, most nutrient amounts in foods, including vitamin A, were formerly expressed in less precise **international units (IUs).** Some food and supplement labels still show the IU value for vitamin A. To compare the older IU standards to current RAE recommendations, assume that for any preformed vitamin A in a food or added to food, 3.3 IU = RAE. The same is true for any beta-carotene added to foods.

There is no easy way to convert IU units to RAE units for foods that naturally contain provitamin A carotenoids, such as carrots, spinach, and apricots. A general rule of thumb is to divide the IU units for foods containing carotenoids by 2, and then divide the result by 3.3 as just discussed.

Average intakes of vitamin A for North American adult men and women meet the RDA. Most adults in North America have liver reserves of vitamin A three to five times greater than needed to provide good health. Thus, the use of vitamin A supplements by most people is unnecessary. At present, there is no separate RDA for beta-carotene or any of the other provitamin A carotenoids.

Deficient vitamin A status in North America may be seen in preschool children who do not eat enough vegetables. The urban poor, older adults, and people with alcoholism or liver disease (which limits vitamin A storage) can also show diminished vitamin A status, especially with respect to stores. Finally, children and adults with severe fat-malabsorption may also experience vitamin A deficiency.

### Upper Level for Vitamin A

The Upper Level for vitamin A intake is established at 3000 micrograms of preformed vitamin A (3000 RAE or 10,000 IU) per day for adult men and women. This is based on the increases in birth defects and liver toxicity that accompany intakes in excess of 3000 micrograms of vitamin A per day. Above the Upper Level, other possible side effects include an increased risk of hip fracture and poor pregnancy outcomes.

During the early months of pregnancy, a high intake of preformed vitamin A is especially dangerous because it may cause **fetal** malformations and spontaneous abortions. This is because vitamin A binds to DNA and so influences cell development. FDA recommends that women of childbearing age limit their overall intake of preformed vitamin A to a total of about 100% of the Daily Value (1000 micrograms RAE or 5000 IU). Therefore, it is important to limit consumption of rich food sources, such as liver. These precautions also apply to women who may possibly become pregnant. Vitamin A is stored in the body for long periods, so women who take large amounts during the months before pregnancy place their fetuses at risk.

The consumption of large amounts of vitamin A–yielding carotenoids does not cause toxic effects. A high carotenoid concentration in the blood can occur if someone consumes large amounts of carrots or takes pills containing beta-carotene (more than 30 milligrams daily) or if infants eat a great deal of squash. This can turn the skin yellow-orange. The palms of the hands and soles of the feet in particular become colored. This condition does not appear to cause harm and disappears when carotenoid intake decreases. Dietary carotenoids do not produce toxic effects because (1) their rate of conversion into vitamin A is relatively slow and regulated, and (2) the efficiency of carotenoid absorption from the small intestine decreases markedly as oral intake increases.

## 8.4 Vitamin D

Vitamin D is not just a vitamin. It is primarily considered a hormone. A cholesterol-like substance in the skin cells is converted to the prohormone vitamin D, when exposed to ultraviolet B (UVB) rays from sunlight or tanning beds (Fig. 8-5). Liver and kidney cells then convert the prohormone to its active hormone form. The skin,

▲ Solar radiation on the skin provides about 80% to 100% of the vitamin D humans use. This is also the most reliable way to maintain vitamin D status. Dietary vitamin D is also effective, but less so.

liver, and kidney cells that participate in vitamin D synthesis are different from the bone and intestinal cells that are responsive to vitamin D. Having a site of synthesis different from the location of action is characteristic of hormones.

For many individuals, UVB exposure provides about 80% to 100% of our vitamin D needs. The amount of sun exposure needed by individuals to produce vitamin D depends on their skin color, age, time of day, season, and location. Experts recommend that people should expose their hands, face, and arms at least two to three times a week for 25% of the time it takes to turn ones skin pink (e.g., 5 to 10 minutes) to make enough vitamin D. Persons with dark skin would need additional exposure, about 3 to 5 times the amount just recommended (or maybe even more). The large amount of melanin pigment in dark-skinned people is a potent natural sunscreen.

Sun exposure is only effective for vitamin D synthesis between about 8:00 A.M. and 4:00 P.M. and without sunscreen over SPF 8. Although excessive exposure to the sun can increase the risk of skin cancer, the minimal amount of UVB exposure needed for vitamin D synthesis is encouraged. Still, this practice is not effective at all when there is little skin exposed to sun in the winter in northern climates. Although some people may have enough vitamin D stored in their adipose cells from summer months, most people in northern climates should find alternate vitamin D sources in the winter months. Overall, anyone who does not receive enough sunshine to synthesize an adequate amount of vitamin D must have a dietary source of the vitamin. About 80% of dietary vitamin D is absorbed.

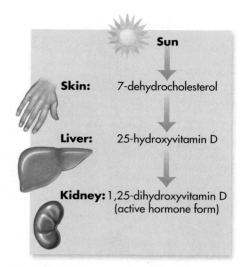

**FIGURE 8-5** ▶ The synthesis of vitamin D can take place in the body.

## Functions of Vitamin D

The main function of the vitamin D hormone (1,25-dihydroxyvitamin D) is to help regulate calcium and bone metabolism. Working with other hormones, especially **parathyroid hormone (PTH),** the vitamin D hormone closely regulates blood calcium so that appropriate amounts of it will be supplied to all cells. This regulation involves two main processes: the vitamin D hormone helps regulate absorption of calcium and phosphorus from the intestine and the deposition of calcium in the bones.

More interestingly, the vitamin D hormone is also capable of ensuring normal development of some cells, such as skin, colon, prostate, ovary, and breast cells, in turn reducing cancer risk in these sites. The vitamin D hormone controls the growth of the parathyroid gland; aids in the function of the immune system; and contributes to skin cell development, muscle and gum health, and blood pressure regulation.

The most obvious result of the vitamin D hormone action is increased calcium and phosphorus deposition in bones. Without adequate calcium and phosphorus deposition during bone synthesis, bones weaken and bow under pressure. A child with these symptoms has the disease **rickets.** Symptoms also include enlarged head, joints, and rib cage and a deformed pelvis (Fig. 8-6).

Studies have shown rickets to be a problem in breastfed infants who receive little sun exposure. For the prevention of rickets, breastfed infants should be provided supplemental vitamin D (under a physician's guidance). Keep in mind that supplements need to be used very carefully to avoid vitamin D toxicity in the infant. Rickets in children is also associated with fat malabsorption, such as that occurring in children with cystic fibrosis.

**Osteomalacia,** which means *soft bones,* is an adult disease comparable to rickets. It results from inefficient calcium absorption in the intestine or poor conservation of calcium by the kidneys. Both of these calcium-related problems can be caused by vitamin D deficiency. Bones then lose their minerals and become porous and weak and break easily. This leads to fractures in the hip and other bones. The risk of vitamin D deficiency increases in older adults. Adults with limited sun exposure may also develop the disease as may many African-American individuals. Combinations of sun exposure, vitamin D intake, or both can prevent this problem. Older people are advised to get sun exposure during early morning and late afternoon to receive the benefit of vitamin D synthesis without also increasing skin cancer risk. Aging decreases production of vitamin D in the skin by about 70% by the time one reaches the age of 70. One study showed that treatment with 10 to 20 micrograms per day

**parathyroid hormone (PTH)** A hormone made by the parathyroid glands that increases synthesis of the vitamin D hormone and aids calcium release from bone and calcium conservation by the kidneys, among other functions.

**rickets** A disease characterized by poor mineralization of newly synthesized bones because of low calcium content. This deficiency disease arises in infants and children from insufficient amounts of the vitamin D hormone in the body.

**osteomalacia** Adult form of rickets. The weakening of the bones seen in this disease is caused by low calcium content. A reduction in the amount of the vitamin D hormone in the body is one cause.

**FIGURE 8-6** ▶ Vitamin D deficiency causes rickets, in which the bones and teeth do not develop normally.

**B**e careful not to confuse osteomalacia with osteoporosis, another type of bone disorder discussed in Chapter 9.

(400 to 800 IU per day) of vitamin D (in conjunction with adequate dietary calcium) greatly decreased fracture risk in older people in nursing homes. Follow-up studies support this role of vitamin D in reducing hip fracture risk.

## MAKING DECISIONS

### New Benefits and Concerns about Vitamin D

Physicians are increasing the testing of blood levels of vitamin D. The jump in vitamin D testing stems from an abundance of emerging research linking vitamin D deficiency not only with osteoporosis and osteomalacia but also with some infectious diseases, cancers, autoimmune disorders, and cardiovascular disease. A recent study found that individuals with low vitamin D levels had a 60% greater risk of cardiac events such as heart attacks and stroke, and when both a vitamin D deficiency and high blood pressure were present, the risk for a serious cardiovascular event was doubled. These results are of concern because vitamin D is becoming more common than previously believed in the United States, especially in people living at higher latitudes where vitamin D is less available from exposure to sunlight. Statistics indicate that 36% of Americans are vitamin D deficient and 40% of infants and toddlers have tested below the optimal blood threshold for vitamin D. A normal vitamin D test result is 30 nanograms/milliliter (ng/ml) or above, whereas under 20 ng/ml is considered deficient. Vitamin D experts suggest that everyone should be taking 1,000 IUs of vitamin D a day, which is greater than the 400 IUs recommended daily for adults. The American Academy of Pediatrics now recommends that all children receive 400 IUs each day which is double the previous recommendation. Children are at risk of vitamin D insufficiency as a result of too little exposure to the sun stemming from concerns about skin cancer and increasing playtime indoors.

## Vitamin D Sources and Needs

Few foods contain significant amounts of vitamin D. Rich sources are fatty fish (e.g., sardines and salmon), fortified milk and yogurt, and some ready-to-eat breakfast cereals (Fig. 8-7). In the United States and Canada, milk usually is fortified with 10 micrograms (400 IU) per quart. Although eggs, butter, liver, and a few brands of margarine contain some vitamin D, large servings must be eaten to obtain an adequate amount of the vitamin from these sources.

The Adequate Intake set for vitamin D is 5 micrograms per day (200 IU per day) for people under age 51 and increases two to three times for older adults. (An RDA could not be set for vitamin D because the amount produced by sunlight exposure is too variable between individuals.) The Daily Value used on food and supplement labels is 10 micrograms (400 IU). As mentioned, young, light-skinned people can synthesize all the vitamin D needed from casual sun exposure. A number of experts suggest older adults, especially those age 70 and over who have limited sun exposure or dark skin, receive about 25 micrograms (1000 IU) from a combination of vitamin D-fortified foods and a multivitamin and mineral supplement. Within the 2005 Dietary Guidelines for Americans, a key recommendation for older adults, people with dark skin, and people exposed to insufficient ultraviolet band radiation (i.e., sunlight) is to consume extra vitamin D from vitamin D-fortified foods and/or supplements.

## Upper Level for Vitamin D

The Upper Level for vitamin D is 50 micrograms per day (2000 IU per day). Too much vitamin D taken regularly can create problems, especially in some infants and young children. For adults, intakes somewhat above the Upper Level appear to be safe. The Upper Level is based on the risk of too much vitamin D, causing the overabsorption of calcium which eventually leads to calcium deposits in the kidneys and other organs. These high intakes of vitamin D would also cause the typical symptoms of high blood calcium: weakness, loss of appetite, diarrhea, vomiting, mental confusion,

## Food Sources of Vitamin D

| Food Item and Amount | Vitamin D (micrograms) Daily Value = 10 micrograms | Vitamin D (IU) | Adult Male and Female AI = 5 micrograms %AI |
|---|---|---|---|
| AI | 5 | 200 | 100% |
| Baked Salmon, 3 ounces | 6.0 | 238 | 119% |
| Sardines, 1 ounce | 3.4 | 136 | 68% |
| Canned tuna, 3 ounces | 3.4 | 136 | 68% |
| 1% milk, 1 cup | 2.5 | 99 | 50% |
| Nonfat milk, 1 cup | 2.5 | 98 | 49% |
| Soft margarine, 1 teaspoon | 1.5 | 60 | 30% |
| Italian pork sausage, 3 ounces | 1.1 | 44 | 22% |
| Soy milk, 1 cup | 1.0 | 40 | 20% |
| Raisin Bran cereal, ¾ cup | 1.0 | 38 | 19% |
| Baked bluefish, 3 ounces | 0.9 | 34 | 17% |
| Special K cereal, ¾ cup | 0.8 | 30 | 15% |
| Cooked egg yolk, 1 | 0.6 | 25 | 13% |

**Key:**
- Grains
- Vegetables
- Fruits
- Oils
- Milk
- Meat & Beans

**FIGURE 8-7** ▶ Food sources of vitamin D compared to the Adequate Intake for adults.

and increased urine output. Calcium deposits in organs cause metabolic disturbances and cell death. However, vitamin D toxicity does not result from tanning in the sun too long because the body regulates the amount made in the skin.

### CONCEPT CHECK

Vitamin A is found in foods as preformed vitamin A and as provitamin A carotenoids. The most fully understood function of vitamin A is its importance in vision. Blindness caused by vitamin A deficiency is a major problem in many parts of the world. Vitamin A is also needed to maintain the health of many types of cells, support the immune system, and promote proper growth and development. Vitamin A and some carotenoids may be important in preventing cancer. However, because taking supplements of preformed vitamin A can be toxic, especially in pregnancy, the best recommendation is to focus primarily on eating plenty of provitamin A–rich foods, such as fruits and vegetables.

Vitamin D is a true vitamin only for people who fail to produce enough from sunlight, such as some older people and those with dark skin. Humans synthesize vitamin D from a cholesterol-like substance by the action of sunlight on their skin. The vitamin D is later acted on by the liver and kidneys to form the hormone 1,25-dihydroxyvitamin D. This hormone increases calcium absorption in the intestine and works with another hormone (parathyroid hormone) to maintain calcium in bones. Rich food sources of vitamin D are fish oils and fortified milk. Megadose vitamin D intake can be toxic, especially in infancy and early childhood.

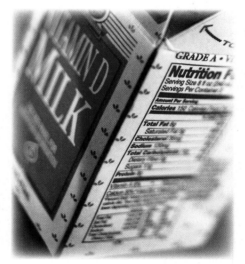

▲ Milk is usually fortified with vitamin D as well as vitamin A.

## 8.5 Vitamin E

North Americans are spending more than $1 billion on vitamin E supplements each year. The following section attempts to sort out fact from fiction in the debate over this high-profile vitamin.

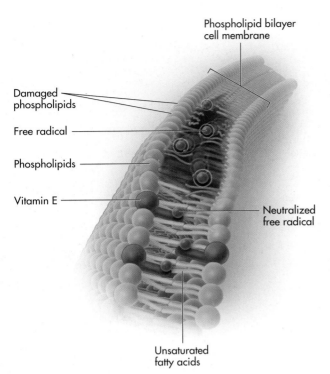

Phospholipid bilayer cell membrane

Damaged phospholipids

Free radical

Phospholipids

Vitamin E

Neutralized free radical

Unsaturated fatty acids

**FIGURE 8-8** ▶ Fat-soluble vitamin E can donate an electron to stop free radical chain reactions. If not interrupted, these reactions cause extensive oxidative damage to cell membranes.

**hemolysis** Destruction of red blood cells. The red blood cell membrane breaks down, allowing cell contents to leak into the fluid portion of the blood.

## Functions of Vitamin E

Acting as a fat-soluble antioxidant, vitamin E resides mostly in cell membranes. As discussed in Chapter 5, an antioxidant can form a barrier between a target molecule—an unsaturated fatty acid in a cell membrane, for example—and a compound seeking its electrons (Fig. 8-8). The antioxidant donates electrons or hydrogens to the electron-seeking compound. This protects other molecules or parts of a cell from having electrons stolen (such as from double bonds of unsaturated fatty acids).

Free radicals are highly reactive compounds containing an unpaired electron. Production of free-radicals is a normal result of cell metabolism and immune system function. For example, white blood cells generate free radicals as part of their action to stop infection. Some exposure to free radicals, then, is an important part of life. If vitamin E is not available to do its job, the electron-seeking free radicals can pull electrons from cell membranes, DNA, and other electron-dense cell components. This either alters the cell's DNA, which may increase the risk for cancer, or injures cell membranes, possibly causing the cell to die. Overall, the body needs antioxidants like vitamin E to carefully regulate exposure to free radicals and thereby prevent cellular damage.

Cells do not rely exclusively on vitamin E for protection from free radicals. Many other antioxidant systems exist in cells, some of which use minerals, such as copper, selenium, and manganese (see Chapter 9 for details). As discussed earlier in this chapter, carotenoids in fruits and vegetables also act as antioxidants. In addition, cells have mechanisms other than antioxidants to repair molecules (such as DNA) that have been damaged by free radicals.

Thus, vitamin E is just one component of the antioxidant system. Recent research has shown that individuals with the highest levels of vitamin E were less likely to die from any cause than those with the lowest blood vitamin E. Specifically, male smokers with high blood levels of vitamin E cut risk of dying from prostate cancer, lung cancer, stroke, and respiratory disease. Consuming vitamin E as a dietary supplement, however, may not be the most effective way to produce these effects. Two large recent studies have shown no benefit from vitamin E supplements on the prevention of certain diseases in males. In the Physician's Health Study II, neither vitamin E nor C had an effect on major cardiovascular events including heart attacks, stroke, or death. The major prostate cancer SELECT trial also found no benefit of vitamin E or selenium supplements on prostate cancer. These results suggest that pulling a nutrient out of the whole diet, may not produce the same effects. Furthermore, there is far stronger evidence to support the benefits of lifestyle changes such as improving diet (especially fruit, vegetable, and whole-grain bread and cereal intake), performing regular physical activity, not smoking, and maintaining a healthy body weight than there is for the postulated benefits of supplemental antioxidants, including vitamin E. Thus, as reviewed in Chapter 5, even if antioxidant supplements are eventually determined to be effective in preventing cardiovascular disease or cancer, they should be used only as an adjunct—not as an alternative—to a healthful lifestyle. In fact, the American Heart Association and a group of leading cardiologists stated that it is premature to recommend vitamin E supplements to the general population, based on current knowledge and the failure of major clinical trials to show any benefit (review Chapter 5). This conclusion is in agreement with the latest report on vitamin E by the Food and Nutrition Board of the National Academy of Sciences. In addition, FDA has denied the request of the supplement industry to make a health claim that vitamin E supplements reduce the risk of cardiovascular disease and cancer. Still, some experts recommend vitamin E supplements (50 IU to 400 IU per day), while at the same time noting that evidence supporting this recommendation is sketchy.

A deficiency of vitamin E causes cell membranes to break down. The double bonds in the unsaturated fatty acids in cell membranes are sensitive to attack by oxidizing compounds. Vitamin E neutralizes these compounds, so it protects cell membranes from damage. When oxidative damage causes the cell membranes of red blood cells to break down, it is called **hemolysis.**

## Vitamin E Sources and Needs

Vitamin E is a family of four **tocopherols,** called alpha, beta, gamma, and delta. Alpha-tocopherol is the main form in the human body, whereas gamma-tocopherol is the main form in foods. Major sources of vitamin E include plant oils, the main components of products such as salad dressings and mayonnaise, ready-to-eat breakfast cereals, some fruits and vegetables (e.g., asparagus, tomatoes, and green leafy vegetables), eggs, and margarine. Also, whole grains, nuts (e.g., almonds), and seeds (e.g., sunflower seeds) are good sources of vitamin E (Fig. 8-9). Plant oils are made up of mainly unsaturated fatty acids, and the vitamin E in plant oils protects these unsaturated fats from oxidation. Animal fats and fish oils, on the other hand, have practically no vitamin E (Fig. 8-10). The actual vitamin E content of a food depends on how it was harvested, processed, stored, and cooked because vitamin E is susceptible to destruction by oxygen, metals, light, and especially repeated use in deep-fat frying.

The RDA of vitamin E for adults is 15 milligrams per day of alpha-tocopherol, the most active form of vitamin E. The 15 milligram allotment is equivalent to 22 IU of a natural source and 33 IU of a synthetic source. Typically, North American adults consume about two-thirds of the RDA for vitamin E from food sources. Daily intake of nuts and seeds, ready-to-eat breakfast cereals containing vitamin E, or use of a multivitamin and mineral supplement would close this gap between needs and actual intakes. A Daily Value of 30 IU is used to express the vitamin E content on food and supplement labels.

The chemical structure of vitamin E varies depending on its source. The dl form or isomer is found in synthetic vitamin E and the d isomer is found in natural sources of vitamin E. Within the older IU system, 1 IU equals about 0.45 milligrams vitamin E,

**tocopherols** The chemical name for some forms of vitamin E. The alpha form is the most potent.

▲ Plant oils are rich sources of vitamin E.

## Food Sources of Vitamin E

| Food Item and Amount | Vitamin E (milligrams) | Vitamin E (IU) | Adult Male and Female RDA = 15 milligrams |
|---|---|---|---|
| | Daily Value = 30 IU | | %RDA |
| **RDA** | 15 | 22-33 | 100% |
| Fortified Bran cereal, ¾ cup | 22.5 | 33.5 | 150% |
| Sunflower oil, 2 tablespoons | 16.3 | 24.3 | 109% |
| Dry-roasted sunflower seeds, 1 ounce | 14.3 | 21.2 | 95% |
| Dry-roasted almonds, 1 ounce | 7.5 | 11.1 | 50% |
| Safflower oil, 1 tablespoon | 5.9 | 8.7 | 39% |
| Canola oil, 2 tablespoons | 5.7 | 8.5 | 38% |
| Wheat germ, ¼ cup | 5.2 | 7.7 | 35% |
| Almonds, 1 ounce | 4.5 | 6.8 | 30% |
| Oil-roasted sunflower seeds, 1 tablespoon | 3.4 | 5.0 | 23% |
| Italian dressing, 2 tablespoons | 3.1 | 4.5 | 21% |
| Mayonnaise, 1 tablespoon | 3.0 | 4.5 | 20% |
| Avocado, 1 | 2.7 | 4.0 | 18% |
| Chunky peanut butter, 2 tablespoons | 2.4 | 3.6 | 16% |
| Mango, 1 | 2.3 | 3.5 | 15% |
| Peanuts, 1 ounce | 2.1 | 3.1 | 14% |

Key:
- Grains
- Vegetables
- Fruits
- Oils
- Milk
- Meat & Beans

**FIGURE 8-9** ▶ Food sources of vitamin E compared to the RDA for adults.

**FIGURE 8-10** ▶ Sources of vitamin E from MyPyramid. The height of the background color (none, 1/3, 2/3, or completely covered) within each group in the pyramid indicates the average nutrient density for vitamin E in that group. Overall, plant oils are the richest source, followed by nuts and seeds in the meat & beans group. With regard to physical activity, vitamin E has no primary role in the related energy metabolism *per se*, but likely limits some oxidant damage during such endeavors.

| Grains | Vegetables | Fruits | Oils | Milk | Meat & Beans |
|---|---|---|---|---|---|
| • Wheat germ (whole grains) • Some fortified breakfast cereals | • Cabbage • Asparagus • Sweet potatoes • Tomatoes | • Apples • Avocados • Mango | • Plant oils • Margarines • Salad dressings | • None | • Nuts • Seeds • Shrimp • Peanut butter |

**isomers** Different chemical structures for compounds that share the same chemical formula.

based on the synthetic form (dl **isomer**) of vitamin E found in most supplements. If vitamin E is from a natural source (d isomer), 1 IU equals 0.67 milligrams, because the natural form of vitamin E is more potent than the synthetic form.

The maximum dose the body can retain on a daily basis is thought to be 200 milligrams. This would represent 300 IU of the d isomer (200/0.67 = 300) to 450 IU of the dl isomer (200/0.45 = 450).

Cell damage by free radicals occurs over an extended period. Therefore, the beneficial effects of vitamin E and other antioxidants in counteracting this damage is most apparent when viewed over the long term. Research on a possible benefit of intakes of vitamin E in excess of the RDA for healthy adults is currently underway.

Several populations are especially susceptible to developing marginal vitamin E status. Preterm infants are born with low vitamin E stores, because this vitamin is transferred from mother to baby during late stages of pregnancy. Hemolysis (described on page 304) is of particular concern for preterm infants, due to red blood cell damage that occurs in the absence of adequate vitamin E. The rapid growth of preterm infants, coupled with the high oxygen needs of their immature lungs, greatly increases the stress on red blood cells. Special formulas and supplements designed for preterm infants can help compensate for their low vitamin E status. Smokers are another group at high risk for vitamin E deficiency, as smoking readily destroys vitamin E in the lungs. Still, one study showed that even using megadoses of vitamin E was ineffective in preventing this damage in smokers. Others at considerable risk of vitamin E deficiency include adults on very low-fat diets or those with fat malabsorption.

## Upper Level for Vitamin E

The Upper Level for vitamin E for a healthy population is 1000 milligrams per day of supplemental alpha-tocopherol. The upper level has been established because excessive amounts of vitamin E can interfere with vitamin K's role in the clotting mechanism, leading to **hemorrhage**. Individuals who are vitamin K deficient or taking anticoagulants (e.g., Coumadin) or heavy doses of aspirin are especially at risk for hemorrhage from megadose vitamin E use. In international units, the Upper Level

**hemorrhage** An escape of blood from blood vessels.

is 1500 IU for vitamin E isolated from natural sources (d isomer; 1000/0.67 = 1500) and 1100 IU for synthetic vitamin E (dl isomer; 1000/0.45/2 = 1100). The lower IU value for the synthetic form reflects the greater number of forms present in the synthetic product, only half or less of which contribute to vitamin E activity in cells, but are still absorbed. This Upper Level is set for a healthy population.

# 8.6 Vitamin K

A family of compounds known collectively as vitamin K is found in plants, plant oils, fish oils, and meats. While most vitamin K comes from our diet, another form is also synthesized by bacteria in the human intestine. This form supplies us with about 10% of the vitamin K we need.

## Functions of Vitamin K

Vitamin K is vital for blood clotting, working along with various proteins and calcium. The *K* stems from the Danish spelling of **coagulation** because a Danish researcher first noted the relationship between vitamin K and blood clotting. Vitamin K is needed for the activation of several blood-clotting factors (Fig. 8-11). Vitamin K

**coagulation** Blood clotting; essentially a transition of blood from a liquid cell suspension into a solid, gel-like form.

**FIGURE 8-11** ▶ Vitamin K works to activate clotting factors, which are then able to bind calcium. This calcium binding to clotting factors is necessary for clot formation.

▲ A salad containing dark greens (or other green vegetables) each day provides abundant vitamin K for a diet.

also activates proteins present in bone, muscle, and kidneys, to give calcium-binding ability to these organs. A poor vitamin K intake has been linked to an increase in hip fractures in women because of its effect on various proteins in bone.

At birth, a newborn's intestinal tract lacks a sufficient amount of bacteria to produce enough vitamin K to allow for effective blood clotting. Therefore, vitamin K also is routinely given by injection shortly after birth to insure blood clotting if the infant is injured or needs surgery. In adults, deficiencies of vitamin K have occurred in the presence of severe, long-standing fat malabsorption or when a person takes long-term antibiotics that destroy many of the intestinal bacteria that produce vitamin K.

## Vitamin K Sources and Needs

Major food sources of vitamin K are liver, green leafy vegetables (e.g., kale, turnip greens, dark green lettuce, and spinach), broccoli, peas, and green beans (Fig. 8-12). Other sources are soybean and canola oils and certain fortified chocolate confections (these also contain extra calcium). Thus, another reason to consume a diet rich in green vegetables is to obtain sufficient vitamin K. Most vitamin K consumed in a day disappears from the body by the next day. Nevertheless, vitamin K is abundant in a balanced diet, and a deficiency is uncommon. Vitamin K is resistant to cooking losses.

The Adequate Intake for vitamin K is 90 to 120 micrograms per day for adults. Most North Americans consume at least this much. A Daily Value of 80 micrograms is used to express vitamin K content on food and supplement labels. Older adults may be at risk of a deficiency because of low consumption of green vegetables.

## Food Sources of Vitamin K

| Food Item and Amount | Vitamin K (micrograms) | Adult Male AI = 120 micrograms %AI | Adult Female AI = 90 micrograms %AI |
|---|---|---|---|
| **RDA** | 90–120 | 100% | 100% |
| Cooked kale, ½ cup | 530 | 442% | 589% |
| Cooked turnip greens, 1 cup | 520 | 433% | 578% |
| Cooked spinach, 1 cup | 480 | 400% | 533% |
| Cooked brussel sprouts, ½ cup | 150 | 125% | 167% |
| Raw spinach, 1 cup | 144 | 120% | 160% |
| Cooked asparagus, 1 cup | 144 | 120% | 160% |
| Cooked broccoli, ½ cup | 110 | 92% | 122% |
| Looseleaf lettuce, 1 cup | 97 | 81% | 108% |
| Cooked green beans, ½ cup | 49 | 41% | 54% |
| Raw cabbage, 1 cup | 42 | 35% | 47% |
| Sauerkraut, ½ cup | 30 | 25% | 33% |
| Green peas, ½ cup | 26 | 22% | 29% |
| Soybean oil, 1 tablespoon | 25 | 21% | 28% |
| Cooked cauliflower, 1 cup | 20 | 17% | 22% |
| Canola oil, 1 tablespoon | 17 | 14% | 19% |

Daily Value = 80 micrograms

Key:
- ■ Grains
- ■ Vegetables
- ■ Fruits
- ☐ Oils
- ■ Milk
- ■ Meat & Beans

**FIGURE 8-12** ▶ Food sources of vitamin K compared to the Adequate Intake for adult males and females.

Oral vitamin K generally poses no risk of toxicity, so no Upper Level has been set. The main problem with megadose use is reduced effectiveness of oral medications used to reduce blood clotting (e.g., Coumadin). These medications are used to lessen blood-clotting especially in those who have undergone recent cardiovascular surgery.

Table 8-2 reviews what we have covered so far regarding the fat-soluble vitamins.

**TABLE 8-2** Summary of the Fat-Soluble Vitamins

| Vitamin | Major Functions | RDA or Adequate Intake | Dietary Sources | Deficiency Symptoms | Toxicity Symptoms |
|---|---|---|---|---|---|
| Vitamin A (preformed vitamin A and provitamin A) | • Promote vision: night and color<br>• Promote growth<br>• Prevent drying of skin and eyes<br>• Promote resistance to bacterial infection and overall immune system function | Females: 700 micrograms RAE<br><br>Males: 900 micrograms RAE<br><br>2300–3000 IU if as preformed (vitamin A) | Preformed Vitamin A:<br>• Liver<br>• Fortified milk<br>• Fortified breakfast cereals<br><br>Provitamin A:<br>• Sweet potatoes<br>• Spinach<br>• Greens<br>• Carrots<br>• Cantaloupe<br>• Apricots<br>• Broccoli | • Night blindness<br>• Xerophthalmia<br>• Poor growth<br>• Dry skin | • Fetal malformations<br>• Hair loss<br>• Skin changes<br>• Bone pain<br>• Fractures<br><br>Upper Level is 3000 micrograms of preformed vitamin A (10,000 IU) based on the risk of birth defects and liver toxicity |
| Vitamin D | • Increase absorption of calcium and phosphorus<br>• Maintain optimal blood calcium and calcification of bone | 5–15 micrograms<br><br>(200–600 IU) | • Vitamin D fortified milk<br>• Fortified breakfast cereals<br>• Fish oils<br>• Sardines<br>• Salmon | • Rickets in children<br>• Osteomalacia in adults | • Growth retardation<br>• Kidney damage<br>• Calcium deposits in soft tissue<br><br>Upper Level is 50 micrograms (2000 IU) based on the risk of elevated blood calcium |
| Vitamin E | • Antioxidant prevents breakdown of vitamin A and unsaturated fatty acids | 15 milligrams alpha-tocopherol<br><br>22 IU natural form, 33 IU (synthetic form) | • Plant oils<br>• Products made from plant oils<br>• Some greens<br>• Some fruits<br>• Nuts and seeds<br>• Fortified breakfast cereals | • Hemolysis of red blood cells<br>• Nerve degeneration | • Muscle weakness<br>• Headaches<br>• Nausea<br>• Inhibition of vitamin K metabolism<br><br>Upper Level is 1000 milligrams (1100 IU synthetic form, 1500 IU natural form) based on the risk of hemorrhage |
| Vitamin K | • Activation of blood-clotting factors<br>• Activation of proteins involved in bone metabolism | Females: 90 micrograms<br><br>Males: 120 micrograms | • Green vegetables<br>• Liver<br>• Some plant oils<br>• Some calcium supplements | • Hemorrhage<br>• Fractures | No Upper Level has been set |

Abbreviations: RAE = retinol activity equivalents; IU = international units

**Inactive enzyme**

**+**

**Vitamin coenzyme**

**Active enzyme**

**FIGURE 8-13** ▶ Coenzymes, such as those formed from B vitamins, aid in the function of various enzymes. Without the coenzyme, the enzyme cannot function, and deficiency symptoms associated with the missing vitamin eventually appear. Health-food stores sell the coenzyme forms of some vitamins. These more expensive forms of vitamins are unnecessary. The body makes all the coenzymes it needs from vitamin precursors.

**bioavailability** The degree to which an ingested nutrient is absorbed and thus is available to the body.

**CONCEPT CHECK**

Vitamin E functions primarily as an antioxidant. It can donate electrons to electron-seeking free radical (oxidizing) compounds. By neutralizing these compounds, vitamin E helps prevent cell destruction, especially the destruction of red blood cell membranes. Vitamin E occurs in a wide variety of foods, but its richest sources are plant oils, foods rich in these oils, and nuts. Studies using dietary supplements of vitamin E have not shown beneficial effects on the risk of diseases including heart disease and cancer.

Vitamin K plays a key role in efficient blood clotting; it contributes to the activation of certain blood-clotting proteins. In addition, vitamin K contributes to the synthesis of the calcium-binding proteins in some organs, such as bones. About 10% of the vitamin K we absorb every day is synthesized by our intestinal bacteria; the rest comes from our diets. The amount in the diet alone generally meets our daily needs. Thus, except for newborns and possibly older adults, a deficiency of vitamin K is unlikely.

## 8.7 The Water-Soluble Vitamins and Choline

Regular consumption of good sources of the water-soluble vitamins is important. Most water-soluble vitamins are readily excreted from the body with any excess generally ending up in the urine or stool and very little being stored. They dissolve in water, so large amounts of these vitamins can be lost during food processing and preparation. Vitamin content is best preserved by light cooking methods, such as stir-frying, steaming, and microwaving (review Table 8-1).

The B vitamins are thiamin, riboflavin, niacin, pantothenic acid, biotin, vitamin B-6, folate, and vitamin B-12. Choline is a related nutrient, but currently is not classified as a vitamin. Vitamin C is also a water-soluble vitamin.

The B vitamins often occur together in the same foods, so a lack of one B vitamin may mean other B vitamins are also low in a diet. The B vitamins function as coenzymes, small molecules that interact with enzymes to enable the enzymes to function. In essence, the coenzymes contribute to enzyme activity (Fig. 8-13).

As coenzymes, the B vitamins play many key roles in metabolism. The metabolic pathways used by carbohydrates, fats, and amino acids all require input from B vitamins. Because of their role in energy metabolism, needs for many B vitamins increase somewhat as energy expenditure increases. Still, this is not a major concern because this increase in energy expenditure usually results in a corresponding increase in food intake, which contributes more B vitamins to a diet. Many B vitamins are interdependent because they participate in the same processes (Fig. 8-14). B vitamin deficiency symptoms typically occur in the brain and nervous system, skin, and GI tract. Cells in these tissues are metabolically active, and those in the skin and GI tract are also constantly being replaced.

After being ingested, the B vitamins are first broken down from their active coenzyme forms into free vitamins in the stomach and small intestine. The vitamins are then absorbed, primarily in the small intestine. Typically, about 50% to 90% of the B vitamins in the diet are absorbed, which means they have relatively high **bioavailability**. Once inside cells, the active coenzyme forms are resynthesized. There is no need to consume the coenzyme forms themselves. Some vitamins are sold in their coenzyme forms but these are broken down during digestion and we activate them when needed.

### B Vitamin Intakes of North Americans

The nutritional health of most North Americans with regard to the B vitamins is generally good. Typical diets contain a good amount and variety of natural sources of

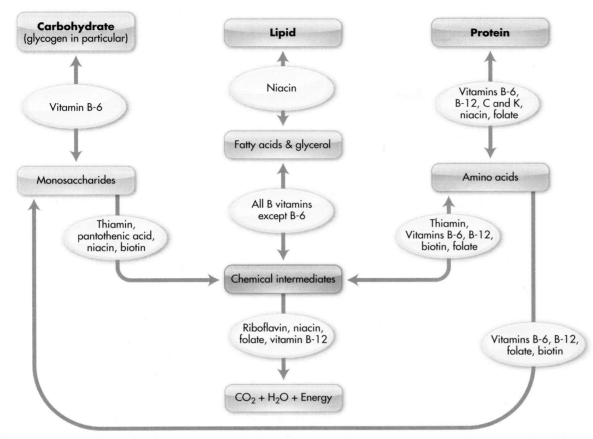

**FIGURE 8-14** ▶ Examples of metabolic pathways for which water soluble vitamins are essential. The metabolism of energy-yielding nutrients requires vitamin input.

these vitamins. In addition, many common foods, such as ready-to-eat breakfast cereals, are fortified with one or more of the water-soluble vitamins. In some developing countries, however, deficiencies of the water-soluble vitamins are more common, and the resulting deficiency diseases pose significant public health problems. (A detailed discussion of nutritional deficiencies worldwide is presented in Chapter 12.)

Despite the generally good B vitamin status of North Americans, marginal deficiencies of the water-soluble vitamins may occur in some cases, especially in older people who eat little food and in people who follow poor dietary patterns. The long-term effects of such marginal deficiencies are unknown, but increased risk of cardiovascular disease, cancer, and cataracts of the eye is suspected. However, in the short run, such a marginal deficiency in most people likely leads only to fatigue or other bothersome and unspecific physical effects. With rare exceptions, healthy adults do not develop the more serious B vitamin deficiency diseases from dietary inadequacies alone. The main exceptions are people with alcoholism. The combination of extremely unbalanced diets and alcohol-induced alterations of vitamin absorption and metabolism creates significant risks for serious nutrient deficiencies among people with alcoholism (see Chapter 16).

**Grains: One Important Source of B-Vitamins** The milling of grains leads to losses of vitamins and minerals. In the milling process, seeds are crushed and the germ, bran, and husk layers are discarded, leaving just the starch-containing endosperm in the refined grains. The starch is used to make flour, bread, and cereal products. Unfortunately, many nutrients are lost along with the discarded germ, bran, and husk materials. To counteract these losses, in the United States, bread and cereal products made from milled grains are enriched with four B vitamins (thiamin, riboflavin, niacin, and folic acid) and with the mineral iron. This addition helps protect us from the common deficiency diseases associated with a dietary lack of these nutrients. Unfortunately, these products remain lower in vitamin E, vitamin B-6, potassium, magnesium, fiber, and other nutrients compared to whole grain products (Fig. 8-15). This is one reason why nutrient experts advocate regular consumption of whole-grain products, such as whole-wheat bread and brown rice, rather than refined grain products.

## 8.8 Thiamin

Thiamin (formerly called *vitamin B-1*) is used, among other purposes, to help release energy from carbohydrate. Its coenzyme form participates in reactions in which a carbon dioxide ($CO_2$) is lost from a larger molecule. This reaction is particularly important in the breakdown of carbohydrates and certain amino acids for energy needs (review Fig. 8-14).

**beriberi** The thiamin deficiency disorder characterized by muscle weakness, loss of appetite, nerve degeneration, and sometimes edema.

The thiamin deficiency disease is called **beriberi,** a word that means "I can't, I can't" in the Sri Lanka language of Sinhalese. The symptoms include weakness, loss of appetite, irritability, nervous tingling throughout the body, poor arm and leg coordination, and deep muscle pain in the calves. A person with beriberi often develops an enlarged heart and sometimes severe edema.

Beriberi results when glucose, the primary fuel for brain and nerve cells, cannot be metabolized to release energy. The thiamin coenzyme participates in glucose metabolism, so problems with body functions associated with brain and nerve action are the first signs of a thiamin deficiency, some after only 10 days on a thiamin-free diet.

Beriberi is seen in areas where rice is a staple and polished (white) rice is consumed rather than brown (whole-grain) rice. In most parts of the world, brown rice has had its bran and germ layer removed to make white rice, a poor source of thiamin, unless it is enriched.

### Thiamin Sources and Needs

Major sources of thiamin include pork products, whole grains (wheat germ), ready-to-eat breakfast cereals, enriched grains, green beans, milk, orange juice, organ meats, peanuts, dried beans, and seeds (Figs. 8-16 and 8-17).

The adult RDA for thiamin is 1.1 to 1.2 milligrams per day. The Daily Value of 1.5 milligrams is used to express the thiamin content on food and supplement labels.

▲ Pork is a good source of thiamin.

**FIGURE 8-15 ▶** When compared with white rice, brown rice has 93% more vitamin B-6, 50% more potassium, 160% more zinc, 435% more magnesium, and 550% more fiber. Similarly, compared with white bread, whole-wheat bread has 200% more vitamin B-6, 250% more potassium, 260% more zinc, 370% more magnesium, and 285% more fiber.

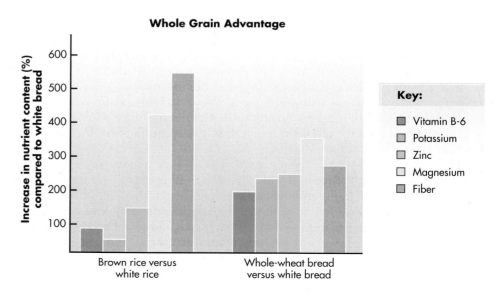

**Whole Grain Advantage**

Increase in nutrient content (%) compared to white bread

Brown rice versus white rice

Whole-wheat bread versus white bread

**Key:**
■ Vitamin B-6
□ Potassium
□ Zinc
□ Magnesium
■ Fiber

## Food Sources of Thiamin

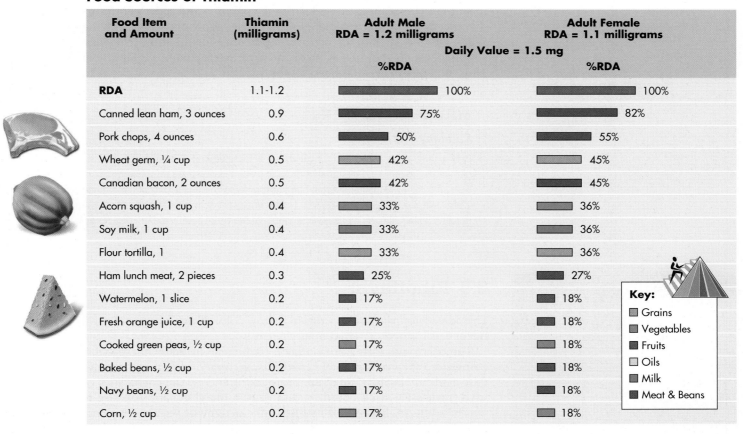

| Food Item and Amount | Thiamin (milligrams) | Adult Male RDA = 1.2 milligrams | | Adult Female RDA = 1.1 milligrams | |
|---|---|---|---|---|---|
| | | Daily Value = 1.5 mg | | | |
| | | %RDA | | %RDA | |
| **RDA** | 1.1–1.2 | | 100% | | 100% |
| Canned lean ham, 3 ounces | 0.9 | | 75% | | 82% |
| Pork chops, 4 ounces | 0.6 | | 50% | | 55% |
| Wheat germ, ¼ cup | 0.5 | | 42% | | 45% |
| Canadian bacon, 2 ounces | 0.5 | | 42% | | 45% |
| Acorn squash, 1 cup | 0.4 | | 33% | | 36% |
| Soy milk, 1 cup | 0.4 | | 33% | | 36% |
| Flour tortilla, 1 | 0.4 | | 33% | | 36% |
| Ham lunch meat, 2 pieces | 0.3 | | 25% | | 27% |
| Watermelon, 1 slice | 0.2 | | 17% | | 18% |
| Fresh orange juice, 1 cup | 0.2 | | 17% | | 18% |
| Cooked green peas, ½ cup | 0.2 | | 17% | | 18% |
| Baked beans, ½ cup | 0.2 | | 17% | | 18% |
| Navy beans, ½ cup | 0.2 | | 17% | | 18% |
| Corn, ½ cup | 0.2 | | 17% | | 18% |

Key:
◼ Grains
◼ Vegetables
◼ Fruits
◻ Oils
◼ Milk
◼ Meat & Beans

**FIGURE 8-16** ▶ Food sources of thiamin compared to the RDA for adult males and females.

## MyPyramid: Sources of Thiamin, Riboflavin, and Niacin

| Grains | Vegetables | Fruits | Oils | Milk | Meat & Beans |

**FIGURE 8-17** ▶ Sources of thiamin, riboflavin, and niacin from MyPyramid. The height of the background color (none, 1/3, 2/3, or completely covered) within each group in the pyramid indicates the average nutrient density for these vitamins in that group. Overall, the meat & beans group and the grains group contain many foods that are nutrient-dense sources of thiamin, riboflavin, and niacin. As well, foods from the milk group are especially rich sources of riboflavin. With regard to physical activity, these vitamins play key roles in the increased energy metabolism that takes place during such endeavors.

Average daily intakes for men exceed this by 50% or more, and women generally meet the RDA. Some groups, such as low-income and older people, may barely meet their needs for thiamin. A diet dominated by highly processed and unenriched foods, sugar, fat, and alcohol also creates a potential for thiamin deficiency. Oral thiamin supplements are typically nontoxic because excess thiamin is rapidly lost in the urine. Thus, no Upper Level has been set for thiamin.

### MAKING DECISIONS

#### Thiamin and Alcohol

People with alcoholism are at the greatest risk for thiamin deficiency because absorption and use of thiamin are profoundly diminished and excretion is increased by consumption of alcohol. Furthermore, the low-quality diet that often accompanies severe alcoholism makes matters worse. There is limited thiamin storage in the body, so an alcoholic binge lasting 1 to 2 weeks may quickly deplete already diminished amounts of the vitamin and result in deficiency symptoms.

(a)

(b)

**FIGURE 8-18** ▶ *(a)* Glossitis is a painful, inflamed tongue that can signal a deficiency of riboflavin, niacin, vitamin B-6, folate, or vitamin B-12. *(b)* Angular cheilitis, also called cheilosis or angular stomatitis, is another result of a riboflavin deficiency. It causes painful cracks at the corners of the mouth. Both glossitis and angular cheilitis can be caused by other medical conditions; thus, further evaluation is required before diagnosing a nutrient deficiency.

## 8.9 Riboflavin

The name *riboflavin* comes from its yellow color (*flavus* means yellow in Latin). Riboflavin was formerly referred to as *vitamin B-2*.

The coenzyme forms of riboflavin participate in many energy-yielding metabolic pathways. When cells generate energy using oxygen-requiring pathways, such as when fatty acids are broken down and burned for energy, the coenzymes of riboflavin are used (review Fig. 8-14). Some vitamin and mineral metabolism also requires riboflavin. In addition, because of its link to the activity of certain enzymes, riboflavin has an antioxidant role in the body.

The symptoms associated with riboflavin deficiency include inflammation of the mouth and tongue, dermatitis, cracking of tissue around the corners of the mouth (called *cheilosis*), various eye disorders, sensitivity to the sun, and confusion (Fig. 8-18). Such symptoms develop after approximately 2 months on a riboflavin-poor diet. In addition, riboflavin deficiencies probably do not exist by themselves. Instead, a riboflavin deficiency would occur with deficiencies of niacin, thiamin, and vitamin B-6 because these nutrients often occur in the same foods.

### Riboflavin Sources and Needs

Major sources of riboflavin are milk and milk products, enriched grains, ready-to-eat breakfast cereals, meat, and eggs (Fig. 8-19). Vegetables such as asparagus, broccoli, and various greens (e.g., spinach) are also good sources.

The adult RDA of riboflavin is 1.1 to 1.3 milligrams per day. The Daily Value used on food and supplement labels is 1.7 milligrams. On average, daily intakes of riboflavin are slightly above the RDA. As with thiamin, people with alcoholism risk riboflavin deficiency because they generally eat nutrient-poor diets. No specific symptoms indicate that riboflavin taken in megadoses is toxic, so no Upper Level has been set.

## 8.10 Niacin

Niacin functions in the body as one of two related compounds: nicotinic acid and nicotinamide. Niacin was formerly referred to as *vitamin B-3*.

The coenzyme forms of niacin function in many cellular metabolic pathways. In general, when energy is being released from the energy nutrients and used by cells,

## Food Sources of Riboflavin

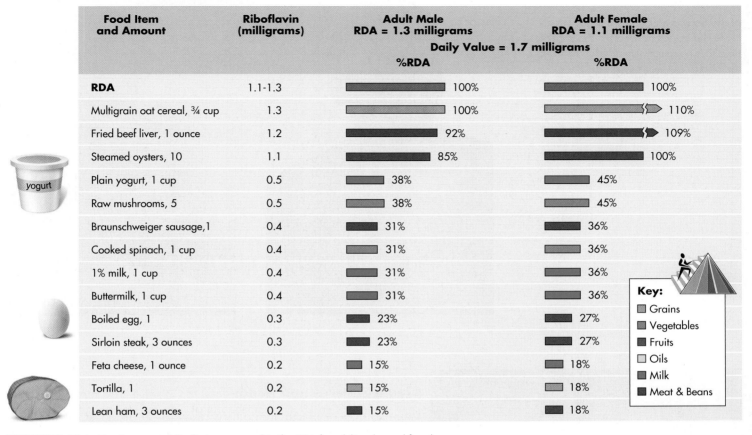

| Food Item and Amount | Riboflavin (milligrams) | Adult Male RDA = 1.3 milligrams %RDA | Adult Female RDA = 1.1 milligrams %RDA |
|---|---|---|---|
| **RDA** | 1.1-1.3 | 100% | 100% |
| Multigrain oat cereal, ¾ cup | 1.3 | 100% | 110% |
| Fried beef liver, 1 ounce | 1.2 | 92% | 109% |
| Steamed oysters, 10 | 1.1 | 85% | 100% |
| Plain yogurt, 1 cup | 0.5 | 38% | 45% |
| Raw mushrooms, 5 | 0.5 | 38% | 45% |
| Braunschweiger sausage,1 | 0.4 | 31% | 36% |
| Cooked spinach, 1 cup | 0.4 | 31% | 36% |
| 1% milk, 1 cup | 0.4 | 31% | 36% |
| Buttermilk, 1 cup | 0.4 | 31% | 36% |
| Boiled egg, 1 | 0.3 | 23% | 27% |
| Sirloin steak, 3 ounces | 0.3 | 23% | 27% |
| Feta cheese, 1 ounce | 0.2 | 15% | 18% |
| Tortilla, 1 | 0.2 | 15% | 18% |
| Lean ham, 3 ounces | 0.2 | 15% | 18% |

Daily Value = 1.7 milligrams

**Key:**
- ■ Grains
- ■ Vegetables
- ■ Fruits
- □ Oils
- ■ Milk
- ■ Meat & Beans

**FIGURE 8-19** ▶ Food sources of riboflavin compared to the RDA for adult males and females.

a niacin coenzyme is used. Synthetic pathways in the cell—those that make new compounds—also often use a niacin coenzyme. This is especially true for fatty acid synthesis (review Fig. 8-14).

Almost every cellular metabolic pathway uses a niacin coenzyme, so a deficiency causes widespread changes in the body. The group of niacin deficiency symptoms is known as *pellagra*, which means rough or painful skin. The symptoms of the disease are **dementia,** diarrhea, and dermatitis (especially on areas of skin exposed to the sun) (Fig. 8-20). Later, death often results. Early symptoms include poor appetite, weight loss, and weakness.

Pellagra is the only dietary deficiency disease ever to reach epidemic proportions in the United States. It became a major problem in the southeastern United States in the late 1800s and persisted until the late 1930s when standards of living and diets improved. Today, pellagra is rare in Western societies, but can be seen in the developing world.

**dementia** A general loss or decrease in mental function.

## MAKING DECISIONS

### Niacin in Corn

Do you enjoy corn tortillas? Niacin in corn is bound by a protein that hampers its absorption. Soaking corn in an alkaline solution, such as lime water (water with calcium hydroxide), releases bound niacin and renders it more usable. Hispanic people in North America traditionally soak corn in lime water before making tortillas. This treatment is one reason this Hispanic population never experienced much pellagra.

**FIGURE 8-20** ▶ The dermatitis of pellagra. *(a)* Dermatitis on both sides (bilateral) of the body is a typical symptom of pellagra. Sun exposure worsens the condition. *(b)* The rough skin around the neck is referred to as Casal's necklace.

(a)

(b)

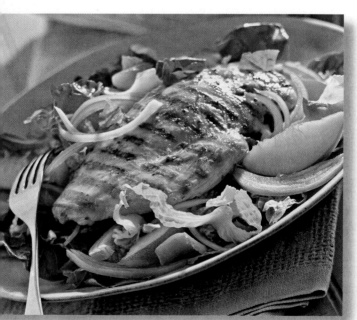

▲ Chicken is a good source of niacin. The tryptophan present can also be metabolized to niacin.

## Niacin Sources and Needs

Major sources of niacin are poultry, ready-to-eat breakfast cereals, beef, wheat bran, tuna and other fish, asparagus, and peanuts (Fig. 8-21). Coffee and tea also contribute some niacin to the diet. Niacin is heat stable; little is lost in cooking.

Besides the preformed niacin found in protein foods, we can synthesize niacin from the amino acid tryptophan: 60 milligrams of tryptophan in a diet yield about 1 milligram of niacin. In this manner, we synthesize about 50% of the niacin we need.

The adult RDA of niacin is 14 to 16 milligrams per day. The RDA is expressed as niacin equivalents (NE) to account for niacin received intact from the diet, as well as that made from tryptophan. A Daily Value of 20 milligrams is used to express niacin content on food and supplement labels. Intakes of niacin by adults are about double the RDA, without considering the contribution from tryptophan. (Tables of food composition values also ignore this contribution.) People with alcoholism and those with rare disorders of tryptophan metabolism are generally the only groups to show a niacin deficiency.

## Upper Level for Niacin

The Upper Level for niacin is 35 milligrams per day of the nicotinic acid form. Effects of high intakes include headache, itching, and increased blood flow to the skin, causing a general blood vessel dilation or flushing in various parts of the body, especially when intakes are above 100 milligrams per day. In the long run, GI tract and liver damage is possible, so any use of megadoses, including large doses recommended for treatment of cardiovascular disease, requires close physician scrutiny (review Chapter 5).

## Food Sources of Niacin

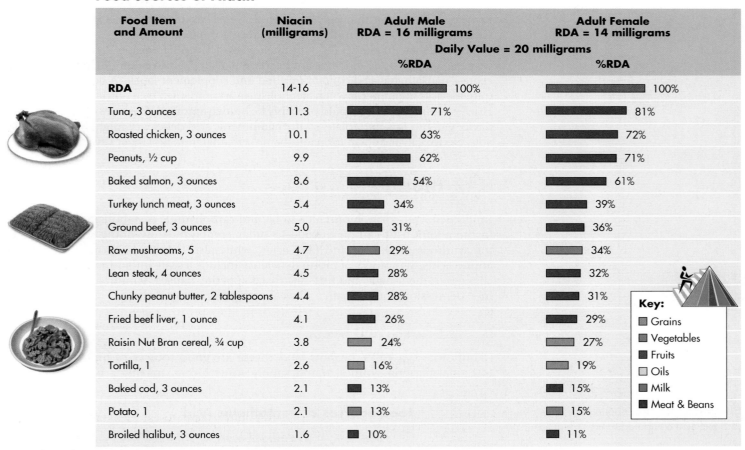

| Food Item and Amount | Niacin (milligrams) | Adult Male RDA = 16 milligrams | Adult Female RDA = 14 milligrams |
|---|---|---|---|
| | | Daily Value = 20 milligrams | |
| | | %RDA | %RDA |
| **RDA** | 14-16 | 100% | 100% |
| Tuna, 3 ounces | 11.3 | 71% | 81% |
| Roasted chicken, 3 ounces | 10.1 | 63% | 72% |
| Peanuts, ½ cup | 9.9 | 62% | 71% |
| Baked salmon, 3 ounces | 8.6 | 54% | 61% |
| Turkey lunch meat, 3 ounces | 5.4 | 34% | 39% |
| Ground beef, 3 ounces | 5.0 | 31% | 36% |
| Raw mushrooms, 5 | 4.7 | 29% | 34% |
| Lean steak, 4 ounces | 4.5 | 28% | 32% |
| Chunky peanut butter, 2 tablespoons | 4.4 | 28% | 31% |
| Fried beef liver, 1 ounce | 4.1 | 26% | 29% |
| Raisin Nut Bran cereal, ¾ cup | 3.8 | 24% | 27% |
| Tortilla, 1 | 2.6 | 16% | 19% |
| Baked cod, 3 ounces | 2.1 | 13% | 15% |
| Potato, 1 | 2.1 | 13% | 15% |
| Broiled halibut, 3 ounces | 1.6 | 10% | 11% |

Key:
- Grains
- Vegetables
- Fruits
- Oils
- Milk
- Meat & Beans

**FIGURE 8-21** ▶ Food sources of niacin compared to the RDA for adult males and females.

### CONCEPT CHECK

The B vitamins thiamin, riboflavin, and niacin are important in the metabolism of carbohydrates, proteins, and fats. Energy metabolism in particular requires adequate amounts of the coenzyme forms of these three vitamins. Deficiency symptoms typically occur in the brain and nervous system, skin, and GI tract. Cells in these tissues are metabolically active, and those in the skin and GI tract are also constantly being replaced. Enriched grains and ready-to-eat breakfast cereals are adequate sources of all three vitamins. Additionally, pork is an excellent source of thiamin, milk is an excellent source of riboflavin, and protein foods in general—such as chicken—are excellent sources of niacin. Deficiencies of all three vitamins can occur with alcoholism; a thiamin deficiency is the most likely of the three.

## 8.11 Pantothenic Acid

Like the other B vitamins, pantothenic acid helps release energy from carbohydrates, fats, and protein. By forming its coenzyme (coenzyme A or CoA) pantothenic acid allows many energy-yielding metabolic reactions to occur (review Fig. 8-14). This coenzyme also activates fatty acids so they can yield energy. It is also used in the beginning steps of fatty acid synthesis. Pantothenic acid is so widespread in foods that a nutritional deficiency among healthy people who eat varied diets is unlikely.

## Pantothenic Acid Sources and Needs

Rich sources of pantothenic acid are sunflower seeds, mushrooms, peanuts, and eggs. Other sources are meat, milk, and many vegetables (Fig. 8-22).

The Adequate Intake set for pantothenic acid is 5 milligrams per day for adults, and we generally consume that amount or more. A Daily Value of 10 milligrams is used to express pantothenic acid content on food and supplement labels. A deficiency of pantothenic acid might occur when alcoholism is accompanied by a nutrient-deficient diet. However, the symptoms would probably be hidden among deficiencies of thiamin, riboflavin, vitamin B-6, and folate, so the pantothenic acid deficiency might be unrecognizable. No toxicity is known for pantothenic acid, therefore no Upper Level has been set.

# 8.12 Biotin

In its coenzyme form, biotin aids in fat and carbohydrate metabolism. Biotin assists in the addition of carbon dioxide to other compounds. By doing so, it promotes the synthesis of glucose and fatty acids, while also helping to break down certain amino acids. Symptoms of biotin deficiency include a scaly inflammation of the skin, changes in the tongue and lips, decreased appetite, nausea, vomiting, a form of anemia, depression, muscle pain and weakness, and poor growth.

## Biotin Sources and Needs

Cauliflower, egg yolks, peanuts, and cheese are good sources of biotin (Fig. 8-23). Intestinal bacteria synthesize and supply some biotin, making a biotin deficiency

**FIGURE 8-22** ► Food sources of pantothenic acid compared to the Adequate Intake for adults.

## Food Sources of Pantothenic Acid

| Food Item and Amount | Pantothenic Acid (milligrams) | Adult Male and Female AI = 5 milligrams Daily Value = 10 milligrams %AI |
|---|---|---|
| **AI** | 5 | 100% |
| Fortified corn flakes cereal, ¾ cup | 11.8 | 236% |
| Power bar, 1 | 10.0 | 200% |
| Luna bar, 1 | 9.9 | 198% |
| Sunflower seeds, ¼ cup | 2.3 | 46% |
| Fried beef liver, 1 ounce | 1.7 | 34% |
| Raw mushrooms, 5 | 1.7 | 34% |
| Plain yogurt, 1 cup | 1.5 | 30% |
| Acorn squash, 1 cup | 1.2 | 24% |
| Peanuts, ½ cup | 1.0 | 20% |
| 1% milk, 1 cup | 0.9 | 18% |
| Roasted chicken breast, 3 ounces | 0.8 | 16% |
| Broccoli, 1 cup | 0.8 | 16% |
| Baked potato, 1 | 0.7 | 14% |
| Legumes, ½ cup | 0.7 | 14% |
| Cooked egg yolk, 1 | 0.6 | 12% |

Key:
■ Grains
■ Vegetables
■ Fruits
□ Oils
■ Milk
■ Meat & Beans

**Food Sources of Biotin**

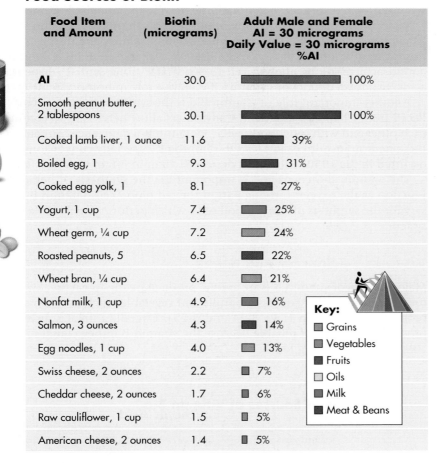

| Food Item and Amount | Biotin (micrograms) | Adult Male and Female AI = 30 micrograms Daily Value = 30 micrograms %AI |
|---|---|---|
| AI | 30.0 | 100% |
| Smooth peanut butter, 2 tablespoons | 30.1 | 100% |
| Cooked lamb liver, 1 ounce | 11.6 | 39% |
| Boiled egg, 1 | 9.3 | 31% |
| Cooked egg yolk, 1 | 8.1 | 27% |
| Yogurt, 1 cup | 7.4 | 25% |
| Wheat germ, ¼ cup | 7.2 | 24% |
| Roasted peanuts, 5 | 6.5 | 22% |
| Wheat bran, ¼ cup | 6.4 | 21% |
| Nonfat milk, 1 cup | 4.9 | 16% |
| Salmon, 3 ounces | 4.3 | 14% |
| Egg noodles, 1 cup | 4.0 | 13% |
| Swiss cheese, 2 ounces | 2.2 | 7% |
| Cheddar cheese, 2 ounces | 1.7 | 6% |
| Raw cauliflower, 1 cup | 1.5 | 5% |
| American cheese, 2 ounces | 1.4 | 5% |

Key:
- Grains
- Vegetables
- Fruits
- Oils
- Milk
- Meat & Beans

**FIGURE 8-23** ▶ Food sources of biotin compared to the Adequate Intake for adults.

unlikely. However, scientists are not sure how much of the bacteria-synthesized biotin in our intestines is absorbed. If intestinal bacterial synthesis is not sufficient, as in people missing a large part of the small intestine or who take antibiotics for many months, special attention should be paid to meeting biotin needs. A protein called *avidin* in raw egg whites binds biotin and inhibits its absorption. Consuming many raw egg whites eventually leads to the deficiency disease. Cooking denatures avidin in eggs such that it cannot bind biotin.

The Adequate Intake set for biotin is 30 micrograms per day for adults. Our food supply is thought to provide 40 to 60 micrograms per person per day. A Daily Value of 30 micrograms is used to express biotin content on food and supplement labels and is 10 times our current estimate of needs. Biotin is relatively nontoxic. Large doses have been given over an extended period without harmful side effects to children who exhibit defects in biotin metabolism. Thus, no Upper Level for biotin has been set.

# 8.13 Vitamin B-6

Vitamin B-6 can exist in three chemical forms, all of which can be changed to the active vitamin B-6 coenzyme. Pyridoxine is the general vitamin name and form added to foods.

## Functions of Vitamin B-6

The coenzymes of vitamin B-6 are needed for the activity of many enzymes involved in carbohydrate, protein, and fat metabolism. Vitamin B-6 is needed in many areas

▲ Bananas are a plant source of vitamin B-6.

of metabolism, so a deficiency results in widespread symptoms, such as depression, vomiting, skin disorders, irritation of the nerves, and impaired immune response.

Vitamin B-6 plays a particularly important role in protein and amino acid metabolism (review Fig. 8-14). The coenzyme helps to remove the nitrogen group ($-NH_2$) from certain amino acids, making nitrogen available to another amino acid. These amino acid reactions allow a cell to synthesize nonessential (dispensable) amino acids. In a related function, vitamin B-6 plays a role in homocysteine metabolism.

Another important role of vitamin B-6 is the synthesis of many neurotransmitters. Recall from Chapter 3 that neurotransmitters allow nerve cells to communicate with each other and with other body cells. A vitamin B-6 deficiency can cause a decrease in these neurotransmitters and lead to symptoms, especially convulsions. This problem occurred in the 1950s when heat destroyed vitamin B-6 in formulas fed to infants.

The vitamin B-6 coenzyme is important for the synthesis of hemoglobin and its function as the oxygen-carrying part of the red blood cell. Vitamin B-6 is also necessary for the synthesis of white blood cells, which perform a major role in the immune system.

## Vitamin B-6 Sources and Needs

Major sources of vitamin B-6 are animal products, ready-to-eat breakfast cereals, potatoes, and milk. Other sources are fruits and vegetables such as bananas, cantaloupes, broccoli, and spinach (Figs. 8-24 and 8-25). Overall, animal sources and fortified products are the most reliable because the vitamin B-6 they contain is more absorbable than that in plant foods.

**FIGURE 8-24** ▶ Food sources of vitamin B-6 compared to the RDA for adults.

### Food Sources of Vitamin B-6

| Food Item and Amount | Vitamin B-6 (milligrams) | Adult Male and Female RDA = 1.3 milligrams<br>Daily Value = 2 milligrams<br>%RDA |
|---|---|---|
| **RDA** | 1.3 | 100% |
| Baked salmon, 3 ounces | 0.8 | 62% |
| Baked potato, 1 medium | 0.7 | 54% |
| Banana, 1 | 0.7 | 54% |
| Avocado, 1 | 0.6 | 46% |
| Roasted chicken breast, 3 ounces | 0.5 | 38% |
| Acorn squash, 1 cup | 0.5 | 38% |
| Special K cereal, ¾ cup | 0.5 | 38% |
| Fried beef liver, 1 ounce | 0.4 | 31% |
| Roasted turkey lunch meat, 3 ounces | 0.4 | 31% |
| Sirloin steak, 3 ounces | 0.4 | 31% |
| Lean ham, 3 ounces | 0.4 | 31% |
| Watermelon, 1 slice | 0.3 | 23% |
| Sunflower seeds, ¼ cup | 0.3 | 23% |
| Cooked spinach, ½ cup | 0.2 | 15% |

**Key:**
- ■ Grains
- ■ Vegetables
- ■ Fruits
- □ Oils
- ■ Milk
- ■ Meat & Beans

**MyPyramid: Sources of Vitamin B-6**

| Grains | Vegetables | Fruits | Oils | Milk | Meat & Beans |
|--------|-----------|--------|------|------|--------------|
| • Fortified break-fast cereals<br>• Wheat germ (whole-wheat products) | • Potatoes<br>• Spinach<br>• Cauliflower | • Avocados<br>• Bananas<br>• Dates<br>• Cantaloupe<br>• Watermelon | • None | • Milk<br>• Yogurt<br>• Cottage cheese | • Meat<br>• Poultry<br>• Fish<br>• Beans<br>• Nuts<br>• Seeds |

**FIGURE 8-25** ▶ Sources of vitamin B-6 from MyPyramid. The height of the background color (none, 1/3, 2/3, or completely covered) within each group in the pyramid indicates the average nutrient density for vitamin B-6 in that group. Overall, the meat group especially contains many foods that are nutrient-dense sources of vitamin B-6. With regard to physical activity, vitamin B-6 participates in the related energy metabolism during such endeavors.

The adult RDA of vitamin B-6 is 1.3 to 1.7 milligrams per day. A Daily Value of 2 milligrams is used to express vitamin B-6 content on food and supplement labels. Average daily consumption of vitamin B-6 for men and women is somewhat above the RDA.

Athletes may need slightly more vitamin B-6 than sedentary adults. The athlete's body processes a great deal of glycogen and ingested protein (in the form of amino acids) for fuel, and the metabolism of these compounds requires vitamin B-6. However, athletes are likely to consume plenty of protein-rich foods—enough to supply needed amounts of vitamin B-6.

People with alcoholism are susceptible to a vitamin B-6 deficiency because a metabolite formed in alcohol metabolism can displace the coenzyme form from enzymes, increasing its tendency to be destroyed. In addition, alcohol decreases the absorption of vitamin B-6 and the synthesis of its coenzyme form. Cirrhosis and hepatitis (both of which may accompany alcoholism) also disable liver tissue from metabolizing vitamin B-6, which decreases synthesis of its coenzyme form.

Nausea is experienced by 70% to 85% of women during the first trimester of pregnancy (see Chapter 14). Sometimes physicians recommend vitamin B-6 supplementation, typically 30 to 75 mg/day, to reduce nausea. A review of the research on treating nausea during pregnancy suggests that this therapy is both safe and likely to help reduce nausea. Even though vitamin B-6 supplements to treat nausea are available over-the-counter without a prescription, pregnant women should first discuss this treatment option with their physicians.

## Upper Level for Vitamin B-6

The Upper Level for vitamin B-6 is 100 milligrams per day, based on the risk of developing nerve damage. Studies have shown that intakes of 2 to 6 grams of vitamin B-6 per day for 2 or more months especially can lead to irreversible nerve damage. Symptoms of vitamin B-6 toxicity include walking difficulties and hand and foot numbness. Some nerve damage in individual sensory neurons is probably reversible, but damage to the ganglia (where many nerve fibers converge) appears to be permanent. With 500 milligram tablets of vitamin B-6 available in health-food stores, taking a toxic dose is easy.

## CONCEPT CHECK

Pantothenic acid and biotin both participate in the metabolism of carbohydrate and fat. A deficiency of either vitamin is unlikely; pantothenic acid is found widely in foods, and our need for biotin is partially met by intestinal synthesis from bacteria. Vitamin B-6 is important for protein metabolism, neurotransmitter synthesis, homocysteine metabolism, and other key metabolic functions. Headache, a form of anemia, nausea, and vomiting can result from a vitamin B-6 deficiency. Increased risk of cardiovascular disease is also likely. Animal protein foods, ready-to-eat breakfast cereals, broccoli, spinach, and bananas are some food sources of vitamin B-6. Megadose supplements of vitamin B-6 can lead to nerve damage.

## 8.14 Folate

The term *folate* encompasses a variety of food forms of the vitamin. Folic acid is the synthetic chemical form added to foods and present in supplements. Folic acid is more readily absorbed (1.7 times greater) than natural forms of folate. The structure of natural food folate differs from folic acid by containing extra units of the amino acid, glutamic acid. These extra units must be removed before absorption, yielding free folic acid.

### Functions of Folate

A key role of the folate coenzymes is to supply or accept single carbon compounds. In this role, the coenzymes help form DNA and also metabolize various amino acids and their derivatives, such as homocysteine.

One major result of a folate deficiency is decreased red blood cell synthesis. Without folate, the immature cells cannot divide because they cannot form new DNA. The cells grow progressively larger because they can still synthesize enough protein and other cell parts to make new cells. When the time comes for the cells to divide, however, the amount of DNA is insufficient to form two nuclei. The cells then remain in a large immature form, known as a **megaloblast** (Fig. 8-26).

The bone marrow of a folate-deficient person, therefore, produces mostly immature megaloblast cells, and very few mature red blood cells (called **erythrocytes**). With fewer mature red blood cells in the bloodstream, the blood's capacity to carry oxygen decreases, causing folate deficiency anemia called **megaloblastic anemia** (also called macrocytic anemia).

The changes in red blood cell formation occur after 7 to 16 weeks on a folate-free diet, depending on the person's folate stores. White blood cell formation is also affected, but to a lesser degree. In addition, cell division throughout the entire body is disrupted. Clinicians focus primarily on red blood cells because they are easy to collect and examine. Other symptoms of folate deficiency are inflammation of the tongue, diarrhea, poor growth, mental confusion, depression, and problems in nerve function.

About 10% of the North American population has a genetic defect in an important aspect of folate metabolism. They may need up to twice the RDA to compensate for the defect. Genetic testing for this defect is not routine in medical practice, but one day it may be.

A maternal deficiency of folate along with this genetic abnormality related to folate metabolism has been linked to development of **neural tube defects** in the fetus (Fig. 8-27). These defects include spina bifida (spinal cord or spinal fluid bulge

**megaloblast** A large, immature red blood cell that results from the particular cell's inability to divide normally.

**erythrocytes** Mature red blood cells. These have no nucleus and a life span of about 120 days; they contain hemoglobin, which transports oxygen and carbon dioxide.

**megaloblastic anemia** Anemia characterized by the presence of abnormally large red blood cells.

**neural tube defect** A defect in the formation of the neural tube occurring during early fetal development. This type of defect results in various nervous system disorders, such as spina bifida. Folate deficiency in the pregnant woman increases the risk that the fetus will develop this disorder.

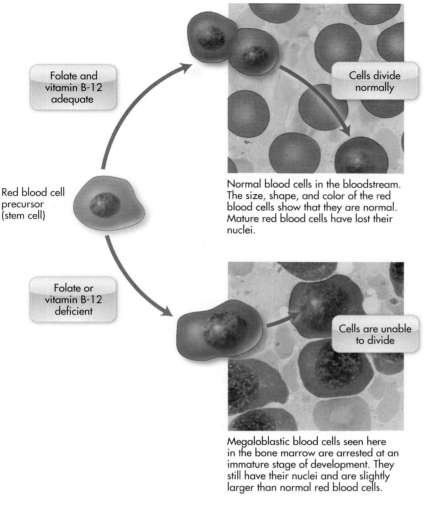

Folate and vitamin B-12 adequate

Cells divide normally

Red blood cell precursor (stem cell)

Normal blood cells in the bloodstream. The size, shape, and color of the red blood cells show that they are normal. Mature red blood cells have lost their nuclei.

Folate or vitamin B-12 deficient

Cells are unable to divide

Megaloblastic blood cells seen here in the bone marrow are arrested at an immature stage of development. They still have their nuclei and are slightly larger than normal red blood cells.

**FIGURE 8-26 ▶** Megaloblastic anemia occurs when blood cells are unable to divide, leaving large, immature red blood cells. Either a folate or vitamin B-12 deficiency may cause this condition. Measurements of blood concentrations of both vitamins are taken to help determine the cause of the anemia.

**Healthy Spine**

Skin on back

Spinal cord
Spinal fluid
Vertebra

**Spine Affected by Spina Bifida**

Skin on back
Spinal fluid

Spinal cord
Vertebra

**FIGURE 8-27 ▶** Neural tube defects result from a developmental failure affecting the spinal cord or brain in the embryo. Very early in fetal development, a ridge of neural-like tissue forms along the back of the embryo. As the fetus develops, this material develops into both the spinal cord and nerves at the lower end and into the brain at the upper end. At the same time, the bones that make up the back gradually surround the spinal cord on all sides. If any part of this sequence goes awry, many defects can appear. The worst case is total lack of a brain (anencephaly). Spina bifida, in which the back bones do not form a complete ring to protect the spinal cord, is much more common. Deficient folate status in the mother during the beginning of pregnancy, especially in combination with a genetic abnormality in folate metabolism, greatly increases the risk of neural tube defects.

through the back) and anencephaly (absence of a brain). About 2000 infants are affected with neural tube defects annually in the United States. Victims of spina bifida exhibit paralysis, incontinence, learning disabilities, and other health problems. Children born with anencephaly die shortly after birth. Adequate folate nutriture is crucial for all women of childbearing age because the neural tube closes within the first 28 days of pregnancy, a time when many women are not even aware that they are pregnant. Research that has been done with synthetic folic acid supplementation has resulted in a recommendation that ample folate, specifically 400 micrograms of synthetic folic acid per day, be consumed at least 6 weeks before conception. It appears that even those women with varied diets may not consume adequate synthetic folic acid to prevent neural tube defects unless specific attention to rich sources is given. Perhaps as many as 70% of these defects could be avoided by adequate folate status before conception. (Women who have had a child with a neural tube defect are advised to consume 4 milligrams per day of folic acid, beginning at least one month before any future pregnancy. This must be done under strict physician supervision.)

Consuming ready-to-eat breakfast cereals that contain 100% of the Daily Value for folate (this is the same as the RDA) is a good practice for meeting the goal for synthetic folic acid intake. A multivitamin and mineral supplement can also be used to supply adequate synthetic folic acid, but women should be careful to monitor the amount of any accompanying preformed vitamin A content (do not exceed 100% of the Daily Value). Since 1992, there has been an effort to get all women of Childbearing age to take daily vitamins containing folic acid. A March of Dimes survey found that 40% of these women did so in 2007.

Research is underway on the link between folate and cancer protection. Folate aids in DNA synthesis, so it is hypothesized that even mild folate deficiency contributes to abnormal DNA integrity, which in turn affects certain cancer-protecting genes. Meeting the RDA for folate is thought to be one way to reduce cancer risk. A recent 7-year study found that, in women, folate supplements in combination with vitamin B-6 and vitamin B-12 did not prevent breast cancer or other invasive cancers.

## MAKING DECISIONS

### Folate and Cancer Therapy

Some forms of cancer therapy provide a vivid example of the effects of a folate deficiency on DNA metabolism. A cancer drug, methotrexate, closely resembles a form of folate but cannot act in its place. Because of this resemblance, when methotrexate is taken in high doses, it hampers folate metabolism. In essence, methotrexate crowds out folate in the metabolic pathways. DNA synthesis and, consequently, cell division, then decrease. Cancer cells are among the most rapidly dividing cells in the body, so they are among those first affected. However, other rapidly dividing cells, such as intestinal cells and skin cells, are also affected. Not surprisingly, typical side effects of methotrexate therapy are diarrhea, vomiting, and hair loss. These are also typical symptoms of folate deficiency. Today when patients are given methotrexate, they need to follow a high-folate diet and/or take folic acid supplements because this reduces the toxic side effects of the drug. High supplemental doses generally have little or no influence on methotrexate's effectiveness as a cancer therapy.

## Folate Sources and Needs

Green, leafy vegetables (*folate* is derived from the Latin word *folium,* which means *foliage* or *leaves*), organ meats, sprouts, other vegetables, dried beans, and orange juice are the richest sources of folate (Figs. 8-28 and 8-29). The vitamin C in orange juice also reduces folate destruction. Ready-to-eat breakfast cereals, milk, and bread also are important sources of folate for many adults.

Folate is susceptible to destruction by heat. Food processing and preparation destroy 50% to 90% of the folate in food. This under-scores the importance of regularly eating fresh fruits and raw or lightly cooked vegetables. As mentioned, vegetables retain their nutrients best when cooked quickly in minimal water—steaming, stir-fry-ing, or microwaving (review Table 8-1).

The RDA of folate for adults is 400 micrograms per day, as is the Daily Value used to express folate content on food and supplement labels. Folate recommendations for all but women of child-bearing age (these women should meet such recommendations with synthetic folic acid), are based on dietary folate equivalents (DFE). To com-pute folate intake in DFE units, one has to determine how much of a day's folate intake comes from food folate and how much comes from synthetic folic acid added to foods. When in doubt, assume all folate in a diet is in the food form, except that coming from ready-to-eat breakfast cereals and refined grain products. Also included in this second category is any folic acid in supplements. To calculate the DFE, multi-ply total synthetic folic acid intake by 1.7, and add that value to the food folate con-sumed. For example, if a person consumed 300 micrograms as food folate and 200 micrograms from a ready-to-eat breakfast cereal, total DFE would be 640 micrograms (300 + [200 × 1.7] = 640). Compared to the RDA of 400 micrograms, this intake would be sufficient.

Prior to 1998, average daily folate intakes in the United States were approximately 320 micrograms for men and 220 micrograms for women. In 1998, the fortification of grain products with folate was mandated in the United States and Canada, with the aim of reducing birth defects of the spine. With this mandate, average intakes have increased by about 200 micrograms per day. Studies have shown this practice has decreased rates of neural tube defects in infants.

## CRITICAL THINKING

Suzanne and Ted are planning to start a fam-ily. They are especially concerned because Suzanne's sister gave birth last year to a baby with spina bifida. In preparation for her pregnancy, Suzanne takes a multivitamin supplement and eats fortified breakfast cereal most days. She also tries to include oranges, orange juice, broccoli, and spinach salads in her diet. What is spina bifida? How do Suzanne's diet and multivitamin supple-ment help prevent this serious disorder?

## Food Sources of Folate

| Food Item and Amount | Folate (micrograms) | Adult Male and Female RDA = 400 micrograms Daily Value = 400 micrograms %RDA |
|---|---|---|
| **RDA** | 400 | 100% |
| Asparagus, 1 cup | 263 | 66% |
| Cooked spinach, 1 cup | 262 | 66% |
| Cooked lentils, ½ cup | 179 | 45% |
| Black-eyed peas, ½ cup | 179 | 45% |
| Romaine lettuce, 1½ cups | 114 | 29% |
| Great Grains cereal, ¾ cup | 114 | 29% |
| Tortilla, 1 | 89 | 22% |
| Cooked turnips, ½ cup | 85 | 21% |
| Cooked broccoli, 1 cup | 78 | 20% |
| Sunflower seeds, ¼ cup | 76 | 19% |
| Fresh orange juice, 1 cup | 75 | 19% |
| Cooked beets, ½ cup | 68 | 17% |
| Kidney beans, ½ cup | 65 | 16% |

**Key:**
■ Grains
■ Vegetables
■ Fruits
□ Oils
■ Milk
■ Meat & Beans

**FIGURE 8-28** ▶ Food sources of folate compared to the RDA for adults.

**FIGURE 8-29** ▶ Sources of folate from MyPyramid. The height of the background color (none, 1/3, 2/3, or completely covered) within each group in the pyramid indicates the average nutrient density for folate in that group. Overall, the vegetables group provides the richest sources, but the fruits group and the grains group contain some foods that are nutrient-dense sources of folate.

**MyPyramid: Sources of Folate**

| Grains | Vegetables | Fruits | Oils | Milk | Meat & Beans |
|---|---|---|---|---|---|
| • Fortified break-fast cereals<br>• Wheat germ (whole-wheat products)<br>• Enriched grains | • Asparagus<br>• Leafy green vegetables | • Oranges<br>• Strawberries<br>• Cantaloupes and other melons | • None | • Cottage cheese<br>• Yogurt | • Liver<br>• Eggs<br>• Beans<br>• Sunflower seeds |

 See *Nutrition and Your Health: Dietary Supplements—Who Needs Them?* at the end of Chapter 8.

Pregnant women need extra folate (a total of 600 micrograms DFE) to accommodate the increased rates of cell division and DNA synthesis in their own bodies and in the developing fetus. A healthy diet easily supplies this much. Although most vitamin supplements have no proven health benefits in most people (See the "Nutrition and Your Health" section at the end of this chapter), supplemental folic acid is effective at preventing birth defects. Prenatal care often includes a specially formulated multivitamin and mineral supplement enriched with synthetic folic acid to help compensate for the extra needs associated with pregnancy. Within the 2005 Dietary Guidelines for Americans, a key recommendation for women of childbearing age who may become pregnant and those in the first trimester of pregnancy is to consume adequate synthetic folic acid daily (from fortified foods or supplements) in addition to food forms of folate from a varied diet.

Older people are also at risk for folate deficiency, possibly due to a combination of inadequate folate intake and decreased absorption. Perhaps these people fail to consume sufficient amounts of fruits and vegetables because of poverty or physical problems, such as poor dental health. In addition, folate deficiencies often occur with alcoholism, due mostly to poor intake and absorption. Symptoms of a folate-related anemia can alert a physician to the possibility of alcoholism.

## MAKING DECISIONS

### Dietary Folate Equivalents

The use of dietary folate equivalents (DFEs) instead of the actual amount of folate in a food has some important implications. Typically, many foods will be richer in folate than the Nutrition Facts label suggests because folate content is due primarily to synthetic folic acid added to the foods, such as in enriched grains and ready-to-eat breakfast cereals. This contributes substantially to the DFE calculation. Another implication is that food composition tables and diet analysis software programs (such as that supplied with this book) also underestimate the true folate contribution of a diet compared to folate needs because these have not been updated to DFE units.

▲ Enriched grains and ready-to-eat breakfast cereals are good sources of synthetic folic acid.

## Upper Level for Folate

The Upper Level for folate is 1 milligram (1000 micrograms) per day but only refers to the synthetic source. This is because folate naturally present in foods has limited absorption. Large doses of folate can hide the signs of vitamin B-12 deficiency and therefore complicate its diagnosis. Specifically, regular consumption of large amounts of folate can prevent the appearance of an early warning sign of vitamin B-12 deficiency—enlarged red blood cell size. To prevent such masking of vitamin B-12 deficiency, the goal of the folate fortification of grains program is, to increase the folate status of women of childbearing age without causing excessive intake (over 1 milligram of synthetic folic acid per day) by other individuals. Also, because of risk of masking a vitamin B-12 deficiency, FDA limits supplements for nonpregnant adults and food fortification to 400 microgram amounts.

# 8.15  Vitamin B-12

Vitamin B-12 represents a family of compounds that contain the mineral cobalt. All vitamin B-12 compounds are synthesized by bacteria, fungi, and other lower organisms.

The body has a complex means of absorbing vitamin B-12. Vitamin B-12 in food enters the stomach and is digested from other materials, especially by stomach acid. The free vitamin B-12 in the stomach binds with a protein produced by the salivary glands in the mouth, and that protects vitamin B-12 from stomach acid. Vitamin B-12 is later freed from this protein in the small intestine. Finally, vitamin B-12 binds in the small intestine with a compound made in the stomach called **intrinsic factor.** The resulting intrinsic factor/vitamin B-12 complex travels to the last portion of the small intestine for absorption. After these digestion steps, approximately 50% of dietary vitamin B-12 is absorbed, depending on the body's need for it.

If a person has a defect in the digestion and absorption of vitamin B-12, the body may only be able to use 1% to 2% of dietary vitamin B-12. Monthly injections of vitamin B-12 or vitamin B-12 nasal gels are used to bypass the need for absorption or megadoses of a supplemental form (300 times the RDA) are needed to overcome the absorption defect by providing enough of the vitamin via simple diffusion across the intestinal tract.

About 95% of all cases of vitamin B-12 deficiencies in healthy people result from defective vitamin B-12 absorption, rather than from inadequate intakes. This is especially true for older people. As we age, our stomachs have a decreased ability to synthesize the intrinsic factor needed for vitamin B-12 absorption.

**intrinsic factor**  A protein-like compound produced by the stomach that enhances vitamin B-12 absorption.

## Functions of Vitamin B-12

Vitamin B-12 participates in a variety of cellular processes. The most important function is in folate metabolism. Vitamin B-12 is required to convert folate coenzymes to the active forms needed for metabolic reactions, such as DNA synthesis. Without vitamin B-12, reactions that require certain active forms of folate do not take place in the cell. Thus, a vitamin B-12 deficiency can result in symptoms of a folate deficiency. Another vital function of vitamin B-12 is maintaining the myelin sheaths that insulate neurons from each other. People with vitamin B-12 deficiencies have destruction of segments of the myelin sheaths. This destruction eventually causes paralysis and, perhaps, death. Vitamin B-12 also participates in homocysteine metabolism and certain minor metabolic pathways.

In the past, the inability to absorb enough vitamin B-12 eventually led to death, mainly because it destroyed nerves. This phenomenon was

▼ As we age, our digestive system absorbs vitamin B-12 from food less efficiently.

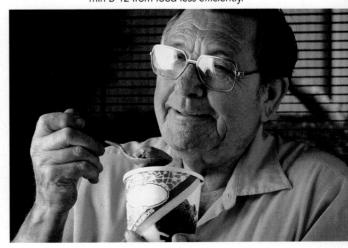

**pernicious anemia** The anemia that results from a lack of vitamin B-12 absorption; it is pernicious because of associated nerve degeneration that can result in eventual paralysis and death.

called **pernicious anemia** (*pernicious* literally means "leading to death"). Clinically, the anemia looks much like a folate-deficiency anemia, characterized by the appearance of many large red blood cells in the bloodstream. However, the true cause of pernicious anemia is poor vitamin B-12 absorption rather than inadequate folate intakes.

Some symptoms of pernicious anemia include weakness, sore tongue, back pain, apathy, and tingling in the extremities. We are able to store significant amounts of vitamin B-12, so symptoms of nerve destruction generally do not develop until at least 3 years after the onset of the deficiency. Unfortunately, significant nerve destruction often occurs before the anemia is detected, and this destruction is irreversible. Pernicious anemia and its accompanying nerve destruction generally start after middle age, affecting up to 10% to 20% of older adults. The explanation for this age-associated pernicious anemia is twofold. First, aging is often associated with low production of stomach acid. Thus, vitamin B-12 is not properly cleaved from other food components during digestion. Second, aging may be accompanied by reduced output of intrinsic factor, resulting in decreased absorption of the vitamin.

Infants who are breastfed by vegetarian or vegan mothers are at risk for vitamin B-12 deficiency accompanied by anemia and long-term nervous system problems, such as diminished brain growth, degeneration of the spinal cord, and poor intellectual development. The problems may have their origins during pregnancy, when the mother is deficient in vitamin B-12. Vegan diets supply little vitamin B-12 unless they include vitamin B-12–enriched food or supplements, so achieving an adequate vitamin B-12 intake is a key diet-planning goal for vegans (review Chapter 6).

## Vitamin B-12 Sources and Needs

Major sources of vitamin B-12 include meat, milk, ready-to-eat breakfast cereals, poultry, seafood, and eggs (Fig. 8-30). Organ meats (especially liver, kidneys, and heart) are especially rich sources of vitamin B-12. Adults over age 50 are encouraged

**FIGURE 8-30** ▶ Food sources of vitamin B-12 compared to the RDA for adults.

### Food Sources of Vitamin B-12

| Food Item and Amount | Vitamin B-12 (micrograms) | Adult Male and Female RDA = 2.4 micrograms Daily Value = 6 micrograms %RDA |
|---|---|---|
| **RDA** | 2.4 | 100% |
| Baked clams, 1 ounce | 15.7 | 654% |
| Boiled oysters, 2 | 14.4 | 600% |
| Lobster, 3 ounces | 2.7 | 113% |
| Pot roast, 3 ounces | 2.5 | 104% |
| Plain yogurt, 1 cup | 1.4 | 58% |
| Corn Flakes cereal, ¾ cup | 1.1 | 46% |
| Shrimp, 3 ounces | 1.0 | 42% |
| 1% milk, 1 cup | 0.9 | 38% |
| Soy milk, 1 cup | 0.8 | 33% |
| Boiled egg, 1 | 0.6 | 25% |
| Lean ham, 3 ounces | 0.6 | 25% |
| Beef hot dog, 1 | 0.5 | 21% |
| Ham lunch meat, 2 ounces | 0.4 | 17% |

**Key:**
- Grains
- Vegetables
- Fruits
- Oils
- Milk
- Meat & Beans

to seek a synthetic vitamin B-12 source to aid absorption, which can be limited due to reduced intrinsic factor and stomach acid output seen in aging, as mentioned. Synthetic vitamin B-12 is not food bound, so it doesn't need stomach acid to release it from foods. Thus, it will be more readily absorbed than the food form. Ready-to-eat breakfast cereals and a multivitamin and mineral supplement are two possible synthetic sources.

The RDA of vitamin B-12 for adults is 2.4 micrograms per day. The Daily Value of 6 micrograms is used on food and supplement labels. On average, adults consume 2 times the RDA or more. This high intake provides the average meat-eating person with storage of vitamin B-12 in the liver for about 2 to 3 years.

It takes a person approximately 20 years of consuming a diet essentially free of vitamin B-12 to exhibit nerve destruction caused by a diet deficiency. Still, vegans, who eat no animal products, should find a reliable source of vitamin B-12, such as fortified soybean milk, ready-to-eat breakfast cereals, and a supplemental form of vitamin B-12 enriched yeast. Use of a multivitamin and mineral supplement containing vitamin B-12 is another option. As noted earlier, older persons are at significant risk for developing pernicious anemia due to the loss of vitamin B-12 absorption capacity. Within the 2005 Dietary Guidelines for Americans, a key recommendation for people over age 50 is to consume vitamin B-12 in its crystalline form (i.e., fortified foods or supplements). Regular physical examinations should test for pernicious anemia in older adults. Vitamin B-12 supplements are essentially nontoxic, so no Upper Level has been set.

**P**eople with HIV/AIDS also are at risk of vitamin B-12 deficiency, linked to long-standing malabsorption that they often experience. In a few studies, adequate vitamin B-12 status has been shown to lessen the decline in health experienced by those with HIV/AIDS.

▲ Seafood, especially clams and lobster, are good sources of vitamin B-12.

## CONCEPT CHECK

Folate is needed for cell division because it influences DNA synthesis. A folate deficiency results in megaloblastic (macrocytic) anemia, as well as elevated blood homocysteine, inflammation of the tongue, diarrhea, and poor growth. Excess folate intake can mask a vitamin B-12 deficiency because these vitamins work together in metabolism. Folate is found in fruits and vegetables, beans, and organ meats. Emphasizing fresh and lightly cooked vegetables in the diet is important because much folate is lost during cooking. Women of childbearing age should meet needs by consuming a source of synthetic folic acid. Folate needs during pregnancy are especially high; a deficiency around the time of conception and in the first month of pregnancy may lead to neural tube defects in the fetus.

Vitamin B-12 is necessary for folate metabolism. Without dietary vitamin B-12, folate deficiency symptoms, such as macrocytic anemia, develop. In addition, vitamin B-12 is necessary for maintaining the nervous system. Paralysis can develop from a vitamin B-12 deficiency. Vitamin B-12 also participates in homocysteine metabolism. The absorption of vitamin B-12 requires a number of specific factors. If absorption is inhibited, the resulting deficiency can lead to pernicious anemia and its associated nerve destruction. Concentrated amounts of vitamin B-12 are found only in animal foods; meat-eaters generally have a 2- to 3-year supply stored in the liver. Vegans need to find an alternate source. Vitamin B-12 absorption may decline as we age. Monthly injections, nasal gels, or megadoses can make up for this.

# 8.16 Vitamin C

Vitamin C (ascorbic acid) is found in all living tissues, and most animals (but not humans) synthesize it from the simple sugar glucose. Vitamin C is absorbed in the small intestine. About 70% to 90% of vitamin C is absorbed when a person eats between 30 and 180 milligrams of it per day. If someone ingests 1 gram (1000 milligrams) per day, absorption efficiency drops to about 50%. A common side effect of megadose vitamin C use is diarrhea. The unabsorbed vitamin C stays in the small intestine and attracts water, resulting in diarrhea (see the section on toxicity of vitamin C).

## Functions of Vitamin C

**Collagen Synthesis** The best understood function of vitamin C is its role in synthesizing the protein collagen. This protein is highly concentrated in connective tissue, bone, teeth, tendons, and blood vessels. It is important for wound healing. Vitamin C increases the cross-connections between amino acids in collagen, greatly strengthening the structural tissues it helps form.

On long sea voyages, captains often lost half or more of their crews to scurvy, the vitamin C deficiency disease. Its symptoms include weakness, slow wound healing, opening of previously healed wounds, bone pain, fractures, bleeding gums, diarrhea, and pinpoint hemorrhages around hair follicles on the back of the arms and legs. In 1740, the Englishman Dr. James Lind first showed that citrus fruits—two oranges and one lemon a day—could cure scurvy. Fifty years after Lind's discovery, rations for British sailors included limes to prevent scurvy (thus their nickname, limeys).

A vitamin C deficiency can cause widespread changes in tissue metabolism. Most symptoms of scurvy are linked to a decrease in collagen synthesis, such as in the skin. About 20 to 40 days with no vitamin C intake are required for the first symptoms of scurvy to appear (Fig. 8-31).

**Antioxidant Activity** Vitamin C has antioxidant properties. This may allow vitamin C to reduce the formation of cancer-causing nitrosamines in the stomach and also keep the folate coenzymes intact, preventing their destruction. Vitamin C may work as a free radical scavenger. Vitamin C also may aid in reactivating oxidized vitamin E so that it can be reused. The extent to which all this antioxidant activity happens in the body, however, is debatable and not proven as of now. Population studies suggest that vitamin C is effective in helping prevent certain cancers (of the esophagus, mouth, and stomach) and cataracts in the eye, probably because of its antioxidant properties.

**Iron Absorption** Vitamin C enhances iron absorption by keeping iron in its most absorbable form, especially as the mineral travels through the small intestine's alkaline environment. This is seen with a vitamin C intake of 75 milligrams or more at a meal. Increasing intake of vitamin C-rich foods is beneficial for those with poor iron stores. Within the 2005 Dietary Guidelines for Americans, a key recommendation for women of childbearing age who may become pregnant is to eat foods high in heme-iron and/or consume iron-rich plant foods or iron-fortified foods with an enhancer of iron absorption, such as vitamin C-rich foods.

**Immune Function** Finally, vitamin C is vital for the function of the immune system, especially for the activity of certain immune cells. Thus, disease states that increase the need for immune function can increase the need for vitamin C, possibly above the RDA. Partly on the basis of this observation, Dr. Linus Pauling gained great notoriety by claiming that vitamin C could combat the common cold. He claimed that 1000 milligrams (1 gram) or more of vitamin C daily could reduce the number of colds for most people by nearly half. As a result of the popularity of his books and the respectability of his scientific credentials, millions of North Americans supplement their diets with vitamin C.

But does vitamin C reliably and effectively work against colds and other infections? Most medical and nutrition scientists disagree with Pauling's views of vitamin C. Numerous well-designed, double-blind studies have not shown megadoses of vitamin C to reliably prevent colds, though it seems to reduce the duration of symptoms by a day or so.

**FIGURE 8-31** ▶ Pinpoint hemorrhages of the skin—an early symptom of scurvy. The spots on the skin are caused by slight bleeding. The person may experience poor wound healing. These are all signs of defective collagen synthesis.

## Vitamin C Sources and Needs

Major sources of vitamin C are citrus fruits, green peppers, cauliflower, broccoli, cabbage, strawberries, papayas, and romaine lettuce. Potatoes, ready-to-eat breakfast cereals, and fortified fruit drinks are also good sources of vitamin C (Figs. 8-32 and 8-33).

## Food Sources of Vitamin C

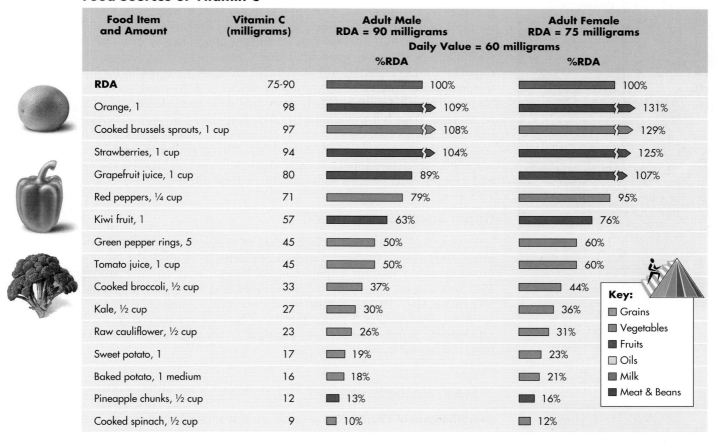

| Food Item and Amount | Vitamin C (milligrams) | Adult Male RDA = 90 milligrams %RDA | Adult Female RDA = 75 milligrams %RDA |
|---|---|---|---|
| | | Daily Value = 60 milligrams | |
| **RDA** | 75-90 | 100% | 100% |
| Orange, 1 | 98 | 109% | 131% |
| Cooked brussels sprouts, 1 cup | 97 | 108% | 129% |
| Strawberries, 1 cup | 94 | 104% | 125% |
| Grapefruit juice, 1 cup | 80 | 89% | 107% |
| Red peppers, ¼ cup | 71 | 79% | 95% |
| Kiwi fruit, 1 | 57 | 63% | 76% |
| Green pepper rings, 5 | 45 | 50% | 60% |
| Tomato juice, 1 cup | 45 | 50% | 60% |
| Cooked broccoli, ½ cup | 33 | 37% | 44% |
| Kale, ½ cup | 27 | 30% | 36% |
| Raw cauliflower, ½ cup | 23 | 26% | 31% |
| Sweet potato, 1 | 17 | 19% | 23% |
| Baked potato, 1 medium | 16 | 18% | 21% |
| Pineapple chunks, ½ cup | 12 | 13% | 16% |
| Cooked spinach, ½ cup | 9 | 10% | 12% |

Key:
- ▇ Grains
- ▇ Vegetables
- ▇ Fruits
- ☐ Oils
- ▇ Milk
- ▇ Meat & Beans

**FIGURE 8-32** ▶ Food sources of vitamin C compared to the RDA for adult males and females.

**FIGURE 8-33** ▶ Sources of vitamin C from MyPyramid. The height of the background color (none, 1/3, 2/3, or completely covered) within each group in the pyramid indicates the average nutrient density for vitamin C in that group. Overall, the vegetables group and the fruits group contain many foods that are nutrient-dense sources of vitamin C. With regard to physical activity, vitamin C has no primary role in the related energy metabolism *per se*, but likely limits some oxidant damage during such endeavors.

## MyPyramid: Sources of Vitamin C

| Grains | Vegetables | Fruits | Oils | Milk | Meat & Beans |
|---|---|---|---|---|---|
| • Fortified breakfast cereals | • Tomatoes<br>• Potatoes<br>• Cauliflower<br>• Green vegetables | • Citrus fruits<br>• Pineapple<br>• Strawberries | • None | • None | • None |

▲ In addition to orange juice, fruits such as strawberries and kiwis are excellent sources of vitamin C.

▲ Oranges are a rich source of vitamin C. The many phytochemicals they provide are an additional benefit and are not found in vitamin C supplements.

Meeting the servings for fruits and vegetables recommended by MyPyramid can easily provide enough vitamin C. Vitamin C is rapidly lost in processing and cooking as it is unstable in the presence of heat, iron, copper, or oxygen and is water soluble.

The adult RDA of vitamin C is 75 to 90 milligrams per day. The Daily Value of 60 milligrams is used to express vitamin C content on food and supplement labels. Cigarette smokers need to add an extra 35 milligrams per day to the RDA because of the great stress on their lungs from oxygen and toxic by-products of cigarette smoke. Nearly all North Americans likely meet their daily needs for vitamin C. We consume an average 70 to 100 milligrams per day. Respected nutrition experts who advocate increased use of vitamin C often recommend intakes of about 200 milligrams per day. Still, this amount can be obtained by sufficient fruit and vegetable intake. Today, vitamin C deficiency appears mostly in alcoholic people who eat nutrient-poor diets and in some older persons with inadequate food intakes.

## Upper Level for Vitamin C

Most vitamin C consumed in large doses in supplements ends up in the feces or the urine. Only a small fraction of such large doses can be used. The kidneys start rapidly excreting excess vitamin C, beginning at intakes of about 100 milligrams per day. This means that if more than that is ingested, much is quickly excreted. At dosages of 500 milligrams per day, almost all of consumed vitamin C is excreted. The Upper Level for vitamin C is 2 grams per day. Regularly consuming more than that may cause stomach inflammation and diarrhea. Other suggested toxicity symptoms have been discounted in healthy people.

### MAKING DECISIONS

#### High Doses of Vitamin C

If people want to experiment with large doses of vitamin C, they should alert their physician. High doses of vitamin C can change reactions to medical tests for blood in the feces and glucose in the urine (test for diabetes). Vitamin C can interact with the testing procedures because much of a high dose of vitamin C will not be absorbed and end up in the feces, or if absorbed, will be rapidly excreted in the urine. Physicians may misdiagnose conditions when large doses of vitamin C are consumed without their knowledge.

### CONCEPT CHECK

Vitamin C is important in the synthesis of collagen, a major connective tissue protein. A vitamin C deficiency, known as scurvy, causes many changes in the skin and gums, such as small hemorrhages. This is mainly because of poor collagen synthesis. Vitamin C also modestly improves iron absorption, is involved in synthesizing certain hormones and neurotransmitters, and likely acts as a general body antioxidant. Citrus fruits, green peppers, cauliflower, broccoli, strawberries, and ready-to-eat breakfast cereals are good sources of vitamin C. As with folate, eating fresh or lightly cooked foods is important because vitamin C loses a lot of its potency in cooking. High doses of vitamin C can lead to diarrhea and foil various medical tests.

## 8.17 Choline

The dietary component choline is the latest addition to the list of essential nutrients. Choline is part of acetylcholine, a neurotransmitter associated with attention, learning and memory, muscle control, and many other functions. It is also part of phospholipids, such as **lecithin,** the major component of the cell membrane. Finally, choline participates in some aspects of homocysteine metabolism.

There has been only one published study examining the effect of inadequate dietary intake of choline in healthy humans. The study of male volunteers showed decreased choline stores and liver damage when humans were fed choline-deficient total parental (intravenous) nutrition solutions. Based on this human study and several laboratory animal studies, choline has been deemed essential, but is not yet classified as a vitamin.

> **lecithin** A group of phospholipid compounds that are major components of cell membranes.

### Choline Sources and Needs

Choline is widely distributed in foods (Fig. 8-34). Milk, liver, and peanuts are sources. Lecithins often are added to food during processing, so this is yet another source. There is so much choline available in ordinary foods that it is unlikely that a dietary deficiency exists naturally. Choline also can be synthesized from the nonessential (dispensable) amino acid serine.

The Adequate Intake for choline for adults is 425 to 550 milligrams per day. We do not know if a dietary supply is needed at all life stages. Although Adequate Intakes are set for choline, it may be that the choline requirement can be met by body synthesis at some or all stages of life. We consume ample choline from food, at least 700 to 1000 milligrams per day.

### Upper Level for Choline

The Upper Level for adults is 3.5 grams per day. This is based on development of a fishy body odor and low blood pressure at excessive intakes.

▲ Nuts, such as peanuts, are a good source of choline. Body cells also produce choline.

## 8.18 Vitamin-Like Compounds

A variety of vitamin-like compounds are found in the body. These include the following:

- Carnitine, needed to transport fatty acids into cell mitochondria
- Inositol, part of cell membranes

### Food Sources of Choline

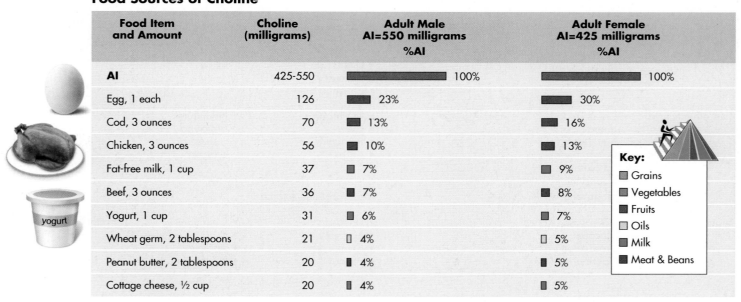

| Food Item and Amount | Choline (milligrams) | Adult Male AI=550 milligrams %AI | Adult Female AI=425 milligrams %AI |
|---|---|---|---|
| **AI** | 425-550 | 100% | 100% |
| Egg, 1 each | 126 | 23% | 30% |
| Cod, 3 ounces | 70 | 13% | 16% |
| Chicken, 3 ounces | 56 | 10% | 13% |
| Fat-free milk, 1 cup | 37 | 7% | 9% |
| Beef, 3 ounces | 36 | 7% | 8% |
| Yogurt, 1 cup | 31 | 6% | 7% |
| Wheat germ, 2 tablespoons | 21 | 4% | 5% |
| Peanut butter, 2 tablespoons | 20 | 4% | 5% |
| Cottage cheese, ½ cup | 20 | 4% | 5% |

Key:
- Grains
- Vegetables
- Fruits
- Oils
- Milk
- Meat & Beans

**FIGURE 8-34** ▶ Food sources of choline compared to the Adequate Intake for adult males and females.

- Taurine, part of bile acids
- Lipoic acid, which participates in carbohydrate metabolism and acts as an antioxidant

These vitamin-like compounds can be synthesized by cells using common building blocks, such as amino acids and glucose. Our diets are also a source. In disease states or periods of active growth, synthesis of vitamin-like compounds may not meet needs, so dietary intake can be crucial. The needs for vitamin-like compounds in certain groups of individuals, such as for preterm infants, are being investigated. Although promoted and sold by health-food stores, these vitamin-like compounds need not be included in the diet of the average healthy adult.

Table 8-3 summarizes much of what we know about the water-soluble vitamins. Now that you have studied the vitamins, review MyPyramid and note how each food group can make an important vitamin contribution (Fig. 8-35).

Figure 8-36 summarizes much of what we have covered about the functions of the fat-soluble and water-soluble vitamins. Many vitamins work together for a common purpose.

**TABLE 8-3** Summary of the Water-Soluble Vitamins and Choline

| Vitamin | Major Functions | RDA or Adequate Intake | Dietary Sources* | Deficiency Symptoms | Toxicity Symptoms |
|---|---|---|---|---|---|
| Thiamin | • Coenzyme of carbohydrate metabolism<br>• Nerve function | 1.1–1.2 milligrams | • Sunflower seeds<br>• Pork<br>• Whole and enriched grains<br>• Dried beans<br>• Peas | *Beriberi*<br>• Nervous tingling<br>• Poor coordination<br>• Edema<br>• Heart changes<br>• Weakness | None |
| Riboflavin† | • Coenzyme of carbohydrate metabolism | 1.1–1.3 milligrams | • Milk<br>• Mushrooms<br>• Spinach<br>• Liver<br>• Enriched grains | • Inflammation of the mouth and tongue<br>• Cracks at the corners of the mouth<br>• Eye disorders | None |
| Niacin | • Coenzyme of energy metabolism<br>• Coenzyme of fat synthesis<br>• Coenzyme of fat breakdown | 14–16 milligrams (niacin equivalents) | • Mushrooms<br>• Bran<br>• Tuna<br>• Salmon<br>• Chicken<br>• Beef<br>• Liver<br>• Peanuts<br>• Enriched grains | *Pellagra*<br>• Diarrhea<br>• Dermatitis<br>• Dementia<br>• Death | Upper Level is 35 milligrams from supplements, based on flushing of skin |
| Pantothenic acid | • Coenzyme of energy metabolism<br>• Coenzyme of fat synthesis<br>• Coenzyme of fat breakdown | 5 milligrams | • Mushrooms<br>• Liver<br>• Broccoli<br>• Eggs<br><br>*Most foods have some* | • No natural deficiency disease or symptoms | None |
| Biotin | • Coenzyme of glucose production<br>• Coenzyme of fat synthesis | 30 micrograms | • Cheese<br>• Egg yolks<br>• Cauliflower<br>• Peanut butter<br>• Liver | • Dermatitis<br>• Tongue soreness<br>• Anemia<br>• Depression | Unknown |

| Vitamin | Major Functions | RDA or Adequate Intake | Dietary Sources* | Deficiency Symptoms | Toxicity Symptoms |
|---|---|---|---|---|---|
| Vitamin B-6[†] | • Coenzyme of protein metabolism<br>• Neurotransmitter synthesis<br>• Hemoglobin synthesis<br><br>*Many other functions* | 1.3–1.7 milligrams | • Animal protein foods<br>• Spinach<br>• Broccoli<br>• Bananas<br>• Salmon<br>• Sunflower seeds | • Headache<br>• Anemia<br>• Convulsions<br>• Nausea<br>• Vomiting<br>• Flaky skin<br>• Sore tongue | Upper Level is 100 milligrams, based on nerve destruction |
| Folate (folic acid)[†] | • Coenzyme involved in DNA synthesis<br><br>*Many other functions* | 400 micrograms (dietary folate equivalents) | • Green leafy vegetables<br>• Orange juice<br>• Organ meats<br>• Sprouts<br>• Sunflower seeds | • Megaloblastic anemia<br>• Inflammation of tongue<br>• Diarrhea<br>• Poor growth<br>• Depression | None likely<br><br>Upper Level for adults set at 1000 micrograms for synthetic folic acid (exclusive of food folate), based on masking of B-12 deficiency |
| Vitamin B-12[†] | • Coenzyme of folate metabolism<br>• Nerve function<br><br>*Many other functions* | 2.4 micrograms<br><br>*Older adults and vegans should use fortified foods or supplements.* | • Animal foods (not natural in plants)<br>• Organ meats<br>• Oysters<br>• Clams<br>• Fortified, ready-to-eat breakfast cereals | • Macrocytic anemia<br>• Poor nerve function | None |
| Vitamin C | • Connective tissue synthesis<br>• Hormone synthesis<br>• Neurotransmitter synthesis<br>• Possible antioxidant activity | 75–90 milligrams<br><br>*Smokers should add 35 milligrams* | • Citrus fruits<br>• Strawberries<br>• Broccoli<br>• Greens | • Scurvy<br>• Poor wound healing<br>• Pinpoint hemorrhages<br>• Bleeding gums | Upper Level is 2 grams, based on development of diarrhea<br><br>Can also alter some diagnostic tests |
| Choline[†] | • Neurotransmitter synthesis<br>• Phospholipid synthesis | 425–550 milligrams | Widely distributed in foods and synthesized by the body | No natural deficiency | Upper Level is 3.5 grams per day based on development of fishy body odor and reduced blood pressure |

*Fortified ready-to-eat breakfast cereals are good sources for most of these vitamins and a common source of B vitamins for many of us.

[†]These nutrients also participate in homocysteine metabolism, which in turn may reduce the risk of developing cardiovascular disease.

**FIGURE 8-35 ▶** Certain groups of MyPyramid are especially rich sources of various vitamins and choline. This is true for those listed. Each may be also found in other groups in the pyramid but in lower amounts. Pantothenic acid is also present in moderate amounts in many groups.

**MyPyramid: Sources of Vitamins and Choline**

| Grains | Vegetables | Fruits | Oils | Milk | Meat & Beans |
|--------|------------|--------|------|------|--------------|
| • Thiamin<br>• Riboflavin<br>• Niacin<br>• Folic acid | • Vitamin A<br>• Vitamin K<br>• Folate<br>• Vitamin C | • Vitamin A<br>• Vitamin C | • Vitamin E | • Vitamin D<br>• Riboflavin<br>• Vitamin B-12<br>• Choline | • Thiamin<br>• Riboflavin<br>• Niacin<br>• Biotin<br>• Vitamin B-6<br>• Vitamin B-12<br>• Choline |

**FIGURE 8-36 ▶** Vitamins and related compounds (e.g., choline) work together to maintain health.

Vitamin B-6
Vitamin B-12
Folate
Vitamin K

**Blood formation (and clotting)**

Thiamin
Riboflavin
Niacin
Pantothenic acid
Biotin
Vitamin B-12

**Energy metabolism**

Vitamin B-6
Folate
Vitamin B-12
Vitamin C
Choline (not a true vitamin)
Riboflavin (indirect)

**Protein and amino acid metabolism**

Vitamin A
Vitamin D
Vitamin K
Vitamin C

**Bone health**

Vitamin A
Vitamin D

**Gene expression**

Vitamin E
Vitamin C (likely)
Carotenoids
Riboflavin (indirect)

**Antioxidant defenses**

# Dietary Supplements—Who Needs Them?

The term *multivitamin and mineral supplement* has been mentioned many times so far in this textbook. Often, these and other supplements are marketed as cures for anything and everything. This cure-all approach is promoted by the supplement industry and countless health-food stores, pharmacies, and supermarkets.

According to the Dietary Supplement Health and Education Act of 1994 (discussed in Chapter 1), a supplement in the United States is a product intended to supplement the diet that bears or contains one or more of the following ingredients:

- A vitamin
- A mineral
- An herb or another botanical
- An amino acid
- A dietary substance to supplement the diet, which could be an extract or a combination of the first four ingredients in this list

The definition is broad and covers a wide variety of nutritional substances. The use of dietary supplements is a common practice among North Americans and generates about $24-25 billion annually for the industry in the United States (Fig. 8-37). Supplements can be sold without proof that they are safe and effective. Unless FDA has evidence that a supplement is inherently dangerous or marketed with an illegal claim, it will not regulate such products closely. (The vitamin folate is an exception.) FDA has limited resources to police supplement manufacturers and has to act against these manufacturers one at a time. Thus, we cannot rely on FDA to protect us from vitamin and mineral supplement overuse and misuse. We bear that responsibility ourselves, with the help of professional advice from a physician or registered dietitian.

The supplement makers can make broad claims about their products under the "structure or function" provision of the law. The products, however, cannot claim to prevent, treat, or cure a disease. Menopause in women and aging are not diseases *per se*, so products alleging to treat symptoms of these conditions can be marketed without FDA approval. For example, a product that claims to treat hot flashes arising during menopause can be sold without any evidence to prove that the product works, but a product that claims to decrease the risk of cardiovascular disease by reducing blood cholesterol must have results from scientific studies that justify the claim.

Why do people take supplements? Frequently given reasons include to:

- Reduce susceptibility to health problems (e.g., colds)
- Prevent heart attacks
- Prevent cancer
- Reduce stress
- Increase "energy"

## Should You Take a Supplement?

The choice to take a supplement is up to you. Opinions vary about the wisdom and safety of supplement use even among knowledgeable scientists. Typically, nutrition scientists have recommended that supplement use is needed only by a few groups. The National Institutes of

**FIGURE 8-37** ▶ The dietary supplement industry is a growing multibillion dollar business.

**Supplement Sales: 1994-2008**

Health State-of-the-Science Conference came to the same conclusion, noting there is insufficient evidence to support the recommendation of use of a multivitamin and mineral supplement by the general population. The experts found that only a few studies of vitamins and minerals demonstrate beneficial effects for the prevention of chronic disease, including increased bone mineral density and decreased fractures in postmenopausal women who use calcium and vitamin D supplements. (See the next section in this feature for more specific examples.) In contrast, several other studies provide disturbing evidence of risk, such as increased lung cancer risk with beta-carotene use among smokers. The NIH report concludes that the present evidence is insufficient to recommend either for or against the use of multivitamin/mineral supplements by Americans to prevent chronic disease.

The rationale for widespread use of a multivitamin and mineral supplement is primarily because many North Americans have been unwilling to change their food habits to include the recommended servings of fruits, vegetables, and whole grains. As for individual vitamins, there are specific cases in which supplements are advised. As discussed in Chapter 8, adequate folate status when a woman becomes pregnant helps reduce the risk of certain birth defects in her offspring (400 micrograms per day of synthetic folic acid is recommended). Folate also limits homocysteine in the blood, a likely risk factor for cardiovascular disease that can affect all of us. In addition, the committee appointed by the Food and Nutrition Board that set current nutrient standards for vitamin B-12 suggested that adults over age 50 consume vitamin B-12 in a synthetic form, such as that added to ready-to-eat breakfast cereals or present in supplements. Synthetic vitamin B-12 is more easily absorbed than that found in food; this helps compensate for the fall in vitamin B-12 absorption often seen in one's older years.

Whether experts support use of a multivitamin and mineral supplement or not, they all emphasize that many of the health-promoting effects of foods cannot be found in a bottle. Recall the discussions of phytochemicals in Chapter 2 and

the benefits of fiber in Chapter 4. Few or no phytochemicals and no fiber are present in supplements. Multivitamin and mineral supplements also contain little calcium to keep the pill size small, and the oxide forms of magnesium, zinc, and copper used in many supplements are not as well absorbed as forms found in foods.

Overall, supplement use cannot fix a poor diet in all respects. Uninformed megadose supplement use also can lead to harm—most cases of nutrient toxicity are a result of supplement use. Thus, we are advised to first take a good look at our dietary habits and then improve them, as outlined in Chapter 2 (Fig. 8-38). Then we should find out which nutrient gaps remain, and identify food sources that can help. Such a source could be ready-to-eat breakfast cereals to increase vitamin E, folic acid, and vitamin B-6 intake, and as well provide highly absorbable forms of vitamin B-12. Calcium-fortified orange juice could be used to increase calcium intake, or milk and yogurt to increase vitamin D and calcium intake. You need to be careful of highly fortified foods, however, as these products may provide the appropriate amount of nutrients in 1 serving, but the typical consumer may eat more than 1 serving. This can lead to an excessive intake of some nutrients, such as vitamin A, iron, and synthetic folic acid.

If supplement use is desired, you should discuss this practice with a physician or registered dietitian, as some supplements can interfere with certain medicines. For example, high intakes of vitamin K or vitamin E alter the action of anticlotting medications. Vitamin B-6 can offset the action of L-dopa (used in treating Parkinson's disease). Large doses of vitamin C can interfere with certain cancer therapy regimens, excessive zinc intake can inhibit copper absorption. Large amounts of folate can mask signs and symptoms of a vitamin B-12 deficiency (review the section on toxicity of folate in this chapter). Remember, you *can* get too much of a good thing.

## People Most Likely to Need Supplements

As you might guess, generally the people who take supplements in our society

▲ The USP (United States Pharmacopeia) label indicates the product meets USP standards.

▶ Because research on a variety of nutrient supplements has revealed a lack of product quality, FDA now requires supplement makers to test the purity, strength, and composition of all their products. The USP (United States Pharmacopeia) designation, which has been extended to an increasing number of nutrient supplements, establishes professionally-accepted standards for these products and can be used to evaluate supplements. The USP standards designate strength, quality, purity, packaging, labeling, speed of dissolution, and acceptable length of storage of ingredients for drugs.

Top Ten Dietary Supplements in 2008

1. Multivitamins
2. Sports Nutrition Supplements
3. Calcium
4. B vitamins
5. Vitamin C
6. Glucosamine and Chondroitin
7. Homeopathic Medicines
8. Vitamin D
9. Fish/animal Oil
10. Coenzyme Q

*Source: Nutrition Business Journal*

▲ Focus first on foods that meet nutrient needs.

▲ Long-term intake of just three times the Daily Value for some fat-soluble vitamins—particularly preformed vitamin A—can cause toxic effects. Know what you are taking if you use supplements.

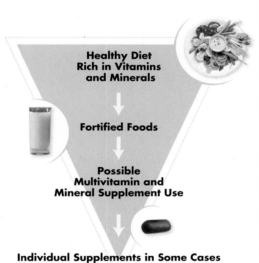

**Healthy Diet Rich in Vitamins and Minerals**

↓

**Fortified Foods**

↓

**Possible Multivitamin and Mineral Supplement Use**

↓

**Individual Supplements in Some Cases**

**FIGURE 8-38** ▶ Supplement savvy—an approach to the use of nutrient supplementation. Emphasizing a healthy diet rich in vitamins and minerals is always the first option.

## Critical Thinking

Believing that supplements provide the nutrition her body needs, Janice regularly takes numerous supplements while paying relatively little attention to daily food choices. How would you explain to her that this practice may lead to health problems?

are already healthy. Various medical and health-related organizations suggest that the following vitamin and mineral supplements can be important for certain groups of healthy people:

- Women of childbearing age may need extra synthetic folic acid if their dietary patterns do not supply the recommended amount (400 micrograms).
- Women with excessive bleeding during menstruation may need extra iron.
- Women who are pregnant or breast-feeding may need extra iron, folate, and calcium.
- People with low calorie intakes (less than about 1200 kcal per day) may need a range of vitamins and minerals. This is true of some women and many older people.
- Strict vegans may need extra calcium, iron, zinc, and vitamin B-12.
- Newborns need a single dose of vitamin K, as directed by a physician.
- Some older infants may need fluoride supplements, as directed by a dentist.
- People with limited milk intake and sunlight exposure may need extra vitamin D. This includes breastfed infants and many African-American and older people.
- People with lactose maldigestion or lactose intolerance, and those with allergies to dairy products, may need extra calcium.
- Adults over age 50 may need a synthetic source of vitamin B-12.
- People on low-fat diets or diets low in plant oils and nuts may need some extra vitamin E.
- People who consume a large part of their diet as refined foods rather than as fruits, vegetables, or whole grains may need a range of vitamins and minerals.

Individuals with certain medical conditions (e.g., vitamin-resistant diseases or longstanding fat malabsorption) and those who use certain medications also may require supplementation with specific vitamins and minerals. Children who are "picky eaters" may require supplementation as well (see Chapter 15). Finally, smokers and alcohol abusers may benefit from supplementation, but cessation of these two activities is far more beneficial than any supplementation.

## Which Supplement Should You Choose?

If you decide to take a multivitamin and mineral supplement, which one should you choose? As a start, choose a nationally recognized brand (from a supermarket or pharmacy) that contains about 100% of the Daily Values for the nutrients present. A multivitamin and mineral supplement should generally be taken with or just after meals to maximize absorption. Make sure also that intake from the total of this supplement, any other supplements used, and highly fortified foods (such as ready-to-eat breakfast cereals) provide no more than the Upper Level for each vitamin and mineral. (See the inside cover of this text book for Upper Levels.) This is especially important with regard to preformed vitamin A intake. Two exceptions are (1) both men and older women should make sure any product used is low in iron or iron-free to avoid possible iron overload (see Chapter 9 for details), and (2) somewhat exceeding the Upper Level for vitamin D is likely a safe practice for adults. One should read the labels carefully to be sure of what is being taken (Fig. 8-39).

Another consideration in choosing a supplement is avoiding superfluous ingredients, such as para-aminobenzoic acid (PABA), hesperidin complex, inositol, bee pollen, and lecithins. These are not needed in our diets. They are especially common in expensive supplements sold in health-food stores and by mail. In addition, use of l-tryptophan and high doses of beta-carotene or fish oils is discouraged.

Five websites to help you evaluate ongoing claims and evaluate safety of supplements are:

www.acsh.org
www.quackwatch.com
www.ncahf.org
dietary-supplements.info.nih.gov
www.eatright.org
www.usp.org/USPVerified/dietarySupplements/

These sites are maintained by groups or individuals committed to providing reasoned and authoritative nutrition and health advice to consumers.

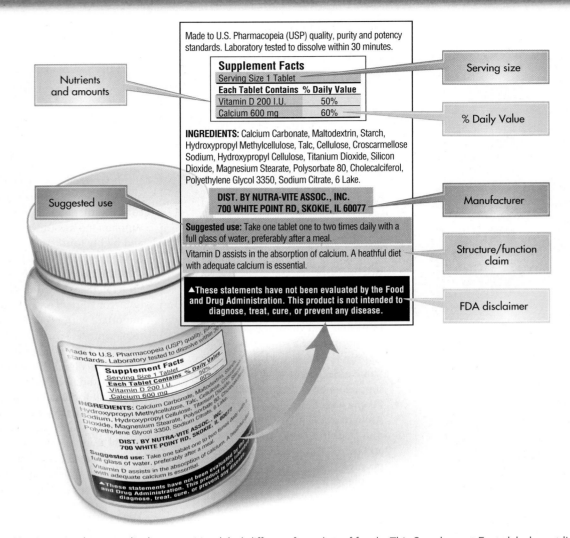

| Nutrients and amounts | | Serving size |
| % Daily Value | | Manufacturer |
| Suggested use | | Structure/function claim |
| | | FDA disclaimer |

Made to U.S. Pharmacopeia (USP) quality, purity and potency standards. Laboratory tested to dissolve within 30 minutes.

**Supplement Facts**
Serving Size 1 Tablet

| **Each Tablet Contains** | **% Daily Value** |
| Vitamin D 200 I.U. | 50% |
| Calcium 600 mg | 60% |

**INGREDIENTS:** Calcium Carbonate, Maltodextrin, Starch, Hydroxypropyl Methylcellulose, Talc, Cellulose, Croscarmellose Sodium, Hydroxypropyl Cellulose, Titanium Dioxide, Silicon Dioxide, Magnesium Stearate, Polysorbate 80, Cholecalciferol, Polyethylene Glycol 3350, Sodium Citrate, 6 Lake.

**DIST. BY NUTRA-VITE ASSOC., INC.
700 WHITE POINT RD, SKOKIE, IL 60077**

**Suggested use:** Take one tablet one to two times daily with a full glass of water, preferably after a meal.

Vitamin D assists in the absorption of calcium. A heathful diet with adequate calcium is essential.

▲These statements have not been evaluated by the Food and Drug Administration. This product is not intended to diagnose, treat, cure, or prevent any disease.

**FIGURE 8-39** ► Nutrient supplements display a nutrition label different from that of foods. This Supplement Facts label must list the ingredient(s), amount(s) per serving, serving size, suggested use, and % Daily Value if one has been established. This label also includes structure/function claims. Thus, it also must include the FDA warning that these claims have not been evaluated by the agency.

► The regular use of individual nutrient supplements could lead to health risks. These should be used with caution.

## Case Study Choosing a Dietary Supplement

Amy works the "pre-dawn" shift as a baker at a popular bistro. Amy is also a full-time student, and the combination of taking a full course load at college and working early hours while her friends are sleeping has created a lot of stress for her. Amy's many commitments also make it important that she not become ill. Recently one of her co-workers suggested that she take *Nutramega* supplements to help prevent colds, flu, and other illnesses. The product's label suggests that *Nutramega* helps prevent such problems, especially those associated with the changing of seasons. The label recommends taking two to three tablets daily for health maintenance and two to three tablets every 3 hours at the first sign of feeling ill. Amy looks at the Supplement Facts label on the bottle and finds that each tablet contains (as percent of the Daily Value): 33% for vitamin A (three-quarters is preformed vitamin A), 700% for vitamin C, 200% for niacin, and 100% for vitamin B-6. A month's supply costs about $50.

Answer the following questions, and check your response in Appendix A.

1. Are there any health risks associated with taking the "maintenance" dose of two to three tablets per day? How does this dose compare with the Upper Tolerable Intake Levels for the four nutrients?

2. How many tablets would be taken per day if Amy was feeling ill?
   a. For vitamin A, use the % Daily Value to calculate the micrograms RAE that would be in this larger dose. How does this compare to the Upper Level for Vitamin A?
   b. Use the % Daily Value to calculate the milligrams of vitamin C in this larger dose. How does this compare to the Upper Level for vitamin C?
   c. Use the % Daily Value to calculate the milligrams of niacin in this larger dose. How does this compare to the Upper Level for niacin?
   d. Use the % Daily Value to calculate the micrograms of vitamin B-6 in this larger dose. How does this compare to the Upper Level for vitamin B-6?
   e. Does the recommended dosage of any of these nutrients pose any health risks?

3. Does the cost of this supplement seem reasonable? How does it compare to the

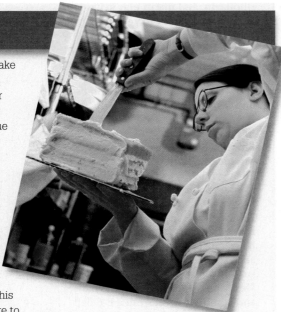

▲ Is a dietary supplement a safe way for Amy to prevent colds and the flu?

cost of a typical multivitamin supplement available at your local drug store?

4. Should Amy be concerned about meeting her nutrient needs? Does the type of stress she is under increase her nutrient needs?

5. After studying Chapter 8, what diet and supplement advice would you offer to Amy?

## Summary

1. Vitamins are carbon-containing compounds we generally need daily in small amounts from foods. They yield no energy directly, but many contribute to energy-yielding chemical reactions in the body and promote growth and development. Many vitamins act as coenzymes, which help enzymes function.

2. Vitamins A, D, E, and K are fat soluble, whereas the B vitamins, vitamin C and choline are water soluble.

3. Vitamin A is a family of compounds that includes several forms of preformed vitamin A. Three forms of carotenoids can also yield vitamin A; some also function as antioxidants. Vitamin A contributes to vision, immune function, and cell development. Vitamin D is both a hormone and a vitamin. It can be synthesized in the human body using sunshine and a cholesterol-like substance in the skin. The active hormone form of vitamin D helps regulate blood calcium in part by increasing calcium absorption from the intestine. Infants and children who don't get enough vitamin D may develop rickets, and adults develop osteomalacia. Vitamin E functions primarily as an antioxidant. By donating electrons to electron-seeking, free-radical (oxidizing) compounds, it neutralizes them. This effect shields cell membranes and red blood cells from breakdown. Vitamin K helps blood clot and increases the calcium-binding potential of some organs. Vitamin K is poorly stored in the body, but our dietary intake alone is usually sufficient to meet needs. People who can't absorb fat well or who are on antibiotics for long periods may need extra vitamin K. Thiamin,

riboflavin, and niacin play key roles as coenzymes in energy-yielding reactions. They help metabolize carbohydrates, fats, and proteins. Alcoholism and a poor diet can create deficiencies of these three nutrients, which often show up as symptoms in the brain and nervous system, skin, and GI tract. Pantothenic acid, which participates in many aspects of cell metabolism. Biotin, which participates in glucose production, fatty acid synthesis, and DNA synthesis, can be synthesized by bacteria in the intestine. Vitamin B-6 performs a vital role in protein metabolism, especially in synthesizing nonessential amino acids. It also helps synthesize neurotransmitters and performs other metabolic roles, such as metabolism of homocysteine. Headaches, a form of anemia, nausea, and vomiting result from a B-6 deficiency. Folate plays an important role in DNA synthesis and homocysteine metabolism. Symptoms of a deficiency include generally poor cell division in various areas of the body, megaloblastic anemia, tongue inflammation, diarrhea, and poor growth. Pregnancy puts high demands for folate on the body; deficiency during the first month of pregnancy can result in neural tube defects in offspring. A deficiency can also occur in people with alcoholism. Vitamin B-12 is needed to metabolize folate and homocysteine, and maintain the insulation surrounding nerves. A deficiency results in anemia (because of its relationship to folate) and nerve degeneration. Older people often suffer from inefficient absorption of vitamin B-12, in which case they can benefit from monthly injections or megadoses of the vitamin. Vitamin C is mainly used to synthesize collagen, a major protein for building connective tissue. A vitamin C deficiency results in scurvy, evidenced by poor wound healing, pinpoint hemorrhages in the skin, and bleeding gums. Vitamin C also modestly enhances iron absorption, is likely a general antioxidant,

and is needed for synthesizing some hormones and neurotransmitters. Deficiencies can occur in people with alcoholism and those whose diets lack sufficient fruits and vegetables. Smoking makes matters worse for people already at risk. Choline is used to form a neurotransmitter, and has other functions, including a role in homocysteine metabolism. Nutritional needs have recently been set. No natural deficiency of choline has been reported. The vitamin-like compounds carnitine, inositol, taurine, and lipoic acid, while participating in many important chemical reactions in the body, are not true vitamins because they can be synthesized in the body from readily available building blocks; they are also obtained from the diet.

4. Vitamin A is found in liver and fish oils; carotenoids are especially plentiful in dark green and orange vegetables. If we don't spend enough time in the sun, such foods as fish and fortified milk can supply vitamin D. Older people, African-Americans, and breast-fed infants often need a supplemental source. Vitamin E is found in plant oils. Claims are made about the curative powers of vitamin E, but more information is needed before megadose vitamin E recommendations for healthy adults can be made with certainty. Some vitamin K absorbed each day comes from bacterial synthesis in the intestine, but most comes from foods, primarily green, leafy vegetables. Enriched grain products are common sources of thiamin, riboflavin, and niacin. Pantothenic acid is widely distributed among foods. Biotin comes from foods such as eggs, peanuts, and cheese. Regular consumption of animal protein foods and rich plant sources such as broccoli provide needed vitamin B-6. Food sources of folate are leafy vegetables, organ meats, and orange juice. Women of child-bearing age need to meet the RDA with synthetic folic acid. Great amounts of folate can be lost in prolonged cooking. Generally, a dietary

deficiency is unlikely because vitamin B-12 is highly concentrated in animal foods, which constitute a major part of the North American diet. Vitamin B-12 does not occur naturally in plant foods. Vegans need a supplemental source, and adults over age 50 should consume a synthetic source, such as that in ready-to-eat breakfast cereals. Fresh fruits and vegetables, especially citrus fruits, are generally good sources. A great amount of vitamin C is lost in cooking, so a diet should emphasize fresh or lightly cooked vegetables. Choline is a dietary component available from a wide variety of foods and is synthesized in the body.

5. Vitamin A can be toxic, even when taken at just 3 times the RDA for preformed vitamin A (the Upper Level). High vitamin A intakes are especially dangerous during pregnancy. Vitamin D is potentially a toxic substance in infancy and early childhood. The Upper Level for vitamin E is set at about 50 times adult needs. Niacin has an Upper Level (2.5 times adult needs). Taking high doses of Vitamin B-6 causes damage to the nervous system. The Upper Level is about 60 times adult needs. Excess folate in the diet can mask a vitamin B-12 deficiency, so an Upper Level has been set at 2½ times adult needs (refers to synthetic folic acid only). The Upper Level of vitamin is set at about 20 times adult needs. The Upper Level of choline is set at about 8 times adult needs.

6. Taking a multivitamin and mineral supplement to help meet nutrient needs is recommended by some experts, while other experts suggest that only some in the population need such supplementation. Taking many nutrient supplements can lead to nutrient-related toxicity, so any such use should be carefully considered. The clearest evidence is for a diet rich in fruits and vegetables and whole-grain breads and cereals, not reliance on supplements.

## Study Questions

1. Why is the risk of toxicity greater with the fat-soluble vitamins A and D than with water-soluble vitamins in general?

2. How would you determine which fruits and vegetables displayed in the produce section of your supermarket are likely to provide plenty of carotenoids?

3. What is the primary function of the vitamin D hormone? Which groups of people likely need to supplement their diets with vitamin D, and on what do you base your answer?

4. Describe how vitamin E functions as an antioxidant. Use the term *free radical*.

5. Describe how the RDA, Daily Value, and Upper Level for vitamin B-6 should be used in everyday life. How do the RDA and Daily Value for vitamin B-6 differ?

6. The need for certain vitamins increases as energy expenditure increases. Name two such vitamins and explain why this is the case.

7. Take one of the B vitamins that might be low in the North American diet and explain why a deficiency might occur.

8. Which vitamins are lost from cereal grains as a result of the "refining" process? Which vitamins must be replaced by law in the subsequent enrichment process?

9. Why does FDA limit the amount of folate that may be included in supplements and fortified foods?

10. Is it necessary for North Americans to consume a great excess of vitamin C to avoid the possibility of a deficiency? Do vitamin C intakes well above the RDA have any negative consequences?

## Check Your Knowledge

Answers to the following multiple choice questions are below.

1. Vitamins are classified as
   a. organic and inorganic.
   b. fat-soluble and water-soluble.
   c. essential and nonessential.
   d. elements and compounds.

2. Vitamin D is called the sunshine vitamin because
   a. it is available in orange juice.
   b. exposure to sunlight converts a precursor to vitamin D.
   c. it can be destroyed by exposure to sunlight.
   d. All of the above.

3. Vitamin E functions as
   a. a coenzyme.
   b. an antioxidant.
   c. a hormone.
   d. a peroxide.

4. A deficiency of vitamin A can lead to the disease called
   a. xerophthalmia.
   b. osteomalacia.
   c. scurvy.
   d. pellagra.

5. A high intake of vitamin E can
   a. inhibit vitamin K metabolism.
   b. lead to lead poisoning.
   c. inhibit copper absorption.
   d. cause baldness.

6. A vitamin synthesized by bacteria in the intestine is
   a. A.
   b. D.
   c. E.
   d. K.

7. Bowed legs, an enlarged and misshapen head, and enlarged knee joints in children are all symptoms of
   a. rickets.
   b. xerophthalmia.
   c. osteoporosis.
   d. vitamin D toxicity.

8. Thiamin, riboflavin, and niacin are called the "energy" vitamins because they
   a. can be broken down to provide energy.
   b. are coenzymes needed for release of energy from carbohydrates, fats, and proteins.
   c. are ingredients in energy drinks such as Powerade.
   d. are needed in large amounts by competitive athletes.

9. A deficient intake of _____ has been shown to increase the risk of having a baby with a neural tube defect such as spina bifida.
   a. vitamin A
   b. vitamin C
   c. vitamin E
   d. folic acid

10. Vitamin C is necessary for the production of
   a. stomach acid.
   b. collagen.
   c. hormones.
   d. clotting factors.

Answers: 1.b, 2.b, 3.b, 4.a, 5.a, 6.d, 7.a, 8.b, 9.d, 10.b

## Further Readings

1. ADA Reports: Position of the American Dietetic Association: Fortification and nutritional supplements. *Journal of the American Dietetic Association* 105:1300, 2005.

   *The best nutritional strategy for promoting optimal health and reducing the risk of chronic disease is to wisely choose a wide variety of foods. Additional vitamins and minerals from fortified foods and/or supplements can help some people meet their nutritional needs as set by science-based nutrition standards (e.g., the Dietary Reference Intakes).*

2. Andres E and others: Food-cobalamin malabsorption in elderly patients: Clinical manifestations and treatments. *American Journal of Medicine* 118:1154, 2005.

   *About 15% of older adults show defective vitamin B-12 absorption. This condition especially affects absorption of the vitamin B-12 found naturally in foods. Consumption of crystalline vitamin B-12 in contrast is not so affected and was found to be a useful form of therapy for the older adults in this study.*

3. Bleys J and others: Vitamin-mineral supplementation and the progression of atherosclerosis: A meta-analysis of randomized controlled trails. *American Journal of Clinical Nutrition* 84(4):880, 2006.

   *The results of previous studies suggest that antioxidant and B vitamin supplementation may prevent atherosclerosis. This meta-analysis showed no evidence of a protective effect of antioxidant or B vitamin supplements on the progression of atherosclerosis as measured by imaging techniques. These results provide an explanation for the lack of effect of these supplements on clinical cardiovascular events.*

4. DeWals P and others: Reduction in neural-tube defects after folic acid fortification in Canada. *New England Journal of Medicine* 357;135, 2007.

   *Changes in the prevalence of neural-tube defects were assessed in Canada before and after food fortification of cereal products with folic acid became mandatory in 1998. A 46% reduction in the prevalence of neural-tube defects occurred during the full-fortification period, with a decrease from 1.58 per 1000 births before fortification to 0.86 per 1000 births after fortification. The reduction rate was greater for spina bifida (a decrease of 53%) than for anencephaly and encephalocele (decreases of 38% and 31%, respectively).*

5. Food and Nutrition Board, Institute of Medicine: *Dietary Reference Intakes for thiamin, riboflavin, niacin, vitamin B-6, folate, vitamin B-12, pantothenic acid, biotin, and choline.* Washington, DC: National Academies Press, 1998.

   *This work outlines how nutrient recommendations were established for the B vitamins and choline, with specific reference to establishing the RDA and related standards. The functions of each of the B vitamins and choline are explained.*

6. Food and Nutrition Board, Institute of Medicine: *Dietary Reference Intakes for vitamin A, vitamin K, arsenic, boron, chromium, copper, iodine, iron, manganese, molybdenum, nickel, silicon, vanadium, and zinc.* Washington, DC: National Academies Press, 2001.

   *Recommendations for vitamin A and vitamin K intake are listed. The rationale used to set the RDA or Adequate Intake and Upper Level for these nutrients is discussed in detail.*

7. Food and Nutrition Board, Institute of Medicine: *Dietary Reference Intakes for vitamin C, vitamin E, selenium, and carotenoids.* Washington, DC: National Academies Press, 2000.

   *The functions of antioxidant nutrients, how RDA and related standards were determined, and deficiency and toxicity symptoms are explained. This is the definitive report by the panel of experts on nutrient needs for dietary antioxidants.*

8. Food and Nutrition Board, Institute of Medicine: *Dietary Reference Intakes for calcium, phosphorus, magnesium, vitamin D, and fluoride.* Washington, DC: National Academies Press, 1997.

   *The RDAs and related standards for vitamin D and some minerals are discussed in detail. A major change in setting these new (and all other) estimates of human needs is the use of a specific biological marker or estimate of current intakes that shows adequacy.*

9. Garland CF and others: Vitamin D and prevention of breast cancer: Pooled analysis. *Journal of Steroid Biochemistry & Molecular Biology* 103:708, 2007.

   *This review of all studies reported risk of breast cancer and assessed the dose—response association between serum 25(OH)D and risk of breast cancer. The conclusion of this review is that daily intake of 2000 IU of Vitamin D3, and, when possible, very moderate exposure to*

   *sunlight, could raise serum 25(OH)D to 52 ng/ml, a level associated with reduction by 50% in incidence of breast cancer, according to observational studies.*

10. Giovannucci E and others: 25-Hydroxyvitamin D and risk of myocardial infarction in men: A prospective study. *Archives Internal Medicine* 168:1174, 2008.

    *Vitamin D deficiency is thought to be involved in the development of atherosclerosis and coronary heart disease in humans. This study found men 40 to 75 years of age with vitamin D levels below normal had a higher risk of heart attack even after controlling for factors known to be associated with coronary artery disease. Even men with intermediate vitamin D levels were at elevated risk of heart disease relative to those with sufficient vitamin D levels.*

11. Gordon CM and others: Prevalence of vitamin D deficiency among healthy infants and toddlers. Archives of Pediatric and Adolescent Medicine 162:505, 2008.

    *The prevalence of vitamin D deficiency was determined and 25-hydroxyvitamin D concentration was examined as a function of skin pigmentation, season, sun exposure, breastfeeding, and vitamin D supplementation. Suboptimal vitamin D status was common among otherwise healthy young children with 40% of infants and toddlers testing below average for vitamin D. One-third of the vitamin D–deficient infant and toddlers exhibited demineralization a hallmark of the deleterious skeletal effects of this condition.*

12. Holick MF: Vitamin D deficiency. *New England Journal of Medicine* 357:266, 2007.

    *This is a review of numerous studies that have shown that vitamin D does more than just enhance bone health in children and adults. Studies show that vitamin D deficiency in adults has been linked to an increased risk for osteoporosis and osteomalacia but also certain cancers.*

13. Lee I and others: Vitamin E in the primary prevention of cardiovascular disease and cancer: The women's health study: A randomized controlled trial. *Journal of the American Medical Association* 294:56, 2005.

    *The data from this large trial indicated that 600 IU of natural-source vitamin E taken every other day provided no overall benefit for major cardiovascular events or cancer. These data do not support recommending vitamin E supplementation for cardiovascular disease or cancer prevention among healthy women, but* more research is warranted, because a decrease in sudden cardiac death was seen in a subset of older women in this study.

14. Lichtenstein AH and Russell RM: Essential nutrients: Food or supplements? Where should the emphasis be? *Journal of the American Medical Association* 294:351, 2005.

    *There is insufficient evidence to justify a shift in public health policy from one that emphasizes a food-based diet to fulfill nutrient requirements and promote optimal health to one that emphasizes dietary supplementation. Targeted nutrient supplementation is appropriate in some cases, however, as reviewed by these authors.*

15. McCormick DB: The dubious use of vitamin-mineral supplements in relation to cardiovascular disease. *American Journal of Clinical Nutrition* 84(4):680, 2006.

    *This editorial supports the finding of recent studies, including the meta-analysis by Bleys and others that antioxidants and B vitamins should not be used to prevent cardiovascular disease. The author hopes that these recent findings, "which carefully separate fact from faith," will decrease the extensive use of vitamin-mineral supplements.*

16. Nield LS and others: Rickets: Not a disease of the past. *American Family Physician* 74(4), 200:619, 2006.

    *This review article emphasizes the current need to screen for rickets even in developed countries. Background and support is given for the recent recommendation by the American Academy of Pediatrics (AAP) to provide a daily vitamin D supplement for all solely breastfed babies beginning in the first two months of life. Until recently, vitamin D supplementation was not advised for breastfed infants. Multiple case reports of nutritional rickets in the United States have promoted the AAP recommendation.*

17. Sesso HD and others: Vitamins E and C in the prevention of cardiovascular disease in men. The Physicians' Health Study II Randomized Controlled Trial. *Journal of American Medical Association* 300:2123, 2008.

    *Men enrolled in the Physician's Health Study II were placed into four groups, which were given vitamin C and a placebo, vitamin E and a placebo, C and E together, and placebo only. Neither C nor E had an effect on major cardiovascular events, which include heart attacks, stroke, or death. The results suggest that when you pull a nutrient out of the whole diet, you don't see the same effects.*

18. Voutilainen S and others: Carotenoids and cardiovascular health. *American Journal of Clinical Nutrition* 83:1265, 2006.

    *This report reviews the role of carotenoids in the prevention of heart disease. Although fruit and vegetables are recognized as having protective effects against cardiovascular disease, the role of a single group of compounds such as carotenoids cannot be ascertained. Therefore, the consumption of carotenoids in supplemental forms cannot be recommended.*

19. Wang TJ and others: Vitamin D deficiency and risk of cardiovascular disease. *Circulation* 117:503, 2008.

    *This study was conducted over five years and examined the vitamin D levels in the blood of 1,739 people with an average age of 59 years and no prior history of cardiovascular disease. Individuals with low vitamin D levels had a 60% greater risk of cardiac events such as heart attacks and stroke. For people with both a vitamin D deficiency and high blood pressure, the risk for a serious cardiovascular event was doubled. These results are of concern because vitamin D is becoming more common, especially in people living at higher latitudes where vitamin D is less available from exposure to sunlight.*

20. Zhang SM and others: Effect of combined folic acid, vitamin B-6, and vitamin B-12 on cancer risk in women: A randomized trial. *Journal of the American Medical Association* 300(17):2012, 2008.

    *Use of a combined supplement of folic acid, vitamin B-6, and vitamin B-12 had no significant effect on overall risk of total invasive cancer or breast cancer in a seven-year study of 5,442 women. This was the longest-running trial of its kind and occurred at the time that background fortification of the food supply with folic acid had begun.*

# RATE YOUR PLATE

## I. Spotting Fraudulent Claims on the Internet

Search for vitamins and vitamin-like substances sold over the Internet. Then write a report concerning any claims made on behalf of these products that you consider fraudulent or misleading. Are the websites selling vitamins, or are they a cover for selling something else? Compare the price of the vitamins from these sites with the price you would pay at the local supermarket or drugstore. Do any of these sites display any disclaimers or warnings about the products?

## II. A Closer Look at Supplement Use

With the current popularity of vitamin and mineral supplements, it is more important than ever to understand how to evaluate a supplement. Study the label of a supplement you use or one readily available from a friend or the supermarket. Then answer the following questions.

1. What is the recommended dosage of this supplement?

   _____

   _____

2. Based on the recommended dosage, are there any individual vitamins for which the intake would be greater than 100% of the Daily Value? List these vitamins.

   _____

   _____

3. Are any suggested intakes above the Upper Level for the nutrient?

   _____

   _____

4. Are there any superfluous ingredients, such as herbs or flavors, in the supplement? You can often determine these by looking for ingredients that do not have a percent of Daily Value.

   _____

   _____

5. Does at least 50% of the vitamin A in the product come from beta-carotene or other provitamin A carotenoids (to reduce risk of preformed vitamin A toxicity)?

   _____

   _____

   _____

6. Are there any warnings on the label as to populations who should not consume this product?

   _____

   _____

7. Are there any other signs that tip you off that this product may not be safe?

   _____

   _____

# CHAPTER 9 Water and Minerals

## Student Learning Outcomes   After studying Chapter 9 you will be able to:

1. List and briefly explain the functions of water in the body.
2. Discuss healthy water intake and output levels to maintain water balance.
3. List safety concerns about our water supply.
4. Classify the minerals as major or trace minerals.

5. List conditions of the body, dietary factors, and other pertinent relationships that influence the absorption, retention, and availability of specific minerals.
6. List key functions and at least two food sources of the major and trace minerals. Identify possible deficiency and toxicity

symptoms associated with the major and trace minerals.
7. Explain the role of nutrition in maintaining a healthy blood pressure.
8. Describe the processes involving minerals that aid in maintaining bone health and preventing osteoporosis.

## Chapter Outline

Student Learning Outcomes
Refresh Your Memory
9.1 Water
9.2 Minerals—An Overview
9.3 Major Minerals
9.4 Sodium (Na)
9.5 Potassium (K)
9.6 Chloride (Cl)
9.7 Calcium (Ca)
9.8 Phosphorus (P)

9. 9 Magnesium (Mg)
9.10 Sulfur (S)
9.11 Trace Minerals—An Overview
9.12 Iron (Fe)
9.13 Zinc (Zn)
9.14 Selenium (Se)
9.15 Iodide (I)
9.16 Copper (Cu)
9.17 Fluoride (F)
9.18 Chromium (Cr)

9.19 Manganese (Mn)
9.20 Molybdenum (Mo)
9.21 Other Trace Minerals
Nutrition and Your Health: *Maintaining a Healthy Blood Pressure*
Nutrition and Your Health: *Preventing Osteoporosis*
Case Study: Giving Up Milk
Summary/Study Questions/Check Your Knowledge/Further Readings
Rate Your Plate

WATER—THE MOST VERSATILE MEDIUM FOR A VARIETY OF CHEMICAL REACTIONS— CONSTITUTES THE MAJOR PORTION OF THE HUMAN BODY. Without water, biological processes necessary to life would cease in a matter of days. We must replenish water regularly, as the comic in the chapter suggests, because the body does not store it *per se*. We recognize this constant demand for water as thirst. Recent beverage guidelines recommend a water intake of approximately 50 fluid ounces (1.7 liters) per day, with other beverages totaling about 48 fluid ounces (1.4 liters).

Many nutrients, including minerals, exist in the body dissolved in water. The functions of several minerals are related to the characteristics of water, so water and its roles in the body are explored first in Chapter 9.

Many minerals, like water, are vital to health. They are considered inorganic because they are typically not bonded to carbon atoms. Minerals are key participants in body metabolism, muscle movement, body growth, water balance, and other wide-ranging processes. We also know that some mineral deficiencies can cause severe health problems. For this reason, the study of minerals in Chapter 9 also is critical to understanding human nutrition.

**Refresh Your Memory**

As you begin your study of water and minerals in Chapter 9, you may want to review:

- Cell structure and function, digestion and absorption of nutrients, cardiovascular function, immunity, and endocrine function in Chapter 3
- The functions of vitamin D and vitamin K related to calcium and bone health in Chapter 8
- The role of vitamin C in collagen synthesis in Chapter 8

## 9.1 Water

**solvent** A liquid substance in which other substances dissolve.

**intracellular fluid** Fluid contained within a cell; it represents about two-thirds of body fluid.

**extracellular fluid** Fluid present outside the cells; represents about one-third of body fluid.

Life as we know it could not exist without water. Acting as a **solvent,** it dissolves many body compounds such as sodium chloride (table salt). Water is the perfect medium for body processes because it enables chemical reactions to occur. Water even participates directly in many of these reactions. It forms the greatest component of the human body, making up 50% to 70% of the body's weight (about 10 gallons or 40 liters). Lean muscle tissue contains about 73% water. Adipose tissue is about 20% water. Thus, as fat content increases (and the percentage of lean tissue decreases) in the body, total body water content drifts downward toward 50%.

Depending on the amount of fat stores present, an adult can survive for about 8 weeks without eating food but only a few days without drinking water. This occurs not because water is more important than carbohydrate, fat, protein, vitamins, or minerals, but rather because we cannot conserve or store water as well as we can the other components of our diet.

### Water in the Body—Intracellular and Extracellular Fluid

Water flows in and out of body cells through cell membranes. Water inside cells forms part of the **intracellular fluid.** When water is outside cells or in the bloodstream, it is part of the **extracellular fluid** (Fig. 9-1). Cell membranes are permeable to water, so

**FRANK & ERNEST by Bob Thaves**

As suggested in the comic, replacing fluids—water as part of foods, beverages, and water itself—is an important daily task. Why is this so critical for maintaining health? And why are infants, athletes, and older adults particularly at risk for dehydration? In addition, how does water interact with some of the minerals used by the body? Chapter 9 provides some answers.

FRANK & ERNEST © Reprinted by permission of Newspaper Enterprise Association, Inc.

water shifts freely in and out of cells. For example, if blood volume decreases, water can move into the bloodstream from the areas inside and around cells to increase blood volume. On the other hand, if blood volume increases, water can shift out of the bloodstream into cells and the surrounding areas, leading to edema (review Fig. 6-8 in Chapter 6).

The body controls the amount of water in the intracellular and extracellular compartments mainly by controlling *ion* movement and concentrations. Ions are minerals that have electrical charges and so are called **electrolytes.** Water is attracted to ions, such as sodium, potassium, chloride, phosphate, magnesium, and calcium. By controlling the movements of ions in and out of the cellular compartments, the body maintains the appropriate amount of water in each compartment using a process called **osmosis.** Overall, where ions go, water follows (Fig. 9-2).

Positive ions, such as sodium and potassium, end up pairing with negative ions, such as chloride and phosphate. Maintenance of intracellular water volume depends primarily on intracellular potassium and phosphate concentrations. Extracellular water volume depends primarily on the extracellular sodium and chloride concentrations.

**electrolytes** Substances that separate into ions in water and, in turn, are able to conduct an electrical current. These include sodium, chloride, and potassium.

**osmosis** The passage of a solvent such as water through a semipermeable membrane from a less concentrated compartment to a more concentrated compartment.

## Water Contributes to Body Temperature Regulation

Water temperature changes slowly because it has a great ability to hold heat. It takes much more energy to heat water than it does to heat fat. Water molecules are attracted to each other, and it takes much energy to separate them. Because water requires so much energy to change states—for example, from a liquid to a gas in the evaporation of perspiration—it forms an ideal medium for removing heat from the body.

When overheated, the body secretes fluids in the form of perspiration, which evaporates through skin pores. To evaporate water, heat energy is required. So, as perspiration evaporates, heat energy is taken from the skin, cooling it in the process.

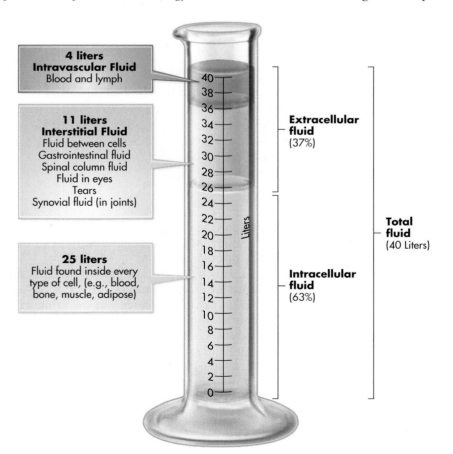

**FIGURE 9-1** ▶ Fluid compartments in the body. Total fluid volume is about 10 gallons (40 liters).

**4 liters**
**Intravascular Fluid**
Blood and lymph

**11 liters**
**Interstitial Fluid**
Fluid between cells
Gastrointestinal fluid
Spinal column fluid
Fluid in eyes
Tears
Synovial fluid (in joints)

**25 liters**
Fluid found inside every type of cell, (e.g., blood, bone, muscle, adipose)

**Extracellular fluid** (37%)

**Intracellular fluid** (63%)

**Total fluid** (40 Liters)

**FIGURE 9-2** ▶ Effects of various ion concentrations in a fluid on red blood cells. This shows the process of osmosis. Fluid is shifting in and out of the red blood cells in response to changing ion concentrations in the flasks.

Red blood cell

$H_2O$

Dilute solution     Normal concentration     Concentrated solution

(a) A dilute solution with a low ion concentration results in swelling (*black arrows*) and subsequent rupture (*puff of red in the lower left part of the cell*) of a red blood cell placed into the solution.

(b) A normal concentration (a concentration of ions outside the cell equal to that inside the cell) results in a typically shaped red blood cell. Water moves into and out of the cell in equilibrium (*black arrows*), but there is no net water movement.

(c) A concentrated solution, with a high ion concentration, causes shrinkage of the red blood cell as water moves out of the cell and into the concentrated solution (*black arrows*).

▲ The evaporation of sweat is an important part of temperature regulation.

**urea** Nitrogen-containing waste product of protein metabolism; major source of nitrogen in the urine.

**F**unctions of water:
- Chemical processes
- Temperature regulation
- Removal of waste products
- Primary component of body fluids, such as in joints

Each quart (liter) of perspiration evaporated represents approximately 600 kcal of energy lost from the skin and surrounding tissues. Similarly the heat lost when we have a fever increases one's need for calories.

About 60% of the chemical energy in food is turned directly into body heat; the other 40% is converted to forms of energy cells can use, and almost all of that energy eventually leaves the body in the form of heat. If this heat could not be dissipated, the body temperature would rise too high, preventing enzyme systems from functioning efficiently. Perspiration is the primary way to prevent this rise in body temperature.

### MAKING DECISIONS

#### Importance of Perspiration

To cool efficiently, perspiration must be allowed to evaporate. If it simply rolls off the skin or soaks into clothing, perspiration doesn't cool the body as much. Evaporation of perspiration occurs quickly when humidity is low. This is why humans can cool off and therefore tolerate hot, dry climates far better than they do hot, humid climates. This is also why increasing air circulation with a fan cools the body during an exercise workout.

### Water Helps Remove Waste Products

Water is an important vehicle for transporting substances throughout the body and for removing waste products from the body. Most unusable substances in the body can dissolve in water and exit the body through the urine.

**Urea** is a major body waste product. This by-product of protein metabolism contains nitrogen. The more protein we eat in excess of needs, the more nitrogen we remove from amino acids and excrete—in the form of urea—in the urine. Likewise, the more sodium we consume, the more sodium we excrete in the urine. Overall, the amount of urine a person needs to produce is determined primarily by excess protein and salt intake. By limiting excess protein and salt intakes, it is possible to limit urine output—a useful practice, for example, in space flights and in the treatment of some kidney diseases wherein the ability to produce urine is hampered.

A typical volume of urine produced per day is about 1 liter (1 quart) or more, depending mostly on the intake of fluid, protein, and sodium. A somewhat greater urine output than that is fine, but less—especially less than 500 milliliters (2 cups)—forces the kidneys to form concentrated urine. The simplest way to determine if water intake is adequate is to observe the color of one's urine. Whereas urine should be clear or pale yellow, concentrated urine is very dark yellow. The heavy ion content of concentrated urine in turn increases the risk of kidney stone formation in susceptible people (generally men). Kidney stones are formed from minerals and other substances that have precipitated out of the urine and accumulate in kidney tissues.

## Other Functions of Water

Water helps form the lubricants found in knees and other joints of the body. It is the basis for saliva, bile, and **amniotic fluid.** Amniotic fluid acts as a shock absorber surrounding the growing fetus in the mother's womb. Ion concentrations vary in each fluid compartment to accommodate Specific needs, such as the ability to transfer nerve impulses.

## How Much Water Do We Need per Day?

The Adequate Intake for total water intake per day is 2.7 liters (11 cups) for adult women and 3.7 liters (15 cups) for adult men. This is based primarily on our typical total water intakes from a combination of fluids and foods. For fluid alone this corresponds to about 2.2 liters (9 cups) for women and about 3 liters (13 cups) for men. (Keep in mind also that it does not indicate that water *per se* must be used to meet fluid needs.) At minimum, adults need 1 to 3 liters of fluid to replace daily water losses.

We consume water in various liquids, such as fruit juice, coffee, tea, soft drinks, and water itself. Note that coffee, tea, and soft drinks often contain caffeine, which increases urine output. However, the fluid consumed from these beverages is not completely lost in urine, so these fluids still help to meet water needs. Foods also supply water; many fruits and vegetables are more than 80% water (Fig. 9.3). Water as a by product of metabolism provides approximately 250 to 350 milliliters (1 to 1½ cups) of additional water.

Much of the water needed is used to produce urine (500 to 1000 milliliters or more). The rest compensates for typical water losses through the lungs (250 to 350 milliliters), feces (100 to 200 milliliters), and skin (450 to 1900 milliliters) (Fig. 9.4). These are just estimates: altitude, caffeine intake, alcohol intake, and humidity can affect these individual losses.

When we consider the large amount of water used to lubricate the gastrointestinal (GI) tract, the loss of only 100 to 200 milliliters of water each day through the feces

**amniotic fluid**  Fluid contained in a sac within the uterus. This fluid surrounds and protects the fetus during development.

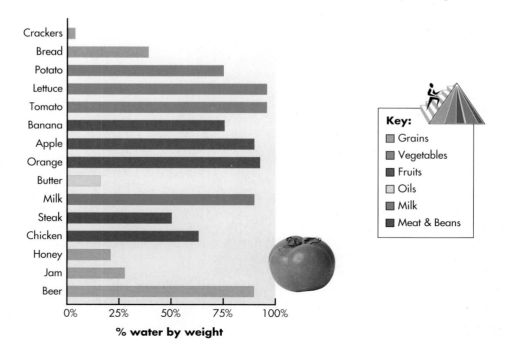

**FIGURE 9-3** ▶ Water content of foods by weight. In addition to the MyPyramid food groups, pink is used for substances that do not fit easily into food groups (e.g., honey, candy, coffee, alcohol, and table salt).

% water by weight

▶ Regular intake of water and water-rich fluids are essential to replace daily fluid losses. One trend in North America is to carry bottles of water with us.

is remarkable. About 8000 milliliters of water enter the GI tract daily through secretions from the mouth, stomach, intestine, pancreas, and other organs, while the diet supplies an additional 30% to 50% or more. The small intestine reabsorbs most of this water, while the large intestine takes up a lesser—but still important—amount. The kidneys also greatly conserve water. They reabsorb about 97% of the water filtered from waste products.

**FIGURE 9-4** ▶ Estimate of water balance—intake versus output—in a woman. We primarily maintain body fluids at an optimum amount by adjusting water output to intake. As you can see for this woman, most water comes from the liquids we consume. Some comes from the moisture in more solid foods, and the remainder is manufactured during metabolism. Water output includes that lost via lungs, urine, skin, and feces.

**Water Intake**

Fluids:
2000 milliliters (8 cups)

+

Water content in food:
500 milliliters (2 cups)

+

Water produced
from metabolism:
300 milliliters (1.25 cups)

**Water Output**

Skin perspiration:
750 milliliters (3 cups)

+

Lung respiration:
300 milliliters (1.25 cups)

+

Urine:
1650 milliliters
(6.75 cups)

+

Feces:
100 milliliters (0.4 cup)

**Total Water Intake**
2800 milliliters
(approximately 10 cups)

**Total Water Output**
2800 milliliters
(approximately 10 cups)

## MAKING DECISIONS

### Hard Water or Soft Water?

Water can be classified by whether it is hard or soft. Hard water generally comes from underground wells and usually contains calcium, magnesium, and iron. The more minerals the water contains, the harder it is. Soft water has a low content of these minerals and is often produced by replacing other minerals with sodium.

## Thirst

If you don't drink enough water, your body eventually lets you know by signaling thirst. Your brain is communicating the need to drink. This thirst mechanism can lag behind actual water loss, however, during prolonged exercise and illness, as well as in one's older years. For this reason, athletes should carefully monitor fluid status—they should weigh themselves before and after training sessions to determine their rate of water loss and, thus, their water needs. The current goal for athletes is to consume 2½ to 3 cups of fluid for every pound lost (see Chapter 10 for details). Sick children—especially those with fever, vomiting, diarrhea, and increased perspiration—and older persons often need to be reminded to drink plenty of fluids (see Chapters 15 and 16 for details). As Chapter 15 discusses in further detail, infants can easily become dehydrated.

## What If the Thirst Message Is Ignored?

Once the body registers a shortage of available water, it increases fluid conservation. Two hormones that participate in this process are **antidiuretic hormone** and **aldosterone.** The pituitary gland releases antidiuretic hormone to force the kidneys to conserve water. The kidneys respond by reducing urine flow. At the same time, as fluid volume decreases in the bloodstream, blood pressure falls. This eventually triggers the release of the hormone aldosterone, which signals the kidneys to retain more sodium and, in turn, more water.

Alcohol inhibits the action of antidiuretic hormone. One reason people feel so weak the day after heavy drinking is that they are dehydrated. Even though they may have consumed a lot of liquid in their drinks, they have lost even more liquid because alcohol has inhibited antidiuretic hormone.

However, despite mechanisms that work to reduce water loss via the kidneys, fluid continues to be lost via the feces, skin, and lungs. Those losses must be replaced. In addition, there is a limit to how concentrated urine can become. Eventually, if fluid is not consumed, the body becomes dehydrated and suffers ill effects.

By the time a person loses 1% to 2% of body weight in fluids, he or she will be thirsty. Even this small water deficit can cause one to feel tired. At a 4% loss of body weight, muscles lose significant strength and endurance. By the time body weight is reduced by 10% to 12%, heat tolerance is decreased and weakness results. At a 20% reduction, coma and death may soon follow. The progression of the symptoms of dehydration are shown in Figure 9-5.

**antidiuretic hormone** A hormone that is secreted by the pituitary gland and that acts on the kidneys to decrease water excretion.

**aldosterone** A hormone produced by the adrenal glands that acts on the kidneys to conserve sodium (and therefore water).

## Healthy Beverage Consumption Guidelines

Water is the key component in the beverage consumption guidelines that have been recently developed (Table 9-1). These recommendations give guidance on the health and nutritional benefits as well as the risks of various beverage categories. The basis of the Beverage Guidance System is that fluids should not provide a significant amount of the energy or nutrients in a healthy diet. More specifically, the system recommends that beverages provide less than 10% of total calories consumed for a 2200 kcal diet.

**FIGURE 9-5 ▶** The effects of dehydration can range from thirst to death, depending on the extent of water weight lost.

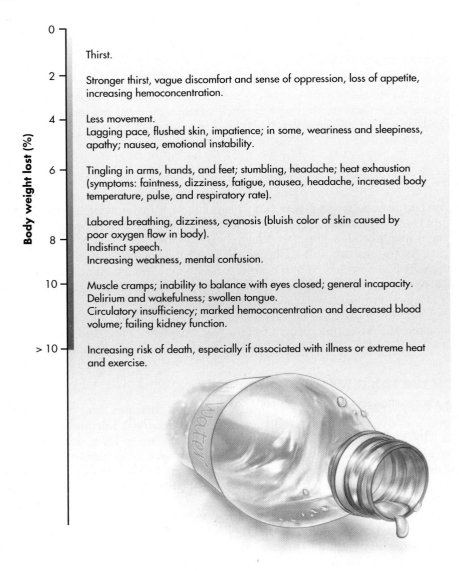

Body weight lost (%)

**0** Thirst.

**2** Stronger thirst, vague discomfort and sense of oppression, loss of appetite, increasing hemoconcentration.

**4** Less movement.
Lagging pace, flushed skin, impatience; in some, weariness and sleepiness, apathy; nausea, emotional instability.

**6** Tingling in arms, hands, and feet; stumbling, headache; heat exhaustion (symptoms: faintness, dizziness, fatigue, nausea, headache, increased body temperature, pulse, and respiratory rate).

Labored breathing, dizziness, cyanosis (bluish color of skin caused by poor oxygen flow in body).
**8** Indistinct speech.
Increasing weakness, mental confusion.

**10** Muscle cramps; inability to balance with eyes closed; general incapacity.
Delirium and wakefulness; swollen tongue.
Circulatory insufficiency; marked hemoconcentration and decreased blood volume; failing kidney function.

**> 10** Increasing risk of death, especially if associated with illness or extreme heat and exercise.

**TABLE 9-1** The Beverage Guidance System

| Level | Category* | Recommended Servings per day |
|-------|-----------|------------------------------|
| 1 | Water | 50 fluid ounces (1.7 liters) |
| 2 | Tea or coffee, unsweetened | 0 to 40 fluid ounces (0 to 1.4 liters) |
| 3 | Low-fat and skim milk and soy beverages | 0 to 16 fluid ounces (0 to 0.5 liter) |
| 4 | Non-calorically sweetened beverages (diet drinks) | 0 to 32 fluid ounces (0 to 1 liter) |
| 5 | Calorie beverages with some nutrients (100% fruit juices, alcoholic beverages, whole milk, sports drinks) | 0 to 8 fluid ounces (0 to 0.25 liter) 0 to 2 alcoholic drinks for men 0 to 8 fluid ounces (0 to 0.25 liter) |
| 6 | Calorically-sweetened beverages (regular soft drinks) | 0 to 1 alcoholic drinks for women, |

*Categories established based on their possible health benefits or risks.

Adapted from Popkin and others: Am J Clin Nutr 83:529,2006.

## Is There Such a Thing as Too Much Water?

Consuming too much water—whatever amount the kidneys are unable to excrete—can also lead to ill health, especially if concentrations of blood electrolytes, notably sodium, become too low. However, an excessive amount would have to approach many quarts (liters) each day. When excessive water intake overwhelms the kidneys' capacity to excrete fluid, blurred vision is one resulting symptom. Such water toxicity risks during athletic events are covered in Chapter 10.

### MAKING DECISIONS

#### Bottled Water

Bottled water has become very popular. In 2008, Americans consumed more than 9.4 billion gallons of bottled water, or about 31 gallons each. The public perception that bottled water is safer and healthier than tap water has stimulated the current bottle-toting habit. But when making a choice between the wide variety of bottled waters and tap water, do we really know what we are drinking? Bottled and tap water are both regulated: bottled water by the FDA and tap water by the Environmental Protection Agency (EPA). The FDA requirements for bottled water mimic those of the EPA for water quality, but neither have to be contaminant-free. Consumers should be aware of the FDA definitions for the various types of bottled water. Artesian water must come from a confined aquifer; mineral water must contain consistent levels of natural elements; spring water must flow naturally to the surface; and purified water is produced through an approved process such as distillation or reverse osmosis. "Pure" is an advertising term and means nothing about the quality of the water. Recent controversy over misleading advertising by major companies such as Pepsico and Coca Cola that use public source water in their respective products, Aquafina and Dansani, has led to the printing of "Public Source Water" or "PSW" on labels. Relying on bottled water is an expensive habit, personally and environmentally. If you use bottled water to meet your recommended fluid needs, you will spend close to $1,500 per year compared with about 50 cents for the same volume of tap water. On a larger scale it is estimated that close to 90% of water bottles end up in the trash, clogging our landfills or being shipped to other countries for recycling. It is well known that America has some of the cleanest, safest tap water in the world. So while following the recommendations to drink more water, consider doing it from the tap in a reusable container such as a drinking glass.

▲ Bottled water is a convenient but relatively expensive source of water. In most cases, tap water is just as healthy a choice to meet our water needs.

### CONCEPT CHECK

The body can neither readily store nor conserve water, so we can survive only a few days without it. Water transports nutrients and waste products, serves as a medium for chemical reactions and as a lubricant, and aids in temperature regulation. Water accounts for 50% to 70% of body weight and distributes itself all over the body—among lean and other tissues (in both intracellular and extracellular fluids) and in urine and other body fluids. The Adequate Intake for total water intake is 2.7 liters (11 cups) for women and 3.7 liters (15 cups) for men per day. Thirst is the body's first sign of dehydration. If this thirst mechanism is faulty, as it may be during illness or vigorous exercise, hormonal mechanisms also help conserve water by reducing urine output. Excess fluid intake can be hazardous to a person's health. Overall, the United States enjoys a safe water supply. However, people with poor immune status should boil water used for drinking and cooking to avoid waterborne illness. Bottled water can also be used if desired.

## Our Water Supply: Safety Issues

Many people choose bottled water over tap water because they doubt the safety of their public drinking water. Some concern over municipal water supplies is warranted. For example, contamination of the public water supply by the parasite *Cryptosporidium* is possible. This parasite is usually found in lakes and rivers; the typical chlorination procedures used to treat public water supplies do not kill *Cryptosporidium*. This parasite poses little risk to healthy people—other than a case of diarrhea—but it can harm people who have AIDS or other diseases that compromise function of the immune system (such as some forms of cancer therapy or organ transplant therapy). High-risk people have been advised to boil for at least 1 minute any tap water they use for cooking or drinking to ensure that the parasite is destroyed. Alternatively, individuals can purchase a water filter that screens out *Cryptosporidium* (the National Sanitation Foundation at (800) 673-8010 can provide a list of manufacturers) or use bottled water certified to be free of the parasite (contact the supplier if in doubt). Generally, distilled water or that which has undergone reverse osmosis is parasite free.

### Monitoring the Safety of Your Water

Under the Safe Water Drinking Act, all public drinking water supplies are monitored for contaminants such as bacteria, various chemicals, and toxic metals (such as lead and mercury). The local municipal water department must mail the results of these tests each year to its consumers. According to the Environmental Protection Agency (EPA), the U.S. water supply ranks among the safest in the world. However, this water does sometimes fail to meet the agency's standards for contaminants such as lead and nitrates. Generally, the public will be warned about the latter, because it is danger-ous to use nitrate-rich water for mixing infant formulas (Chapter 15). Some studies indicate that in one year, about one in five Americans consumes water not up to standards, especially in rural areas. These people could consider using a home water filter or bottled water. The local water department can help a person evaluate whether health risks are worth the cost of home water filters or bottled water.

As a safeguard against contamination, chlorine and ammonia are added to kill bacteria. The addition of such chemicals has raised concern that drinking water may increase rectal and bladder cancer risk, though there is no conclusive proof of such risk. If chlorine in tap water does increase cancer risk, the risk is likely extremely small (perhaps two cases of cancer in 1 million people).

If you find the taste of chlorinated tap water unpleasant or are concerned about the possible cancer risk, you can remove the chlorine from tap water by boiling it or by letting a large container filled with water stand uncovered overnight. In both cases, the chlorine will evaporate, taking its characteristic flavor with it. Alternatively, you can install a filter on the household spigot from which you obtain your water. It should be designed to remove trihalomethanes, common chlorine by-products.

### Options Regarding Your Water Source

Keep in mind that by most standards, bottled water ranges from moderately expensive to expensive. In many cases, you are paying for water not much different from the water you get from your tap. If you are concerned about the safety of your tap water, you can ask the municipal water department for its most recent test results, or you can have the water tested. A local testing laboratory or state health department can be of service, as can the EPA at (800) 426-4791, if local information is not available (for example, if you have a well). This testing can point out whether there are health risks associated with your water supply. Compared with the cost of bottled water, the testing fee will be insignificant. Letting cold water run for a minute or so before taking a drink or before using it in meal preparation is a good way to limit possible lead exposure, especially if the water has been off for more than two hours. In addition, do not use hot tap water for food preparation. For more information, see the website www.epa.gov/safewater.

## 9.2 Minerals—An Overview

**cofactor** A mineral or other substance that binds to a specific region on a protein, such as an enzyme, and is necessary for the protein's function.

The metabolic roles of minerals and the amounts of them in the body vary consid-erably (Fig. 9-6). Some minerals, such as copper and selenium, work as **cofactors,** enabling various proteins, such as enzymes, to function. Minerals also contribute to

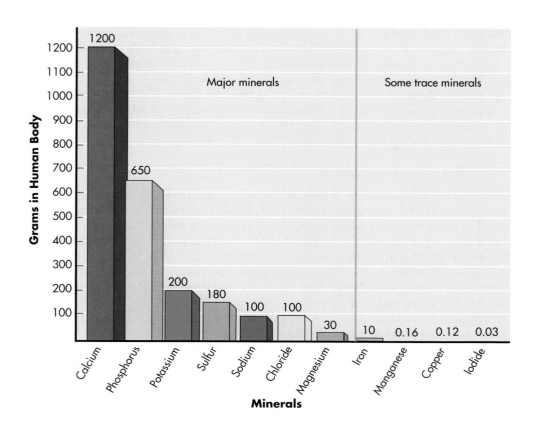

**FIGURE 9-6** ▶ Approximate amounts of various minerals present in the average human body. Other trace minerals of nutritional importance not listed include chromium, fluoride, molybdenum, selenium, and zinc.

many body compounds. For example, iron is a component of red blood cells. Sodium, potassium, and calcium aid in the transfer of nerve impulses throughout the body. Body growth and development also depend on certain minerals, such as calcium and phosphorus. Water balance requires sodium, potassium, calcium, and phosphorus. At all levels—cellular, tissue, organ, and whole body—minerals clearly play important roles in maintaining body functions.

Minerals are categorized based on the amount we need per day. Recall from Chapter 1 that if we require greater than 100 milligrams (1/50 of a teaspoon) of a mineral per day, it is considered a **major mineral**; otherwise, it is considered a **trace mineral**. For example, calcium and phosphorus are major minerals and iron and zinc are trace minerals.

The roles and nutritional significance of both the major and the trace minerals are discussed in this chapter. But before examining the properties of the individual minerals, let's consider some topics that apply to all these nutrients.

## Mineral Bioavailability

Foods offer us a plentiful supply of many minerals, but the ability of our bodies to absorb and use them varies. The degree to which an ingested nutrient is absorbed from food sources and is available to the body is called **bioavailability.** The bioavailability of minerals depends on many factors. The mineral content listed in a food composition table for the amount of a mineral in a food is just a starting point for estimating the actual contribution the food will make to our mineral needs. Spinach, for example, contains plenty of calcium, but only about 5% of it can be absorbed because of the vegetable's high concentration of **oxalic acid (oxalate),** a calcium-binder. Usually, about 25% of dietary calcium is absorbed by adults.

The average North American diet derives minerals from both plant and animal sources. Overall, minerals from animal products are better absorbed than those from plants because binders such as fiber are not present to hinder absorption. The mineral content of plants greatly depends on mineral concentrations of the soil in which they are grown. Vegans must be aware of the potentially poor mineral content of

**major mineral** A mineral vital to health that is required in the diet in amounts greater than 100 milligrams per day.

**trace mineral** A mineral vital to health that is required in the diet in amounts less than 100 milligrams per day.

**bioavailability** The degree to which an ingested nutrient is absorbed and available to the body.

**oxalic acid (oxalate)** An organic acid found in spinach, rhubarb, and other leafy green vegetables that can depress the absorption of certain minerals present in the food, such as calcium.

▲ Spinach is often touted as a rich source of calcium, but little of the calcium present is available to the body.

some plant foods and choose some concentrated sources of minerals (review "Nutrition and Your Health" in Chapter 6). Soil conditions have less of an influence on the mineral content of animal products because livestock usually consume a variety of plant products grown from soils of differing mineral contents.

In general, the more refined a plant food—as in the case of white flour—the lower its content of minerals. During the enrichment of refined grain products, iron is the only mineral added, whereas the selenium, zinc, copper, and other minerals lost during refinement are not replaced.

### Fiber-Mineral Interactions

Mineral bioavailability can be greatly affected by nonmineral substances in the diet. Components of fiber, especially **phytic acid (phytate)** in grain fiber, can limit absorption of some minerals by binding to them. Oxalic acid, mentioned in the previous section, is another substance in plants that binds minerals and makes them less bioavailable. High-fiber diets can decrease the absorption of iron, zinc, and probably other minerals. An intake above the current recommendation of 25 (adult women) to 38 (adult men) grams of fiber per day may cause problems with mineral status of the body, but the actual degree of this effect is uncertain.

If grains are leavened with yeast, as they are in breadmaking, enzymes produced by the yeast can break some of the bonds between phytic acid and minerals. This increases mineral absorption. The zinc deficiencies found among some Middle Eastern populations are attributed partly to their consumption of unleavened breads, resulting in low bioavailability of dietary zinc. Zinc bioavailability is discussed in greater detail in a later section.

### Mineral-Mineral Interactions

Many minerals, such as magnesium, calcium, iron, and copper, are of similar sizes and electrical charges. Having similar sizes and the same electrical charge causes these minerals to compete with each other for absorption, and therefore they affect each other's bioavailability. Simply stated, an excess of one mineral decreases the absorption and metabolism of other minerals. For example, a large intake of zinc decreases copper absorption. Because of this, people should avoid taking individual mineral supplements unless a dietary deficiency or medical condition specifically warrants it. Food sources, however, pose little risk for these mineral interactions, giving us another reason to emphasize foods in meeting nutrient needs.

### Vitamin-Mineral Interactions

Several beneficial vitamin-mineral interactions occur during nutrient absorption and metabolism. When consumed in conjunction with vitamin C, absorption of certain forms of iron—such as that in plant products—improves. The active vitamin D hormone improves calcium absorption. Many vitamins require specific minerals to act as components in their structure and function. For example, the thiamin coenzyme requires magnesium or manganese to function efficiently.

### Mineral Toxicities

An excessive mineral intake, especially of trace minerals, such as iron and copper, can have toxic results. For many trace minerals, the gap between just enough and too much is small. Taking minerals as supplements poses the biggest threat for mineral toxicity, whereas food sources are unlikely culprits. Mineral supplements exceeding current standards for mineral needs—especially those that supply more than 100% of the Daily Values on supplement labels—should be taken only under a physician's supervision. The Daily Values are for the most part higher than our current standards (e.g., RDA) for mineral needs. Without close monitoring, doses of minerals should not exceed any Upper Level set on a long-term basis.

**phytic acid (phytate)**  A constituent of plant fibers that binds positive ions to its multiple phosphate groups.

▲ Mineral supplements pose a high risk for toxicity. Generally, mineral intake from a supplement should not exceed 100% of the Daily Value, unless otherwise specified by a physician.

The potential for toxicity is not the only reason to carefully consider the use of mineral supplements. Harmful interactions with other nutrients are possible. Also, contamination of mineral supplements—with lead, for example—is a possibility. Use of brands approved by the United States Pharmacopeia (USP) lessens this risk (review "Nutrition and Your Health" in Chapter 8). In summary, even with the best intentions, people may harm themselves using mineral supplements.

## CONCEPT CHECK

Minerals are vital to the functioning of many body processes. Their bioavailability depends on many factors, including a mineral's interaction with fiber, vitamins, and other minerals. Animal products often yield better mineral absorption than do plants. Still, both animal and plant sources help us meet our mineral needs. Taking megadoses of an individual mineral supplement can greatly diminish the absorption and metabolism of other minerals. In addition, some minerals are potentially toxic in amounts not much in excess of body needs. These are two good reasons to carefully consider any use of mineral supplements exceeding the Daily Value on the label, particularly long-term use of supplements that lead to intakes in excess of the Upper Level set for any mineral.

# 9.3 Major Minerals

Up to now, some general characteristics of minerals and how some of them interact with water in the body have been covered. Now let us review the individual properties of the major minerals (also called macrominerals) in the context of the North American diet.

# 9.4 Sodium (Na)

**F**or your information, the chemical symbols for the minerals discussed are given next to each mineral heading.

Our primary dietary source of sodium is table salt, chemically known as sodium chloride, added during food processing. This mineral is an essential part of our diets and adds flavor to our foods, but there is concern that an overabundance of sodium in the diet may cause harm. Table salt is 40% sodium and 60% chloride. For example, dietary intake of 10 grams of salt translates into about 4 grams of sodium. A teaspoon of salt contains about 2 grams of sodium (2000 milligrams).

The human body absorbs almost all sodium that gets eaten. Once absorbed, sodium becomes the major positive ion outside of cells in extracellular fluid and a key factor for retaining body water. Fluid balance throughout the body depends partly on the variation in the sodium and other ion concentrations among the water-containing compartments in the body. Sodium ions also function in nerve impulse conduction and absorption of some nutrients (e.g., glucose).

A dietary deficiency of sodium is rare. However, a diet low in sodium—coupled with excessive perspiration, persistent vomiting, or diarrhea—has the ability to deplete the body of sodium. This state can lead to muscle cramps, nausea, vomiting, dizziness, and later, shock and coma. The likelihood of this happening, however, is low because the kidney responds early to low sodium status, eventually triggering the body to conserve sodium. This conservation of sodium by the body demonstrates how important small amounts of sodium are to body functions.

Only when perspiration leads to weight loss exceeding 2% to 3% of total body weight (or about 5 to 6 pounds) should sodium losses raise concern. Even then, merely salting foods is sufficient to restore body sodium for most people. Certain endurance athletes, however, may need to consume sports drinks during competition to replace sodium losses from perspiration in order to avoid depletion of sodium (see Chapter 10). Although perspiration tastes salty on the skin, sodium is not highly concentrated in perspiration. Rather, water evaporating from the skin leaves concentrated

▲ Table salt is our primary source of the minerals sodium and chloride.

sodium behind. Perspiration contains about two-thirds the sodium concentration found in blood.

## Sodium Sources and Needs

About 80% of the sodium we consume is added to foods during manufacturing and preparation at restaurants (Fig. 9-7). Sodium added in cooking provides about 10% of our intakes, and sodium naturally present in foods provides the rest, about another 10%. Almost all foods naturally contain a little sodium; the higher amount found in milk (about 120 milligrams per cup) is one exception.

The more processed and restaurant food one consumes, generally the higher one's sodium intake. Conversely, the more home cooking one does, the more sodium control that person has. The foods that contribute most of the sodium in the adult diet (white bread and rolls, hot dogs and lunch meats, cheese, soups, and foods with tomato sauce) do so partly because they are eaten so often. Other foods that generally are especially high in sodium include salted snack foods, French fries and potato chips, and sauces and gravies (Fig. 9-8).

If we ate only unprocessed foods and added no salt, we would consume about 500 milligrams of sodium per day. In comparison, the Adequate Intake for sodium for adults under age 51 is 1500 milligrams, a generous amount; this is reduced by 100 to 200 milligrams for older adults. (See the inside back cover for references to mineral needs for various age groups.) The 2005 Dietary Guidelines for Americans recommends that the general population consume less than 2300 milligrams (approximately 1 teaspoon of salt) of sodium per day and choose and prepare foods with little salt. The Dietary Guidelines for individuals with hypertension, blacks, and middle-aged and older adults are to aim to consume no more than 1500 milligrams of sodium per day. We really need only about 200 milligrams per day to maintain physiological functions. (Additional sodium above needs was added to establish the Adequate Intake to allow for a more varied diet where not all foods are low in sodium.)

If we compare 500 milligrams of sodium from unprocessed food with the amount typically eaten by adults (2300 to 4700 milligrams or more), it is clear that food processing and cooking contribute most of our dietary sodium. As discussed in Chapter 2, nutrition labels list a food's sodium content. When dietary sodium must be severely restricted, attention to food labels is of utmost importance. Under FDA food and supplement labeling rules, the Daily Value for sodium is 2400 milligrams (2.4 grams).

Most humans can adapt somewhat to various dietary salt intakes, though very high intakes can be toxic. For most people, today's sodium intake simply will be in tomorrow's urine output. However, approximately 10% to 15% of adults, such as African-Americans and people who have diabetes and/or are overweight, are especially *sodium sensitive*. For these people, high sodium intakes can increase blood pressure, whereas lower-sodium diets (about 2000 milligrams daily) often help correct

▲ Deli meats, such as ham, are high in sodium (salt).

**FIGURE 9-7** ▶ Salt arrives in the American diet largely as a result of food processing.

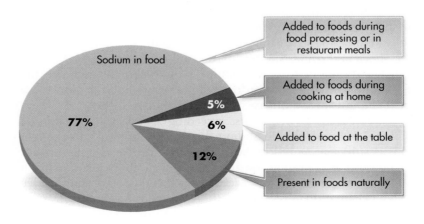

## Food Sources of Sodium

| Food Item and Amount | Sodium Content (milligrams) | Daily Value = 2400 milligrams %AI |
|---|---|---|
| AI* | 1500 | 100% |
| Pepperoni pizza, 2 slices | 2045 | 136% |
| Ham, sliced, 1 ounce | 1215 | 81% |
| Chicken noodle soup, canned, 1 cup | 1106 | 74% |
| V8 vegetable juice, 8 ounces | 620 | 41% |
| Macaroni salad, ½ cup | 561 | 37% |
| Hard pretzels, 1 ounce | 486 | 32% |
| Hamburger with bun, 1 each | 474 | 32% |
| Green beans, canned, ½ cup | 390 | 26% |
| Saltine crackers, 6 each | 234 | 16% |
| Cheddar cheese, 1 ounce | 176 | 12% |
| Peanut butter, 2 tablespoons | 156 | 10% |
| Nonfat milk, 1 cup | 127 | 8% |
| Seven grain bread, 1 slice | 126 | 8% |
| Animal crackers, 1 ounce | 112 | 7% |
| Grape juice, 1 cup | 10 | 1% |

Key:
- Grains
- Vegetables
- Fruits
- Oils
- Milk
- Meat & Beans

* For adults; See the DRI table in the back of this book for age-specific recommendations.

**FIGURE 9-8** ▶ Food sources of sodium compared to the Adequate Intake.

the problem (see the following "Nutrition and Your Health" section on minerals and hypertension). Still, keep in mind that other lifestyle factors, such as being overweight and inactive, are more likely to contribute to hypertension.

Scientific groups typically suggest that adults in general reduce sodium intake, mostly to limit the risk of developing hypertension later. It is also a good idea to have your blood pressure checked regularly. If you have hypertension, you should try to reduce your sodium intake as you follow a comprehensive plan to treat this disease. Reducing sodium intake also helps to maintain healthy calcium status, because urinary calcium loss is increased along with sodium when sodium intake is greater than about 2000 milligrams per day.

It is not that hard to follow a low-sodium diet, but many typical food choices such as processed meats and salty snacks will have to be limited (see the first "Rate Your Plate" activity at the end of this chapter). At first, foods may also taste bland, but eventually you will perceive more flavor as the tongue becomes more sensitive to the salt content of foods. By slowly reducing dietary sodium and substituting lemon juice, herbs and spices, you can eventually become accustomed to a diet that contains minimal sodium but does not result in much of a flavor trade-off. Many new cookbooks offer excellent recipes for flavorful low-sodium foods.

The FDA is considering whether to remove salt (sodium chloride) from its list of foods categorized as "generally recognized as safe" or GRAS.

### Upper Level for Sodium

The Upper Level for sodium for adults is 2300 milligrams (2.3 grams). Intakes exceeding this amount are common but are not recommended because they typically increase blood pressure. About 95% of North American adults have sodium intakes that exceed the Upper Level.

## CRITICAL THINKING

Mrs. Massa has recently seen and heard a lot about the amount of salt (sodium) in foods. She has been surprised by the number of articles that advise the public to decrease the amount of salt in their food. If sodium is such a bad thing, Mrs. Massa wonders, why do you need to have any at all? How would you respond to her question?

## CONCEPT CHECK

Sodium is the major positive ion in the extracellular fluid. It is important for maintaining fluid balance and conducting nerve impulses. Sodium depletion is unlikely, because the typical North American's diet has abundant sources of sodium and most of it gets absorbed. Compared to dining out or buying commercially-prepared foods, preparation of foods in the home allows greater control over sodium intake. The Adequate Intake for sodium for adults is 1500 milligrams per day. The average adult consumes 2300 to 4700 milligrams or more daily. About 10% to 15% of the population is especially sensitive to sodium, such as overweight individuals and African-Americans. In these people, hypertension can develop as a result of high-sodium diets, but many other lifestyle habits also contribute to hypertension. Nutrition experts suggest that for young adults, sodium intake should be about 1500 milligrams (1.5 grams) and not exceed 2300 milligrams (2.3 grams) on a regular basis. Sodium in the North American diet is provided predominantly through processed and restaurant foods.

## 9.5 Potassium (K)

Potassium performs many of the same functions as sodium, such as fluid balance and nerve impulse transmission. However, it operates inside, rather than outside cells. Intracellular fluids—those inside cells—contain 95% of the potassium in the body. Also, unlike sodium, increasing potassium intake is associated with lower rather than higher blood pressure values. We absorb about 90% of the potassium we eat.

Low blood potassium is a life-threatening problem. Symptoms often include a loss of appetite, muscle cramps, confusion, and constipation. Eventually, the heart beats irregularly, which decreases its capacity to pump blood.

▲ Vegetables in general are a rich source of potassium, as are fruits.

### Potassium Sources and Needs

Generally, unprocessed foods are rich sources of potassium. This includes fruits, vegetables, milk, whole grains, dried beans, and meats (Fig. 9-9). Major contributors of potassium to the adult diet include milk, potatoes, beef, coffee, tomatoes, and orange juice (Fig. 9-10).

The Adequate Intake for potassium for adults is 4700 milligrams (4.7 grams) per day. The Daily Value used to express potassium content on food and supplement labels is 3500 milligrams. On average, North Americans consume 2000 to 3000 milligrams per day. Thus, many of us need to increase our potassium intakes, preferably by increasing fruit and vegetable intake.

Diets are more likely to be lower in potassium than sodium because we generally do not add potassium to foods. Some **diuretics** used to treat high blood pressure also deplete the body's potassium. Thus, people who take potassium-wasting diuretics need to monitor their potassium intakes carefully. For these people, high-potassium foods are good additions to the diet, as are potassium chloride supplements if prescribed by a physician.

**diuretic** A substance that increases the volume of urine.

A chronically deficient food intake, as may be the case in alcoholism, can result in a severe potassium deficiency that requires medical attention. People with certain eating disorders, whose diets are poor and whose bodies can be depleted of nutrients because of vomiting, are also at risk for severe potassium deficiency (see Chapter 11).

## Food Sources of Potassium

| Food Item and Amount | Potassium (milligrams) | Daily Value = 3500 milligrams %AI | |
|---|---|---|---|
| **AI*** | 4700 | ████████████████████ | 100% |
| Kidney beans, 1 cup | 715 | ██ | 15% |
| Winter squash, ¾ cup | 670 | ██ | 14% |
| Plain yogurt, 1 cup | 570 | ██ | 12% |
| Orange juice, 1 cup | 495 | ██ | 11% |
| Cantaloupe, 1 cup | 495 | ██ | 11% |
| Lima beans, ½ cup | 480 | ██ | 10% |
| Banana, 1 medium | 470 | ██ | 10% |
| Zucchini, 1 cup | 450 | ██ | 10% |
| Soybeans, ½ cup | 440 | ██ | 9% |
| Artichoke, 1 medium | 425 | ██ | 9% |
| Tomato juice, ¾ cup | 400 | ██ | 9% |
| Pinto beans, ½ cup | 400 | ██ | 9% |
| Baked potato, 1 small | 385 | ██ | 8% |
| Buttermilk, 1 cup | 370 | ██ | 8% |
| Sirloin steak, 3 ounces | 345 | ██ | 7% |

Key:
- ▢ Grains
- ▢ Vegetables
- ▢ Fruits
- ▢ Oils
- ▢ Milk
- ▢ Meat & Beans

* For adults; See the DRI table in the back of this book for age-specific recommendations.

**FIGURE 9-9** ▶ Food sources of potassium compared to the Adequate Intake.

# MyPyramid: Sources of Potassium

| Grains | Vegetables | Fruits | Oils | Milk | Meat & Beans |
|---|---|---|---|---|---|
| • Whole-wheat bread<br>• Whole-grain products | • Spinach<br>• Squash<br>• Potatoes<br>• Tomatoes<br>• Lettuce<br>• Lima beans | • Pears<br>• Prunes<br>• Peaches<br>• Avocados<br>• Cantaloupes<br>• Bananas | • None | • Milk<br>• Yogurt<br>• Cottage cheese<br>• Ricotta cheese | • Meat<br>• Chicken<br>• Fish<br>• Shrimp<br>• Beans |

**FIGURE 9-10** ▶ Sources of potassium from MyPyramid. The height of the background color (none, 1/3, 2/3, or completely covered) within each group in the pyramid indicates the average nutrient density for potassium in that group. Overall, the vegetables group and the fruits group contain many foods that are nutrient-dense sources of potassium, with the milk group and meat & beans group following close behind. With regard to physical activity, potassium is especially needed for cardiovascular function.

Other populations especially at risk for a severe potassium deficiency include people on very low-calorie diets and athletes who exercise heavily. As covered in Chapters 7 and 10, all of these people should compensate for potentially low body potassium by consuming potassium-rich foods.

If the kidneys function normally, typical food intakes will not lead to potassium toxicity. Thus, no Upper Level for potassium has been set. When the kidneys function poorly, potassium builds up in the blood. This inhibits heart function, causing slowed heartbeat. If untreated, this can be fatal, as the heart eventually stops beating. Consequently, in cases of reduced kidney function, close control of potassium intake becomes critical.

## 9.6 Chloride (Cl)

In our bodies, chloride—an ion form of chlorine—is an important negative ion for the extracellular fluid. Chlorine, on the other hand, is a poisonous gas. Chloride ions are a component of the acid produced in the stomach and are also used during immune responses as white blood cells attack foreign cells. In addition, nerve function relies on the presence of chloride. As is the case with sodium, most of the body's chloride is excreted by the kidneys; some is lost in perspiration. It is also thought to contribute to the blood pressure-raising ability of sodium chloride.

A chloride deficiency is unlikely because our dietary sodium chloride (salt) intake is so high. Frequent and lengthy bouts of vomiting—if coupled with a nutrient-poor diet—can, however, contribute to a deficiency because stomach secretions contain much chloride.

### Chloride Sources and Needs

A few fruits and some vegetables are naturally good sources of chloride. Chlorinated water is also a source. However, the chloride we consume is mostly in the salt added to foods. Knowing a food's salt content allows for a close prediction of its chloride content; recall salt is 60% chloride.

The Adequate Intake for chloride for adults is 2300 milligrams per day. This is based on the 40:60 ratio of sodium to chloride in salt (1500 milligrams of sodium in a diet is accompanied by 2300 milligrams of chloride). The Daily Value used to express chloride content on food and supplement labels is 3400 milligrams. If the average adult consumes about 9 grams of salt daily, that yields 5.4 grams (5400 milligrams) of chloride.

### Upper Level for Chloride

The Upper Level is 3600 milligrams. The average adult typically consumes an excess amount of this ion.

▲ Chloride is likely part of the blood pressure-raising property of sodium chloride (salt).

---

### CONCEPT CHECK

The functions of potassium closely parallel those of sodium, but whereas sodium is found outside cells, potassium is the main positive ion found inside cells. Potassium is vital to fluid balance and nerve transmission. A potassium deficiency—caused by an inadequate intake of potassium, persistent vomiting, or use of some diuretics—can eventually lead to loss of appetite, muscle cramps, confusion, and heartbeat irregularities. Fruits and vegetables are generally rich sources of potassium. Potassium intake can be toxic if a person's kidneys do not function properly. Chloride is the major negative ion of extracellular fluid. Chloride also functions in digestion as part of stomach acid and in immune and nervous system responses. Deficiencies of chloride are highly unlikely because we eat so much sodium chloride (salt).

# 9.7 Calcium (Ca)

All cells need calcium, but more than 99% of the calcium in the body is used to strengthen bones and teeth. This calcium represents 40% of all the minerals present in the body and equals about 2.5 pounds (1200 grams). The calcium circulating in the bloodstream supplies the calcium needs of body cells. Growth and bone development require an adequate calcium intake.

Unlike sodium, potassium, and chloride, the amount of calcium in the body depends greatly on its absorption from the diet. Calcium requires an acidic environment in the GI tract to be absorbed efficiently. Absorption occurs primarily in the upper part of the small intestine. This area tends to be the most acidic portion of the small intestine because it receives the acidic stomach contents. Calcium absorption in the upper small intestine also depends on the active vitamin D hormone.

Adults absorb about 25% of the calcium in the foods eaten, but during times when the body needs extra calcium—such as in infancy and pregnancy—absorption increases to as high as 60%. Young people tend to absorb calcium better than do older people, especially those older than 70.

Many factors enhance calcium absorption, including:

- Blood levels of parathyroid hormone
- The presence of glucose and lactose in the diet
- The gradual flow (motility) of digestive contents through the intestine

On the other hand, several factors limit calcium absorption, such as:

- Large amounts of phytic acid in fiber from grains
- Great excess of phosphorus (and possibly magnesium) in the diet
- Polyphenols (tannins) in tea
- Vitamin D deficiency
- Diarrhea
- Old age

We have excellent hormonal systems to control blood calcium, so a normal blood calcium value can be maintained despite an inadequate calcium intake. The bones, however, pay the price. Bones can be seen as a calcium bank to which calcium can be added or withdrawn. Bone loss caused by a net calcium loss from this bank proceeds slowly. Only after many years of calcium loss are clinical symptoms apparent. By not meeting calcium needs, some people—especially women—are most likely setting the stage for future bone fractures.

▲ Ninety-nine percent of calcium in the body is in bones.

## Functions of Calcium

Forming and maintaining bones are calcium's major roles in the body. This is discussed in detail in the second "Nutrition and Your Health" section on minerals and **osteoporosis** found at the end of this chapter. However, calcium is important in many other processes as well. Calcium is essential for blood clotting and for muscle contraction. If blood calcium falls below a critical point, muscles cannot relax after contraction; the body stiffens and shows involuntary twitching, called **tetany.** In nerve transmission, calcium assists in the release of neurotransmitters and permits the flow of ions in and out of nerve cells. Without sufficient calcium, nerve function fails, which can also cause tetany. Finally, calcium helps regulate cellular metabolism by influencing the activities of various enzymes and hormonal responses. It is the hormonal regulation of blood calcium that keeps all of these processes going, even if a person fails to consume enough calcium on a daily basis.

**osteoporosis**  Decreased bone mass related to the effects of aging, genetic background, and poor diet in both genders, and hormonal changes at menopause in women.

**tetany**  A body condition marked by sharp contraction of muscles and failure to relax afterward; usually caused by abnormal calcium metabolism.

## Other Possible Health Benefits of Calcium

Researchers have been examining links between calcium intake and risks for a variety of diseases including certain cancers, kidney stones, hypertension, high blood cholesterol, and most recently, obesity. An adequate calcium intake can reduce the risk of colon cancer, especially in people who consume a high-fat diet. A decreased risk of some forms of kidney stones and reduced lead absorption are other possible benefits when calcium is part of a meal. Calcium intakes of 800 to 1200 milligrams per day can also decrease blood pressure, compared with intakes of 400 milligrams per day or less. As covered in Chapter 5, calcium intakes of 1200 milligrams per day in combination with a low-fat, low-cholesterol diet can help people with elevated LDL cholesterol improve their blood lipid profiles. A link between a low calcium intake and overweight/obesity is also under study. Although the true benefit in this regard is not clear, studies suggest that an adequate calcium intake (compared to a very low intake [e.g., 400 milligrams per day]), coupled with a low calorie intake, may promote even more weight loss than the low calorie diet alone. Focusing on dairy sources of calcium is recommended because other components in dairy foods, such as some of the specific dairy proteins, contribute to this potential weight loss benefit. For women, an adequate calcium in-take might also reduce the risk of premenstrual syndrome and high blood pressure that can develop during pregnancy. Overall, the benefits of a diet providing adequate calcium extend beyond bone health.

## Calcium Sources and Needs

Dairy products, such as milk and cheese, provide about 75% of the calcium in North American diets. The exception is cottage cheese, because most calcium is lost during production. Bread, rolls, crackers, and other foods made with milk products are secondary contributors. Other calcium sources are leafy greens (such as spinach), broccoli, sardines, and canned salmon (Fig. 9-11). It is important to remember that much of the calcium in some leafy green vegetables, notably spinach, is not absorbed because of the presence of oxalic acid. This effect is not as strong, however, in kale, collard,

**FIGURE 9-11 ▶** Food sources of calcium compared to the Adequate Intake.

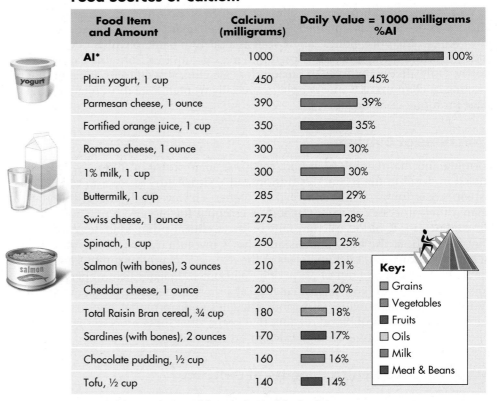

## Food Sources of Calcium

| Food Item and Amount | Calcium (milligrams) | Daily Value = 1000 milligrams %AI |
|---|---|---|
| AI* | 1000 | 100% |
| Plain yogurt, 1 cup | 450 | 45% |
| Parmesan cheese, 1 ounce | 390 | 39% |
| Fortified orange juice, 1 cup | 350 | 35% |
| Romano cheese, 1 ounce | 300 | 30% |
| 1% milk, 1 cup | 300 | 30% |
| Buttermilk, 1 cup | 285 | 29% |
| Swiss cheese, 1 ounce | 275 | 28% |
| Spinach, 1 cup | 250 | 25% |
| Salmon (with bones), 3 ounces | 210 | 21% |
| Cheddar cheese, 1 ounce | 200 | 20% |
| Total Raisin Bran cereal, ¾ cup | 180 | 18% |
| Sardines (with bones), 2 ounces | 170 | 17% |
| Chocolate pudding, ½ cup | 160 | 16% |
| Tofu, ½ cup | 140 | 14% |

**Key:**
- Grains
- Vegetables
- Fruits
- Oils
- Milk
- Meat & Beans

*For adults; See the DRI table in the back of this book for age-specific recommendations.

turnip, and mustard greens. Overall, fat-free milk is the most nutrient-dense (milligrams per kcal) source of calcium because of its high bioavailability and low calorie content, with some of the vegetables just noted following close behind (Fig. 9-12). The new calcium-fortified versions of orange juice and other beverages (e.g., soy milk), as well as calcium-fortified cottage cheese, breakfast cereals, breakfast bars, snacks, and certain chewable candies, also follow as close competitors. Another source of calcium is soybean curd (tofu) if it is made with calcium carbonate (check the label). Also, the bones in canned fish, such as salmon and sardines, supply calcium.

Information about calcium is mandatory on food labels. The Daily Value used to express the calcium content on food and supplement labels is 1000 milligrams.

The Adequate Intake for calcium for adults ranges from 1000 to 1200 milligrams per day and is based on the amount of calcium needed each day to offset calcium losses in urine, feces, and other routes. The Adequate Intake for young people includes an additional amount to allow for increases in bone mass during growth and development. In the United States, average calcium intakes are approximately 800 milligrams for women and 1000 milligrams for men. Thus, dietary intakes of calcium by many women, especially young women, are below the Adequate Intake, whereas intakes by most men are roughly equivalent to the Adequate Intake. It is also important for vegans to focus on eating good plant sources of calcium as well as on the total amount of calcium ingested.

To estimate your calcium intake, use the rule of 300s. Count 300 milligrams for the calcium provided by foods scattered throughout the diet. Add to that another 300 milligrams for every cup of milk or yogurt or 1.5 ounces of cheese. If you eat a lot of tofu, almonds, or sardines, or drink calcium-fortified beverages, use the second "Rate Your Plate" activity at the end of this chapter or your diet analysis software to get a more accurate calculation of your calcium intake.

## Calcium Supplements

Calcium supplements can be used by people who do not like milk or who cannot incorporate enough calcium-containing foods into their diets. Calcium carbonate,

▲ Milk is a rich as well as convenient source of calcium.

**MyPyramid: Sources of Calcium**

| Grains | Vegetables | Fruits | Oils | Milk | Meat & Beans |
|---|---|---|---|---|---|
| • Calcium-fortified snack foods<br>• Calcium-fortified flour tortillas<br>• Calcium-fortified breakfast cereals | • Greens<br>• Spinach<br>• Broccoli<br>• Green beans | • Calcium-fortified orange juice | • None | • Milk<br>• Yogurt<br>• Cheese | • Tofu<br>• Almonds<br>• Shrimp<br>• Sardines<br>• Canned salmon |

**FIGURE 9-12** ▶ Sources of calcium from MyPyramid. The height of the background color (none, 1/3, 2/3, or completely covered) within each group in the pyramid indicates the average nutrient density for calcium in that group. Overall, foods from the milk group and many fortified foods are nutrient-dense and bioavailable sources of calcium. Additional calcium-fortified foods appear in stores each year and thus will add to the food sources listed for various groups. With regard to physical activity, calcium is especially important for related muscle contraction and as well to maintain a strong skeleton to support the body.

the form found in calcium-based antacid tablets, is the most common supplement used. People should take this supplement with or just after meals in doses of about 500 milligrams so that stomach acid produced during digestion can aid with absorption of this mineral. On the other hand, a supplement containing calcium citrate, which is acidic itself, can be taken without regard to meals.

With calcium supplements, interactions with other minerals are a valid concern. Perhaps most importantly, there is some evidence that calcium supplements may decrease zinc absorption. Therefore, calcium supplements should not be taken with meals rich in zinc. An effect of calcium supplementation on iron absorption is possible; however, this appears to be small over the long term. To be safe, people should notify their physician if using a calcium supplement on a regular basis.

Some calcium supplements also contain lead. FDA has no standards for lead content in food supplements, but does plan to regulate the lead content of supplements, including calcium, in the future. Until then, it is important to avoid supplements made from bonemeal, the worst offender when it comes to lead. Tablet or liquid calcium supplements with the USP seal of approval are less likely than others to contain high concentrations of contaminants.

No form of natural calcium, such as coral calcium, is superior to typical supplement forms. People making such claims of superiority have been prosecuted by the U.S. Federal Trade Commission for false advertising.

### Upper Level for Calcium

The Upper Level for calcium intake is 2500 milligrams per day, based on the observation that greater intakes increase the risk for some forms of kidney stones. Excessive calcium intakes by some people also can cause high blood and urinary calcium concentrations, irritability, headache, kidney failure, soft tissue calcification, and decreased absorption of other minerals, as noted above.

So, which is better: calcium from food or supplements? Taking 1000 milligrams of calcium carbonate or calcium citrate daily in divided doses (about 500 milligrams per tablet) is probably safe in many instances. However, people often have difficulty adhering to a supplement regimen. If possible, modification of eating habits to include foods that are good sources of calcium is a better plan. In addition to this important mineral, foods that contain calcium also supply other vitamins, minerals, phytochemicals, and fats needed to support health. Plus, problems associated with excessive consumption of calcium are not likely when foods are one's sources of calcium.

### CONCEPT CHECK

About 99% of calcium in the body is found in the bones. Aside from its critical role in bone, calcium also functions in blood clotting, muscle contraction, nerve-impulse transmission, and cell metabolism. Calcium requires a slightly acid pH and the vitamin D hormone for efficient absorption. Factors that reduce calcium absorption include a vitamin D deficiency, large amounts of fiber (especially excess wheat bran), and old age in general. Blood calcium is regulated primarily by hormones and does not closely reflect daily intake.

Dairy products are rich food sources of calcium. Other foods, such as calcium-fortified beverages, are rich sources as well. Supplemental forms, such as calcium carbonate, are well-absorbed by most people. However, overzealous supplementation can also result in the development of kidney stones and other health problems.

## 9.8 Phosphorus (P)

Although no disease is currently associated with an inadequate phosphorus intake, a deficiency may contribute to bone loss in older women. The body efficiently absorbs phosphorus, at about 70% of dietary intake. This high absorption, plus the wide availability of phosphorus in foods, makes this mineral less important than is calcium in diet planning. The active vitamin D hormone enhances phosphorus absorption, as it does for calcium. Blood phosphorus concentration is regulated primarily by kidney excretion and also by changes in the degree of absorption.

Phosphorus is a component of enzymes, other key compounds, DNA (genetic material), cell membranes, and bone. About 85% of the body's phosphorus is inside bone. The remaining phosphorus circulates freely in the bloodstream and functions inside cells.

## Phosphorus Sources and Needs

Milk, cheese, meat, and bread provide most of the phosphorus in the adult diet. Breakfast cereals, bran, eggs, nuts, and fish are also good sources (Fig. 9-13). About 20% to 30% of dietary phosphorus comes from food additives, especially in baked goods, cheeses, processed meats, and many soft drinks with about 75 milligrams per 12-ounce ($\frac{1}{3}-$ liter) serving of soft drinks. Next time you have a soft drink, look for a listing of phosphoric acid on the label.

The RDA for phosphorus for adults over age 18 is 700 milligrams daily, based on the amount needed to maintain normal blood concentrations of phosphorus. The Daily Value used to express phosphorus content on food and supplement labels is 1000 milligrams. Adults consume about 1000 to 1600 milligrams of phosphorus per day. Thus, deficiencies of phosphorus are unlikely in healthy adults, especially because it is so efficiently absorbed.

▲ Meats are rich in phosphorus.

## Food Sources of Phosphorus

| Food Item and Amount | Phosphorus (milligrams) | Daily Value = 1000 milligrams %RDA |
|---|---|---|
| **RDA*** | 700 | 100% |
| Plain yogurt, 1 cup | 350 | 50% |
| Swiss cheese, 2 ounces | 345 | 49% |
| Almonds, ½ cup | 340 | 49% |
| Sunflower seeds, 1 ounce | 330 | 47% |
| 1% milk, 1 cup | 235 | 34% |
| Cheddar cheese, 1.5 ounces | 220 | 31% |
| Salmon, 3 ounces | 220 | 31% |
| Raisin Bran cereal, 1 cup | 215 | 31% |
| Sirloin steak, 3 ounces | 210 | 30% |
| Egg, 2 hard boiled | 200 | 29% |
| Chicken breast, 3 ounces | 180 | 26% |
| Roasted turkey, 3 ounces | 180 | 26% |
| Pot roast, 3 ounces | 170 | 24% |
| Lean ham, 3 ounces | 165 | 24% |
| American cheese, 1 slice | 155 | 22% |

**Key:**
- ☐ Grains
- ☐ Vegetables
- ☐ Fruits
- ☐ Oils
- ☐ Milk
- ☐ Meat & Beans

*For adults; See the DRI table in the back of this book for age-specific recommendations.

**FIGURE 9-13** ▶ Food sources of phosphorus compared to the RDA.

Marginal phosphorus status can be found in preterm infants, vegans, people with alcoholism, older people on nutrient-poor diets, and people with long-term bouts of diarrhea.

### Upper Level for Phosphorus

The Upper Level for phosphorus intake is 3 to 4 grams per day. Intakes greater than this impair kidney function. High intakes are especially a problem in people with certain kidney diseases. In addition, a chronically high phosphorus intake coupled with a low calcium intake can cause an imbalance in the calcium-to-phosphorus ratio in the diet, which can contribute to bone loss. This situation most likely arises when the Adequate Intake for calcium is not met, as can occur in adolescents and adults who regularly substitute soft drinks for milk or otherwise underconsume calcium.

## 9.9 Magnesium (Mg)

Magnesium is important for nerve and heart function and aids many enzyme reactions. It is found mostly in the plant pigment chlorophyll, where it functions in respiration. We normally absorb about 40% to 60% of the magnesium in our diets, but absorption efficiency can increase up to about 80% if intakes are low.

Bone contains 60% of the body's magnesium. The rest circulates in the blood and operates inside cells. Over 300 enzymes use magnesium, and many energy-yielding compounds in cells require magnesium to function properly, as does the hormone insulin.

In humans, a magnesium deficiency causes an irregular heartbeat, sometimes accompanied by weakness, muscle pain, disorientation, and seizures. Adequate magnesium intakes decrease cardiovascular disease risk by decreasing blood pressure by dilating arteries and preventing heart rhythm abnormalities. People with cardiovascular disease should closely monitor magnesium intake, especially because they are often on medications such as diuretics that reduce magnesium status. Keep in mind that a magnesium deficiency develops slowly because our bodies store it readily.

### Magnesium Sources and Needs

Rich sources for magnesium are plant products, such as whole grains (like wheat bran), broccoli, potatoes, squash, beans, nuts, and seeds (Fig. 9-14). Animal products, such as milk and meats, and even chocolate supply some magnesium, although less than the foods in the magnesium pyramid (Fig. 9-15). Two other sources of magnesium are hard tap water, which contains a high mineral content, and coffee.

The adult RDA for magnesium is about 400 milligrams per day for men and about 310 milligrams per day for women. This is based on the amount needed to offset daily losses. The Daily Value used to express magnesium content on food and supplement labels is 400 milligrams. Adult men consume an average of 320 milligrams daily, whereas women consume closer to 220 milligrams daily. This suggests that many of us should improve our intakes of magnesium-rich foods, such as whole-grain breads and cereals. The refined grain products that dominate the diets of many North Americans are poor sources of this mineral. If dietary means are not enough, a balanced multivitamin and mineral supplement containing approximately 100 milligrams of magnesium can help to close the gap between intake and needs. The typical form used in supplements (magnesium oxide) is not as well absorbed as the forms of magnesium found in foods, but still contributes to meeting magnesium needs.

Poor magnesium status is especially found among users of certain diuretics. In addition, heavy perspiration for weeks in hot climates and bouts of long-standing diarrhea or vomiting cause significant magnesium loss. Alcoholism also increases the risk of a deficiency because dietary intake may be poor and because alcohol increases

**D**iabetes and hypertension have both been linked with low levels of magnesium in the blood. However, the cause for low magnesium in people with these diseases is unclear. Research is underway to uncover the potential role of magnesium in treatment and/or prevention of these chronic diseases.

## Food Sources of Magnesium

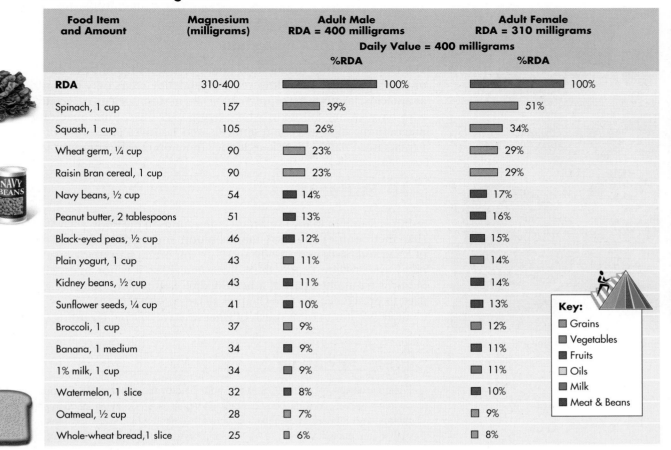

| Food Item and Amount | Magnesium (milligrams) | Adult Male RDA = 400 milligrams | Adult Female RDA = 310 milligrams |
|---|---|---|---|
| | | Daily Value = 400 milligrams | |
| | | %RDA | %RDA |
| **RDA** | 310-400 | 100% | 100% |
| Spinach, 1 cup | 157 | 39% | 51% |
| Squash, 1 cup | 105 | 26% | 34% |
| Wheat germ, ¼ cup | 90 | 23% | 29% |
| Raisin Bran cereal, 1 cup | 90 | 23% | 29% |
| Navy beans, ½ cup | 54 | 14% | 17% |
| Peanut butter, 2 tablespoons | 51 | 13% | 16% |
| Black-eyed peas, ½ cup | 46 | 12% | 15% |
| Plain yogurt, 1 cup | 43 | 11% | 14% |
| Kidney beans, ½ cup | 43 | 11% | 14% |
| Sunflower seeds, ¼ cup | 41 | 10% | 13% |
| Broccoli, 1 cup | 37 | 9% | 12% |
| Banana, 1 medium | 34 | 9% | 11% |
| 1% milk, 1 cup | 34 | 9% | 11% |
| Watermelon, 1 slice | 32 | 8% | 10% |
| Oatmeal, ½ cup | 28 | 7% | 9% |
| Whole-wheat bread, 1 slice | 25 | 6% | 8% |

**Key:**
- Grains
- Vegetables
- Fruits
- Oils
- Milk
- Meat & Beans

**FIGURE 9-14** ► Food sources of magnesium compared to the RDA for adult males and females.

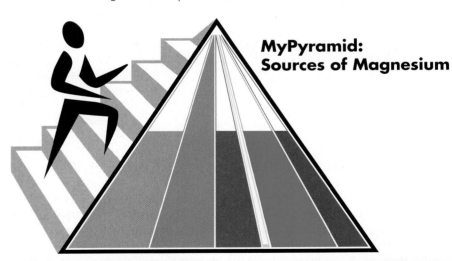

## MyPyramid: Sources of Magnesium

**FIGURE 9-15** ► Sources of magnesium from MyPyramid. The height of the background color (none, 1/3, 2/3, or completely covered) within each group in the pyramid indicates the average nutrient density for magnesium in that group. Overall, the vegetables group provides the richest sources. Whole grain choices in the grains group are also rich sources. With regard to physical activity, magnesium is especially needed for the carbohydrate metabolism that takes place in such endeavors.

| Grains | Vegetables | Fruits | Oils | Milk | Meat & Beans |
|---|---|---|---|---|---|
| • Wheat bran<br>• Wheat germ<br>• Whole-grain products | • Spinach<br>• Greens<br>• Broccoli<br>• Lima beans<br>• Potatoes<br>• Squash | • Figs<br>• Peaches<br>• Avocados<br>• Bananas<br>• Berries | • None | • Milk<br>• Yogurt | • Tofu<br>• Nuts<br>• Shrimp<br>• Kidney beans<br>• Sunflower seeds |

▲ Protein-rich foods supply sulfur in the diet.

▲ Seafood, such as scallops, is a good source of many trace minerals.

magnesium excretion in the urine. The disorientation and weakness associated with alcoholism closely resemble the behavior of people with low blood magnesium.

### Upper Level for Magnesium

The Upper Level for magnesium intake is 350 milligrams per day, based on the risk of developing diarrhea. However, this guideline refers only to nonfood sources such as antacids, laxatives, or supplements. Magnesium toxicity especially occurs in people who have kidney failure or who overuse over-the-counter medications that contain magnesium, such as certain antacids and laxatives (e.g., milk of magnesia). Older people are at particular risk, as kidney function may be compromised.

## 9.10 Sulfur (S)

Sulfur is found in many important compounds in the body, such as some amino acids (like methionine) and the vitamins biotin and thiamin. Sulfur helps in the balance of acids and bases in the body and is an important part of the liver's drug-detoxifying pathways. Proteins supply the sulfur we need, so it is not an essential nutrient *per se*. Sulfur is naturally a part of a healthy diet. Sulfur compounds (e.g., sulfites) are also used to preserve foods (see Chapter 13).

Table 9-2 summarizes much of what we have covered regarding the major minerals.

### CONCEPT CHECK

Phosphorus absorption is efficient and enhanced by the active vitamin D hormone. Urinary excretion mainly controls body content. Phosphorus aids enzyme function and is part of key metabolic compounds and cell membranes. No distinct deficiency symptoms caused by an inadequate phosphorus intake have been reported. Food sources for phosphorus include dairy products, baked goods, and meat. The RDA is met by most North Americans. An excess intake of phosphorus can compromise bone health, if sufficient calcium is not consumed, and can impair kidney function. Magnesium is required for nerve and heart function; it also aids activity for many enzymes. Food sources of magnesium are whole grains (wheat bran), vegetables, beef, coffee, beans, nuts, and seeds. People using certain diuretics and people with alcoholism are at greatest risk of developing a deficiency. Magnesium toxicity is most likely in people with kidney failure or people using certain forms of laxatives and antacids. Sulfur is a component of certain vitamins and amino acids. The protein we consume supplies sufficient sulfur for the body's needs.

## 9.11 Trace Minerals—An Overview

Information about trace minerals (also called microminerals) is perhaps the most rapidly expanding area of knowledge in nutrition. With the exceptions of iron and iodide, the importance of trace minerals to humans has been recognized only within the last 40 years. Although we need 100 milligrams or less of each trace mineral daily, they are as essential to good health as major minerals.

In some cases, discovering the importance of a trace mineral reads like a detective story, and the evidence is still unfolding. In 1961, researchers linked dwarfism among Middle Eastern villagers to a zinc deficiency. Other scientists recognized that a rare form of heart disease in an isolated area of China was linked to a selenium deficiency. In North America, some trace mineral deficiencies were first observed in the late 1960s and early 1970s when the minerals were not added to newly developed synthetic formulas used for intravenous feeding.

**TABLE 9-2** Summary of the Major Minerals

| Mineral | Major Functions | RDA, or Adequate Intake | Dietary Sources | Deficiency Symptoms | Toxicity Symptoms |
|---|---|---|---|---|---|
| Sodium | • Major positive ion of the extracellular fluid<br>• Aids nerve impulse transmission<br>• Water balance | *Age 19–50 years:* 1500 milligrams<br>*Age 51–70 years:* 1300 milligrams<br>*Age > 70 years* 1200 milligrams | • Table salt<br>• Processed foods<br>• Condiments<br>• Sauces<br>• Soups<br>• Chips | • Muscle cramps | • Contributes to hypertension in susceptible individuals<br>• Increases calcium loss in urine<br>• Upper Level is 2300 milligrams |
| Potassium | • Major positive ion of intracellular fluid<br>• Aids nerve impulse transmission<br>• Water balance | 4700 milligrams | • Spinach<br>• Squash<br>• Bananas<br>• Orange juice<br>• Milk<br>• Meat<br>• Legumes<br>• Whole grains | • Irregular heart beat<br>• Loss of appetite<br>• Muscle cramps | • Slowing of the heartbeat, as seen in kidney failure |
| Chloride | • Major negative ion of extracellular fluid<br>• Participates in acid production in stomach<br>• Aids nerve impulse transmission<br>• Water balance | 2300 milligrams | • Table salt<br>• Some vegetables<br>• Processed foods | • Convulsions in infants | • Linked to hypertension in susceptible people when combined with sodium<br>• Upper Level is 3600 milligrams |
| Calcium | • Bone and tooth structure<br>• Blood clotting<br>• Aids in nerve impulse transmission<br>• Muscle contractions<br>• Other cell functions | *Age 9–18 years:* 1300 milligrams<br><br>*Age > 18 years:* 1000–1200 milligrams | • Dairy products<br>• Canned fish<br>• Leafy vegetables<br>• Tofu<br>• Fortified orange juice (and other fortified foods) | • Increased risk of osteoporosis | • May cause kidney stones and other problems in susceptible people<br>• Upper Level is 2500 milligrams |
| Phosphorus | • Major ion of intracellular fluid<br>• Bone and tooth strength<br>• Part of various metabolic compounds<br>• Acid/base balance | *Age 9–18 years:* 1250 milligrams<br><br>*Age > 18 years:* 700 milligrams | • Dairy products<br>• Processed foods<br>• Fish<br>• Soft drinks<br>• Bakery products<br>• Meats | • Possibility of poor bone maintenance | • Impairs bone health in people with kidney failure<br>• Poor bone mineralization if calcium intakes are low<br>• Upper Level is 3 to 4 grams |
| Magnesium | • Bone formation<br>• Aids enzyme function<br>• Aids nerve and heart function | *Men:* 400–420 milligrams<br><br>*Women:* 310–320 milligrams | • Wheat bran<br>• Green vegetables<br>• Nuts<br>• Chocolate<br>• Legumes | • Weakness<br>• Muscle pain<br>• Poor heart function | • Causes diarrhea and weakness in people with kidney failure<br>• Upper Level is 350 milligrams, but refers to nonfood sources (e.g., supplements) only |
| Sulfur | • Part of vitamins and amino acids<br>• Aids in drug detoxification<br>• Acid/base balance | None | • Protein foods | • None observed | • None likely |

It is difficult to precisely define our trace mineral needs because we need only minute amounts. Highly sophisticated technology is required to measure such small amounts in both food and body tissues.

# 9.12 Iron (Fe)

Although the importance of dietary iron has been recognized for centuries, today, iron deficiency is still one of the most common nutrient deficiencies worldwide. Iron is the only nutrient for which young women have a greater RDA than do adult men. Iron is found in every living cell, adding up to about 5 grams (1 teaspoon) for the entire body.

## Absorption and Distribution of Iron

Controlling absorption is important because our bodies cannot easily eliminate excess iron once it is absorbed. The body uses several mechanisms to regulate iron absorption. Overall, iron absorption depends on its form in the food, the body's need for it, and a variety of other factors. Healthy people absorb about 18% of that present in food, whereas people with iron deficiency absorb somewhat more.

The form of iron in foods especially influences how much is absorbed. About 40% of the total iron in animal flesh is in the form of **hemoglobin** (the same form as in red blood cells) and **myoglobin** (pigment found in muscle cells). This type of iron, called **heme iron,** is absorbed about two to three times more efficiently than the simple elemental iron, called **nonheme iron.** Nonheme iron is added to grain products during the enrichment process and is also present in animal flesh, as well as in eggs, milk, vegetables, grains, and other plant foods.

Consuming heme iron and nonheme iron together increases nonheme iron absorption. A protein factor in meats may also aid nonheme absorption. Overall, eating meat with vegetables and grain products enhances the absorption of all nonheme iron present.

Vitamin C in amounts of about 75 milligrams can also increase nonheme iron absorption. Drinking a glass of orange juice when taking an iron supplement, therefore, will enhance the iron absorbed from the supplement. Consuming more foods rich in vitamin C is particularly desirable if dietary iron is inadequate or if blood iron is low. Iron use in the body is also aided by copper, as explained in the later section on copper.

In contrast, several dietary factors interfere with our ability to absorb nonheme iron. Phytic acid and other factors in grain fibers and oxalic acid in vegetables can all bind this iron and reduce its absorption. Polyphenols (tannins) found in tea also reduce nonheme iron absorption. It is a good idea to moderate intake of tannins if one has iron deficiency and keep fiber intake within current recommendations. Taking zinc supplements will also interfere with nonheme iron because zinc will compete with iron for absorption.

Overall, the most important factor influencing nonheme iron absorption is the body's need for it. Iron needs are increased during pregnancy and growth. At high altitudes, the need for iron is also increased because the lower oxygen concentration of the air causes an increase in the hemoglobin concentration of blood. During an iron deficiency state, nonheme iron absorption can increase. When iron stores are inadequate, the main protein that carries iron in blood readily binds more iron from intestinal cells and shifts it into the bloodstream. When iron stores are adequate and the iron-binding protein in the blood is fully saturated with iron, iron stays bound in the intestinal cells and little will be absorbed.

By this mechanism, under normal circumstances, iron, especially the nonheme form, is absorbed as needed. If not needed, iron stored in intestinal cells will be excreted when intestinal cells are shed at the end of their 2- to 5-day life cycle. High doses of iron can still be toxic, but absorption is carefully regulated under typical dietary conditions in most people.

**hemoglobin** The iron-containing part of the red blood cell that carries oxygen to the cells and some carbon dioxide away from the cells. The heme iron portion is also responsible for the red color of blood.

**myoglobin** Iron-containing protein that binds oxygen in muscle tissue.

**heme iron** Iron provided from animal tissues in the form of hemoglobin and myoglobin. Approximately 40% of the iron in meat is heme iron; it is readily absorbed.

**nonheme iron** Iron provided from plant sources and animal tissues other than in the forms of hemoglobin and myoglobin. Nonheme iron is less efficiently absorbed than heme iron; absorption is closely dependent on body needs.

▲ Pregnancy greatly increases iron needs, as does growth in childhood.

Most iron in the body is contained in the hemoglobin molecules of the red blood cells. Some iron is stored in the bone marrow, and a small portion goes to other body cells, such as the liver, for storage. As iron is needed, it can be mobilized from these body stores. If dietary intake is chronically inadequate, these iron stores become depleted. Only then do signs of an iron deficiency appear.

## Functions of Iron

Iron is part of the hemoglobin in red blood cells and myoglobin in muscle cells. Hemoglobin molecules in red blood cells transport oxygen ($O_2$) from the lungs to cells and assist in the return of some carbon dioxide ($CO_2$) from cells to the lungs for excretion. In addition, iron is used as part of many enzymes, some proteins, and compounds that cells use in energy production. Iron is also needed for brain and immune function and contributes to drug detoxification in the liver and to bone health.

If neither the diet nor body stores can supply the iron needed for hemoglobin synthesis, the number of red blood cells decreases in the bloodstream. The blood hemoglobin concentration also falls. Physicians use both the percentage of red blood cells (called the **hematocrit**) and the hemoglobin concentration in blood to assess iron status, along with the amount of iron and iron-containing proteins in the bloodstream. When hematocrit and hemoglobin fall, an iron deficiency is suspected. In severe deficiency, hemoglobin and hematocrit fall so low that the amount of oxygen carried in the bloodstream is decreased. Such a person has **anemia,** defined as a decreased oxygen-carrying capacity of the blood.

While there are many types of anemia, iron-deficiency anemia is the major type worldwide. About 30% of the world's population is anemic, and about half of those cases are caused by an iron deficiency. Probably about 10% of North Americans in high-risk categories have iron-deficiency anemia. This appears most often in infancy, the preschool years, and at puberty for both males and females. Growth, with accompanying expansion of blood volume and muscle mass, increases iron needs, making it difficult to consume enough iron. Women are also vulnerable during childbearing years from blood loss during menstruation. In addition, anemia is often found in pregnant women, as discussed in Chapter 14. Iron-deficiency anemia in adult men is usually caused by blood loss from ulcers, colon cancer, or hemorrhoids. Finally, athletes can develop iron-deficiency anemia, as discussed in Chapter 10.

Clinical symptoms of iron-deficiency anemia primarily include pale skin, fatigue upon exertion, poor temperature regulation, loss of appetite, and apathy. Insufficient iron for the synthesis of red blood cells and key cell compounds may cause the fatigue. Poor iron stores may also decrease learning ability, attention span, work performance, and immune status even before a person is anemic.

More North Americans have an iron deficiency without anemia than have iron-deficiency anemia. Their blood hemoglobin values are still normal, but they have no stores to draw from in times of pregnancy or illness, and basic functioning may be at decreased levels. These effects could range from having too little energy to perform everyday tasks in an efficient manner to difficulties staying alert in school or on the job.

To speed the cure of iron-deficiency anemia, a person needs to take iron supplements. A physician should determine the cause of the anemia, be it an inadequate diet or a bleeding ulcer, for example, so that the anemia does not recur. Changes in diet may prevent iron-deficiency anemia, but supplemental iron is the only reliable cure once it has developed.

## Iron Sources and Needs

Because animal sources contain some heme iron, the most bioavailable form, they are our best iron sources. The major iron sources in the adult diet are ready-to-eat breakfast cereals, animal products, and bakery items, such as bread (Figs. 9-16 and 9-17). Most of the iron in bakery items has been added to refined flour in the enrichment

**hematocrit** The percentage of blood made up of red blood cells.

**anemia** Generally refers to a decreased oxygen-carrying capacity of the blood. This can be caused by many factors, such as iron deficiency or blood loss.

▲ Red meat is a major source of iron in the North American diet. The heme iron present is better absorbed than the nonheme iron found in meats and plants.

## Food Sources of Iron

| Food Item and Amount | Iron (milligrams) | Adult Male RDA = 8 milligrams %RDA | Adult Female RDA = 18 milligrams Daily Value = 18 milligrams %RDA |
|---|---|---|---|
| **RDA** | | 100% | 100% |
| Oat bran cereal, 1 cup | 15 | 188% | 83% |
| Baked clams, 3 ounces | 14 | 175% | 78% |
| Spinach, 1 cup | 6.4 | 80% | 36% |
| Kidney beans, 1 cup | 5.3 | 66% | 29% |
| Pot roast, 4 ounces | 3.9 | 49% | 22% |
| Sirloin steak, 4 ounces | 3.8 | 48% | 21% |
| Parsley, 1 cup | 3.7 | 46% | 21% |
| Fried beef liver, 2 ounces | 3.6 | 45% | 20% |
| Shrimp, 3 ounces | 2.7 | 34% | 15% |
| Braunschweiger sausage, 1 piece | 2.7 | 34% | 15% |
| Flour tortilla, 1 | 2.4 | 30% | 13% |
| Garbanzo beans, ½ cup | 2.4 | 30% | 13% |
| Navy beans, ½ cup | 2.3 | 29% | 13% |
| Baked potato, 1 | 1.7 | 21% | 9% |
| Artichoke, 1 | 1.6 | 20% | 9% |

**Key:**
- Grains
- Vegetables
- Fruits
- Oils
- Milk
- Meat & Beans

**FIGURE 9-16** ▶ Food sources of iron compared to the RDA for adult males and females.

**FIGURE 9-17** ▶ Sources of iron from MyPyramid. The height of the background color (none, 1/3, 2/3, or completely covered) within each group in the pyramid indicates the average nutrient density for iron in that group. Overall, the meat & beans group and the grains group contain many foods that are nutrient-dense sources of iron. Still, the iron content of a food containing mostly nonheme iron is only an approximate measure of the amount delivered to body cells, as body need greatly influences the absorption of nonheme iron. With regard to physical activity, iron is especially needed as part of the hemoglobin that carries oxygen in the red blood cells to muscle (and other) cells.

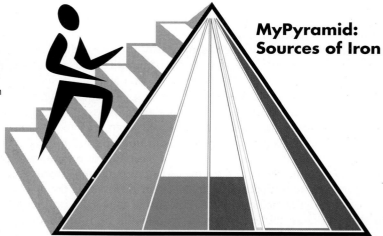

**MyPyramid: Sources of Iron**

| Grains | Vegetables | Fruits | Oils | Milk | Meat & Beans |
|---|---|---|---|---|---|
| • Whole grains<br>• Enriched grains<br>• Wheat germ<br>• Oatmeal | • Spinach<br>• Peas<br>• Potatoes<br>• Green beans<br>• Broccoli | • Peaches<br>• Prune juice<br>• Dried apricots | • None | • None | • Beef<br>• Tofu<br>• Beans<br>• Seafood<br>• Organ meats |

process. Other iron sources are spinach, peas, and legumes, but the iron is less available from these foods than from animal products.

Milk is a poor source of iron. A common cause of iron-deficiency anemia in children is an overreliance on milk, coupled with an insufficient meat intake. Total vegetarians (vegans) are particularly susceptible to iron-deficiency anemia because of their lack of dietary heme iron.

The daily adult RDA for iron for men, and for women over 50 years, is 8 milligrams. For women ages 19 to 50 years the RDA is 18 milligrams. The higher RDA for young and middle-age women is primarily because of menstrual blood loss. The variation in menstrual blood loss, and hence, loss of iron, makes it difficult to set an RDA for iron for women. Women who menstruate more heavily and longer than average may need even more dietary iron than those who have lighter and shorter flows. The Daily Value used to express iron content on food and supplement labels is 18 milligrams.

Most women do not consume 18 milligrams of iron daily. The average daily intake is closer to 13 milligrams, while in men it is about 18 milligrams per day. Women can close this gap between average daily intakes and needs by seeking out iron-fortified foods, such as ready-to-eat breakfast cereals that contain at least 50% of the Daily Value. Use of a balanced multivitamin and mineral supplement containing up to 100% of the Daily Value for iron is another option. Consuming more than that much iron is not advised unless a physician suggests otherwise (e.g., compensating for heavy menstrual loss).

## MAKING DECISIONS

### Blood Donation

The adult human body contains about 21 cups (5 liters) of blood. Blood donations are generally 2 cups (500 milliliters). Thus, a blood donor gives about a tenth of his or her total supply with each donation. Healthy people generally can donate blood two to four times a year without harmful consequences. As a precaution, blood banks first screen potential donors' blood for the presence of anemia.

## Upper Level for Iron

The Upper Level for iron is 45 milligrams per day. Higher amounts can lead to stomach irritation. Although iron overload is not as common as iron deficiency, it can be a serious result of misuse because iron can easily build up in the body and lead to toxic symptoms. Even a large single dose of 60 milligrams of iron can be life-threatening to a 1-year-old. Children are frequently victims of iron poisoning because iron pills and nutrient supplements containing iron are tempting when accessible on kitchen tables and even from cabinets.

FDA has ruled that all iron supplements must carry a warning about toxicity and that tablets with 30 milligrams of iron or more must be individually wrapped. Smaller doses of iron (but still greater than what is needed) over a long period can also cause problems. Repeated blood transfusions can also lead to iron toxicity.

**Hemochromatosis.** Iron toxicity can occur as a result of the genetic disease called hereditary **hemochromatosis.** The disease is associated with a substantial increase in iron absorption. Heme iron poses the greatest risk as body needs do not influence its absorption to a great extent. For people with this disease, iron in the body eventually builds up to dangerous amounts, especially in the blood and liver. Some iron is deposited in the muscles, pancreas, and heart. If not treated, the excess iron deposits contribute to severe organ damage, especially in the liver and heart.

Development of hereditary hemochromatosis requires that a person carry two defective copies of a particular gene. People with one defective gene and one normal

**C**hapter 8 noted that if men, in general, and older women take a multivitamin and mineral supplement, it should be low in iron or iron-free because of their increased risk for iron toxicity.

**hemochromatosis** A disorder of iron metabolism characterized by increased iron absorption and deposition in the liver and heart tissue. This eventually poisons the cells in those organs.

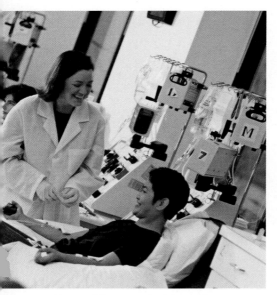

▲ Young adult women should avoid frequent blood donations because a significant amount of iron is lost in each donation. Blood donation, however, is an effective treatment for hemochromatosis.

gene, called carriers, may also absorb too much dietary iron but not to the same extent as those with two defective genes. About 5% to 10% of North Americans of Northern European descent are carriers of hemochromatosis. Approximately 1 in 250 North Americans has both hemochromatosis genes. These numbers are high considering that many physicians regard hemochromatosis as a rare disease and thus do not routinely test for it.

A reasonable approach is for you to ask to be screened for iron overload at your next visit to a physician (ask for a transferrin saturation test or a ferritin test to assess iron stores). Hemochromatosis can go undetected until a person is in their fifties or sixties, so some experts recommend screening for anyone over the age of 20. If the disease goes untreated, many organs will have become irreversibly damaged by one's middle years. If you show evidence of hemochromatosis, it would be wise to undergo therapy. This includes regular blood donations and avoidance of iron-rich foods and iron supplements (see the website www.americanhs.org).

Ideally, consent of a physician should precede any intake of iron from supplements, especially by men. When iron supplements are advised, there should be adequate follow-up so that supplementation does not exceed what is necessary. Probably the only factor keeping many people with hemochromatosis and carriers of one gene from experiencing serious effects of the disease is that they consume only a moderate amount of iron.

---

### CONCEPT CHECK

Iron is absorbed depending mostly on its form and the body's need for it. Absorption is affected by iron needs but excess iron intake can override the system, leading to toxicity. Nonheme iron absorption increases somewhat in the presence of vitamin C and meat protein and decreases in the presence of large amounts of some components of grain fiber, such as phytic acid. Iron is used in synthesizing hemoglobin and myoglobin, in supporting immune function, and in energy metabolism. An iron deficiency can cause decreased red blood cell synthesis, which can lead to anemia. It is particularly important for women of childbearing age to consume adequate iron, primarily to replace that lost in menstrual blood. Sources include red meat, pork, liver, enriched grains and cereals, and oysters. Iron toxicity usually results from a genetic disorder called hemochromatosis. This disease causes overabsorption and accumulation of iron, which can result in severe liver and heart damage. Any use of iron supplements should be supervised by a physician because of the risk of toxicity.

## 9.13 Zinc (Zn)

Zinc deficiency was first recognized in humans in the early 1960s in Egypt and Iran. Zinc deficiencies were determined to cause growth retardation and poor sexual development in some groups of people, even though the zinc content of their diets was fairly high. The zinc bioavailability of the customary diet however, was decreased by the lack of animal protein and almost exclusive use of unleavened bread. Unleavened bread is very high in phytic acid and other factors that decrease zinc bioavailability.

In North America, zinc deficiencies were first observed in the early 1970s in hospitalized patients who were fed only intravenously via total parenteral nutrition containing individual amino acids as the protein source. Zinc deficiency symptoms quickly developed because amino-acid formulas are low in trace minerals compared to whole proteins.

Like iron, zinc absorption is influenced by the foods a person ingests. About 40% of dietary zinc is absorbed, especially when animal protein sources are used and when the body needs more zinc. Most people worldwide rely on cereal grains (low in zinc) for their sources of protein and calories. This makes consuming adequate zinc

▲ Low intakes of zinc limit growth in people worldwide. On the right, an Egyptian farm boy, age 16 years old and 49 inches tall, with limited growth and sexual development associated with zinc deficiency.

a problem. In addition, high-dose calcium supplementation with meals decreases zinc absorption. Finally, zinc competes with copper and iron for absorption, and vice versa, when supplemental sources are taken.

## Functions of Zinc

Up to 200 or so enzymes, such as alcohol dehydrogenase, require zinc as a cofactor for optimal activity. Adequate zinc intake is necessary to support many bodily functions, such as:

- DNA synthesis and function
- Protein metabolism, wound healing, and growth
- Immune function (intakes in excess of the RDA do not provide any extra benefit to immune function)
- Development of sexual organs and bones
- Storage, release, and function of insulin
- Cell membrane structure and function
- Indirect antioxidant as a component of two forms of superoxide dismutase, an enzyme that aids in the prevention of oxidative damage to cells.

Other possible functions of zinc are slowing the progression of macular degeneration of the eye and reducing the risk for developing certain forms of cancer. One study has shown that megadose zinc supplements (80 milligrams per day of zinc oxide) reduces the progression of macular degeneration by 25% in people who had a moderate case of the disease. The zinc supplements worked even better when provided in combination with 400 IU of vitamin E, 500 milligrams of vitamin C, and 15 milligrams of beta-carotene. (Copper oxide [2 milligrams] was also included because zinc decreases copper absorption.) Experts suggest that adults who have evidence of moderate macular degeneration talk to their physicians and eyecare specialists about the possibility of following such a protocol.

Symptoms of adult zinc deficiency include an acnelike rash, diarrhea, lack of appetite, reduced sense of taste and smell, and hair loss. In children and adolescents with zinc deficiency, growth, sexual development, and learning ability may also be hampered.

▲ Peanuts are a plant source of zinc.

## Zinc Sources and Needs

In general, protein-rich diets are also rich in zinc. Animal foods supply almost half of an individual's zinc intake. Major sources of zinc are beef, fortified breakfast cereals, milk, poultry, and bread. As with iron, bioavailability is also important to consider for zinc. Animal foods are again our prime sources because zinc from animal sources is not bound by phytic acid. However, good plant sources of zinc—such as whole grains, peanuts, and legumes (beans)—should not be discounted. They can deliver substantial amounts of zinc to body cells (Figs. 9-18 and 9-19). Also, the form generally used in multivitamin and mineral supplements (zinc oxide) is not as well absorbed as zinc found naturally in foods, but still contributes to meeting zinc needs.

The adult RDA for zinc is 11 milligrams for men and 8 milligrams for women, based on the amount to cover daily losses of zinc. The Daily Value used to express zinc content on food and supplement labels is 15 milligrams. The average North American takes in 10 to 14 milligrams of zinc per day, with men consuming the higher values. There are no indications of moderate or severe zinc deficiencies in an otherwise healthy adult population. It is likely, however, that some North Americans—especially some women, poor children, vegans, older people, and people with alcoholism—have a marginal zinc status. These and other people who show deterioration in taste sensation, recurring infections, poor growth, or depressed wound healing should have zinc status checked.

**FIGURE 9-18** ▶ Sources of zinc from MyPyramid. The height of the background color (none, 1/3, 2/3, or completely covered) within each group in the pyramid indicates the average nutrient density for zinc in that group. Overall, the meat & beans group and the grains group contain many foods that are nutrient-dense sources of zinc. With regard to physical activity, zinc is especially needed to support muscle growth and muscle healing.

**MyPyramid: Sources of Zinc**

| Grains | Vegetables | Fruits | Oils | Milk | Meat & Beans |
|---|---|---|---|---|---|
| • Whole-grain breads and cereals<br>• Fortified breakfast cereals | • Spinach<br>• Peas<br>• Asparagus | • Avocados<br>• Dried fruit | • None | • Milk<br>• Yogurt<br>• Cheese | • Beef<br>• Eggs<br>• Beans<br>• Nuts<br>• Shellfish<br>• Poultry |

## Food Sources of Zinc

| Food Item and Amount | Zinc (milligrams) | Adult Male RDA = 11 milligrams %RDA | Adult Female RDA = 8 milligrams %RDA |
|---|---|---|---|
| **RDA** | | 100% | 100% |
| Steamed oysters, 3 | 24.9 | 226% | 311% |
| Sirloin steak, 4 ounces | 7.4 | 67% | 93% |
| Pot roast, 3 ounces | 4.6 | 42% | 58% |
| Special K cereal, 1 cup | 3.8 | 35% | 48% |
| Wheat germ, ¼ cup | 3.5 | 32% | 44% |
| Lamb chops, 3 ounces | 2.7 | 25% | 34% |
| Peanuts, ½ cup | 2.4 | 22% | 30% |
| Black-eyed peas, 1 cup | 2.2 | 20% | 28% |
| Plain yogurt, 1 cup | 2.2 | 20% | 28% |
| Lean ham, 3 ounces | 1.9 | 17% | 24% |
| Swiss cheese, 1.5 ounces | 1.7 | 15% | 21% |
| Ricotta cheese, ½ cup | 1.7 | 15% | 21% |
| Sunflower seeds, 1 ounces | 1.5 | 14% | 19% |
| Cheddar cheese, 1.5 ounces | 1.3 | 12% | 16% |
| Enriched white rice, ½ cup | 1.1 | 10% | 14% |

Daily Value = 15 milligrams

**Key:**
- ▢ Grains
- ▢ Vegetables
- ▢ Fruits
- ▢ Oils
- ▢ Milk
- ▢ Meat & Beans

**FIGURE 9-19** ▶ Food sources of zinc compared to the RDA for adult males and females.

## Upper Level for Zinc

The Upper Level for zinc is 40 milligrams per day based on the potential interference with copper metabolism. Excessive zinc intakes over time can lead to problems by interfering with copper metabolism. An increased risk for prostate cancer with high intakes of zinc is also under study. Overall, if a person uses megadose zinc supplements (e.g., to try to slow macular degeneration), he or she should be under close medical supervision and also take a supplement containing copper (2 milligrams per day). Zinc intakes over 100 milligrams per day also result in diarrhea, cramps, nausea, vomiting, and depressed immune system function, especially if intake exceeds 2 grams per day.

### MAKING DECISIONS

### Zinc and the Common Cold

Many companies are singing the praises of zinc as a cold remedy. Products such as Cold-EEZE are lozenges that contain zinc, and their claims are based largely on one study done with 100 participants. The 50 individuals in the experimental group took 13 milligrams of zinc via the lozenges every 2 hours for the duration of their symptoms. Cold symptoms subsided after 4 days in the experimental group and 7 days in the control group. Nausea was a common side effect of the zinc lozenges. Of 10 other follow-up studies, however, only half have shown beneficial results from zinc. This may be due to differences in the bioavailability of various forms of zinc. Experts also note that we also have no idea of how the zinc would treat a cold, if it did. Adults can determine if the benefits outweigh the taste. Zinc expert Dr. Ananda Prasad recommends discontinuing use of zinc lozenges after 3 to 4 days unless they are showing evidence of effectiveness. Any use of such amounts beyond a week or so is potentially dangerous.

## 9.14 Selenium (Se)

Selenium exists in many readily absorbed forms. Like zinc, selenium has an indirect antioxidant function. Selenium's best understood role is as part of the enzyme (glutathione peroxidase) that works to reduce damage to cell membranes from electron-seeking, free-radical (oxidizing) compounds. Selenium also contributes to thyroid hormone metabolism and other functions.

In Chapter 8 you saw that vitamin E helps prevent attacks on cell membranes by donating electrons to electron-seeking compounds. Thus, vitamin E and selenium work together toward the same goal. The potential for free-radical compounds to cause cancer was also discussed in Chapter 8. Although selenium could prove to have a role in prevention of cancers, such as prostate cancer, it is premature to recommend megadose selenium supplementation for this purpose. Animal studies in this area are conflicting; recent studies with humans using supplemental intakes of 200 micrograms per day have shown no benefit of selenium in cancer prevention.

Selenium deficiency symptoms in humans include muscle pain and wasting and a certain form of heart damage. In some areas of China, people develop characteristic muscle and heart disorders associated with inadequate selenium intake. Other factors probably also contribute.

## Selenium Sources and Needs

Fish, meats (especially organ meats), eggs, and shellfish are good animal sources of selenium (Fig. 9-20). Grains and seeds grown in soils containing selenium are good plant sources. Major selenium contributors to the adult diet are animal and grain

▲ Pasta made from North American wheat is generally a good source of selenium, as is any meat in the accompanying sauce.

### CRITICAL THINKING

Tammy read an article about antioxidants and their role in preventing free-radical damage to cells. When Tammy went to the drugstore to take a closer look at such supplements, she saw that selenium was one of the antioxidants in the supplements. Why does selenium deserve consideration as an antioxidant?

**FIGURE 9-20 ▶** Food sources of selenium compared to the RDA.

## Food Sources of Selenium

| Food Item and Amount | Selenium (micrograms) | Daily Value = 70 micrograms %RDA |
|---|---|---|
| **RDA*** | 55 | 100% |
| Tuna, 3 ounces | 68 | 124% |
| Sirloin steak, 5 ounces | 47 | 85% |
| Lean ham, 3 ounces | 42 | 76% |
| Clams, 3 ounces | 41 | 75% |
| Salmon, 3 ounces | 40 | 73% |
| Egg noodles, 1 cup | 35 | 64% |
| Chicken breast, 3 ounces | 20 | 36% |
| Special K cereal, 1 cup | 17 | 31% |
| Oat bran cereal, 1 cup | 14 | 25% |
| Whole-wheat bread, 1 slice | 10 | 18% |
| Cooked oatmeal, 1 cup | 10 | 18% |
| White bread, 1 slice | 9 | 16% |
| Raisin bran cereal, 1 cup | 4 | 7% |

**Key:**
- ■ Grains
- ■ Vegetables
- ■ Fruits
- □ Oils
- ■ Milk
- ■ Meat & Beans

*For adults; See DRI table in the back of this book for gender- and age-specific recommendations.

products. We eat a varied diet of foods supplied from many geographic areas, so it is unlikely that low soil selenium in a few locations will mean inadequate selenium in our diets.

The RDA for selenium is 55 micrograms per day for adults. This intake maximizes the activity of selenium-dependent enzymes. The Daily Value used to express selenium content on food and supplement labels is 70 micrograms. In general, adults meet the RDA, consuming on average 105 micrograms of selenium each day.

## Upper Level for Selenium

The Upper Level for selenium is 400 micrograms per day for adults. This is based on overt signs of selenium toxicity, such as hair loss.

▲ Iodide deficiency leads to a goiter. The mother on the left has a goiter, but is otherwise normal. Her daughter on the right has a goiter and is mentally retarded, deaf, and mute.

### CONCEPT CHECK

Zinc functions as a cofactor for many enzymes (including those that act as antioxidants) and is important for growth, cell membrane structure and function, immune function, and sense of taste. Beef, seafood, and whole grains are good food sources. As in the case of iron, zinc absorption is regulated according to the body's needs for the mineral. If taken in excess amounts, zinc competes with copper for absorption. Selenium activates an enzyme that helps change electron-seeking, free-radical (oxidizing) compounds into less toxic compounds so these do not attack and break down cell membranes. By helping to dismantle the free-radical compounds, selenium works toward the same goal as vitamin E in providing antioxidant protection to the body. A selenium deficiency results in muscle and heart disorders. Animal products and grains are good selenium sources; however, the selenium content in plants depends on the selenium concentration in the soil. The misuse of both selenium and zinc supplements can readily lead to toxic results.

# 9.15 Iodide (I)

Iodine in foods is found in an ion form, called iodide. During World War I, a link was discovered between a deficiency of iodide and the production of a **goiter,** an enlarged thyroid gland. Men drafted from areas such as the Great Lakes Region of the United States had a much higher rate of goiter than did men from some other areas of the country. The soils in these areas have low iodide contents. In the 1920s, researchers in Ohio found that low doses of iodide given to children over a 4-year period could prevent goiter. That finding led to the addition of iodide to salt beginning in the 1920s.

Today, many nations such as Canada require iodide fortification of salt. In the United States, salt can be purchased either iodized or plain. Iodized salt is clearly marked on the label of a package of salt. Some areas of Europe, such as northern Italy, have low levels of iodide in soil, but have yet to adopt an iodide fortification program. People in these areas, especially women, still suffer from goiter, as do people in areas of Latin America, the Indian subcontinent, Southeast Asia, and Africa. About 2 billion people worldwide are at risk of iodide deficiency, and approximately 800 million of these people have suffered the widespread effects of the deficiency. Eradication of iodide deficiency is a goal of many health-related organizations worldwide.

## Function of Iodide

The thyroid gland actively accumulates and traps iodide from the bloodstream to support thyroid hormone synthesis. Thyroid hormones are synthesized using iodide and the amino acid tyrosine. These hormones help regulate metabolic rate and promote growth and development throughout the body, including the brain.

If a person's iodide intake is insufficient, the thyroid gland enlarges as it attempts to take up more iodide from the bloodstream. This eventually leads to goiter. Simple goiter is a painless condition, but if uncorrected can lead to pressure on the trachea (windpipe), which may cause difficulty in breathing. Although iodide can prevent goiter formation, it does not significantly shrink a goiter once it has formed. Surgical removal may be required in severe cases.

If a woman has an iodide-deficient diet during the early months of her pregnancy, the fetus suffers iodide deficiency because the mother's body uses up the available iodide. The infant then may be born with short length and develop mental retardation. The stunted growth and mental retardation that results is known as **cretinism.** Cretinism appeared in North America before iodide fortification of table salt began. Today, cretinism still appears in Europe, Africa, Latin America, and Asia.

## Iodide Sources and Needs

Saltwater fish, seafood, iodized salt, dairy products, and grain products contain various forms of iodide (Fig. 9-21). Sea salt found in health-food stores, however, is not a good source because the iodide is lost during processing.

The RDA for iodide for adults is 150 micrograms to support thyroid gland function. This is the same as the Daily Value used to express iodide content on food and supplement labels. A half teaspoon of iodide-fortified salt (about 2 grams) supplies that amount. Most adults consume more iodide than the RDA—an estimated 190 to 300 micrograms daily, not including that from use of iodized salt at the table. The iodide in our diets adds up because dairies and fast-food restaurants use it as a sterilizing agent, bakeries use it as a dough conditioner, food producers use it as part of food colorants, and it is added to salt. There is concern, however, that vegans may not consume enough unless iodized salt is used.

## Upper Level for Iodide

The Upper Level for iodide is 1.1 milligrams per day. When high amounts of iodide are consumed, thyroid hormone synthesis is inhibited, as in a deficiency. This can appear

**goiter**  An enlargement of the thyroid gland; this is often caused by insufficient iodide in the diet.

**cretinism**  The stunting of body growth and poor mental development in the offspring that results from inadequate maternal intake of iodide during pregnancy.

**FIGURE 9-21** ▶ Food sources of Iodide compared to the RDA.

**Food Sources of Iodide**

| Food Item and Amount | Iodide (micrograms) | Daily Value = 150 micrograms %RDA |
|---|---|---|
| **RDA*** | 150 | 100% |
| Iodized table salt, ½ cup | 195 | 130% |
| Plain yogurt, ½ cup | 87 | 56% |
| Buttermilk, 1 cup | 60 | 40% |
| 1% milk, 1 cup | 59 | 39% |
| Luna bar, 1 | 38 | 25% |
| Soy protein bar, 1 | 38 | 25% |
| Egg, 1 large | 35 | 23% |
| 1% cottage cheese, ½ cup | 28 | 19% |
| Mozzarella cheese, 1 ounce | 10 | 7% |

Key:
- Grains
- Vegetables
- Fruits
- Oils
- Milk
- Meat & Beans

*For adults; See the DRI table in the back of this book for gender- and age-specific recommendations.

in people who eat a lot of seaweed, because some seaweeds contain as much as 1% iodide by weight. Total iodide intake then can add up to 60 to 130 times the RDA.

## 9.16  Copper (Cu)

Copper is involved in the metabolism of iron by functioning in the formation of hemoglobin and transport of iron. A copper-containing enzyme aids in the release of iron from storage. Copper is needed by enzymes that create cross-links in connective tissue proteins. Copper is also needed by other enzymes, such as those that defend the body against free-radical (oxidizing) compounds (e.g., a form of superoxide dismutase) and those that act in the brain and nervous system. Finally, copper performs in immune system function, blood clotting, and blood lipoprotein metabolism. About 12% to 75% of dietary copper is absorbed, with higher intakes associated with lower absorption. Absorption takes place primarily in the stomach and upper small intestine. Copper is excreted in the bile made by the liver and released by the gallbladder. Phytates, fiber, as well as zinc and iron supplements, may all interfere with copper absorption. Symptoms of copper deficiency include a form of anemia, low white blood cell count, bone loss, poor growth, and some forms of cardiovascular disease.

### Copper Sources and Needs

Copper is found primarily in liver, seafood, cocoa, legumes, nuts, seeds, and whole-grain breads and cereals (Fig. 9-22).

The RDA for copper is 900 micrograms daily for adults, based on the amount needed for activity of copper-containing proteins and enzymes in the body. The Daily Value used to express copper content on food and supplement labels is 2 milligrams. The average adult intake is about 1 to 1.6 milligrams per day. Women generally consume the smaller amount. The form of copper typically found in multivitamin and mineral supplements (copper oxide) is not readily absorbed. It is best to rely on food sources to meet copper needs. The copper status of adults appears to be good, though we lack sensitive measures to determine copper status.

The groups most likely to develop copper deficiencies are preterm infants, infants recovering from semistarvation on a milk-dominated diet (a poor source of copper),

▲ Seafood is one source of copper in the diet

## Food Sources of Copper

| Food Item and Amount | Copper (micrograms) | Daily Value = 2 milligrams %RDA |
|---|---|---|
| **RDA*** | 900 | 100% |
| Fried beef liver, 3 ounces | 3800 | 422% |
| Power bar, 1 | 700 | 78% |
| Walnuts, ½ cup | 600 | 67% |
| Kidney beans, ½ cup | 500 | 56% |
| Lobster, 3 ounces | 400 | 44% |
| Molasses, 3 tablespoons | 300 | 33% |
| Sunflower seeds, 2 tablespoons | 300 | 33% |
| Shrimp, 3 ounces | 300 | 33% |
| Raisin Bran cereal, 1 cup | 300 | 33% |
| Great Grains cereal, 1 cup | 300 | 33% |
| Black-eyed peas, ½ cup cooked | 200 | 22% |
| Wheat germ, ¼ cup | 200 | 22% |
| Milk chocolate, 1 ounce | 110 | 12% |
| Whole-wheat bread, 1 slice | 80 | 9% |

**Key:**
- Grains
- Vegetables
- Fruits
- Oils
- Milk
- Meat & Beans

*For adults, See the DRI table in the back of this book for gender- and age-specific recommendations.

**FIGURE 9-22** ▶ Food sources of copper compared to the RDA.

and people recovering from intestinal surgery (during which time copper absorption decreases). Recall that a copper deficiency can also result from overzealous supplementation of zinc, because zinc and copper compete with each other for absorption.

### Upper Level for Copper

The Upper Limit for copper is 10 milligrams per day. High doses of copper can cause toxicity, including vomiting, at single doses of greater than 10 milligrams. Other effects, such as liver toxicity, are also possible with megadose uses.

## 9.17 Fluoride (F)

The fluoride ion ($F^-$) is the form of this trace mineral essential for human health. Like chlorine, fluorine ($F_2$) is a poisonous gas. This link was found as dentists in the early 1900s noticed a lower rate of dental caries (cavities) in the southwestern United States. These areas contained high amounts of fluoride in the water. The amounts of fluoride were sometimes so high that small spots on the teeth, called **mottling,** appeared. Even though mottled teeth were quite discolored, they contained very few dental caries. After experiments showed that fluoride in the water did indeed decrease the rate of dental caries, controlled fluoridation of water in parts of the United States began in 1945.

Those who grew up drinking fluoridated water generally have 40% to 60% fewer dental caries than people who did not drink fluoridated water as children. Dentists can provide topical fluoride treatments, and schools can provide fluoride tablets, but it is much less expensive and more reliable to add fluoride to a community's drinking

**mottling** The discoloration or marking of the surface of teeth from fluorosis.

▲ Example of mottling in a tooth caused by overexposure to fluoride.

▲ Fluoridated water is responsible for much of the decrease in dental caries throughout North America.

water. State and private water sources do not always contain enough fluoride, however. When in doubt, contact your local water plant or have the water in your home analyzed for fluoride content. If it is less than 1 part fluoride per million parts of water (e.g., 1 milligram per kilogram or liter of water), talk to your dentist about the best means to obtain the fluoride.

### Functions of Fluoride

Dietary fluoride consumed during childhood, when bones and teeth are developing, aids the synthesis of a form of tooth enamel that strongly resists acid. Therefore, teeth become resistant to dental caries. Fluoride also inhibits metabolism and growth of the bacteria that cause dental caries, and fluoride present in saliva directly inhibits tooth demineralization and enhances tooth remineralization.

Fluoride applied to the surface of the teeth by dentists or from toothpaste or rinses adds additional protection against dental caries. Thus, people of all ages benefit from the topical effects of fluoride, whether they consumed fluoridated water or fluoride supplements as children.

### Fluoride Sources and Needs

Tea, seafood, seaweed, and some natural water sources are the only good food sources of fluoride. Most of our fluoride intake comes from fluoride added to drinking water and toothpaste and from fluoride treatments performed by dentists. Fluoride is not added to bottled water. Therefore, if people such as children consume bottled water, they won't receive fluoride from such water intake.

The Adequate Intake for fluoride for adults is 3.1 to 3.8 milligrams per day. This range of intake provides the benefits of resistance to dental caries without causing ill effects. Typical fluoridated water contains about 1 milligram per liter, which works out to about 0.25 milligrams per cup.

### Upper Level for Fluoride

The Upper Level for fluoride is set at 1.3 to 2.2 milligrams per day for young children, and 10 milligrams per day for children over 9 years of age and adults, based on skeletal and tooth damage seen with higher doses. If children swallow large amounts of fluoridated toothpaste as part of daily tooth care, tooth mottling may develop. Not swallowing toothpaste and limiting the amount used to "pea" size are the best ways to prevent this problem. In addition, children under 6 years should have toothbrushing supervised by an adult. Fluoride-related mottling only occurs during tooth development, so adults do not develop mottling from their fluoride exposure.

### CONCEPT CHECK

Iodide is vital for the synthesis of thyroid hormones. A prolonged insufficient intake causes the thyroid gland to enlarge, resulting in a goiter. The use of iodized salt in North America has virtually eliminated this condition. Copper functions mainly in iron and free-radical metabolism, and in the cross-bonding of connective tissue. A deficiency can result in a type of anemia. Good food sources of copper are seafoods, legumes, nuts, dried fruits, and whole grains. Fluoride becomes incorporated into teeth during development and is present in salivary secretions. The presence of this trace mineral makes teeth resistant to acid and bacterial growth, in turn reducing development of dental caries. Fluoride also aids in remineralization of teeth once decay begins. Most of us receive adequate amounts of fluoride from that added to drinking water and toothpaste. An excessive fluoride intake during tooth development can lead to spotted (i.e., mottled) teeth and possibly bone damage.

# 9.18 Chromium (Cr)

The importance of chromium in human diets has been recognized only in the past 40 years. The most-studied function of chromium is the maintenance of glucose uptake into cells. Our current understanding is that chromium enters the cell and acts to enhance the transport of glucose across the cell membrane by aiding insulin function. Marginal to low chromium intakes may contribute to an increased risk for developing type 2 diabetes, but opinions are mixed on the true degree of this effect.

A chromium deficiency is characterized by impaired blood glucose control and elevated blood cholesterol and triglycerides. The mechanism by which chromium influences cholesterol metabolism is not known but may involve enzymes that control cholesterol synthesis. Chromium deficiency originally appeared in people maintained on intravenous total parenteral nutrition solutions not supplemented with chromium and in children with malnutrition. Sensitive measures of chromium status are not available, so marginal chromium deficiencies may go undetected.

## Chromium Sources and Needs

Specific data regarding the chromium content of various foods are limited, and most food composition tables do not include values for this trace mineral. Egg yolks, whole grains (bran), organ meats, other meats, mushrooms, nuts, and beer are good sources. Yeast is also a source. The amount of chromium in foods is closely tied to the local soil content of chromium. To provide yourself with a good chromium intake, regularly choose whole grains in place of mostly refined grains.

The Adequate Intake for chromium is 25 to 35 micrograms per day, based on the amount present in a balanced diet. The Daily Value used to express chromium content on food and supplement labels is about 4 times greater at 120 micrograms. Average adult intakes in North America are estimated at about 30 micrograms per day, but could be somewhat higher.

No Upper Level for chromium has been set because toxicity for that present in foods has not been observed. Chromium toxicity, however, has been reported in people exposed to industrial waste and in painters who use art supplies with a high chromium content. Liver damage and lung cancer can result. Use of any supplement should normally not exceed the Daily Value set unless supervised by a physician, because of the risk of toxicity.

▲ Mushrooms are a good source of chromium.

**C**hromium supplements have been touted to help with exercise-induced increases in muscle mass and weight loss. Careful research, however, does not support this assertion.

# 9.19 Manganese (Mn)

The mineral manganese is easily confused with magnesium. Not only are their names similar, but they also often substitute for each other in metabolic processes. Manganese is needed by enzymes used in carbohydrate metabolism and by a form of superoxide dismutase used in free-radical metabolism. Manganese is also important in bone formation.

No human deficiency symptom is associated with a low manganese intake. Our need for manganese is low, and our diets tend to be adequate in this trace mineral.

Good food sources of manganese are nuts, rice, oats and other whole grains, beans, and leafy vegetables. The Adequate Intake for manganese is 1.8 to 2.3 milligrams to offset daily losses. Average intakes generally fall within this range. The Daily Value used to express manganese content on food and supplement labels is 2 milligrams.

▲ Nuts are rich in manganese.

## Upper Level for Manganese

Manganese is toxic at high doses. The Upper Level is 11 milligrams per day and is based on the development of nerve damage.

## 9.20 Molybdenum (Mo)

Several human enzymes use molybdenum. No molybdenum deficiency has been noted in people who consume normal diets, though deficiency symptoms have appeared in people maintained on intravenous total parenteral nutrition feedings. These symptoms include increased heart and respiration rates, night blindness, mental confusion, edema, and weakness.

Good food sources of molybdenum include milk and milk products, beans, whole grains, and nuts. The RDA for molybdenum is 45 micrograms to offset daily losses. The Daily Value used to express molybdenum content on food and supplement labels is 75 micrograms. Our daily intakes average 75 to 110 micrograms.

### Upper Level for Molybdenum

The Upper Level for molybdenum is 2 milligrams per day. When consumed in high doses, molybdenum causes toxicity in laboratory animals, resulting in weight loss and decreased growth.

Table 9-3 summarizes what we have covered regarding the trace minerals, as does Figure 9-23. Figure 9-24 summarizes the various contributions of groups in MyPyramid to mineral needs.

**FIGURE 9-23 ▶** Water and minerals are involved in many processes in the body.

**TABLE 9-3**  A Summary of Key Trace Minerals

| Mineral | Major Functions | RDA, or Adequate Intake | Dietary Sources | Deficiency Symptoms | Toxicity Symptoms |
|---|---|---|---|---|---|
| Iron | • Components of hemoglobin and other key compounds used in respiration<br>• Immune function<br>• Cognitive development | *Men:* 8 milligrams<br><br>*Premenopausal Women:* 18 milligrams | • Meats<br>• Seafood<br>• Broccoli<br>• Peas<br>• Bran<br>• Enriched breads | • Fatigue<br>• Anemia<br>• Low blood hemoglobin values | • Liver and heart damage (extreme cases)<br>• GI upset<br>• Upper Level is 45 milligrams |
| Zinc | • Required for nearly 200 enzymes<br>• Growth<br>• Immunity<br>• Alcohol metabolism<br>• Sexual development<br>• Reproduction<br>• Antioxidant protection | *Men:* 11 milligrams<br><br>*Women:* 8 milligrams | • Seafood<br>• Meats<br>• Greens<br>• Whole grains | • Skin rash<br>• Diarrhea<br>• Decreased appetite and sense of taste<br>• Hair loss<br>• Poor growth and development<br>• Poor wound healing | • Reduced copper absorption<br>• Diarrhea<br>• Cramps<br>• Depressed immune function<br>• Upper Level is 40 milligrams |
| Selenium | • Part of an antioxidant system | 55 micrograms | • Meats<br>• Eggs<br>• Fish<br>• Seafood<br>• Whole grains | • Muscle pain<br>• Weakness<br>• Form of heart disease | • Nausea<br>• Vomiting<br>• Hair loss<br>• Weakness<br>• Liver disease<br>• Upper Level is 400 micrograms |
| Iodide | • Component of thyroid hormones | 150 micrograms | • Iodized salt<br>• White bread<br>• Saltwater fish<br>• Dairy products | • Goiter<br>• Mental retardation<br>• Poor growth in infancy when mother is iodide deficient during pregnancy | • Inhibition of thyroid gland function<br>• Upper Level is 1.1 milligrams |
| Copper | • Aids in iron metabolism<br>• Works with many antioxidant enzymes<br>• Involved with enzymes of protein metabolism and hormone synthesis | 900 micrograms | • Liver<br>• Cocoa<br>• Beans<br>• Nuts<br>• Whole grains<br>• Dried fruits | • Anemia<br>• Low white blood cell count<br>• Poor growth | • Vomiting<br>• Nervous system disorders<br>• Upper Level is 8–10 milligrams |
| Fluoride | • Increases resistance of tooth enamel to dental caries | *Men:* 3.8 milligrams<br><br>*Women:* 3.1 milligrams | • Fluoridated water<br>• Toothpaste<br>• Tea<br>• Seaweed<br>• Dental treatments | • Increased risk of dental caries | • Stomach upset<br>• Mottling (staining) of teeth during development<br>• Bone pain<br>• Upper Level is 10 milligrams for adults |
| Chromium | • Enhances insulin action | 25–35 micrograms | • Egg yolks<br>• Whole grains<br>• Pork<br>• Nuts<br>• Mushrooms<br>• Beer | • High blood glucose after eating | Caused by industrial contamination, not dietary excesses, so no Upper Level has been set |
| Manganese | • Cofactor of some enzymes, such as those involved in carbohydrate metabolism<br>• Works with some antioxidant systems | 1.8–2.3 milligrams | • Nuts<br>• Oats<br>• Beans<br>• Tea | None observed in humans | • Nervous system disorders<br>• Upper Level is 11 milligrams |
| Molybdenum | • Aids in action of some enzymes | 45 micrograms | • Beans<br>• Grains<br>• Nuts | None observed in healthy humans | • Poor growth in laboratory animals<br>• Upper Level is 2 milligrams |

**FIGURE 9-24** ▶ Certain groups of MyPyramid are especially rich sources of various minerals. This is true for the minerals listed. Each mineral may also be found in other groups, but in lower amounts. Other trace minerals are also present in moderate amounts in many groups. With regard to the grains group, whole-grain varieties are the richest sources of most trace minerals listed.

## MyPyramid: Sources of Minerals

| Grains | Vegetables | Fruits | Oils | Milk | Meat & Beans |
|---|---|---|---|---|---|
| • Sodium chloride<br>• Calcium (fortified products)<br>• Phosphorus<br>• Magnesium<br>• Iron<br>• Zinc<br>• Copper<br>• Selenium<br>• Chromium | • Potassium<br>• Magnesium | • Potassium<br>• Boron | • None | • Calcium<br>• Phosphorus<br>• Zinc | • Sodium chloride (processed foods)<br>• Potassium<br>• Phosphorus<br>• Magnesium<br>• Selenium<br>• Iron<br>• Zinc<br>• Copper |

## 9.21 Other Trace Minerals

Although a variety of other trace minerals is found in humans, many of them have not yet been shown to be required. The list of minerals in this category includes boron, nickel, vanadium, arsenic, and silicon. Widespread deficiency symptoms in humans have never been noted, probably because typical diets provide adequate amounts of these minerals and they are needed by very few enzymes and metabolic systems. Their potential for toxicity should make one question any supplementation not supervised by a physician. These trace minerals may achieve more importance as more research is reported.

### CONCEPT CHECK

Chromium contributes to insulin function. The amount of chromium found in food depends on chromium content of the soil on which it was grown. Meats, whole grains, and egg yolks are good sources. Manganese is a component of bone and is used by many enzymes, including those involved in glucose production. Our need for manganese is low, so deficiencies are rare. Nuts, rice, oats, and beans are good food sources. Molybdenum is another trace mineral required by a few enzymes. Good sources include milk, beans, whole grains, and nuts. Deficiencies have appeared only in people nourished by unsupplemented total parenteral nutrition. The needs for some other trace minerals—such as boron, nickel, arsenic, and vanadium—have not been fully established in humans. If required, these minerals are needed in such small amounts that our current diets are probably adequate sources of them.

# Maintaining a Healthy Blood Pressure

Among North Americans, an estimated 1 in 5 adults has hypertension. Over the age of 65, the number rises to 1 in every 2 adults. Only about half of cases are being treated. Blood pressure is expressed by two numbers. The higher number represents systolic blood pressure, the pressure in the arteries when the heart muscle is contracting and pumping blood into the arteries. Optimal systolic blood pressure is 120 millimeters of mercury (mm Hg) or less. The second value is diastolic blood pressure, the artery pressure when the heart is relaxed. Optimal diastolic blood pressure is 80 mm Hg or less. Elevations in both systolic and diastolic blood pressure are strong predictors of disease (Fig. 9-25).

Hypertension is defined as sustained systolic pressure exceeding 139 mm Hg or diastolic blood pressure exceeding 89 mm Hg. Most cases of hypertension (about 95% of cases) have no clear-cut cause. It is described as primary, or essential (i.e., essential hypertension). Kidney disease, sleep-disordered breathing (sleep apnea), and other causes often lead to the other 5% of cases, known as secondary hypertension. African-Americans are more likely than Caucasians to develop hypertension and to do so earlier in life.

Unless blood pressure is periodically measured, the development of hypertension is easily overlooked. Thus, it's described as a silent disorder, because it usually does not cause symptoms.

## Why Control Blood Pressure?

Blood pressure needs to be controlled mainly to prevent cardiovascular disease, kidney disease, strokes and related declines in brain function, poor blood circulation in the legs, problems with vision, and sudden death. These conditions are much more likely to be found in individuals with hypertension than in people with normal blood pressure. Smoking and elevated blood lipoproteins make these diseases even more likely. Individuals with hypertension need to be diagnosed and treated as soon as possible, as the condition generally progresses to a more serious stage over time and even resists therapy if it persists for years.

## Causes Of Hypertension

A family history of hypertension is a risk factor, especially if both parents have (or had) the problem. In addition, blood pressure usually increases as a person ages. Some increase is caused by atherosclerosis. As plaque builds up in the arteries, the arteries become less flexible and cannot expand. When vessels remain rigid, blood pressure remains high. Eventually, the plaque begins to decrease the blood supply to the kidneys, decreasing their ability to control blood volume and, in turn, blood pressure.

An enzyme secreted by the kidneys and some hormone-like compounds are designed to maintain a healthy blood pressure. When blood pressure is elevated, the effect of these compounds can be reduced by anti-hypertension medications.

Overweight people have six times greater risk of having hypertension than lean people. Overall, obesity is considered the number one lifestyle factor related to hypertension.

**FIGURE 9-25** ▶ The cut-off for hypertension is 140/90 mm Hg, but the risk of heart attacks and stroke precedes the rise in blood pressure.

## How High is High?

If your systolic and diastolic pressures fall into different categories, your risk depends on the higher category

SYSTOLIC | DIASTOLIC

**Hypertension (High)**

140 | 90

**Pre-hypertension**

120 | 80

**Normal**

Numbers (in millimeters of mercury) apply to adults who aren't taking drugs to lower their blood pressure.

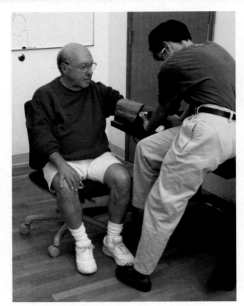

▲ Older adults are particularly at risk of hypertension.

This is especially the case in minority populations. Additional blood vessels develop to support excess tissue in overweight and obese individuals, and these extra miles of associated blood vessels increase work by the heart and also blood pressure. Hypertension is linked to obesity if elevated blood insulin levels result from insulin-resistant adipose cells. This increased insulin level increases sodium retention in the body and accelerates atherosclerosis. A weight loss of as little as 10 to 15 pounds often can help treat hypertension.

Inactivity is considered the number two lifestyle factor related to hypertension. If an obese person can engage in regular physical activity (at least 5 days per week for 30 to 60 minutes) and lose weight, blood pressure often returns to normal.

Third, excess alcohol intake is responsible for about 10% of all cases of hypertension, especially in middle-aged males and among African-Americans in general. When hypertension is caused by excessive alcohol intake, it is usually reversible. A sensible alcohol intake for people with hypertension is two or fewer drinks per day for men and one or no drinks per day for women and all older adults. Did you recognize that this is the same recommendation given in the 2005 Dietary Guidelines for Americans? Some studies suggest that such a minimal alcohol intake may reduce the risk of ischemic stroke. These data, however, should not be used to encourage alcohol use.

In some people, particularly African-Americans and older overweight persons, blood pressure is especially sensitive to sodium. In these people, excess salt leads to fluid retention by the kidney and a corresponding increase in blood volume, which therefore increases blood pressure. It is not clear whether the sodium ion or the chloride ion is most responsible for the effect. Still, as reviewed in this chapter, if one reduces sodium intake, chloride intake naturally falls; the opposite is also true. For the most part, a recommendation to consume less sodium is equivalent to a call for less salt in the diet. Only some North Americans are very susceptible to increases in blood pressure from salt intake, so it is only the number four lifestyle factor related to hypertension. It is unfortunate that salt intake receives the major portion of public attention with regard to hypertension. Efforts to prevent hypertension should also focus on obesity, inactivity, and alcohol abuse.

## Other Minerals and Blood Pressure

Minerals such as calcium, potassium, and magnesium also deserve attention when it comes to prevention and treatment of hypertension. Studies show that a diet rich in these minerals and low in salt can decrease blood pressure within days of beginning this type of diet, especially among African-Americans. The response is even similar to that seen with

▲ Opting for the fruits, vegetables, and low-fat foods recommended by the DASH diet represents a sound approach to nutrition for most people regardless of hypertension risk.

commonly used medications. The diet is called the Dietary Approaches to Stop Hypertension (DASH) diet (Table 9-4). The diet, rich in calcium, phosphorus, and magnesium and low in salt, takes a standard MyPyramid food plan and adds 1 to 2 extra vegetables and fruits servings and a serving of nuts, seeds, or legumes (beans) 4 to 5 days of the week. In DASH studies, participants also consumed no more than 3 grams of sodium and no more than one to two alcoholic drinks per week. A DASH 2 diet trial tested three daily sodium intakes (3300 milligrams, 2400 milligrams, and 1500 milligrams). People showed a steady decline in blood pressure on the DASH diet as sodium

**TABLE 9-4** What Is the DASH Diet?

The DASH diet is characterized as low in fat and sodium and rich in fruits, vegetables, and low-fat dairy products. Here is the breakdown:

| Per Day | Per Week |
|---|---|
| 6–8 servings of grains and grain products | 4–5 servings of nuts, seeds, or legumes |
| 4–5 servings of fruit | 5 servings of sweets and added sugars |
| 4–5 servings of vegetables | |
| 2–3 servings of low-fat or fat-free dairy products | |
| 2 or less servings of meats, poultry, and fish | |
| 2–3 servings of fats/oils | |

intake declined. Over all, the DASH diet is seen as a total dietary approach to treating hypertension. It is not clear which of the many healthful practices of this diet are responsible for the fall in blood pressure.

Other studies also show a reduction in stroke risk among people who consume a diet rich in fruits, vegetables, and vitamin C (recall that fruits and vegetables are rich vitamin C sources). Overall, a diet low in salt and rich in low-fat and fat-free dairy products, fruits, vegetables, whole grains, and some nuts can substantially reduce hypertension and stroke risk in many people, especially those with hypertension.

## Medications to Treat Hypertension

Diuretic medications are one class of drugs used to treat hypertension. These "water pills" work to reduce blood volume (and therefore blood pressure) by increasing fluid output in the urine. Other medications act by slowing heart rate or by causing relaxation of blood vessels. A combination of two or more medications is commonly required to treat hypertension that does not respond to diet and lifestyle therapy.

## Prevention of Hypertension

Many of the risk factors for hypertension and stroke are controllable, and appropriate lifestyle changes can reduce a person's risk (Fig. 9-26). Experts also recommend that those with hypertension lower blood pressure through diet and lifestyle changes before resorting to blood pressure medications.

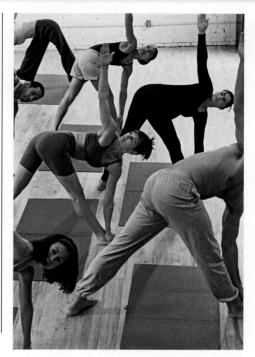

▲ Regular, moderate physical activity contributes to better blood pressure control.

**FIGURE 9-26** ▶ What works? If your blood pressure is high, here's how much lifestyle changes should lower it.

| Advice | Details | Drop in Systolic Blood Pressure |
| --- | --- | --- |
| **Lose excess weight** | For every 20 pounds you lose | 5 to 20 points |
| **Follow a DASH diet** | Eat a lower-fat diet rich in vegetables, fruits, and low-fat dairy foods | 8 to 14 points |
| **Exercise daily** | Get 30 minutes a day of aerobic activity (such as brisk walking) | 4 to 9 points |
| **Limit sodium** | Eat no more than 2400 mg per day (1500 mg per day is better) | 2 to 8 points |
| **Limit alcohol** | Have no more than 2 drinks per day for men, 1 drink per day for women<br><br>(1 drink = 12 oz. beer, 5 oz. wine, or 1.5 oz. 80-proof whiskey) | 2 to 4 points |

Source: *The Seventh Report of the Joint National Committee on Prevention, Detection, Evaluation, and Treatment of High Blood Pressure, May 2003* (www.nhibl.hih.gov/guidelines/hypertension).

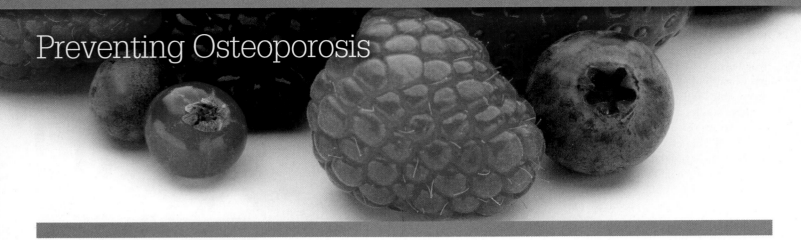

# Preventing Osteoporosis

Widespread media attention has made it almost impossible for women to ignore osteoporosis. The crippling effect this disease has on older persons is now recognized as a major medical problem. Osteoporosis leads to approximately 1.5 million bone fractures per year in the United States, usually in the hip, spine, or wrist, leading to about $18 billion per year in health-care costs. Many older women in North America experience osteoporosis-related fractures in their lifetimes.

The slender, inactive woman who smokes is most susceptible to osteoporosis, but any person who lives long enough can suffer from the disease, including men. About 25% of women older than age 50 develop osteoporosis. Among people older than age 80, osteoporosis becomes the rule—not the exception. The spine fractures commonly found in women with osteoporosis cause considerable pain and deformity and decrease physical ability (Fig. 9-27); hip fractures are seen in both men and women with osteoporosis. Not only is this disease debilitating, it also can be fatal. Almost one-quarter of older persons who suffer hip fractures die within the first year from fracture-related complications.

## Bone Structure and Strength

To better understand the role calcium plays in bone health and osteoporosis, it is important to understand how bone is constructed. Visual observation of the cross-sections of a bone reveals two primary bone structural types: **cortical bone** and **trabecular bone.** These interact

within each bone to form an engineering marvel of strength (Fig. 9-28).

The entire outer surface of all bones is composed of cortical bone, also known as compact bone, which is very dense. The shafts of long bones, such as those of the arm, are almost entirely cortical bone. Trabecular bone, also known as spongy bone, is found in the ends of the long bones, inside the spinal vertebrae, and inside the flat bones of the pelvis.

**cortical bone** Dense, compact bone that comprises the outer surface and shafts of bone; also called compact bone.

**trabecular bone** The spongy, inner matrix of bone, found primarily in the spine, pelvis, and ends of bones; also called spongy or cancellous bone.

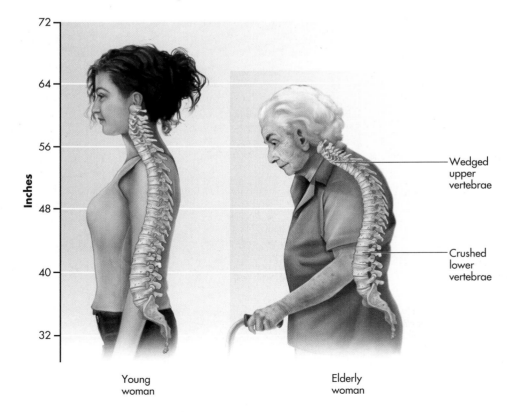

Young woman          Elderly woman

**FIGURE 9-27 ▶** Normal and osteoporotic woman. Osteoporotic bones have less substance, so osteoporosis generally leads to loss of height, distorted body shape, fractures, and loss of teeth. Monitoring changes in adult height is one way to detect early evidence of osteoporosis.

Trabecular bone is porous and forms an internal scaffolding-like network for a bone. It supports the outer cortical shell of the bone, especially in heavily stressed areas, such as joints. Like the beams of a building, the trabecular bone adds strength to the bone without the added weight of a more solid matrix. It is especially critical for the horizontal and vertical trabecular beams to extend continuously—without breaks. Any break in the trabecular beams weakens the support system of a bone and increases the risk for bone fracture. Once these beams are broken, there is no way to rebuild them. This is why it is so important to limit bone loss as people age.

## Bone Mass Is Related to Age and Gender

Bone strength depends on a person's **bone mass** and **bone mineral density**. The more bone there is, and especially the more densely packed bone crystals are in the bone, the stronger the bone structure. Rapid and continual bone growth and calcification occur throughout the adolescent years, ultimately resulting in what is called *peak bone mass*. In the adolescent growth spurt, bone mass is increasing at the rate of about 8.5% per year. Small increases in bone mass then continue between 20 and 30 years of age.

The ultimate amount of bone built by a person is clearly dependent on gender; race; familial patterns seen in the mother and father; and probably other genetically–determined factors, such as the degree of calcium absorption. In addition, men have higher bone mass than women, and African-Americans have heavier skeletons than Caucasians. As a direct consequence, men and African-Americans in general have a somewhat lower risk of osteoporosis-related fractures than do other populations. Slender,

**bone mass** Total mineral substance (such as calcium or phosphorus) in a cross section of bone, generally expressed as grams per centimeter of length.

**bone mineral density** Total mineral content of bone at a specific bone site divided by the width of the bone at that site, generally expressed as grams per cubic centimeter.

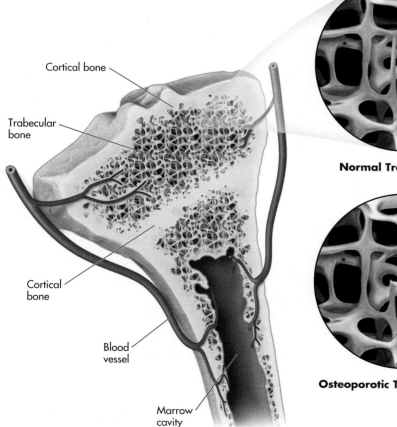

Cortical bone

Trabecular bone

Cortical bone

Blood vessel

Marrow cavity

**Normal Trabecular Bone**

**Osteoporotic Trabecular Bone**

**FIGURE 9-28 ▶** Cortical and trabecular bone. Cortical bone forms the shafts of bones and their outer mineral covering. Trabecular bone supports the outer shell of cortical bone in various bones of the body, as in the illustration. Note how the osteoporotic bone has much less trabecular bone. This leads to a more fragile bone and is not reversible to any major extent with current therapies.

small-framed Caucasian and Asian women show the lowest bone mass values. Peak bone mass is also related to dietary intake of calcium and other nutrients, such as protein, phosphorus, vitamin A, vitamin D, vitamin K, magnesium, iron, zinc, and copper (Table 9-5). Thus, osteoporosis is not just a calcium story—many minerals and other nutrients play a part.

Bone mass varies among young adults; some have much denser bone than others, perhaps because they built more bone when they were young. Some people also may adapt more easily to lower-calcium diets. People who have developed more bone by early adulthood can sustain greater age-related bone loss with less risk of osteoporosis compared with those who reach adulthood with less bone. Thus, osteoporosis is considered to be a "pediatric disease" with geriatric (old age) consequences (Fig. 9-29).

For women, bone loss begins at age 30 and proceeds slowly and continuously to menopause (approximately age 50). It often speeds up at menopause with the decline in estrogen output and continues at a high rate of loss for the next 10 years. By age 65 to 70, the rate of bone loss falls to about the same rate as before menopause. In men, bone loss is slow and steady from around age 30. Overall, this bone loss in both males and females progresses without noticeable short-term symptoms.

## Osteoporosis

Failure to maintain enough bone mass in the body is generally diagnosed as osteoporosis. Bone loss can also be caused by the vitamin D deficiency disease osteomalacia, the use of certain medications (such as cortisol and anti-seizure drugs), and cancer.

All women age 65 and older should be screened for this disease. The most accurate screening involves a **dual energy X-ray absorptiometry (DEXA) bone scan** of the whole body. (Somewhat less accurate instruments measure bone mineral density at a single site, such as the heel.) Younger women with associated risk factors are advised to do the same at menopause, because the results of the screening would help them decide whether medical therapy for bone loss is an appropriate plan for menopause.

▲ Women with osteoporosis typically develop abnormal curvature of the upper spine. This results from fractures of the weakened vertebrae. This can lead to both physical and emotional pain.

**Dual energy X-ray absorptiometry (DEXA) bone scan**  Method to measure bone density that uses small amounts of X-ray radiation. The ability of a bone to block the path of the radiation is used as a measure of bone density at that bone site.

**TABLE 9-5** Diet and Lifestyle Factors Associated with Bone Status

| Positive Diet and Lifestyle Factors | Call to Action |
|---|---|
| Adequate diet containing a sufficient amount of protein, calcium, phosphorus, magnesium, potassium, vitamin A, vitamin C, vitamin D, vitamin K, iron, zinc, copper, fluoride, and manganese and possibly boron. | • Follow MyPyramid with special emphasis on adequate amounts of fruits, vegetables, and low-fat and fat-free dairy products.<br>• Consider use of fortified foods (or supplements) to make up for specific nutrient shortfalls, such as vitamin D and calcium. |
| Healthy body weight | • Be aware that low body weight (slender figure) increases the risk for low bone mass. |
| Normal menses | • During childbearing years, seek medical advice if menses cease (such as in cases of anorexia nervosa or extreme athletic training).<br>• Women at menopause and beyond should consider use of current medical therapies to reduce bone loss linked to the fall in estrogen output. |
| Weight-bearing physical activity | • Perform weight-bearing activity as this contributes to bone maintenance, whereas bed rest and a sedentary lifestyle lead to bone loss. Strength training is especially helpful for bone maintenance. |
| **Negative Diet and Lifestyle Factors** | **Call to Action** |
| Excessive intake of protein, phosphorus, sodium, caffeine, wheat bran, and alcohol | • Moderate intake of these dietary constituents is recommended. Problems primarily arise if adequate calcium is not consumed.<br>• Excessive soft drink consumption is especially discouraged. |
| Smoking | • Smoking lowers estrogen output in women, so smoking cessation is advised. |

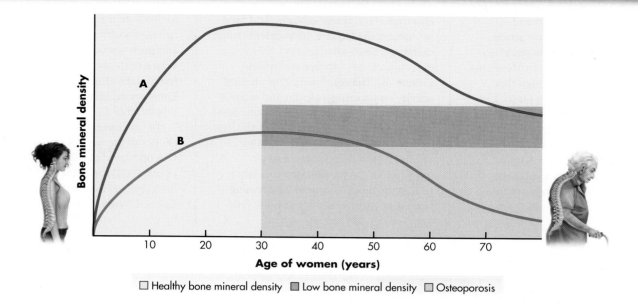

**FIGURE 9-29** ▶ The relationship between peak bone mass and the ultimate risk of developing osteoporosis and related bone fractures
• **Woman A** had developed a high peak bone mass by age 30. Her bone loss was slow and steady between ages 30 and 50 and sped up somewhat after age 50 because of the effects of menopause. At age 75, the woman had a healthy bone mineral density value and did not show evidence of osteoporosis.
• **Woman B** with low peak bone mass experienced the same rate of bone loss as woman A. By age 50, she already had low mineral density and by age 70 kyphosis and spinal fractures had occurred.
Given the low calcium intakes that are common among young women today, line B is a sobering reality. Following a diet and lifestyle pattern that contributes to maximal bone mineral density can help women follow line A and significantly reduce their risk of developing osteoporosis.

For the DEXA test, a person will lie down on his or her back on a padded table while a movable imaging arm moves over the length of the body. The procedure usually takes about 20 to 30 minutes. The ability of a bone to block the path of radiation is used as a measure of bone mineral density at that bone site. A low dose of radiation is used for the DEXA—about one-tenth of the exposure from a chest X-ray.

From the DEXA measurement of bone density, a T score is generated, which compares the observed bone density to that of a person at peak bone strength (e.g., age 30). Such a T score is interpreted as follows:

| | |
|---|---|
| 0 to −1 | Normal |
| −1 to −2.4 | Low bone mineral density |
| −2.5 or lower | Osteoporosis |

## Preventing Osteoporosis

Once osteoporosis is present, there is no way to repair the bone damage. This makes prevention important. Strategies for prevention of osteoporosis vary based on age and individual risk factors.

For young women, osteoporosis prevention involves three main elements. First, young women should focus on meeting calcium, vitamin D, protein, and other nutrient needs. Second, because the hormones of regular menstruation contribute to bone maintenance in young women, any sign of menstrual irregularities is reason to see a physician. Some non-menstruating female athletes and other women with irregular menstrual cycles (e.g., women with anorexia nervosa) already exhibit low bone mineral density. Third, an active lifestyle that includes weight-bearing physical activity is also important. The increased muscle mass that stems from weight-bearing physical activity is associated with greater bone mineral density, as muscle keeps tension on bone. However, physical activity cannot prevent the bone loss associated with irregular menstruation. Even though female athletes may do plenty of weight-bearing physical activity, they should be closely monitored by a physician if they have irregular menstrual cycles.

Once they have reached menopause, women should discuss approved osteoporosis-related therapies with a physician. The most common medications are **bisphosphonates**. These lessen bone breakdown. Estrogen replacement previously was the most common therapy for bone protection, but it has been shown to increase the risks in some women for cardiovascular disease and strokes, as well as cancers of the breast and ovaries. Estrogen replacement is now reserved for short-term use to control menopausal symptoms in most cases.

**bisphosphonates** Compounds primarily composed of carbon and phosphorus that bind to bone mineral and in turn reduce bone breakdown. Examples are alendronate (Fosamax), risedronate (Actonel), and ibandronate (Boniva).

As age advances, both men and women need to take preventive action. First, adults need to accurately track their height. A decrease of more than 1½ inches from young adult height is a sign that significant bone loss is taking place.

Older adults especially need to stay physically active—including some weight-bearing and resistance activities—and they should meet the Adequate Intake for calcium set for their particular age. Regular sun exposure and the consumption of food sources of vitamin D are also important. If sun exposure and food sources are inadequate, supplements containing up to 25 micrograms (1000 IU) of vitamin D are appropriate (review Chapter 8). The combination of physical activity and meeting calcium and vitamin D needs are most likely to limit bone loss in some areas of the body, such as the hip.

At any age, smoking and excessive alcohol intake decrease bone mass. Smoking lowers the estrogen concentration in the blood in women, increasing bone loss. Alcohol is toxic to bone cells for both men and women, and alcoholism is probably a major undiagnosed and unrecognized cause of osteoporosis. Excessive intakes of phosphorus, caffeine, and sodium are also discouraged. These are especially problematic when insufficient calcium is consumed.

To find out more about osteoporosis, check out the website of the National Osteoporosis Foundation (www.nof.org) or call (800)464-6700. Another helpful website is that of the National Dairy Council (www.nationaldairycouncil.org).

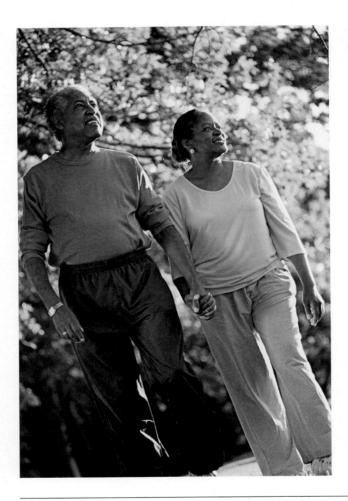

◀ Regular, moderate, weight-bearing physical activity contributes to bone health in both men and women. Note that men can also develop osteoporosis as they age.

## Case Study Giving Up Milk

Ashley, a 19-year-old sophomore in college, recently gave up drinking milk. She thought this would help her stay slim by avoiding the calories in milk. Ashley's mother is concerned about her diet change. One of her primary concerns is the future risk of osteoporosis. Ashley also started smoking, and her only physical activity is practice for Women's Glee Club.

Ashley's typical diet consists of oatmeal made with water, a banana and a cup of fruit juice for breakfast. At midmorning, she buys a snack cake or candy bar from the vending machine. At lunch, she has pasta with vegetables, bread with olive oil, a side salad, 1 ounce of mixed nuts, and a soft drink. For dinner, she has a chicken or hamburger sandwich along with mixed vegetables and another soft drink. As an evening snack, she has some cookies and hot tea.

Answer the following questions about Ashley's situation and check your responses in Appendix A.

1. What nutrients are low in Ashley's typical diet that put her at risk of osteoporosis in the future?
2. Which of Ashley's lifestyle factors contribute to this increased risk of osteoporosis?
3. Is there any evidence that consumption of milk or other dairy products leads to weight gain?
4. What changes to her current diet could reduce the risk of osteoporosis and also help Ashley maintain her weight?
5. What lifestyle changes (other than the dietary changes) could Ashley make to decrease her risk of osteoporosis and maintain a healthy weight?

## Summary

1. Water constitutes 50% to 70% of the human body. Its unique chemical properties enable it to dissolve substances as well as serve as a medium for chemical reactions, temperature regulation, and lubrication. Water also helps regulate the acid-base balance in the body.

2. For adults, daily water needs are estimated at 9 cups (women) to 13 cups (men) per day; fluid intake contributes to meeting this need.

3. Overall, the United States enjoys a safe water supply. However, people with poor immune status should boil water used for drinking and cooking to avoid waterborne illness. Bottled water can be used, but reliance on it to meet fluid needs is costly to the environment and our personal budgets.

4. Minerals are categorized based on the amount we need per day. If we require greater than 100 milligrams of a mineral per day, it is considered a major mineral; otherwise it is considered a trace mineral.

5. Many minerals are vital for sustaining life. For humans, animal products are the most bioavailable sources of most minerals. Supplements of minerals exceeding 100% of the Daily Values listed on the label should be taken only under a physician's supervision. Toxicity and nutrient interactions are especially likely if the Upper Level (when set) is exceeded on a long-term basis.

6. Sodium, the major positive ion found outside cells, is vital in fluid balance and nerve impulse transmission. The North American diet provides abundant sodium through processed foods and table salt. About 10% to 15% of the adult population, such as overweight people, is especially sodium-sensitive and at risk for developing hypertension from consuming excessive sodium.

Potassium, the major positive ion found inside cells, has a similar function to sodium. Milk, fruits, and vegetables are good sources.

Chloride is the major negative ion found outside cells. It is important in digestion as part of stomach acid and in immune and nerve functions. Table salt supplies most of the chloride in our diets.

Calcium forms a part of bone structure and plays a role in blood clotting, muscle contraction, nerve transmission, and cell metabolism. Calcium absorption is enhanced by stomach acid and the active vitamin D hormone. Dairy products are important calcium sources. Women are particularly at risk for not meeting calcium needs.

Phosphorus aids enzyme function and forms part of key metabolic compounds, cell membranes, and bone. It is efficiently absorbed, and deficiencies are rare, although there is concern about possible poor intake by some older women. Good food sources are dairy products, bakery products, and meats.

Magnesium is a mineral found mostly in plant food sources. It is important for nerve and heart function and as an activator for many enzymes. Whole-grain breads and cereals (bran portion), vegetables, nuts, seeds, milk, and meats are good food sources. Sulfur is incorporated into certain vitamins and amino acids.

Iron absorption depends mainly on the form of iron present and the body's need for it. Heme iron from animal sources is better absorbed than the nonheme iron obtained primarily from plant sources. Consuming vitamin C or meat simultaneously with nonheme iron increases absorption. Iron operates mainly in synthesizing hemoglobin and myoglobin and in the action of the immune system. Women are at great risk for developing iron deficiency, which decreases blood hemoglobin and hematocrit. When this condition is severe, iron-deficiency anemia develops. This decreases the amount of oxygen carried in the blood. Iron toxicity usually results from a genetic disorder called hemochromatosis. This disease causes overabsorption

and accumulation of iron, which can result in severe liver and heart damage.

Zinc aids in the action of up to 200 enzymes important for growth, development, cell membrane structure and function, immune function, antioxidant protection, wound healing, and taste. A zinc deficiency results in poor growth, loss of appetite, reduced sense of taste and smell, hair loss, and a persistent rash. Zinc is best absorbed from animal sources. The richest sources of zinc are oysters, shrimp, crab, and beef. Good plant sources are whole grains, peanuts, and beans.

An important role of selenium is decreasing the action of free-radical (oxidizing) compounds. In this way, selenium acts along with vitamin E in providing antioxidant protection. Muscle pain, muscle wasting, and a form of heart damage may result from a selenium deficiency. Meats, eggs, fish, and shellfish are good animal sources of selenium. Good plant sources include grains and seeds.

Iodide forms part of the thyroid hormones. A lack of dietary iodide results in the development of an enlarged thyroid gland or goiter. Iodized salt is a major food source.

Copper is important for iron metabolism, cross-linking of connective tissue, and other functions, such as enzymes that provide antioxidant protection. A

copper deficiency can result in a form of anemia. Copper is found mainly in liver, seafood, cocoa, legumes, and whole grains.

Fluoride as part of regular dietary intake or toothpaste use makes teeth resistant to dental caries. Most North Americans receive the bulk of their fluoride from fluoridated water and toothpaste.

Chromium aids in the action of the hormone insulin. Egg yolks, meats, and whole grains are good sources of chromium. Manganese and molybdenum are used by various enzymes. One enzyme that uses manganese provides antioxidant protection. Clear deficiencies in otherwise healthy people are rarely seen for any of these three nutrients. Human needs for other trace minerals are so low that deficiencies are uncommon.

7. Controlling weight and alcohol intake; exercising regularly; decreasing salt intake; and ensuring adequate potassium, magnesium, and calcium in the diet all can play a part in controlling high blood pressure.

8. Women are particularly at risk for developing osteoporosis as they age. Numerous lifestyle and medical options can help reduce this risk, including an adequate intake of calcium and many other minerals.

## Study Questions

1. Approximately how much water do you need each day to stay healthy? Identify at least two situations that increase the need for water. Then list three sources of water in the average person's diet.

2. What is the relationship between sodium and water balance, and how is that relationship monitored as well as maintained in the body?

3. Identify four factors that influence the bioavailability of minerals from food.

4. What are two similarities and differences between sodium and potassium? Sodium and chloride?

5. In terms of total amounts in the body, calcium and phosphorus are the first and second most abundant minerals, respectively. What function do these minerals have in common?

6. What are the best food sources for zinc and copper?

7. Describe the symptoms of iron-deficiency anemia and explain possible reasons they occur.

8. Which trace minerals are lost from cereal grains when they are refined? Are any of these nutrients replaced by enrichment?

9. Describe the chief functions of fluoride, copper, and chromium in the body.

10. What are the practical consequences of the Daily Values on food and supplement labels exceeding the RDA or Adequate Intake for many trace minerals?

# Check Your Knowledge

Answers to the following questions are found below.

1. Dietary heme iron is derived from
   a. elemental iron in food.
   b. animal flesh.
   c. breakfast cereal.
   d. vegetables.

2. Chloride is
   a. a component of hydrochloric acid.
   b. an intracellular fluid ion.
   c. a positively charged ion.
   d. converted to chlorine in the intestinal tract.

3. Minerals involved in fluid balance are
   a. calcium and magnesium.
   b. copper and iron.
   c. calcium and phosphorus.
   d. sodium and potassium.

4. In a situation where there is an insufficient intake of dietary iodide, the thyroid-stimulating hormone promotes the enlargement of the thyroid gland. This condition is called
   a. Graves' disease.
   b. goiter.
   c. hyperparathyroidism.
   d. cretinism.

5. Ninety-nine percent of the calcium in the body is found in
   a. intracellular fluid.
   b. bones and teeth.
   c. nerve cells.
   d. the liver.

6. At the end of long bones, inside the spinal vertebrae, and inside the flat bones of the pelvis, is a spongy type of bone known as _____ bone.
   a. osteoclastic
   b. osteoblastic
   c. trabecular
   d. compact

7. Which compartment contains the greatest amount of body fluid?
   a. intracellular
   b. extracellular
   c. They contain the same amount.

8. The primary function of sodium is to maintain
   a. bone mineral content.
   b. hemoglobin concentration.
   c. immune function.
   d. fluid distribution.

9. Hypertension is defined as a blood pressure greater than
   a. 110/60.
   b. 120/65.
   c. 140/90.
   d. 190/80.

10. Which of the following individuals are most likely to develop osteoporosis?
    a. premenopausal women athletes
    b. women taking estrogen replacement therapy
    c. slender, inactive women who smoke
    d. women who eat a lot of high-fat dairy products

Answer Key: 1. b, 2. a, 3. d, 4. b, 5. b, 6. c, 7. a, 8. d, 9. c, 10. c

# Further Readings

1. ADA Reports: Position of the American Dietetic Association: The impact of fluoride on health. *Journal of the American Dietetic Association* 105:1620, 2005.

   *The American Dietetic Association reaffirms that fluoride is an important element for all mineralized tissues in the body. Appropriate fluoride in-take is beneficial to bone and tooth health.*

2. America's pressure cooker. *Nutrition Action HealthLetter* July/August:3, 2005.

   *This article summarizes three recent trials (TOHP II, TONE, and DASH) on diet and hypertension and provides lists of the sodium content of several common foods and of many restaurant foods. Healthy lifestyle changes are outlined, including losing excess weight, following a DASH diet, and limiting sodium and alcohol. Finally, foods rich in potassium are suggested as a "sodium antidote."*

3. Appel LJ and others: Dietary approaches to prevent and treat hypertension: A scientific statement from the American Heart Association. *Hypertension* 47:296, 2006.

   *Latest advice from the American Heart Association on diet and hypertension. Key preventive factors are to avoid overweight and inactivity and to moderate alcohol and salt intake.*

4. Cook NR and others: Joint effects of sodium and potassium intake on subsequent cardiovascular disease. *Archives of Internal Medicine* 169: 32, 2009.

   *This study suggests that potassium is effective in lowering blood pressure. Furthermore, the combination of a higher intake of potassium and a lower intake of sodium seems to be more effective than either on its own in reducing the risk of cardiovascular disease. The sodium-to-potassium ratio in subjects' urine was a stronger predictor of cardiovascular disease than sodium or potassium alone.*

5. Elliott P and others: Dietary phosphorus and blood pressure: International study of macro- and micro-nutrients and blood pressure. *Hypertension* 51:669, 2008.

   *Little attention has been given to the possible effects of phosphorus intake on blood pressure. The results of this study indicate that increased phosphorus intake, as well as calcium and magnesium intake, have the potential to lower blood pressure. This may be an important recommendation for prevention and control of prehypertension and hypertension.*

6. Flores-Mateo G and others: Selenium and coronary heart disease: A meta-analysis. *American Journal of Clinical Nutrition* 84 (4):762, 2006.

   *The meta-analysis of studies of selenium and coronary heart disease show an inverse association between selenium concentrations and coronary heart disease risk in observational studies. The validity of this association is uncertain because the results of observational studies have been misleading for other antioxidants. Only a few randomized trials that have addressed the efficacy of selenium supplementation on* cardiovascular health and their findings are inconclusive. Large ongoing trials are needed to establish if low selenium concentrations are a cardiovascular disease risk factor. Therefore, selenium supplements are not currently recommended for cardiovascular disease prevention.

7. Food and Nutrition Board, Institute of Medicine: *Dietary Reference Intakes for water, potassium, sodium, chloride, and sulfate.* Washington, DC: National Academies Press, 2004.

   *Dietary standards for water, potassium, sodium, and chloride are discussed. The rationale used to derive the Adequate Intakes, as well as the Upper Levels, are presented along with information on function, intake, and deficiency.*

8. Food and Nutrition Board, Institute of Medicine: *Dietary Reference Intakes for calcium, phosphorus, magnesium, vitamin D, and fluoride.* Washington, DC: National Academies Press, 1997.

   *Dietary standards for many major minerals are discussed. The rationale used to set RDA or Adequate Intakes and Upper Levels for these nutrients is discussed in detail.*

9. Food and Nutrition Board, Institute of Medicine: *Dietary Reference Intakes for vitamin A, vitamin K, arsenic, boron, chromium, copper, iodine, iron, manganese, molybdenum, nickel, silicon, vanadium, and zinc.* Washington, DC: National Academies Press, 2001.

   *Dietary standards for many trace minerals are discussed. The rationale used to set RDA or Adequate Intakes and Upper Levels for these nutrients is discussed in detail.*

10. Havas S and others: The urgent need to reduce sodium consumption. *Journal of the American Medical Association* 298:1439, 2007.

    *In the US, 77% of sodium comes from processed and restaurant foods, with many processed foods containing 1000 mg or more per serving. There is a general consensus that sodium levels should be reduced substantially in processed and restaurant foods. Policy developments and possible solutions to address this problem are presented in this article.*

11. Heaney RP: Absorbability and utility of calcium in mineral waters. *American Journal of Clinical Nutrition* 84(2):371, 2006.

    *Published absorbability and utility of high-calcium mineral waters is summarized and integrated in this article. The absorbability of all the high-calcium mineral waters was equal to or slightly better than milk calcium. The utility of calcium as measured by increased urinary*

calcium, decreased serum parathyroid hormone, decreased bone resorption biomarkers, and protection of bone mass indicated that a significant quantity of calcium was absorbed. High-calcium mineral waters, therefore, appear to provide useful quantities of bioavailable calcium.

12. Hollenberg NK: The influence of dietary sodium on blood pressure. *Journal of the American College of Nutrition* 25:240S, 2006.

    *Evidence relating salt intake to blood pressure is reviewed. The merit of mandating a reduction in salt intake is discussed. The author indicates that the evidence supporting such a policy is inconsistent and small. The importance of antihypertensive drugs is emphasized.*

13. Jackson RD and others: Calcium plus vitamin D supplementation and the risk of fractures. *New England Journal of Medicine* 354 (7):669, 2006.

    *Postmenopausal women, 50 to 79 years of age, who were enrolled in a Women's Health Initiative (WHI) clinical trial were assigned to receive 1000 mg of elemental calcium as calcium carbonate with 400 IU of vitamin $D_3$ daily or a placebo. The occurrence of fractures and bone density was determined for 7 years. Calcium with vitamin D supplementation resulted in a small but significant increase in hip bone density, but did not significantly reduce hip fracture and increased the risk of kidney stones.*

14. Lanham-New SA. The balance of bone health: Tipping the scales in favor of potassium-rich, bicarbonate-rich foods. *Journal of Nutrition* 137:1725, 2008.

    *About 10 million Americans have osteoporosis. This review article summarizes the current evidence linking potassium-rich, bicarbonate-rich foods (e.g., fruits and vegetables) to osteoporosis prevention.*

15. Lippman SM and others: Effect of selenium and vitamin E on risk of prostate cancer and other cancers: The Selenium and vitamin E cancer prevention trial (SELECT). *Journal of the American Medical Association* 301:39, 2009.

    *The results of this study showed no benefit to taking a supplement of selenium or vitamin E alone or in combination for the prevention of prostate cancer, colon cancer, lung cancer, all cancers, and cardiovascular disease and for overall survival.*

16. Palmer S: Busting bottled water. *Today's Dietitian* 9(12): 60, 2007.

    *This article highlights several reasons why consumers have been wrong in assuming that*

bottled water is always better than tap water. The ecological, environmental, and economic problems with relying on bottled water for our fluids needs. The laws regulating bottled and tap water are also compared, suggesting that bottled water is generally not safer and healthier than tap water. The author recommends that we drink more water, but do it from the tap.

17. Park Y and others: Dairy food, calcium, and risk of cancer in the NIH-AARP diet and health study. *Archives of Internal Medicine* 169: 391, 2009.

    *The 7-year study of 493,000 older men and women provides evidence that diets rich in calcium may lower risk of total cancer and cancers of the digestive system, especially colorectal cancer. Benefits were mostly associated with foods high in calcium, rather than calcium supplements. Getting more than the recommended 1200 milligrams of calcium for older people did not result in greater cancer protection.*

18. Popkin BM and others: A new proposed guidance system for beverage consumption in the United States. *American Journal of Clinical Nutrition* 83:529, 2006.

    *Drinking water is recommended as the preferred beverage to fulfill water needs, with tea, coffee, and low-fat and skim milk also ranked high. The Beverage Guidance Panel suggests that beverages with no or few calories should be consumed more often than calorie-containing beverages. An intake of 98 fluid ounces is recommended daily for a person consuming 2200 calories.*

19. Reid IR and others: Randomized controlled trial of calcium in healthy older women. *American Journal of Medicine* 119(9):777, 2006.

    *In this study of postmenopausal women receiving 1 g/day as calcium citrate over 5 years, height loss was reduced by calcium but constipation was more common. The authors conclude that calcium results in a sustained reduction in bone loss and turnover, but its effect on fracture is uncertain.*

20. Van Dam RM and others: Dietary calcium and magnesium, major food sources, and risk of type 2 diabetes in U.S. black women. *Diabetes Care* 29:2238, 2006.

    *Magnesium and calcium intakes have been inversely associated with risk of type 2 diabetes in predominantly white populations. The results of this study of 41,186 participants of the Black Women's Health Study indicated that a diet high in magnesium-rich foods, particularly whole grains, is associated with a significantly lower risk of type 2 diabetes in U.S. black women.*

## I. How High Is Your Sodium Intake?

Complete this questionnarie to evaluate your sodium habits with respect to typically rich sources.

| How Often Do You... | Rarely | Occasionally | Often | Regularly (Daily) |
|---|---|---|---|---|
| 1. Eat cured or processed meats, such as ham, bacon, sausage, frankfurters, and other luncheon meats? | ☐ | ☐ | ☐ | ☐ |
| 2. Choose canned or frozen vegetables with sauce? | ☐ | ☐ | ☐ | ☐ |
| 3. Use commercially-prepared meals, main dishes, or canned or dehydrated soups? | ☐ | ☐ | ☐ | ☐ |
| 4. Eat cheese, especially processed cheese? | ☐ | ☐ | ☐ | ☐ |
| 5. Eat salted nuts, popcorn, pretzels, corn chips, or potato chips? | ☐ | ☐ | ☐ | ☐ |
| 6. Add salt to cooking water for vegetables, rice, or pasta? | ☐ | ☐ | ☐ | ☐ |
| 7. Add salt, seasoning mixes, salad dressings, or condiments—such as soy sauce, steak sauce, catsup, and mustard—to foods during preparation or at the table? | ☐ | ☐ | ☐ | ☐ |
| 8. Salt your food before tasting it? | ☐ | ☐ | ☐ | ☐ |
| 9. Ignore labels for sodium content when buying foods? | ☐ | ☐ | ☐ | ☐ |
| 10. When dining out, choose obviously salty sauces or foods? | ☐ | ☐ | ☐ | ☐ |

The more checks you put in the "often" or "regularly" columns, the higher your dietary sodium intake is. However, not all the habits in the table contribute the same amount of sodium. For example, many natural cheeses such as cheddar are relatively moderate in sodium, whereas processed cheeses and cottage cheese are much higher. To moderate sodium intake, choose lower-sodium foods from each food group more often and balance high-sodium food choices with low-sodium ones.

Adapted from *USDA Home and Garden Bulletin* No. 232–6, April 1986.

## II. Working for Denser Bones

Osteoporosis and related low bone mass affect many adults in North America, especially older women. One-third of all women experience fractures because of this disease, amounting to about 2 million bone fractures per year.

Osteoporosis is a disease you can do something about. Some risk factors can't be changed, but others, such as a poor calcium intake, can. Is this true for you? To find out, complete this tool for estimating your current calcium intake. For all the following foods, write the number of servings you eat in a day. Total the number of servings in each category and then multiply the total number of servings by the amount of calcium for each category. Finally, add the total amount for each food category to estimate your calcium intake for that day.

Does your intake meet your AI set for calcium?

| Food | Serving Size | Number of Servings | Calcium (mg) | Total Calcium (mg) |
|------|-------------|--------------------|--------------| -------------------|
| Plain low-fat yogurt | 1 cup | _____ | | |
| Fat-free dry milk powder | 1/2 cup | _____ | | |
| | Total servings | _____ | × 400 | = _____ mg |
| Canned sardines (with bones) | 3 ounces | _____ | | |
| Fruit-flavored yogurt | 1 cup | _____ | | |
| Milk: fat-free, reduced-fat, whole, chocolate, buttermilk | 1 cup | _____ | | |
| Calcium-fortified soy milk (e.g., Silk) | 1 cup | _____ | | |
| Parmesan cheese (grated) | 1/4 cup | _____ | | |
| Swiss cheese | 1 ounce | _____ | | |
| | Total servings | _____ | × 300 | = _____ mg |
| Cheese (all other hard cheese) | 1 ounce | _____ | | |
| Pancakes | 3 | _____ | | |
| | Total servings | _____ | × 200 | = _____ mg |
| Canned pink salmon | 3 ounces | _____ | | |
| Tofu (processed with calcium) | 4 ounces | _____ | | |
| | Total servings | _____ | × 150 | = _____ mg |
| Collards or turnip greens, cooked | 1/2 cup | _____ | | |
| Ice cream or ice milk | 1/2 cup | _____ | | |
| Almonds | 1 ounce | _____ | | |
| | Total servings | _____ | × 75 | = _____ mg |
| Chard, cooked | 1/2 cup | _____ | | |
| Cottage cheese | 1/2 cup | _____ | | |
| Corn tortilla | 1 medium | _____ | | |
| Orange | 1 medium | _____ | | |
| | Total servings | _____ | × 50 | = _____ mg |
| Kidney, lima, or navy beans, cooked | 1/2 cup | _____ | | |
| Broccoli | 1/2 cup | _____ | | |
| Carrot, raw | 1 medium | _____ | | |
| Dates or raisins | 1/4 cup | _____ | | |
| Egg | 1 large | _____ | | |
| Whole-wheat bread | 1 slice | _____ | | |
| Peanut butter | 2 tablespoons | _____ | | |
| | Total servings | _____ | × 25 | = _____ mg |
| Calcium-fortified orange juice | 6 ounces | _____ | | |
| Calcium-fortified snack bars | 1 each | _____ | | |
| Calcium-fortified breakfast bars | 1/2 bar | _____ | | |
| | Total servings | _____ | × 200 | = _____ mg |
| Calcium-fortified chocolate candies | 1 each | _____ | | |
| Calcium supplements* | 1 each | _____ | × 500 | = _____ mg |
| | Total servings | _____ | Total calcium intake | = _____ mg |

Other calcium sources to consider include many breakfast cereals (100 to 250 mg per cup) and some vitamin/mineral supplements (200 to 500 mg or more per tablet).

*Amount varies, so check the label for the amount in a specific product and then adjust the calculation as needed.

Reprinted with permission from *Topics in Clinical Nutrition*, "Putting Calcium into Perspective for Your Clients," G. Wardlaw and N. Weese, 11:1, p. 29. © 1995 Aspen Publishers, Inc.

# CHAPTER 10 Nutrition: Fitness and Sports

## Student Learning Outcomes After studying Chapter 10, you will be able to:

1. List five positive health-related outcomes of a physically active lifestyle.

2. Design a fitness regimen.

3. Describe when and how glycogen, blood glucose, fat, and protein are used to meet energy needs during different types of physical activity.

4. Differentiate between anaerobic and aerobic use of glucose, and identify advantages and disadvantages of each.

5. Show how muscles and related organs adapt to an increase in physical activity.

6. Outline how to estimate an athlete's calorie needs and discuss the general principles for meeting overall nutrient requirements in the training diet.

7. Examine the problems associated with rapid weight loss by dehydration and outline the importance of water and/or sports drinks during exercise.

8. Understand the importance of staying well nourished with carbohydrate, protein, and various vitamins and minerals during training.

9. List several ergogenic aids and describe their effects, if any, on an athlete's performance.

## Chapter Outline

Student Learning Outcomes

Refresh Your Memory

10.1 The Close Relationship Between Nutrition and Fitness

10.2 Guidelines for Achieving and Maintaining Physical Fitness

10.3 Energy Sources for Exercising Muscles

10.4 Power Food: Dietary Advice for Athletes

10.5 A Focus on Fluid Needs

10.6 Specialized Dietary Advice for Before, During, and After Endurance Exercise

Nutrition and Your Health: *Ergogenic Aids and Athletic Performance*

Case Study: Planning a Training Diet

Summary/Study Questions/Check Your Knowledge/Further Readings

Rate Your Plate

**ATHLETES INVEST A LOT OF TIME AND EFFORT IN TRAINING.** Most athletes don't want to miss out on any advantage, whether real or perceived, that might give them the winning edge. Athletes often seek ways to enhance their diets to improve performance, so they make easy targets for purveyors of nutrition misinformation.

Although good eating habits can't substitute for physical training and genetic endowment, proper food and beverage choices are crucial for top-notch performance, contributing to endurance and helping to speed the repair of injured tissues.

Although experts might disagree on how much carbohydrate, protein, and fat we should consume, there is no argument over the health benefits of regular physical activity. It is even beneficial for overweight people who remain at that excess weight. As the comic in this chapter suggests, it takes a strong commitment to reap the benefits.

In Chapter 10, you will discover how physical fitness benefits the entire body and how nutrition relates to fitness and sports performance.

## Refresh Your Memory

As you begin your study of nutrition for fitness and sports in Chapter 10, you may want to review:

- The current trend of consuming "energy bars" in Chapter 1
- Components of the cell in Chapter 3
- Concept of glycemic load in Chapter 4
- Various food sources of carbohydrates, proteins, and lipids in Chapters 4–7
- Food sources of calcium and iron in Chapter 9

# 10.1 The Close Relationship Between Nutrition and Fitness

**physical fitness** The ability to perform moderate to vigorous activity without undue fatigue.

The ability to engage routinely in vigorous physical activity requires good health. Peak performance also depends on a diet that supplies all the needed nutrients.

The type of fuel used by muscles depends on how physically fit the athletes are and how hard each one performs. This **physical fitness**—defined as the ability to perform moderate to vigorous activity without undue fatigue—especially affects fat use by the body. As one's level of physical fitness improves, so does one's ability to mobilize fat stores for energy needs—especially during activities that last for 20 minutes or more.

Beyond affecting fuel use, the benefits of regular physical activity include enhancement of several aspects of heart function, less injury, better sleep habits, and improvement in body composition (less body fat, more muscle mass). Physical activity also can reduce stress and positively affect blood pressure, blood cholesterol, blood glucose regulation, and immune function. In addition, physical activity aids in weight control, both by raising resting energy expenditure for a short time after exercise and by increasing overall energy expenditure. See Figure 10-1 for a further look at these and other benefits of a physically active lifestyle.

Unfortunately, as noted in Chapter 7, many North American adults lead sedentary lives. Most adults do not practice moderate to vigorous physical activity on a

**Sherman's Lagoon** by J.P. Toomey

Why is regular physical activity—including some strength-building activities—generally advocated for all of us? What benefits accrue from this practice? How do strength-training and endurance athletes need to tailor their diets to support their vigorous physical activities? Chapter 10 provides some answers.

**FIGURE 10-1** ▶ The benefits of regular, moderate physical activity and exercise.

regular basis, and about half of all adults quit an exercise program within 3 months of initiation.

*Healthy People 2010* has set a number of specific objectives for U.S. adults, related to physical activity and exercise:

- Reduce by 50% the proportion of adults engaging in no leisure time physical activity (currently 27% of adults).
- Double the proportion of adults engaging regularly, preferably daily, in moderate exercise for at least 30 minutes per day (currently 45% of adults).
- Increase by 50% the proportion of adults who perform physical activities that enhance and maintain muscular strength and endurance (currently 19% of adults).

To help yourself stay with an exercise program, experts recommend the following:

- Start slowly.
- Vary your activities; make it fun.
- Include friends and others.
- Set specific attainable goals and monitor progress.
- Set aside a specific time each day for exercise; build it into your routine, but make it convenient.
- Reward yourself for being successful in keeping up with your goals.
- Don't worry about occasional setbacks; focus on the long-term benefits to your health.

▲ Visit **exerciseismedicine.org** to learn about an initiative spearheaded by the American College of Sports Medicine to incorporate fitness goals as part of routine medical care.

▶ One day in December 2000, Joe Decker:

bicycled 100 miles,

ran 10 miles, hiked 10 miles,

power-walked 5 miles,

kayaked 6 miles,

skied on a NordicTrack 10 miles,

rowed 10 miles, swam 2 miles,

did 3000 abdominal crunches,

did 1100 jumping jacks,

did 1000 leg lifts, did 1100 push-ups,

and he lifted weights for a cumulative total of 278,540 lb.

For his efforts (and pains), he earned a place in the *Guinness Book of World Records* as the fittest man alive.

The *2005 Dietary Guidelines for Americans* recommends three different time goals for physical activity (review Chapter 2).

- 30 minutes/day of moderate-intensity physical activity, in addition to usual activity, for individuals trying to reduce their risk of chronic disease in adulthood. Doing more than 30 minutes or increasing the intensity of the workout could lead to even greater benefits.
- 60 minutes/day of moderate- to vigorous-intensity physical activity to help adults manage body weight and prevent gradual weight gain.
- 90 minutes/day of moderate-intensity physical activity may be needed for some adults to sustain weight loss; at the same time, these individuals also need to monitor their calorie intakes.

## MAKING DECISIONS

### Planning Your Exercise

Consider applying the dietary principles of variety, balance, and moderation to your exercise plan:

- Variety: Enjoy many different activities to exercise different muscles.
- Balance: Different activities have different benefits, so balance your exercise pattern. For overall fitness, you need exercises that build cardiovascular endurance, muscular strength, and flexibility.
- Moderation: Exercise to keep fit without overdoing it. You don't need a heavy workout every day to achieve fitness.

## CONCEPT CHECK

Regular physical activity is a vital part of a healthy lifestyle, ideally consisting of a total of at least 30 minutes (and preferably 60, especially if weight loss/weight control is an issue) of aerobic activity on most (or all) days. Physically active people benefit from lower risks of cardiovascular disease, type 2 diabetes, obesity, and other common chronic diseases.

# 10.2 Guidelines for Achieving and Maintaining Physical Fitness

For healthy people, a gradual increase to a goal of regular physical activity is recommended. Men 40 years of age or older and women 50 years of age or older who have been inactive for many years, or who have an existing health problem, should discuss their fitness goals with their physician before increasing activity. Health problems that require medical evaluation before beginning an exercise program are obesity, cardiovascular disease (or family history of it), hypertension, diabetes (or family history), shortness of breath after mild exertion, and arthritis.

During the first phase of a fitness program to promote health, you should begin to incorporate short periods of physical activity into the daily routine. This includes walking, taking the stairs instead of the elevator, house cleaning, gardening, and other activities that cause you to "huff and puff" a bit. The goal is a total of 30 minutes of this moderate type of physical activity on most (and preferably all) days. If necessary, this can be broken up into increments lasting at least 10 minutes. Experts suggest starting with short intervals, building up to a total of 30 minutes of activity incorporated into each day's tasks. If there is not much time for activity, you can even go for more intensity in the activities over shorter periods to get the same benefits. Clearly, many of the activities just recommended are not very vigorous.

Once you can perform physical activity for 30 minutes per day, turn your attention to more specific goals, such as increasing muscle mass and strength, to reap even more benefits. Guidelines for designing a fitness program are listed in Table 10-1. Aerobic, strength, and stretching activities are included, as well as considerations for duration, frequency, intensity, and progression.

Begin by warming up with 5 to 10 minutes of low-intensity exercises, such as walking, slow jogging, or any slow version of the anticipated activity. This warms up your muscles so that muscle filaments more easily slide over one another to increase range of motion and decrease the risk of injury.

## Aerobic Workout

Daily aerobic activity is recommended. Health benefits from regular physical activity are especially seen when you can achieve a moderate level of intensity of exercise.

There are a few ways to determine the intensity of exercise. A popular and simple method is to use a percentage of your age-predicted maximum heart rate (Fig. 10-2). To find maximum heart rate, subtract your age from 220. Multiplying maximum heart rate by 0.60 and 0.90 will result in a range of heart rates, sometimes called the *target zone*. For a 20-year-old person beginning an exercise program, maximum heart rate equals 200 beats per minute (220 − 20 = 200). Then, (200 × 0.6) and (200 × 0.9) yields a target zone of 120 to 180 beats per minute. Measuring heart rate (pulse) is easy: Stop and count your pulse for 10 seconds and then multiply that number by 6 to determine your heart rate for one minute. Some exercise equipment and high-tech watches contain heart rate monitors.

At the initiation of an exercise program, aim for the lower end of the target zone. As you progress and become more physically fit, you can work up to a higher heart rate. As with many of the prediction formulas, calculation of maximum heart rate is just an estimate. Medications, such as those for hypertension and other health conditions, may impact heart rate. If you have health concerns, a physician can help to personalize your target zone.

▲ What is the best exercise? One you want to continue to do.

**TABLE 10-1** Designing a Fitness Program

| Type of Activity | Aerobic (uses large muscle groups in rhythmic fashion) | Strength (resistance activity) | Stretching (uses major muscle groups; important during warm-up and cooldown) |
|---|---|---|---|
| Examples | Brisk walking, running, cycling, swimming, basketball, tennis, soccer | Weight-lifting, pilates, push-ups, pull-ups | Yoga |
| Duration (time spent in exercise session) | 20 to 60 minutes | 8 to 12 repetitions of 8 to 10 different exercises | 4 repetitions of 10 to 30 seconds per muscle group |
| Frequency (times activity is performed) | 5 days per week | 2 to 3 days per week | 2 to 3 days per week and during warm-up and cooldown |
| Intensity (level of exertion) | 55% to 90% maximum heart rate or RPE of 4 or above (see Figure 10-3) | Enough to condition major muscle groups of the upper and lower body | 5 to 10 minutes during warm-up and cooldown |
| Progression (increase in frequency, intensity, and duration over time) | **Initiation phase:** 3 to 6 weeks **Improvement phase:** 5 to 6 months **Maintenance phase:** plateau in gains in fitness | | Start with smaller muscle groups (e.g., arms) and work toward large muscle groups (e.g., legs and abdomen) |

**FIGURE 10-2** ▶ Heart rate training chart. This chart shows the number of heart beats per minute that corresponds to various exercise intensities.

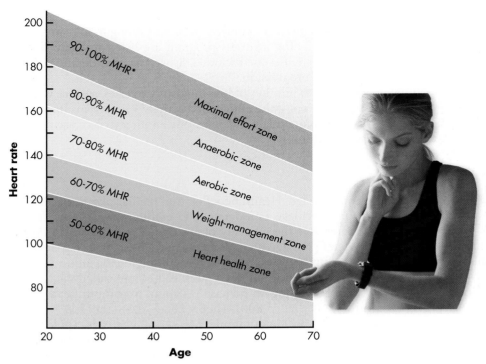

*MHR (maximum heart rate) = 220 − Age in years

High-energy bonds

**Structure of ATP**

Another way of determining the intensity of exercise is the Rating of Perceived Exertion scale (RPE). One version includes a range of 1 to 10, with each number corresponding to a subjective feeling of exertion. For example, the number 0 is "nothing at all" (sitting at a table) and the number 10 is considered close to maximal effort or "very, very strong" (all-out sprint) (Fig. 10-3).

When using the RPE scale, the goal is to aim for the number 4, which corresponds to the beginning of "somewhat strong." This is the point at which you begin to see significant fitness results. You should be working hard, but still be able to talk to an exercise partner (sometimes called the "talk test").

During cooldown, follow a reverse pattern of the warm-up: 5 to 10 minutes of low-intensity activity and add 5 to 10 minutes of stretching. The same exercises performed during warm-up are appropriate. The cooldown is essential to the prevention of injury and soreness.

## 10.3 Energy Sources for Exercising Muscles

Like other cells, muscle cells cannot directly use the energy released from breaking down glucose or triglycerides. Muscle cells need a specific form of energy for contraction. Body cells must first convert food energy (i.e., calories) to **adenosine triphosphate (ATP).**

The chemical bonds between phosphates in ATP and related molecules are high-energy bonds. Using the energy obtained from foodstuffs, cells make ATP from its breakdown product **adenosine diphosphate (ADP)** and a phosphate group (abbreviated $P_i$).

$$ADP + \text{Energy from food} + P_i \rightarrow ATP$$

Conversely, to release energy from ATP, cells partially break the compound down into ADP and $P_i$. The released energy is used for many cell functions.

$$ATP \rightarrow \text{Energy to do work} + ADP + P_i$$

**adenosine triphosphate (ATP)** The main energy currency for cells. ATP energy is used to promote ion pumping, enzyme activity, and muscular contraction.

**adenosine diphosphate (ADP)** A breakdown product of ATP. ADP is synthesized into ATP using energy from foodstuffs and a phosphate group (abbreviated $P_i$).

**RPE Scale\***

Nothing at all · Very weak · Weak · Moderate · Somewhat strong · Strong · Very strong · Very, very strong

0  1  2  3  4  5  6  7  8  9  10

\* Rating of Perceived Exertion (RPE) beyond 10 is considered maximal

**FIGURE 10-3** ▶ Rating of Perceived Exertion scale. When exercising, a rating of 4 or above is advocated for building/maintaining physical fitness.

Essentially, ATP is the immediate source of energy for body functions (Table 10-2). The primary goal in the use of any fuel, whether carbohydrate, fat, or protein, is to make ATP. A resting muscle cell contains only a small amount of ATP that can be used immediately. This amount of ATP could keep the muscle working maximally for only about 2 to 4 seconds if no resupply of ATP were possible. Fortunately, another type of high-energy compound—**phosphocreatine (PCr)**—is also present in muscle cells and can be quickly broken down to release enough energy to make more ATP. This supports the working muscle cells until metabolism of carbohydrate and fat for fuel begins in earnest. Overall, cells must constantly and repeatedly use and then re-form ATP, using a variety of energy sources.

**phosphocreatine (PCr)** A high-energy compound that can be used to re-form ATP. It is used primarily during bursts of activity, such as lifting and jumping.

**creatine** An organic (i.e., carbon-containing) molecule in muscle cells that serves as a part of a high-energy compound (termed creatine phosphate or phospho-creatine) capable of synthesizing ATP from ADP.

## Phosphocreatine Is the First Line of Defense for Resupplying ATP in Muscles

As soon as ATP stored in muscle cells begins to be used, another source of energy just mentioned, PCr, is used to produce ATP. An enzyme in the muscle cell is activated to split PCr into phosphate and **creatine**. This releases energy that can be used to re-form ATP from its breakdown products. If no other source of energy for ATP resupply were available, PCr could probably maintain maximal muscle contractions

**TABLE 10-2** Energy Sources Used by Resting and Working Muscle Cells

| Energy Source\* | When in Use | Activity |
| --- | --- | --- |
| ATP | At all times | All types |
| Phosphocreatine (PCr) | All exercise initially; short bursts of exercise thereafter | Shotput, high jump, bench press |
| Carbohydrate (anaerobic) | High-intensity exercise, especially lasting 30 seconds to 2 minutes | 200-yard (about 200 meters) sprint |
| Carbohydrate (aerobic) | Exercise lasting 2 minutes to 3 hours or more; the higher the intensity (for example, running a 6-minute mile), the greater the use | Basketball, swimming, jogging, power walking, soccer, tennis |
| Fat (aerobic) | Exercise lasting more than a few minutes; greater amounts are used at lower exercise intensities | Long-distance running, long-distance cycling; much of the fuel used in a 30-minute brisk walk is fat |
| Protein (aerobic) | Low amount during all exercise; slightly more in endurance exercise, especially when carbohydrate fuel is depleted | Long-distance running |

\*At any given time, more than one source is used. The relative amount of use differs during various activities.

▲ Bursts of muscle activity use a variety of energy sources, including PCr and ATP.

See the *Nutrition and Your Health Section: Ergogenic Aids and Athletic Performance* at the end of Chapter 10.

for about 10 seconds. Other sources of ATP resupply kick in, however, so PCr ends up as a source of energy for events lasting about 1 minute or less.

$$PCr + ADP \rightarrow ATP + Cr$$

The main advantage of PCr is that it can be activated instantly and can replenish ATP at rates fast enough to meet the energy demands of the fastest and most powerful actions, including jumping, lifting, throwing, and sprinting. The disadvantage of PCr is that not much of it is made and stored in the muscles. Strength-training athletes have begun to use creatine supplements in an effort to increase PCr in muscles.

## Carbohydrate Fuel for Muscles

Carbohydrates are an important fuel for muscles. The most useful form of carbohydrate fuel is the simple sugar glucose, available to all cells from the bloodstream. As you will recall from Chapter 4, glucose is stored as glycogen in the liver and muscle cells. Blood glucose is maintained by the breakdown of liver glycogen. Breakdown of glycogen stored in a specific muscle also helps meet the carbohydrate demand of that muscle, but the actual amount of glycogen stored in muscle is limited (about 350 grams for all the muscles in the body, which would yield about 1400 kcal).

Depending on whether oxygen is available to exercising muscles, use of glucose to make ATP can be either anaerobic or aerobic.

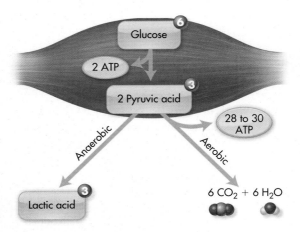

**FIGURE 10-4** ▶ ATP yield from aerobic versus anaerobic glucose use. Encircled numbers indicate the number of carbons in each molecule.

**pyruvic acid** A three-carbon compound formed during glucose metabolism; also called *pyruvate*.

**lactic acid** A three-carbon acid formed during anaerobic cell metabolism; a partial breakdown product of glucose; also called *lactate*.

**Anaerobic Glucose Breakdown Yields Energy Fast.** When oxygen supply in the muscle is limited (anaerobic conditions), glucose is broken down into a three-carbon compound called **pyruvic acid.** The pyruvic acid accumulates in the muscle and is then converted to **lactic acid.** Only about 5% of the total amount of ATP that could be formed from complete breakdown of glucose, is released through this anaerobic process (glucose → → lactic acid).

The advantage of anaerobic glucose breakdown is that it is the fastest way to resupply ATP, other than PCr breakdown. It therefore provides most of the energy needed for events that require a quick burst of energy, ranging from about 30 seconds to 2 minutes. Examples of activities that primarily rely on anaerobic glucose breakdown include sprinting 400 meters or swimming 100 meters.

The two major disadvantages of the anaerobic process are that (1) the high rate of ATP production cannot be sustained for long periods, and (2) the rapid accumulation of lactic acid greatly increases the acidity of the muscle. Acidity inhibits the activities of key enzymes in the muscle cells, slowing anaerobic ATP production and causing short-term fatigue. The acidity also leads to a net potassium loss from muscle cells, providing another cause of fatigue. We learn by trial-and-error a pace that will control muscle lactic acid concentrations during these anaerobic events.

For the most part, lactic acid builds up in active muscle cells until it is released into the bloodstream. The liver (and the kidneys, to some extent) takes up the lactic acid and resynthesizes it into glucose. Glucose can then reenter the bloodstream, where it is available for cell uptake and breakdown.

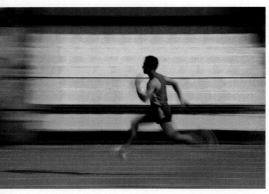

▲ Sprinting relies primarily on anaerobic glucose breakdown.

**Aerobic Glucose Breakdown Is a Sustained Energy Source.** If plenty of oxygen is available in the muscle (aerobic conditions), such as when the exercise is of low to moderate intensity, the bulk of the three-carbon pyruvic acid is shuttled to the mitochondria of the cell, where it is fully metabolized into carbon dioxide ($CO_2$) and water ($H_2O$) (Fig. 10-5). This aerobic breakdown of glucose yields approximately 95% of the ATP made from complete glucose metabolism (glucose → → $CO_2$ + $H_2O$).

Aerobic glucose breakdown supplies more ATP than does the anaerobic process, but it releases the energy more slowly. This slower rate of aerobic energy supply can be sustained for hours. One reason is that the products are carbon dioxide and water, not lactic acid. Aerobic glucose breakdown makes a major energy contribution to activities that last anywhere from 2 minutes to 3 hours or more. Examples of such activities include jogging or distance swimming (review Table 10-2).

Many researchers have studied the ability of various types of carbohydrate feeding regimens to maximize glucose supply to muscles during prolonged exercise. Overall, the techniques have succeeded. Consuming about 30 to 60 grams of carbohydrate per hour during strenuous endurance exercise that lasts 1 hour or more, such as cycling, can aid in maintaining adequate blood glucose, resulting in a delay of fatigue by 30 to 60 minutes. This attention to carbohydrate intake also helps one tolerate vigorous training on a daily basis.

As blood glucose declines during exercise, so does mental function. Cyclists refer to this diminished mental ability as "bonking." The fall in blood glucose is related to depletion of liver glycogen, not muscle glycogen, because liver glycogen is used to maintain blood glucose. See the later section, "Sports Drinks," to learn more about carbohydrate replacement during exercise (see Figure 10-7 on page 429).

## CRITICAL THINKING

Marty started going to the gym about 8 weeks ago. At first, he noticed that he began "huffing and puffing" about 7 minutes into his aerobic workout. Now, however, he can work out for about 25 minutes without tiring. What is a possible explanation for this ability to work out longer?

**FIGURE 10-5** ▶ Simplified view of ATP formation from carbohydrate, fat, and protein. Along with phosphocreatine (PCr), all three nutrients may be used for ATP synthesis, but glucose and fatty acids are primary sources. Glucose may be broken down anaerobically or may undergo complete aerobic metabolism. The products of fatty acid breakdown are channeled into aerobic metabolism. Although limited, products of amino acid breakdown are channeled into the aerobic pathway as well. Recall also from Chapters 8 and 9 that many vitamins and minerals participate in these metabolic pathways.

16-carbon
fatty acid

about 108 ATP
for cell use

$CO_2 + H_2O$

ATP yield from aerobic fatty acid utilization.

▲ ATP yield from aerobic fatty acid utilization.

▲ Fatty acids can come from all over the body, not necessarily from fat stored near the active muscles. *This is why spot reducing does not work.* Exercise can tone the muscles near adipose tissue but does not preferentially use those stores.

Carbohydrate intake during exercise is not as important in shorter events (e.g., 30 minutes or so) because the muscles do not take up much blood glucose during short-term exercise, relying instead primarily on their glycogen stores for fuel.

## Fat: The Main Fuel for Prolonged Low-Intensity Activity

When fat stores in body tissues begin to be broken down for energy, each triglyceride first yields three fatty acids and a glycerol. The majority of the stored energy is found in the fatty acids. During physical activity, fatty acids are released from various adipose tissue depots into the bloodstream and travel to the muscles, where they are taken into each cell and broken down aerobically to carbon dioxide and water. Some of the fat stored in muscles also is used, especially as activity increases from a low to a moderate pace.

The rate at which muscles use fatty acids partly depends on the concentration of fatty acids in the bloodstream. In other words, the more fatty acids released from adipose tissue stores into the bloodstream, the more fat will be used by the muscles. Some cyclists and other endurance athletes have attempted to raise their blood concentrations of fatty acids by consuming caffeinated beverages. This practice can actually increase fatty acid release from the adipose tissue depots and is therefore helpful to certain athletes, but it is illegal under NCAA rules if the amount of caffeine in the body exceeds the equivalent of 6 to 8 cups of coffee (see the "Nutrition and Your Health" section at the end of this Chapter).

Fat is not a very useful muscle fuel for intense, brief exercise, but it becomes a progressively more important energy source as duration increases, especially when exercise remains at a low or moderate (aerobic) rate for more than 20 minutes (Fig. 10-6). The reason for this is that some of the steps involved in fat breakdown cannot occur fast enough to meet the ATP demands of short-duration, high-intensity exercise. If fat were the only available fuel, we would be unable to exercise beyond a fast walk or jog.

The advantage of fat fuel is that it provides stores of energy in a relatively concentrated form, and we generally have a lot of it stored. For a given weight of fuel, fat supplies more than twice as much energy as carbohydrate does. For lengthy activities at a moderate pace (for example, hiking) or even sitting at a desk for 8 hours a day, fat supplies about 70% to 90% of the energy required. Carbohydrate use is much less. As intensity increases, such as in a 3-hour marathon run at a competitive pace, muscles use about a 50:50 ratio of fat to carbohydrate. In comparison, for short events, such as a 100-meter sprint or even a 1500-meter race, the contribution of fat to resupply ATP is minimal. To summarize, remember that the only fast-paced (anaerobic) fuel we eat is carbohydrate; slow and steady (aerobic) activity uses fat in addition to carbohydrate.

### MAKING DECISIONS

#### Training Effect

As people start exercising regularly four or five times per week, they experience a "training effect." Initially, these individuals might be able to exercise for 20 minutes before tiring. Months later, exercise can be extended to an hour before they feel tired. During the months of training, muscle cells have produced more mitochondria and thus can burn more fat. Training also increases the number of capillaries in muscles, which increases oxygen supply to the muscles. As a result, lactic acid production from anaerobic glucose metabolism decreases. Lactic acid contributes to short-term muscle fatigue, so the less lactic acid produced, the longer the exercise can be sustained. Other contributors to the training effect include increased aerobic efficiency of the heart and muscles and elevations in muscle triglyceride content, with an enhanced ability of muscles to use triglycerides for energy needs.

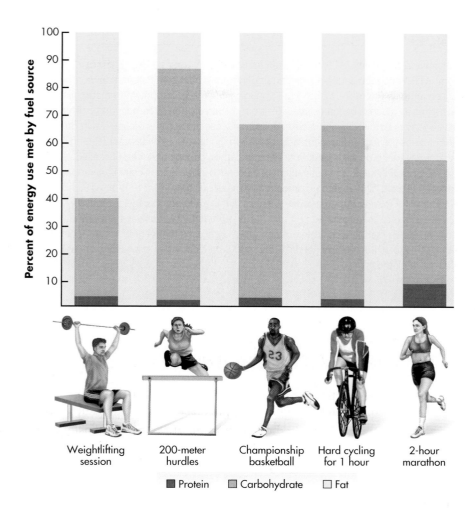

**FIGURE 10-6** ▶ Rough estimates of fuel use during various forms of physical activity. With regard to the weightlifting session, carbohydrate use could be somewhat greater and fat use somewhat less if the session is intense and fast-paced (e.g., circuit training). Fat use generally is higher because much of the time spent weight lifting is for rest periods and equipment-related activities.

## Protein: A Minor Fuel Source, Primarily for Endurance Exercise

Although amino acids derived from protein can be used to fuel muscles, their contribution is relatively small, compared with that of carbohydrate and fat. As a rough guide, only about 5% of the body's general energy needs, as well as the typical energy needs of exercising muscles, is supplied by the metabolism of amino acids.

During endurance exercise, proteins can contribute importantly to energy needs, perhaps as much as 10% to 15%, especially as glycogen stores in the muscle are exhausted. Most of the energy supplied from protein comes from metabolism of the branched-chain amino acids—leucine, isoleucine, and valine. A normal diet provides ample branched chain amino acids to supply this amount of fuel, so protein or amino acid supplements are not needed. Contrary to what many athletes believe, protein is used for fuel less in resistance types of exercise (e.g., weightlifting) than in endurance exercise (e.g., running) (review Fig. 10-6). The primary muscle fuels for weightlifting are phosphocreatine (PCr) and carbohydrate for the brief bursts of activity, with fat providing energy during the resting stages, and with little use of protein overall. Despite this, high-protein products such as Pro-Complex, Amino Fuel 2000, High Voltage Protein Drink, and Instant Egg Protein are marketed specifically to weightlifters and bodybuilders in nearly every health-food and fitness store. Consuming high-carbohydrate, moderate-protein foods immediately after a weight-training workout enhances the muscle-building effect of the activity, most likely by increasing the concentrations of insulin and growth hormone released into the blood and contributing to protein synthesis. Still, it is impossible to increase muscle mass simply by eating protein. Putting physical strain on muscle through strength training or other physical activity is needed.

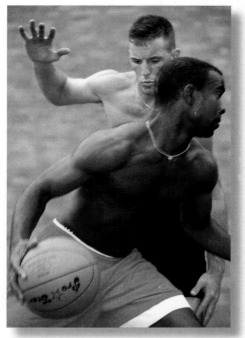

▲ The calories needed to perform come from carbohydrate, fat, and protein. The relative mix depends on the pace.

## CONCEPT CHECK

Adenosine triphosphate (ATP) is the main form of energy used by cells. Cells use food energy to form ATP. Phosphocreatine (PCr) can rapidly re-form ATP from its breakdown product adenosine diphosphate (ADP), but PCr supplies are limited. Carbohydrate metabolism to form ATP begins as glucose becomes available from the absorption of carbohydrates from the diet or glycogen breakdown. In a muscle cell, each glucose molecule is broken down through a series of steps to yield either lactic acid or carbon dioxide ($CO_2$) plus water ($H_2O$). The process that occurs when glucose is broken down into carbon dioxide and water is called *aerobic* because oxygen is used. The conversion of glucose to lactic acid is called *anaerobic* because no oxygen is used. The anaerobic process allows the cell to quickly re-form ATP and supports the demand for energy during intense exercise. Fat is a key aerobic fuel for muscle cells, especially at low exercise outputs. At rest and during light activity, muscles burn primarily fat for energy needs. In comparison, little protein generally is used to fuel muscles. At most, protein supplies 10% to 15% of energy needs during endurance activities, especially when glycogen stores are depleted.

▲ Intense athletic training may require thousands of additional calories. This increased food intake should easily provide ample protein and other nutrients to support activity.

**R**eview Table 7-4 in Chapter 7, which listed the energy costs of typical forms of physical activity.

## 10.4 Power Food: Dietary Advice for Athletes

Athletic training and genetic makeup are two important determinants of athletic performance. A good diet won't substitute for either factor, but diet can help to enhance and maximize an athlete's potential. On the other hand, a poor diet can seriously reduce performance.

### Calorie Needs

Athletes need varying amounts of calories, depending on each athlete's body size, body composition, and the type of training or competition being considered. A small person may need only 1700 kcal daily to sustain normal daily activities without losing body weight; a large, muscular man may need 4000 kcal. These rough estimates can be viewed as starting points that need to be individualized by trial and error for each athlete.

An estimate of the calories required to sustain moderate activity is 5 to 8 kcal per minute. The calories required for sports training or competition then have to be added to those used to carry on normal activities. For example, an hour of bowling requires few calories in addition to that required to sustain normal daily living. At the other extreme, a 12-hour endurance bicycle race over mountains can require an additional 4000 kcal per day. Therefore, some athletes may need as much as 7000 kcal or more daily to maintain body weight while training, whereas others may need 1700 kcal or less. If an athlete experiences daily fatigue, the first consideration should be whether he or she is consuming enough food. Up to six meals per day may be needed, including one before each workout.

How can we know if an athlete is getting enough calories? Estimating daily intake from a food diary kept by the athlete is one way. Another step is to estimate the athlete's body fat percentage via skinfold measurements, bioelectrical impedance, or underwater weighing (review Chapter 7). Body fat should be the typical amount found for athletes in the specific sport practiced. This corresponds to 5% to 18% for most male athletes and 17% to 28% for most female athletes. The next step is to monitor body weight changes on a daily or weekly basis. If body weight starts to fall, calories should be increased; if weight rises and it is because of increases in body fat, the athlete should eat less.

## MAKING DECISIONS

### Making Weight

Wrestlers, boxers, judoists, jockeys, and oarsmen often try to lose weight before a competition, so that they can be certified to compete in a lower weight class. This helps them gain a mechanical advantage over an opponent of smaller stature. They usually lose this weight before stepping on the scale for weight certification. Athletes can lose up to 22 pounds (10 kilograms) of body weight as water in 1 day by sitting in a sauna, exercising in a plastic sweat suit, or taking diuretic drugs, which speed water loss from the kidneys. Losing as little as 2% of body weight by dehydration, however, can adversely affect endurance and performance, especially in hot weather. A pattern of repeated weight loss or gain of more than 5% of body weight by dehydration carries risk of kidney malfunction and heat-related illness. Death is also a possibility.

To prevent future deaths from such weight loss in athletes, the National Collegiate Athletic Association and many states have authorized physicians or athletic trainers to set safe weight and body fat content minimums (e.g., 7% or more of total body weight for male athletes and 12% or more for females) in weight-class sports. Under new guidelines, athletes are assigned to weight classes at the beginning of the season and are not allowed to "cut weight" to gain a competitive advantage. Weight gain in the days after a competition (reflecting regain of body water) can now be no greater than 2 pounds. If athletes, such as wrestlers, wish to compete in a lower-bodyweight class and have enough extra fat stores, they should begin a gradual, sustained reduction in calorie intake long before the competitive season starts.

If the body composition test shows that an athlete has too much body fat, the athlete should lower food intake by about 200 to 500 kcal per day, while maintaining a regular exercise program, until the desirable fat percentage is achieved. Reducing fat intake is the best nutrient-related approach. On the other hand, if an athlete needs to gain weight, increasing food intake by 500 to 700 kcal per day will eventually lead to the needed weight gain. A mix of carbohydrate, fat, and protein is advised, coupled with exercise to make sure this gain is mostly in the form of lean tissue and not fat stores.

## Carbohydrate Needs

Anyone who exercises vigorously, especially for more than 1 hour per day on a regular basis, needs to consume a diet that includes moderate to high amounts of carbohydrates. The diet should provide a variety of foods, such as those recommended by MyPyramid. Numerous servings of grains, starchy vegetables, and fruits provide enough carbohydrate to maintain adequate liver and muscle glycogen stores, especially for replacing glycogen losses from workouts on the previous day. Relatively low-carbohydrate/high-protein diets, such as *The Zone Diet*, are not recommended. Recall that Chapter 7 discussed the Zone Diet. The carbohydrate content of this diet is only 40% of calories, rather than the 60% or more typically recommended for athletes.

Carbohydrate intake should be at least 5 grams per kilogram body weight. People engaged in aerobic training and endurance activities (60 minutes or more per day) may need as much as 7 grams per kilogram body weight. When exercise duration approaches several hours per day, the carbohydrate recommendation increases to up to 10 grams per kilogram of body weight. In other words, triathletes and marathoners should consider eating close to 500 to 600 grams of carbohydrates daily, and even more if necessary, to (1) prevent chronic fatigue and (2) load the muscles and liver with glycogen. Attention to carbohydrate intake is especially important when performing multiple training bouts in a day, such as swim practices, or heavy training on successive days, as in cross-country running. Depletion of carbohydrate ranks just behind depletion of fluid and electrolytes as a major cause of fatigue. Table 10-3 shows sample menus, based on MyPyramid, for diets providing food energy ranging from

▲ High-carbohydrate foods should form the basis of the diet for athletes.

**TABLE 10-3** Sample Daily Menus Based on MyPyramid That Provide Various Total Calorie Intakes

| 1500 kcal | 2000 kcal | 3000 kcal | 4000 kcal | 5000 kcal |
|---|---|---|---|---|
| **Breakfast**<br>Fat-free milk, 1 cup<br>Cheerios, 1/2 cup<br>Bagel, 1/2<br>Cherry jam, 2 tsp<br>Margarine, 1 tsp | **Breakfast**<br>Fat-free milk, 1 cup<br>Cheerios, 1 cup<br>Bagel, 1/2<br>Cherry jam, 1 tbsp<br>Margarine, 1 tsp | **Breakfast**<br>Fat-free milk, 1 cup<br>Cheerios, 2 cups<br>Bagel, 1<br>Cherry jam, 2 tsp<br>Margarine, 1 tsp<br>Oat bran muffins, 2 | **Breakfast**<br>Fat-free milk, 1 cup<br>Cheerios, 2 cups<br>Orange, 1<br>Bran muffins, 2 | **Breakfast**<br>Fat-reduced milk, 1 cup<br>Cheerios, 2 cups<br>Bran muffins, 2<br>Orange, 1 |
| | | | **Snack**<br>Chopped dates, 3/4 cup | **Snack**<br>Low-fat yogurt, 1 cup<br>Chopped dates, 1 cup |
| **Lunch**<br>Chicken breast (roasted),<br> 2 oz<br>Figs, 1<br>Fat-free milk, 1/2 cup<br>Banana, 1 | **Lunch**<br>Chicken breast (roasted),<br> 2 oz<br>Wheat bread, 2 slices<br>Mayonnaise, 1 tsp<br>Raisins, 1/4 cup<br>Cranberry juice,<br> 1 1/2 cups<br>Banana, 1 | **Lunch**<br>Chicken breast (roasted),<br> 2 oz<br>Wheat bread, 2 slices<br>Provolone cheese, 1 oz<br>Mayonnaise, 1 tsp<br>Raisins, 1/3 cup<br>Cranberry juice,<br> 1 1/2 cups<br>Low-fat fruit yogurt, 1 cup | **Lunch**<br>Romaine lettuce, 1 cup<br>Garbanzo beans, 1 cup<br>Grated carrots, 1/2 cup<br>French dressing, 2 tbsp<br>Macaroni and cheese,<br> 3 cups<br>Apple juice, 1 cup | **Lunch**<br>Apple juice, 1 cup<br>Chicken enchilada, 1<br>Romaine lettuce, 1 cup<br>Garbanzo beans, 1 cup<br>Shredded carrots, 3/4 cup<br>Chopped celery, 1/2 cup<br>Seasoned croutons, 1 oz<br>French dressing, 2 tbsp<br>Wheat bread, 2 slices<br>Margarine, 1 tbsp |
| **Snack**<br>Oatmeal-raisin cookie, 1<br>Low-fat fruit yogurt, 1 cup | **Snack**<br>Oatmeal-raisin cookies, 3<br>Low-fat fruit yogurt, 1 cup | **Snack**<br>Banana, 1<br>Oatmeal-raisin cookies, 3 | **Snack**<br>Wheat bread, 2 slices<br>Margarine, 1 tsp<br>Jam, 2 tbsp | **Snack**<br>Banana, 1<br>Bagel, 1<br>Cream cheese, 1 tbsp |
| **Dinner**<br>Spaghetti w/meatballs,<br> 1 cup<br>Romaine lettuce, 1 cup<br>Italian dressing, 2 tsp<br>Green beans, 1/2 cup<br>Cranberry juice, 1 1/2 cups | **Dinner**<br>Broiled beef sirloin, 3 oz<br>Romaine lettuce, 1 cup<br>Italian dressing, 2 tsp<br>Green beans, 1 cup<br>Fat-free milk, 1/2 cup | **Dinner**<br>Broiled beef sirloin, 3 oz<br>Romaine lettuce, 1 cup<br>Garbanzo beans, 1 cup<br>Italian dressing, 2 tsp<br>Spinach pasta noodles,<br> 1 1/2 cups<br>Margarine, 1 tsp<br>Green beans, 1 cup<br>Fat-free milk, 1/2 cup | **Dinner**<br>Skinless turkey breast, 2 oz<br>Mashed potatoes, 2 cups<br>Peas and onions, 1 cup<br>Banana, 1<br>Fat-free milk, 1 cup | **Dinner**<br>Fat-reduced milk, 1 cup<br>Beef sirloin, 5 oz<br>Mashed potatoes, 2 cups<br>Spinach pasta noodles,<br> 1 1/2 cups<br>Grated parmesan cheese,<br> 2 tbsp<br>Green beans, 1 cup<br>Oatmeal-raisin cookies, 3 |
| | | | **Snack**<br>Pasta, 1 cup cooked<br>Margarine, 2 tsp<br>Parmesan cheese, 2 tbsp<br>Cranberry juice, 1 cup | **Snack**<br>Cranberry juice, 2 cups<br>Air-popped popcorn,<br> 4 cups<br>Raisins, 1/3 cup |
| 18% protein (68 grams)<br>64% carbohydrate<br>(240 grams)<br>19% fat (32 grams) | 17% protein (85 grams)<br>63% carbohydrate<br>(315 grams)<br>20% fat (44 grams) | 17% protein (128 grams)<br>62% carbohydrate<br>(465 grams)<br>21% fat (70 grams) | 14% protein (140 grams)<br>61% carbohydrate<br>(610 grams)<br>26% fat (116 grams) | 14% protein (175 grams)<br>63% carbohydrate<br>(813 grams)<br>24% fat (136 grams) |

1500 to 5000 kcal per day. In addition, the Exchange System described in Appendix D is a very useful tool for planning all types of diets, including high-carbohydrate diets for athletes.

As noted, athletes should obtain at least 60% of their total energy needs from carbohydrate (rather than the 50% typical of most North American diets), especially if exercise duration is expected to exceed 2 hours and total caloric intake is about 3000 kcal per day or less. Diets providing 4000 to 5000 kcal per day can be as low as 50% carbohydrate, as these will still provide sufficient carbohydrate (e.g., 500 to 600 grams or so per day).

One does not have to give up any specific food when planning a high-carbohydrate diet. The focus is to include more high-carbohydrate foods while moderating concentrated fat sources. Sports nutritionists emphasize the difference between a high-carbohydrate meal and a high-carbohydrate/high-fat meal. Before endurance events, such as marathons or triathlons, some athletes seek to increase their carbohydrate reserves by eating foods such as potato chips, French fries, banana cream pie, and pastries. Although such foods provide carbohydrate, they also contain a lot of fat. Better high-carbohydrate food choices include pasta, rice, potatoes, bread, fruit and fruit juices, and many breakfast cereals (check the label for carbohydrate content) (Table 10-4). Sports drinks appropriate for carbohydrate loading, such as GatorLode and UltraFuel, can also help. Consuming a moderate rather than a high amount of fiber during the final day of training is a good precaution to reduce the chances of bloating and intestinal gas during the next day's event.

## Carbohydrate Loading

For athletes who compete in continuous, intense aerobic events lasting more than 60 to 90 minutes (or in shorter events taking place more than once within a 24-hour period), a **carbohydrate-loading** regimen can help to maximize the amount of energy stored in the form of muscle glycogen for the event. (However, this amount of activity applies to few athletes.) In one possible regimen, during the week prior to the event, the athlete gradually reduces the intensity and duration of exercise ("tapering") while simultaneously increasing the percentage of total calories supplied by carbohydrate.

For example, consider the carbohydrate-loading schedule of a 25-year-old man preparing for a marathon. His typical calorie needs are about 3500 kcal per day. Six days before competition, he completes a final hard workout of 60 minutes. On that day, carbohydrates contribute 45% to 50% of his total calorie intake. As he goes through the rest of the week, the duration of his workouts decreases to 40 minutes, and then to about 20 minutes by the end of the week. Meanwhile, he increases the amount of carbohydrate in his diet to reach 70% to 80% of total calorie intake as the week continues. Total calorie intake should decrease as exercise time decreases throughout the week. On the final day before competition, he rests while maintaining the high-carbohydrate intake.

Carbohydrate Loading Regimen

| Days Before Competition | 6 | 5 | 4 | 3 | 2 | 1 |
|---|---|---|---|---|---|---|
| Exercise time (minutes) | 60 | 40 | 40 | 20 | 20 | Rest |
| Carbohydrate (grams) | 450 | 450 | 450 | 600 | 600 | 600 |

This carbohydrate-loading technique usually increases muscle glycogen stores by 50% to 85% over typical conditions (that is, when dietary carbohydrate constitutes only about 50% of total calorie intake).

A potential disadvantage of carbohydrate loading is that additional water (about 3 grams) is incorporated into the muscles along with each gram of glycogen. Although the additional water aids in maintaining hydration, for some individuals this additional water weight and related muscle stiffness detract from their sports performance, making carbohydrate loading inappropriate. Athletes considering a carbohydrate-loading regimen should try it during training (and well before an important competition) to experience its effects on performance. They can then determine whether it is worth the effort. Also, consuming carbohydrates during a competition provides about the same advantage as carbohydrate loading prior to the event. Expert advice is shifting away from carbohydrate loading and more toward this second method, coupled with a daily diet high in carbohydrate. In addition, remember the importance of the "training effect" discussed in " Making Decisions: Training Effect " on page 418.

## CRITICAL THINKING

Joe is a wrestler who qualified for the 125-pound weight classification in the annual state high school competition. After a few matches, Joe began to feel dizzy and faint. He was disqualified because he was unable to continue the match. Later, the coach found out that Joe had spent 2 hours in the sauna before weighing in, which had made him dehydrated. What are the consequences of dehydration? What can you suggest as a safer alternative for weight loss?

**carbohydrate loading**  A process in which a high carbohydrate intake is consumed for 6 days before an athletic event while tapering exercise duration in an attempt to increase muscle glycogen stores.

▶ **Carbohydrate Loading May Be Beneficial for These activities**

Marathons

Long-distance swimming

Cross-country skiing

30-kilometer runs

Triathlons

Tournament-play basketball

Soccer

Cycling time trials

Long-distance canoe racing

**Carbohydrate Loading Is Not Beneficial for These Activities**

American football games

10-kilometer or shorter runs

Walking and hiking

Most swimming events

Single basketball games

Weightlifting

Most track and field events

**TABLE 10-4** Grams of Carbohydrate Based on Serving Size of Typical Carbohydrate-Rich Foods

### Starches—15 grams Carbohydrate per Serving (80 kcal)

**One Serving**

| | |
|---|---|
| dry breakfast cereal*, 1/2–3/4 cup | baked potato, 1/4 large |
| cooked breakfast cereal, 1/2 cup | bagel, 1/4 (4 oz) |
| cooked grits, 1/2 cup | English muffin, 1/2 |
| cooked rice, 1/3 cup | bread, 1 slice |
| cooked pasta, 1/3 cup | pretzels, 3/4 oz |
| baked beans, 1/3 cup | saltine crackers, 6 |
| cooked corn, 1/2 cup | pancake, 4 inches in diameter, 1 |
| cooked dry beans, 1/2 cup | taco shells, 2 (add 45 kcal) |

### Vegetables—5 grams Carbohydrate per Serving (25 kcal)

**One Serving**
cooked vegetables, 1/2 cup
raw vegetables, 1 cup
vegetable juice, 1/2 cup
Examples: carrots, green beans, broccoli, cauliflower, onions, spinach, tomatoes, vegetable juice

### Fruits—15 grams Carbohydrate per Serving (60 kcal)

**One Serving**

| | |
|---|---|
| canned fruit or berries, 1/2 cup | grapes (small), 17 |
| fruit juice, 1/2 cup | grapefruit, 1/2 |
| figs (dried), 1 1/2 | dates, 3 |
| apple or orange, 1 small | peach, 1 |
| apricots (dried), 8 | watermelon cubes, 1 1/4 cups |
| banana, 1 small | |

### Milk—12 grams Carbohydrate per Serving

**One Serving**                    soymilk, 1 cup
milk, 1 cup
plain low-fat yogurt, 2/3 cup

### Sweets—15 grams Carbohydrate per Serving (variable calories)

**One Serving**

| | |
|---|---|
| cake, 2-inch square | ice cream, 1/2 cup |
| cookies, 2 small | sherbet, 1/2 cup |

*The carbohydrate content of dry cereal varies widely. Check the labels of the ones you choose and adjust the serving size accordingly.

Modified from *Choose Your Foods: Exchange Lists for Diabetes* by the American Diabetes Association and American Dietetic Association, 2008, Chicago, American Dietetic Association.

▲ Fruits provide a good source of carbohydrate, especially starch and natural sugars, for athletes.

▲ Carbohydrate loading is appropriate only for endurance activities such as a long-distance race.

## Fat Needs

A diet containing up to 35% of calories from fat is generally recommended for athletes. Rich sources of monounsaturated fat, such as canola oil, should be emphasized, and saturated fat and *trans* fat intake should be limited.

## Protein Needs

For most athletes, typical recommendations for protein intake range from 1.0 to 1.6 grams of protein per kilogram of body weight. This is considerably higher than the RDA of 0.8 grams per kilogram body weight for nonathletes recommended by the Food and Nutrition Board for all adults, including athletes (Table 10-5).

For athletes beginning a strength-training program, some experts recommend up to 1.7 grams of protein per kilogram of body weight. That is more than twice the RDA

**TABLE 10-5** Recommendations for Protein Intake Based on Kilograms Body Weight*

| Activity Group | grams/kilograms | Amount for a 70-kilogram (154 lb) Person (grams) |
|---|---|---|
| Sedentary | 0.8 | 56 |
| Strength trained, maintenance | 1.0–1.2 | 70–84 |
| Strength trained, gain muscle mass | 1.5–1.7 | 105–119 |
| Moderate intensity endurance activities | 1.2 | 84 |
| High-intensity endurance training | 1.6 | 112 |

*Calculate kilograms by dividing pounds by 2.2.

Source: Burke L, Deakin V: Clinical Sports Nutrition, McGraw-Hill, Roseville NSW2069, Australia, 2000.

for protein. To date, the value of such an excessive protein intake during the initial phases of strength training has not been supported by sufficient research. In addition, protein intakes above this amount result in an increased use of amino acids for energy needs; no further increase in muscle protein synthesis is seen. Recall from earlier in this chapter that phosphocreatine and carbohydrate (not extra protein) primarily fuel the body during strength-training activities. The extra protein, theoretically, is required for the synthesis of new muscle tissue brought on by the loading effect of strength training. Once the desired muscle mass is achieved, protein intake need not exceed 1.2 grams per kilogram of body weight.

Table 10-5 summarizes recommended ranges of protein intakes for various types of activity. Any athlete not specifically on a low-calorie regimen can easily meet these protein recommendations by eating a variety of foods (review Table 10-3). To illustrate, a 123-pound (53-kilogram) woman performing endurance activity can consume 64 grams of protein (53 × 1.2) during a single day by including 3 ounces of chicken (one chicken breast), 3 ounces of beef (a small, lean hamburger), and two glasses of milk in her diet. Similarly, a 180-pound (77-kilogram) man who aims to gain muscle mass through strength training needs to consume only 6 ounces of chicken (a large chicken breast), ½ cup of cooked beans, a 6-ounce can of tuna, and three glasses of milk to achieve an intake of 130 grams of protein (77 × 1.7) in a day. And, for both athletes, these calculations do not even include the protein present in grains or vegetables they will also eat. As you can see, by meeting their calorie needs, many athletes consume much more protein than is required. Despite marketing claims, protein supplements are an expensive and unnecessary part of a fitness plan.

Consuming excessive amounts of protein has drawbacks. As noted in Chapter 6, it increases calcium loss somewhat in the urine. It also leads to increased urine production, possibly compromising body hydration. It also may lead to kidney stones in people with a history of this or other kidney problems. Finally, enough carbohydrate fuel may not be consumed on such a diet, leading to fatigue. Athletes who either feel they must significantly limit their calorie intake or are vegetarians should specifically determine how much protein they eat. They should make sure to follow a diet that provides at least 1.2 grams of protein per kilogram of body weight per day, the upper recommendation for most athletes.

## Vitamin and Mineral Needs

Vitamin and mineral needs are the same or slightly higher for athletes, compared with those of sedentary adults. Athletes usually have high calorie intakes, so they tend to consume plenty of vitamins and minerals. An exception is athletes consuming low-calorie diets (about 1200 kcal or less), such as seen with some female athletes participating in events in which maintaining a low body weight is crucial. These diets may not meet B-vitamin and other micronutrient needs. Vegetarian athletes are also a

▲ High-protein products, often marketed to athletes, are unnecessary. The same holds true for high-protein bars, a trend in marketing products to athletes.

▲ Weight-restricted athletes especially should make sure they are consuming enough protein as well as other essential nutrients.

concern. In these cases, consuming fortified foods, such as ready-to-eat breakfast cereals or a balanced multivitamin and mineral supplement is recommended.

Athletes' needs for antioxidants such as vitamin E and vitamin C may be somewhat greater because of the potential protection these nutrients provide; this effect could be especially important in the face of high oxygen use by muscles. The use of large doses of vitamin E and vitamin C, however, requires more study and is not currently an accepted part of the dietary guidance for athletes. Experts suggest consuming a diet containing foods rich in antioxidants, such as fruits, vegetables, whole-grain breads and cereals, and vegetable oils. In addition, there is evidence that antioxidant systems in the body increase in activity as exercise training progresses. There is also speculation that the "oxidative stress" produced during exercise might have benefits, such as for muscle adaptation to exercise, and so trying to block this process may not be advantageous.

**Iron Deficiency Impairs Performance.** Iron is involved in red blood cell production, oxygen transport, and energy production, so a deficiency of this mineral can noticeably detract from optimal athletic performance. The potential causes for iron deficiency in athletes vary. As in the general population, female athletes are most susceptible to low iron status due to monthly menstrual losses. Special diets followed by athletes, such as low-calorie and vegetarian (especially vegan) diets are likely to be low in iron. Distance runners should pay special attention to iron intake, because their intense workouts may lead to gastrointestinal bleeding. Another concern is *sports anemia*—which occurs because exercise causes blood plasma volume to expand, particularly at the start of a training regimen before the synthesis of red blood cells increases. This results in dilution of the blood. In this case, even if iron stores are adequate, blood iron tests may appear low.

Sports anemia is not detrimental to performance, but it is hard to differentiate between sports anemia and true anemia. If iron status is low and not replenished, iron-deficiency anemia and markedly impaired endurance performance can eventually result. Although true anemia (a depressed blood hemoglobin level) is not that common among athletes, it is a good idea for athletes (especially adult women), to have their iron status checked at the beginning of a training season and at least once during midseason and to monitor dietary iron intake.

Any blood test indicating low iron status—sports anemia or not—is cause for follow-up. For some, the use of iron supplements may be advisable. However, indiscriminate use of iron supplements is not advised because toxic effects are possible. It is important that physicians investigate the cause of the deficiency because iron deficiency can be caused by blood loss. If caught early, some serious medical conditions such as this can be treated or prevented.

Some studies have suggested that iron deficiency without anemia may also have a negative effect on physical activity and performance. Also, once depleted, iron stores can take months to replenish. For this reason, athletes must be especially careful to meet iron needs.

**Calcium Intake Is Important, Especially in Women.** Athletes, especially women trying to lose weight by restricting their intake of dairy products, can have marginal or low dietary intakes of calcium. This practice compromises optimal bone health. Of still greater concern are women athletes who have stopped menstruating because their arduous training and low body fat content interferes with the normal secretion of reproductive hormones. Disturbing reports show that female athletes who do not menstruate regularly have spinal bones far less dense than those of both nonathletes and female athletes who menstruate regularly. This places them at increased risk for bone fractures during training and competition and osteoporosis in later life. The negative impacts of low dietary calcium intake and irregular menses in female athletes outweigh the benefits of weight-bearing exercise on bone density. This topic is discussed further in Chapter 11, with respect to the female athlete triad, and in Chapter 9, where osteoporosis was reviewed in detail.

**R**ecall from Chapter 8 that nutrients in dietary supplements should not exceed any Upper Levels set over the long term. As well, men should be cautious about any use of supplements containing iron.

**"B**lood doping" is the injection of red blood cells, naturally containing iron, to enhance aerobic capacity. This is an illegal practice under Olympic guidelines.

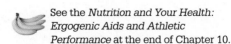

See the *Nutrition and Your Health: Ergogenic Aids and Athletic Performance* at the end of Chapter 10.

Research has clearly documented the importance of regular menstruation to maintain bone mineral density. Studies show that a woman runner who does not menstruate regularly may also have a higher risk for the development of a **stress fracture.** Thus, female athletes whose menstrual cycles become irregular should consult a physician to determine the cause. Decreasing the amount of training or increasing energy intake and body weight often restores regular menstrual cycles. If irregular menstrual cycles persist, severe bone loss (much of which is not reversible) and osteoporosis can result. Extra calcium in the diet does not necessarily compensate for these damaging effects of menstrual irregularities, but inadequate dietary calcium can make matters worse.

> **stress fracture** A fracture that occurs from repeated jarring of a bone. Common sites include bones of the foot.

## 10.5 A Focus on Fluid Needs

Fluid needs for an average adult are about 9 cups per day for women and 13 cups per day for men. Athletes generally need even more water to maintain the body's ability to regulate internal temperature and to keep cool. Most energy released during metabolism appears immediately as heat. Furthermore, heat production in contracting muscles can rise 15 to 20 times above that of resting muscles. Unless this heat is quickly dissipated, heat exhaustion, heat cramps, and potentially fatal heat-stroke may ensue.

Athletes must avoid becoming dehydrated not only for the sake of athletic performance, but also to prevent heat exhaustion, heat cramps, and fatal heatstroke. Fluid intake during exercise, when possible, should be adequate to minimize body-weight loss; following this practice is a good idea even when sweating can go unnoticed, such as when swimming or during the winter. To replace fluids lost in sweat, regulate body temperature, and prevent dehydration and low blood sodium levels, the American College of Sports Medicine recommends appropriate fluid intake before, during, and after physical activity. Fluid and electrolyte needs vary widely, based on differences in body mass, environmental conditions, level of training, event duration, and even genetics. Because fluid needs are highly individualized and dynamic, it is not appropriate to make general recommendations for fluid replacement. Rather, an athlete should aim to replace the total amount of fluid lost during exercise. This can be accomplished by knowing the body's hourly sweat rate, which can be calculated from the weight lost during exercise per hour plus the fluid consumed during exercise per hour.

The recommended fluid status goal is a loss of no more than 2% of body weight during exercise, especially in hot weather. Athletes should first calculate 2% of their body weight and then by trial and error determine how much fluid they must take in to avoid losing more than this amount of weight during exercise. This determination will be most accurate if an athlete is weighed before and after a typical workout. For every 1 pound (½ kilogram) lost, 2½ to 3 cups (about 0.75 liters) of water should be consumed during exercise or immediately afterward. The fluid recommendations replace the previous recommendation of 2 cups per pound, as some of the fluid replacement will quickly be lost via increased sweating after exercise and increased urine output. Much of this fluid replacement will have to take place after exercise because it is difficult to consume enough fluid during exercise to prevent weight loss. If weight change can't be monitored, urine color is another measure of hydration status. Urine color should be no more yellow than lemonade.

Thirst is a late sign of dehydration and so is not a reliable indicator of an athlete's need to replace fluid during exercise. An athlete who drinks only when thirsty is likely to take 48 hours to replenish fluid losses. After several days of training, an athlete relying on thirst as an indicator can build up a fluid debt that will impair performance. The following fluid replacement approach can meet athletes' fluid needs in most cases:

- Freely drink beverages (e.g., water, diluted fruit juice, sports drinks) during the 24-hour period before an event, even if not particularly thirsty.
- Drink 1½ to 2½ cups of fluid (400 to 600 milliliters) 2 to 3 hours before exercise. This allows time for both adequate hydration and excretion of excess fluid.

▲ Dehydration, which can lead to illness and death, is a problem that must be avoided during physical activity in hot, humid environments.

▲ Fluid intake before, during, and after physical activity is important.

- During events lasting more than 30 minutes, consume about ½ to 1½ cups (150 to 350 milliliters) of fluid every 15 to 20 minutes throughout the exercise. Consuming more than 1 quart (1 liter) per hour can cause discomfort. On hot days, cold drinks are preferable to help cool the body. Again, the athlete should not wait until he or she feels thirsty. In many cases, athletes, especially children and teenagers, need to be reminded to consume fluids during exercise.
- Within 4 to 6 hours after exercise, about 2½ to 3 cups of fluid should be consumed for every pound lost, as mentioned. It is also important that weight be restored before the next exercise period. Skipping fluids before or during events will almost certainly impair performance. Both caffeine and alcohol have purported diuretic effects. However, recent research shows that moderate caffeine consumption is not detrimental for athletes and may, in fact, improve performance in endurance events. Alcohol, on the other hand, is not a good choice for hydration.

The popularity of caffeine-containing energy drinks has surged in recent years. Some studies show that caffeine improves athletic performance during endurance events (e.g., cycling) or sports that require a high level of mental alertness (e.g., archery). However, excessive caffeine consumption can lead to shakiness, nervousness, anxiety, nausea, and insomnia. In addition, the diuretic effect of caffeine does not support optimal hydration. Compare the caffeine contents of several top-selling energy drinks.

| | |
|---|---|
| Amp (8.4 oz) | 75 mg |
| Full Throttle (16 oz) | 144 mg |
| Monster (16 oz) | 160 mg |
| No Fear (16 oz) | 174 mg |
| Red Bull (8.3 oz) | 80 mg |
| Rockstar (16 oz) | 160 mg |
| SoBe Adrenaline Rush (8.3 oz) | 79 mg |
| Tab Energy (10.5) | 95 mg |

**Heat exhaustion** occurs when heat stress causes loss of body fluid and then depletion of blood volume. Maintaining adequate body fluid is important. As environmental temperature rises above 95°F (35°C), virtually all body heat is lost through the evaporation of sweat from the skin. Sweat rates during prolonged exercise range from 3 to 8 cups (750 to 2000 milliliters) per hour. However, as the humidity rises, especially above 75%, evaporation slows and sweating becomes an inefficient way to cool the body. The result is rapid fatigue, increased work for the heart, and difficulty with prolonged exertion. Clearly, the combination of high heat and humidity (e.g., 95°F and 90% humidity) can be as dangerous as extreme cold.

Increased body temperature associated with dehydration is evident when the amount of water loss exceeds only 2% of body weight, especially in hot weather. This dehydration then leads to a decline in endurance, strength, and overall performance. Wearing football equipment in hot weather can lead to a loss of 2% of body weight in 30 minutes. Marathon runners have been shown to lose 6% to 10% of body weight during a race.

Common symptoms of heat exhaustion include profuse sweating, headache, dizziness, nausea, vomiting, muscle weakness, visual disturbances, and flushing of the skin. A person with heat exhaustion should be taken to a cool environment immediately, and excess clothing should be removed. The body should be sponged with tap water. Fluid replacement, as tolerated, then should suffice to correct the condition.

**Heat cramps** are a frequent complication of heat exhaustion, but they may appear without other symptoms of dehydration. Cramps usually occur in individuals who have exercised for several hours in a hot climate, experienced significant sweating, and have consumed a large volume of water without replacing sodium losses. It is important not to confuse heat cramps with other forms of muscle cramps, such as those caused by GI tract upset. Heat cramps occur in skeletal muscles, including those of the abdomen and extremities. They consist of a contraction lasting 1 to 3 minutes at a time. The cramp moves down the muscle and is associated with excruciating pain. To prevent heat cramps exercise moderately at first; aim to have adequate salt intake before engaging in long, strenuous activity in the heat; and avoid dehydration.

**Heatstroke** can occur when the internal body temperature reaches 104°F or more. Related symptoms include nausea, confusion, irritability, poor coordination, seizures, and coma. Exertional heatstroke results from high blood flow to exercising muscles, which overloads the body's cooling capacity. Sweating generally ceases, and the body temperature may become dangerously high. If left untreated, circulatory collapse, nervous system damage, and death are likely. The death rate from heatstroke is high, approximately 10%. Typically, three to five athletes die each year of heatstroke. In 2001, both college and professional football players died this way.

Many individuals faint during heatstroke, and their skin becomes hot and dry. Cooling the skin with ice packs or cold water is the usual recommended immediate treatment until medical help can be summoned. To decrease the risk of developing heatstroke, athletes should watch for rapid body-weight changes (2% or more of body weight), replace lost fluids, and avoid exercising under extremely hot, humid conditions.

## Sports Drinks

A question that often arises is whether to drink water or a sports-type carbohydrate-electrolyte drink (e.g., All Sport, Exceed Energy Drink, Gatorade, PowerAde, and Amino Force) during competition (Fig. 10-7). For sports that require less than 60 minutes of exertion or when total weight loss is less than 5 to 6 pounds, the primary concern is replacing the water lost in sweat, because losses of carbohydrate stores and electrolytes (sodium, chloride, potassium, and other minerals) are not usually very great. Although electrolytes are lost in sweat, the quantities lost in exercise of brief to moderate duration can be easily replaced later by consuming normal foods, such as orange juice, potatoes, and tomato juice. Keep in mind that sweat is about 99% water and only 1% electrolytes and other substances.

When exercise extends beyond 60 minutes, electrolyte (especially sodium) and carbohydrate replacement becomes increasingly important. Use of sports drinks during these longer bouts of exercise—even more so in hot weather—offers several distinct advantages over water alone.

Water by itself, as you have learned, increases blood volume to allow for efficient cooling and transport of fuels and waste products to and from cells. The addition of carbohydrate to a sports drink supplies glucose to muscles as they become depleted of glycogen, and thus can enhance performance when administered during endurance activities (see the later section on carbohydrate replacement). Carbohydrate also adds flavor, which encourages athletes to drink. Finally, the electrolytes in sports drinks help to maintain blood volume, enhance the absorption of water and carbohydrate from the intestine, and stimulate thirst. For these reasons, some experts prefer sports drinks over water for all athletes.

Overall, the decision to use a sports drink hinges primarily on the duration of the activity. As the projected duration of continuous activity approaches 60 minutes or longer, the advantages of the use of a sports drink over plain water clearly emerge. However, athletes should first experiment with sports drinks during practice, instead of trying them for the first time during competition.

It is also possible for some athletes to drink too much water and thereby develop water intoxication (hyponatremia). Endurance athletes (especially poorly trained individuals) may compete at relatively low exercise intensities for prolonged periods and therefore may not sweat as much as one might predict. Thus, water losses are not high. Drinking less fluid, choosing a sports drink containing sodium (usually in the form of sodium chloride), and not gaining weight during the activity can help prevent this problem. (A drop in blood sodium can occur in both hot and cold weather.)

**heatstroke** Heatstroke can occur when internal body temperature reaches 104°F. Sweating generally ceases if left untreated, and blood circulation is greatly reduced. Nervous system damage may ensue, and death is likely. Often the skin of individuals who suffer heatstroke is hot and dry.

**FIGURE 10-7** ▶ Sports drinks for fluid and electrolyte replacement typically contain a form of simple carbohydrate plus sodium and potassium. The various sugars in this product total 14 grams per 1 cup (240 milliliters) serving. In percentage terms based on weight, the sugar content is about 6% ([14 grams sugar per serving ÷ 240 grams per serving] × 100 = 5.8%). Sports drinks typically contain about 6% to 8% sugar. This provides ample glucose and other monosaccharides to aid in fueling working muscles, and it is well tolerated. Drinks with a sugar content above 10%, such as soft drinks or fruit juices, may cause stomach distress and so are not recommended.

**General Guide for Approximate Pre-event Carbohydrate Intake**

| Hours Before | Grams per kilogram Body Weight | For a 70-kilogram Person |
|---|---|---|
| 1 | 1 | 70 |
| 2 | 2 | 140 |
| 3 | 3 | 210 |
| 4 | 4 | 280 |

▲ Carbohydrate intake during endurance exercise helps maintain this source of energy for the body.

## 10.6 Specialized Dietary Advice for Before, During, and After Endurance Exercise

A light meal supplying up to 1000 kcal should be eaten about 2 to 4 hours before an endurance event to top off muscle and liver glycogen stores, prevent hunger during the event, and provide extra fluid. The longer the period before an event, the larger the meal can be, because there will be more time available for digestion. A pre-event meal should consist primarily of carbohydrate (about 200 grams), contain little fat or fiber, and include a moderate amount of protein (Table 10-6). A meal eaten 1 hour or so before an event should be blended or liquid to promote rapid stomach emptying. Examples are low-fat smoothies, juices, and sports drinks.

Good food choices for a pre-event meal include spaghetti, muffins, bagels, pancakes with fresh fruit topping, oatmeal with fruit, baked potato topped with yogurt or a small amount of sour cream, toasted bread with jam, bananas, apples, oranges, pears, plums, nuts, and low-sugar breakfast cereals with reduced-fat or fat-free milk. Liquid meal-replacement formulas, such as Carnation Instant Breakfast, also can be used. Foods especially rich in fiber should be eaten the previous day to help empty the colon before an event, but they should not be eaten the night before or in the morning before the event. Avoid fatty or fried foods, such as sausage, bacon, sauces, and gravies.

**TABLE 10-6** Convenient Pre-event Meals

| **Breakfast** | |
|---|---|
| Cheerios, ¾ cup<br>Reduced-fat milk, 1 cup<br>Blueberry muffin, 1<br>Orange juice, 4 oz | 450 kcal<br>92 grams (82%) carbohydrate |
| or | |
| Low-fat fruit yogurt, 1 cup<br>Plain bagel, ½<br>Apple juice, 4 oz<br>Peanut butter (for bagel), 1 tbsp | 482 kcal<br>84 grams (68%) carbohydrate |
| or | |
| Whole-wheat toast, 1 slice<br>Jam, 1 tsp<br>Apple, 1 large<br>Reduced-fat milk, 1 cup<br>Oatmeal, ½ cup (with reduced-fat milk, ½ cup) | 507 kcal<br>98 grams (73%) carbohydrate |
| **Lunch or Dinner** | |
| Chili with beans, 8 oz<br>Baked potato with sour cream and chives<br>Chocolate milk shake | 900 kcal<br>150 grams (65%) carbohydrate |
| or | |
| Spaghetti noodles, 2 cups<br>Spaghetti sauce, 1 cup<br>Reduced-fat milk, 1½ cups<br>Green beans, 1 cup | 761 kcal<br>129 grams (66%) carbohydrate |
| or | |
| Orange, 1 large<br>Reduced-fat milk, 1½ cups<br>Chicken noodle soup, 1 cup<br>Saltine crackers, 12<br>Buttered beans, 1 cup<br>Corn, 1 cup<br>Angel food cake, 1 slice | 829 kcal<br>160 grams (70%) carbohydrate |

With regard to the timing of pre-activity meals, a general guide is to allow 4 hours for a big meal (about 1200 kcal), 3 hours for a moderate meal (about 800 to 900 kcal), 2 hours for a light meal (about 400 to 600 kcal), and an hour or less for a snack (about 300 kcal).

## Replenishing Fuel During Endurance Exercise

We've already established the importance of consuming adequate fluids during endurance exercise. For sporting events longer than 60 minutes, consumption of carbohydrate during activity can also improve athletic performance. This is because prolonged exercise depletes muscle glycogen stores and low levels of blood glucose lead to fatigue, both physical and mental. When the supply of carbohydrate calories runs low, athletes often complain of "hitting the wall," the point at which maintaining a competitive pace seems impossible. One way to overcome this obstacle is to maintain normal blood glucose concentrations by carbohydrate feedings. As mentioned, a general guideline for endurance events is to consume 30 to 60 grams of carbohydrate per hour; however, an athlete should experiment during training sessions to establish the level that leads to optimal performance.

In the previous section on fluid needs, you learned that sports drinks are a good source of carbohydrate calories during endurance events. They supply the necessary fluid, electrolytes, and carbohydrate to keep an athlete performing at his or her best. As an alternative to sports drinks, some athletes have begun to use carbohydrate gels (e.g., PowerGel and Clif Shot) and energy bars (e.g., PowerBar). Check the label on these products to gauge the amount of gel or bar that provides 30 to 60 grams of carbohydrate per hour. Gels contain about 25 grams of carbohydrate per serving, and depending on the type, popular energy bars range from 2 to 45 grams of carbohydrate per serving (Table 10-7). Sports drinks, by comparison, contain about 14 grams of carbohydrate per 8-oz serving. The wide range of carbohydrate content in energy bars is due to a variety of marketing trends in the sports supplement industry. Overall, choosing a bar with about 40 grams of carbohydrate and no more than 10 grams of protein, 4 grams of fat, and 5 grams of fiber is recommended. The bars are also typically fortified with vitamins and minerals, often up to 100% of the Daily Values. As such, these bars can be seen as a convenient, although somewhat expensive, source of nutrients. Caution should be exercised, however, because the highly fortified nature of these bars may also lead to nutrient toxicities, such as with vitamin A, if overused.

> **I**t cannot be emphasized enough that any nutrition strategies should be tested during practice and trial runs before being used in a meet or key event. An athlete should never try a new food or beverage on the day of competition. Some food items and beverages may not be well tolerated, and the day of competition is not the time to find out.

### MAKING DECISIONS

#### Fat for Endurance?

Why hasn't fat been mentioned as a way to improve athletic performance during an endurance event? While fat is used along with carbohydrate as fuel during prolonged aerobic activity, the processes of digestion, absorption, and metabolism of fat are relatively slow. Therefore, consumption of fat during activity is not likely to translate into better athletic performance.

If solid sources of carbohydrate are one's preference, fig cookies, Gummy Bears, and jellybeans can also yield a quick source of glucose and with a much lower cost. However, any carbohydrate-containing food, including energy bars and gels, must be accompanied by fluid to ensure adequate hydration.

### MAKING DECISIONS

#### Energy Bars

As discussed, food manufacturers have begun to promote meal replacement bars (also called "energy" bars) to all kind of athletes. These bars typically contain about 180 to 250 kcal, with a macronutrient distribution typical of common diets. However, some bars replace much of the carbohydrate with protein. The bars are fortified with vitamins and minerals in amounts ranging from about 25% to 100% of typical human needs. Some people find these bars provide a convenient way to consume a meal (or snack) on the run, while also focusing on certain nutrients they may underconsume, such as the B vitamin folate or the mineral calcium. These bars generally cost $1 to $2. The energy and nutrient contents of popular energy bars are shown in Table 10-7. Critics suggest these products are essentially the nutritional equivalent of a cup of low-fat yogurt and piece of fruit.

▲ Elite athletes such as Olympic beach volleyball gold medal winner Kerri Walsh are well aware that modifying their diet and training regimen to match the specific needs of their sport is key to optimum performance. Replenishing carbohydrate and fluids is especially important when training.

**TABLE 10-7** Energy and Macronutrient Contents of Popular Energy Bars and Gels

| Product | Energy (kcal) | Carbohydrates (g) | Fiber (g) | Protein (g) | Fat (g) |
|---|---|---|---|---|---|
| Balance Bar (chocolate) | 200 | 22 | <1 | 14 | 6 |
| Clif Bar (chocolate chip) | 250 | 45 | 5 | 10 | 5 |
| Clif Shot (vanilla) | 100 | 25 | 0 | 0 | 0 |
| Gatorade Nutrition Bar (peanut butter crunch) | 250 | 38 | 2 | 15 | 5 |
| Genisoy Bar (cookies & cream) | 240 | 35 | 1 | 14 | 4.5 |
| GU Energy Gel (lemon sublime) | 100 | 25 | 0 | 0 | 0 |
| Kashi GoLean Bar (malted chocolate crisp) | 290 | 49 | 6 | 13 | 6 |
| LARABAR (coconut cream pie) | 200 | 27 | 5 | 3 | 10 |
| LUNA Bar (cherry-covered chocolate) | 180 | 28 | 3 | 9 | 5 |
| MET-Rx Big 100 Bar (super cookie crunch) | 410 | 43 | 3 | 32 | 14 |
| PowerBar Gel (strawberry banana) | 110 | 27 | 0 | 0 | 0 |
| PowerBar Performance (chocolate) | 230 | 45 | 3 | 10 | 2 |
| PowerBar Pria (French vanilla crisp) | 110 | 17 | 5 | 5 | 3 |
| PowerBar ProteinPlus (cookies & cream) | 300 | 38 | 1 | 23 | 6 |
| Power Crunch Bar (peanut butter crème) | 200 | 10 | 1 | 13 | 12 |
| Promax Energy Bar (black forest cake) | 280 | 38 | 2 | 20 | 6 |
| Snickers Marathon (multigrain crunch) | 220 | 32 | 2 | 10 | 7 |
| Soldier Fuel (apple cinnamon) | 280 | 42 | 1 | 10 | 8 |
| Tiger's Milk (peanut butter and honey) | 140 | 19 | 1 | 5 | 5 |
| Zone Perfect (apple cinnamon) | 210 | 21 | 1 | 15 | 7 |

Overall, choosing energy bars is preferable to choosing candy bars and packaged cakes. When used in sports situations, energy bars can be handy. Better yet, however, is to eat a variety of wholesome foods; these offer more health-protective compounds. This is also a less expensive choice, especially for day-to-day snacking. An additional concern is that micronutrient toxicity might occur if numerous bars are eaten in a day, as many are highly fortified. Vitamin A and iron are two nutrients of special concern in this regard.

## Carbohydrate Intake During Recovery from Prolonged Exercise

Carbohydrate-rich foods providing 1 to 2 grams of carbohydrate per kilogram body weight should be consumed within 2 hours after extended (endurance) exercise, and the sooner the better (Table 10-8). Immediately after exercise is when glycogen synthesis is greatest, because the muscles are insulin-sensitive at this point. This process should then be repeated over the next 2-hour interval. Athletes training hard can consume a sugar candy, sugared soft drink, fruit or fruit juice, or a sports-type carbohydrate supplement right after training as they attempt to reload their muscles with glycogen.

Later, enriched bread, mashed potatoes, and short-grain white rice can contribute to additional carbohydrate consumption. These high-glycemic-load carbohydrates especially contribute to glycogen synthesis. Recall that Table 4-4 shows the glycemic load for various foods. Adding an appropriate amount of protein (3 grams of carbohydrate: 1 gram of protein) during recovery can be especially helpful for meeting overall calorie

**TABLE 10-8** Sample Postexercise Meals for Rapid Muscle Glycogen Replacement

**Option 1**
1 regular bagel
2 tbsp peanut butter, smooth
8 fl oz fat-free milk
1 medium banana
562 kcal, 77 grams carbohydrate, 23 grams protein, 18 grams fat

**Option 2 blend until smooth**
1 packet Carnation Instant Breakfast
8 oz fat-free milk
1 medium banana
1 tbsp peanut butter
438 kcal, 70 grams carbohydrate, 17 grams protein, 10 grams fat

**Option 3**
1.5 cans GatorPro (11 fl oz per can)
559 kcal, 89 grams carbohydrate, 26 grams protein, 11 grams fat

**F**or more information on sports nutrition, visit the Gatorade Sport Science Institute webpage (www.gssiweb.com). For more information on sports medicine, visit www.physsportsmed.com. This homepage of *The Physician and Sportsmedicine* journal details current issues in sports medicine, including injury prevention, nutrition, and exercise. Also helpful are the webpages of the American College of Sports Medicine (www.acsm.org), Centers for Disease Control and Prevention Division of Nutrition and Physical Activity (www.cdc.gov/nccdphp/dnpa), and the American Council on Exercise (www.acefitness.org).

and nutrient needs. For a 154-pound (70-kilogram) athlete, this corresponds to about 70 grams of carbohydrate and 25 grams of protein in each 2-hour interval (Table 10-8 contains sample meals of this composition). In summary, the following are key factors for achieving the most rapid replenishment of muscle glycogen after exercise: (1) availability of adequate carbohydrate, (2) ingestion of carbohydrate as soon as possible after completion of exercise, and (3) selection of high-glycemic-load carbohydrates.

Fluid and electrolyte (i.e., sodium and potassium) intake is also an essential component of an athlete's recovery diet. This helps replenish body fluids as quickly as possible. This is especially important if two workouts a day are performed or if the environment is hot and humid. If food and fluid intake is sufficient to restore weight loss, it generally will also supply enough electrolytes to meet needs during recovery from endurance activities.

## CONCEPT CHECK

All athletes would do well to plan a diet following MyPyramid. High-carbohydrate foods should be emphasized, and these should dominate in pre-event meals. Protein intake above 1.7 grams per kilogram of body weight is not supported by scientific evidence. Most athletes easily consume enough protein from typical food choices. If nutrient supplements are used, dosages generally should not exceed the Upper Level set for each nutrient. Fluid should be consumed as liberally as possible before, during, and after an event. Carbohydrate and electrolytes in the fluid are especially helpful to help delay fatigue and maintain electrolyte balance when exercise duration exceeds 60 minutes.

# Ergogenic Aids and Athletic Performance

## Ergogenic Aids to Enhance Athletic Performance

Extreme diet manipulation to improve athletic performance is not a recent innovation. As long as 30 years ago, American football players were encouraged on hot practice days to "toughen up" for competition by liberally consuming salt tablets before and during practice and by not drinking water. Now it is widely recognized that this practice can be fatal. Today's athletes are as likely as their predecessors to experiment with any substance that promises a competitive advantage. In 2007, consumers spent more than $18.2 billion on sports nutrition and weight loss supplements. Artichoke hearts, bee pollen, dried adrenal glands from cattle, seaweed, freeze-dried liver flakes, gelatin, and ginseng are just some of the ineffective substances used by athletes in hopes of gaining an **ergogenic** (work-producing) edge.

Based on what is known at this time, today's athletes can benefit from scientific evidence documenting the ergogenic properties of a few dietary substances. These ergogenic aids include sufficient water and electrolytes, lots of carbohydrates, and a balanced and varied diet consistent with MyPyramid. Protein and amino acid supplements are not among those aids because athletes can easily meet protein needs from foods,

> **ergogenic** Work-producing. An ergogenic aid is a mechanical, nutritional, psychological, pharmacological, or physiological substance or treatment intended to directly improve exercise performance.

as Table 10-3 demonstrated. The use of nutrient supplements should be designed to meet a specific dietary shortcoming, such as an inadequate iron intake. These and other aids, which often have dubious benefits and may pose health risks, must be given close scrutiny before use. The risk-benefit ratio of any ergogenic aid merits careful evaluation.

As summarized in Table 10-9, no scientific evidence supports the effectiveness of many substances touted as performance-enhancing aids. Many are useless; some are dangerous. Athletes should be skeptical of any substance until its ergogenic effect is scientifically validated. FDA has a limited ability to regulate these dietary supplements (review Chapter 1), and the manufacturing processes for dietary supplements are not as tightly regulated by FDA as they are for prescription drugs. Some supplements may contain substances that will cause athletes to "test positive" for various banned substances. This was demonstrated in the 2002 Winter

Olympics. Studies also have called into question the quality control associated with the manufacturing of dietary supplements. Many do not contain the substance and/or the amount listed on the label.

These results add yet another worry for the athlete. Not only must he or she determine whether there is evidence that a dietary supplement is safe and effective, but must also question if the dietary supplement contains what it is supposed to contain.

Even substances whose ergogenic effects have been supported by systematic scientific studies should be used with caution, as the testing conditions may not match those of the intended use.

Finally, rather than waiting for a magic bullet to enhance performance, athletes are advised to concentrate their efforts on improving their training routines and sport techniques, while consuming well-balanced diets as described in this chapter.

### MAKING DECISIONS

#### NCAA and Supplements

The NCAA's Committee on Competitive Safeguards and Medical Aspects of Sports has developed lists of permissible and nonpermissible supplements for athletic departments to dispense. Following are key examples:

| Permissible | Nonpermissible |
|---|---|
| Vitamins and minerals | Amino acids |
| "Energy" bars (if no more than 30% protein) | Creatine |
| Sports drinks | Glycerol |
| Meal replacement drinks such as Ensure Plus or Boost | HMB |
| | L-carnitine |
| | Protein powders |

**TABLE 10-9** An Evaluation of Current Ergogenic Aids

| Substance/Practice | Rationale | Reality |
|---|---|---|
| **Useful in Some Circumstances** | | |
| Creatine | Increase phosphocreatine (PCr) in muscles to keep ATP concentration high | Use of 20 grams per day for 5 to 6 days and then a maintenance dose of 2 grams per day may improve performance in those who undertake repeated bursts of activity, such as in sprinting and weightlifting. Vegetarian athletes benefit the most because their diets are low in or void of creatine. Some of the muscle weight gain noted with use results from water contained in muscles. Endurance athletes do not benefit from use. Little is known about the safety of long-term creatine use. Continual use of high doses has led to kidney damage in a few cases. Cost: $25 to $65 per month. |
| Sodium Bicarbonate (baking soda) | Counter lactic acid buildup | Partially effective in some circumstances (when lactic acid is rapidly produced), such as wrestling, but induces nausea and diarrhea. The dose used is 300 milligrams/kilogram, given 1 to 3 hours before exercise. Cost: nil. |
| Caffeine | Increase use of fatty acids to fuel muscles, promote mental alertness | Drinking two to three 5-ounce cups of coffee (equivalent to 3 to 9 milligrams of caffeine per kilogram of body weight) about 1 hour before events lasting about 5 minutes or longer is useful for some athletes; benefits are less apparent in those who have ample stores of glycogen, are highly trained, or habitually consume caffeine; intake of more than about 600 milligrams (six to eight cups of coffee) elicits a urine concentration illegal under NCAA rules (greater than 15 micrograms per milliliter). Possible side effects include shakiness, nervousness, nausea, anxiety, and insomnia. Cost: $0.08 per 300 milligrams. |
| **Possibly Useful, Still Under Study** | | |
| Beta-hydroxy-beta methylbutyric acid (HMB) | Decrease protein catabolism, causing a net growth-promoting effect | Research in livestock and humans suggests that supplementation with this substance may increase muscle mass. Still, safety and effectiveness of long-term HMB use in humans is unknown. Cost: $100 per month. |
| Glutamine (an amino acid) | Enhance immune function, preserve lean body mass | Some preliminary studies show decreased occurrence of upper respiratory tract infections in athletes with use. It also may promote muscle growth, but long-term studies are lacking. Protein foods are a rich source of glutamine. Cost: $10 to $20 per month for 1 to 2 grams per day. |
| Branched-chain amino acids (BCAA) (leucine, isoleucine, valine) | Important energy source, especially when carbohydrate stores are depleted | Supplementation of BCAA (10 to 30 grams per day) during exercise can increase BCAA in the blood when it has been lowered due to exercise, but there is no consistent evidence of improved performance. Carbohydrate feeding, by delaying use of BCAA as fuel, may negate the need for BCAA supplementation. Preliminary studies show that BCAA use increases muscle mass more than does carbohydrate supplementation alone in swimmers, but there are no studies regarding resistance training. Protein-rich foods (especially dairy proteins) are also rich in BCAA. Cost: $20 per month. |
| **Dangerous or Illegal Substances/Practices** | | |
| Anabolic steroids (and related substances, such as androstenedione and tetrahydrogestrinone) | Increase muscle mass and strength | Although effective for increasing protein synthesis, anabolic steroids are illegal in the United States unless prescribed by a physician. They have numerous potential side effects, such as premature closure of growth plates in bones (thus possibly limiting the adult height of a teenage athlete), bloody cysts in the liver, increased risk of cardiovascular disease, increased blood pressure, and reproductive dysfunction. Possible psychological consequences include increased aggressiveness, drug dependence (addiction), withdrawal symptoms (such as depression), sleep disturbances, and mood swings (known as "roid rage"). Use of needles for injectable forms adds further health risk. Banned by the International Olympic Committee. |
| Growth hormone | Increase muscle mass | At critical ages, may increase height; may also cause uncontrolled growth of the heart and other internal organs and even death; potentially dangerous; requires careful monitoring by a physician. Use of needles for injections adds further health risk. Banned by the International Olympic Committee. |

**TABLE 10-9** *(continued)*

| Substance/Practice | Rationale | Reality |
|---|---|---|
| Blood doping | To enhance aerobic capacity by injecting red blood cells harvested previously from the athlete, or alternately the athlete may use the hormone erythropoietin (Epogen) to increase red blood cell number | May offer aerobic benefit; very serious health consequences are possible, including thickening of the blood, which puts extra strain on the heart; is an illegal practice under Olympic guidelines. |
| Gamma hydroxybutyric acid (GHB) | Promoted as a steroid alternative for bodybuilding | FDA has never approved it for sale as a medical product; is illegal to produce or sell GHB in the United States. GHB-related symptoms include vomiting, dizziness, tremors, and seizures. Many victims have required hospitalization, and some have died. Clandestine laboratories produced virtually all of the chemical accounting for GHB abuse. FDA is working with the U.S. Attorney's office to arrest, indict, and convict individuals responsible for the illegal operations. |

◀ Attention to carbohydrate and fluid needs—along with meeting overall nutrient needs—is the most important ergogenic aid.

## Case Study Planning a Training Diet

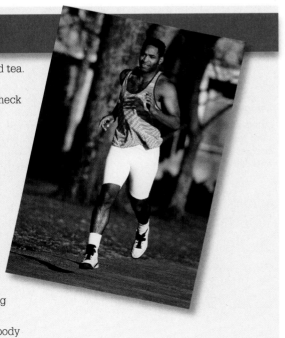

Michael is training for a 10K run coming up in 3 weeks. He has read a lot about sports nutrition and especially about the importance of eating a high-carbohydrate diet while in training. He also has been struggling to keep his weight in a range that he feels contributes to better speed and endurance. Consequently he is also trying to eat as little fat as possible. Unfortunately, over the past week his workouts in the afternoon have not met his expectations. His run times are slower, and he shows signs of fatigue after just 20 minutes into his training program.

His breakfast yesterday was a large bagel, a small amount of cream cheese, and orange juice. For lunch, he had a small salad with fat-free dressing, a large plate of pasta with marinara sauce and broccoli, and a diet soft drink. For dinner, he had a small broiled chicken breast, a cup of rice, some carrots, and iced tea. Later, he snacked on fat-free pretzels.

Answer the following questions, and check your responses in Appendix A.

1. Is the high-carbohydrate diet a good idea during Michael's training?
2. Are there any important components missing in Michael's diet? Are missing components contributing to his fatigue?
3. Describe some changes that should be made in Michael's diet including some specific foods that should be emphasized.
4. How should fluid needs be met during workouts?
5. Should Michael focus on fueling his body before, during, or after workouts?

# Summary

1. A gradual increase in regular physical activity is recommended for all healthy persons in order to reap the benefits illustrated in Figure 10-1.

2. A minimum fitness plan includes 30 minutes of physical activity on most (or all) days; 60 minutes per day provides even more benefit, especially if weight control is an issue. An intense program lasting about 60 to 90 minutes should begin with warm-up exercises to increase blood flow and warm the muscles and end with cooldown exercises. Regular resistance activities and stretching add further benefits.

3. Human metabolic pathways extract chemical energy from food and transform it into ATP, the compound that provides energy for body functions.

4. In carbohydrate fuel use, glucose is broken down into the three-carbon compound pyruvic acid, yielding some ATP. This is metabolized further via the aerobic pathway to form carbon dioxide ($CO_2$) and water ($H_2O$) or via the anaerobic pathway to form lactic acid.

5. At rest, muscle cells mainly use fat for fuel. For intense exercise of short duration, muscles mostly use phosphocreatine (PCr) for energy. During more sustained intense activity, muscle glycogen breaks down to lactic acid, providing a small amount of ATP. For endurance exercise, both fat and carbohydrate are used as fuels; carbohydrate is used increasingly as activity intensifies. Little protein is used to fuel muscles.

6. Anyone who exercises regularly should consume a diet that meets calorie needs and is moderate to high in carbohydrates and fluid and adequate in other nutrients such as iron and calcium.

7. Athletes should consume enough fluid to both minimize loss of body weight and ultimately restore pre-exercise weight. Sports drinks help replace fluid, electrolytes, and carbohydrates lost during workouts. Their use is especially appropriate when continuous activity lasts beyond 60 minutes.

8. Plenty of carbohydrates should be in the pre-event meal, especially for endurance athletes. High-glycemic-load carbohydrates should be consumed by an athlete within 2 hours after a workout to begin restoration of muscle glycogen stores. Some protein in the meal is also helpful.

9. Athletes can benefit from ergogenic properties of sufficient water and electrolytes, lots of carbohydrates, and a balanced and varied diet consistent with MyPyramid. Protein and amino acid supplements are not among beneficial aids because athletes meet protein needs from foods.

# Study Questions

1. How does greater physical fitness contribute to better overall health? Explain the process.

2. The store of ATP in muscle is rapidly depleted once muscle contraction begins. For physical activity to continue, ATP must be resupplied immediately. Describe how this occurs after initiation of exercise and at various times thereafter.

3. What is the difference between anaerobic and aerobic exercise? Explain why aerobic metabolism is increased by a regular exercise routine.

4. What is glycogen? How is it used during exercise?

5. Is fat from adipose tissue used as an energy source during exercise? If so, when?

6. What are some typical measures used to assess whether an athlete's calorie intake is adequate?

7. List five specific nutrients that athletes need and the appropriate food sources from which these nutrients can be obtained.

8. What conditions might contribute to the inability to get all required nutrients from food, thus requiring use of a multivitamin and mineral supplement?

9. What advice would you give your neighbor, planning to run a 5-kilometer (km) race, concerning fluid intake before and during the event?

10. One of your friends, a competitive athlete, asks your opinion about an amino acid supplement sold in a local sporting-goods store. She has read that such supplements can help improve athletic performance. What would you tell her about the general effectiveness of such products?

# Check Your Knowledge

Answers to the following questions are below.

1. An energy-rich compound, phosphocreatine (PCr), is found in _____ tissue.
   a. adipose
   b. muscle
   c. liver
   d. kidney

2. Carbohydrate loading is a process designed to increase
   a. fat stores.
   b. blood glucose concentrations.
   c. liver glucose levels.
   d. muscle glycogen stores.

3. During muscle-building regimes, athletes should consume _____ grams of protein per kilogram body weight.
   a. 0.5 to 0.7
   b. 0.8
   c. 1.5 to 1.7
   d. 2 to 2.5

4. Which of these foods is the best choice for carbohydrate loading before endurance events?

   a. potato chips
   b. French fries
   c. All-Bran (high-fiber) cereal
   d. rice

5. It is a good idea, especially for adult women athletes, to have blood hemoglobin checked regularly to detect for a possible deficiency of what mineral?
   a. calcium
   b. potassium
   c. copper
   d. iron

6. Additional fluid should be consumed _____ an athletic event.
   a. before
   b. during
   c. after
   d. a, b, and c.

7. How many cups of fluid are required to replace each pound of weight lost during an athletic event or workout?
   a. 0.5 to 0.75
   b. 1 to 1.5
   c. 2.5 to 3
   d. 4 to 5

8. The benefit of a "sports" drink is to provide
   a. water to hydrate.
   b. electrolytes to enhance water absorption in the intestine and maintain blood volume.
   c. carbohydrate for energy.
   d. All of the above.

9. A light meal is best eaten _____ before participating in a sporting event.
   a. immediately
   b. 2 to 4 hours
   c. 4 to 6 hours
   d. 8 to 10 hours

10. Caffeine is used as an ergogenic aid by some athletes because it is thought to
    a. increase use of fatty acids.
    b. decrease the buildup of lactic acid.
    c. serve as an energy source.
    d. increase muscle mass and strength.

Answers: 1. b, 2. d, 3. c, 4. d, 5. d, 6. d, 7. c, 8. d, 9. b, 10. a

# Further Readings

1. Adamidou J, Bell-Wilson J: Iron deficiency anemia and exercise. *IDEA Fitness Journal* May:82, 2006.

   *This article reviews why athletes may have increased iron requirements. The best food sources to prevent iron depletion and sports anemia are also suggested.*

2. Bell-Wilson J, Nisevich P: Eating for endurance: Nutrition needs of power players. *Today's Dietitian* 8:3, 2006.

   *Endurance athletes need fuel for their rigorous workouts. Guidelines for proper carbohydrate and fluid intake at all stages of activity—before, during, and after—are offered.*

3. Casa DJ and others: American College of Sports Medicine Roundtable on Hydration and Physical Activity: Consensus Statements. *Current Sports Medicine Reports* 4:115, 2005.

   *This report by an international panel of experts concludes that appropriate fluid intake before, during, and after physical activity is important to replace fluids lost in sweat and to regulate*

body temperature. An athlete should aim to replace the total amount of fluid lost during exercise. This can be accomplished by knowing their body's hourly sweat rate, which can be calculated from the weight lost during exercise per hour + fluid consumed during exercise per hour.

4. De Jonge L, Smith SR: Macronutrients and exercise. *Obesity Management* February:11, 2008.

   *Body stores of carbohydrate and fat are used preferentially as fuel for exercising muscles, whereas protein is conserved. This article reviews the importance of exercise for weight management because of its role in increasing fat oxidation. Exercise not only leads to increased fat oxidation during exercise, but also in the post-exercise period. Furthermore, the body's ability to burn fat is improved by training.*

5. Denny S: What are the guidelines for prevention of hyponatremia in individuals training for endurance sports, as well as other physically active adults? *Journal of the American Dietetic Association* 105:1323, 2005.

To decrease the risk of hyponatremia (low blood sodium levels), experts agree that endurance athletes should replace body fluids by drinking beverages, such as sports drinks, that contain carbohydrate and electrolytes in addition to water.

6. Glazer JL: Management of heat stroke and heat exhaustion. *American Family Physician* 71:2133, 2005.

   *Heat exhaustion and heat stroke are common and preventable conditions that affect athletes (and other individuals such as older adults). Treatment of heat exhaustion involves putting the person in a cool shady environment and ensuring adequate hydration. Treating heat stroke is much more complicated, as outlined in the article.*

7. Gleeson M: Can nutrition limit exercise-induced immunodepression? *Nutrition Reviews* March:119, 2006.

   *Intense or prolonged exercise can lead to immunodepression, resulting in increased incidence of infections (e.g., upper respiratory infections) among athletes. These effects are* due to the activity of stress hormones, such as adrenaline and cortisol, on immune cells. Optimal nutrition can attenuate immunodepression. Adequate habitual dietary intake of protein, essential fatty acids, zinc, iron, and antioxidants supports immune function. Acutely (e.g., during endurance exercise), consuming carbohydrate and staying hydrated are important strategies to prevent the stress response that leads to immune dysfunction.

8. Harber VJ: Energy balance and reproductive function in active women. *Canadian Journal of Applied Physiology* 29:48, 2004.

It is important for female athletes engaged in rigorous training programs to meet their calorie needs. If not, the resulting negative calorie balance will likely lead to a variety of menstrual cycle disturbances that can lead to other health problems. The article discusses this problem in detail and provides treatment strategies for problems that may develop.

9. Hew-Butler T and others: Updated fluid recommendation: Position statement from the International Marathon Medical Directors Association (IMMDA). *Clinical Journal of Sport Medicine* 16:283, 2006.

This position statement is the result of an extensive review by the IMMDA of current scientific evidence regarding the physiological processes that regulate fluid balance in marathon runners. Studies have shown that thirst is a more dynamic cue to maintaining fluid balance than are static approaches such as estimating fluid or weight loss. To prevent dehydration due to fluid loss while exercising, the key recommendation is to drink when thirsty. Avoiding drinking when not thirsty is recommended to avoid the risk of dangerously low sodium levels caused by excessive fluids. Runners are also advised to follow their body's cues as to whether to drink plain water or sports drinks, which provide sodium and other minerals.

10. Kunstel K: Calcium requirements for the athlete. *Current Sports Medicine Reports* 4:203, 2005.

Adequate calcium intake is needed to maintain bone health and prevent osteoporosis in all individuals. This article points out that the increased physical activity of athletes does not necessarily require an increased intake of dietary calcium or other micro-nutrients. Calcium may be lost in sweat, however, so athletes are advised to replenish it by consuming a diet including calcium-rich foods or by taking a calcium supplement.

11. Laaksonen DE and others: Physical activity in the prevention of type 2 diabetes: The Finnish Diabetes Prevention Study. *Diabetes* 54:158, 2005.

Regular physical activity can substantially reduce the risk of developing type 2 diabetes in high risk individuals. People who increased their activity from moderate to vigorous amounts reduced their risk of developing type 2 diabetes by 65% compared to people who remained inactive. Even typical low intensity activities, such as walking, conferred similar benefits in this study.

12. Maughan RJ, Shirreffs SM: Development of individual hydration strategies for athletes. *International Journal of Sport and Nutrition and Exercise Metabolism* 18:457, 2008.

Both dehydration and hyperhydration are detrimental to athletic performance and can be lethal. Despite the popular devaluation of thirst as an indicator of dehydration, recent research demonstrates that adherence to physiologic cues for consumption of fluid and electrolytes supports optimal athletic performance even when 100% body weight is not maintained. Individual fluid needs are determined by a combination of factors, including genetics, body size, duration and intensity of activity, level of athletic training, and environment. This article reviews several methods for assessing hydration status, from high-tech measures of plasma osmolality to the low-tech method of observing urine color. For optimal performance, hydration strategies should account for carbohydrate and electrolyte replacements in addition to fluid intake.

13. McCaffree J: Managing the diabetic athlete. *Journal of the American Dietetic Association* 106:8, 2006.

Compared to other athletes and other diabetics, the athlete with diabetes faces challenges in terms of balancing their insulin/medications, food, and exercise. This article offers advice for diabetic athletes and their health care providers on when and what to eat. In addition, the difference between type 1 and type 2 diabetes is addressed. Guidelines are also provided for specific nutrients and for hydration.

14. Rosenbloom C, Rosbruck M: Popular dietary supplements used in sports. *Nutrition Today* 43:60, 2008.

The authors review four dietary supplements that are popular as ergogenic and weight loss aids. Creatine, with its demonstrated ability to modestly improve performance in events requiring short bursts of activity, leads the article. The benefits of caffeine for endurance athletes are also explored, although the authors point out that effectiveness is dependent on prior caffeine consumption. Recent research on caffeine reveals that concern over its negative impact on hydration is unwarranted. Epigallocatechin gallate (EGCG) is discussed as a potential weight loss aid, particularly in combination with caffeine. Finally, nitric oxide and its metabolite, L-arginine, are reviewed as potentially increasing aerobic capacity. However, more research in human athletes is needed before nitric oxide can be recommended as an ergogenic aid.

15. Sawka MN and others: Human water needs. *Nutrition Reviews* 63:S30, 2005.

This review summarizes the water intake recommendations for healthy humans, emphasizing that hydration is well maintained as long as food and fluid are readily available. The effect of strenuous physical exercise and heat stress on water needs is also reviewed. The review concludes that exercise and heat can greatly increase water needs, and that the individual variability between athletes can be significant.

16. Sinclair LM, Hinton PS: Prevalence of iron deficiency with and without anemia in recreationally active men and women. *Journal of the American Dietetic Association* 105:975, 2005.

Both male and female athletes are at risk of exhibiting poor iron stores and even iron deficiency anemia, with females being at much higher risk. The authors recommend that athletes be screened for iron deficiency anemia, and as well have their current state of iron storage tested. Poor iron status can lead to poor work performance, and therefore should be avoided.

17. Spano M: Ergogenic aids: Fueling the sports nutrition industry. *Today's Dietitian* 8:3, 2006.

This article reviews the trends in sports nutrition and the influence of research, consumer demand, and legislation. The industry is improving with the top companies basing new products on scientific research and with more qualified sports nutritionists positioning themselves as professionals.

18. Suedekum NA, Dimeff RJ: Iron and the athlete. *Current Sports Medicine Reports* 4:1999, 2005.

Iron deficiency can occur in the athlete at different levels with a higher incidence in female athletes compared with males. Symptoms can range from none to severe fatigue. Iron deficiency can occur without anemia and may decrease athletic performance. This article discusses various causes of iron deficiency including poor intake, menstrual losses, gastrointestinal and genitourinary losses due to exercise-induced ischemia or organ movement, foot strike hemolysis, thermohemolysis, and sweat losses.

19. William SL and others: Antioxidant requirements of endurance athletes: Implications for health. *Nutrition Reviews* 64:93, 2006.

Exercise increases production of reactive oxygen species, which are associated with cell damage and numerous chronic diseases. Results of the limited number of studies of antioxidant supplements (primarily vitamins C or E) in athletes are equivocal; indeed, some studies show a pro-oxidant effect of these supplements. Furthermore, the increased production of reactive oxygen species during exercise may be part of beneficial physiological adaptations to exercise. Current evidence does not support the use of supplements of antioxidant nutrients. Rather, dietary guidance for athletes should emphasize the importance of consuming a variety of fruits and vegetables as sources of antioxidants.

20. Williams MH: *Nutrition for health, fitness & sport.* 7th ed. Boston: McGraw-Hill, 2005.

Excellent textbook for reviewing nutrient needs of athletes, as well as learning more about ergogenic aids; also provides a detailed look at metabolism in exercise.

## I. Evaluating Protein Intake—A Case Study

Mark is a college student who has been lifting weights at the student recreation center. The trainer at the center recommended a protein drink to help Mark build muscle mass. Answer the following questions about Mark's current food intake and determine whether a protein drink is needed to supplement Mark's diet.

1. The following is a tally of yesterday's intake.

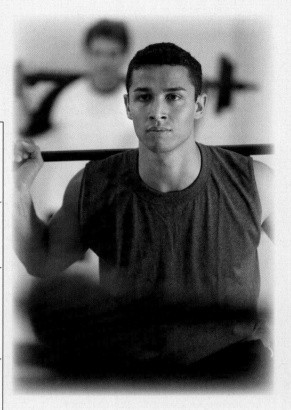

| Breakfast | Frosted Mini-Wheats cereal, 2 oz<br>1% milk, 1½ cups<br>Orange juice, chilled, 6 oz<br>Glazed yeast doughnut, 1<br>Brewed coffee, 1 cup |
|---|---|
| Lunch | Double hamburger with condiments, 1<br>French fries, 30<br>Cola, 12 oz<br>Medium apple, 1 |
| Dinner | Frozen lasagna w/meat, 2 pieces<br>1% milk, 1 cup<br>Looseleaf lettuce, chopped, 1 cup<br>Creamy Italian salad dressing, 2 tsp<br>Medium tomato, ½<br>Whole carrot, raw, 1 |
| Evening snack | Vanilla ice milk, 1 cup<br>Hot fudge chocolate topping, 2 tsp<br>Soft chocolate chip cookies, 2 |

Evaluate Mark's diet using NutritionCalc Plus—is he meeting the minimum recommendations of MyPyramid?

_____

2. Mark's weight has been stable at 70 kilograms (154 pounds). Determine his protein needs based on the RDA (0.8 grams per kilogram).
   a. Mark's estimated protein RDA: _____
   b. What are the maximum recommendations for protein intake for strength-training athletes (see p. 425)? _____
   c. Calculate the maximum protein recommendation for Mark. _____

_____

3. An analysis of the total calorie and protein content of Mark's current diet is 3470 kcal, 125 grams of protein (14% of total calories supplied by protein). This diet is representative of the food choices and amounts of food that Mark chooses on a regular basis.
   a. What is the difference between Mark's estimated protein needs as an athlete (from number 2) and the amount of protein that his current diet provides? _____
   b. Is his current protein intake inadequate, adequate, or excessive? _____

4. Mark takes his trainer's advice and goes to the supermarket to purchase a protein drink to add to his diet. Four products are available; they contain the following label information.

| | Amino Fuel | Joe Weider's Sugar-Free 90% Plus Protein | Joe Weider's Dynamic Muscle Builder | Victory Super Mega Mass 2000 |
|---|---|---|---|---|
| Serving size | 3 tbsp | 3 tbsp | 3 tbsp | ¼ scoop |
| Kcal | 104 | 110 | 103 | 104 |
| Protein (grams) | 15 | 24 | 10 | 5 |

The trainer recommends adding the supplement to Mark's diet two times a day. Mark chooses the Muscle Builder protein drink.

a. How much protein would be added to Mark's diet daily from two servings of the supplement alone (prior to mixing it with a beverage)?

b. Mark mixes the powder with the milk he already consumes at breakfast and dinner. How much protein total would Mark now consume in 1 day? (Add the protein amount from the nutrition analysis to the value from question 4a.)

c. What is the difference between Mark's estimated protein needs as an athlete and this total value?

5. What is your conclusion—does Mark need the protein supplement?

**Answers to Calculations**

2a. Mark's estimated protein RDA: 70 kilograms × 0.8 grams per kilogram = 56 grams.
2b. Maximum recommendation for protein intake for athletes = 1.7 grams per kilogram.
2c. Applied to Mark: 1.7 × 70 = 119 grams.
3a. Difference between Mark's estimated maximum protein needs for muscle mass gain and the amount of protein provided by his current diet:
125−119 = 6 grams protein.
3b. Mark's current protein intake exceeds maximum protein needs.
4a. Two servings of protein supplement alone = 20 grams of protein.
4b. Mark's total protein consumption: 125 grams + 20 grams = 145 grams protein.
4c. Difference between Mark's estimated maximum protein needs for muscle mass gain and total protein consumption with protein supplement (from above): 145 grams−119 grams = 26 grams protein.

# II. How Physically Fit Are You?

The fitness assessments presented here are easy to do and require little equipment. Also included are charts to compare your results to those typical of your peers.

### Cardiovascular Fitness: One-Mile Walk

Measure a mile on a running track (usually four laps) or on a little-trafficked neighborhood street (use a car's odometer to get the right distance). With a stopwatch or watch with a second hand, walk the mile as fast as you can. Note the time it took.

### Strength: Push-ups

Men: Get up on your toes and hands. Keep your back straight, with hands flat on the floor directly below your shoulders.
Women: Same position, but you can support your body on your knees if necessary.
   Lower your body, bending your elbows, until your chin grazes the floor. Push back up until your arms are straight. Continue until you can't do any more push-ups (you can rest when in the up position).

### Strength: Curl-ups

Lie on the floor on your back with your knees bent, feet flat. Your hands should rest on your thighs. Now squeeze your stomach muscles, push your back flat, and raise your upper body high enough for your hands to touch the tops of your knees. Don't pull with your neck or head, and keep your lower back on the floor. Count how many curl-ups you can do in one minute.

### Flexibility: Sit-and-Reach

Place a yardstick on the floor and apply a two-foot piece of tape on the floor perpendicular to the yardstick, crossing at the 15-inch mark. Sit on the floor with your legs extended and the soles of your feet touching the tape at the 15-inch mark, the zero-inch facing you. Your feet should be about 12 inches apart. Put one hand on the other, exhale, and very slowly reach forward as far as you can along the yardstick, lowering your head between your arms. Don't bounce! Note the farthest inch mark you reach. Don't hurt yourself by reaching farther than your body wants to. Relax, and then repeat two more times.
   Now check your results. Want to improve? You know the answer:

- Do aerobic exercise that makes you breathe hard for at least half an hour on most or all days of the week.
- Lift weights that challenge you two to three times per week.
- Stretch after activity at least a couple of times per week.
- Walk more.

### Cardiovascular: One-mile walk (time, in minutes)

|  | Under 40 Years | | Over 40 Years | |
|---|---|---|---|---|
|  | Men | Women | Men | Women |
| Excellent | 13:00 or less | 13:30 or less | 14:00 or less | 14:30 or less |
| Good | 13:01–15:30 | 13:31–16:00 | 14:01–16:30 | 14:31–17:00 |
| Average | 15:31–18:00 | 16:01–18:30 | 16:31–19:00 | 17:01–19:30 |
| Below average | 18:01–19:30 | 18:31–20:00 | 19:01–21:30 | 19:31–22:00 |
| Poor | 19:31 or more | 20:01 or more | 21:31 or more | 22:01 or more |

Source: Copper Institute

**Strength: Push-ups (number completed without rest)**

| | Men | | | | | |
|---|---|---|---|---|---|---|
| **Age** | **17–19** | **20–29** | **30–39** | **40–49** | **50–59** | **60–65** |
| Excellent | >56 | >47 | >41 | >34 | >31 | >30 |
| Good | 47–56 | 39–47 | 34–41 | 28–34 | 25–31 | 24–30 |
| Above average | 35–46 | 30–39 | 25–33 | 21–28 | 18–24 | 17–23 |
| Average | 19–34 | 17–29 | 13–24 | 11–20 | 9–17 | 6–16 |
| Below average | 11–18 | 10–16 | 8–12 | 6–10 | 5–8 | 3–5 |
| Poor | 4–10 | 4–9 | 2–7 | 1–5 | 1–4 | 1–2 |
| Very poor | <4 | <4 | <2 | 0 | 0 | 0 |

| | Women | | | | | |
|---|---|---|---|---|---|---|
| **Age** | **17–19** | **20–29** | **30–39** | **40–49** | **50–59** | **60–65** |
| Excellent | >35 | >36 | >37 | >31 | >25 | >23 |
| Good | 27–35 | 30–36 | 30–37 | 25–31 | 21–25 | 19–23 |
| Above average | 21–27 | 23–29 | 22–30 | 18–24 | 15–20 | 13–18 |
| Average | 11–20 | 12–22 | 10–21 | 8–17 | 7–14 | 5–12 |
| Below average | 6–10 | 7–11 | 5–9 | 4–7 | 3–6 | 2–4 |
| Poor | 2–5 | 2–6 | 1–4 | 1–3 | 1–2 | 1 |
| Very poor | 0–1 | 0–1 | 0 | 0 | 0 | 0 |

Source: Golding LA: *YMCA Fitness Testing and Assessment Manual*. YMCA of the USA, 4th ed, 2000. **topendsports.com**

## Strength: Curl-ups (number completed in 60 seconds)

| | Men | | | | | |
|---|---|---|---|---|---|---|
| Age | 18–25 | 26–35 | 36–45 | 46–55 | 56–65 | 65+ |
| Excellent | >49 | >45 | >41 | >35 | >31 | >28 |
| Good | 44–49 | 40–45 | 35–41 | 29–35 | 25–31 | 22–28 |
| Above average | 39–43 | 35–39 | 30–34 | 25–28 | 21–24 | 19–21 |
| Average | 35–38 | 31–34 | 27–29 | 22–24 | 17–20 | 15–18 |
| Below average | 31–34 | 29–30 | 23–26 | 18–21 | 13–16 | 11–14 |
| Poor | 25–30 | 22–28 | 17–22 | 13–17 | 9–12 | 7–10 |
| Very poor | <25 | <22 | <17 | <13 | <9 | <7 |

| | Women | | | | | |
|---|---|---|---|---|---|---|
| Age | 18–25 | 26–35 | 36–45 | 46–55 | 56–65 | 65+ |
| Excellent | >43 | >39 | >33 | >27 | >24 | >23 |
| Good | 37–43 | 33–39 | 27–33 | 22–27 | 18–24 | 17–23 |
| Above average | 33–36 | 29–32 | 23–26 | 18–21 | 13–17 | 14–16 |
| Average | 29–32 | 25–28 | 19–22 | 14–17 | 10–12 | 11–13 |
| Below average | 25–28 | 21–24 | 15–18 | 10–13 | 7–9 | 5–10 |
| Poor | 18–24 | 13–20 | 7–14 | 5–9 | 3–6 | 2–4 |
| Very poor | <18 | <13 | <7 | <5 | <3 | <2 |

Source: Golding LA: *YMCA Fitness Testing and Assessment Manual*. YMCA of the USA, 4th ed, 2000.

**Flexibility: Sit-and-reach (in inches)**

|  | Men | Women |
|---|---|---|
| Super | >+27 | >+30 |
| Excellent | +17–+27 | +21–+30 |
| Good | +6–+16 | +11–+20 |
| Average | 0–+5 | +1–+10 |
| Fair | –8––1 | –7–0 |
| Poor | –19––9 | –14––8 |
| Very poor | <–20 | <–15 |

Source: Golding LA: *YMCA Fitness Testing and Assessment Manual.* YMCA of the USA, 4th ed, 2000.

These charts are typical charts used by health and fitness experts. For a more thorough assessment of fitness or for development of an exercise plan appropriate for your fitness level, consult a certified personal trainer or other fitness professional.

# CHAPTER 11 Eating Disorders:
## Anorexia Nervosa, Bulimia Nervosa, and Other Conditions

## Student Learning Outcomes After studying Chapter 11, you will be able to

1. Contrast healthy attitudes toward uses of food with behavior patterns that could lead to unhealthy uses of food.

2. Outline the causes of, effects of, typical persons affected by, and treatment for anorexia nervosa.

3. Outline the causes of, effects of, typical persons affected by, and treatment for bulimia nervosa.

4. Describe still other forms of eating disorders: binge-eating disorder, night eating syndrome, and the female athlete triad.

5. Relate the presence of eating disorders to current social trends.

6. Describe methods to reduce the development of eating disorders, including the use of warning signs to identify early cases.

## Chapter Outline

Student Learning Outcomes

Refresh Your Memory

11.1 From Ordered to Disordered Eating Habits

11.2 A Closer Look at Anorexia Nervosa

11.3 A Closer Look at Bulimia Nervosa

11.4 Other Disordered Eating Patterns

11.5 Prevention of Eating Disorders

Nutrition and Your Health: *Eating Disorder Reflections*

Case Study: Eating Disorders—Steps to Recovery

Summary/Study Questions/Check Your Knowledge/Further Readings

Rate Your Plate

MANY OF US OCCASIONALLY EAT UNTIL WE'RE STUFFED AND UNCOMFORTABLE, SUCH AS AT THANKSGIVING DINNER. Faced with savory and tempting foods, we find that we can't easily stop eating. Usually we forgive ourselves, vowing not to overeat the next time. Nevertheless, many of us have problems controlling our food intake and body weight. The combination of too many instances of simple overeating, and too little physical activity eventually leads to progressive weight gain.

Actually, obesity, now considered a chronic disease, is the most common eating disorder in our society; however, the eating disorders explored in Chapter 11 involve much more severe distortions of the eating process. The eating disorders discussed here are just as serious, if not more, than obesity, and can develop into life-threatening conditions if left untreated. What's most alarming about these disorders—anorexia nervosa, bulimia nervosa, binge-eating disorder, and the female athlete triad—is the increasing number of cases reported each year.

Some people are more susceptible to these eating disorders than other people are—for genetic, psychological, and physical reasons. Successful treatment of eating disorders, therefore, is complex and must go beyond nutritional therapy. And keep in mind that eating disorders are not restricted to any socioeconomic class or ethnicity. They can also strike, as suggested in the comic in this chapter, at any age in both females and males. Let's examine the causes and treatments of these conditions in detail, because eating disorders touch many of our lives.

### Refresh Your Memory

As you begin your study of eating disorders, such as anorexia nervosa and bulimia nervosa, in Chapter 11, you may want to review:

- The effects of neurotransmitters on food intake in Chapter 1
- The role of genetic risk in disease susceptibility in Chapter 3
- Calculation of BMI in Chapter 7
- The effects and treatment of osteoporosis in Chapter 9
- The effects and treatment of iron-deficiency anemia in Chapter 9

## 11.1 From Ordered to Disordered Eating Habits

Eating—a completely instinctive behavior for animals—serves an extraordinary number of psychological, social, and cultural purposes for humans. Eating practices may take on religious meanings; signify bonds within families and ethnic groups; and provide a means to express hostility, affection, prestige, or class values. Within the family, supplying, preparing, and distributing food may be a means of expressing love, hatred, or even power.

We are bombarded daily with images of our society's portrayal of the "ideal" body. Dieting is promoted to achieve this ideal body—eternally young and admired. Television programs, billboard advertisements, magazine pictures, movies, and newspapers suggest that an ultraslim body will bring happiness, love, and ultimately, success. This fantasy notion is contradictory to the fact that much of society is becoming fatter, even obese. In response to this social pressure, some of us take an extreme approach—the pathological pursuit of weight control or weight loss.

Early in life, we develop images of "acceptable" and "unacceptable" body types. Of the attributes that constitute attractiveness, many people view body weight as the most important, partly because we can control our weight somewhat. Fatness is the most dreaded deviation from our cultural ideals of body image, the one most derided and shunned, even among schoolchildren.

It is difficult to resist comparing ourselves to the "ideal" body. Not everyone can look like a fashion model. People who are overly impressed by these messages,

**FOR BETTER OR FOR WORSE**

Concern with body image often starts early in life. Why do you think this is so? What societal trends have fostered this concern? Are some people more vulnerable, based on genetics and environment? Chapter 11 provides some answers.

especially those with genetic, psychological, and environmental influences, may be more likely than others to develop eating disorders in an effort to close the gap between reality and the perceived ideal.

Given the multiple functions associated with normal eating and the media bombardment with the ideal body image, it is not surprising that some people progress from typical responses to hunger and satiety cues to obsessive weight-loss behaviors, and then to a full-blown eating disorder.

## Food: More than Just a Source of Nutrients

From birth, we link food with personal and emotional experiences. As infants, we associate milk with security and warmth so the breast or bottle becomes a source of comfort as well as food. As noted in Chapter 1, even when older, most people continue to derive comfort and great pleasure from food. This is both a biological and a psychological phenomenon. Food can be a symbol of comfort, but eating can also stimulate the release of certain neurotransmitters (e.g., serotonin) and *natural opioids* (including **endorphins**), which produce a sense of calm and euphoria in the human body. Thus, in times of great stress, some people turn to food for a druglike, calming effect.

Food is also used as a reward or a bribe. Haven't you heard or spoken something similar to the following comments?

You can have your dessert if you eat five more bites of your vegetables.
You can't play until you clean your plate.
I'll eat the broccoli if you let me watch TV.
If you love me, you'll eat your dinner.

On the surface, using food as a reward or bribe seems harmless enough. Eventually, however, this practice encourages both caregivers and children to use food to achieve goals other than satisfying hunger and nutrient needs. Food may then become much more than a source of nutrients. Regularly using food as a bargaining chip can contribute to abnormal eating patterns. Carried to the extreme, these patterns can lead to **disordered eating.**

Disordered eating can be defined as mild and short-term changes in eating patterns that occur in response to a stressful event, an illness, or even a desire to modify the diet for a variety of health and personal appearance reasons. The problem may be no more than a bad habit, a style of eating adapted from friends or family members, or an aspect of preparing for athletic competition. While disordered eating can lead to weight loss or weight gain, as well as certain nutritional problems, it rarely requires in-depth professional attention. If, however, disordered eating becomes sustained, distressing, or starts to interfere with everyday activities and is linked to physiological changes, it may require professional intervention.

## Overview of Anorexia Nervosa and Bulimia Nervosa

Given the common practice of dieting in North America, it can sometimes be difficult to tell where disordered eating stops and an **eating disorder** begins. Indeed, many eating disorders start with a simple diet. Eating disorders then go on to involve physiological changes associated with food restriction, binge eating, purging, and fluctuations in weight. They also involve a number of emotional and cognitive changes that affect the way a person perceives and experiences his or her body, such as feelings of distress or extreme concern about body shape or weight. Eating disorders are not due to a failure of will or behavior; rather, they are real, treatable medical illnesses in which certain maladaptive patterns of eating take on a life of their own.

The main types of eating disorders are **anorexia nervosa** and **bulimia nervosa.** Other types, including **binge-eating disorder** and night eating syndrome, have been suggested but have not yet been approved as formal psychiatric diagnoses. More

▲ Maintaining an anorexic body type is an all too common goal in today's culture. The media and the fashion world bombard us with body images that are unrealistic for most people.

**endorphins** Natural body tranquilizers that may be involved in the feeding response and function in pain reduction.

**disordered eating** Mild and short-term changes in eating patterns that occur in relation to a stressful event, an illness, or a desire to modify one's diet for a variety of health and personal appearance reasons.

**eating disorder** Severe alterations in eating patterns linked to physiological changes. The alterations are associated with food restriction, binge eating, purging, and fluctuations in weight. They also involve a number of emotional and cognitive changes that affect the way a person perceives and experiences his or her body.

**anorexia nervosa** An eating disorder involving a psychological loss or denial of appetite, followed by self-starvation; related in part to a distorted body image and to various social pressures commonly associated with puberty.

**bulimia nervosa** An eating disorder in which large quantities of food are eaten at one time (binge eating) and then purged from the body by vomiting, or misuse of laxatives, diuretics, or enemas. Alternate means to counteract the binge behavior are fasting and excessive exercise.

**binge-eating disorder** An eating disorder characterized by recurrent binge eating and feelings of loss of control over eating that have lasted at least 6 months. Binge episodes can be triggered by frustration, anger, depression, anxiety, permission to eat forbidden foods, and excessive hunger.

▲ Self-image is an important part of adolescence. For people with eating disorders, the difference between the real and desired body images may be too difficult to accept. See the website www.4women.gov/bodyimage.

**Progression from Ordered to Disordered Eating**

Attention to hunger and satiety signals; limitation of calorie intake to restore weight to a healthful level

↓

Some disordered eating habits begin as weight loss is attempted, such as very restricted eating

↓

Clinically evident eating disorder recognized

than 5 million people in North America have one of these disorders; females outnumber males 5 to 1. Eating disorders frequently (85% of the time) develop during adolescence or early adulthood but some reports indicate their onset can occur during childhood or later in adulthood. Eating disorders frequently co-occur with other psychological disorders such as depression, substance abuse, and anxiety disorders. *People who suffer from eating disorders, especially anorexia nervosa and bulimia nervosa, can experience a wide range of physical health complications, including serious heart conditions and kidney failure, which may even lead to death.* Recognition of eating disorders as important and treatable diseases, therefore, is critical.

Currently, up to 5% of women in North America develop some form of anorexia nervosa or bulimia nervosa in their lifetimes. This section provides a brief description of the characteristics and diagnoses of the two primary eating disorders that primarily afflict those of college age and younger. A detailed discussion of these and related disorders, including treatment, then follows.

Anorexia nervosa is characterized by extreme weight loss, a distorted body image, and an irrational, almost morbid, fear of obesity and weight gain. Anorexic patients irrationally believe they are fat, even though others constantly comment on their thin physique. Some anorexics realize they are thin but continue to be haunted by certain areas of their bodies that they believe to be fat (such as thighs, buttocks, and stomach).

Common to both eating disorders, *nervosa* refers to an attitude of disgust with one's body. The term *anorexia* implies a loss of appetite; however, a denial of one's appetite more accurately describes the behavior of people with anorexia nervosa. By rough estimate, approximately 1 in 200 (0.5%) adolescent girls in North America eventually develops anorexia nervosa. This high number may be due to the tendency for females to blame themselves for weight gain typical of their age group. Men only account for approximately 10% of the cases of anorexia nervosa, partly because the ideal image conveyed for men is big and muscular. Among men, athletes are most prone to develop this and other eating disorders, especially those who participate in sports that require weight classes, such as boxers, wrestlers, and jockeys. Other activities that may foster eating disorders in men include swimming, dancing, and modeling.

Bulimia nervosa (*bulimia* means "great [ox] hunger") is characterized by episodes of binge eating followed by attempts to purge the calories consumed by vomiting or misusing laxatives, diuretics, or enemas. People with this disorder may be difficult to identify because they keep their binge-purge behaviors secret, and their symptoms are not obvious. Four percent or more of adolescent and college-age women suffer from bulimia nervosa. And, as with anorexia nervosa, about 10% of the cases occur in men.

Specific criteria are used by clinicians to diagnose eating disorders (e.g., *Diagnostic and Statistical Manual of Mental Disorders* of the American Psychiatric Association). Some characteristics are listed in Table 11-1. It is possible that people exhibit some symptoms of eating disorders but not enough to enable a medical worker to diagnose one of the two diseases. Also, as suggested in the diagnostic criteria, some people show characteristics of both anorexia nervosa and bulimia nervosa because the diseases overlap considerably. About half of the women diagnosed as having anorexia nervosa eventually develop bulimic symptoms. As shown in Table 11-1, bulimic characteristics also can be seen in anorexia nervosa, which blurs the distinction. Still, appreciating the differences between the disorders helps us to understand the various approaches to prevention and treatment.

Until recently, most researchers have reported that eating disorders primarily affect middle- and upper-class Caucasian women. Now, studies show greater similarities in the rates of body dissatisfaction and disordered eating behaviors across ethnic and cultural groups. Perhaps minorities with eating disorders have been less likely to seek help in the past due to fear of shame or stigma, lack of resources, or language barriers.

**TABLE 11-1** Typical Characteristics of Anorexic and Bulimic Persons

| Anorexia Nervosa | Bulimia Nervosa |
|---|---|
| • Rigid dieting causing dramatic weight loss, generally to less than 85% of what would be expected for one's age (or BMI of 17.5 or less)<br>• False body perception—thinking "I'm too fat," even when extremely underweight; relentless pursuit of control<br>• Rituals involving food, excessive exercise, and other aspects of life<br>• Maintenance of rigid control in lifestyle; security found in control and order<br>• Feeling of panic after a small weight gain; intense fear of gaining weight<br>• Feelings of purity, power, and superiority through maintenance of strict discipline and self-denial<br>• Preoccupation with food, its preparation, and observing another person eat<br>• Helplessness in the presence of food<br>• Lack of menstrual periods (after what should be the age of puberty) for at least 3 months<br>• Possible presence of bingeing and purging practices | • Secretive binge eating; generally not overeating in front of others<br>• Eating when depressed or under stress<br>• Bingeing on a large amount of food, followed by fasting, laxative or diuretic abuse, self-induced vomiting, or excessive exercise (at least twice a week for 3 months)<br>• Shame, embarrassment, deceit, and depression; low self-esteem and guilt (especially after a binge)<br>• Fluctuating weight (±10 pounds or 5 kilograms) resulting from alternate bingeing and fasting<br>• Loss of control; fear of not being able to stop eating<br>• Perfectionism, "people pleaser"; food as the only comfort/escape in an otherwise carefully controlled and regulated life<br>• Erosion of teeth, swollen glands<br>• Purchase of syrup of ipecac, a compound sold in pharmacies that induces vomiting |

Those who exhibit only one or a few of these characteristics may be at risk but probably do not have either disorder. They should, however, reflect on their eating habits and related concerns and take appropriate action, such as seeking a careful evaluation by a physician.

▲ Anorexia nervosa is characterized by a feeling of panic after only a small weight gain; bulimia nervosa is characterized by frequent weight fluctuations from alternate bingeing and fasting.

It seems more likely, however, that health care workers are less likely to diagnose non-Caucasians as having eating disorders. Previously, it seemed that non-Caucasian cultures were more accepting of larger body shapes, but mainstream pressures for thinness now seem to cut across racial differences. Our overall cultural change may be associated with increased vulnerability to eating disorders.

Do you know someone who is at risk of these eating disorders? If so, suggest that the person seek a professional evaluation because, the sooner treatment begins, the better the chances for recovery. However, do not try to diagnose eating disorders in your friends or family members. Only a professional can exclude other possible diseases and correctly evaluate the diagnostic criteria required to make a diagnosis of anorexia nervosa or bulimia nervosa. Once an eating disorder is diagnosed, immediate treatment is advisable. As a friend, the best you can do is to encourage an affected person to seek professional help. Such help is commonly available at student health centers and student guidance/counseling facilities on college campuses.

There are no simple causes of eating disorders, and there are no simple treatments. Stress may have an especially strong role in the development of eating disorders. An underlying commonality seems to be the lack of appropriate coping mechanisms as individuals begin to reach adolescence and young adulthood, coupled with dysfunctional family relationships.

A few research studies have investigated the influence of genetics on the development of eating disorders. These studies have involved a comparison of identical twins with fraternal twins and the incidence of eating disorders. In general, these studies have shown that identical twins have a higher likelihood of sharing eating disorders

**O**ur passion for thinness may have its roots in the Victorian era of the nineteenth century, which specialized in denying "unpleasant" physical realities, such as appetite and sexual desire. Flappers of the 1920s cemented the twentieth century trend for thinness. Since 1922, the BMI values of Miss America winners have steadily decreased; during the last three decades, most winners had a BMI in the "underweight" range (less than 18.5).

than do fraternal twins. This indicates that genetics is a strong risk factor in development of such disorders, because identical twins share the same DNA. One study found genetic background to describe 50% of the overall risk of developing anorexia nervosa. Identifying genes that cause eating disorders eventually could help in tailoring prevention efforts to those who are at risk, but affected individuals would still need the same counseling that is part of therapy today.

## 11.2 A Closer Look at Anorexia Nervosa

Anorexia nervosa evolves from a dangerous mental state to an often life-threatening physical condition. As first described in the early medical literature in 1689, people suffering from this disorder think they are fat and intensely fear obesity and weight gain. They lose much more weight than is healthful. Although food is entwined in this disease, it stems more from psychological conflict.

About 10% of people with anorexia nervosa eventually die from the disease—from suicide, heart ailments, and infections. About one quarter of those with anorexia nervosa recover within 6 years, whereas the rest simply exist with the disease or go on to develop another form of eating disorder. The longer someone suffers from this eating disorder, the poorer the chances for complete recovery. A young patient with a brief episode and a cooperative family has a better outlook than those without these factors. Overall, prompt and vigorous treatment with close follow-up improves the chances for success.

Anorexia nervosa may begin as a simple attempt to lose weight. A comment from a well-meaning friend, relative, or coach suggesting that the person seems to be gaining weight or is too fat may be all that is needed. The stress of having to maintain a certain weight to look attractive or competent on a job can also lead to disordered eating. Physical changes associated with puberty, the stress of leaving childhood, or the loss of a friend are examples of triggers for extreme dieting. Leaving home for boarding school or college or starting a job can reinforce the desire to appear more "socially acceptable." Still, looking "good" does not necessarily help people deal with anger, depression, low self-esteem, or past experiences with sexual abuse. If these issues are behind the disorder and are not resolved as weight is lost, the individual may intensify efforts to lose weight "to look even better," rather than work through unresolved psychological concerns.

During adolescence, a period of turbulent sexual and social tensions, teenagers seek—and are often expected—to establish separate and independent lives. While declaring independence, they seek acceptance and support from peers and parents and react intensely to how they think others perceive them. At the same time, their bodies are changing, and much of the change is beyond their control. In response to the adolescent's or teenager's lack of control and coping mechanisms, dieting may start and then lead to a failure to gain appropriate weight-for-height. This may not be readily identified as a problem because the child has not actually lost any weight. Stunting (failure to grow in height) may also occur if inadequate calories are ingested during a period of growth. If anorexia develops before puberty, sexual maturation and menstruation also may be delayed.

Teens with chronic illnesses, such as type 1 diabetes or asthma, are at even greater risk for disordered eating. Any evidence of poor weight gain/maintenance or excessive exercise among these individuals needs to be investigated as a possible sign of disordered eating.

Extreme dieting is the most important predictor of an eating disorder. (Adolescents expressing concern about their weight should be advised to focus on exercise, which does not appear to impart a risk for subsequent problems.) Once dieting begins, a person developing anorexia nervosa does not stop. The result is a long period of rigidly self-enforced semistarvation, practiced almost with a vengeance, in a relentless pursuit of control. Anorexia nervosa may eventually lead to bingeing on large amounts of

▲ Eating disorders are commonly seen in people who must maintain low body weight, such as ballet dancers.

**L**inks exist between disordered eating behaviors and substance abuse, particularly alcohol abuse. Some people may use food restriction or purging to offset the calories consumed during drinking binges. Popularly called "drunkorexia," this practice can lead to severe nutrient deficiencies and dehydration.

food in a short time, then purging. Purging occurs primarily through vomiting, but laxatives, diuretics, and enemas are also used. Thus, a person with anorexia nervosa may exist in a state of semistarvation or may alternate periods of starvation with periods of bingeing and purging.

## Profile of the Typical Person with Anorexia Nervosa

A person with anorexia nervosa refuses to eat enough food to maintain an acceptable weight. This refusal is a hallmark of the disease, whether or not other practices, such as binge-purge cycles, appear. The most typical anorexic person is a Caucasian female from the middle or upper socioeconomic class. Perhaps her mother also has distorted views of desirable body shape and acceptable food habits. The girl is often described by parents and teachers as responsible, meticulous, and obedient.

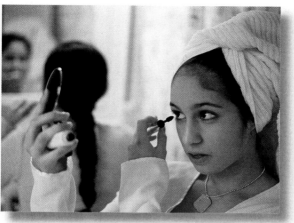

▲ Concern over appearance begins early in life; a focus on a healthful outlook with regard to body weight should also begin at this time.

She is competitive and often obsessive. Her parents set high standards for her. At home, she may not allow clutter in her bedroom. Physicians note that, after a physical examination, she may fold her examination gown very carefully and clean up the examination room before leaving. Even though such behavior may seem odd, only a skilled professional can tell the difference between anorexia nervosa and other adolescent complaints, such as delayed puberty, fatigue, and depression.

A common thread underlying many—but not all—cases of anorexia nervosa is conflict within the family structure, typically with an overbearing mother and an emotionally absent father. When family expectations are always too high—including those regarding body weight—frustration results and leads to fighting. Overinvolvement, rigidity, over-protection, and denial are typical daily transactions of such families.

Issues of control are central to the development of anorexia nervosa. Often, the eating disorder allows an anorexic person to exercise control over an otherwise powerless existence. Losing weight may be the first independent success the person has had. People with anorexia evaluate their self-worth almost entirely in terms of self-control. Some sexually abused children develop anorexia nervosa, believing that if they control their appetite for food, sexual relations, and human contact, they will feel in control and competent and will eliminate shameful feelings. Moreover, food restriction, which arrests development and shuts down sexual impulses, may be a strategy to prevent future victimization and guilt feelings. Often anorexic persons feel hopeless about human relationships and socially isolated because of their dysfunctional families. They focus on food, eating, and weight instead of human relationships.

**B**y severely limiting calorie intake for long periods, adolescent girls and young adult women greatly compromise their nutritional status, impair their reproductive systems, and restrict growth. The harm produced by milder, shorter periods of diet restriction is not clear. Evidence, however, suggests that even moderate diet restriction, if continued, contributes to the risks for various forms of anemia, future pregnancy complications and delivery of low-birth-weight infants, and permanently reduced bone mass.

## Early Warning Signs

A person developing anorexia nervosa exhibits important warning signs. At first, dieting becomes the life focus. The person may think, "The only thing I am good at is dieting. I can't do anything else." This innocent beginning often leads to very abnormal self-perceptions and eating habits, such as cutting a pea in half before eating it. Other habits include hiding and storing food and or spreading food around a plate to make it look as if much has been eaten. An anorexic person may cook a large meal and watch others eat it while refusing to eat anything. Anorexic persons may also exercise compulsively to the point that it is obsessive and driven. Exercise can interfere with life activities or occur at unusual times or settings—for example, doing squats while brushing teeth.

As the disorder progresses, the range of foods may narrow and be rigidly divided into safe and unsafe ones, with the list of safe foods becoming progressively shorter. For people developing anorexia nervosa, these practices say "I am in control." These people may be hungry, but they deny it, driven by the belief that good things will happen by just becoming thin enough. It becomes a question of willpower.

▲ Anorexia nervosa occurs much more frequently in young women than in young men.

**P**arents may not consider a teenager mature enough to make decisions. If the teen disagrees and the situation is very tense, she may turn to purging or starving as a way to show her power: "You may try to control my life, but I can do anything I want with my body."

In the words of one young woman, "I couldn't get angry, because it would be like destroying someone else, like my mother. It felt like she would hate me forever. I got angry through anorexia nervosa. It was my last hope. It's my own body and this was my last-ditch effort."

**lanugo** Down-like hair that appears after a person has lost much body fat through semi-starvation. The hair stands erect and traps air, acting as insulation for the body to compensate for the relative lack of body fat, which usually functions as insulation.

People with anorexia become irritable and hostile and begin to withdraw from family and friends. School performance generally crumbles. They refuse to eat out with family and friends, thinking, "I won't be able to have the foods I want to eat," or "I won't be able to throw up afterward."

Anorexic persons see themselves as rational and others as irrational. They also tend to be excessively critical of themselves and others. Nothing is good enough. Because it cannot be perfect, life appears meaningless and hopeless. A sense of joylessness pervades everything.

As stress increases in the person's life, sleep disturbances and depression are common. Many of the psychological and physical problems associated with anorexia nervosa arise from insufficient calorie intake, as well as deficiencies of nutrients, such as thiamin and vitamin B-6. For a female, the combination of problems—coupled with lower and lower body weight and fat stores—causes menstrual periods to cease. This may be the first sign of the disease that a parent notices and represents an additional hallmark of the disease.

Ultimately, an anorexic person eats very little food; 300 to 600 kcal daily is not unusual. In place of food, the person may consume up to 20 cans of diet soft drinks and chew many pieces of sugarless gum each day.

## Physical Effects of Anorexia Nervosa

Rooted in the emotional state of the victim, anorexia nervosa produces profound physical effects. The anorexic person often appears to be skin and bones. Body weight less than 85% of that expected is one clinical indicator of anorexia nervosa. This percentage can be calculated using the Metropolitan Life Insurance Company tables (see Appendix G), but body build and weight history should also be used when estimating an appropriate weight. BMI is a more reliable indicator of the degree of malnourishment; generally, a BMI of 17.5 or less indicates a severe case (review Chapter 7 for more on BMI). For children under age 18, growth charts should be used to assess weight status (see Chapter 15).

The state of semistarvation disturbs many body systems as it forces the body to conserve energy stores as much as possible (Fig. 11-1). This attempt to conserve energy stores is the cause of most of the physical effects. Thus, many complications can be reversed by returning to a healthy weight, provided the duration of the insult has not been too long. The following are predictable effects caused by hormonal responses to and deficient nutrient intakes from semistarvation:

- Lowered body temperature and cold intolerance from loss of insulating fat layer
- Slowed metabolic rate from decreased synthesis of thyroid hormones
- Decreased heart rate as metabolism slows, leading to premature fatigue, fainting, and an overwhelming need for sleep. Other changes in heart function may occur as well, including loss of heart tissue and irregular heart rhythm.
- Iron-deficiency anemia, which leads to further weakness
- Rough, dry, scaly, and cold skin, which may show multiple bruises because of the loss of the protective fat layer normally present under the skin
- Low white blood cell count, which increases the risk of infection—one cause of death in people with anorexia nervosa
- Abnormal feeling of fullness or bloating, which can last for several hours after eating
- Loss of hair
- Appearance of **lanugo**—downy hairs on the body that trap air to partially counteract heat loss that occurs with loss of fat tissue
- Constipation due to deterioration of the gastrointestinal tract and abuse of laxatives

- Low blood potassium, worsened by potassium losses during vomiting and use of some types of diuretics. This increases the risk of heart rhythm disturbances, another leading cause of death in anorexic people.
- Loss of menstrual periods because of low body weight, low body fat content, and the stress of the disease. Accompanying hormonal changes cause a loss of bone mass and increase the risk of osteoporosis later in life.
- Changes in neurotransmitter function in the brain, which lead to depression
- Eventual loss of teeth caused by acid erosion of tooth enamel if frequent vomiting occurs. Until vomiting ceases, one way to reduce this effect on teeth is to rinse the mouth with water right away and brush the teeth as soon as possible. Loss of teeth (along with low bone mass) can be lasting signs of the disease, even if the other physical and mental problems are resolved.
- Muscle tears and stress fractures in athletes because of decreased bone and muscle mass.

A person with this disorder is psychologically and physically ill and needs help.

## CRITICAL THINKING

Jennifer is an attractive 13-year-old. However, she's very compulsive. Everything has to be perfect—her hair, her clothes, even her room. Her body is beginning to mature, so she's obsessed with having perfect physical features as well. Her parents are worried about her behavior. Given her behavioral traits, what symptoms of an eating disorder should they watch for? What should Jennifer's parents do if they suspect an eating disorder?

## CONCEPT CHECK

Anorexia nervosa is an eating disorder characterized by semistarvation. It is found primarily—but not exclusively—in adolescent girls, starting at or around puberty. People with anorexia dwindle essentially to skin and bones yet still believe they are fat. Semistarvation produces hormonal changes and nutrient deficiencies, which lower body temperature; slow the heart rate; decrease immune response; stop menstrual periods; and contribute to hair, muscle, and bone loss. It is a serious disease, which often produces lifelong consequences and may be fatal.

**E**rika Goodman, former dancer with the Joffrey Ballet, became crippled from osteoporosis resulting from years of restricting food intake to maintain a low body weight. Her food restriction led to irregular or absent menstrual periods for many years. She died in 2004 at the age of 59 after falling in her Manhattan apartment.

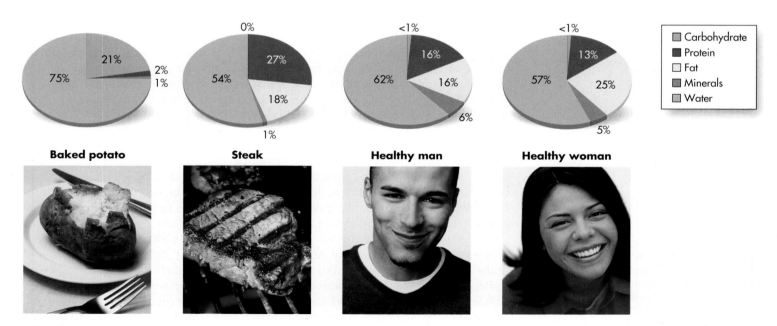

**FIGURE 11-1** ▶ Signs and symptoms of eating disorders. A vast array of physical effects are associated with anorexia nervosa and bulimia nervosa. This figure contains many but is not an exhaustive list of all potential consequences. These physical effects can also serve as warning signs that a problem exists. Professional evaluation is then indicated.

**S**inger Karen Carpenter's death from complications of anorexia nervosa in 1983 increased awareness of the serious nature of this disease. Currently, the average time for recovery from anorexia nervosa is 7 years; many insurance companies cover only a fraction of the estimated $150,000 cost of treatment.

**A** young woman in a self-help group for those with anorexia nervosa explained her feelings to the other group members: "I have lost a specialness that I thought it gave me. I was different from everyone else. Now I know that I'm somebody who's overcome it, which not everybody does."

**A** disturbing trend is the attempt to promote eating disorders as a way of life. Some anorexic individuals have personified their illness into a role model named "Ana," who tells them what to eat and mocks them when they don't lose weight. Ana websites reject the serious health risks of anorexia behaviors and instead dispense unsafe "thinspiration" to vulnerable individuals.

## Treatment of Anorexia Nervosa

People with anorexia often sink into shells of isolation and fear. They deny that a problem exists. Frequently, their friends and family members meet with them to confront the problem in a loving way. This is called an *intervention*. They present evidence of the problem and encourage immediate treatment. Treatment then requires a multidisciplinary team of experienced physicians, registered dietitians, psychologists, and other health professionals working together. An ideal setting is an eating disorders clinic in a medical center. Outpatient therapy generally begins first. This may be extended to 3 to 5 days per week. Day hospitalization (6 to 12 hours) is another option, as is total hospitalization. Hospitalization is necessary once a person falls below 75% of expected weight, experiences acute medical problems, and/or exhibits severe psychological problems or suicidal risk. Still, even in the most skilled hands at the finest facilities, efforts may fail. This tells us that the prevention of anorexia nervosa is of utmost importance.

Once a medical team has gained the cooperation and trust of an anorexic person, the team attempts to work together to restore a sense of balance, purpose, and future possibilities. As previously stated, anorexia nervosa is usually rooted in psychological conflict. However, the anorexic person who has been barely existing in a state of semi-starvation cannot focus on much besides food. Dreams and even morbid thoughts about food will interfere with therapy until sufficient weight is regained.

**Nutrition Therapy.** The first goal of nutrition therapy is to gain the person's cooperation and trust, with the ultimate objective of increasing oral food intake. Ideally, weight gain must be enough to raise the metabolic rate to normal and reverse as many physical signs of the disease as possible. Food intake is designed first to minimize or stop any further weight loss. Then, the focus shifts to restoring appropriate food habits. After this, the expectation can be switched to slowly gaining weight. A gain of 2 to 3 pounds per week is appropriate. Tube and/or intravenous (IV) feeding is used only if immediate renourishment is required, as this can frighten the person and cause him or her to distrust medical staff.

Persons with anorexia nervosa need considerable reassurance during the refeeding process because of uncomfortable and unfamiliar effects—such as bloating, increase in body heat, and increase in body fat. This is a frightening process because these changes can symbolize a loss of control. Rapid changes in electrolytes and minerals in the blood associated with refeeding, especially potassium, phosphorus, and magnesium, can be dangerous. Therefore, monitoring blood levels of these minerals is of critical importance during the process of incorporating more food into the diet.

In addition to helping persons with anorexia nervosa reach and maintain adequate nutritional status, the registered dietitian on the medical team provides accurate nutrition information throughout the treatment, promotes a healthy attitude toward food, and helps the person learn to eat in response to natural hunger and satiety cues. The focus then turns to identifying healthy and adequate food choices that promote weight gain to achieve and maintain a clinically estimated goal weight (e.g., BMI of 20 or more). As noted, nutrient deficiencies are commonly seen in anorexic persons. A multivitamin and mineral supplement will be added, as well as enough calcium to raise intake to about 1500 milligrams per day.

Excessive physical activity prevents weight gain, so professionals must help anorexic persons moderate their activity. At many treatment centers, moderate bed rest is used in the early stages of treatment to help promote weight gain.

Experienced professional help is the key. An anorexic person may be on the verge of suicide and starvation. In addition, anorexic people are often very clever and resistant to therapy. They may try to hide weight loss by wearing many layers of clothes, putting coins in their pockets or underwear, and drinking numerous glasses of water.

**Psychological and Related Therapy.** Once the physical problems of anorexia nervosa are addressed, the treatment focus shifts to the underlying emotional problems that led to excessive dieting and other symptoms of the disorder. To heal, these anorexic persons must reject the sense of accomplishment they have associated with an emaciated body and begin to accept themselves at a healthy body weight. If therapists can discover reasons for the disorder, they can develop strategies for restoring normal weight and eating habits that involve resolving psychological conflicts. Education about the medical consequences of semistarvation is also helpful. A key aspect of psychological treatment is showing affected individuals how to regain control of other facets of their lives and cope with difficult situations. As eating evolves into a normal routine, they can turn to previously neglected activities.

Therapists may use **cognitive behavior therapy,** which involves helping the person confront and change irrational beliefs about body image, eating, relationships, and weight. Underlying issues that may be the cause for the disease, such as sexual abuse, also must be identified and addressed by the therapist.

Family therapy often is important in treating anorexia nervosa, especially for younger persons who still live with their families. It focuses on the role of the illness among family members, the reactions of individual family members and ways in which their subconscious behavior might contribute to the abnormal eating patterns. Frequently, a therapist finds family struggles at the heart of the problem. As the disorder resolves, patients must relate to family members in new ways to gain the attention that was needed and previously tied to the disease. For example, the family may need to help the young person ease into adulthood and accept its responsibilities as well as its advantages. Self-help groups for anorexic (and bulimic) people, as well as their families and friends, represent nonthreatening first steps into treatment.

Food is the drug of choice in the treatment of anorexic patients. Generally, medications are not effective in management of the primary symptoms of anorexia nervosa. Fluoxetine (Prozac®) and related medications may stabilize recovery once 85% of expected body weight has been attained. These medications work by prolonging serotonin activity in the brain, which in turn regulates mood and feelings of satiety. A variety of other pharmacologic agents, such as olanzapine (Zyprexa®), may have some role in treating mood changes, anxiety, or psychotic symptoms associated with anorexia nervosa, but they have limited value unless weight gain is also achieved.

With professional help, many people with anorexia nervosa can lead normal lives. Although they may not be totally cured, anorexic individuals do not have to depend on unusual eating habits to cope with daily problems. They recover a sense of normalcy in their lives. No universal approach exists, because each case is unique. Establishing a strong relationship with either a therapist or another supportive person is an especially important key to recovery. Once anorexic persons feel understood and accepted by another person, they can begin to build a sense of self and exercise some autonomy. As they learn alternative coping mechanisms, they can relinquish their dysfunctional relationships with food and instead develop healthy personal relationships.

**cognitive behavior therapy** Psychological therapy in which the person's assumptions about dieting, body weight, and related issues are confronted. New ways of thinking are explored and then practiced by the person. In this way, an individual can learn new ways to control disordered eating behaviors and related life stress.

▲ Early treatment for an eating disorder, such as anorexia nervosa, improves chances of success.

### CONCEPT CHECK

To relieve the semistarved condition of most anorexic persons, the initial treatment focuses on moderately increased food intake and slow weight gain. Once this is accomplished, psychotherapy can begin to uncover the causes of the disease and help the individual develop the skills needed to return to a healthy life. Family therapy can be an important tool in treatment, whereas medications have a limited role.

## 11.3 A Closer Look at Bulimia Nervosa

Bulimia nervosa involves episodes of binge eating followed by various means to purge the food. It is most common among young adults of college age, although some high school students are also at risk. Susceptible people often have genetic factors and

**B**ingeing and purging (via vomiting) was evident in pre-Christian Roman times, but was practiced in a group setting. The eating disorder bulimia nervosa is generally practiced in private. It was first described in the medical literature in 1979.

▲ Excessive exercising can be one component of bulimia if it is used as a way to offset the calorie intake from a binge. Exercise is considered excessive when it is done at inappropriate times or settings or when a person does it despite injury or other medical complications.

lifestyle patterns that predispose them to becoming overweight, and many try frequent weight-reduction diets as teenagers. Like people with anorexia nervosa, those with bulimia nervosa are usually female and successful. Unlike anorexic individuals, however, they are usually at or slightly above a normal weight. Females with bulimia nervosa are also more likely to be sexually active than those with anorexia nervosa.

The person with bulimia nervosa may think of food constantly. But unlike the anorexic person, who turns away from food when faced with problems, the bulimic person turns toward food in critical situations. Also, unlike those with anorexia nervosa, people with bulimia nervosa recognize their behavior as abnormal. These people often have low self-esteem and are depressed. Approximately half of the people with bulimia nervosa have major depression. Lingering effects of child abuse may be one reason for these feelings. Many bulimic persons report that they have been sexually abused. They appear competent to outsiders, while they actually feel out of control, ashamed, and frustrated.

Bulimic people tend to be impulsive, which may be expressed in behaviors such as stealing, increased sexual activity, drug and alcohol abuse, self-mutilation, or attempted suicide. Some experts have suggested that part of the problem may actually arise from an inability to control responses to impulse and desire. Some studies have demonstrated that bulimic people tend to come from disengaged families—ones that are loosely organized. In these families, roles for family members are not clearly defined, rules are disregarded, and a great deal of conflict exists. (In contrast, anorexic people tend to have families so actively engaged that roles may be too well defined.)

## Typical Behavior in Bulimia Nervosa

It is likely that many people with bulimic behavior are never diagnosed; the diagnostic criteria specify that a person must binge and purge at least twice a week for 3 months. People with bulimia nervosa lead secret lives, hiding their abnormal eating habits. Moreover, it is impossible to recognize the disorder simply by appearance. Most diagnoses of bulimia nervosa rely on self-reports, so estimates of the number of cases are probably low. The disorder, especially in its milder forms, may be much more widespread than commonly thought.

For intake to qualify as a binge, an atypically large amount of food must be consumed in a short time and the person must exhibit a lack of control over his or her behavior. Among sufferers of bulimia nervosa, bingeing often alternates with attempts to rigidly restrict food intake. Elaborate food rules are common, such as avoiding all sweets. Thus, eating just one cookie or donut may cause individuals with this disorder to feel as though they have broken a rule. At that point, in the mind of a bulimic person, the objectionable food must be eliminated. Usually this leads to further overeating, partly because it is easier to regurgitate a large amount of food than a small amount.

Binge-purge cycles may be practiced daily, weekly, or across longer intervals. A specific time often is set aside. Most binge eating occurs at night, when other people are less likely to interrupt, and usually lasts from ½ to 2 hours. A binge can be triggered by a combination of stress, boredom, loneliness, and depression. It often follows a period of strict dieting and thus can be linked to intense hunger. The binge is not at all like normal eating; once begun, it seems to propel itself. The person not only loses control, but generally doesn't even taste or enjoy food during a binge. This separates the practice from overeating.

Most commonly, bulimic people consume cakes, cookies, ice cream, and other high-carbohydrate convenience foods during binges because these foods can be purged relatively easily and comfortably by vomiting. In a single binge, foods supplying 3000 kcal or more may be eaten. Purging follows in hopes that no weight will be gained. However, even when vomiting follows the binge, 33% to 75% of the calories taken in is still absorbed, inevitably causing some weight gain. When laxatives or enemas are used, about 90% of the calories are absorbed, as laxatives act in the large intestine, beyond the point of most nutrient absorption. The belief that purging soon after bingeing will prevent excessive calorie absorption and weight gain is a misconception.

At the onset of bulimia nervosa, sufferers often induce vomiting by placing their fingers deep into the mouth. They may bite down on these fingers inadvertently, resulting in bite marks and scars around the knuckles, a characteristic sign of this disorder. Once the disease is established, however, a person may be able to vomit simply by contracting the abdominal muscles. Vomiting may also occur spontaneously.

Another way bulimic persons attempt to compensate for a binge and control their weight is by engaging in excessive exercise to expend a large amount of calories. In this practice, referred to as "debting," bulimic individuals try to estimate the amount of calories eaten during a binge, and then exercise to counteract the excess.

People with bulimia nervosa are not proud of their behavior. After a binge, they usually feel guilty and depressed. Over time, they experience low self-esteem, feel hopeless about their situation, and are caught in a vicious cycle of obsession (Fig. 11-2). Compulsive lying, shoplifting to obtain food, and drug abuse can further intensify these feelings. Bulimic people discovered in the act of bingeing by a friend or family member may order the intruder to "get out" and "go away." Sufferers gradually distance themselves from others, spending more time preoccupied by and engaging in bingeing and purging.

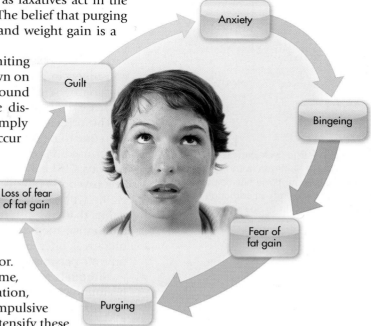

**FIGURE 11-2** ▶ Bulimia nervosa's vicious cycle of obsession.

## Health Problems Stemming from Bulimia Nervosa

The vomiting that many bulimic sufferers induce is a physically destructive method of purging. Indeed, the majority of health problems associated with bulimia nervosa, as noted here, arise from vomiting:

- Repeated exposure of teeth to the acid in vomit causes demineralization, making the teeth painful and sensitive to heat, cold, and acids. Eventually, the teeth may decay severely, erode away from fillings, and finally fall out (Fig. 11-3). Dental professionals are sometimes the first health professionals to notice signs of bulimia nervosa. As noted, it is important to rinse the mouth with water after any vomiting episode, especially before brushing the teeth.
- Blood potassium can drop significantly with regular vomiting or the use of certain diuretics. This can disturb the heart's rhythm and even produce sudden death.
- Salivary glands may swell as a result of infection and irritation from persistent vomiting.
- Stomach ulcers and bleeding and tears in the esophagus develop in some cases.
- Constipation may result from frequent laxative use.
- Ipecac syrup, sometimes used to induce vomiting, is toxic to the heart, liver, and kidneys. It has caused accidental poisoning when taken repeatedly.

Overall, bulimia nervosa is a potentially debilitating disorder that can lead to death, usually from suicide, low blood potassium, or overwhelming infections.

**FIGURE 11-3** ▶ Excessive tooth decay is common in bulimic patients.

## Treatment of Bulimia Nervosa

Therapy for bulimia nervosa, as for anorexia nervosa, requires a team of experienced clinicians. Bulimic individuals are less likely than those with anorexia to enter treatment in a state of semistarvation. However, if a bulimic person has lost significant weight, this must be treated before psychological treatment begins. Although clinicians have yet to agree on the best therapy for bulimia nervosa, they generally agree that treatment should last at least 16 weeks. Hospitalization may be indicated in cases of extreme laxative abuse, regular vomiting, substance abuse, and depression, especially if physical harm is evident.

The first goal of treatment for bulimia nervosa is to decrease the amount of food consumed in a binge session to decrease the risk of esophageal tears from related purging by vomiting. A decrease in the frequency of this type of purging will also decrease damage to the teeth.

The primary aim of psychotherapy is to improve a persons' self-acceptance and help one to be less concerned about body weight. Cognitive behavior therapy is generally used. Psychotherapy helps correct the all-or-none thinking typical of bulimic persons: "If I eat one cookie, I'm a failure and might as well binge." The premise of this psychotherapy is that, if abnormal attitudes and beliefs can be altered, normal eating will follow. In addition, the therapist guides the person in establishing food habits that will minimize bingeing: avoiding fasting, eating regular meals, and using alternative methods—other than eating—to cope with stressful situations. Group therapy is often useful to foster strong social support. One goal of therapy is to help bulimic persons accept some depression and self-doubt as normal.

Although pharmacological agents should not be used as the sole treatment for bulimia nervosa, studies indicate that some medications may be beneficial in conjunction with other therapies. Fluoxetine (Prozac®) is the only antidepressant that has been approved by FDA for use in the treatment of bulimia nervosa, but physicians also may prescribe other similar forms of antidepressants, other classes of psychiatric medications, or certain antiseizure medications, (e.g., topiramate [Topamax®]).

Nutritional counseling has two main goals: correcting misconceptions about food and re-establishing regular eating habits. Bulimic persons are given information about bulimia nervosa and its consequences. Avoiding binge foods and not constantly stepping on a scale may be recommended early in treatment. The primary goal, however, is to develop a normal eating pattern. To achieve this goal, some specialists encourage these individuals to develop daily meal plans and keep a food diary in which they record food intake, internal sensations of hunger, environmental factors that precipitate binges, and thoughts and feelings that accompany binge-purge cycles. Keeping a food diary not only is an accurate way to monitor food intake but also may help identify situations that seem to trigger binge episodes. With the help of a therapist, bulimic persons can develop alternative coping strategies.

In general, the focus is not on stopping bingeing and purging *per se* but on developing regular eating habits. Once this is achieved, the binge-purge cycle should start to break down. Individuals are discouraged from following strict rules about healthy food choices, because this mimics the typical obsessive attitudes associated with bulimia nervosa. Rather, encouraging a mature perspective on nutrient intake—that is, regular consumption of moderate amounts of a variety of foods balanced among the food groups—helps one overcome this disorder.

Setting time limits for the completion of meals and snacks is important for people with eating disorders. Many bulimic persons eat quickly, reflecting their difficulties with satiety. Suggesting that the person put his or her utensil down after each bite is a behavioral technique that a therapist might try during recovery for bulimia. (In comparison, many anorexic persons eat in an excessively slow manner—for example, taking 1 hour to eat a muffin cut into tiny, bite-size pieces.)

People with bulimia nervosa must recognize that they have a serious disorder that can have grave medical complications if not treated. Relapse is likely, so therapy should be long term. Those with bulimia nervosa need professional help because they can be very depressed and are at a high risk for suicide. About 50% of people with bulimia nervosa recover completely from the disorder. Others continue to struggle with it to varying degrees for the rest of their lives. This underscores the need for prevention because treatment is difficult.

**T**he binge-purge cycle can create an initial state of euphoria in the person. Giving up this euphoria has been equated to giving up an addiction. Still, it is important to do so.

▲ Developing regular eating habits helps a person with bulimia nervosa to stop the binge-purge cycle.

# 11.4 Other Disordered Eating Patterns

In recent years, other patterns of disordered eating have been recognized. Several of these patterns fall under the diagnosic category, *eating disorder not otherwise specified* (EDNOS). EDNOS is described in the American Psychiatric Association diagnostic manual as a "category [of] disorders of eating that do not meet the criteria for any specific eating disorder."

The EDNOS category is frequently used for people who have some, but not all, of the characteristics of anorexia nervosa or bulimia nervosa. Each EDNOS has distinctive qualities. For example, a person may experience episodes of bingeing and purging, but not frequently enough to meet the diagnosis of bulimia nervosa. A person may also engage in bingeing episodes without the use of inappropriate compensatory behaviors; this is referred to as binge-eating disorder. Another disordered eating pattern under study is night eating syndrome. **Night eating syndrome** is characterized by eating a lot of food in the late evening and nocturnal awakening with ingestion of food. Finally, the **female athlete triad** is a condition characterized by disordered eating, lack of menstrual periods, and osteoporosis. These conditions have been recognized as requiring professional treatment and are discussed in the following sections.

**night eating syndrome** Eating a lot of food in the late evening and nocturnal awakenings with ingestion of food.

**female athlete triad** A condition characterized by disordered eating, lack of menstrual periods (amenorrhea), and osteoporosis.

## Binge-Eating Disorder

The typical characteristics for binge-eating disorder are listed in Table 11-2. Generally, it can be defined as binge-eating episodes not accompanied by purging (as typifies bulimia nervosa) at least two times per week for at least 6 months. First officially described in 1994, today health care professionals recognize binge-eating disorder as a growing, complex, and potentially serious problem.

Approximately 30% of subjects in organized weight-control programs have binge-eating disorder, whereas among the general U.S. population, about 4 million have this disorder. However, many more people in the general population are likely to have less severe forms of the disorder that do not meet all the criteria that describe the problem. The number of cases of binge-eating disorder is far greater than that of either anorexia nervosa or bulimia nervosa. This disorder is also more common among the severely obese and those with a long history of frequent restrictive dieting, although obesity is not a criterion for having binge-eating disorder.

**Development and Characteristics of Binge-Eating Disorder.** Individuals with binge-eating disorder (about 40% of whom are males) often perceive themselves as hungry more often than normal. They usually started dieting at a young age, began bingeing during adolescence or in their early twenties, and did not succeed in commercial weight-control programs. Almost half of those with severe binge-eating disorder exhibit clinical depression. Some people also may have a genetic predisposition for this disorder.

▲ Binge-eating disorder is seen in both men and women.

▲ Professional help is advised for people with a binge-eating disorder.

**A**s noted in Chapter 2, spreading one's dietary intake into numerous, small meals (grazing) over a day provides some health advantages if overall calorie intake remains appropriate.

**P**eople with binge-eating disorder may come from families with alcoholism or may have suffered sexual abuse. Members of such dysfunctional families often do not know how to deal effectively with emotions. They cope by turning to substances. Family members learn to cover up dysfunctional patterns for the alcoholic person and to nurture him or her at the expense of each other and their own needs.

**TABLE 11-2** Some Characteristics of Binge-Eating Disorder

A. Recurrent episodes of binge eating, which is characterized by:
  (1) Eating, in a discrete period (e.g., within any 2-hour period), an amount of food definitely larger than most people would eat during a similar period in similar circumstances
  (2) A sense of lack of control during the episodes (e.g., a feeling that one can't stop eating or control what or how much one is eating)

B. During most binge episodes, at least three of the following occur:
  (1) Eating much more rapidly than usual
  (2) Eating until feeling uncomfortably full
  (3) Eating large amounts of food when not feeling physically hungry
  (4) Eating alone because of being embarrassed by how much one is eating
  (5) Feeling disgusted with oneself, depressed, or guilty after overeating

C. Marked distress regarding binge eating

D. The binge eating occurs, on average, at least 2 days a week for 6 months.

E. The behavior does not occur only during the course of bulimia nervosa or anorexia nervosa.

Based on information from the *Diagnostic and Statistical Manual of Mental Disorders*, Fourth Edition (DSM-IV-TR). Washington DC: American Psychiatric Association, 2000.

Typical binge eaters isolate themselves and eat large quantities of a favorite food. Stressful events and feelings of depression or anxiety can trigger this behavior. Giving themselves permission to eat a forbidden food can also precipitate a binge. Other triggers include loneliness, anxiety, self-pity, depression, anger, rage, alienation, and frustration. They sometimes binge on whatever is easy to eat in large amounts—noodles, rice, bread, leftovers. Characteristically, however, binge eaters consume foods that carry the social stigma of "junk" or "bad" foods—ice cream, cookies, sweets, potato chips, and similar snack foods.

In general, people engage in binge eating to induce a sense of well-being and perhaps even numbness, usually in an attempt to avoid feeling and dealing with emotional pain and anxiety. They eat without regard to biological need and often in a recurrent, ritualized fashion. Some people with this disorder eat food continually over an extended period, called *grazing*; others cycle episodes of bingeing with normal eating. For example, someone with a stressful or frustrating job might come home every night and graze until bedtime. Another person might eat normally most of the time but find comfort in consuming large quantities of food when an emotional setback occurs.

Although people with anorexia nervosa and bulimia nervosa exhibit persistent preoccupation with body shape, weight, and thinness, binge eaters do not necessarily share these concerns. Thus, neither purging nor prolonged food restriction is characteristic of binge-eating disorder. Some physicians classify binge-eating disorder as an addiction to food, involving psychological dependence. The person becomes attached to the behavior and has a drive to continue it, senses only limited control over it, and needs to persist at it despite negative consequences. Food is used to reduce stress, produce feelings of power and well-being, avoid feelings of intimacy with others, and avoid life problems. Obesity and binge eating are not necessarily linked. Not all obese people are binge eaters, and, although obesity may result from trying to numb emotional pain with food, it is not necessarily an outcome of binge eating.

Binge-eating disorder is most likely to develop in people who never learned to express and deal appropriately with their feelings. Rather than face their frustration, anger, and pain, they turn to food. The frustration will continue because they never confront the basic problem. Binge eating makes them feel they cannot control the behavior pattern and therefore cannot control their lives. Worse, the binge eating usually increases feelings of guilt, embarrassment, and shame.

Often, people who practice binge eating have been shaped by families who do not address and express feelings in healthful ways. The parents nurture and comfort their children with food rather than engage in healthy exchanges of self-disclosure of feelings and potential solutions. Members of such families learn to eat in response to emotional needs and pain instead of hunger. Those who regularly practice binge eating may grow up nurturing others instead of themselves, avoiding their own feelings and taking little time for themselves. Not knowing how to satisfy their personal and emotional needs in more healthful ways, people in these families turn to food.

For some people, frequent dieting beginning in childhood or adolescence is a precursor to binge-eating disorder. During periods when little food is eaten, they get very hungry and obsessive about food. When allowed to eat more food, they feel driven to eat in a compulsive, uncontrolled way. The pattern of strict dieting alternating with binge eating may continue over time.

**Help for the Person with Binge-Eating Disorder.** Those with binge-eating disorder must learn to eat in response to hunger—a biological signal—rather than in response to emotional needs or external factors (such as the time of day or the simple presence of food). Counselors often direct binge eaters to record their perceptions of physical hunger throughout the day and at the beginning and end of every meal. These people must learn to respond to a prescribed amount of fullness at each meal. They should initially avoid weight-loss diets because feelings of food deprivation can lead to more disruptive emotions and a greater sense of unmet needs. Diets are likely to encourage more intense problems, such as extreme hunger. Many people with binge-eating disorder may experience difficulty in identifying personal emotional needs and expressing emotions. This problem is a common predisposing factor in binge eating, so communication issues should be addressed during treatment. Binge eaters often must be helped to recognize their buried emotions in anxiety-producing situations, and then encouraged to share them with their therapist or therapy group. Learning simple but appropriate phrases to say to oneself can help stop bingeing when the desire is strong.

Self-help groups, such as Overeaters Anonymous, aim to help recovery from binge-eating disorder. Their treatment philosophy, which parallels that of Alcoholics Anonymous, attempts to create an environment of encouragement and accountability to overcome this eating disorder. Dietary advice typically ranges from avoiding restraint in eating in general to limiting binge foods. Some experts feel that learning to eat all foods—but in moderation—is an effective goal for binge eaters. This practice can prevent the feelings of desperation and deprivation that come from limiting particular foods. Antidepressants, such as fluoxetine (Prozac®), and other types of medications (e.g., topiramate [Topamax®]) also have been found to help reduce binge eating in these individuals by decreasing depression. Overall, people who have this disorder are usually unsuccessful in controlling it on their own. Professional help is advised.

▼ Night eating syndrome is characterized by waking at least once during the night and needing to eat to be able to fall asleep again.

## Night Eating Syndrome

Night eating syndrome is characterized by evening hyperphagia (eating more than one-third of total daily calories after the evening meal) and nighttime awakening accompanied by the ingestion of food. Although night eating syndrome was first observed among obese patients, it also occurs among nonobese persons. It has been estimated to occur in 1.5% of the general population and in 8.9% of persons treated in obesity clinics.

### Signs and Symptoms of Night Eating Syndrome
- Not feeling hungry in the morning and delaying the first meal until several hours after waking

- Overeating in the evening with more than one-third of daily food intake after dinner
- Difficulty falling asleep and a need to eat something to help fall asleep faster
- Waking at least once during the night with a need to eat to be able to fall asleep again
- Eating produces feelings of guilt and shame
- Feeling depressed, especially at night

Research shows that the cause of night eating syndrome may be an abnormal food cycle in the body, resulting in a delayed intake of food during the day. The circadian rhythm (your body's 24-hour clock) of food intake appears to be disturbed in night eating syndrome. Studies have also shown that night eating syndrome is prevalent among outpatients with psychiatric conditions and that the symptoms, including nocturnal ingestion and evening hyperphagia, are significantly improved with use of the antidepressant setraline (Zoloft®).

## Female Athlete Triad

Women participating in appearance-based and endurance sports are at risk of developing an eating disorder. One study of college-age female athletes found that 15% of swimmers, 62% of gymnasts, and 32% of varsity athletes exhibited disordered eating patterns. Estimates of eating disorders for college women not involved in competitive sports are much lower.

In addition to disordered eating, college women athletes tend to experience irregular menstruation more frequently than other college women. Disordered eating, particularly food restriction, and stress can precipitate this, causing women to have less dense and weaker bones than normal because of lower estrogen concentrations in the blood. Some of these young women have bone mass values equivalent to those of 50- to 60-year-olds, increasing their risk for bone and stress fractures during sports as well as general activities. Much of the bone loss is irreversible.

The American College of Sports Medicine (ACSM) has named this syndrome "female athlete triad" because it consists of three parts: disordered eating, lack of menstrual periods, and osteoporosis (Fig. 11-4). The ACSM has issued a plea to teachers, coaches, health professionals, and parents to educate female athletes about the triad and its health consequences.

Many coaches/trainers and even some health professionals wrongly believe that loss of menstrual periods is a normal consequence of a high level of physical activity. However, loss of menstrual periods in female athletes stems from a dramatic decrease in female reproductive hormones, particularly estrogen. Loss of estrogen has other negative consequences on the body, such as fragile bones, as mentioned. Correcting the hormonal imbalance and menstrual irregularities by increasing caloric intake should stabilize bone mass. During therapy, a physician may prescribe a multivitamin and mineral supplement as well as calcium supplements as needed to maintain an intake of 1200 to 1500 milligrams.

Those exhibiting symptoms of the female athlete triad should seek treatment from a multidisciplinary team of health professionals. Involving the coach or trainer in therapy is usually a key factor in the success of the treatment plan. Suggestions for treatment are as follows:

- Reduce preoccupation with food, weight, and body fat.
- Gradually increase meals and snacks to an appropriate amount.
- Achieve an appropriate weight-for-height.
- Establish regular menstrual periods.
- Decrease training time and/or intensity by 10% to 20%.

The tragic case of Christy Henrich illustrates why anyone at risk for the female athlete triad should seek professional help. As a young teenager, Christy weighed

It is often difficult to get female athletes to accept necessary treatment plans. They frequently have a single-minded approach to their sport, while ignoring future health consequences.

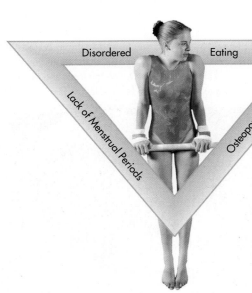

**FIGURE 11-4** ▶ The female athlete triad occurs when the athlete has disordered eating, lack of menstrual periods, and osteoporosis. Stress fractures and chronic fatigue also occur. This triad often is seen in appearance-related sports, such as gymnastics. Long-term health is at risk; thus, prevention and early treatment is crucial.

95 pounds and was 4 feet 11 inches tall. She showed promise as a gymnast but was told that she was too fat to excel in gymnastics. Christy continued her training but often starved herself, some days consuming just an apple and frequently purging by vomiting. Her success in gymnastics continued, but at age 22 her weight had fallen to 52 pounds, and she died from the effects of long-term semistarvation.

## 11.5 Prevention of Eating Disorders

A key to developing and maintaining healthful eating behavior is to realize that some concern about diet, health, and weight is normal. It is also normal to experience variation in what we eat, how we feel, and even how much we weigh. For example, it is normal to experience some minimal weight change (up to 2 to 3 pounds) throughout the day and even more over the course of a week. A large weight fluctuation or ongoing weight gain or weight loss is more likely to indicate that a problem is present. If you notice a large change in your eating habits, how you feel, or your body weight, it is a good idea to consult your personal physician. Treating physical and emotional problems early helps lead you to peace of mind and good health.

With a view on society as a whole, many people begin to form opinions about food, nutrition, health, weight, and body image prior to or during puberty. Parents, friends, and professionals working with young adults should consider the following advice for preventing eating disorders:

- Discourage restrictive dieting and meal skipping. Fasting is also discouraged (except for religious occasions).
- Provide information about normal changes that occur during puberty.
- Correct misconceptions about nutrition, healthy body weight, and approaches to weight loss.
- Carefully phrase any weight-related recommendations and comments.
- Don't overemphasize numbers on a scale. Instead, primarily promote healthful eating.
- Encourage normal expression of disruptive emotions.
- Encourage children to eat only when they're hungry.
- Teach the basics of proper nutrition and regular physical activity in school and at home.
- Provide adolescents with an appropriate, but not unlimited, degree of independence, choice, responsibility, and self-accountability for their actions.
- Increase self-acceptance and appreciation of the power and pleasure emerging from one's body.
- Enhance tolerance for diversity in body weight and shape.
- Build respectful environments and supportive relationships.
- Encourage coaches to be sensitive to weight and body-image issues among athletes.
- Emphasize that thinness is not necessarily associated with better athletic performance.

Our society as a whole can benefit from a fresh focus on nutritious food practices and a healthful outlook toward food and body weight. Not only is treatment of eating disorders far more difficult than prevention, these disorders also have devastating effects on the entire family. For this reason, caregivers and health care professionals must emphasize the importance of an overall healthful diet that focuses on moderation, as opposed to restriction and perfection. Restricted diets are especially detrimental to children because they do not supply enough calories to sustain growth. In response, nutritional counseling can assure caregivers that including some sweets and fast-food in a child's diet is appropriate (see Chapter 15 for more details).

**A** female high school athlete recently admitted her 3-year struggle with anorexia nervosa and bulimia nervosa. Even after her athletic performance declined and she suffered a sports-related injury, which sidelined her for a year and required surgery, she continued to think that controlling her weight and eating behaviors would make her the best—academically and physically. This example demonstrates several important points about eating disorders: certain groups of people are at greater risk for developing eating disorders; these people are often high achievers and are careful about concealing their eating disorder; and eating disorders such as the female athlete triad, bulimia nervosa, and anorexia nervosa frequently overlap.

## CRITICAL THINKING

Tom, a high school teacher, is concerned about eating disorders. He wants to try to prevent young adults from falling into the discouraging traps of anorexia nervosa and bulimia nervosa. What are some of the topics and issues he should discuss with students in his health classes?

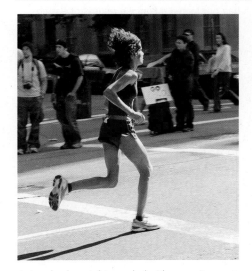

▲ Low body weight coupled with excessive exercise can lead to amenorrhea and ultimately the female athlete triad.

▲ Bulimia nervosa affects many college students. Counselors are aware of this and are available to help.

**F**or further information on eating disorders, contact:

Academy for Eating Disorders, 111 Deer Lake Road, Suite 100, Deerfield, IL 60015 847-498-4274; **www.aedweb.org**

The National Eating Disorders Association, 603 Stewart St., Suite 803, Seattle, WA 98101; 206-382-3587 or 800-931-EDAP; **www.nationaleatingdisorders.org**

The National Institute of Mental Health has published a concise review of eating disorders (**www.nimh.nih.gov/publicat/ eatingdisorders.cfm**).

Overall, the challenge facing many North Americans is achieving a healthy body weight without excessive dieting. This means adopting and maintaining sensible eating habits, a physically active lifestyle, and realistic and positive attitudes and emotions while practicing creative ways to handle stress. Eating disorders develop in part from certain cultural values; changing these values might reduce the pressures predisposing some people to various types of disordered eating behavior. Some feminists, for example, assert that true liberation means being free to find one's natural weight. Women who combine careers and motherhood are saying that they have more important things to worry about; some fashion leaders are tolerating more curves; exercise programs are encouraging regular brisk walking, rather than high-intensity activities such as jogging. Finally, writers, therapists, and registered dietitians are working to help women accept their bodies, as noted in the "size acceptance" approach discussed in Chapter 7.

## MAKING DECISIONS

### Polycystic Ovary Syndrome and Eating Disorders

Polycystic ovary syndrome (PCOS) is a complex hormonal disorder and is the leading cause of infertility. PCOS is characterized by hormonal imbalances in women with high levels of male hormones such as testosterone secreted by the ovaries. The hormonal imbalance causes tiny cysts to surround the ovaries like a strand of pearls. The signs and symptoms of PCOS include difficulty losing weight, intense cravings for carbohydrates, and irregular or absent periods. Most of these have a direct effect on body image and self-esteem, so a relationship between PCOS and eating disorders is suspected. The overlap in symptoms means it is important that persons with these characteristics be screened for both PCOS and eating disorders before recommendations for treatment are made.

## CONCEPT CHECK

Food bingeing (without purging) and grazing are two characteristic behaviors of binge-eating disorder. Treatment addresses the deeper emotional issues that undermine healthy eating practices, while shifting the person's focus away from food deprivation and restrictive diets and toward more normal eating behaviors. Night eating syndrome involves overeating in the evening and a need to eat to be able to fall asleep. The female athlete triad consists of disordered eating, amenorrhea, and osteoporosis, and most commonly affects those in appearance-related and endurance sports. Parents, coaches, teachers, and health professionals need to initiate efforts to prevent and treat this problem.

# Eating Disorder Reflections

## Thoughts of an Anorexic Woman

It was the spring of my freshman year of high school, and I had just turned 15. I wanted to get a leading role in the upcoming high school musical *West Side Story*. I thought I should lose some weight to look more attractive to the student director Shawn, so I decided to give up "junk" food. The next day my friend Sandra looked at my lunch, spread out neatly on a napkin before me, and squawked, "Dill pickles?! Who brings dill pickles for lunch in a zip-lock baggie?" The other girls at the table fell into a fit of hysterics. "Casting for *West Side Story* is coming up," I said, "and I gave up 'junk' food to try to

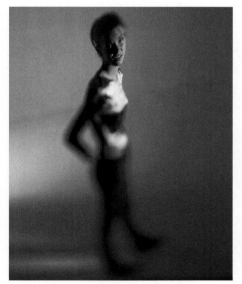

▲ A history of anorexia nervosa can harm physical as well as mental health.

lose a few pounds." One of my friends thought it would be funny to give me an M&M—just to smell. Ha, ha. I put it in a little Tupperware container and kept it for days in my backpack as a reminder. Every once in a while, I did smell it.

For the next few weeks there were times when I would find myself cracking open the refrigerator door and just staring down what I knew to be a deliciously crunchy, crisp, and cold Kit Kat bar in the dairy bin. I didn't eat it though. At the mall with my friends (since at 15, that's about all my parents allowed me to do), Bridgette and Nora wanted to stop and get a cinnamon bun. They chided me, but I didn't budge. The cinnamon bun smelled so good. But as I sat opposite them in the food court and watched them over-dramatize its ooey-gooey goodness, I felt a sense of pride that I could make a decision and stick with it. I could see that they were jealous of my willpower.

When Easter came around, I took a look at the contents of the Easter basket my mom insisted on preparing and turned up my nose at it. I had proven to myself that I could resist temptation . . why stop now?

I was eventually offered only a minor part in the musical, but I wasn't that disappointed. I was looking so much better as the pounds kept coming off. Every morning, just after going to the bathroom and before getting any breakfast, I would pop onto the scale in my mom's bathroom. One hundred and fifteen pounds and still going. At 5 feet 7 inches, that wasn't too bad.

Also at this time, I started running, and my friend Laura became my running partner. She was getting in shape for the next season of field hockey. After school, we met in the locker room, changed out of our school clothes, and out we went. I had never been much of an athlete—I thought that being part of a team, whether in sports or academics, diluted the excellence I could achieve on my own. Running, however, could just be me and the road—no mediocrity there.

Cheese and butter had made it to the "no" list by the time I was 16 and down to 105 pounds. Fat-free was my mantra. For my 16th birthday, my friends threw a little surprise party for me. Nora, knowing I would put up a fight, made me a cake. "It's your birthday! You can have a piece of cake!" I politely said no, that I would cut it for everyone else, but I really didn't want any. They pestered me and Nora started to feel offended, so finally I took a few bites so she wouldn't burst into tears. It had been so long since I'd had so much sugar. I felt bloated and sick. I ate nothing for the rest of the day, and only 6 saltines, 1 apple, and 2 stalks of celery the next day. Those foods were on the "yes" list. Salads also were okay, but only lettuce with salt and vinegar. I told my parents that the dissections in biology class had given me a distaste for meat, but really, I just didn't want all those calories. For a while, I craved food day and night, but I was getting better and better at holding my ground.

By my senior year, I was skipping lunches altogether, opting instead to hang out in the library and read over my AP Bio text. "Where were you at lunch today?" Bridgette would ask later. "Oh, I had some reading to do. The AP exam is going to be tough." At 100 pounds, I was getting closer to finding out what "tough" really meant.

Even though Laura moved out of state, I didn't give up on exercising. Now, the stair stepper in the gym was my favorite. I'd take my microbiology notes, prop them up in front of me, and step-step-step until I had burned 400 kcal. I felt so efficient being that I could multi-task. Sometimes I'd go twice a day. As senior year wore on, though, it got harder and harder to get up in the morning and put on my tennis shoes. And then one morning, in the shower, I just collapsed under the stream of hot water.

I ended up in this hospital bed with an IV tube in my arm. At 92 pounds, my body was starving. As it turns out, if you don't give your body any fuel, you start to cannibalize yourself, in a sense. My body had been so hungry, my muscles had been wasting away, and the episode in the shower was due to a problem with my heart. It's a problem I have created . . . not my parents or my distant group of friends . . . just me. My mom was there, next to me, caressing the arm with the IV tube, putting her whole life on hold because of me. Isn't this what I'd wanted—to be in control of my own destiny?

Where do I go from here?

## Thoughts of a Bulimic Woman

From Hall L, Cohn L: *Bulimia—A Guide to Recovery.* Gurze Books: Carlsbad, CA, 1992.

I am wide awake and immediately out of bed. I think back to the night before, when I made a new list of what I wanted to get done and how I wanted to be. My husband is not far behind me on his way into the bathroom to get ready for work. Maybe I can sneak onto the scale to see what I weigh this morning before he notices me. I am already in my private world. I feel overjoyed when the scale says that I stayed the same weight as I was the night before, and I can feel that slightly hungry feeling. Maybe it will stop today; maybe today everything will change. What were the projects I was going to get done?

We eat the same breakfast, except that I take no butter on my toast, no cream in my coffee, and never take seconds (until Doug gets out the door). Today I am going to be really good, and that means eating certain predetermined portions of food and not taking one more bite than I think I am allowed. I am very careful to see that I don't take more than Doug. I judge myself by his body. I can feel the tension building. I wish Doug would hurry up and leave so I can get going!

As soon as he shuts the door, I try to get involved with one of the myriad responsibilities on my list. I hate them all! I just want to crawl into a hole. I don't want to do anything. I'd rather eat. I am alone; I am nervous; I am no good; I always do everything wrong anyway; I am not in control; I can't make it through the day, I know it. It has been the same for so long. I remember the starchy cereal I ate for breakfast. I am into the bathroom and onto the scale. It measures the same, but I don't want to stay the same! I want to be thinner! I look into the mirror. I think my thighs are ugly and deformed looking. I see a lumpy, clumsy, pear-shaped wimp. There is always something wrong with what I see. I feel frustrated, trapped in this body, and I don't know what to do about it.

I float to the refrigerator knowing exactly what is there. I begin with last night's brownies. I always begin with the sweets. At first I try to make it look like nothing is missing, but my appetite is huge and I resolve to make another batch of brownies. I know there is half of a bag of cookies in the bathroom, thrown out the night before, and I polish them off immediately. I take some milk so my vomiting will be smoother. I like the full feeling I get after downing a big glass. I get out six pieces of bread and toast one side of each in the broiler, turn them over and load them with pats of butter, and put them under the broiler again until they are bubbling. I take all six pieces on a plate to the television and go back for a bowl of cereal and a banana to have along with them. Before the last piece of toast is finished, I am already preparing the next batch of six more pieces. Maybe another brownie or five, and a couple of large bowls full of ice cream, yogurt, or cottage cheese.

My stomach is stretched into a huge ball below my rib cage. I know I'll have to go into the bathroom soon, but I want to postpone it. I am in never-never land. I am waiting, feeling the pressure, pacing the floor in and out of the rooms. Time is passing. Time is passing. It is getting to be time. I wander aimlessly through each of the rooms again, tidying, making the whole house neat and put back together. I finally make the turn into the bathroom. I brace my feet, pull my hair back and stick my finger down my throat, stroking twice, and get up a huge pile of food. Three times, four times, and another pile of food. I can see everything come back. I am so glad to see those brownies because they are so fattening. The rhythm of the emptying is broken and my head is beginning to hurt. I stand up feeling dizzy, empty, and weak. The whole episode has taken about an hour.

▲ Bulimic episodes add to the despair felt in this disorder.

## Case Study Eating Disorders—Steps to Recovery

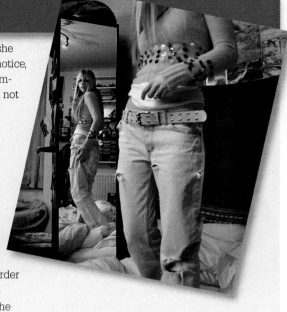

At age 16, Sarah suddenly became self-conscious about her body when her peers teased her about being overweight. She began exercising to an aerobics video for an hour each day and found that she had success in losing weight; this was the beginning of her obsession to be thin. Next, Sarah turned to eating less food to lose even more weight and began eliminating certain foods from her diet, such as candy and meat. She increased her water and vegetable intake and chewed sugarless gum to curb her appetite. Once she began dieting, it was impossible for her to stop. She enjoyed having a high degree of self-control over her body. Still, she was literally obsessed with food, even staring at others while they were eating a meal. She occasionally cooked large meals and then refused to eat all but a few bites. By the time Sarah was 19 years old and 5 feet 6 inches tall, her weight had dropped from 150 pounds to 85 pounds in 20 months. Her family was concerned about her weight status, demanding that she go to a physician for an evaluation. Sarah was not happy about this idea but believed that her family would stop pestering her if she went. Sarah did not think she had a problem; she thought she was still grotesquely overweight. She did notice, however, that she was intolerant of cold temperatures and was concerned that she had not menstruated in a year.

Answer the following questions, and check your responses in Appendix A.

1. Sarah appears to have an eating disorder. Which eating disorder best describes her behavior?
2. List the behaviors that Sarah developed between age 16 and 19 years that are signs of the development of this eating disorder.
3. What physical symptoms of this disorder does Sarah have (review Fig. 11-1)?
4. What types of therapy do you think the physician will suggest for Sarah?
5. Do you think Sarah has developed any vitamin or mineral deficiencies? Which ones would be most likely? How could these deficiencies be best treated?
6. Where could she go for the therapy she needs?
7. What type of professionals would most likely provide therapy for Sarah's condition?
8. What is the likelihood that she will fully recover from her condition?

## Summary

1. Anorexia nervosa is most common among high-achieving, perfectionist girls from families marked by conflict, high expectations, rigidity, and denial. The disorder usually starts with dieting in early puberty and proceeds to the near-total refusal to eat. Early warning signs include intense concern about weight gain and dieting, as well as abnormal food habits, such as cooking food that they won't allow themselves to eat.

2. Anorexia nervosa may be defined as a denial of appetite. Anorexic persons become irritable, hostile, overly critical, and joyless; they tend to withdraw from family and friends. Eventually, anorexia nervosa can lead to numerous physical effects, including a profound decrease in body weight and body fat, a fall in body temperature and heart rate, iron-deficiency anemia, a low white blood cell count, hair loss, constipation, low blood potassium, and the loss of menstrual periods. Those with anorexia nervosa are in a state of physical illness. Treatment of anorexia nervosa includes increasing food intake to support gradual weight gain. Psychological counseling attempts to help establish regular food habits and to find means of coping with the life stresses that led to the disorder. Hospitalization may be necessary, as well as use of certain medications.

3. Bulimia nervosa is characterized by secretive bingeing on large amounts of food within a short time span, and then purging by vomiting or misusing laxatives, diuretics, or enemas. Alternately, fasting and excessive exercise may be used. Both men and women are at risk. Vomiting as a means of purging is especially destructive to the body; it can cause severe tooth decay, stomach ulcers, irritation of the esophagus, low blood potassium, and other problems. Bulimia nervosa poses a serious health problem and is associated with significant risk of suicide. Treatment of bulimia nervosa includes psychological as well as nutritional counseling. During treatment, bulimic persons learn to accept themselves and to cope with problems in ways that do not involve food. Regular eating patterns are developed as these bulimic persons begin to plan meals in an informed, healthful manner. Certain medications can be a helpful addition to the regimen.

4. Binge-eating disorder, more widespread than either anorexia nervosa or bulimia nervosa, is most common among people with a history of frequent, unsuccessful dieting. Binge eaters typically either practice bingeing (without purging) or grazing (i.e., eating continually over extended periods). Emotional disturbances are often at the root of this disordered form of eating. Night eating syndrome is overeating in the evening with more than one-third of daily food intake after

dinner, difficulty falling asleep and a need to eat something to help fall asleep faster, and waking at least once during the night and a need to eat to be able to fall asleep again. The female athlete triad consists of disordered eating, loss of menstrual periods, and osteoporosis. It is particularly common in appearance-related and endurance sports. If not corrected, this disorder eventually leads to decreased athletic performance and general health problems.

5. Prevention of eating disorders is crucial because treatments are expensive and lengthy and are not 100% effective. Encouraging healthy attitudes about eating and exercise from a young age will aid in preventing the development of eating disorders. Those who work closely with children and young adults should encourage acceptance of diversity in body sizes and carefully phrase comments about body weight. Helping children to develop healthy ways to cope with emotions is also important.

## Study Questions

1. What are the typical characteristics of a person with anorexia nervosa? What may influence a person to begin rigid, self-imposed dietary patterns?

2. List the detrimental physical and psychological side effects of bulimia nervosa. Describe important goals of the psychological and nutrition therapy used to treat bulimic patients.

3. What is the current thinking concerning medication use for anorexia nervosa and bulimia nervosa?

4. Explain the role of excessive exercise in eating disorders.

5. How might parents significantly contribute to the development of an eating disorder? Suggest an attitude that a

parent or an adult friend of yours displayed that may not have been conducive to developing a normal relationship to food.

6. Based on your knowledge of good nutrition and sound dietary habits, answer the following questions:
   a. How can repeated bingeing and purging lead to significant nutrient deficiencies?
   b. How can significant nutrient deficiencies contribute to major health problems in later life?
   c. A friend asks you, the nutrition expert, if it is okay to "cleanse" the body by eating only grapefruit for a week. What is your response?

7. How, in your opinion, has society contributed to the development of various forms of disordered eating? Provide an example.

8. List the three symptoms that constitute the female athlete triad. What is the major health risk associated with loss of menstrual periods in the female athlete?

9. How does binge-eating disorder differ from bulimia nervosa? Describe the factors that contribute to the development and treatment of binge-eating disorder.

10. Provide two recommendations to reduce the problem of eating disorders in our society.

## Check Your Knowledge

Answers to the following multiple choice questions are below.

1. Anorexia nervosa generally is a disease of
   a. children.
   b. middle-aged women.
   c. young boys.
   d. teenage women.

2. Anorexia nervosa can be defined as
   a. compulsive eating.
   b. hyperactivity.
   c. psychological denial of appetite.
   d. purging.

3. A long-term health consequence of anorexia nervosa could be
   a. fractures resulting from bone loss.
   b. atherosclerotic heart disease.
   c. esophageal ulcers.
   d. cancer.

4. Bulimia is most frequently diagnosed by a
   a. dietitian.
   b. physician.
   c. dentist.
   d. physical therapist.

5. The *major* health risk from frequent vomiting due to bulimia nervosa is
   a. a drop in blood potassium.
   b. constipation.
   c. weight gain.
   d. a swelling of salivary glands.

6. Initial treatment of bulimia nervosa includes all of the following *except*
   a. psychotherapy to improve body image.
   b. emphasis on regular eating habits.
   c. nutritional counseling.
   d. refeeding via tube feedings.
   e. Both a and c.

7. Binge-eating disorder can be characterized as
   a. bingeing accompanied by purging.
   b. secretive eating.
   c. eating to avoid feeling and dealing with emotional pain.
   d. the early phase of bulimia nervosa.

8. Binge-eating disorder is different from anorexia nervosa, and particularly bulimia nervosa, because it doesn't necessarily involve
   a. females.
   b. a persistent concern with body shape, weight, and thinness.

c. purging, such as regular vomiting.
d. health risks.
e. Both b and c.

9. Night eating syndrome is characterized by
   a. eating dinner but no breakfast or lunch.
   b. the need to eat to fall asleep.
   c. waking at night to purge by vomiting.
   d. consuming all of the daily calories at night.

10. Female athlete triad consists of
    a. anorexia nervosa, lack of family support, and overtraining.
    b. disordered eating, overtraining, and lack of menstrual periods.
    c. osteoporosis, lack of menstrual periods, and disordered eating.
    d. osteoporosis, lack of sleep, and disordered eating.

Answers: 1. d, 2. c, 3. a, 4. c, 5. a, 6. d, 7. c, 8. e, 9. b, 10. c

# Further Readings

1. ADA Reports: Position of the American Dietetic Association: Nutrition intervention in the treatment of anorexia nervosa, bulimia nervosa, and other eating disorders. *Journal of the American Dietetic Association* 106: 2073, 2006.

   *Eating disorders are complex and serious illnesses that exist across a continuum from extreme dieting to diagnosed conditions, as described in detail in this article. To be effective in treating individuals who suffer from these illnesses, the expert interaction between professionals in many disciplines, including dietetics, is required.*

2. American Academy of Pediatrics: Identifying and treating eating disorders. *Pediatrics* 111:204, 2003.

   *Eating disorders are becoming more common in our society. This article reviews the current diagnostic and treatment options for such disorders.*

3. American Psychiatric Association: Treatment of patients with eating disorders, 3rd ed. *American Journal of Psychiatry* 163(suppl):4, 2006.

   *People with eating disorders display a broad range of symptoms that occur along a continuum between those of anorexia nervosa and those of bulimia nervosa. The care of these people requires a comprehensive array of approaches to provide the best chance of treatment success.*

4. Bonci CM: National athletic trainers' association position statement: Preventing, detecting, and managing disordered eating in athletes. *Journal of Athletic Training* 43: 80, 2008.

   *Disordered eating practices are common among athletes, particularly those participating in sports with weight classifications or those in which appearance is related to success. At the same time, training intensity increases nutrient needs and nutrient deficiencies impair athletic performance. Because of their frequent interaction with athletes, athletic trainers are in a unique position for detection, referral, and treatment for eating disorders. Coaches and others who work closely with athletes should be trained to promote healthful dietary behaviors and recognize signs of eating disorders and should be sensitive to weight issues.*

5. Couturier J, Lock J: What is recovery in adolescent anorexia nervosa? *International Journal of Eating Disorders* 39:550, 2006.

   *A range of definitions are used to define recovery from anorexia nervosa including percent ideal body weight, psychological recovery, and combinations of these variables. In this study of adolescents treated for anorexia nervosa, the recovery rates ranged from 57% to 94% depending on the definition used. Mean time to remission for weight ranged from 11 to 22 months. A consistent definition of recovery is needed that includes both weight and psychological symptoms.*

6. Goebel-Fabbri AE: Eating disorders in type 1 diabetes: Clinical significance and treatment recommendations. *Current Diabetes Reports* 9:133, 2009.

   *Girls and women with type 1 diabetes are at increased risk for eating disorders. Dietary restrictions necessary for diabetes control and a fear of hypoglycemia may precipitate binge eating. Some individuals may restrict insulin therapy as a means of purging calories without regard to the detrimental outcomes of impaired glucose control. This review highlights the importance of screening girls and women with diabetes for the presence of eating disorders.*

7. Grassi A: Are polycystic ovary syndrome & eating disorders related? *Today's Dietitian* p. 32, October 2006.

   *Polycystic ovary syndrome (PCOS) is a complex hormonal disorder and is the leading cause of infertility. The symptoms of polycystic ovary syndrome and certain eating disorders are similar. In addition, the symptoms of PCOS have a direct effect on body image and self-esteem and may lead to the development of eating disorders. This article discusses these relationships.*

8. Jackson K: Exercise abuse: Too much of a good thing. *Today's Dietitian* p. 51, March 2005.

   *Regularly performing an excessive amount of exercise has deleterious effects on the body, including the skeleton. This author discusses the problem of exercise abuse and reviews treatment options.*

9. Kouba S and others: Pregnancy and neonatal outcomes in women with eating disorders. *Obstetrics and Gynecology* 105: 255, 2005.

   *Pregnant women with past or ongoing eating disorders such as anorexia nervosa and bulimia nervosa have a greater risk for delivering infants with low birth weight. The authors suggest that these women receive careful medical follow up during pregnancy.*

10. Lundgren JD and others: Prevalence of the night eating syndrome in a psychiatric population. *American Journal of Psychiatry* 163 (1):156, 2006.

    *The night eating syndrome is a pattern of disordered eating characterized by evening hyperphagia (eating more than one-third of total daily calories after the evening meal) and nocturnal awakening with ingestion of food. The results of this study show that night eating syndrome is a common disorder among psychiatric outpatients and is associated with substance use and obesity.*

11. Mathieu J: What is orthorexia? *Journal of the American Dietetic Association* 105:1510, 2005.

*"Orthorexia," although not currently classified as an eating disorder, describes an emerging condition in which healthful eating becomes an obsession. A need for perfection or purity lies at the heart of orthorexia. Healthful or not, strict dietary practices become a problem when they interfere with a person's ability take part in society. Such extreme perfectionism in dietary practices may be related to a psychiatric diagnosis of obsessive-compulsive disorder. Registered dietitians are in a unique position to recognize orthorexia and direct individuals to seek psychiatric help.*

12. Mehler PS: Bulimia nervosa. *The New England Journal of Medicine* 349:875, 2003.

    *The combination of cognitive behavior therapy and antidepressant medications provides the best hope for treatment of bulimia nervosa. Nutritional counseling also has a role, such as addressing concerns about specific "forbidden" foods.*

13. Mond JM and others: An update on the definition of "excessive exercise" in eating disorders research. *International Journal of Eating Disorders* 39:147, 2006.

    *The relationship between exercise behavior and eating-disordered behavior was studied in 3,472 women aged 18–42 years who exercised regularly. The results of the study indicated that exercise was excessive when its postponement was followed by intense guilt and when it was undertaken solely to influence weight or shape. Women who reported these exercise characteristics had significantly greater levels of eating disorder psychopathology. Therefore these variables could be a useful indicator of eating disorders.*

14. Norris ML and others: Ana and the Internet: A review of pro-anorexia websites. *International Journal of Eating Disorders* 39:443, 2006.

    *Searching for "anorexia" using common search engines results in hundreds of links, many of which are "pro-anorexia." These websites provide information that is supportive of anorexia nervosa but is largely controversial and dangerous. This study was conducted to identify key characteristics of pro-anorexia websites. Themes that were most common were control, success, and perfection. Photo galleries are prevalent that serve as motivators for weight loss. It is important that health care providers and caregivers be aware of these websites and their content.*

15. Ringham R and others: Eating disorder symptomatology among ballet dancers. *International Journal of Eating Disorders* 39:503, 2006.

    *Ballet dancers are at high risk of developing eating disorders. In this study, 29 female ballet dancers were compared to women with anorexia nervosa, bulimia nervosa, and not eating pathology. The results showed that the eating patterns of dancers were more similar to eating-disordered individuals than to control individuals. The majority of the dancers (83%) met lifetime criteria for eating disorders.*

16. Robinson-O'Brien R and others: Adolescent and young adult vegetarianism: Better dietary intake and weight outcomes but increased risk of disordered eating behaviors. *Journal of the American Dietetic Association* 109: 648, 2009.

    *This study of more than 2500 young men and women contributes to the body of evidence demonstrating that appropriately planned vegetarian and vegan lifestyles can be healthfully practiced by people of all ages. However, some young adults may use these socially-acceptable eating patterns as a means of unhealthful dietary restriction for extreme weight loss. A history of vegetarian dietary practices is associated with disordered eating practices, such as binge eating. If weight loss is the primary motive for choosing a vegetarian lifestyle, parents should be on alert for warning signs of eating disorders.*

17. Spear BA: Does dieting increase the risk for obesity and eating disorders? *Journal of the American Dietetic Association* 106:523, 2006.

    *This editorial summarizes the results of recent studies on dieting and other unhealthful weight control methods in adolescents that appear to predict and be associated with later weight gain, overweight, and eating disorders.*

18. Stuppy P: Eating disorders in women at midlife. *Today's Dietitian* p. 12, January 2006.

    *Several emotional changes that occur in middle age, such as death of a spouse, divorce, the "empty nest" syndrome, and caring for aging parents, may precipitate eating disorders. Women, who already experience a high level of dissatisfaction with their bodies, may use dietary restriction or bingeing behaviors as coping mechanisms. Registered dietitians can help clients by facilitating recognition of the emotional underpinnings of clients' eating problems and by appropriately referring clients to mental health professionals, when needed.*

19. Wolfe BE: Reproductive health in women with eating disorders. *Journal of Obstetric, Gynecologic, and Neonatal Nursing* 34:255, 2005.

    *Medical complications from eating disorders include symptoms associated with reproductive health. This review discusses the reproductive health issues that may occur in women with anorexia nervosa and bulimia nervosa as well as the clinical implications.*

20. Yager J, Andersen AA: Anorexia nervosa. *The New England Journal of Medicine* 353:1481, 2005.

    *Excellent review of eating disorders by noted experts. Both diagnosis and treatment are highlighted.*

## I. Assessing Risk of Developing an Eating Disorder

British investigators have developed a five-question screening tool called the **SCOFF** Questionnaire for recognizing eating disorders:[†]

1. Do you make yourself **S**ick because you feel full?
2. Do you lose **C**ontrol over how much you eat?
3. Have you lost more than **O**ne stone (about 13 pounds) recently?
4. Do you believe yourself to be **F**at when others say you are thin?
5. Does **F**ood dominate your life?

Two or more positive responses suggest an eating disorder.

1. After completing this questionnaire, do you feel that you might have an eating disorder or the potential to develop one?

   _____

   _____

2. Do you think any of your friends might have an eating disorder?

   _____

   _____

3. What counseling and education resources exist in your area or on your campus to help with a potential eating disorder?

   _____

   _____

4. If a friend has an eating disorder, what do you think is the best way to assist him or her in getting help?

   _____

   _____

[†]Morgan JF and others: The SCOFF Questionnaire, *British Medical Journal* 319:1467, 1999.

## II. Helping Prevent Eating Disorders

You have been asked to speak to a junior high school class about eating disorders. What are four major points that you would make to help prevent disordered eating in this population?

1. _____
2. _____
3. _____
4. _____

Here are points you may consider:

1. Extreme thinness is oversold in the media. Extremely low weight (i.e., BMI of less than 17.5) is generally not healthy.
2. Self-induced vomiting is dangerous. Damage to the teeth, stomach, and esophagus often results.
3. Loss of menstrual periods is a sign of illness. It is important to see a physician about this. Bone deterioration is a common result.
4. The treatment of eating disorders in early phases aids success. These diseases are difficult to treat once firmly established.

# CHAPTER 12 Undernutrition Throughout the World

## Student Learning Outcomes After studying this chapter you will be able to:

1. Define and characterize the terms *hunger, malnutrition,* and *undernutrition.*

2. Examine undernutrition in the United States and highlight several programs established to combat this problem.

3. Examine undernutrition in the developing world and evaluate the major obstacles that hinder a solution.

4. Outline some possible solutions to undernutrition in the developing world.

5. Evaluate the consequences of undernutrition during critical periods in a person's life.

## Chapter Outline

Student Learning Outcomes

Refresh Your Memory

12.1 World Hunger: A Crisis on the Rise

12.2 Undernutrition in the United States

12.3 Undernutrition in the Developing World

12.4 The Role of Sustainable Agriculture and Biotechnology in Worldwide Food Availability

Nutrition and Your Health: Undernutrition at Critical Life Stages

Case Study: Undernutrition During Childhood

Summary/Study Questions/Check Your Knowledge/Further Readings

Rate Your Plate

**TODAY, NEARLY ONE IN SIX PEOPLE WORLDWIDE IS CHRONICALLY UNDERNOURISHED—** too hungry to lead a productive, active life. Over the past 10 years, this problem has worsened. Throughout the world, the problems of poverty and undernutrition are widespread and growing—even though there is enough food available to sufficiently feed all of us.

Within the developing world, approximately 1 billion people are malnourished, with Asia having the largest number. Malnutrition is the main cause of lowered resistance to disease, infection, and death, with children under 5 years being the most susceptible.

Chapter 12 examines the problem of undernutrition, the conditions that create it, and some possible solutions. If we are to eradicate undernutrition, we all have to understand the problem. As the comic in the chapter suggests, we must begin to assume responsibility today, not tomorrow, to work on solutions to hunger close to home and in faraway nations. It is important to recognize that many political, economic, and social factors worldwide contribute directly and indirectly to the hunger problem.

▲ Malnutrition is associated with or exacerbated by overpopulation in some developing countries.

**food insecure** Condition in which the quality, variety, and/or desirability of the diet is reduced and there is difficulty at times providing enough food for everyone in the household.

**hunger** The primarily physiological (internal) drive to find and eat food.

 **Refresh Your Memory**

As you begin your study of world hunger in Chapter 12, you may want to review:

- The health effects of protein-calorie malnutrition in Chapter 6
- The role of vitamin A and rich food sources in Chapter 8
- The roles and rich food sources of iron, zinc, and iodide in Chapter 9

## 12.1 World Hunger: A Crisis on the Rise

Uncertainty regarding the source of one's next meal remains a daily experience for close to 1 billion people around the world. This situation is troubling considering that worldwide agriculture produces more than enough food to meet the energy requirements of each of the nearly 7 billion persons. Even with this abundance, in 2008, 963 million people were unable to access enough food to lead active, healthy lives—that is, they were **food insecure.** The serious problems of food insecurity and malnutrition exist in virtually every nation. They are most common in the developing world, with Asia having the largest number, along with sub-Saharan Africa, Latin America, and the Caribbean. Nearly all people suffering from food insecurity, hunger, or malnutrition are poor.

Let's begin our look at the problem of world hunger and malnutrition by defining some key terms.

### Hunger

The physiological state that results when not enough food is eaten to meet energy needs is **hunger.** It also describes an uneasiness, a discomfort, a weakness, or a pain caused by lack of food. The medical and social costs of the undernutrition that can result from hunger are high—preterm births, mental disabilities, inadequate growth and development in childhood, poor school performance, decreased work output in adulthood, and chronic disease. Although malnutrition does occur in North America, it is not due to extreme poverty over a large section of the population. Instead, there are usually specific causes such as an eating disorder, alcoholism, problems in nursing home settings, or homelessness. There is also some degree of moderate malnutrition in some of the poorer segments of North American society (i.e., those earning less than the current poverty level). Fortunately, there are resources such as food banks and food stamps, though sometimes there are bureaucratic obstacles to getting these

THE PRESENT IS WHAT SLIPS BY US WHILE WE'RE PONDERING THE PAST AND WORRYING ABOUT THE FUTURE.

Millions of people worldwide die each year from health problems related to undernutrition. Rising food prices, war, and environmental catastrophe combine with the global threat of AIDS as important causes. Why must we act today to stem this tide of undernutrition? Why is Ziggy's concern an important one? Chapter 12 provides some answers.

resources to the people who need them. In addition, there is the problem known as **food insecurity** which describes a state of anxiety about running out of food or running out of money to buy more food. In 2008, 12.6% of households in the United States reported that they experienced food insecurity. Food insecurity is also a problem in Canada with 7% living in food insecure households in 2008.

Around the world, poverty is a primary cause of malnutrition. In the United States, at least 13 million children, 18% of all children under the age of 18 are in families living below the federal poverty level, defined as a family of four having an income less than $21,200 a year in 2008 (more information available at www.neep.org). Research, however, estimates that families need an income of about twice that level to cover basic expenses. Using this income standard, 39% of children live in low-income families. Living in poverty impairs a child's ability to learn and contributes to behavioral problems and poor health. The risks of poverty are greatest for young children. Fortunately, the United States does have food assistance programs for low-income families, and therefore most children in the United States are shielded from hunger.

## Malnutrition and Micronutrient Deficiences

A condition of impaired development or function caused by either a long-term deficiency or excess in calorie and/or nutrient intake is **malnutrition.** When food supplies are low and the population is large, **undernutrition** is common, leading to nutritional deficiency diseases, such as goiter (from an iodide deficiency) and xerophthalmia (eye problems caused by poor vitamin A intake). However, when the food supply is ample or overabundant, incorrect food choices coupled with an excessive intake can lead to overnutrition and its related chronic diseases, such as type 2 diabetes.

Undernutrition is the most common form of malnutrition among the poor in both developing and developed countries. Undernutrition is also the primary cause of specific nutrient deficiencies that can result in muscle wasting, blindness, scurvy, pellagra, beriberi, anemia, rickets, goiter, and a host of other problems (Table 12-1).

The most critical micronutrients missing from diets worldwide (see Fig. 12-1) are iron, vitamin A, iodide, zinc, and various B vitamins (e.g., folate), as well as selenium and vitamin C. About 1 billion people, mostly in the developing world, are affected by iron deficiency. The same is true for zinc deficiencies. With poor iron status, cognitive development will likely be impaired, particularly if prolonged deficiency occurs during early infancy. An estimated 50 million people worldwide also suffer brain damage from preventable maternal iodide deficiency. Although severe vitamin A deficiency, which causes blindness, is on the decline, up to 500,000 preschool-age children are still blinded by it each year. UNICEF reports that the lives of 1 million to 3 million children could be saved annually in the developing world if vitamin A supplements were provided a few times each year. The annual cost per child would be about 6 cents.

Of the 6.4 billion people in the world, about 2 billion may experience episodes of food shortages and be affected by some form of micronutrient malnutrition. Death and disease from infections, particularly those causing acute and prolonged diarrhea or respiratory disease, increase dramatically when the infections occur during a state of chronic undernutrition. Chronic undernutrition leaves many people in the developing world in a continual state of depressed immune function, in turn greatly increasing the risk of death, especially in childhood.

Protein-calorie malnutrition (PCM) is a form of undernutrition caused by an extremely deficient intake of calories or protein generally accompanied by an illness. The dramatic results of PCM—kwashiorkor and marasmus—were described in Chapter 6. This chapter focuses on the more subtle effects of a chronic lack of food.

## Famine

The extreme form of chronic hunger is **famine.** Periods of famine are characterized by large-scale loss of life, social disruption, and economic chaos that slows food

**food insecurity** A condition of anxiety regarding running out of either food or money to buy more food.

**malnutrition** Failing health that results from longstanding dietary practices that do not coincide with nutritional needs.

**undernutrition** Failing health that results from a longstanding dietary intake that is not enough to meet nutritional needs.

**famine** An extreme shortage of food, which leads to massive starvation in a population; often associated with crop failures, war, and political unrest.

**T**he Irish potato famine of 1840 to 1850 caused an estimated 2 million deaths and resulted in nearly as many people emigrating to other countries, such as the United States and Canada. More than 3 million people may have perished in the great famine of 1943 in Bengal, India. China suffered a famine from 1959 to 1961—estimates of mortality range from 16 million to 64 million. In 1974, another 1.5 million starved in the country of Bangladesh.

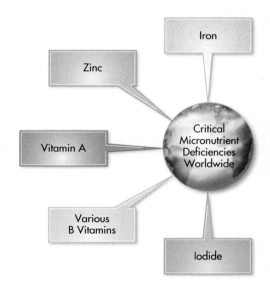

**FIGURE 12-1** ▶ Critical micronutrient deficiencies worldwide.

**TABLE 12-1** Nutrient-Deficiency Diseases That Commonly Accompany Undernutrition

| Disease and Key Nutrient Involved | Typical Effects | Foods Rich in Deficient Nutrient | Target Populations for Intervention |
|---|---|---|---|
| **Xerophthalmia** Vitamin A | Blindness from chronic eye infections, restricted growth, dryness and keratinization of epithelial tissues | Fortified milk, sweet potatoes, spinach, greens, carrots, cantaloupe, apricots | Asia, Africa |
| **Rickets** Vitamin D | Poorly calcified bones, bowed legs, other bone deformities | Fortified milk, fish oils, sun exposure | Asia, Africa, and parts of the world where religious dress codes prevent women and children from receiving adequate sun exposure; older adults in developed nations |
| **Beriberi** Thiamin | Nerve degeneration, altered muscle coordination, cardiovascular problems | Sunflower seeds, pork, whole and enriched grains, dried beans | Victims of famine in Africa |
| **Ariboflavinosis** Riboflavin | Inflammation of tongue, mouth, face and oral cavity, nervous system disorders | Milk, mushrooms, spinach, liver, enriched grains | Victims of famine in Africa |
| **Pellagra** Niacin | Diarrhea, dermatitis, dementia | Mushrooms, bran, tuna, chicken, beef, peanuts, whole and enriched grains | Victims of famine in Africa, survivors of war-torn Eastern Europe |
| **Megaloblastic anemia** Folate | Enlarged red blood cells, fatigue, weakness | Green leafy vegetables, legumes, oranges, liver | Asia, Africa |
| **Scurvy** Vitamin C | Delayed wound healing, internal bleeding, abnormal formation of bones and teeth | Citrus fruits, strawberries, broccoli | Victims of famine in Africa |
| **Iron-deficiency anemia** Iron | Reduced work output, retarded growth, increased health risk in pregnancy | Meats, seafood, broccoli, peas, bran, whole-grain and enriched breads | Worldwide |
| **Goiter** Iodide | Enlarged thyroid gland in teenagers and adults, possible mental retardation, cretinism | Iodized salt, saltwater fish | South America, Eastern Europe, Africa |

Although the nutrients are listed separately to illustrate the important role of each one, often two or more nutrition-deficiency diseases are found in an undernourished person in the developing world.

production. As a result of these extreme events, the affected community experiences a downward spiral characterized by human distress; sales of land, livestock, and other farm assets; migration; division and impoverishment of the poorest families; crime; and the weakening of customary moral codes, as seen in Sudan and Rwanda. In the midst of all this, undernutrition rates soar; infectious diseases, such as cholera, spread; and many people die.

Special efforts are needed to eradicate the fundamental causes of famine. Causes vary by region and decade, but the most common is crop failure. The most obvious reasons for crop failure are extreme weather conditions such as floods or drought, war, and civil strife. War deserves a special focus and will be specifically addressed in a separate section on war and political/civil unrest.

## General Effects of Semistarvation

In the initial stages, the results of undernutrition from semistarvation are often so mild that physical symptoms are absent and blood tests do not usually detect the slight metabolic changes. Even in the absence of clinical symptoms, however, undernourishment may affect reproductive capacity, resistance to and recovery from disease, and physical activity and work output, and lead to fatigue and behavior problems. Recall from Chapter 2 that, as tissues continue to be depleted of nutrients, blood tests eventually detect biochemical changes, such as a drop in blood hemoglobin concentration. Physical symptoms, such as body weakness, appear with further depletion. Finally, the full-blown symptoms of the predominating deficiency are recognizable, such as when blindness accompanies a vitamin A deficiency.

When a few people in a population develop a severe deficiency, this may represent only the "tip of the iceberg." Typically, a much greater number have milder degrees of undernutrition. These deficiencies should not, therefore, be dismissed as trivial, especially in the developing world. It is becoming clear that combined deficiencies of specific vitamins and the minerals iron and zinc can seriously reduce work performance, even when they do not cause obvious physical symptoms. This resulting state of ill health, in turn, diminishes the ability of individuals, communities, and even whole countries to perform at peak levels of physical and mental capacity (Fig. 12-2).

Added to their lack of nourishment, the inhabitants of poorer countries must also contend with recurrent infections, poor sanitation, extreme weather conditions, and regular exposure to infectious diseases. They require greater amounts of certain nutrients—especially iron—to combat rampant parasite and other infections. Deficiencies of both iron and zinc can lead to reduced immune function and thereby increase the risk of diseases, such as diarrhea and pneumonia.

**T**he effects of hunger are widespread:
- Reduced energy and strength
- Diminished concentration
- Impaired ability to learn
- Lowered productivity
- Worsening of chronic health conditions
- Increased susceptibility to infectious diseases
- Deterioration of mood
- Slowed recovery from illness and injury

**H**istorical Research on Undernutrition

In the 1940s a group of researchers led by Dr. Ansel Keys examined the general effects of undernutrition on adults. Previously healthy men were fed a diet averaging about 1800 kcal daily for 6 months. During this time, the men lost an average of 24% of their body weight. After about 3 months, the participants complained of fatigue, muscle soreness, irritability, intolerance to cold, and hunger pains. They exhibited a lack of ambition, self-discipline, and concentration, and were often moody, apathetic, and depressed. Their heart rate and muscle tone decreased, and they developed edema. When the men were permitted to eat normally again, feelings of recurrent hunger and fatigue persisted even after 12 weeks of rehabilitation. Full recovery required about 8 months. This study helps us understand the general state of undernourished adults worldwide.

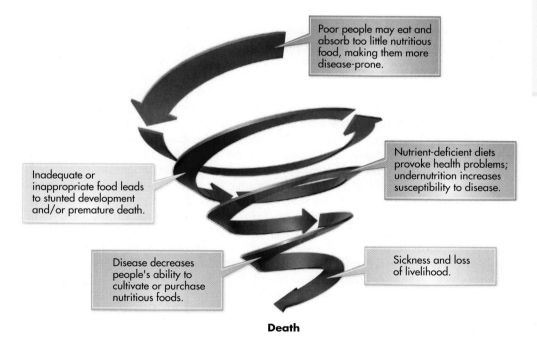

Poor people may eat and absorb too little nutritious food, making them more disease-prone.

Nutrient-deficient diets provoke health problems; undernutrition increases susceptibility to disease.

Inadequate or inappropriate food leads to stunted development and/or premature death.

Disease decreases people's ability to cultivate or purchase nutritious foods.

Sickness and loss of livelihood.

**Death**

**FIGURE 12-2 ▶** The downward spiral of poverty and illness can ultimately end in death (based on World Food Program graphic).

**CONCEPT CHECK**

Hunger provokes uneasiness and pain when insufficient food is eaten to meet calorie needs. Food insecurity is anxiety about running out of food or money to buy more food. Chronic hunger leads to undernutrition, which can cause growth failure in children and physical weakness in adults. Risk of infection increases, and nutrient-deficiency diseases result. The primary cause of undernutrition is poverty. The critical periods for undernutrition occur during pregnancy, infancy, childhood, and old age. Chronic undernutrition decreases work performance, motivation, and immune function. The adverse effects in pregnancy and infancy are dramatic, as evidenced by mortality rates much higher than those of healthy populations. Irreversible developmental damage in surviving children is also common.

## 12.2 Undernutrition in the United States

About 36.5 million (12.3%) people in the United States live at or below the poverty level, estimated at about $21,200 annually for a family of four. Of those 36.5 million, 13 million (36%) are children.

Ten percent of Caucasians, 24% of African-Americans, and 20.6% of Hispanics live in poverty. Many Native Americans are also poor, as are 18% of Asian Americans. (Many Native Americans in Canada also live in poverty.)

The poor often face difficult choices: whether to buy groceries for the family or pay this month's rent; whether to have dental work done or pay the current utility bill; whether to replace clothes the children have outgrown or pay for transportation to apply for a job. Food is one of the few flexible items in a poor person's budget. Whereas housing and utility costs, medical care, and transportation fares are non-negotiable, a person can always eat less. The short-term consequences of eating less may be less dramatic than getting evicted, but the long-term cumulative effects are significant.

▲ Food insecurity is part of the North American landscape. A "safety net" of programs exists, but it is "porous."

### Helping the Hungry in the United States

Until the twentieth century, individuals and a wide variety of charitable, often church-related organizations, provided most of the help to poor, undernourished people in the United States. Early programs rarely distributed direct cash payments to poor people because these were thought to reduce recipients' motivation to improve their circumstances or change behaviors, such as excessive drinking, that contributed to their poverty. Beginning in the early 1900s, the involvement of local, county, and state governments in providing assistance to the poor has steadily increased.

After observing extensive hunger and poverty during his presidential campaign in the 1960s, John F. Kennedy revitalized the Food Stamp Program, which had begun two decades earlier, and expanded commodity distribution programs. As of October 1, 2008, Supplemental Nutrition Assistance Program (SNAP) is the new name for the Food Stamp Program. The new name reflects the program's focus on nutrition and putting healthy food within reach for low-income households. SNAP helps low-income people and families buy food they need for good health. The program allows recipients to use an Electronic Benefit Transfer (EBT) card to purchase food and garden seeds—but not tobacco, cleaning items, alcoholic beverages, and nonedible products—at stores authorized to accept them. In recent years, each participating household received about $190 per month, on average. About 28 million people in the United States participate in this program (Table 12-2). The American Recovery and Reinvestment Act of 2009 increased benefits for SNAP participants. The increase for a participating household of four was $80 in monthly benefits.

The U.S. Congress established the School Breakfast Program in 1965 as politicians became aware of the number of hungry children coming to school. School breakfast

**TABLE 12-2** Some Current Federally Subsidized Programs That Supply Food for People in the United States

| Program | Eligibility | Description |
| --- | --- | --- |
| Supplemental Nutrition Assistance Program (formerly Food Stamp Program)* | Low-income families | Electronic Benefit Transfer (debit) cards are given to purchase food at grocery stores; the amount is based on size of household and income. |
| The Emergency Food Assistance Program (TEFAP)* | Low-income families | Provides nutrition assistance to needy Americans through distribution of USDA food commodities. |
| Commodity Supplemental Food Program | Certain low-income populations, such as pregnant women, children until the age of 6 years, and seniors | USDA surplus foods are distributed by county agencies; not found in all states; may be based on nutritional risk. |
| Special Supplemental Nutrition Program for Women, Infants, and Children (WIC)* | Low-income pregnant/lactating women, infants, and children less than 5 years old at nutritional risk | Coupons are given to purchase milk, cheese, fruit juice, cereal, infant formula, and other specific food items at grocery stores; includes nutrition education component. |
| National School Lunch Program* | Low-income children of school age | Free or reduced-price lunch is distributed by the school; meal follows USDA pattern based on MyPyramid; cost for the child depends on family income. For students who do not participate in the lunch program, special milk program may be available. |
| School Breakfast Program | Low-income children of school age | Free or reduced-price breakfast is distributed by the school; meal follows USDA pattern; cost for the child depends on family income. |
| Child and Adult Care Food Program | Child enrolled in organized child-care program and seniors in adult-care programs; income guidelines are the same as those for the School Lunch Program | Reimbursement is given for meals supplied to children at the site; meals must follow USDA guidelines based on MyPyramid. |
| Congregate Meals for the Elderly | Age 60 or over (no income guidelines) | Free noon meal is furnished at a site; meal follows specific pattern based on one-third of nutrient needs. |
| Home-Delivered Meals | Age 60 or over, homebound | Noon meal is delivered at no cost or for a donation at least 5 days a week. Sometimes additional meals for later consumption are delivered at the same time; often referred to as "Meals on Wheels." |
| Summer Food Service Program | Residence in a low-income neighborhood or participation in a program | Free, nutritious meals and snacks are given to children in a low-income area at a central site, such as a school or a community center during long school vacations. |
| Food Distribution Program on Indian Reservations* | Low-income American Indian and non-Indian households on reservations; members of federally recognized tribes | Alternative to Food Stamp Program, distribution of monthly food packages; includes nutrition education component. |

* Benefits increased through the American Recovery and Reinvestment Act of 2009.

and lunch programs still enable low-income students—8.1 million for breakfast and 30.5 million for lunch—to receive meals free or at reduced cost if certain income guidelines are met (under $27,560 to $39,220, respectively, for annual income of a family of four). In the same year, the U.S. Congress funded group noontime (called *congregate*) meals and home-delivered meals for all citizens over 60 years of age, regardless of income (donations are requested, however). Both remain active programs, serving about 1 million meals each day, but they still do not reach all who need help. In addition, in 1972, the Special Supplemental Nutrition Program for Women, Infants, and Children (WIC) was authorized. This program provides food vouchers and nutrition

## CRITICAL THINKING

While studying early childhood development, Nakia was surprised to learn that some children in the United States are undernourished. What evidence might Nakia observe in children that would suggest undernourishment?

education to low-income pregnant and lactating women and their young children. It serves about 8.7 million people.

Between 1969 and 1971, some already large federal food programs were expanded and others were created. For example, the Food Stamp Program served only 2 million people in 1968, but by 1971 it was serving 11 million. The National School Lunch Program, which served only 2 million poor children before 1970, was serving 8 million children by 1971. Soon after, the School Breakfast Program, a pilot program for children living in impoverished areas, became available nationally.

Sometimes, severe undernutrition due to involuntary hunger does occur in the United States. More often, though, Americans experience periodic episodes of hunger and food insecurity. Unemployment, medical and housing expenses, and even occasional holiday shopping can cause a household to be hungry or food insecure.

Government food assistance programs are like a "safety net"—they are strong, yet porous. The Recovery Act that was signed by President Obama in February 2009 was an unprecedented effort to increase benefits and services offered by the federal food and nutrition programs (Table 12-2). The enhancement of these programs has helped those workers and families hardest hit by the economic crisis. Privately funded programs have stepped in to add to state and federal efforts to combat hunger and related food insecurity in the United States. There are more than 150,000 charitable food providers (such as food banks and food pantries) helping to cope with this problem. They serve about 23 million Americans. Many low-income U.S. households rely on food pantries, and one survey found that slightly more than two of every three people requesting such emergency food assistance are members of families—children and their parents.

## MAKING DECISIONS

### Food Insecurity and Overweight?

Undernutrition in North America is a much more subtle problem than in developing countries. To the untrained eye, undernourished children may just seem skinny, when, in fact, their growth is being stunted by insufficient nutrients. More likely, though, children from food-insecure households are prone to be overweight. This may be the result of considerable reliance on convenience foods that provide mostly fat and sugar. Also, food-insecure families may buy candies and snack foods as treats when expensive toys and clothing aren't affordable.

The availability of cooking facilities affects nutrient intake among the poor. Without cooking facilities, people may buy expensive convenience foods that require no preparation. These are typically highly processed snack foods, which provide calories but are often lacking in nutrients.

## Socioeconomic Factors Related to Undernutrition

In the United States, persistent hunger and food insecurity are largely associated with two interrelated conditions: poverty and homelessness. Thus, the economic, social, and political changes that lead to an increase in the number of poor or homeless people also tend to intensify the problem of undernutrition.

**Poverty.** Underemployment leads to poverty. This relationship has increased significantly with the economic recession that began late in 2007. The recent economic crisis is the worst in decades and has caused unemployment to soar. Between December 2007 and September 2009, 7.6 million jobs were lost. These job losses occurred across all major private-sector industries, including manufacturing, retail trade, leisure and hospitality, financial, transportation, and warehousing. In September 2009 the number of unemployed persons was 15.1 million resulting in an unemployment rate of 8.9%. The impact of the increase in unemployment has been enhanced because, at the same time that millions more have become unemployed, the number of people receiving public aid has been the lowest in more than 40 years. Fewer

▲ Food pantries and soup kitchens are important sources of nutrients for a growing number of people in the United States. Consider volunteering some of your time to a local program.

people are receiving aid during the economic downturn because many states have cut their welfare assistance. This combination of events has resulted in more people living in poverty and in need of food assistance, at risk of homelessness, and without sufficient healthcare.

**Homelessness.** Homelessness stems from a lack of affordable housing and is much more evident now than a few decades ago. The growing shortage of affordable rental housing and a simultaneous increase in poverty are the two trends largely responsible for the rise in homelessness over the past 25 years. The more recent foreclosure and economic crises have added to this situation and created a significant increase in homelessness and the number of families at risk of homelessness across the country. In 2009, data from major cities indicated increases of homelessness by as much as 20% since the foreclosure crisis began in 2007. A study done by the National Law Center on Homelessness and Poverty estimates that 3.5 million people, including 1.35 million children are likely to experience homelessness in a given year. Families with children are one of the fastest growing homeless groups, especially in rural areas, and make up about 23% of the homeless population. Single mothers in their late 20s with approximately two children are the most common heads of homeless families. Poor people must make difficult choices when limited resources cover only some necessities such as housing, food, childcare, health care, and education. Because housing absorbs a high percentage of income, it is often given up. The median wage needed to afford a two-bedroom apartment is now more than twice the minimum wage. This combined with the decline in wages has made housing out of reach for many families. Currently the largest gap on record exists between the number of affordable housing units and the number of people needing them. The homelessness created by this gap impacts the health and well-being of all individuals. Homeless children are most vulnerable and are twice as likely to experience hunger compared to children with a home.

▲ Homelessness can be the result of many problems, including poverty.

## Possible Solutions to Poverty and Hunger in the United States

Few would dispute the importance of supporting physically and mentally challenged adults and the multitude of poor children in the United States. Government-funded food assistance programs have helped to alleviate some problems of undernutrition in the United States. The question is, *Can government programs provide a permanent solution to poverty and undernutrition . . . and should they?*

It is documented that an increasing number of people who are experiencing poverty are accessing the Supplemental Nutrition Assistance Program (SNAP; formerly called the Food Stamp Program) benefits as well as other federal programs. As a result of the American Recovery and Reinvestment Act of 2009 (www.recovery.gov), more federal funds have been infused into assistance programs. There is no guarantee, however, that benefits from these programs will suitably meet the needs of the poor. In addition, there is a growing sentiment that state and federal support programs and policies are ineffective and inappropriate. These concerns are especially expressed by those who are falling deeper into poverty and those who are at increased risk of poverty and homelessness.

Obtaining food to survive is a tremendous challenge, especially when homeless people are forced to live outside. Surveys on hunger and homelessness in U.S. cities indicate that indoor food programs are not adequate to meet the need in some cities. Homeless persons in other cities may not be able to travel to indoor food programs due to work conflicts, illness, disability, or lack of adequate public transportation. A national survey by the Interagency Council on Homelessness also revealed that 40% of homeless people did not have anything to eat on one or more days during the month previous to the survey.

Although many people assume that food pantries and soup kitchens are abundant and accessible enough for every needy person to get the food they desire, there are many obstacles to these resources. Food pantries are often ineffective because they can give only one box of food to families per month, which does not meet their needs. Furthermore, homeless people lack the cooking facilities necessary to prepare the food. Food availability through soup kitchens is also limited in many cities. An additional challenge is that cities have recently begun to use a variety of measures such as ordinances and policies to discourage or prohibit the sharing of food with poor or homeless persons by individuals and groups. These laws are troubling, considering that most cities do not have adequate food resources to meet the need of their poor and homeless. Advocacy groups raise questions about individual rights and freedoms and have challenged these practices in court cases. Advocates and food providers appear eager to work with cities and other government agencies to help address the problems of hunger and homelessness by improving access to federal food benefits and other food resources.

Despite even the highest motivation, the outlook is bleak for many people who attempt to gain independence from assistance programs. Teen pregnancy may have cut short the education or vocational training of one or both parents, thwarting efforts to earn adequate income. Often, the expense of reliable and safe child care far exceeds the meager income from a minimum-wage job. Illness of either the parents or children may prevent the adults from holding steady employment. Poor communication skills, inability to relocate, and a lack of economic reserves also complicate financial independence. Regardless of how wasteful government assistance appears to some people, it will probably always be necessary to some extent.

Many in the United States consider an increase in individual responsibility as a critical goal. Government programs cannot easily fix poverty and the resulting hunger that stem from irresponsible individual behavior. Government programs can, however, help reduce or prevent the poverty that results largely from lack of education or opportunity.

Long-term undernutrition—especially among children—has both individual and societal consequences, so everyone in the United States is affected by this problem, either directly or indirectly. As government programs are redesigned, it is likely that some will suffer. The hope is that these new approaches will lead to long-term progress and the eventual relief of poverty and hunger.

**O**ne goal of *Healthy People 2010* is to increase food security among U.S. households from the current 88% to 94%. Another is to reduce growth retardation to 5% among low-income children under age 5.

### CONCEPT CHECK

In response to reports of widespread poverty and hunger during the 1960s, the U.S. Congress established several food assistance programs and substantially increased funding for already existing programs. Largely as a result of these federal programs, undernutrition had decreased substantially by the mid-1970s. The presence of poverty, homelessness, and undernutrition is influenced by economic, cultural, and individual factors, as well as government policies. The serious questions about the long-term effectiveness of many government assistance programs are causing major changes in their program design. All citizens can help reduce the problem of undernutrition.

## 12.3 Undernutrition in the Developing World

Undernutrition in the developing world is also tied to poverty, and any true solution must address this problem. However, these countries have a multitude of problems so complex and interrelated that they cannot be treated separately. Programs that have proved immensely helpful in the United States (and throughout the rest of North America) are only a starting point in this context. The following major obstacles challenge those seeking a solution:

- Extreme imbalances in the food/population ratio in different regions of a country
- War and political/civil unrest, especially in Africa

- The rapid depletion of natural resources, such as farmland, fish, and water
- The disease AIDS, especially in sub-Saharan Africa and Asia
- High external (foreign) debt, much of which is owed to developed nations
- Poor **infrastructure**, especially poor housing, sanitation and storage facilities, education, communications, and transportation systems

Each problem deserves individual consideration (Fig. 12-3).

> **infrastructure** The basic framework of a system of organization. For a society, this includes roads, bridges, telephones, and other basic technologies.

## Food/Population Ratio

The world has 6.8 billion inhabitants. Population growth exceeds economic growth in much of the developing world, and as a result, poverty is increasing. This disrupts the balance in the food/population ratio, tipping it toward food shortages. If we want to ensure a decent life for a widening segment of humanity, many experts suggest that the growth in the earth's most vulnerable populations should slow. If not, by 2050 the world may have 1 to 3 billion more people than it does today—most of them in countries where the average person earns less than $2 per day. In Africa's poorest countries, nearly 65% of people live on less than $1 per day. Unless a catastrophe occurs, more than 9 of 10 infants in the next generation will be born in the poorest parts of the world.

More than three-quarters of people in the world live in developing countries, and more than half live in Asia. A United Nations report on worldwide hunger revealed that almost two-thirds of the world's undernourished live in Asia and the Pacific Rim. The world's food supplies also are not distributed equally among consumers. Gross disparities exist between developed and developing countries, among the rich and the poor within countries, and even within families (males may be fed before females).

Still, economists estimate that world food production will continue to increase more rapidly than the world population in the near future, allowing the food/population ratio to increase through the year 2020. This will come at a high cost, however, in terms of the water, fertilizer, and pesticides needed to allow for this production. Overall, in the short run, the primary problem appears not to be food production *but* distribution and use, especially in poverty-stricken areas of developing nations.

Eventually, though, food production will begin to lag behind population growth. Most good farmland in the world is already in use, and because of poor farming practices or competing land-use demands, the number of farmable acres worldwide decreases annually. For many reasons, sustainable world food output—an amount that doesn't deplete the earth's resources—is now running well behind food consumption. This discrepancy suggests that food production in less-developed countries will barely keep up with population growth and will soon lag behind.

▲ Poverty aggravates the problem of hunger in the developing world

**FIGURE 12-3** ▶ Many factors contribute to undernutrition in the developing world. Any solutions to the problem must take these factors into consideration.

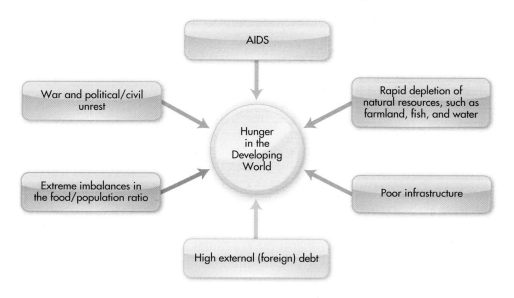

AIDS

War and political/civil unrest

Rapid depletion of natural resources, such as farmland, fish, and water

Hunger in the Developing World

Extreme imbalances in the food/population ratio

Poor infrastructure

High external (foreign) debt

Birth control programs, an obvious brake on population expansion, have been effective in developed countries but relatively ineffective in many developing countries that could really benefit from them. Among women, family planning and contraceptive use worldwide has increased to 60% today, up from 10% in 1969. If the United Nations, voluntary organizations, and governments had not started promoting family planning and contraceptive use, the population today might be as high as 7 or 8 billion. However, women (and men) in many developing countries are still lacking adequate access to contraceptives. The United Nations estimates that at least 200 million women want to use safe and effective family planning methods, but they lack access to information and services or the support of their husbands and communities. Organizations such as Population Services International are trying to keep distribution costs low and make the products available to as many people as possible by subsidizing condoms and oral contraceptives to areas such as Bangladesh.

## MAKING DECISIONS

### Benefits of Breastfeeding

Promoting breastfeeding also contributes to the goal of birth control. Although it is not a completely reliable method of contraception, exclusively breastfeeding an infant lessens ovulation, thereby lowering the likelihood of fertilization, for an average of six months. (Women who do not breastfeed generally begin to ovulate within a month or so after giving birth.) When childbirths are more widely spaced, not only do fewer total births occur, but the mother has a longer chance to recover from pregnancy, and the infant receives feeding priority for a longer time. One possible exception to the healthful nature of breastfeeding occurs, however, when mothers are infected with the **human immunodeficiency virus (HIV).** The risk of transferring the virus through human milk is about 10%. Depending on the circumstances, this may outweigh the benefits of breastfeeding.

**human immunodeficiency virus (HIV)** The virus that leads to acquired immune deficiency syndrome (AIDS).

**acquired immune deficiency syndrome (AIDS)** A disorder in which a virus (human immunodeficiency virus [HIV]) infects specific types of immune system cells. This leaves the person with reduced immune function and, in turn, defenseless against numerous infectious agents; typically contributes to the person's death.

Experience with family planning programs in developing countries and historical changes in birth rates in many developed countries suggest an important conclusion. Generally, only when people have enough to eat and are financially secure do they feel confident that having fewer children will still result in enough surviving sons and/or daughters to provide for their care in later years. Increasing per capita income and improving education, especially for women in developing nations, are considered to be the most likely long-term solutions to excessive population growth. In the last few years, this effort has led to a decline in family size in Brazil, Egypt, India, and Mexico. A major concern is whether there are enough resources worldwide to raise per capita income and provide enough education to slow population growth.

## CONCEPT CHECK

World food production is sufficient to meet the calorie needs of the world's population. Despite these adequate food resources, undernutrition continues to exist because of poverty, politics, and unequal food distribution. In addition, projected population growth may soon overwhelm food production. Most scientists and world leaders recommend limiting population growth, especially in developing countries where birth rates are high.

▲ Lasting gains have come slowly in the world's battle against undernutrition.

**T**he conflicts in the Darfur region of Sudan have led to high rates of death and undernutrition among people displaced by war.

## War and Political/Civil Unrest

The Millennium Summit of the United Nations in September 2000 resulted in the Millennium Declaration that included the resolution to "spare no effort to free our peoples from the scourge of war." Against that background stands the reality that worldwide military spending is reported to be over $1.2 trillion in annual expenditure and has been rising in recent years since 2001. The entire budget of the United Nations is only a fraction of the world's military expenditure at approximately 1.5%. In the twentieth century, deadly weapons of war took an enormous toll on civilians living in poor, politically vulnerable, war-torn nations. Less than one-half of 1% of the world's yearly production of goods and services is devoted to economic development assistance, whereas approximately 6% goes to military expenditures.

Aside from the economic impact of military spending, civil disruptions and wars are setting back the progress of the poor and contributing to massive undernutrition. Many regions of Africa have been involved in numerous civil wars and conflicts in recent years. These include conflicts in the countries directly involved in the Democratic Republic of Congo, the Sierra Leone crisis, and the war in Ethiopia/Eritrea. These conflicts have resulted in millions of deaths as well as over 9 million refugees and internally displaced people. While war has raged, health, education, and public services have declined for African people, and poverty has increased in Sub-Saharan Africa. War-related famine affects at least 20 million people in southern and northeastern Africa. The border war between Ethiopia and neighboring Eritrea has had a tremendous negative impact on food resources. A World Bank official stated that the food shortage in Ethiopia is a problem that will persist until political changes are made. Approximately 12.4 million people in Ethiopia, Eritrea, Djibouti, Kenya, Somalia, and Zimbabwe are at risk for food shortages. Other conflicts continue between Congo (formerly Zaire) and the Republic of Congo, as well as in Angola and Sudan, where millions have been put at risk of starvation. In the capitol of war-torn Iraq, Baghdad, child malnutrition has increased dramatically. Disruptions in infrastructure from bombing and looting limit the safety of water, and as a result, health officials have observed a 250% increase in cases of diarrhea. Furthermore, health facilities needed to cope with undernutrition and dehydration have been damaged and looted throughout Baghdad and the surrounding area. Overall, most people in war-torn areas are without sufficient shelter, clothing, food, or means of obtaining them. Worldwide, this entire problem is projected to worsen over the next 15 years.

Even when food is available, political divisions may impede its distribution to the point that undernutrition will plague many people for years. Especially during emergencies, programs designed to help the poor have been undermined by unstable administration, corruption, and political influence. During such political chaos, relief agencies are often caught between warring factions and those they are trying to help. This has been the case in Sudan where non-governmental relief organizations, such as the Children's Hunger Relief Fund, have been expelled in recent years. This has caused continued deterioration in the Darfur region, and hundreds of thousands of refugees are left without the help they depended on from relief organizations.

During the 1960s and 1970s, the problem of undernutrition in developing countries was perceived as a technical one: how to produce enough food for the growing world population. The problem is now seen as largely political: how to achieve cooperation among and within nations, so that gains in food production and infrastructure are not wiped out by war. The best answer lies in a combination of approaches—finding technical solutions to help with the problems of chronic hunger and poverty and resolving political crises that have pushed developing nations into a state of acute hunger and chaos.

## Rapid Depletion of Natural Resources

As we quickly deplete the earth's resources, population control grows increasingly critical. Agriculture production is approaching its limits in many areas worldwide. Environmentally unsustainable farming methods are undermining food production, especially in developing countries.

The **green revolution** was a phenomenon that began in the 1960s when crop yields rose dramatically in some countries, such as the Philippines, India, and Mexico (countries in Africa did not benefit because climates were not compatible with the

▲ Homes and infrastructure are often damaged during times of war and political unrest.

**green revolution** This refers to increases in crop yields that accompanied the introduction of new agricultural technologies in less-developed countries, beginning in the 1960s. The key technologies were high-yielding, disease-resistant strains of rice, wheat, and corn; greater use of fertilizer and water; and improved cultivation practices.

crops used). The increased use of fertilizers, irrigation, and the development of superior crops through careful plant breeding made this boost in agricultural production possible. Many of the technologies associated with the green revolution have now achieved their potential. Rice yields, for example, have not increased significantly since the release of superior varieties in 1966. (The green revolution was intended as a stopgap measure until world leaders could control population growth.)

Future gains in productivity may be much harder to accomplish because of the existence of less productive farmland. Until the introduction of another superior strain of rice or other grain, developing countries will not benefit greatly from recent, more modest breakthroughs in biotechnology (see the section on use of biotechnology).

Areas of the world that remain uncultivated or ungrazed are mostly too rocky, steep, infertile, dry, wet, or inaccessible to sustain farming. Nearly all irrigation water available worldwide is being used, and groundwater supplies are becoming depleted at rapid rates in many regions. An eventual water shortage is projected to increase war and civil unrest in arid areas of the world, such as Northern Africa and the Middle East. China, which has more than 20% of the world's irrigated land, is also plagued with a growing scarcity of fresh water. In the future, billions of people will face ongoing water shortages.

The prospects of obtaining substantially more food from the oceans are also poor. In recent years, the amount of fish caught worldwide has leveled off. Fish was once considered the poor person's protein, but this is not likely to continue because farming of fish does not come close to compensating for the degree of reduction in wild fish populations.

Clearly, we can exploit the earth's resources only so far—the world population probably cannot continue to expand as it does today without the potential for serious famine and death. The Food and Agriculture Organization (FAO) of the United Nations works on this principle: "The fight to ensure that all people have enough nutritious food to eat is worthy of our greatest efforts, but it must be fought with the full recognition that it cannot be won unless agricultural, fishery, and forestry production returns to the earth as much as—or more than—it takes." Thus, if food production is to keep up with the expanding population, immediate action is needed to protect the earth's already deteriorated environment from further destruction.

## Inadequate Shelter and Sanitation

When people die from undernutrition in developing countries, other factors, such as inadequate shelter and sanitation, almost always contribute. Poor sanitation along with undernutrition particularly raises the risk of infection. Inadequate and deteriorating shelters threaten the lives of more than 500 million people. Many of the 15 million annual deaths of children—half of them under 5 years old—in developing countries could be prevented by improving the standards of environmental hygiene. Urban populations of some developing countries are growing at an annual rate of 5% to 7%. Such a skewed population distribution will result in more poverty. The urban explosion is the result of both high birth rates and continuing migration of people to the cities from rural areas. People go to the cities to find employment and resources the countryside can no longer provide. Worldwide, 38% of people lived in urban areas in 1975. The figure is now about 50% and is expected to reach 70% by 2050. Nine of the world's 10 largest cities will be in poor countries 20 years from now. The World Bank reports that 16 of the 20 most polluted cities in the world are in China.

In developing countries, the poor make up most of the urban population, and their needs for housing and community services often go beyond available governmental resources. Most of these urban poor live in overcrowded, self-made shelters, which lack a safe and adequate water supply and are only partially served by public utilities. The shantytowns and ghettos of the developing world are often worse than

▲ Rich agricultural resources in North America, seen in the wheat fields above, results in a bounty of food to enjoy, such as these loaves of fresh bread.

In Brazil, migrants displaced by multinational land developers have flooded from the north and northeast into Rio de Janeiro and São Paulo, attracted by the prospect of jobs. There they have built shantytowns next to apartment towers and affluent suburbs, but the jobs do not materialize, and urban poverty replaces rural impoverishment.

the rural areas the people left behind. The urban poor need cash to purchase food, so they often subsist on diets even more meager than the homegrown rural fare. Making matters worse, haphazard shelters often lack facilities to protect food from spoilage or damage by insects and rodents. This inability to protect food supplies in some developing countries leads to the loss of as much as 40% of all perishable foods.

The shift from rural to urban life takes its greatest toll on infants and children. Infants are often weaned early from the breast to infant formula, partly because the mother must find employment and partly because she may be influenced by advertisements depicting images of sophisticated, formula-feeding women. Unfortunately, because infant formulas are relatively expensive, poor parents may try to conserve the formula by either overdiluting the mixture or using too little to meet the infant's needs. The water supply may not be safe, so the prepared formula is also likely to be contaminated with bacteria. Human milk, in contrast, is much more hygienic, readily available, and nutritious. It also provides infants with immunity to some ailments. Promoting breastfeeding is important when it is safe for the infant (review the earlier discussion of AIDS, HIV, and breastfeeding).

Overall, the single most effective health advantage for people, wherever they live, is a safe and convenient water supply. Inadequate sanitation and the consumption of contaminated water cause 75% of all diseases and more than one-third of deaths in developing countries. The World Health Organization (WHO) estimates that 1.1 billion people, about one-sixth of all people, have an unsafe and inadequate water supply. In addition, up to 90% of the diseases seen in developing countries may be attributed to contaminated water.

Poor sanitation, another example of inadequate infrastructure in the developing world, creates a critical public health problem. Human feces, rotting garbage, and associated insect and rodent infestations are potent sources of disease organisms commonly seen in urban areas of the developing world. Two of the most dangerous substances encountered in routine daily living are human urine and feces. The inability to dispose of the massive numbers of dead people (and dead animals) resulting from civil wars causes additional sanitation problems. In some developing countries, diarrheal diseases account for as many as one-third of all deaths in children under 5 years of age. WHO estimates that even with improvements in housing, 2 billion people in the world still lack proper sanitation facilities.

## High External Debt

Since the 1970s many developing countries have become trapped in a cycle of borrowing repeatedly from foreign countries and international banks. Servicing these external debts has brought several countries to the verge of economic collapse. About $6 billion is owed to the United States. The external debt of Latin America represents 45% of the region's gross regional output of goods and services.

Many African nations also carry large debt burdens. This problem is made worse by drops in prices for the raw commodities they export, higher prices for imported oil, and embezzlement of funds by high-ranking officials. To make up the difference between export income and import expenses, countries have been forced to borrow millions of dollars from international banks. Although the African debts are much smaller in absolute terms than those of Brazil, Argentina, and Mexico, for example, the burden is greater when national incomes and export earnings are considered. Nearly half the money African nations earn from exports goes to paying off the continent's multibillion-dollar debt. Much of the rest goes to fund imports of machinery, concrete, trucks, and consumer goods from developed countries. This leaves little for domestic programs, necessitating cutbacks that translate into fewer resources to counter already widespread undernutrition.

**B**lood loss caused by intestinal and blood-borne parasite infections is another common cause of anemia among poor populations, especially when people do not wear shoes. Parasites, such as hookworms, can easily penetrate the soles of the feet and legs and enter the bloodstream. Although hookworm disease has been largely eradicated through improved sanitation in the United States and other industrialized nations, it continues to plague more than one-eighth of the world's population, mostly in tropical regions.

▲ Inadequate sanitation facilities and the consumption of contaminated water cause the majority of all diseases. About 1 billion people in developing countries often lack access to a safe water supply.

**I**n 2005 the Group of Eight most industrialized nations announced plans to forgive some external debt owed by developing countries. The debt repayment promise has been criticized and depended on the developing country's agreement to practice good governance and to use the money saved to support health care, education, and infrastructure improvements.

**CONCEPT CHECK**

War and civil strife, along with a decline in the world's natural resources, contribute to the difficulty of ending undernutrition in many developing countries. In addition, substandard housing conditions, impure water, and inadequate sanitation worldwide increase the risk for infection and disease. Infection then combines with undernutrition to compromise further the health of impoverished people. Finally, many developing countries are burdened by extremely high external debts, which severely limit their ability to implement programs to reduce undernutrition.

## The Impact of AIDS Worldwide

About 33 million people around the world are infected with the human immunodeficiency virus (HIV) or have gone on to develop acquired immune deficiency syndrome (AIDS) from the infection. The male to female ratio is about 1:1 but is now increasing faster in women than in men in several countries. Although the annual number of AIDS deaths has declined worldwide since 2005, over 2 million adults and children died with AIDS in 2007.

An individual can be infected with HIV through contact with bodily fluids including blood, semen, vaginal secretions, and human milk. Thus the virus can be transmitted through sexual contact; through blood-to-blood contact; as well as from a mother to an infant during pregnancy, delivery, or breastfeeding. The virus has a very limited ability to exist outside the body.

Once infected with HIV, the individual is said to be HIV-positive. If untreated, the viral disease progresses over the next few years, and the individual develops symptoms of opportunistic infections such as diarrhea, lung disease, weight loss, and a form of cancer. Once the individual has developed these symptoms, they are said to have AIDS. Without treatment, an individual will likely die from AIDS within 4 to 5 years.

Global efforts are having some effect in that the HIV epidemic worldwide is stabilizing and the rate of new HIV infections has decreased in several countries. From 2001 to 2007 the annual number of new HIV infections decreased from 3.0 to 2.7 million. In Africa, particularly sub-Saharan countries, HIV is rampant throughout the entire population, both in men and women. This region contains over 60% of the world's HIV-positive people (Fig. 12-4). In most areas of sub-Saharan Africa, AIDS is reducing life expectancy by one-half, especially if the person also has tuberculosis. In many countries, AIDS is also creating orphans, with an estimated 12 million in Africa alone.

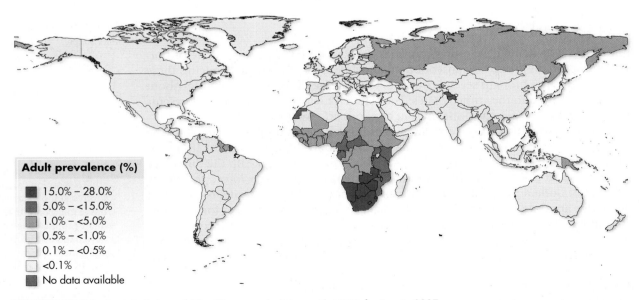

**Adult prevalence (%)**

- 15.0% – 28.0%
- 5.0% – <15.0%
- 1.0% – <5.0%
- 0.5% – <1.0%
- 0.1% – <0.5%
- <0.1%
- No data available

**FIGURE 12-4** ▶ A global view of 33 million people living with HIV infection in 2007.

*Source: Report on the Global HIV/AIDS Epidemic 2008: executive Summary, July 2008.*

North America also has an AIDS problem. In the United States, it is estimated that about 1.2 million people (1 in every 280 persons) are infected with HIV, many of whom are unaware of their infections. (Reports show 1 in every 100 persons in New York City is infected with HIV.) About 580,000 people in the United States have died from the disease since it surfaced in the early 1980s, and each year about 50,000 new cases are reported. HIV affects a greater percentage of minority populations in the United States.

The face of AIDS is quickly becoming the face of a child. In 2007, 2 million children under 15 years were living with HIV/AIDS globally.

Although no vaccine is available to prevent AIDS, the latest antiviral drugs can significantly slow the progression of the disease. However, there are many barriers to the use of these drugs in the developing world. For example, the newest therapies require a person to take at least three different drugs in the form of about 14 pills each day. A few missed doses can significantly reduce the effectiveness of the drugs and result in faster disease progression. Another barrier is economic: a typical drug regimen can cost approximately $14,000 per year, not including unforeseen hospital stays. Certain drug companies and governments are working to lower the cost of AIDS drugs for developing nations. Still, in most cases, the drugs will remain out of reach to those who need them. It has been suggested that developed nations should step in and cover most or all of the costs. The United Nations is spearheading an effort to raise the $8 to $10 billion needed to fight the disease.

## MAKING DECISIONS

### Nutrition and AIDS

Can eating a balanced diet prevent AIDS? The answer, unfortunately, is no. Healthy eating does not cure the disease, but it can help to lessen the impact of infections associated with AIDS. Poor nutritional status, such as a low status of vitamin A and vitamin E, contributes to a quicker onset of symptoms such as body wasting and fever, and a more rapid demise. This explains why daily use of a balanced vitamin and mineral supplement was shown to slow health declines in such people in one study. Overall, maintenance of nutritional status should be an integral part of the treatment for AIDS.

The devastating effects of AIDS on our civilization have been rapid when measured by earth's scale of time. One study warns us that 57 countries risk major HIV outbreaks. Reported HIV cases are increasing rapidly in Africa, the Indian subcontinent, Southeast Asia, China, the Caribbean, Russia, and much of Eastern Europe. The main goal for addressing the problem of AIDS in the developing world is prevention of new cases through education regarding safer sex and the importance of clean needles, and other behavior-linked approaches. Providing AIDS drugs to pregnant women is also important. If a woman begins taking AIDS drugs such as zidovudine (AZT) by the fourteenth week of pregnancy, the risk of transferring the virus to her offspring is greatly reduced. Providing the drug immediately before birth also helps.

Behind the mind-boggling statistics on AIDS are less obvious costs to businesses, families, schools and universities, and society in general. For example, worker productivity will plummet because AIDS victims produce less and demand more, especially in the latter stages of the disease. Business productivity drops even further when relatives take time away from work and school to care for family members afflicted with AIDS. Furthermore, AIDS demands a considerable amount of family income. Hard-pressed families, who have to devote much of their income to doctors and medicines, have little left for living expenses. Other family members must struggle to keep up with daily duties because they must care for orphans left behind in the disease's wake. To learn more about AIDS, check out the website www.unaids.org.

▲ A particularly sad consequence of AIDS in Africa is the number of AIDS orphans, children whose parents have both died of AIDS. The United Nations reports that about 15 million AIDS orphans have become responsible for the care of their siblings and other family members.

## CONCEPT CHECK

About 40 million people around the world are infected with the human immunodeficiency virus (HIV) or have gone on to develop acquired immunodeficiency syndrome (AIDS) from the infection. The virus can be transmitted through sexual contact; through blood-to-blood contact; or from a mother to a baby during pregnancy, delivery, and breastfeeding. Without treatment, an individual once infected will likely die from AIDS within 4 to 5 years. The main hope for addressing the problem of AIDS in the developing world is prevention of new cases.

## Reducing Undernutrition in the Developing World

As you have probably guessed, greatly reducing undernutrition in the developing world will be complicated and will take considerable time to accomplish (Fig. 12-5). It is a common practice for the more affluent nations to supply famine areas with direct food aid. However, direct food aid is not a long-term solution. Although it reduces the number of deaths from famine, it can also reduce incentives for local production by driving down prices. In addition, the affected countries may have little or no means of transporting the food to those who need it most, and the donated foods may not be culturally acceptable.

In the short run, there is no choice—aid must be given because people are starving. Still, improving the infrastructure for poor people, especially rural people, needs to be the long-term focus. This future-minded approach is necessary because the most

**FIGURE 12-5** ▶ Possible solutions to the puzzle of hunger in the developing world. Putting all the pieces together employs the action steps that contribute to meeting the overall goal.

significant factor affecting the undernutrition of people in impoverished areas of the world is their reliance on outside sources for basic needs. Their dependence makes them constantly vulnerable.

Three basic approaches to counteract micronutrient deficiencies are suggested by the World Bank: increase diversity of the food supply; fortify specific foods with nutrients; and provide nutrient supplementation for individuals when necessary.

**Development Tailored to Local Conditions Is Important.** Recall that, in the past 40 years, world food supplies have grown faster than the population. Thus, the increase in undernutrition during this period has been caused by an increase in the number of people cut off from their share of this supply. Millions of farmers are losing access to resources they need to be self-reliant. There is a growing realization that unless economic opportunities can be created as part of a plan for sustainable development, rural people who own no land will flock to the overcrowded cities. In response, careful, small-scale regional development is one option.

For the most part, the solution lies in helping people meet their own needs and directing them to resources and employment opportunities, rather than giving them resources. Experience has shown that the provision of credit—along with training, food storage facilities, and marketing support—allows rural people to actively participate in their development, which will benefit their families and communities.

One U.S. program, the Peace Corps, has helped improve conditions in developing nations by providing education, distributing food and medical supplies, and building structures for local use. The aim of the Peace Corps is to help create independent, self-sustaining economies around the world.

Impoverished women are a special concern. In addition to working longer hours than men, they grow most of the food for family consumption and make up three-fourths of the labor force in the informal sector of the economy and an increasing proportion in the formal sector. Economic opportunities for women and education regarding family planning must be augmented. Of the 3 billion people in the world living on less than $2 a day, 70% are women. Moreover, among the developing world's 900 million illiterate people, women outnumber men 2 to 1. Thus, an important means of propelling nations out of poverty is to end the cycle of female neglect.

Suitable technologies for processing, preserving, marketing, and distributing nutritious local staples also need to be encouraged, so that small farmers can flourish. Education on how to use these foods to create healthful diets, such as preparing vitamin A-rich vegetables, adds further benefit. Supplementing indigenous foods with nutrients that are in short supply, such as iron, various B vitamins, zinc, and iodide, also deserves consideration. One program involves adding iron to sugar in various parts of the world. The next section examines the role of biotechnology in improving nutrient quality and other plant and animal characteristics, another possible positive step in lessening undernutrition. In addition, advances in water purification need to be employed.

Promoting extensive land ownership may also be one part of the solution. Increasing the availability of food is one of its many advantages. If food resources are concentrated among a minority of people, as often happens with unequal land ownership, food is not likely to be equally distributed unless efficient transportation systems are in place. Inequitable distribution then proves to be a difficult problem to resolve.

Raising the economic status of impoverished people by employing them is as important as expanding the food supply. If an increase in food supply is achieved without an accompanying rise in employment, there may be no long-term change in the number of undernourished people. Although food prices may fall with increased mechanization, use of fertilizers, and other modern technologies, it needs to be realized that these advances can also displace people from jobs, a result that worsens rather than helps the population.

▲ Food security is fostered by communities raising and distributing locally grown food.

## CRITICAL THINKING

Stan has read about various relief efforts to help undernourished people in developing countries, especially the emergency food aid programs for famine-ravaged areas. Many of these efforts appear to be only temporary, and he wonders what long-range approaches might help alleviate the problem of undernutrition. What suggestions would you give Stan about possible long-term solutions for undernutrition in developing countries?

**sustainable development** Economic growth that will simultaneously reduce poverty, protect the environment, and preserve natural capital.

**gender and development (GAD) approach** Understanding the roles and responsibilities of both men and women in the process of sustainable development.

## MAKING DECISIONS

### Sustainable Development and the Gender and Development (GAD) Approach

**Sustainable development** is economic growth that will reduce poverty while at the same time protect the environment and preserve natural capital. In its 2005 World Summit Outcome Document, the United Nations cites economic development, social development, and environmental protection as the "reinforcing pillars" of sustainable development. During the past 20 years, an understanding of the roles and responsibilities of both women and men in the community and the relationship of men and women to each other have been important components of sustainable development. The **gender and development (GAD) approach** works toward improving the status of women through the active participation of both men and women. By increasing women's access to education, information and communication technologies, economic resources, and governance, the GAD approach reduces poverty, promotes development, achieves gender equality, protects women's human rights, and eliminates violence against women.

## 12.4 The Role of Sustainable Agriculture and Biotechnology in Worldwide Food Availability

### Sustainable Agriculture

Over the years, changes in agricultural practices have had many positive results on the availability of food around the world. Along with the positive effects on farming, however, there have been significant negative impacts. Most significant among these are depletion of topsoil, contamination of groundwater, the decline of family farms, neglect of living and working conditions for farm laborers, increasing costs of production, and the lack of integration of economic and social conditions in rural communities.

During the past two decades, the role of the agriculture industry in promoting practices that contribute to environmental and social problems has been debated. As a result, interest in alternative farming practices has grown and a movement toward **sustainable agriculture** has emerged. Sustainable agriculture describes farming systems that can indefinitely maintain their productivity and usefulness to society. Sustainable agriculture depends on the integration of several goals including environmental health, economic profitability, and social and economic equity. It addresses many environmental and social concerns, and offers innovative and economically viable opportunities for many in the food system including growers, laborers, consumers, and policymakers. Today sustainable agriculture is gaining support and acceptance from conventional farmers in many countries.

**sustainable agriculture** Agricultural system that provides a secure living for farm families; maintains the natural environment and resources; supports the rural community; and offers respect and fair treatment to all involved, from farm workers to consumers to the animals raised for food.

Sustainable agriculture involves maintaining or enhancing the land and natural resources for use long into the future. In addition, the social responsibilities of human resources, including working and living conditions of laborers, the needs of rural communities, and consumer health and safety, must be considered both in the present and the future. The potential of sustainability is best understood when the consequences of farming practices on both human communities and the environment are considered.

Farmers around the globe can succeed in their transition to sustainable agriculture by taking small realistic steps based on their personal goals and family economics. Reaching the goal of worldwide sustainable agriculture will require participation by all stakeholders including farmers, laborers, retailers, consumers, researchers, and policymakers.

The ability of humans to manipulate nature has enabled us to improve the production and yield of many important foods. Traditional **biotechnology** is almost as old as agriculture. The first farmer to improve stock by selectively breeding the best bull with the best cows was implementing biotechnology in a simple sense. The first baker to use yeast to make bread rise took advantage of biotechnology.

By the 1930s, biotechnology made possible the selective breeding of better plant hybrids. As a result, corn production in the United States quickly doubled. Through similar methods, agricultural wheat was crossed with wild grasses to confer more desirable properties, such as greater yield, increased resistance to mildew and bacterial diseases, and tolerance to salt or adverse climatic conditions.

Another type of biotechnology uses hormones rather than breeding. In the last decade, Canadian salmon have been treated with a hormone that allows them to mature three times faster than normal—without changing the fish in any other way. In general terms, biotechnology can be understood as the use of living things—plants, animals, bacteria—to manufacture products.

## Biotechnology

The new biotechnology used in agriculture includes several methods that directly modify products. It differs from traditional methods because it more directly changes some of the genetic material (DNA) of organisms to improve characteristics. Cross-breeding plants or animals is no longer the only tool. Development of the new process, called **genetic engineering,** began in the 1970s. The field now features a wide range of cell and subcell techniques for the synthesis and placement of genetic material in organisms (Fig. 12-6).

This process of **recombinant DNA technology** allows access to a wider gene pool, and it permits faster and more accurate production of new and more useful microbial, plant, and animal species. Conventional breeding is inefficient and has inconsistent results; biotechnology uses genetic material more precisely. Scientists select the traits they want and genetically engineer or introduce the gene that produces the desired trait into plants or animals (now called a **genetically modified organism [GMO]** or **transgenic**). Genetic engineering has not replaced conventional breeding practices; both work together.

Biotechnology has been used to enhance crops in three main categories. The primary category is the addition of a unique characteristic called an *input trait* to a crop. These enhanced input traits include herbicide tolerance, insect and virus protection, and tolerance to environmental stressors such as drought. Other categories are

**biotechnology** A collection of processes that involves the use of biological systems for altering and, ideally, improving the characteristics of plants, animals, and other forms of life.

**genetic engineering** Manipulation of the genetic makeup of any organism with recombinant DNA technology.

**recombinant DNA technology** A test tube technology that rearranges DNA sequences in an organism by cutting the DNA, adding or deleting a DNA sequence, and rejoining DNA molecules with a series of enzymes.

**genetically modified organism (GMO)** Any organism created by genetic engineering.

**transgenic** Organism that contains genes originally present in another organism.

DNA of the host plant, corn.

Gene from bacteria (Bt gene) that produces a protein toxic to the European corn borer.

Bt gene inserted into DNA of corn plant. Now the corn plant is genetically modified. It makes the Bt toxin and, so, is resistant to the European corn borer.

**FIGURE 12-6 ▶** Biotechnology involves various techniques for transferring foreign DNA into an organism. In this diagram, a sample of DNA is cleaved out of a larger DNA fragment and inserted into the DNA of a host cell. Thus, the host cell contains new genetic information, with the potential of providing the cell with new capabilities. For corn, this could mean resistance to the European corn borer. The corn plant is now referred to as a genetically modified organism (GMO). In another application, bacteria can be engineered to produce the human form of the hormone insulin.

▲ Both traditional plant breeding and biotechnology have produced high-yielding and disease-resistant plant varieties, including new varieties of corn.

value-added output traits, such as plant oils with increased levels of omega-3 fatty acids, and crops that produce pharmaceuticals. Scientists have engineered plants that grow with the use of less pesticides and new forms of potatoes that can be stored longer without preservatives. In addition, biotechnology allows scientists to create fruits and grains with greater amounts of nutrients such as beta-carotene (e.g., "golden rice") and vitamins E and C. Biotechnology is being used cautiously and conservatively, so benefits of the new biotechnology will strike us as only subtly different. The ultimate benefits, however, could be important if foods eaten by people in the developing world can be so enhanced.

Few consumers in the United States realize that at least 50% of corn and 90% of soybeans produced in the United States have been genetically engineered to either resist certain insects, thereby reducing pesticide use, and/or survive when sprayed with herbicides that kill surrounding weeds. Papaya plants have been genetically engineered for viral resistance.

Genetic modification of corn has received a lot of media attention. Corn can be genetically altered by inserting a gene from the bacterium *Bacillus thuringiensis*, usually referred to as the Bt gene, into the corn DNA (Fig. 12-6). The gene allows the corn plant to make a protein lethal to certain caterpillars that destroy the plant. The Bt protein in the corn, however, is present in the plant in low concentrations and has no effect on humans—it is digested along with the other proteins in corn. For many years organic farmers have used the Bt bacteria as a dust on plants to destroy pests. (Dusting crops, however, does not change the DNA of the plant.)

FDA is confident that approved varieties of genetically engineered foods are safe to consume. Food manufacturers, therefore, are not required to disclose the genetically modified ingredient content on food labels. FDA does not believe labeling of GMO products is needed because they pose no health risk.

Public response to use of GMO biotechnology, however, has been mixed. Even the scientific community has conflicting opinions about this technology, with supporters as convinced about the benefits as opponents are of the risks. The biggest debate in the United States surrounds the potential environmental hazards of introducing genes from one species to another. Some challengers even question the reduction in pesticide use that accompanies the cultivation of genetically modified crops. Although the use of genetically modified crops may reduce the need for environmentally harmful activities, such as spraying crops with pesticides, critics point out that seeds produced with additional insecticide potentially will lead to rapid insect resistance because the insecticides are continuously emitted. Use of traditional pesticides involves prudent application, in part to avoid insect resistance. In addition, accidental release of genetically modified animals, such as fish, may go on to harm wild varieties.

Although the risks of biotechnology may appear to be momentarily negligible, they may be cumulative and therefore of concern in the long run. FDA carefully examines all products developed using this technology and will enforce labeling of potential allergens that may be newly present in food altered by biotechnology.

The public has long been opposed to processes perceived as harmful to the environment, such as producing unnatural products. Food reserves are high in the United States, Canada, and Europe, so some question the need to increase food production. Skepticism surrounds unnatural products, as exemplified by Western Europe's ban of hormones used in beef and milk production, and of almost all genetically modified foods.

## Role of the New Biotechnology in the Developing World

Twenty-three countries planted 282 million acres of crops enhanced through biotechnology in 2007. These crops included improved varieties of soybeans, corn, cotton, canola, papaya, and squash. In 2005, seven countries, the United States, Canada, Brazil, Argentina, Uruguay, Paraguay, and Australia planted 94% of these crops on 208.7 million acres. Small-scale farms in China, India, South Africa, Mexico, Philippines,

Columbia, Honduras, and Iran were the second leading producers of biotechnology crops with acreage of 13.2 million. These countries aimed to increase crop production in rural areas to improve incomes and supply growing urban populations.

Whether applications of genetic engineering will help to significantly reduce undernutrition in the developing world remains to be seen. Unless price cuts accompany the increased production, only landowners and suppliers of biotechnology will enjoy the benefits. Small farmers may benefit if they can afford to purchase the genetically modified seeds. This point deserves emphasis: The person who cannot afford to buy enough food today will still face that same predicament in the future.

As with most innovations, the more successful farmers—often those with larger farms—will adopt the new biotechnology first. Because of this, the present trend toward fewer and larger farms will continue in the developing world, a movement that undermines the solution to one of the most pressing undernutrition issues there. Furthermore, biotechnology does not promise dramatic increases in the production of most grains and cassava, the primary food resources in developing parts of the world.

With the introduction of drought- and pest-resistant, as well as self-fertilizing crops, agricultural biotechnology may help to lessen world hunger. Perhaps the most promising potential of genetically modified foods today lies within the realm of plant breeding for micronutrients. Developing countries will then have a tool to treat and prevent selected nutrient deficiencies among their populations if they have access to farming resources to augment the micronutrient composition of crops. In addition, greater yields for indigenous plants, such as tomatoes that tolerate high soil salinity, are another hopeful outcome. Biotechnology will likely be a useful tool against the complex scourge of world undernutrition. Improved crops produced by this technology, together with political and other efforts, can contribute to success in the battle against worldwide undernutrition.

▲ Soybeans are a common GMO food in the marketplace. Over 90% of the soybeans grown in the United States are genetically modified.

## Some Concluding Thoughts

The economic loss from undernutrition is staggering, and the amount of human pain and suffering is incalculable. With all the international relief efforts and assistance from governments and private organizations combined, we are still failing in our battle against undernutrition.

Ultimately, the depletion of world resources, the massive debt incurred by poorer countries, the threat of danger to more prosperous countries nearby, and the toll taken in human lives affect the world economy and well-being. The resulting instability can go on to affect the developing world, as has been apparent in recent years. Life is not necessarily fair, but the aim of civilization should be to make it more so. The world has both enough food and the technical expertise to end hunger. What is lacking is the concerted political will to do so.

## CONCEPT CHECK

Overall, one important strategy to reducing undernutrition in the developing world lies in providing sufficient employment, so that people can purchase the food their families need. Providing access to land and other food production resources will also counteract undernutrition. Development programs must be sensitive to regional conditions to ensure that the new technologies introduced do not intensify existing problems for the poorest people.

# Undernutrition at Critical Life Stages

## Critical Life Stages When Undernutrition is Particularly Devastating

Prolonged undernutrition is detrimental to many aspects of human health (Fig. 12-7). It is particularly damaging during some periods of growth and old age. The United Nations Children's Fund developed a conceptual framework of malnutrition in 1990 (Fig. 12-8). According to this framework, the immediate causes of malnutrition (inadequate dietary intake and unsatisfactory health) affect individuals. The underlying causes relate to families and include inadequate access to food, inadequate care for women and children, and insufficient health services. Basic causes relate to human and economic resources and have their effect on communities and nations.

### Pregnancy

Undernutrition poses the greatest health risk during pregnancy. About 500,000 women worldwide die each year from complications of pregnancy and childbirth. A pregnant woman needs extra nutrients to meet both her own needs and those of her developing offspring. Nourishing the fetus may deplete maternal stores of nutrients. Maternal iron deficiency anemia is one possible consequence (Chapter 14).

In Africa, women in their lifetimes give birth, on average, to more than six live babies. Coupled with chronic undernutrition, these high birth rates result in a 1 in 20 in chance that a woman will die from pregnancy-related causes. In contrast, North American women only face a risk of 1 death in about 8000 births from pregnancy-related causes. Pregnancy-related death is the social indicator showing the largest disparity between the developing and industrialized worlds. Smaller differences exist for literacy, life expectancy, and infant mortality.

### Fetal and Infant Stages

The fetus faces major health risks from undernutrition during gestation. To support growth and development of the brain and other body tissues, a growing fetus requires a rich supply of protein, vitamins, and minerals. When these needs are not met, the infant is often born before 37 weeks of gestation, well before the ideal 40 weeks of gestation. The consequences of this pre-term birth include reduced lung function and a weakened immune system. These conditions not only compromise health but also increase the likelihood of premature death. Long-term problems in growth and development can result if the infant survives. In extreme cases, low-birth-weight infants (about 5.5 pounds [2.5 kilograms] or less) face 5 to 10 times the normal risk of dying before the age of 1 year, primarily because of reduced lung development. When low birth weight is accompanied by other physical abnormalities, medical intervention can cost $200,000 or more. These costs can be met only in developed countries.

Worldwide, more than 30 million infants are born each year with low birth weight. About 8% of infants born in the United States and 6% in Canada have low birth weights. In the United States, low birth weight accounts for more than half of all infant deaths and 75% of deaths of infants younger than 1 month old. Whereas undernutrition is a major contributor to low birth weight in developing countries, the primary cause for this problem in industrialized countries is cigarette smoking. Pregnancy during the teenage years, while a girl's body is still growing, contributes to low birth weight in developing and industrialized countries alike.

The percentage of infants born with low birth weight in the United States has been increasing steadily during the past 20 years. One reason is that more twins, triplets, and higher-order multiple births are being born because of improvements in medicine and fertility procedures. Rates of low birth weight also vary by race. About 13% of infants born to African-American women have low birth weights. Among Hispanics in the United States, infants of Mexican origin have the lowest rate of low birth weight (6%), while infants of Puerto Rican heritage have the highest (9%). Among Asian subgroups, low-birth-weight rates range from 5% for infants of Chinese heritage to nearly 9% for Filipino infants.

### Childhood

Early childhood, when growth is rapid, is another period when undernutrition is extremely risky. The central nervous system— including the brain—continues to be vulnerable because of rapid growth through early childhood. After the

Reduced intellectual and social development

Increased maternal, infant, and child mortality

**Undernutrition**

Human suffering, especially in a famine

Reduced work capacity

Increased maternal mortality in pregnancy

Loss of parents, especially linked to AIDS

Exploitation of women

**FIGURE 12-7** ▶ Undernutrition results from and affects many aspects of human health and humanity.

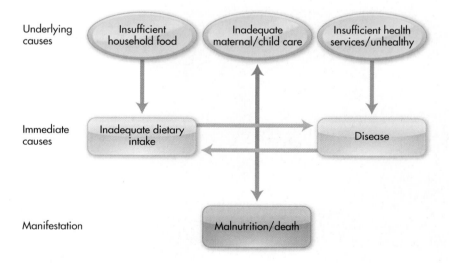

Underlying causes

Insufficient household food

Inadequate maternal/child care

Insufficient health services/unhealthy

Immediate causes

Inadequate dietary intake

Disease

Manifestation

Malnutrition/death

**FIGURE 12-8** ▶ The UNICEF conceptual framework of the causes of malnutrition takes into account food, health, and caring practices. The causes are separated into three causes: immediate, underlying, and basic (not shown). Basic causes include human, economic, and organizational resources. The framework is used as a guide in health policy decision making.

preschool years, brain growth and development slow dramatically until maturity. Nutritional deprivation, especially in early infancy, can lead to permanent brain impairment. Without an effective intervention, it is projected that ongoing undernutrition could leave more than 1 billion children with mental impairment by 2020.

In general, poor children are at the greatest risk for nutritional deprivation and subsequent illness. Stunted growth is an obvious effect, seen in about one-third of children under 5 years of age worldwide. In addition, iron-deficiency anemia is much more common among low-income children than children from less deprived families. This deficiency can lead to fatigue upon exertion, reduced stamina, stunted growth, impaired motor development, and learning problems. Undernutrition in childhood can also weaken resistance to infection because immune function decreases when nutrients such as protein, vitamin A, and zinc are low in a diet. Clearly, undernutrition and illness have a cyclical relationship. Not only does undernutrition lead to illness, but illness, particularly diarrhea and infectious diseases, worsens undernutrition. For this reason, many children in developing countries are dying from the combination of malnutrition and infection. Conversely, when missing nutrients such as vitamin A and zinc are restored to children's diets, improvements in health can be obvious.

## Later Years

Older adults, especially older women living alone in poverty, are also at risk for undernutrition. Older adults in general require nutrient-dense foods, in amounts dependent on their state of health and degree of physical activity. Many of them have fixed incomes and incur significant medical costs, so food often becomes a low-priority item. In addition, depression, social isolation, and declining physical and mental health can compound the problem of undernutrition in older adults.

▶ Compared to other children, homeless children suffer higher rates of many medical problems, some of which include:

- Upper respiratory tract infections
- Scabies and lice
- Tooth decay
- Ear and skin infections
- Diaper rash
- Eye infections
- Developmental delays
- Trauma-related injuries

◀ Minimal intakes of protein and zinc limit the growth of children worldwide. About 30% of children in developing countries show evidence of poor growth rates.

## Case Study Undernutrition During Childhood

Jamal traveled to the Philippines with his church group last summer. During their stay, they helped build shelters for people in a village where, a few weeks before, a storm had destroyed several houses. Jamal noticed that many of the children were very short, much shorter than the children in his neighborhood in the United States. His group worked in a remote, low-elevation area where the storm and subsequent flooding had caused the most damage. On several occasions he noticed young mothers crouched on curbs or in doorways, holding their children. These children rarely moved—they appeared pale and listless. In contrast to the children Jamal's group had met at a church in the capital city, most of the children in this village were not active and lively. One evening a nurse from the local clinic came to speak to Jamal's group. She said that many children in this area do not get enough to eat and that health problems were rampant. She considered the recent storm a blessing in disguise, hoping it would spur the Philippine government to send supplies to the village, particularly food and medicines. Jamal is shocked by such a degree of suffering. He wonders why children in the Philippines can be starving to death while many children in his hometown in the United States are overweight.

Answer the following questions, and check your responses in Appendix A.

1. Should Jamal have been surprised by widespread disease and general listlessness in the Philippine children?
2. Which nutrients are likely to be deficient in the diets of these children?
3. Which nutrient deficiencies contribute to poor growth or "stunting" of growth?
4. Which nutrient deficiencies may be causing diarrhea and illness?
5. Are these children likely to be consuming adequate calories? What effect does consumption of inadequate calories have on growth?
6. Why might the recent storm be a blessing for this small village?

7. List some reasons why the children in Jamal's neighborhood at home are more likely to be overweight

## Summary

1. Poverty is commonly linked to chronic or periodic undernutrition. Malnutrition can occur when the food supply is either scarce or abundant. The resulting deficiency conditions and degenerative diseases contribute to poor health.

    Undernutrition is the most common form of malnutrition in developing countries. It results from inadequate intake, absorption, or use of nutrients or food energy. Many deficiency conditions consequently appear, and infectious diseases thrive because the immune system cannot function properly.

    Undernutrition diminishes both physical and mental capabilities. In poor countries, this is worsened by recurrent infections, unsanitary conditions, extreme weather, inadequate shelter, and exposure to diseases.

2. In North America, famine is not seen but food insecurity and undernutrition remain problems. Soup kitchens, food stamps, the school lunch and breakfast programs, and the Special Supplemental Nutrition Program for Women, Infants, and Children (WIC) have focused on improving the nutritional health of poor and at-risk people. When adequately funded, these programs have proved effective in reducing undernutrition. The need to reduce out-of-wedlock pregnancies remains a national priority because single parents and their children are much more likely to live in poverty.

3. Multiple factors contribute to the problem of undernutrition in the developing world. In densely populated countries, food resources, as well as the means for distributing food, may be inadequate. Farming methods often encourage erosion, which deprives the soil of valuable nutrients and thereby hampers future efforts to grow food. Limited water availability hinders food production. Naturally occurring devastation from droughts, excessive rainfall, fire, crop infestation, and human causes—such as urbanization, war and civil unrest, debt, poor sanitation, and AIDS—all contribute to the major problem of undernutrition.

4. Proposed solutions to world undernutrition must consider multiple interacting factors, many thoroughly embedded in cultural traditions. Family planning efforts, for example, may not succeed until life expectancy increases. Through education, efforts should be made to upgrade farming methods, improve crops, limit

pregnancies, encourage breastfeeding when it is safe to do so, and improve sanitation and hygiene.

Direct food aid is only a short-term solution. In what may appear to be a step backward, many experts recommend more sustainable subsistence-level farming. Small-scale industrial

development is another way to create meaningful employment and purchasing power for vast numbers of the rural poor. Various biotechnology applications may also prove beneficial.

5. The greatest risk of undernutrition occurs during critical periods of growth and development: gestation, infancy,

and childhood. Low birth weight is a leading cause of infant deaths worldwide. Many developmental problems are caused by nutritional deprivation during critical periods of brain growth. People in their later years are also at great risk.

## Study Questions

1. Describe the difference between malnutrition and undernutrition.

2. Describe in a short paragraph any evidence of undernutrition that you saw while you were growing up, such as on television. What are/were the likely roots of these problems?

3. What do you believe are the major factors contributing to undernutrition in wealthy nations, such as the United States? What are some solutions to this problem?

4. What three points would you make to a group of seventh grade girls

concerning the economic perils of teen pregnancy and parenting?

5. What federal programs are available to address the problem of under nutrition in the United States?

6. Outline how war and civil unrest in developing countries have worsened problems of chronic hunger over the past few years.

7. How important is population control in addressing the problem of world hunger now and in the future? Support your answer with three main points.

8. Why is solving the problem of undernutrition a key factor in the ability of developing countries to reach their full potential?

9. Name three nutrients often lacking in the diets of undernourished people. What effects can be expected with each deficiency?

10. Describe how sustainable agriculture and biotechnology can improve food availability worldwide.

## Check Your Knowledge

Answers to the following multiple choice questions are below.

1. There are an estimated _____ chronically undernourished people in the world.
   a. 14 million
   b. 800 million to 1.1 billion
   c. 3 billion
   d. 6 billion

2. The number one killer of children in developing countries is
   a. xerophthalmia.
   b. iron deficiency anemia.
   c. iodide deficiency.
   d. diarrhea.

3. The human organism is particularly susceptible to the effects of undernutrition during
   a. pregnancy.
   b. infancy.
   c. childhood.
   d. All of the above.

4. A barrier to solving undernutrition in the developing world is NOT
   a. external debt.
   b. poor infrastructure.
   c. a lack of manpower.
   d. expanding population

5. Many of the child deaths each year in developing countries could be prevented if
   a. technology was improved.
   b. doctors were more specialized.
   c. mothers would learn more about nutrition.
   d. sanitation and hygiene were improved.

6. The food stamp program, recently renamed the Supplemental Nutrition Assistance Program, allows
   a. low-income families to buy surplus food at government stores with government-issued Electronic Benefit Transfer cards.
   b. low-income people to purchase food, cleaning supplies, alcoholic

beverages, and anything else sold in supermarkets with Electronic Benefit Transfer cards.
   c. low-income people to turn in government-issued Electronic Benefit Transfer cards for cash to buy food.
   d. low-income people to purchase food and seeds with government-issued Electronic Benefit Transfer cards.

7. A long-term solution to world hunger is
   a. the green revolution.
   b. cash crops.
   c. jobs and self-sufficiency.
   d. government/private aid.

8. Bt corn has been genetically modified to make
   a. the bacterium *Bacillus thuringiensis*.
   b. a protein toxic to caterpillars that can destroy the corn plant.
   c. a sugar that makes the corn sweeter.
   d. a fat that makes corn oil healthier.

9. Genetically modified soybeans make up _____% of the soybeans grown in the United States.
   a. 50
   b. 75
   c. 80
   d. 90

10. FDA requires the statement "contains genetically modified ingredients" on the label of all foods containing genetically modified ingredients.
    a. True          b. False

Answer Key: 1. b, 2. d, 3. d, 4. c, 5. d, 6. d, 7. c, 8. b, 9. d, 10. b

# Further Readings

1. ADA Reports: Position of the American Dietetic Association: Agricultural and food bio-technology. *Journal of the American Dietetic Association* 106:285, 2006.

   *It is the position of the American Dietetic Association that agricultural and food biotechnology techniques can enhance the quality, safety, nutritional value, and variety of food available for human consumption and increase the efficiency of food production, food processing, food distribution, and environmental and waste management.*

2. ADA Reports: Position of the American Dietetic Association: Food insecurity and hunger in the United States. *Journal of the American Dietetic Association* 106:446, 2006.

   *It is the position of the American Dietetic Association that systematic and sustained action is needed to bring an end to domestic food insecurity and hunger and to achieve food and nutrition security for all in the United States. Interventions are needed, including adequate funding for and increased use of food and nutrition assistance programs, the inclusion of food and nutrition education in all programs providing food and nutrition assistance, and innovative programs to promote and support the economic self-sufficiency of individuals and families, to end food insecurity and hunger in the United States.*

3. ADA Reports: Position of the American Dietetic Association: Addressing world hunger, malnutrition and food security. *Journal of the American Dietetic Association* 103:1046, 2003.

   *It is the position of the American Dietetic Association that access to adequate amounts of safe, nutritious, and culturally appropriate foods is a fundamental human right. Still, hunger continues to be a worldwide problem of staggering proportions. In response, it is important to encourage programs and practices that combat hunger and malnutrition, increase food security, promote self-sufficiency, and are environmentally and economically sustainable.*

4. ADA Reports: Position of the American Dietetic Association: Child and adolescent food and nutrition programs. *Journal of the American Dietetic Association* 106:1467, 2006.

   *Food programs targeted to low-income households, such as the Food Stamp Program, have gone a long way to increasing the nutrient intake of children and adolescents. It is important that these food programs are supported by adequate funding because the health of many children and adolescents is dependent upon these resources to provide sufficient nutrients to promote optimal physical, social, and cognitive growth and development.*

5. Coutsoudis A: Infant feeding dilemmas created by HIV: South African experiences. *Journal of Nutrition* 135:956, 2005.

   *This paper discusses the dilemma surrounding the risks and benefits of breastfeeding by an HIV-infected mother. The impact of the South African Safer Breastfeeding Programme, implemented to reduce some of the risk factors associated with HIV transmission, is reported.*

6. Darton-Hill I and others: Micronutrient deficiencies and gender: Social and economic costs. *American Journal of Clinical Nutrition* 81:1198S, 2005.

   *Micronutrient deficiencies, such as for vitamin A, iodine, iron, and zinc, in developing countries, lead to health problems, especially in females. Addressing these micronutrient deficiencies is important in order to improve economic status at the personal, community, and national level in developing countries.*

7. Doherty T and others: A longitudinal qualitative study of infant-feeding decision making and practices among HIV-positive women in South Africa. *Journal of Nutrition* 136:2421, 2006.

   *HIV-positive women face challenges regarding infant-feeding decisions. This study examined these challenges and found that successful breastfeeding resulted from a supportive home environment, a strong belief in the benefits of breastfeeding, and the ability to resist pressure to introduce other fluids.*

8. Dworkin SL, Ehrhardt AA: Going beyond "ABC" to include "GEM": Critical reflections on progress in the HIV/AIDS epidemic. *American Journal of Public Health* 97:13, 2007.

   *This article discusses the feminization of HIV/AIDS and the limitations of the "ABC" (abstinence, be faithful, condom use) strategy. Strategies focused on gender relation, economics, and migration (GEM) are suggested as more appropriate prevention measures.*

9. Food and Agriculture Organization of the United Nations: *The state of food insecurity in the world 2008: High food prices and food security-threats and opportunities.* FAO, Rome, Italy, 2008

   *This report of the FAO food security meeting in Rome, Italy in June 2008, emphasizes that in 2008 alone, millions more became food-insecure, demanding urgent action and substantial investments. The worldwide concern about threats to global food security, largely triggered by soaring food prices, is discussed. Representatives of 180 countries plus the European Union met to express their conviction "that the international community needs to take urgent and coordinated action to combat the negative impacts of soaring food prices on the world's most vulnerable countries and populations."*

10. Gibson RS: Zinc: The missing link in combating micronutrient malnutrition in developing countries. *Proceedings of the Nutrition Society* 65:51, 2006.

    *Although zinc deficiency is included as a major risk factor in the global burden of disease, zinc is still not included in the United Nations micronutrient priority list. Certain countries are at risk of zinc deficiency and should be targeted for zinc interventions. Zinc intervention strategies are discussed in this article.*

11. Grandesso F and others: Mortality and malnutrition among populations living in South Darfur, Sudan. *Journal of the American Medical Association* 293:1490, 2005.

    *The conflicts in the Darfur region of Sudan have led to high rates of death and undernutrition among people displaced by war. This article describes what has been seen numerous times in the last 50 years—undernutrition and related death is a typical casualty of war.*

12. Joint United Nations Programme on HIV/ AIDS (UNAIDS) and World Health Organization. 2008 Report on the Global AIDS epidemic July 2008.

*This UNAIDS report contains the 2008 global estimates on the scale of the AIDS pandemic. It is reported that approximately 33 million people were living with HIV in 2007. Forty five percent of the new infections in 2007 occurred in young people aged 15-24.*

13. Milman A and others: Differential improvement among countries in child stunting is associated with long-term development and specific interventions. *Journal of Nutrition* 135:1415, 2005.

*Poor nutrition and health during the pre- and postnatal periods can result in the growth failure known as stunting. Factors that have reduced malnutrition and the resulting growth retardation were studied. National factors found to be most important were changes in immunization rate, safe water rate, female literacy rate, government consumption, income distribution, and the proportion of the economy devoted to agriculture. The results of this study indicate that it is possible to reduce the high prevalence of stunting by investing in specific interventions.*

14. Nord M, Hopwood H: A comparison of household food security in Canada and the United States. Economic Research Report, No. 67, December 2008, http://www.ers. usda.gov/publications/err67/.

*Differences in the prevalence of household food insecurity between Canada and the United States are described in this report. The percentage of the population living in food insecure households was lower in Canada (7.0 percent) than in the United States (12.6 percent). The difference between the percentage of children living in food-insecure households in Canada vs. the US was greater (8.3 percent vs. 17.9 percent) than that for adults (6.6 percent vs. 10.8 percent).*

15. Palmer S: GE foods under the microscope. *Today's Dietitian* p. 34, May 2005.

*About 70% of processed foods sold in the United States have contents that have undergone some genetic alteration. This article explores some of the benefits and concerns regarding use of this fairly recent technology in our food supply.*

16. Palmer S: Water of life in peril. *Today's Dietitian* 9(10):55, 2007.

*This article summarizes the water shortage crisis the world is facing. It provides alarming statistics about our dwindling water supply and the rise in poor sanitation. The crisis of water safety and supply is going to take a global effort focusing on conservation and sanitation. Efforts of the United Nations to bring together governments to take immediate action are reviewed.*

17. Shetty P: Achieving the goal of halving global hunger by 2015. *Proceedings of the Nutrition Society* 65:7, 2006.

*This article reviews the goal of the FAO World Food Summit (WFS) and the United Nations Millennium Development Goals (MDG) to halve the numbers of the global population suffering from hunger by the year 2015. To date, the efforts have fallen short of the pace needed to achieve this goal. Developing countries are facing new challenges of hunger co-existing with new epidemics of diet-related diseases.*

18. Steinbrook R: After Bangkok—Expanding the global response to AIDS. *The New England Journal of Medicine* 351:738, 2004.

*The advances in treatment of AIDS have largely benefited developed countries. There is an urgent need to provide the benefits to those infected with AIDS in the developing world.*

19. United Nations: *Tackling a global crisis: International year of sanitation 2008.* UN-Water, 2008, www.unwater.org.

*The International Year of Sanitation in 2008 focused global attention on the need for improved health and hygiene. It is estimated that around the world, 2.6 billion people do not have a clean and safe place to perform their bodily functions because they lack access to a basic necessity, a toilet. This report helps to expose the scandal of human indignity, unnecessary child death, and lost economic opportunities associated with the sanitation crisis and provides a call to action for organizations to redouble their efforts and bring this silent crisis to an end.*

20. Yach D and others: The global burden of chronic diseases: Overcoming impediments to prevention and control. *Journal of the American Medical Association* 291:2616, 2004.

*Nutrient deficiencies are common in the developing world. Such areas also experience the greatest burden of deaths from diarrhea, HIV and AIDS, and various childhood diseases. There needs be more attention to this enormous problem in the developing world.*

## I. Fighting World Undernutrition on a Personal Level

If you want to do something about world and domestic undernutrition, consider the following activities. It is a noble act to try to make a difference, even if you make only one small step. As with any change in behavior, do not try to do too many things at once. Try one or two activities that represent your commitment to solving this problem.

1. Volunteer at a local soup kitchen or homeless shelter for a time (1 month, for example). What insights did you gain?

2. Coordinate the efforts of a campus organization to donate some money to a voluntary agency that does antihunger work, such as the following:

| | | | |
|---|---|---|---|
| Bread for the World | Catholic Relief Services | Oxfam America | Feeding America |
| 50 F Street NW, Suite 500 | 228 W. Lexington St | 226 Causeway St., 5th Floor | 35 E. Wacker Dr., #2000 |
| Washington, DC 20001 | Baltimore, MD 21201 | Boston, MA 02114 | Chicago, IL 60601 |
| http://www.bread.org/ | www.crs.org | http://www.oxfamamerica.org/ | feedingamerica.org |
| | | | |
| CARE USA | EarthSave International | Save the Children Foundation | |
| 151 Ellis Street, NE | PO Box 96 | 54 Wilton Rd. | |
| Atlanta, GA 30303 | New York, NY 10108 | Westport, CT 06880 | |
| http://www.care.org/ | http://www.earthsave.org/ | http://www.savethechildren.org/ | |

3. Make a contribution of nonperishable foods to the ongoing offering at a place of worship near you. If such an offering does not exist, start one.

4. Get on a food recovery program's mailing list, read its newsletters for information on upcoming fund-raisers and other activities, and become involved.

5. Participate in food drives organized by local grocery stores by contributing food or services. Food-drive organizers may need volunteers to transport the donations from the store to a food pantry. Pay special attention to events around World Food Day, October 16.

6. Point, click, and fight hunger. Internet users can find information on hunger at several sites, including the following:

- Someone somewhere dies of hunger every 3.6 seconds. You can help stop the clock: go to www.thehungersite.com and click on Donate Free Food to send a meal to a needy someone. This site is affiliated with the UN World Food Program, which tracks the number of clicks and then sends a bill to one of its corporate or nonprofit sponsors.

- HungerWeb, at Tufts University, offers information on hunger research, programs, mailing lists, education, and advocacy. This site contains weblinks to Internet sites run by the UN, U.S. AID, and the World Bank. http://nutrition.tufts.edu/academic/hungerweb/

- The Food and Agriculture Organization of the United Nations has worked to alleviate poverty and hunger by promoting agricultural development, improved nutrition, and the pursuit of food security. This website will keep you up-to-date on recent issues and provides an extensive list of publications related to food security. www.fao.org

- America's Second Harvest, the largest domestic hunger-relief organization, shows you how to help online and has information about the latest updates. www.secondharvest.org

- Bread for the World is a nationwide Christian citizens' movement seeking justice for the world's hungry people by lobbying our nation's decision makers. www.bread.org

- CARE is one of the world's largest private international relief and development organizations, with the goal of saving lives, building opportunities, and bringing hope to people in need. www.care.org

## II. Joining the Battle Against Undernutrition

Imagine that you recently spent your summer vacation in a developing country and saw evidence of undernutrition and hunger. Then imagine that you are now asking a large corporation to support your efforts to ease hunger and suffering in this area. Develop a two-paragraph statement outlining why addressing hunger issues in this area is important. Include how you think a large corporation could assist you in your efforts.

# CHAPTER 13 Safety of Our Food Supply

## Student Learning Outcomes After reading Chapter 13, you will be able to:

1. List some of the types and common sources of viruses, bacteria, fungi, and parasites that can make their way into food.

2. Compare and contrast food-preservation methods.

3. Describe the main reasons for using chemical additives in foods, the general classes of additives, and the functions of each class.

4. Identify sources of toxic environmental contaminants in food and the consequences of their ingestion.

5. Understand the reasons behind pesticide use, the possible long-term health complications, and the safety limits set for their use.

6. Understand the effects of conventional and sustainable agriculture on our food choices.

7. Describe the procedures that can be used to limit the risk of foodborne illness.

## Chapter Outline

Student Learning Outcomes

Refresh Your Memory

13.1 Food Safety: Setting the Stage

13.2 Food Preservation—Past, Present, and Future

13.3 Foodborne Illness Caused by Microorganisms

13.4 Food Additives

13.5 Substances That Occur Naturally in Foods and Can Cause Illness

13.6 Environmental Contaminants in Food

13.7 Food Production Choices

Nutrition and Your Health: Preventing Foodborne Illness

Case Study: Preventing Foodborne Illness at Gatherings

Summary/Study Questions/Check Your Knowledge/Further Readings

Rate Your Plate

OVER 100 YEARS AGO, IN 1906, INCREASING PUBLIC PRESSURE FORCED THE PASSAGE OF THE FIRST FOOD AND DRUG ACT IN THE UNITED STATES AND GENERALLY IMPROVED FOOD PREPARATION STANDARDS. Today, warnings about the safety of food and water appear everywhere. Attention has turned to more contemporary concerns, such as microbial and chemical contamination. On the one hand, we are told to eat more fruits, vegetables, fish, and poultry and to drink more water; on the other hand, we are warned that these may contain dangerous substances, so we still must ask, "How safe is our food and water?"

Scientists and health authorities agree that North Americans enjoy a relatively safe food supply, especially if foods are stored and prepared properly. Over the past 100 or so years, tremendous progress has been made to allow for this. Nonetheless, microorganisms and certain chemicals in foods still can pose a health risk. Thus, the nutritional and health benefits of food must be balanced against any food-related hazards. Chapter 13 focuses on these hazards—how real they are and how you can minimize their effect on your life. As the comic in the chapter suggests, you bear some responsibility for this—government agencies and industry can only do so much. Recall from Chapter 2 that the 2005 Dietary Guidelines for Americans encourage us to prepare and store foods safely.

**pasteurizing** The process of heating food products to kill pathogenic microorganisms and reduce the total number of bacteria.

**virus** The smallest known type of infectious agent, many of which cause disease in humans. A virus is essentially a piece of genetic material surrounded by a coat of protein. They do not metabolize, grow, or move by themselves. They reproduce only with the aid of a living cellular host.

**bacteria** Single-cell microorganisms; some produce poisonous substances, which cause illness in humans. Bacteria can be carried by water, animals, and people. They survive on skin, clothes, and hair and thrive in foods at room temperature. Some can live without oxygen and survive by means of **spore** formation.

**spores** Dormant reproductive cells capable of turning into adult organisms without the help of another cell. Various bacteria and fungi form spores.

**fungi** Simple parasitic life forms, including molds, mildews, yeasts, and mushrooms. They live on dead or decaying organic matter. Fungi can grow as single cells, like yeast, or as a multicellular colony, as seen with molds.

**parasite** An organism that lives in or on another organism and derives nourishment from it.

**foodborne illness** Sickness caused by the ingestion of food containing harmful substances.

## Refresh Your Memory

As you begin your study of food safety in Chapter 13, you may want to review:

- Alternative sweeteners in Chapter 4
- The disease phenylketonuria (PKU) in Chapter 4
- Fat substitutes in Chapter 5
- Food biotechnology in Chapter 12

## 13.1 Food Safety: Setting the Stage

During the early stages of urbanization in North America, contaminated water and food—notably, milk—were responsible for many large outbreaks of typhoid fever, septic sore throat, scarlet fever, diphtheria, and other devastating human diseases. These experiences led to the development of processes for purifying water, treating sewage, and **pasteurizing** milk. Since that time, safe water and milk have become universally available, with only occasional problems from either.

The greatest health risk from food today is contamination by **viruses** and **bacteria** and, to a lesser extent, by various forms of **fungi** and **parasites**. These microorganisms can all cause **foodborne illness**. In a recent outbreak, 199 persons in 26 states were infected with *Escherichia coli* (*E. coli*) bacteria O157:H7 from fresh spinach. Of these ill persons, 102 were hospitalized, 31 developed kidney failure, and 22 were children under 5 years. Three deaths were associated with the outbreak.

Although microbial contamination is the cause of most incidents of foodborne illness, North Americans seem more concerned about health risks from chemicals in foods. In the long run, this concern has some merit. On a day-to-day basis, however, food additives cause only about 4% of all cases of foodborne illness in North America. Microbial contamination of food is by far the more important issue for our day-to-day health, so it will be discussed first. Chapter 13 will then cover chemical food safety hazards, including the use and safety of food additives, and discuss the risks of pesticides in foods.

**Garfield ® by Jim Davis**

Which foods pose the greatest risk for foodborne illness? Is any food safe after being stored in the refrigerator for 6 months? Are food additives and pesticides an even greater day-to-day concern? Chapter 13 provides some answers.

## Effects of Foodborne Illness

According to the U.S. Centers for Disease Control and Prevention, foodborne illness causes 76 million illnesses, 325,000 hospitalizations, and 5000 deaths in the United States each year. Hospital costs for foodborne illnesses are estimated at more than $3 billion per year; costs from related lost productivity are estimated at $8 billion per year. Some people are particularly susceptible to foodborne illness, including the following:

- Infants and children
- Older adults
- Those with liver disease, diabetes, HIV infection (and AIDS), or cancer
- Postsurgical patients
- Pregnant women
- People taking immunosuppressant agents (e.g., transplant patients)

It is estimated that in the United States alone about 30 million people with health problems have episodes of foodborne illness. Some bouts of foodborne illness, especially when coupled with ongoing health problems, are lengthy and lead to food allergies, seizures, blood poisoning (from **toxins** or microorganisms in the bloodstream), or other illnesses.

Foodborne illnesses often result from the unsafe handling of food at home, so we each bear some responsibility for preventing them. You can't usually tell so by taste, smell, or sight that a particular food contains harmful microorganisms; therefore, you might not even be aware that food has caused your distress. In fact, your last case of diarrhea may have been caused by foodborne illness (Table 13-1). Government agencies are at work on problems regarding food safety, but this does not substitute for individual safety efforts (Table 13-2).

**toxins** Poisonous compounds produced by an organism that can cause disease.

## Why Is Foodborne Illness So Common?

Foodborne illness is carried or transmitted to people by food. Most foodborne illnesses are transmitted through food in which microorganisms are able to grow rapidly. These foods are generally moist, rich in protein, and have a neutral or slightly acidic pH. Unfortunately, this describes many of the foods we eat every day, such as meats, eggs, and dairy products.

Our food industry tries whenever possible to increase the shelf life of food products; however, a longer shelf life allows more time for bacteria in foods to multiply. Some bacteria even grow at refrigeration temperatures. Partially cooked—and some fully cooked—products pose a particular risk because refrigerated storage may only slow, not prevent, bacterial growth. The risk of contracting foodborne illness also is high because of consumer trends. First, there is greater consumer interest in eating raw or undercooked animal products. In addition, more people receive medication that suppresses their ability to combat foodborne infectious agents. Another factor is the continuing increase in the number of older adults in the population.

The risk of illness from foodborne microorganisms increases as more of our foods are prepared in kitchens outside the home. Supermarkets have become an alternative to cooking at home by offering a variety of prepared foods from specialty meat shops, salad bars, and bakeries. With the increasing number of two-income families, more people are looking for convenient, easy-to-prepare, nutritious foods. Supermarkets offer entrées that can be served immediately or reheated. The foods are usually prepared in central kitchens or processing plants and shipped to individual stores.

This centralization of food production by the food-processing and restaurant industry enhances the risk of foodborne illness. If a food product is contaminated in

▲ Some restaurants that serve requested undercooked food are now warning patrons (on the menu) of the health risks of ordering such foods, particularly with undercooked eggs and meats.

**TABLE 13-1** Some Examples of Cases of Foodborne Illness. We generally have a safe food supply, but there are occasional instances of foodborne illnesses, such as those listed.

### Viruses

- *Norovirus:* During a Caribbean cruise, more than 380 passengers and crew members of the world's largest cruise ship, Royal Caribbean's Freedom of the Seas, were sickened by *Norovirus*. The ship, which carries 3900 passengers, was cleaned and sanitized, but one week later a second outbreak of the gastrointestinal illness afflicted 97 passengers and 11 crew members.

- *Hepatitus A:* Over 500 adults in the United States contracted hepatitis A after eating raw green onions in a Mexican restaurant. These were contaminated during growth in Mexico and not properly washed by food service workers.

### Bacteria

- *Salmonella:* In 2008–2009, two nationwide outbreaks of salmonella received widespread media attention and cost their respective industries millions of dollars. The first outbreak, initially linked to tomatoes, was finally traced to imported jalapeno and serrano peppers from one Mexican farm. Illnesses led to 282 hospitalizations and 2 deaths. The second outbreak, which may have contributed to at least eight deaths, was traced to peanut butter from a processing plant in Georgia.
- *Shigella:* Six persons were reported ill from a *Shigella* infection after eating chopped, uncooked parsley served on chicken sandwiches and in coleslaw. In another incident, a cruise ship returned to port when more than 600 people developed shigellosis and one person died.
- *Listeria:* Forty-eight deaths were associated with foodborne illness caused by *Listeria* organisms in soft, Mexican-style cheeses. A listeriosis outbreak associated with undercooked hot dogs and cold cuts resulted in more than 82 illnesses and 17 deaths in 19 states.
- *E. coli:* One of the largest *E. coli* 0157:H7 outbreaks on record infected more than 1000 people in upstate New York at a county fair. The bacterium was found in infected well water. It killed a 79-year-old man and a 4-year-old girl, and it caused 10 other children

to undergo kidney dialysis. Six adults and a 2-year-old child were killed after an *E. coli* outbreak from contaminated drinking water in Canada. The bacteria entered the water supply from animal manure after flooding from a heavy storm. In northeastern Oklahoma, five children were infected with *E. coli* after consuming unpasterized apple cider. In the recent outbreak of 199 persons infected with *E. coli* from fresh spinach, *E. coli* 0157:H7 was isolated from 13 packages of fresh spinach in 10 states. At least 11 of the packages came from the same manufacturing plant on the same day.
- *C. botulinum:* A man in Arkansas developed botulism after eating stew that was cooked and then kept at room temperature for 3 days. He spent 49 days in the hospital—42 of them on mechanical ventilation.
- *Vibrio:* Since 1992, 17 people in Florida have died of *Vibrio vulnificus* infections after eating raw oysters.
- *B. cereus:* A teenage boy and his father experienced abdominal pain, vomiting, and diarrhea within 30 minutes of eating 4-day-old homemade pesto. The pesto had been reheated and left out a number of times during the 4-day period. It was apparently contaminated with *Bacillus cereus*. As a result, the boy died of liver failure.

### Parasites

- *Cryptosporidium:* A group attending a dinner banquet developed diarrhea 3 to 9 days after eating green onions, the likely cause of the outbreak. Eight of 10 stool specimens obtained from the group

with foodborne illness were positive for *Cryptosporidium*. Food workers at the restaurant reported they did not consistently wash green onions before using them.

### Risks from Seafood

- *Scombroid:* Four adults became ill with scombroid fish poisoning after eating tuna-spinach salad at a restaurant in Pennsylvania.
- *Ciguatera:* An outbreak of ciguatera fish poisoning involved 17 crew members of a cargo ship that caught, cooked, and ate a barra-

cuda in the Bahamas. All 17 men became ill with nausea, vomiting, abdominal cramps, and diarrhea within hours of eating the fish. Within 2 days, all of the men suffered from muscle pain and weakness; dizziness; and numb or itchy feet, hands, and mouth.

▲ Food contaminated in a central plant can go on to produce illness in people across the nation. In the case of juices, pasteurization is an effective method of reducing the risk of foodborne illness.

a central processing plant, consumers over a wide area can suffer foodborne illness. For example, a malfunction in an ice cream plant in Minnesota resulted in 224,000 suspected cases of *Salmonella* bacterial infections, which were linked to use of contaminated ice cream mix. At least 4 people died and 700 became ill in Washington and surrounding western states after eating at a chain of fast-food restaurants. The source of the problem was undercooked hamburger contaminated with the bacterium *E. coli* 0157:H7. Restaurants generally encounter inspection by local health departments only about every 6 months. We must primarily rely on each restaurant to practice good food safety.

Greater consumption of ready-to-eat foods imported from foreign countries is still another cause of increased foodborne illness in North America. In the past, food imports were mostly raw products processed here under strict sanitation standards. Now, however, we import more ready-to-eat processed foods—such as berries from

**TABLE 13-2** Agencies Responsible for Monitoring the Food Supply in the United States

| Agency Name | Responsibilities | Methods | How to Contact |
|---|---|---|---|
| United States Department of Agriculture (USDA) | • Enforces wholesomeness and quality standards for grains and produce (while in the field), meat, poultry, milk, eggs, and egg products | • Inspection<br>• Grading<br>• "Safe Handling Label" | www.fsis.usda.gov |
| Bureau of Alcohol, Tobacco, Firearms and Explosives (ATF) | • Enforces laws on alcoholic beverages | • Inspection | www.atf.treas.gov |
| Environmental Protection Agency (EPA) | • Regulates pesticides<br>• Establishes water quality standards | • Approval required for all U.S. pesticides<br>• Sets pesticide residue limits in food | www.epa.gov |
| Food and Drug Administration (FDA) | • Ensures safety and wholesomeness of all foods in interstate commerce (except meat, poultry, and processed egg products)<br>• Regulates seafood<br>• Controls product labels | • Inspection<br>• Food sample studies<br>• Sets standards for specific foods | www.fda.gov or call 1-800-FDA-4010 |
| Centers for Disease Control and Prevention (CDC) | • Promotes food safety | • Responds to emergencies concerning foodborne illness<br>• Surveys and studies environmental health problems<br>• Directs/enforces quarantines<br>• National programs for prevention and control of foodborne and other diseases | www.cdc.gov |
| National Marine Fisheries Service or NOAA Fisheries | • Domestic and international conservation and management of living marine resources | • Voluntary seafood inspection program<br>• Can use mark to show federal inspection | www.nmfs.noaa.gov |
| State and local governments | • Milk safety<br>• Monitors food industry within their borders | • Inspection of food-related establishments | Government pages of telephone book |

Government agencies responsible for monitoring food safety in Canada and the specific laws followed are listed in Appendix C.

Guatemala and shellfish from Asia—some of which are contaminated. U.S. authorities are re-examining inspection procedures for these imports.

The use of antibiotics in animal feeds is also increasing the severity of cases of foodborne illness. This antibiotic use encourages bacteria to develop antibiotic-resistant strains, those that can grow even if exposed to typical antibiotic medicines. This issue is receiving considerable attention by scientists in the field.

Finally, more cases of foodborne disease are reported now because scientists are more aware of the roles of various players in the process. Every decade the list of microorganisms suspected of causing foodborne illness lengthens. In addition, physicians are more likely to suspect foodborne contaminants as a cause of illness. Furthermore, we now know that food, besides serving as a good growth medium for some microorganisms, transmits many others as well. Seafood is receiving greater scrutiny and surveillance by FDA as a cause of foodborne illness. For more information about food safety, contact FDA's Center for Food Safety and Applied Nutrition information line at 1-888-SAFEFOOD or log on to www.FoodSafety.gov.

One tool in the battle against foodborne illness is HACCP, or Hazard Analysis Critical Control Point. By applying the principles of HACCP, food handlers critically analyze how they approach food preparation and what conditions may exist that might allow pathogenic microorganisms to enter and thrive in the food system. Once specific hazards and critical control points (potential problems) are identified, preventive measures can be used to reduce specific sources of contamination.

## 13.2 Food Preservation—Past, Present, and Future

For centuries, salt, sugar, smoke, fermentation, and drying have been used to preserve food. Ancient Romans used sulfites to disinfect wine containers and preserve wine. In the age of exploration, European adventurers traveling to the New World preserved their meat by salting it. Most preserving methods work on the principle of decreasing water content. Bacteria need abundant stores of water to grow; yeasts and molds can grow with less water, but some is still necessary. Adding sugar or salt binds water and so decreases the water available to these microbes. The process of drying evaporates off free water.

Decreasing the water content of some high-moisture foods, however, would cause them to lose essential characteristics. To preserve such foods—cucumber pickles, sauerkraut, milk (yogurt), and wine—fermentation has been a traditional alternative. Selected bacteria or yeast are used to ferment or pickle foods. The fermenting bacteria or yeast make acids and alcohol, which minimize the growth of other bacteria and yeast.

Today we can add pasteurization, sterilization, refrigeration, freezing, food **irradiation,** canning, and chemical preservation to the list of food preservation techniques. An additional method of food preservation—**aseptic processing**—simultaneously sterilizes the food and package separately before the food enters the package. Liquid foods, such as fruit juices, are especially easy to process in this manner. With aseptic packaging, boxes of sterile milk and juices can remain on supermarket shelves, free of microbial growth, for many years.

Food irradiation uses minimal doses of radiation to control pathogens such as *E. coli* O157:H7 and *Salmonella*. The radiation energy used does not make the food radioactive. The energy essentially passes through the food, as in microwave cooking, and no radioactive residues are left behind. However, the energy is strong enough to break chemical bonds, destroy cell walls and cell membranes, break down DNA, and link proteins together. Irradiation thereby controls growth of insects, bacteria, fungi, and parasites in foods.

FDA approved the use of irradiation for raw red meat to reduce risk of *E. coli* and other infectious microorganisms. Other additions to the approved list are shell eggs and seeds. Prior to this, the only animal products so treated were pork and chicken. Irradiation also extends the shelf life of spices, dry vegetable seasonings, meats, and fresh fruits and vegetables.

Irradiated food, except for dried seasonings, must be labeled with the international food irradiation symbol, the Radura, and a statement that the product has been treated by irradiation. Foods treated in this way are safe in the opinion of FDA and many other health authorities, including the American Academy of Pediatrics. Although the demand for irradiated foods is still low in the United States, other countries, including Canada, Japan, Italy, and Mexico, all use food irradiation technology widely. Certain consumer groups continually try to block its use in the United States, claiming that irradiation diminishes the nutritional value of food and that it can lead to the formation of harmful compounds, such as carcinogens. Future research should be able to sort out this controversy, but in any case the risk is very low. Keep in mind that, even when foods, especially meats, have been irradiated, it is still important to follow basic food-safety procedures, as later contamination during food preparation is possible.

## 13.3 Foodborne Illness Caused by Microorganisms

Most cases of foodborne illness are caused by specific viruses, bacteria, and other fungi. Prions—proteins involved in maintaining nerve cell function—can also turn infectious and lead to diseases such as mad cow disease. Bacteria specifically cause health problems either directly by invading the intestinal wall and producing an *infection* via a toxin contained in the organism, or indirectly by producing a toxin

**irradiation** A process in which **radiation** energy is applied to foods, creating compounds (free radicals) within the food that destroy cell membranes, break down DNA, link proteins together, limit enzyme activity, and alter a variety of other proteins and cell functions of microorganisms that can lead to food spoilage. This process does not make the food radioactive.

**radiation** Literally, energy that is emitted from a center in all directions. Various forms of radiation energy include X-rays and ultraviolet rays from the sun.

**aseptic processing** A method by which food and container are separately and simultaneously sterilized; it allows manufacturers to produce boxes of milk that can be stored at room temperature.

▲ This is the Radura, the international label denoting prior irradiation of the food product.

secreted into the food, which later harms us (called an *intoxication*). The main way to distinguish an infectious route from an intoxication is time: If symptoms appear in 4 hours or less, it is an intoxication.

## Bacteria

Bacteria are single-cell organisms found in the food we eat, the water we drink, and the air we breathe. Many types of bacteria cause foodborne illness, including *Bacillus, Campylobacter, Clostridium, Escherichia, Listeria, Vibrio, Salmonella,* and *Staphylococcus* (Table 13-3). Bacteria are everywhere: each teaspoon of soil contains about 2 billion bacteria. Luckily, only a small number of all bacteria pose a threat. Some foodborne bacteria cause infections, whereas others cause intoxications. *Salmonella,* for example causes an infection because the bacteria causes the illness. *Clostridium botulinum, Staphylococcus aureus,* and *Bacillus cereus* produce toxins and therefore cause illness from intoxication. In addition, while most strains of *E. coli* are harmless, *E. coli* O157: H7 produces a toxin that can cause severe illness, including severe bloody diarrhea and hemolytic uremic syndrome (HUS). Bacterial foodborne illnesses typically cause gastrointestinal symptoms such as vomiting, diarrhea, and abdominal cramps. *Salmonella, Listeria, E. coli* O157:H7, and *Campylobacter* are the bacterial foodborne illnesses of particular interest because they are the ones most often associated with death. *E. coli* O157:H7 has caused deaths when HUS has developed. Of the 2,500 cases of Listeriosis in the United States each year, 500 cases are fatal. Listeriosis is of particular concern for pregnant women because they are about 20 times more likely to get this infection than other healthy adults, and Listeriosis can cause spontaneous abortion or stillbirth because the *Listeria* bacteria can cross the placenta and infect the fetus.

To proliferate, bacteria require nutrients, water, and warmth. Most grow best in **danger zone** temperatures of 41° to 135°F (5° to 57°C) (Fig. 13-1). Pathogenic bacteria

▲ Ground meats are a typical source of foodborne infection because bacteria on the surface of whole meats are distributed throughout the meat during grinding.

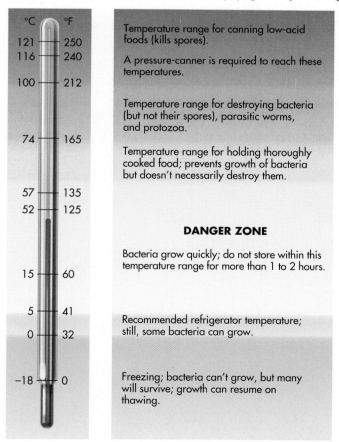

**FIGURE 13-1 ▶** Effects of temperature on microbes that cause foodborne illness.

**TABLE 13-3** Bacterial Causes of Foodborne Illness

| Bacteria | Typical Food Sources | Symptoms | Additional Information |
|---|---|---|---|
| *Salmonella* species | Raw and undercooked meats, poultry, eggs, and fish; produce, especially raw sprouts; peanut butter; unpasteurized milk | Onset: 12–72 hours; nausea, fever, headache, abdominal cramps, diarrhea, and vomiting; can be fatal in infants, the elderly, and those with impaired immune systems; lasts 4–7 days | Estimated 1.4 million infections/year; bacteria live in the intestines of animals and humans; food is contaminated by infected water and feces; about 2,000 strains of *Salmonella* bacteria can cause disease, but 3 strains account for almost 50% of cases; *Salmonella enteritidis* infects the ovaries of healthy hens and contaminates eggs; almost 20% of cases are from eating undercooked eggs or egg-containing dishes; reptiles, such as turtles, also spread the disease |
| *Campylobacter jejuni* | Raw and undercooked meat and poultry (more than half of raw poultry in the U.S. is contaminated), unpasteurized milk, contaminated water | Onset: 2–5 days; muscle pain, abdominal cramping, diarrhea (sometimes bloody), fever; lasts 2–7 days | Estimated 1 million infections/year; produces a toxin that destroys intestinal mucosal surfaces; can cause Guillain-Barré syndrome, a rare neurological disorder that causes paralysis |
| *Escherichia coli* (O157:H7 and other strains) | Undercooked ground beef; produce—lettuce, spinach, sprouts; unpasteurized juice and milk | Onset: 1–8 days; bloody diarrhea, abdominal cramps; in children under age 5 and the elderly, hemolytic uremic syndrome (HUS) is a serious complication; red blood cells are destroyed and kidneys fail; can be fatal; lasts 5–10 days | Leading cause of bloody diarrhea in the U.S.; estimated 73,000 cases/year; lives in the intestine of healthy cattle; cattle and cattle manure are chief sources; illness caused by a powerful toxin made by the bacteria; petting zoos, lakes, and swimming pools can contain pathogenic *E. coli* |
| *Shigella* species | Fecal/oral transmission; water supplies, produce, and other foods contaminated by infected food handlers with poor hygiene | Onset: 1–3 days; abdominal cramps, fever, diarrhea (often bloody); lasts 5–7 days | Estimated 448,000 cases/year; humans and primates are the only sources; common in day-care centers and custodial institutions from poor hygiene; traveler's diarrhea often caused by *Shigella dysenteriae* |
| *Staphylococcus aureus* | Ham, poultry, egg salads, cream-filled pastries, custards, whipped cream | Onset: 1–6 hours; diarrhea, vomiting, nausea, abdominal cramps; lasts 1–3 days | Bacteria on skin and nasal passages of up to 25% of people; can be passed to foods; multiplies rapidly when contaminated foods are held for extended time at room temperature; illness caused by a heat-resistant toxin that cannot be destroyed by cooking |

**TABLE 13-3** *(continued)*

| Bacteria | Typical Food Sources | Symptoms | Additional Information |
|---|---|---|---|
| *Clostridium perfringens* | Beef, poultry, gravy, Mexican food | Onset: 8–24 hours; abdominal pain and diarrhea, usually mild; can be more serious in elderly or ill persons; lasts 1 day or less | Estimated 10,000 cases/year; anaerobic bacteria widespread in soil and water; multiplies rapidly in prepared foods, such as meats, casseroles, and gravies, held for extended time at room temperature |
| *Listeria monocytogenes* | Unpasteurized milk and soft cheeses, raw meats, uncooked vegetables, ready-to-eat deli meats and hotdogs, refrigerated smoked fish | Onset: 9–48 hours for early symptoms, 14–42 days for severe symptoms; fever, muscle aches, headache, vomiting; can spread to nervous system, resulting in stiff neck, confusion, loss of balance, or convulsion; can cause premature birth and stillbirth | Estimated 2500 cases with 500 fatalities/year; widespread in soil and water and can be carried in healthy animals; grows at refrigeration temperatures; about one-third of cases occur during pregnancy; high-risk persons should avoid uncooked deli meats, soft cheeses (e.g., feta, Brie, and Camembert), blue-veined cheeses, Mexican-style cheeses (e.g., queso blanco made from unpasteurized milk), refrigerated meat spreads or pates, uncooked refrigerated smoked fish |
| *Clostridium botulinum* | Incorrectly home-canned vegetables, meats, and fish; incorrectly canned commercial foods; herb-infused oils; bottled garlic; potatoes baked in foil and held at room temperature; honey | Onset: 18–36 hours but can be 6 hours to 10 days; neurological symptoms—double and blurred vision, drooping eyelids, slurred speech, difficulty swallowing, muscle weakness, and paralysis of face, arms, respiratory muscles, trunk, and legs; can be fatal; lasts days to weeks | Estimated 100 cases/year; caused by a neurotoxin; *C. botulinum* grows only in the absence of air in non-acidic foods; incorrect home canning causes most botulism, but in 2007 commercially canned chili sauce caused an outbreak; honey can contain botulism spores and should not be given to infants younger than 1 year of age |
| *Vibrio* | *V. parahemolyticus:* raw and undercooked shellfish, especially oysters | Onset: 24 hours; watery diarrhea, nausea, vomiting, fever, chills; lasts 3 days | Found in coastal waters; more infections in summer; number of infections hard to determine because it is difficult to isolate in the lab |
| | *V. vulnificus:* raw and undercooked shellfish, especially oysters | Onset: 1–2 days; vomiting, diarrhea, abdominal pain; in more severe cases, bloodstream infection with fever, chills, decreased blood pressure, blistering skin lesions; lasts 3 or more days | Estimated 95 cases/year; found in coastal waters; more infections in summer; those with impaired immune systems and liver disease at higher risk of infection; fatality rate of 50% with bloodstream infection |
| | *V. cholerae:* contaminated water and food, human carriers | Onset: 2–3 days; severe, dehydrating diarrhea, vomiting; dehydration, cardiovascular collapse, and death can occur | Occurs mainly in countries without adequate water purification and sewage treatment |
| *Yersinia enterocolitica* | Raw or undercooked pork, particularly pork intestines (chitterlings); tofu; water; unpasteurized milk | Onset: 4–7 days; fever, abdominal pain, diarrhea (often bloody); lasts 1–3 weeks or longer | Yersinosis most common in children under age 5 years; relatively rare; bacteria live mainly in pigs but can be found in other animals |

typically do not multiply when food is held at temperatures above 135°F (57°C) or stored at safe refrigeration temperatures, 32° to 40°F (0° to 4.4°C). One important exception is *Listeria* bacteria, which can multiply at refrigeration temperatures. Also note that high temperatures can kill toxin-producing bacteria, but any toxin produced in the food will not be inactivated by high temperatures. Most pathogenic bacteria also require oxygen for growth, but *Clostridium botulinum* and *Clostridium perfringens* grow only in anaerobic (oxygen-free) environments, such as those found in tightly sealed cans and jars. Food acidity can affect bacterial growth, too. Although most bacteria do not grow well in acidic environments, some, such as disease-causing *E. coli*, can grow in acidic foods, such as fruit juice.

## Viruses

Viruses, like bacteria, are widely dispersed in nature. Unlike bacteria, however, viruses can reproduce only after invading body cells, such as those that line the intestines. Experts speculate that about 70% of foodborne illness cases go un-diagnosed because they result from viral causes, and there is no easy way to test for these pathogens. Table 13-4 describes the two most common viral causes of foodborne illness and describes typical food sources and symptoms of the illnesses they cause. Norovirus causes an illness commonly misdiagnosed as the "stomach flu." Norovirus infection has a sudden onset and usually a short duration of only one to two days. Noroviruses have become a problem on cruise ships. They are hardy and survive freezing, relatively high temperatures, and chlorination up to 10 ppm. A website coordinating the U.S. efforts on food safety is the **www.FoodSafety.gov** site mentioned earlier. Another useful website is **www.homefoodsafety.org.**

▲ Norovirus epidemics commonly occur on cruise ships. Noroviruses were originally called "Norwalk viruses" from Norwalk, Ohio, where they were first known to cause an epidemic of gastroenteritis.

▲ Raw shellfish, especially bivalves (e.g., oysters and clams), present a particular risk related to foodborne viral disease. These animals filter feed, a process that concentrates viruses, bacteria, and toxins present in the water as it is filtered for food. Adequate cooking of shellfish will kill viruses and bacteria, but toxins may not be affected. It's important to buy shellfish from reliable sources who have harvested these foods from safe areas.

**TABLE 13-4** Viral Causes of Foodborne Illness

| Viruses | Typical Food Sources | Symptoms | Additional Information |
| --- | --- | --- | --- |
| **Norovirus (Norwalk and Norwalk-like viruses), human rotavirus** | Foods prepared by infected food handlers; shellfish from contaminated waters; vegetables and fruits contaminated during growing, harvesting, and processing | Onset: 1–2 days; "stomach flu"— severe diarrhea, nausea, vomiting, stomach cramping, low-grade fever, chills, muscle aches; lasts 1–2 days or longer | Viruses found in stool and vomit of infected persons; food handlers can contaminate foods or work surfaces; noroviruses are very infectious—as few as 10–100 particles can lead to infection; workers with norovirus symptoms should not work until 2 or 3 days after they feel better |
| **Hepatitis A virus** | Foods prepared by infected food handlers, especially uncooked foods or those handled after cooking, such as sandwiches, pastries, and salads; shellfish from contaminated waters; vegetables and fruits contaminated during growing, harvesting, and processing | Onset: 15–50 days; anorexia, diarrhea, fever, jaundice, dark urine, fatigue; may cause liver damage and death; lasts several weeks up to 6 months | Infected food handlers contaminate food and transmit the disease to dozens of persons; children and young adults are more susceptible; a vaccine is available, decreasing the number of infections dramatically; immunoglobulin given within 1 week to those exposed to hepatitis A virus can also decrease infection |

<u>**CONCEPT CHECK**</u>

Viruses and bacteria pose the greatest risk for foodborne illness. In the past, the addition of sugar and salt to foods, as well as smoking and drying, were used to prevent the growth of microorganisms. Commercial processes, such as pasteurization and irradiation, offer protection from foodborne illness. Treat all raw animal products, cooked food, and raw fruits and vegetables as potential sources of foodborne illness.

### Parasites

Parasites live in or on another organism, known as the host, from which they absorb nutrients. Humans may serve as a host to parasites. These tiny ravagers rob millions of people around the globe of their health and, in some cases, their lives. Those hardest hit live in tropical countries where poor sanitation fosters the growth of parasites.

The more than 80 foodborne parasites known to affect humans include mainly **protozoa** (one-celled animals), such as *Cryptosporidium* and *Cyclospora,* and **helminths,** such as tapeworms and the roundworm *Trichinella spiralis.* Table 13-5 describes common parasites and typical food sources and symptoms of the illnesses they cause. Parasitic infections spread via person-to-person contact and contaminated food, water, and soil.

## 13.4 Food Additives

By the time you see a food on the market shelf, it usually contains substances added to make it more palatable or increase its nutrient content or shelf life. Manufacturers also add some substances to foods to make them easier to process. Other substances may have accidentally found their way into the foods you buy. All of these extraneous substances are known as **additives,** and, although some may be beneficial, others, such as sulfites, may be harmful for some people. All purposefully added substances must be evaluated by FDA.

### Why Are Food Additives Used?

Most additives are used to limit food spoilage. Common food additives serve the general function of **preservatives,** including acidic or alkaline agents, antioxidants, antimicrobial agents, curing and pickling agents, and **sequestrants.** Table 13-6 helps you to understand exactly why these are used and to learn more about the specific substances used. Food additives, such as potassium sorbate, are used to maintain the safety and acceptability of foods by retarding the growth of microbes implicated in foodborne illness.

Additives are also used to combat some enzymes that lead to undesirable changes in color and flavor in foods but don't cause anything as serious as foodborne illness. This second type of food spoilage occurs when enzymes in a food react to oxygen—for example, when apple and peach slices darken or turn rust color as they are exposed to air. Antioxidants are a type of preservative that slow the action of oxygen-requiring enzymes on food surfaces. These preservatives are not necessarily novel chemicals. They include vitamins E and C and a variety of sulfites.

Without the use of some food additives, it would be impossible to produce massive quantities of foods and safely distribute them nationwide or worldwide, as is now done. Despite consumer concerns about the safety of food additives, many have been extensively studied and proven safe when FDA guidelines for their use are followed.

**protozoa** One-celled animals that are more complex than bacteria. Disease-causing protozoa can be spread through food and water.

**helminth** Parasitic worm that can contaminate food, water, feces, animals, and other substances.

**additives** Substances added to foods, such as preservatives.

**preservatives** Compounds that extend the shelf life of foods by inhibiting microbial growth or minimizing the destructive effect of oxygen and metals.

**sequestrants** Compounds that bind free metal ions. By so doing, they reduce the ability of ions to cause rancidity in foods containing fat.

**TABLE 13-5** Parasitic Causes of Foodborne Illness

| Parasite | Typical Food Sources | Symptoms | Additional Information |
|---|---|---|---|
| **Trichinella spiralis** | Pork, wild game | Onset: weeks to months; GI symptoms followed by muscle weakness, fluid retention in the face, fever, flulike symptoms | The number of trichinosis infections has decreased greatly because pigs are now less likely to harbor this parasite; cooking pork to 160°F (72°C) will kill *trichinella*, as will freezing it for 3 days at −4°F (−20°C) |
| **Anisakis** | Raw or undercooked fish | Onset: 12 hours or less; violent stomach pain, nausea, vomiting | Caused by eating the larvae of roundworms; the infection is more common where raw fish is routinely consumed |
| **Tapeworms** | Raw beef, pork, and fish | Abdominal discomfort, diarrhea | |
| **Toxoplasma gondii** | Raw or undercooked meat, unwashed fruits and vegetables | Onset: 5–20 days; most people are asymptomatic; those with symptoms have fever, headache, sore muscles, diarrhea; can be fatal to the fetus of pregnant women | Parasite is spread to humans from animals, including cats, the main reservoir of the disease; humans acquire the disease from ingesting contaminated meat or from fecal contamination from handling cat litter |
| **Cyclospora cayetanensis** | Water, contaminated food | Onset: 1 week; watery diarrhea, vomiting, muscle aches, fatigue, anorexia, weight loss; lasts 10–12 weeks | Most common in tropical and subtropical areas, but since 1990 about a dozen outbreaks, affecting 3600 people, have occurred in the U.S. and Canada |
| **Cryptosporidium** | Water, contaminated food | Onset: 2–10 days; watery diarrhea, abdominal pain, fever, nausea, vomiting, weight loss; those with impaired immune systems become more ill; lasts 1–2 weeks in otherwise healthy persons | Outbreaks occur worldwide; the largest U.S. outbreak was in 1993 in Milwaukee, with more than 443,000 persons affected; also can be spread in water parks and community swimming pools |

**TABLE 13-6** Types of Food Additives—Sources and Related Health Concerns

| Food Additive Class | Attributes | Health Risks |
|---|---|---|
| **Acidic or alkaline agents,** such as citric acid, calcium lactate, and sodium hydroxide | Acids impart a tart taste to soft drinks, sherbets, and cheese spreads; inhibit mold growth; lessen discoloration and rancidity. They also reduce the risk of botulism in naturally low-acid vegetables, such as canned green beans. Alkaline agents neutralize acids produced during fermentation, and so improve flavor. | No known health risks when used properly |
| **Alternative low-calorie sweeteners,** such as saccharin, sucralose, ascesulfame potassium, aspartame, neotame, and tagatose | Sweeten foods without adding more than a few calories | Moderate use of these alternative sweeteners is considered safe (except for use of aspartame by people with the disease PKU) |
| **Anticaking agents,** such as calcium silicate, magnesium stearate, and silicon dioxide | Absorb moisture to keep table salt, baking powder, or powdered sugar and powdered food products free-flowing and prevent caking and lumping | No known health risks when used properly |
| **Antimicrobial agents,** such as salt, sodium benzoate, sorbic acid, and calcium propionate | Inhibit mold and fungal growth | Salt increases the risk of developing hypertension, especially in some individuals. No known health risks from other agents when used properly |
| **Antioxidants,** such as BHA (butylated hydroxyanisole), BHT (butylated hydroxytoluene), alpha-tocopherol (vitamin E), ascorbic acid (vitamin C), and sulfites | Delay food discolorations from oxygen exposure; Reduce rancidity from the breakdown of fats; Maintain the color of luncheon meats; Prevent the formation of cancer-causing nitrosamines | Sulfites can cause an allergic reaction in about 1 in every 100 people. Symptoms include difficulty breathing, wheezing, hives, diarrhea, abdominal pain, cramps, and dizziness. Salad bars, dried fruit, and wine are typical sources of sulfites. |
| **Color additives,** such as tartrazine | Make foods more appealing | Tartrazine (FD&C yellow number 5) can cause allergic symptoms such as hives and nasal discharge in some people, especially those allergic to aspirin. FDA requires manufacturers to list all forms of synthetic colors on the labels of foods that contain them. |
| **Curing and pickling agents,** such as salt, nitrates, and nitrites | Nitrates and nitrites act as preservatives, especially to prevent the growth of *Clostridium botulinium*; often used in conjunction with salt | Salt increases the risk of developing hypertension, especially in some individuals. Nitrate and nitrite consumption from both cured foods and that found naturally in some vegetables has been associated with synthesis of nitrosamines. (An adequate |

**S**ugar, salt, corn syrup, and citric acid constitute 98% of all additives (by weight) used in food processing.

▲ Soft drinks are typical sources of alternative sweeteners for many of us. Moderate use of these products generally poses no health risk in most people.

**Y**ou might wonder why, if nitrates and nitrites form chemical substances that can cause cancer, they aren't banned by the Delaney Clause. In the United States, USDA regulates the use of chemicals in meats. The laws that govern USDA regulation of foods are separate from those that govern FDA regulation. Because of this, the Delaney Clause does not apply to USDA actions. USDA sees no clear threat to public safety from the regulated use of nitrates and nitrites in meats, so no action has been taken.

**TABLE 13-6** *(continued)*

| Food Additive Class | Attributes | Health Risks |
|---|---|---|
| | | vitamin C intake may reduce this synthesis.) Some nitrosamines are cancer-causing agents, particularly for the stomach, esophagus, and colon, but the risk is low. The National Cancer Institute advises consuming these foods in moderation. |
| **Emulsifiers,** such as mono-glycerides and lecithins | Suspend fat in water to improve uniformity, smoothness, and body of foods, such as baked goods, ice cream, and mayonnaise | No known health risks when used properly |
| **Fat replacements,** such as Paselli SA2, Dur-Low, Oatrim, Sta-Slim 143, Stellar, and Olean | Limit calorie content of foods by reducing some of the fat content | Generally no known health risks when used properly |
| **Flavor and flavoring agents** (such as natural and artificial flavors), sugar, and corn syrup | Impart more or improve flavor of foods | Sugar and corn syrup can increase risk for dental caries. Generally no known health risks for flavoring agents when used properly. |
| **Flavor enhancers,** such as monosodium glutamate (MSG) and salt | Help bring out the natural flavor of foods, such as meats | Some people (especially infants) are sensitive to the glutamate portion of MSG and after exposure experience flushing, chest pain, facial pressure, dizziness, sweating, rapid heart rate, nausea, vomiting, increase in blood pressure, and headache. Those so affected should look for the word glutamate on food labels, as well as isolated protein, yeast extract, bullion, and soup stock. Salt increases the risk of developing hypertension, especially in some people. |
| **Humectants,** such as glycerol, propylene glycol, and sorbitol | Retain more moisture, texture, and fresh flavor in foods such as candies, shredded coconut, and marshmallows | No known health risk when used properly |
| **Leavening agents,** such as yeast, baking powder, and baking soda | Introduce carbon dioxide into food products | No known health risk when used properly |
| **Maturing and bleaching agents,** such as bromates, peroxides, and ammonium chloride | Shorten the time needed for maturation of flour to become usable for baking products | No known health risk when used properly |
| **Nutrient supplements,** such as vitamin A, vitamin D, and potassium iodide | Enhance the nutrient content of foods such as margarine, milk, and ready-to-eat breakfast cereals | No known health risk if intake from such supplemental sources combined with other natural food sources of a nutrient does not exceed the Upper Level set for a particular nutrient (iron may be one exception; review Chapter 9) |

▲ Emulsifiers improve the texture of foods such as ice cream, baked goods, and cookies.

## CRITICAL THINKING

Recognizing that Joseph is taking a nutrition class, his roommate asks him, "What is more risky: the bacteria that can be present in food or the additives listed on the label of my favorite snack cake?" How should Joseph respond? On what information should he base his conclusions?

**TABLE 13-6** *(continued)*

| Food Additive Class | Attributes | Health Risks |
|---|---|---|
| **Stabilizers and thickeners,** such as pectins, gums, gelatins, and agars | Impart a smooth texture and uniform color and flavor to candies, ice cream and other frozen desserts, chocolate milk, and beverages containing alternative sweeteners. Prevent evaporation and deterioration of flavorings used in cakes, puddings, and gelatin mixes | No known health risk when used properly |
| **Sequestrants,** such as EDTA and citric acid | Bind free ions, helping preserve food quality by reducing ability of ions to cause rancidity in products containing fat | No known health risk when used properly |

## Intentional versus Incidental Food Additives

Food additives are classified into two types: **intentional food additives** (directly added to foods) and **incidental food additives** (indirectly added as contaminants). Both types of agents are regulated by FDA in the United States. Currently, more than 2800 different substances are intentionally added to foods. As many as 10,000 other substances enter foods as contaminants. This includes substances that may reasonably be expected to enter food through surface contact with processing equipment or packaging materials.

## The GRAS List

In 1958, all food additives used in the United States and considered safe at that time were put on a **generally recognized as safe (GRAS)** list. The U.S. Congress established the GRAS list because it believed manufacturers did not need to prove the safety of substances that had been used for a long time and were already generally recognized as safe. Since that time, FDA has been responsible for proving that a substance does not belong on the GRAS list. Substances may be added to the GRAS list if data and information about the use of the substance are known and accepted widely by qualified experts, and establish that the substance is safe under the conditions of its intended use.

Since 1958, some substances on the list have been reviewed. A few, such as cyclamates, failed the review process and were removed from the list. The additive red dye #3 was removed because it is linked to cancer. Many chemicals on the GRAS list have not yet been rigorously tested, primarily because of expense. These chemicals have received a low priority for testing, mostly because they have long histories of use without evidence of toxicity or because their chemical characteristics do not suggest they are potential health hazards.

## Are Synthetic Chemicals Always Harmful?

Nothing about a natural product makes it inherently safer than a synthetic product. Many synthetic products are laboratory copies of chemicals that also occur in nature (see the discussion in Chapter 12 on biotechnology for some examples). Moreover, although human endeavors contribute some toxins to foods, such as synthetic pesticides and industrial chemicals, nature's poisons are often even more potent and

**intentional food additives** Additives knowingly (directly) incorporated into food products by manufacturers.

**incidental food additives** Additives that appear in food products indirectly, from environmental contamination of food ingredients or during the manufacturing process.

**generally recognized as safe (GRAS)** A list of food additives that in 1958 were considered safe for consumption. Manufacturers were allowed to continue to use these additives, without special clearance, when needed for food products. FDA bears responsibility for proving they are not safe, but can remove unsafe products from the list.

**S**ome important definitions:

| | |
|---|---|
| toxicology | Scientific study of harmful substances |
| safety | Relative certainty that a substance won't cause injury |
| hazard | Chance that injury will result from use of a substance |
| toxicity | Capacity of a substance to produce injury or illness at some dosage |

▲ Color additives make some foods more desirable.

**T**he 100-fold margin of safety is 25 times less than that for vitamin A, when you compare the RDA for healthy women (700 micrograms) to a potentially harmful dose of vitamin A for pregnant women (3000 micrograms).

**Delaney Clause** A clause to the 1958 Food Additives Amendment of the Pure Food and Drug Act in the United States that prevents the intentional (direct) addition to foods of a compound shown to cause cancer in laboratory animals or humans.

widespread. Some cancer researchers suggest that we ingest at least 10,000 times more (by weight) natural toxins produced by plants than we do synthetic pesticide residues. (Plants produce these toxins to protect themselves from predators and disease-causing organisms.) This comparison does not make synthetic chemicals any less toxic, but it does put them in a more accurate perspective.

Consider vitamin E, often added to food to prevent rancidity of fats. This chemical is safe when used within certain limits. However, high doses have been associated with health problems, such as interfering with vitamin K activity in the body (review Chapter 8). Thus, even well-known chemicals we are comfortable using can be toxic in some circumstances and at some concentrations.

## Tests of Food Additives for Safety

Food additives are tested by FDA for safety on at least two animal species, usually rats and mice. Scientists determine the highest dose of the additive that produces *no observable effects* in the animals. These doses are proportionately much higher than humans are ever exposed to. The maximum dosage that produced no observable effects is then divided by at least 100 to establish a margin of safety for human use. This 100-fold margin is used because it is assumed that we are at least 10 times more sensitive to food additives than are laboratory animals and that any one person might be 10 times more sensitive than another. This broad margin essentially ensures that the food additive in question will cause no harmful health effects in humans. In fact, many synthetic chemicals are probably less dangerous at these low doses than some of the natural compounds in common foods such as apples or celery.

One important exception applies to the schema for testing intentional food additives: If an additive is shown to cause cancer, even though only in high doses, no margin of safety is allowed. The food additive cannot be used, because it would violate the **Delaney Clause** in the 1958 Food Additives Amendment. This clause prohibits intentionally adding to foods a compound introduced after 1958 and that causes cancer at any level of exposure. Evidence for cancer could come from either laboratory animal or human studies. Few exceptions to this clause are allowed; exceptions are discussed regarding curing and pickling agents in Table 13-6.

Incidental food additives are another matter. FDA cannot ban various industrial chemicals, pesticide residues, and mold toxins from foods, even though some of these contaminants can cause cancer. These products are not purposely added to foods. FDA sets an acceptable level for these substances. An incidental substance found in a food cannot contribute to more than one cancer case during the lifetimes of 1 million people. If a higher risk exists, the amount of the compound in a food must be reduced until the guideline is met.

In general, if you consume a variety of foods in moderation, the chances of food additives jeopardizing your health are minimal. Pay attention to your body. If you suspect an intolerance or a sensitivity, consult your physician for further evaluation. Remember that in the short run, you are more likely to suffer either from foodborne illness due to poor food-handling practices that allow viral and bacterial contamination in food, or from the consumption of raw animal foods, than from consuming additives. Excess calories, saturated fat, cholesterol, *trans* fat, salt, and other potential "problem" nutrients in our diets pose the greatest long-term health risk.

## Approval for a New Food Additive

Before a new food additive can be added to foods, FDA must approve its use. Besides rigorously testing an additive to establish its safety margins, manufacturers must give FDA information that (1) identifies the new additive, (2) gives its chemical composition, (3) states how it is manufactured, and (4) specifies laboratory methods used to measure its presence in the food supply at the amount of intended use.

Manufacturers must also offer proof that the additive will accomplish its intended purpose in a food, that it is safe, and that it is to be used in no higher amount than needed. Additives cannot be used to hide defective food ingredients, such as rancid oils; to deceive customers; or replace good manufacturing practices. A manufacturer must establish that the ingredient is necessary for producing a specific food product.

## MAKING DECISIONS

### Processed or Whole Foods?

If you are bewildered or concerned about all the additives in your diet, you can easily avoid most of them by consuming unprocessed whole foods. However, no evidence shows that this will necessarily make you healthier, nor can you avoid all additives, because some are used even on whole foods, such as with pesticides. It amounts to a personal decision. Do you have confidence that FDA and food manufacturers are adequately protecting your health and welfare, or do you want to take more personal control by minimizing your intake of compounds not naturally found in foods?

## CONCEPT CHECK

Food additives are used to reduce spoilage from microbial growth, oxygen, metals, and other compounds. Additives are also used to adjust acidity, improve flavor and color, leaven, provide nutritional fortification, thicken, and emulsify food components. Additives are classified as intentional (direct; purposely added to foods), and incidental (indirect; present in foods from environmental contamination or various manufacturing practices). The amount of an additive allowed in a food is limited to one-one-hundredth of the highest amount that has no observable effect when fed to animals. The Delaney Clause allows FDA to limit intentional addition of cancer-causing compounds to food in the United States under its jurisdiction. Also set by law in the United States are the permissible amounts of carcinogens that incidentally enter foods.

▲ Depending on whether you choose fresh versus processed foods, a diet can be either essentially free of or contain food additives. For most of us, this specific concern regarding food choice is not worth worrying about.

## 13.5 Substances that Occur Naturally in Foods and Can Cause Illness

Foods contain a variety of naturally occurring substances that can cause illness. Here are some of the more important examples:

- *Safrole*—found in sassafras, mace, and nutmeg; causes cancer when consumed in high doses
- *Solanine*—found in potato shoots and green spots on potato skins; inhibits the action of neurotransmitters
- *Mushroom toxins*—found in some species of mushrooms such as aminita; can cause stomach upset, dizziness, hallucinations, and other neurological symptoms. The more lethal varieties can cause liver and kidney failure, coma, and even death. FDA regulates commercially grown and harvested mushrooms. These are cultivated in concrete buildings or caves. However, there are no systematic controls on individual gatherers harvesting wild species, except in Illinois and Michigan.
- *Avidin*—found in raw egg whites (cooking destroys avidin); binds the vitamin biotin in a way that prevents its absorption, so a biotin deficiency may ultimately develop over the long term
- *Thiaminase*—found in raw fish, clams, and mussels; destroys the vitamin thiamin
- *Tetrodotoxin*—found in puffer fish; causes respiratory paralysis
- *Oxalic acid*—found in spinach, strawberries, sesame seeds, and other foods; binds calcium and iron in the foods, and so limits absorption of these nutrients
- *Herbal teas* containing senna or comfrey—can cause diarrhea and liver damage

▲ When hunting wild mushrooms, know what you are looking for. Many varieties contain deadly toxins.

People have coexisted for centuries with these naturally occurring substances and have learned to avoid some of them and limit intake of others. They pose little health risk. Farmers know potatoes must be stored in the dark, so that solanine won't be synthesized. Furthermore, we've developed cooking and food-preparation methods to limit the potency of other substances, such as thiaminase. Spices are used in such small amounts that health risks don't result. Nevertheless, it's important to understand that some potentially harmful chemicals in foods occur naturally.

## Is Caffeine a Cause for Concern?

Why all the controversy over a cup of coffee? Researchers have spent a great deal of time on the study of caffeine, the substance of greatest concern in the favorite beverage of many of us. So why do caffeine recommendations change from year to year?

Caffeine is a stimulant found as a natural or added ingredient in many beverages and chocolate. On average, we consume 75% of our caffeine intake as coffee, 15% as tea, 10% as soft drinks, and 2% as chocolate (Table 13-7). (For teenagers and young adults this ratio is often relatively higher for soft drinks and lower for coffee.)

Caffeine is not often consumed by itself. With the popularity of trendy coffee shops that serve everything from mocha java to flavored lattes, it is difficult to separate caffeine intake from cream, sugar, alternative sweeteners, and flavorings. So what is the conscientious coffee drinker to think? Let's explore the myths and facts of caffeine intake.

Caffeine does not accumulate in the body and is normally excreted within several hours following consumption. Caffeine can cause anxiety, increased heart rate, insomnia, increased urination (possibly resulting in dehydration), diarrhea, and gastrointestinal upset in high doses. In addition, those already suffering from ulcers may experience irritation due to increased acid production; those who have anxiety

**TABLE 13-7** Caffeine Content of Common Sources

| Item | Milligrams of Caffeine | |
| --- | --- | --- |
| | Typical | Range* |
| **Coffee** (8 fl oz) | | |
| Brewed, drip method | 85 | 65–120 |
| Brewed, percolator | 75 | 60–85 |
| Decaffeinated, brewed | 3 | 2–4 |
| Espresso (1 fl oz serving) | 40 | 30–50 |
| **Teas** (8 fl oz) | | |
| Brewed, Black tea | 40 | 20–90 |
| Brewed, Green tea | 20 | 8–30 |
| Iced | 25 | 9–50 |
| Instant | 28 | 24–31 |
| **Some soft drinks** (8 fl oz) | 24 | 20–40 |
| **"Energy drinks" such as Red Bull** (8.3 fl oz) | 80 | 0–80 |
| **Cocoa beverage** (8 fl oz) | 6 | 3–32 |
| **Chocolate milk beverage** (8 fl oz) | 5 | 2–7 |
| **Milk chocolate** (1 oz) | 6 | 1–15 |
| **Dark chocolate, semi-sweet** (1 oz) | 20 | 5–35 |
| **Baker's chocolate** (1 oz) | 26 | 26 |
| **Chocolate-flavored syrup** (1 fl oz) | 4 | 4 |

*For the coffee and tea products, the range varies due to brewing method, plant variety, brand of product, and so on.

Source: International Food Information Council. *Caffeine and women's health*, August 2002.

or panic attacks may find that caffeine worsens their symptoms; and those prone to heartburn may find that caffeine worsens this symptom because it relaxes sphincter muscles in the esophagus. Some people need little caffeine to feel such effects, and the dosage for children is likely even lower than that for adults.

Withdrawal symptoms are also real. Former coffee drinkers may experience headache, nausea, and depression for a short time after discontinuing use. These symptoms can be expected to peak at 20 to 48 hours following the last intake of caffeine. Symptoms hold true even for those trying to quit as little as one cup of coffee per day. Slow tapering of use over a few days is recommended to avoid these problems.

Are there more serious consequences of consuming caffeine regularly? It has been hypothesized that caffeine consumption can lead to certain types of cancer, such as pancreatic and bladder cancers. The association of caffeine with cancer has not been supported in recent literature. In fact, regular coffee consumption has been linked to a decreased risk of colon cancer.

Negative press has dwindled with regard to a link between cardiovascular disease and moderate coffee consumption. Heavy use does increase blood pressure for a short period of time. Coffee consumption also has been linked to increased LDL-cholesterol and triglycerides in the blood. This association was found to be caused by cafestol and kahweol, two oils in ground coffee. However, filtered and instant coffees do not contain the harmful oils. It is prudent, though, to limit the amount of coffee in general, especially from French coffee presses and from espresso as these beverages are not filtered.

Women are thought to be at higher risk for a variety of deleterious effects with caffeine consumption, including miscarriages, osteoporosis, and birth defects in their offspring. It is true that heavy caffeine use mildly increases the amount of calcium excreted in urine. For this reason, it is important that heavy coffee drinkers check their diets for adequate calcium sources. Some studies do show a higher likelihood for miscarriages in women consuming more than 500 milligrams of caffeine per day (about five 8 ounce cups of coffee). FDA warns women to consume caffeine in moderation (no more than the equivalent of one to two 8 ounce cups of coffee per day).

In contrast to these possibly harmful effects of caffeine consumption, many people are convinced of the benefits of a "cup of joe." Though some women testify to the idea that caffeine improves premenstrual symptoms, no study proves this theory. Some weight-loss drugs previously contained caffeine, under the assumption that it made the drugs more effective. FDA has since banned this use as it was found to be ineffective. Some newer research findings suggest caffeine may reduce the risk of developing headaches, cirrhosis of the liver, some forms of kidney stones, gallbladder stones, some nerve-related diseases, and furthermore, that it aids in blood glucose regulation. You may have heard that caffeine can improve physical performance. This has been shown in highly trained athletes; recall that use of large amounts of caffeine is banned by the NCAA (review Chapter 10). For those below professional status, though, no benefit has been shown. Also keep in mind that coffee will not "sober up" a person who is drunk.

Though the debate over caffeine will likely continue as long as North Americans drink coffee, research does not support many of the concepts previously thought of as fact. These studies are reinforcing the idea of moderation—the equivalent of about two to three 8 ounce cups of coffee per day. A prudent dose of caffeine is 200 to 300 milligrams per day. Review Table 13-7 concerning the caffeine content of typical sources.

▲ Coffee is a common source of caffeine for many adults.

## 13.6 Environmental Contaminants in Food

A variety of environmental contaminants can be found in foods. Aside from pesticide residues, other potential contaminants that deserve attention are listed in Table 13-8. To reduce exposure to environmental toxins present in our foods that cause disease, find out which foods pose a risk. In addition, emphasize variety and moderation in food selection. Tips provided in Tables 13-8 and 13-9 also apply to reducing exposure to environmental contaminants.

**G**enetic alteration of foods such as corn and soybeans has created concern, especially in Europe. FDA considers genetically altered products safe if approval for human use has been granted (see Chapter 12 for details).

**TABLE 13-8** Potential Environmental and Other Contaminants in Our Food Supply

| Chemical Substance | Sources | Toxic Effects | Preventive Measures |
|---|---|---|---|
| Acrylamide | Fried foods rich in carbohydrate cooked at high temperatures for extended periods, such as French fries and potato chips | Potential neurotoxin and carcinogen. Known carcinogen for laboratory animals; however, studies have not clearly proven the relationship between acrylamide ingestion and the development of cancer in humans. | Limit intake of deep-fat fried foods rich in carbohydrate. |
| Cadmium | Plants in general if much cadmium is in the soil<br><br>Clams, shellfish, tobacco smoke<br><br>Occupational exposure in some cases | Kidney disease<br><br>Liver disease<br><br>Prostate cancer (debatable)<br><br>Bone deformities<br><br>Lung disease (when inhaled) | Consume a wide variety of foods, including seafood sources. |
| Dioxin | Trash-burning incinerators<br><br>Bottom-feeding fish from the Great Lakes<br><br>Animal fats from animals exposed to such contamination via water or soil | Abnormal reproduction and fetal/infant development<br><br>Immune suppression<br><br>Cancer (to date only clearly shown in laboratory animals) | Pay attention to warnings of dioxin risks from local fish; if risk exists, limit intake as suggested on the fishing license.<br><br>Consume a variety of fish from local waters rather than mostly one specific species. |
| Lead | Lead-based paint chips and related dust in older homes<br><br>Occupational exposure (e.g., radiator repair)<br><br>Lead caps on wine bottles<br><br>Fruit juices and pickled vegetables stored in galvanized or tin containers or leaded glass<br><br>Some types of solder used in joining copper pipes (mostly in older homes)<br><br>Mexican pottery dishes<br><br>Koo Soo herbal remedies<br><br>Leaded glass containers | Anemia<br><br>Kidney disease<br><br>Nervous system damage (tiredness and changes in behavior are symptoms)<br><br>Reduced learning capacity in childhood (even from mild lead exposure) | Avoid paint chips and related dust in older homes; regular cleaning of these homes is also important (see **www.nud. gov/offices/lead**).<br><br>Meet iron and calcium needs to reduce lead absorption.<br><br>Wipe the inside and outside neck of wine bottles before use if the bottle has a lead cap.<br><br>Store fruit juices and pickled vegetables in glass or plastic or waxed paper containers.<br><br>Let water run 1 minute or so if off for more than 2 hours, and use only cold water for cooking; do not soften drinking water.<br><br>Do not store alcoholic beverages in leaded glass containers. |
| Mercury | Swordfish, shark, king mackerel, and tilefish. Fresh and canned albacore tuna also is a possible source. (In contrast, the more typical light chunk tuna is very low in mercury.) | Reduced fetal/child development and birth defects; toxic to nervous system | Consume these sources no more than once per week, no more than two times per week for albacore tuna. Pregnant women should avoid these species of fish, but some albacore tuna consumption is fine. Two to three fish meals per week is appropriate for pregnant (and nursing) women if different types of fish are eaten. |
| Polychlorinated biphenyls (PCBs) | Fish from the Great Lakes and Hudson River Valley (e.g., coho salmon)<br><br>Farmed salmon are a possible source, but less so | Cancer (to date only clearly shown in laboratory animals), as well as a potential for liver, immune, and reproductive disorders | Pay attention to warnings of PCB contamination from local fish; if risk exists, limit intake as suggested on the fishing license or on state advisories. Vary the type of fish eaten during a specific week. |
| Urethane | Alcoholic beverages such as sherry, bourbon, sake, and fruit brandies | Cancer (to date only clearly shown in laboratory animals) | Avoid generous amounts of typical sources. |

## Pesticides in Food

Pesticides used in food production produce both beneficial and unwanted effects. Most health authorities believe that the benefits outweigh the risks. Pesticides help ensure a safe and adequate food supply and help make foods available at reasonable cost. However, there is sentiment nationwide that pesticides pose avoidable health risks. Consumers have come to assume that synthetic is dangerous and organic is safe. Some researchers believe this sentiment is grounded in fear and fueled by unbalanced reports. Other researchers say concern about pesticides is valid and overdue.

Most concern about pesticide residues in food appropriately focuses on chronic rather than acute toxicity because the amounts of residue present, if any, are extremely small. These low concentrations found in foods are not known to produce adverse effects in the short term, although harm has been caused by the high amounts that occasionally result from accidents or misuse. For humans, pesticides pose a danger mainly in their cumulative effects, so their threats to health are difficult to determine. However, growing evidence, including the problems of the contamination of underground water supplies and destruction of wildlife habitats, indicates that North Americans would probably be better off if we could reduce our use of pesticides. Both the U.S. federal government and many farmers are working toward that end. Chapter 12 discussed the lastest use of biotechnology to reduce pesticide use.

## What Is a Pesticide?

Federal law defines a pesticide as any substance or mixture of substances intended to prevent, destroy, repel, or mitigate any pest. The built-in toxic properties of pesticides lead to the possibility that other, nontarget organisms, including humans, might also be harmed. The term *pesticide* tends to be used as a generic reference to many types of products, including insecticides, herbicides, fungicides, and rodenticides. A pesticide product may be chemical or bacterial, natural or synthetic. For agriculture, EPA allows about 10,000 pesticides to be used, containing some 300 active ingredients. About 1.2 billion pounds of pesticides are used each year in the United States, much of which is applied to agricultural crops.

Once a pesticide is applied, it can turn up in a number of unintended and unwanted places. It may be carried in the air and dust by wind currents, remain in soil attached to soil particles, be taken up by organisms in the soil, decompose to other compounds, be taken up by plant roots, enter groundwater, or invade aquatic habitats. Each is a route to the food chain; some are more direct than others.

## Why Use Pesticides?

In the United States, pests destroy nearly $20 billion of food crops yearly, despite extensive pesticide use. The primary reason for using pesticides is economic—the use of agricultural chemicals increases production and lowers the cost of food, at least in the short run. Many farmers believe that it would be impossible to stay in business without pesticides, which help protect farmers from ruinous losses.

Consumer demands also have changed over the years. At one time, we wouldn't have thought twice about buying an apple with a worm hole; we took it home, cut out

One of the problems with pesticides is that they create new pests because they destroy the predators (spiders, wasps, and beetles) that naturally keep most plantfeeding insect populations in check. The brown plant hopper, which has plagued Indonesian rice fields, was not a serious problem before heavy pesticide use began to kill its predators in the early 1970s. In the United States, such major pests as spider mites and the cotton bollworm were merely nuisances until pesticides decimated their predators.

▲ Pesticide use poses a risk-versus-benefit question. Each side has points that deserve to be considered. Rural communities, where exposure is more direct, experience the greatest short-term risk.

the wormy part, and ate the apple. Today, consumers find worm holes less acceptable, so farmers rely more on pesticides to produce cosmetically attractive fruits and vegetables. On the practical side, pesticides can protect against the rotting and decay of fresh fruits and vegetables. This is helpful because our food distribution system doesn't usually permit consumer purchase within hours of harvest. Also, food grown without pesticides can contain naturally occurring organisms that produce carcinogens at concentrations far above current standards for pesticide residues. For example, fungicides help prevent the carcinogen aflatoxin (caused by growth of a fungus) from forming on some crops. Thus, although some pesticides may do little more than improve the appearance of food products, others help keep foods fresher and safer to eat.

### Regulation of Pesticides

The responsibility for ensuring that residues of pesticides in foods are below amounts that pose a danger to health is shared by FDA, EPA, and the Food Safety and Inspection Service of USDA in the United States. Table 13-2 listed the roles of various food protection agencies. FDA is responsible for enforcing pesticide tolerances in all foods except meat, poultry, and certain egg products, which are monitored by USDA. A newly proposed pesticide is exhaustively tested, perhaps over 10 years or more, before it is approved for use. EPA must decide that the pesticide causes no unreasonable adverse effects on people and the environment and that benefits of use outweigh the risks of using it. However, there is concern about older chemicals registered before 1970, when less stringent testing conditions were permitted. EPA is now asking chemical companies to retest the old compounds using more rigorous tests. Unfortunately, inadequate funding at EPA has hampered the review of older pesticides. The slow pace of this retesting has angered the critics of pesticide use. When weighing whether to approve or cancel a pesticide, EPA considers how much more it would cost the farmer to use an alternative pesticide or process and whether cancellation would decrease productivity. After determining the dollar cost to the farmer, EPA then looks at costs to processors and consumers. Once a pesticide is approved for use, it must follow the margin of safety provisions required of food additives (see previous section, " Tests of Food Additives for Safety").

### How Safe Are Pesticides?

Dangers from exposure to pesticides through food depend on how potent the chemical toxin is, how concentrated it is in the food, how much and how frequently it's eaten, and the consumer's resistance or susceptibility to the substance. Accumulating information links pesticide use to increased cancer rates in farm communities. For rural counties in the United States, the incidence of lymph, genital, brain, and digestive tract cancers increases with higher-than-average pesticide use. Respiratory cancer cases increase with greater insecticide use. In tests using laboratory animals, scientists have found that some of the chemicals present in pesticide residues cause birth defects, sterility, tumors, organ damage, and injury to the central nervous system. Some pesticides persist in the environment for years.

Still, some researchers argue that the cancer risk from pesticide residues is hundreds of times less than the risk from eating such common foods as peanut butter, brown mustard, and basil. Plants manufacture toxic substances to defend themselves against insects, birds, and grazing animals (including humans). When plants are stressed or damaged, they produce even more of these toxins. Because of this, many foods contain naturally occurring chemicals considered toxic, and some are even carcinogenic. Other scientists argue that if natural carcinogens are already in the food supply, then we should reduce the number of added carcinogens whenever possible. In other words, we should do what we can to decrease our overall exposure.

### Tests of the Amounts of Pesticides in Foods

FDA tests thousands of raw products each year for pesticide residues. (A pesticide is considered illegal in this case if it is not approved for use on the crop in question or

▲ Fruits and vegetables grown without use of pesticides are available and may bear an "organic" label (see Table 2-10 for rules regarding the use of the term "organic" on food labels). These products generally are more expensive than those grown using pesticides. Consumers need to decide if the potential benefits of the products are worth the extra cost.

if the amount used exceeds the allowed tolerance.) The latest FDA studies show no residues in about 60% of samples. Less than 1% of domestic and about 3% of import samples have residues continually over tolerance. These findings continue to support previous FDA studies over the past 10 years that pesticide residues in food are generally well below EPA tolerances, and they confirm the safety of the food supply relative to pesticide residues.

## Personal Action

We often take risks in our lives, but we prefer to have a choice in the matter after weighing the pros and cons. With regard to pesticides in food, however, someone else is deciding what is acceptable and what is not. Our only choice is whether to buy or avoid pesticide-containing foods. In reality, it's almost impossible to avoid pesticides entirely, because even organic produce often contains traces of pesticides, probably as the result of cross-contamination from nearby farms.

Short-term studies of the effects of pesticides on laboratory animals cannot precisely pinpoint long-term cancer risks in humans. It should be clearly understood, however, that the presence of minute traces of an environmental chemical in a food does not mean that any adverse effect will result from eating that food.

FDA and other scientific organizations believe that the hazards are comparatively low and in the short run are less dangerous than the hazards of foodborne illness created in our kitchens. We cannot avoid pesticide risks entirely, but we can limit exposure by following some simple advice (Table 13-9).

We can also encourage farmers to use fewer pesticides to reduce exposure to our foods and water supplies, but we'll have to settle for produce that isn't perfect in appearance or that has been grown with the aid of biotechnology (again, see Chapter 12 for details). Are you concerned enough about pesticides on food to change your shopping habits or take more political action?

## 13.7 Food Production Choices

Agriculture, the production of food and livestock, has supplied humans with food for millennia. At one time, nearly everyone was involved in food production. Only about 1 in 3 people around the globe and far fewer in the U.S. (less than 1%), is now involved in farming. Today, numerous advances in agricultural sciences are affecting our food supply; of particular note are organic food production and sustainable agriculture.

▲ FDA's yearly evaluation of a "market basket" of typical foods shows that pesticide content is minimal in most foods.

▲ Wash fresh fruits and vegetables under running water to remove bacteria and soil. Special antibacterial washing products are not necessary.

**TABLE 13-9** What You Can Do to Reduce Exposure to Pesticides

FDA's sampling and testing show that pesticide residues in foods do not pose a health hazard. Nevertheless, if you want to reduce dietary exposure to pesticides, follow this advice from the Environmental Protection Agency:

- Consume a wide variety of foods, especially regarding fruits, vegetables, and fish.
- Thoroughly rinse and scrub (with a brush if possible) fruits and vegetables. Peel them, if appropriate—although some nutrients will be peeled away.
- Remove the outer leaves of leafy vegetables, such as lettuce and cabbage.
- Residues of some pesticides in animal feed concentrate in the animals' fat, so trim fat from meat, poultry, and fish; remove skin (which contains most of the fat) from poultry and fish; and discard fats and oils in broths and pan drippings.
- When fishing, throw back the big fish—the little ones have had less time to take up and concentrate pesticides and other harmful residues. In addition, pay attention to any warnings by local authorities (and on the fishing license) about the high risk for contamination in specific waters or species of fish.
- Avoid lawns, gardens, and flower beds that have recently been treated with pesticides and herbicides.

Adapted from Food and Drug Administration: Safety first: Protecting America's food supply, *FDA Consumer,* p. 26, November 1988.

▲ The USDA organic seal identifies organic foods grown on USDA-certified organic farms.

## Organic Foods

Organic foods are increasingly available in supermarkets, specialty stores, farmers' markets, and restaurants. Consumers can select organic fruits, vegetables, grains, dairy products, meats, eggs, and many processed foods, including sauces and condiments, breakfast cereals, cookies, and snack chips. Interest in personal and environmental health has contributed to the increasing availability and sales of organic foods. According to the Organic Trade Association, U.S. sales of organic foods reached $22.9 billion by the end of 2008. This was a 15.8% increase over 2007 sales, despite tough economic times. Despite this rapid growth, less than 3.5% of foods sold are organic. Organic foods, because they often cost more to grow and produce, are typically more expensive than comparable conventional foods.

The term **organic** refers to the way agricultural products are produced. Organic production relies on farming practices such as **biological pest management,** composting, manure applications, and crop rotation to maintain healthy soil, water, crops, and animals. Synthetic pesticides, fertilizers, and hormones; antibiotics; sewage sludge (used as fertilizer); genetic engineering; and irradiation are not permitted in the production of organic foods. Additionally, organic meat, poultry, eggs, and dairy products must come from animals allowed to graze outdoors and are fed only organic feed.

The Organic Foods Production Act of 1990 established standards for the production of foods that bear the USDA organic seal. Foods labeled and marketed as organic must be grown on farms that are certified by the USDA as following all of the rules established in the 1990 act. Foods made from multiple ingredients (e.g., breakfast cereal) labeled as organic must have at least 95% of their ingredients (by weight) meet organic standards. The term "made with organic" can be used if at least 70% of the ingredients are organic. Small organic producers and farmers with sales less than $5000 per year are exempt from the certification regulation. Some farmers use organic production methods but choose not to be USDA certified. Their foods cannot be labeled as organic, but many of these farmers market and sell to those seeking organic foods.

The organic food market received a boost in 2009 when USDA offered $50 million in new funding to encourage greater production of organic food in the United States. The Organic Trade Association (http://www.ota.com/index.html) believes that this funding will further encourage farmers to use organic practices and help increase the U.S. production of organic food to meet growing consumer demand. With tough economic times, consumers have used various strategies in continuing to buy organic products. Because most stores now offer organic products, consumers have the opportunity to shop around. Increased availability and use of coupons, the proliferation of private label and store brands, and better value products offered by major organic brands all have contributed to increased sales.

**Organic Foods and Health** Consumers may choose to eat organic foods to reduce their pesticide intake, to protect the environment, and to improve the nutritional quality of their diets. Those who consume organic produce do ingest lesser amounts of pesticides (only 1 in 4 organically grown fruits and vegetables contains pesticides and in lower amounts than conventional produce), but it's still not known whether or how this affects the health of most consumers. However, organic foods may be a wise choice for young children because pesticide residues may pose a greater risk to them. Consumers also may opt for organic foods to encourage environmentally friendly **sustainable agriculture** practices.

Most studies do not show that organic foods have higher amounts of vitamins and minerals. However, researchers have found that, in some cases, organic fruits and vegetables contain more vitamin C and antioxidants that help protect cells against

**biological pest management** Control of agricultural pests by using natural predators, parasites, or pathogens. For example, ladybugs can be used to control an aphid infestation.

**sustainable agriculture** Agricultural system that provides a secure living for farm families; maintains the natural environment and resources; supports the rural community; and offers respect and fair treatment to all involved, from farm workers to consumers to the animals raised for food.

damage. At this point, it's not possible to recommend organic foods over conventional foods based on nutrient content—both can meet nutritional needs. A healthy dose of common sense also is important—an "organic" label does not change a less healthy food into a more healthy food. Organic potato chips have the same calorie and fat content as conventional potato chips.

One concern raised about organic foods is that food safety may be jeopardized because animal manures used for fertilizers might cause more pathogen contamination of food. However, research does not show that certified organic food has higher contamination with bacterial pathogens. Consumers should wash or scrub all produce—organic as well as conventional—under running water.

The term "natural" is not regulated. Products labeled as "natural" are generally those derived from natural ingredients, such as a plant source, which retain their natural properties in the finished product. Meat or poultry labeled "natural" must be minimally processed, and contain no artificial flavoring, coloring, chemical preservative, or other artificial or synthetic ingredient. No one is really checking these products, and there is some debate over what constitutes "minimally processed." Although all organic products fit this definition of natural, not all natural products are necessarily organic.

## Sustainable Agriculture

Conventional agriculture focuses on maximizing production through the use of large acreages, powerful machines, chemicals to control pests, and petroleum-based fertilizers to boost growth. In contrast, sustainable agriculture is an integrated system of plant and animal production that will, over the long-term, satisfy human food needs, enhance environmental quality, efficiently use nonrenewable resources, sustain the economic viability of farm operations, and enhance the quality of life for farmers and society as a whole. A culture of sustainability has emerged, including a clear trend for sustainable food choices manufactured in an environmentally responsible way. The food industry has responded with a move toward "green" initiatives that should be sustainable for the long-term. A new demographic term, LOHAS (Lifestyle of Health and Sustainability), describes a growing demographic group focused on sustainable living. An increasing number of today's college students are joining this market segment and developing behaviors associated with social responsibility. These consumers are driving changes in many areas, including the food industry. Slow Food Nation is an example of a non-profit group dedicated to creating a framework for a deeper environmental connection to our food and aiming to inspire and empower Americans to build a food system that is sustainable, healthy, and delicious.

## Locally Grown Foods

With people everywhere more interested in the origins of their food, more grocery store shelves are devoted to "locally grown" products. Consumers are demanding increased transparency with the food supply, and local food helps answer questions about where food comes from and how it was grown. Retailers are using the "locally grown" label to respond to consumer desires for fresh, safe products that also support small, local farmers and help the environment. Local products provide fresher options, do not have the added costs of long transportation, and thus, use less fossil fuel. Foodservice establishments are giving greater emphasis to local producers, focusing on where food was grown and how it was handled.

The interest in "local" foods has become such a phenomenon that the term "locavore" was the 2007 Word of the Year in the New Oxford American Dictionary. **Locavore** is defined as someone who eats food grown or produced locally or within a certain radius such as 50, 100, or 150 miles. The locavore movement has gained prominence due to food-safety concerns by consumers and the search for local, sustainable foods. It encourages consumers to buy from farmers' markets or even to

▲ The locavore movement is based on the assumption that local products are more nutritious and taste better and encourages consumers to buy from farmers' markets or even to produce their own food.

**locavore** Someone who eats food grown or produced locally or within a certain radius such as 50, 100, or 500 miles.

produce their own food, with the argument that fresh, local products are more nutritious and taste better.

There is no evidence, however, that locally grown products are safer. Although many small producers have good food-safety practices, they often lack the expensive food-safety audits more common among big producers. Food-safety auditors determine such things as whether or not there is evidence of insects on produce and whether or not producers have enough bathrooms for workers. In addition, undetected foodborne illness outbreaks are more likely with "local" products delivered in small quantities and sold in a small area. Local products are not necessarily pesticide-free and may not be cheaper, given that smaller growers lack the economic advantages of bigger growers.

Unlike organic products, there are no regulations specifying the meaning of "locally grown." Whole Foods Market, Inc. is the biggest retailer of natural and organic food and probably the best-known for buying and selling locally grown produce. Whole Foods considers local to be anything produced within seven hours of one of its stores, with most local producers within 200 miles of a store. Wal-Mart, the world's largest retailer, has also become a large buyer of locally grown fruits and vegetables and considers anything local if it is grown in the same state as it is sold. Searchable databases and mapping resources such as MarketMaker (http://national.marketmaker.uiuc.edu/) are now available to connect growers with buyers, restaurants with distributors, and consumers with local farmers' markets. These tools make it easier for people to find and sell locally grown foods.

## Community Supported Agriculture

Consumers are not only taking comfort in knowing where their food comes from, but are also starting to have interest in community connections with local/regional farmers. Stemming from the interest in locally grown food, there is growing national support for local food collaboratives and community supported agriculture. Community Supported Agriculture programs (CSA) involve a partnership between local food producers and local consumers. During each growing season, CSA farmers offer a share of foods to individuals, families, or companies who have pledged support to the CSA either financially and/or by working for the CSA.

Another example of a farm-community partnership is the National Farm to School Program (http://www.farmtoschool.org/), a non-profit effort to connect farmers with nearby school cafeterias. Between 1997 and 2009, this program grew from only six local programs to 2,051 programs in 41 states resulting in 8,864 schools incorporating the local bounty into their menus. Administrators of the program have found that if kids can meet the farmer who actually grew the food, they are much more likely to eat it.

▲ Farmers participating in community supported agriculture (CSA) offer a share of foods from each growing season, to individuals, families or companies who support the CSA financially and/or by working for the CSA.

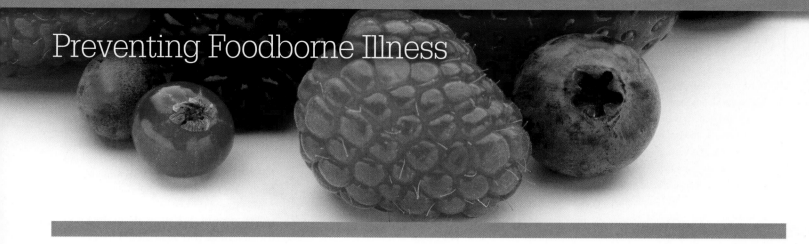

# Preventing Foodborne Illness

## General Rules for Preventing Foodborne Illness

You can greatly reduce the risk of food-borne illness by following some important rules. It's a long list, because many risky habits need to be addressed.

## Purchasing Food

- When shopping, select frozen foods and perishable foods, such as meat, poultry, or fish, last. Always have these products put in separate plastic bags, so that drippings don't contaminate other foods in the shopping cart. Don't let groceries sit in a warm car; this allows bacteria to grow. Get the perishable foods such as meat and egg and dairy products home and promptly refrigerate or freeze them.
- Don't buy or use food from damaged containers that leak, bulge, or are severely dented or from jars that are cracked or have loose or bulging lids. Don't taste or use food that has a foul odor or spurts liquid when the can is opened; the deadly *Clostridium botulinum* toxin may be present.
- Purchase only pasteurized milk and cheese (check the label). This is especially important for pregnant women because highly toxic bacteria and viruses that can harm the fetus thrive in unpasteurized milk.
- Purchase only the amount of produce needed for a week's time. The longer you keep fruits and vegetables, the more time is available for bacteria to grow.
- When purchasing precut produce or salads, avoid those that look slimy, brownish, or dry; these are signs of improper holding temperatures.

- Observe sell-by and expiration dates on food labels.

## Preparing Food

- Thoroughly wash your hands for 20 seconds with hot, soapy water before and after handling food. This practice is especially important when handling raw meat, fish, poultry, and eggs, after using the bathroom, after playing with pets, or after changing diapers.
- Make sure counters, cutting boards, dishes, and other equipment are thoroughly sanitized and rinsed before use. Be especially careful to use hot, soapy water to wash surfaces and equipment that have come in contact with raw meat, fish, poultry, and eggs as soon as possible to remove *Salmonella* bacteria that may be present. Otherwise, bacteria on the surfaces will infect the next foods that come in contact with the surface, a process called cross-contamination. In addition, replace sponges and wash kitchen towels frequently. (Microwaving sponges for 30 to 60 seconds also helps rid them of live bacteria.)
- If possible, cut foods to be eaten raw on a clean cutting board reserved for that purpose. Then clean this cutting board using hot, soapy water. If the same board must be used for both meat and other foods, cut any potentially contaminated items, such as meat, last. After cutting the meat, wash the cutting board thoroughly.

FDA recommends cutting boards with unmarred surfaces made of easy-to-clean, non-porous materials, such as plastic, marble, or glass. If you prefer a wooden board, make sure it is made of a nonabsorbent

hardwood, such as oak or maple, and has no obvious seams or cracks. Then reserve it for a specific purpose; for example, set it aside for cutting raw meat and poultry. Keep a separate wooden cutting board for chopping produce and slicing bread to prevent these products from picking up bacteria from raw meat. Many foods are served raw, so any bacteria clinging to them are not destroyed.

Furthermore, FDA recommends that all cutting boards be replaced when they become streaked with hard-to-clean grooves or cuts, which may harbor bacteria. In addition, cutting boards should be sanitized once a week in a dilute bleach solution. Flood the board with the solution, let it sit a few minutes, then rinse thoroughly.

- When thawing foods, do so in the refrigerator, under cold potable running water, or in a microwave oven. Also, cook foods immediately after thawing under cold water or in the microwave. Never let frozen foods thaw unrefrigerated all day or night. Also, marinate food in the refrigerator.
- Avoid coughing or sneezing over foods, even when you're healthy. Cover cuts on hands with a sterile bandage. This helps stop *Staphylococcus* from entering food.
- Carefully wash fresh fruit and vegetables under running water to remove dirt and bacteria clinging to the surface, using a vegetable brush if the skin is to

▶ Regularly cleaning surfaces and equipment with a dilute bleach solution (1:10) is helpful in reducing the risk of cross-contamination of foods.

▶ The World Health Organization's Golden Rules for Safe Food Preparation

1. Choose foods processed for safety.
2. Cook food thoroughly.
3. Eat cooked foods immediately.
4. Store cooked foods carefully.
5. Reheat cooked foods thoroughly.
6. Avoid contact between raw and cooked foods.
7. Wash hands repeatedly.
8. Keep all kitchen surfaces meticulously clean.
9. Protect foods from insects, rodents, and other animals.
10. Use pure water.

The USDA simplified these rules into four actions as a part of their Fight BAC! Program (check out **www.fightbac.org**):

1. Clean. Wash hands and surfaces often.
2. Separate. Don't cross-contaminate.
3. Cook. Cook to proper temperatures.
4. Chill. Refrigerate promptly.

The 2005 Dietary Guidelines for Americans also stress the importance of these four actions.

▲ Washing hands thoroughly (for at least 20 to 30 seconds) with hot water and soap should be the first step in food preparation. The 4 "F's" of food contamination are fingers, foods, feces, and flies. Handwashing especially combats the finger and fecal routes.

▲ Food safety logo of USDA.

be eaten. People have become ill from *Salmonella* introduced from melons used in making a fruit salad and from oranges used for fresh-squeezed orange juice. The bacteria were on the outside of the melons and oranges.

- Completely remove moldy portions of food or don't eat the food. *When in doubt, throw the food out.* Mold growth is prevented by properly storing food at cold temperatures and using the food promptly.
- Use refrigerated ground meat and patties in 1 to 2 days and frozen meat and patties within 3 to 4 months. The 6-month interval mentioned in the comic at the beginning of this chapter is too long a time to be safe.

### Cooking Food

- Cook food thoroughly using a bimetallic thermometer to check for doneness, especially for beef and fish (145°F [63°C]), pork (160°F [71°C]), and poultry (165°F [74°C]) ( Fig. 13-2). Eggs should be cooked until the yolk and white are hard. Alfalfa sprouts and other types of sprouts should be cooked until they are steaming. Cooking is by far the most reliable way to destroy foodborne viruses and bacteria, such as Norovirus and toxic strains of *E. coli*. Freezing only halts viral and bacterial growth. FDA does not recommend that eggs be prepared sunny-side-up.

As noted, many restaurants now include an advisory on menus stating that an increased risk of foodborne illness is associated with eating undercooked eggs.

As long as restaurants provide this warning on their menus, however, they are allowed to cook eggs to any temperature requested by the consumer. FDA warns us not to consume homemade ice cream, eggnog, and mayonnaise if made with unpasteurized, raw eggs because of the risk of *Salmonella* foodborne illness. It is safer to use eggs or egg products that have been pasteurized, which kills *Salmonella* bacteria. Overall, a good general precaution is to eat no raw animal products. USDA answers questions about the safe use of animal products (800-535-4555, 10 A.M. to 4 P.M. weekdays, Eastern time).

Seafood also poses a risk of foodborne illness, especially oysters. Properly cooked seafood should flake easily and/or be opaque or dull and firm. If it's translucent or shiny, it's not done.

- Cook stuffing separately from poultry (or wash poultry thoroughly, stuff immediately before cooking, and then transfer the stuffing to a clean bowl immediately after cooking). Make sure the stuffing reaches 165°F (74°C). *Salmonella* is the major concern with poultry.
- Once a food is cooked, consume it right away, or cool it to 41°F (5°C) within 2 hours. If it is not to be eaten immediately, in hot weather (80°F and above) make sure this cooling is done within 1 hour. Do this by separating the food into as many shallow pans as needed to provide a large surface area for cooling. Be careful not to recontaminate cooked food by contact with raw meat or juices from hands, cutting boards, dirty utensils, or in other ways.
- Serve meat, poultry, and fish on a clean plate—never the same plate used to hold the raw product. For example, when grilling hamburgers, don't put cooked items on the same plate used to carry the raw product out to the grill.
- For outdoor cooking, cook food completely at the picnic site, with no partial cooking in advance.

### Storing and Reheating Cooked Food

- Keep foods out of the "danger zone" (Fig .13-1) by keeping hot foods hot and cold foods cold. Hold food below 41°F (5°C) or above 135°F (57°C).

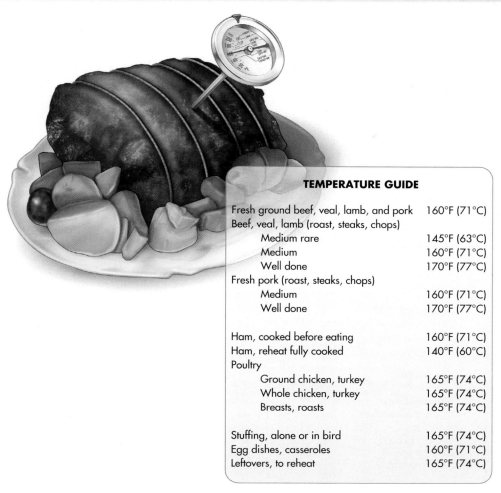

**TEMPERATURE GUIDE**

| | |
|---|---|
| Fresh ground beef, veal, lamb, and pork | 160°F (71°C) |
| Beef, veal, lamb (roast, steaks, chops) | |
|     Medium rare | 145°F (63°C) |
|     Medium | 160°F (71°C) |
|     Well done | 170°F (77°C) |
| Fresh pork (roast, steaks, chops) | |
|     Medium | 160°F (71°C) |
|     Well done | 170°F (77°C) |
| | |
| Ham, cooked before eating | 160°F (71°C) |
| Ham, reheat fully cooked | 140°F (60°C) |
| Poultry | |
|     Ground chicken, turkey | 165°F (74°C) |
|     Whole chicken, turkey | 165°F (74°C) |
|     Breasts, roasts | 165°F (74°C) |
| | |
| Stuffing, alone or in bird | 165°F (74°C) |
| Egg dishes, casseroles | 160°F (71°C) |
| Leftovers, to reheat | 165°F (74°C) |

▲ Sushi, like all raw fish or meat dishes, is a high-risk food. For maximum protection from food-borne illness, animal foods should be cooked thoroughly before eating.

**FIGURE 13-2** ▶ Minimum internal temperatures when cooking or reheating foods.
*Source: USDA "Kitchen's Companion", February 2008.*

Foodborne microorganisms thrive in more moderate temperatures (60°F to 110°F [16°C to 43°C]). Some microorganisms can even grow in the refrigerator. Again, don't leave cooked or refrigerated foods, such as meats and salads, at room temperature for more than 2 hours (or 1 hour in hot weather) because that gives microorganisms an opportunity to grow. Store dry food at 60°F to 70°F (16°C to 21°C).

- Reheat leftovers to 165°F (74°C); reheat gravy to a rolling boil to kill *Clostridium perfringens* bacteria, which may be present. Merely reheating to a good eating temperature isn't sufficient to kill harmful bacteria.
- Store peeled or cut-up produce, such as melon balls, in the refrigerator.
- Make sure the refrigerator stays below 41°F (5°C). Either use a refrigerator ther-

mometer or keep it as cold as possible without freezing milk and lettuce.
- Keep leftovers in the refrigerator only for the recommended length of time (Fig. 13-3).

Cross-contamination is not only a threat during food preparation; it can also become a problem during food storage.

**MAKING DECISIONS**

### Raw Fish

Raw fish dishes, such as sushi, can be safe for most people to eat if they are made with very fresh fish that has been commercially frozen and then thawed. The freezing is important to eliminate potential health risks from parasites. FDA recommends that the fish be frozen to an internal temperature of −10°F for 7 days. If you choose to eat uncooked fish, purchase the fish from reputable establishments that have high standards for quality and sanitation. If you are at high risk for foodborne illness, it is wise to avoid raw fish products.

Make sure all foods, including leftovers, are contained and covered in the refrigerator to prevent drippings from uncooked and potentially hazardous foods from tainting other foods. It is a good idea to store foods likely to pose risk of foodborne illness on lower shelves of the refrigerator, beneath other foods to be eaten raw.

FIGURE 13-3 ▶ Length of time to keep leftovers in the refrigerator.

▶ **Current Safe Handling Instructions Issued by USDA for Labeling Meat and Poultry Products**

This product was prepared from inspected and passed meat and/or poultry. Some food products may contain bacteria that could cause illness if the product is mishandled or cooked improperly. For your protection, follow these handling instructions.

Keep refrigerated or frozen.

Thaw in refrigerator or microwave.

Keep raw meat and poultry separate from other foods.

Wash working surfaces (including cutting boards), utensils, and hands after touching raw meat or poultry.

Cook thoroughly.

Keep hot foods hot. Refrigerate leftovers immediately or discard.

▶ **Safe Handling Instructions for Eggs**

To prevent illness from bacteria: keep eggs refrigerated, cook eggs until yolks are firm, and cook foods containing eggs thoroughly.

▶ To reduce the risk of bacteria surviving during microwave cooking,

- Cover food with glass or ceramic when possible to decrease evaporation and heat the surface.

- Stir and rotate food at least once or twice for even cooking. Then, allow microwaved food to stand, covered, after heating is completed to help cook the exterior and equalize the temperature throughout.

- Use the oven temperature probe or a meat thermometer to check that food is done. Insert it at several spots.

- If thawing meat in the microwave, use the oven's defrost setting. Ice crystals in frozen foods are not heated well by the microwave oven and can create cold spots, which later cook more slowly.

## When in doubt, throw it out!

| Food | Refrigerator Storage Time (days) |
|---|---|
| **Meats** | |
| Cooked ground beef/turkey | 3-4 |
| Deli meat | 2-3 |
| Cooked pork | 3-4 |
| Cooked poultry | 3-4 |
| Cooked beef, bison, lamb | 3-4 |
| **Seafood** | |
| Raw (e.g. sushi/sashimi) | Must consume on day of purchase |
| Cooked | 2 |
| **Other Entrees** | |
| Pizza | 1-2 |
| Pasta/rice | 1-2 |
| Casserole | 3-4 |
| **Soups and Chili** | |
| Chili with meat | 2-3 |
| Chili without meat | 3-4 |
| Soup/stew | 3-4 |
| **Side Dishes** | |
| Fresh salad | 1-2 |
| Fresh vegetables | 1-2 |
| Pasta or potato salad | 2-3 |
| Deviled egg | 2-3 |
| Hard boiled egg | 7 |
| Potato (any style) | 3-4 |
| Cooked vegetables | 3-4 |
| **Dessert** | |
| Cream pie | 2-3 |
| Fruit pie | 2-3 |
| Pastries | 7 |
| Cake | 7 |
| Cheesecake | 7 |

## CONCEPT CHECK

Thoroughly cook all meat and poultry to reduce the risk of foodborne illness from *E. coli*, and *Salmonella*. In addition, always separate raw meats and poultry products from cooked foods. To prevent foodborne intoxication from *Staphylococcus* organisms, cover cuts on hands and avoid sneezing on foods. To avoid intoxication from *Clostridium perfringens*, rapidly cool leftover foods and thoroughly reheat them. To avoid intoxication from *Clostridium botulinum*, carefully examine canned foods. Overall, don't allow cooked food to stand for more than 1 to 2 hours at room temperature. For other causes of foodborne illness, precautions already mentioned generally apply as well. In addition, thoroughly cook fish and other seafood; consume only pasteurized dairy products; wash all fruits and vegetables; and thoroughly wash your hands with soap and water before and after preparing food and after using the bathroom.

## Case Study Preventing Foodborne Illness at Gatherings

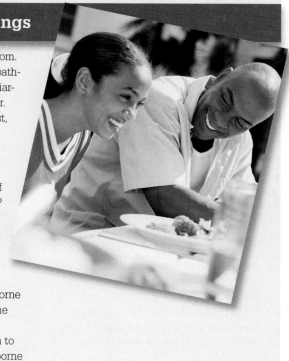

Nicole attended a gathering of her co-workers on a warm Saturday in July. The theme of the party was international dining. Nicole and her husband were asked to bring an Argentinian dish, potato and beef empanadas. They followed the recipe and cooking time carefully, removing the dish from the oven at 1 P.M. and keeping it warm by wrapping the pan in a towel. They traveled in their car to the party and set the dish out on the buffet table at 3 P.M. Dinner was to be served at 4 P.M. However, the guests were enjoying themselves so much lounging around the host's pool and drinking ginger beer (also on the menu) that no one began to eat until 6 P.M. Nicole made sure she sampled the empanadas that she and her husband made, while her husband did not. She also had some salad, garlic bread, and a sweet dessert made with coconut.

The couple returned home at 11 P.M. and went to bed. At about 2 A.M., Nicole knew something was wrong. She had severe abdominal pain and had to make a dash to the bathroom. She spent most of the next 3 hours in the bathroom with severe diarrhea. By dawn, the diarrhea subsided and she started to feel better. After a few cups of tea and a light breakfast, she was feeling like herself by noon.

Answer the following questions, and check your responses in Appendix A.

1. Based on her symptoms, what type of foodborne illness did Nicole contract?
2. Why is the beef the most likely vehicle for this type of foodborne illness?
3. Why is consuming food at large gatherings risky?
4. What precautions for avoiding foodborne illness were ignored by Nicole and the rest of the people at the party?
5. How could this scenario be rewritten to substanitally reduce the risk of foodborne illness?

## Summary

1. Viruses, bacteria, and other microorganisms in food pose the greatest risk for foodborne illness. Major causes of foodborne illness are Norovirus and the bacteria *Campylobacter jejuni, Salmonella, Staphylococcus aureus*, and *Clostridium perfringens*. In addition, such bacteria as *Clostridium botulinum, Listeria monocytogenes*, and *Escherichia coli* have been found to cause illness.

2. In the past, salt, sugar, smoke, fermentation, and drying were used to protect against foodborne illness. Today, careful cooking, pasteurization, keeping hot foods hot and cold foods cold, and thorough hand-washing provide additional insurance.

3. Food additives are used primarily to extend shelf life by preventing microbial growth and the destruction of food components by oxygen, metals, and other substances. Food additives are classified as those intentionally added to foods and those that incidentally appear in foods. An intentional additive is limited to no more than one-one-hundredth of the greatest amount that causes no observed symptoms in animals. Under its jurisdiction in the United States, the Delaney Clause allows FDA to ban the use of any intentional food additive that causes cancer.

Antioxidants, such as BHA, BHT, vitamins E and C, and sulfites, prevent oxygen and enzyme destruction of food products. Emulsifiers suspend fat in water, improving the uniformity, smoothness, and body of foods such as ice cream. Common preservatives include salt, sodium benzoate, and sorbic acid, which prevent bacterial growth. Sequestrants bind metals and thus prevent spoilage of food from metal contamination. Various natural products such as natural flavors, sugar, and corn syrup, as well as artificial flavors and sweeteners, such as aspartame, improve the flavor of food.

4. Toxic substances occur naturally in a variety of foods, such as green potatoes, raw fish, mushrooms, and raw egg whites. Cooking foods limits their toxic effects in some cases; others are best to avoid altogether, such as toxic mushroom species and the green parts of potatoes.

5. A variety of environmental contaminants and pesticide residues can be found in foods. It is helpful to know which foods pose the greatest risks and act accordingly to reduce exposure, such as washing fruits and vegetables before use.

6. Conventional agriculture focuses on maximizing production through the use of large farms, machines, and chemicals. A more recent culture of sustainability demands food choices produced in an environmentally responsible way. U.S. sales of organic foods have grown dramatically in recent years, despite tough economic times. Consumers are more interested in the origins of their

food, resulting in grocery stores providing more "locally grown" products. Although there is no evidence that locally grown products are safer, local products provide fresher options and do not have the added transportation costs. Consumers also have an interest in connecting with local/regional farmers, resulting in growing national support for community-supported agriculture.

7. To protect against viruses and bacteria, cook susceptible foods thoroughly. In addition, cover cuts on the hands, do not sneeze or cough on foods, avoid contact between raw meat or poultry products and other food products, rapidly cool and thoroughly reheat leftovers, and use pasteurized dairy products. Overall, be careful when foods are in the "danger zone" (41°F to 135°F).

Cross-contamination commonly causes foodborne illness. It occurs particularly when bacteria on raw animal products contact foods that can support bacterial growth. Because of the risk of cross-contamination, no perishable food should be kept in the "danger zone" for more than 1 to 2 hours (depending on the environmental temperature), especially if it may have come in contact with raw animal products.

## Study Questions

1. Identify three major classes of microorganisms responsible for foodborne illness.

2. Which types of foods are most likely to be involved in foodborne illness? Why are they targets for contamination?

3. What three trends in food purchasing and production have led to a greater number of cases of foodborne illness?

4. Why is thoroughly cooking food an important practice for reducing the risk of foodborne illness?

5. List four techniques other than thorough cooking that are important in preventing foodborne illness.

6. Define the term *food additive,* and give examples of four intentional food additives. What are their specific functions in foods? What is their relationship to the GRAS list?

7. Describe the federal process that governs the use of food additives, including the Delaney Clause.

8. Put into perspective the benefits and risks of using additives in food. Point out an easy way to reduce the consumption of food additives. Do you think this is worth the effort in terms of maintaining health? Why or why not?

9. Describe four recommendations for reducing the risk of toxicity from environmental contaminants.

10. How do various U.S. federal agencies work together to maintain the safety of food?

## Check Your Knowledge

Answers to the following multiple choice questions are below.

1. Nitrite prevents the growth of
   a. *Clostridium botulinum.*
   b. *Escherichia coli.*
   c. *Staphylococcus aureus.*
   d. yeasts.

2. Substances used to preserve foods by lowering the pH are
   a. smoke and irradiation.
   b. baking powder and soda.
   c. salt and sugar.
   d. vinegar and citric acid.

3. Food additives widely used for many years without apparent ill effects are on the _____ list.
   a. FDA          c. USDA
   b. GRAS          d. Delaney

4. The foodborne illness organism often associated with small cuts and boils is
   a. *Listeria.*          c. *C. botulinum.*
   b. *Staphylococcus.*          d. *Salmonella.*

5. Salmonella bacteria are usually spread via
   a. raw meats, poultry, and eggs.
   b. pickled vegetables.
   c. home-canned vegetables.
   d. raw vegetables.

6. It is unwise to thaw meats or poultry
   a. in a microwave oven.
   b. in the refrigerator.
   c. under cool running water.
   d. at room temperature.

7. Milk that can remain on supermarket shelves, free of microbial growth, for many years has been processed by which of the following methods?
   a. use of humectants
   b. using antibiotics in animal feed
   c. use of sequestrants
   d. aseptic processing

8. Those at greatest risk for food-borne illness include
   a. pregnant women.
   b. infants and children.

   c. immunosuppressed individuals.
   d. All of the above.

9. Pasteurization involves the
   a. exposure of food to high temperatures for short periods to destroy harmful microorganisms.
   b. exposure of food to heat to inactivate enzymes that cause undesirable effects in foods during storage.
   c. fortification of foods with vitamins A and D.
   d. use of irradiation to destroy certain pathogens in foods.

10. Food can be kept for long periods by adding salt or sugar because these substances
   a. make the food too acidic for spoilage to occur.
   b. bind to water, thereby making it unavailable to the microorganisms.
   c. effectively kill microorganisms.
   d. dissolve the cell walls in plant foods.

Answers: 1. a, 2. d, 3. b, 4. b, 5. a, 6. d, 7. d, 8. d, 9. a, 10. b

## Further Readings

1. Acheson DWK, Fiore AE: Preventing food-borne illness—What clinicians can do. *The New England Journal of Medicine* 350:437, 2004.

   *The food supply in the United States is mostly safe, but more could be done to lessen the risk for developing foodborne illness. This article discusses strategies to do so, as well as summarizes the characteristics of the major organisms that cause foodborne illness.*

2. ADA Reports: Position of the American Dietetic Association: Food and water safety. *Journal of the American Dietetic Association* 103:1203, 2003.

   *It is the position of the American Dietetic Association that the public has a right to a safe food and water supply. Still, it is estimated that on an annual basis, there are 76 million cases of foodborne illness in the United States, with significant economic cost. Thus, more work needs to be done with regard to food safety.*

3. Anderson JB and others: A camera's view of consumer food-handling behaviors. *Journal of the American Dietetic Association* 104:186, 2004.

   *Improper food handling practices were common in the households studied in this survey. Implementing the Fight BAC! Campaign recommendations, such as using a thermometer to test for doneness in meats, would improve food handling practices.*

4. Calvert GM: Health effects of pesticides. *American Family Physician* 69:1613, 2004.

   *Clear cases of disease from pesticide exposure are seen from acute exposures with high amounts. The true effects of low dose, chronic exposure have been hard to quantify, but most adults have detectable pesticide levels in their blood. Thus, efforts should be made to reduce pesticide exposure when possible, especially with use in and around the house.*

5. Consumers Union: Dirty birds: Even "premium" chickens harbor dangerous bacteria. *Consumer Reports* p. 20, January 2007.

   *An analysis of fresh, whole chickens bought throughout the United States revealed that 83% contained Campylobacter or Salmonella, two leading causes of foodborne disease. This article describes the details of the investigation and findings.*

6. Food Safety and Inspection Service: A century of progress in food safety. *Be Food Safe* Fall:12, 2006.

   *The Federal Meat Inspection Act became law in 1906. This article summarizes the 100-year history of federal inspection of meat and poultry.*

7. Gerner-Smidt P and others: Invasive listeriosis in Denmark 1994-2003: A review of 299 cases with special emphasis on risk factors for mortality. *Clinical Microbiological Infections* 11:618, 2005.

   *Listeria infections lead to death primarily in older people and those with underlying cases of cancer. It is therefore especially important for these people to be careful of exposure to Listeria.*

8. Hillers VN and others: Consumer food handling behaviors associated with prevention of 13 foodborne illnesses. *Journal of Food Protection* 66:1893, 2003.

   *Handwashing is highly recommended by experts for the prevention of foodborne illness. The importance of not eating certain foods, such as raw seafood, is another important habit to consider. The use of a thermometer in cooking is also an important practice, as is avoidance of cross-contamination of food products.*

9. McCabe-Sellers BJ, Beattie SF: Food safety: emerging trends in foodborne illness surveillance and prevention. *Journal of the American Dietetic Association* 104:1708, 2004.

   *Detailed discussion of prevention of foodborne illness, such as paying attention to fresh produce as a source of the primary causative agents—viruses and bacteria. Recommendations for consumers and food handlers are given to reduce risk of foodborne illness, with proper personal hygiene being a major focus.*

10. Musher DM, Musher BL: Contagious acute bacterial infections. *The New England Journal of Medicine* 351:2417, 2004.

    *Detailed discussion of the viruses and bacteria associated with foodborne illness. Handwashing is one important method mentioned to reduce exposure. Use of diluted bleach solutions (1:10) on surfaces is also recommended when possible.*

11. Schardt D: Get the lead out—What you don't know can hurt you. *Nutrition Action Healthletter* p. 1, March 2005.

    *There is evidence that hypertension, kidney disease, declines in brain function, and cataracts are linked to lead exposure. Testing your water supply for lead as outlined in the article is one inexpensive way to be alerted to a possible source. Using only cold tap water for cooking is also advised.*

12. Scheier LM: The safety of beef in the United States. *Journal of the American Dietetic Association* 105:339, 2005.

    *Bovine spongiform encephalopathy, better known as mad cow disease, continues to be of interest to the general public. The protocols involved in testing and keeping beef safe for the public are discussed in this article, as well as current legislation.*

13. Sivapalasingam S and others: Fresh produce: A growing cause of outbreaks of foodborne illness in the United States. *Journal of Food Protection* 67:2342, 2004.

    *Fresh produce such as lettuce, juices, melons, sprouts, and berries have been highlighted as sources of agents that lead to foodborne illness. Caution should be used with these items, just as one would with raw meat and dairy products.*

14. Spano M: Organics in overdrive—the explosion of natural food products. *Today's Dietitian* 9: 66, October 2007.

    *The increased availability of organic products in mainstream stores, along with consumer fear of hormones and antibiotics, has led to a dramatic growth in organic food sales. Conventional farming is compared to organic farming relative to the issues of stimulating plant growth, pests, weeds, and growth.*

15. U.S. Food and Drug Administration: *Food Code.* U.S. Department of Health and Human Services, Public Health Service, Food and Drug Administration: College Park, MD, 2005.

    *FDA Food Code provides scientifically sound technical and legal basis for regulating the retail and food service segment of the food industry, including restaurants, grocery stores, and institutions, such as nursing homes. The Food Code serves as a model for local, state, tribal, and federal regulators to develop or update their food safety rules and to be consistent with national food regulatory policy.*

16. Widdowson MA and others: Norovirus and foodborne disease, United States, 1991–2000. *Emerging Infectious Diseases* 11:95, 2005.

    *The Norovirus leads to more causes of foodborne illness than any other agent. What is now needed is better surveillance for this organism so better estimates of cases can be made.*

17. Yates J: Traveler's diarrhea. *American Family Physician* 71:2095, 2005.

    *Millions of people who travel are affected by acute diarrhea each year. The contamination of food and water with fecal matter are the main sources of the infection. Escherichia coli, enteroaggregative E. coli, Campylobacter, Salmonella, and Shigella are common causes of traveler's diarrhea, whereas parasites and viruses are less common causes.*

18. Yeager D: Got organic? *Today's Dietitian* 10:60, October 2008.

    *Regulation of the organic milk industry is discussed. The United States Department of Agriculture now regulates the organic industry. The National Organic Program certifies that food is produced using organic practices. Most milk companies follow the regulations stringently when it comes to producing organic milk.*

## I. Can You Spot the Improper Food Safety Practices?

In this chapter you learned that (1) foodborne illness strikes up to 76 million U.S. citizens each year and (2) about 5000 deaths each year in the United States are caused by foodborne organisms.

Carefully preparing foods to prevent foodborne illness can minimize its occurrence for most of us. Read the following excerpt and find the food safety violations that could lead to illness.

### A Local Health Department Inspector Gives the Following Account of His Visit to a Local Diner

As I walked through the kitchen of the Morningside Diner, I noticed that all food handlers washed their hands thoroughly with hot, soapy water before handling the food, especially after handling raw meat, fish, poultry, or eggs. Before preparing raw foods, they also thoroughly washed the cutting boards, dishes, and other equipment. As they used their cutting boards after cutting foods, they wiped them with a damp rag and used them again to cut more food.

When preparing fresh fruits and vegetables, they washed them but were careful to leave a little dirt on for fear of washing important nutrients from the outside. The cooks generally cooked meats to an internal temperature of 180°F (82°C). However, to preserve the flavor, pork was cooked to an internal temperature of 140°F (60°C). Some cooked foods to be served later were cooled to below 41°F (5°C) within 2 hours, and foods like beef stew were cooled in shallow pans.

The diner served canned foods, even when the cans were dented. When leftovers were reheated, they were raised to an internal temperature of 130°F (55°C) and served immediately. Food handlers took great care to remove moldy portions of food. The cooks prepared stuffing separately from the poultry. The temperature of refrigerators was approximately 45°F (7°C).

1. List the violations of food safety practices that could contribute to foodborne illness.

   _____

   _____

   _____

   _____

2. If you were writing a report describing ways to correct these practices, what would you say?

   _____

   _____

   _____

   _____

   _____

3. List the food safety practices that follow the general rules for preventing foodborne illness.

   _____

   _____

   _____

   _____

## II. Take a Closer Look at Food Additives

Evaluate a food label of a convenience food item (e.g., frozen entree, ready-to-eat baked good) either in the supermarket or one you have available.

1. Write out the list of ingredients.

   _____

   _____

   _____

   _____

2. Identify the ingredients that you think may be food additives.

   _____

   _____

   _____

   _____

3. Based on the information available in this chapter, what are the functions of these food additives?

   _____

   _____

   _____

   _____

4. How might this food product differ without these ingredients?

   _____

   _____

   _____

   _____

## III. Take a Closer Look at Organic Foods

Visit one or more supermarkets to see what organic foods are available. Note your findings below.

| | Available | Not Available |
|---|---|---|
| Meat | | |
| Poultry | | |
| Milk | | |
| Eggs | | |
| Cheese | | |
| Lettuce | | |
| Apples | | |
| Bananas | | |
| Broccoli | | |
| Other produce | | |
| Breakfast cereal | | |
| Snack chips | | |
| Crackers | | |
| Bread | | |
| Pasta | | |
| Beer | | |

Do you currently purchase organic foods? Why or why not?

# CHAPTER 14 Pregnancy and Breastfeeding

## Student Learning Outcomes  After studying Chapter 14 you will be able to:

1. List major physiological changes that occur in the body during pregnancy and how nutrient needs are altered.

2. List factors that predict a successful pregnancy outcome and some that do not.

3. Specify the optimal weight gain during pregnancy for a healthy adult woman.

4. Design an adequate, balanced meal plan for a pregnant or lactating woman using MyPyramid as a basis.

5. Identify the nutrients that may need to be supplemented during pregnancy and explain the reason for each.

6. Explain the typical discomforts of pregnancy that can be minimized by dietary changes.

7. Describe the physiological processes involved in breastfeeding, as well as some advantages of breastfeeding for both the infant and mother.

## Chapter Outline

Student Learning Outcomes

Refresh Your Memory

14.1 Planning for Pregnancy

14.2 Prenatal Growth and Development

14.3 Success in Pregnancy

14.4 Increased Nutrient Needs to Support Pregnancy

14.5 Food Plan for Pregnant Women

14.6 Physiological Changes of Concern During Pregnancy

14.7 Breastfeeding

Nutrition and Your Health: Preventing Birth Defects

Case Study: Preparing for Pregnancy

Summary/Study Questions/Check Your Knowledge/Further Readings

Rate Your Plate

**PREGNANCY CAN BE A SPECIAL TIME.** Exhilaration and amazement accompany parents' tremendous responsibility of helping a child develop and grow. Parents-to-be often feel an overriding desire to produce a healthy baby, which can arouse new interest in nutrition and health information. They usually want to do everything possible to maximize their chances of having a robust, lively newborn.

Despite these intentions, the infant mortality rate in North America is higher than that seen in many other industrialized nations. In Canada, about 6.1 of every 1000 infants per year die before their first birthday, while in the United States, it is 6.9. These are alarming statistics for two countries that have such a high per capita expenditure for health care compared to many other countries in the world. Comparatively, the rate of infant mortality in Sweden is roughly 3 of every 1000 infants. In addition, in the United States, about 20% of pregnant women receive inadequate prenatal care in the early months of pregnancy. Expectant teenagers are at the highest risk for this.

Producing a healthy baby is not just a matter of luck. True, some aspects of fetal and newborn health are beyond our control. Still, as the comic in this chapter suggests, conscious decisions about social, health, environmental, and nutritional factors during pregnancy significantly affect the baby's future.

Choosing to breastfeed the infant adds further benefits. Let's examine how eating well during pregnancy and breastfeeding can help a baby to have a healthy start in life.

 **Refresh Your Memory**

As you begin your study of nutrition in pregnancy and breastfeeding in Chapter 14, you may want to review:

- Typical fortification in meal replacement bars in Chapter 1 and ready-to-eat breakfast cereals in Chapter 2
- Causes and effects of ketosis in Chapter 4
- Components of the macronutrient classes—carbohydrates, proteins, and lipids—in Chapters 4 to 6, especially omega-3 fatty aids
- Calculation of body mass index in Chapter 7
- Food sources of folate in Chapter 8 and calcium, iron, and zinc in Chapter 9

## 14.1 Planning for Pregnancy

**I**n an effort to reduce the occurrence of neural tube defects, *Healthy People 2010* includes a goal of increasing to 80% the number of pregnancies that begin with optimal folate status. This is a significant increase from the current estimate of 21%.

Controlling or correcting existing health conditions and modifying potentially harmful habits before conception can improve the chances for a successful pregnancy. About 50% of all pregnancies are unplanned. Even when planned, women often do not suspect they are pregnant during the first few weeks after conception. They may not seek medical attention until after the first 2 to 3 months of pregnancy. Still, even without fanfare, the child-to-be grows and develops daily. For that reason, the health and nutrition habits of a woman who is trying to become pregnant—or who has the ability to become pregnant—are particularly important. Although some aspects of fetal and newborn health are beyond the parents' control, a woman's conscious decisions about social, health, environmental, and nutritional factors affect her infant's health and future.

The time to address ongoing health concerns is before conception. Poor control of existing diabetes, hypertension, phenylketonuria, and HIV-positive status or AIDS may lead to serious complications in pregnancy, including birth defects and fetal death. In

Which diet and lifestyle habits contribute to a successful pregnancy? Which are likely to be harmful?

Why should a woman begin to prepare for pregnancy months before conception of her new baby?

When pregnant, does the mother need to "eat for two"? Chapter 14 provides some answers.

addition, women should aim to achieve a healthy weight prior to becoming pregnant. Prepregnancy weight and nutrient stores affect the woman's ability to become pregnant. Many underweight women experience amenorrhea, which may reduce their ability to ovulate. The chance of ovulating and becoming pregnant improve when body fat increases to a healthy level.

Infants born to women who began pregnancy substantially above or below a healthy weight are more likely to experience problems than women who began pregnancy at a normal weight. For instance, babies born to obese women are at increased risk of having birth defects, death in the first few weeks after birth, and obesity in childhood. Many obese pregnant women experience high blood pressure, gestational diabetes, and difficult deliveries. At the other extreme, women who begin pregnancy underweight (BMI < 19.8) are more likely to have infants who are low birth weight and premature than women at a normal weight. These differences may be because underweight women tend to have lighter placentas and lower nutrient stores, especially iron, than heavier women, which can affect fetal growth negatively. An underweight woman can improve her nutrient stores and pregnancy outcome by gaining weight before pregnancy or gaining extra weight during pregnancy.

Figure 14-1 depicts how and when toxic agents can harm the developing fetus. To prepare for a healthy pregnancy, the mother should undoubtedly eliminate tobacco, alcohol, and illicit drugs (e.g., marijuana and cocaine). Certain medicines, such as aspirin and related NSAIDs (e.g., ibuprofen [Advil]), as well as typical medicines to treat the common cold and many herbal therapies, have the potential to damage the fetus. Lower doses and/or safer alternatives should be used when planning for pregnancy. Health hazards in the mother's environment, including job-related hazards and exposure to x-rays, should be minimized. Caffeine intake also should be limited.

Much research suggests that an adequate vitamin and mineral intake at least 8 weeks before conception and then during pregnancy can improve outcomes of pregnancy. In particular, meeting folate needs (400 micrograms of synthetic folic acid per day) helps to prevent birth defects such as neural tube defects (review Fig. 8-27 in Chapter 8) and decrease the risk of preterm delivery. Recall from Chapter 8 that adequate folate status before and during pregnancy reduces the risk of neural tube defects by about 70%. Low intakes of calcium and iron or excessive intakes of vitamin A also are cause for concern during pregnancy. Careful dietary choices, often with the help of a balanced multivitamin and mineral supplement, will contribute to a healthy pregnancy for both mother and infant.

▲ The time to begin thinking about prenatal nutrition is before becoming pregnant. This includes making sure folic acid intake is adequate (400 micrograms of synthetic folic acid per day) and that any supplemental intake of preformed vitamin A does not exceed 100% of the Daily Value (1000 micrograms RAE or 5000 IU).

## MAKING DECISIONS

### Folate Supplements

Women who have previously given birth to an infant with a neural tube defect such as spina bifida should consult their physician about the need for folate supplementation; an intake of 4 milligrams of synthetic folic acid per day at least one month prior to conception is recommended for these women, but must be taken under a physician's supervision.

## 14.2 Prenatal Growth and Development

For 8 weeks after conception, a human **embryo** develops from a fertilized **ovum** into a **fetus.** For about another 32 weeks, the fetus continues to develop. When its body finally matures, the infant is born. Until birth, the mother nourishes it via a **placenta,** an organ that forms in her uterus to accommodate the growth and development of the fetus (Fig. 14-2). The role of the placenta is to exchange nutrients, oxygen and other gases, and waste products between the mother and the fetus.

**embryo** In humans, the developing offspring in utero from about the beginning of the third week to the end of the eighth week after conception.

**ovum** The egg cell from which a fetus eventually develops if the egg is fertilized by a sperm cell.

**fetus** The developing life form from about the beginning of the ninth week after conception until birth.

**placenta** An organ that forms in the uterus in pregnant women. Through this organ, oxygen and nutrients from the mother's blood are transferred to the fetus, and fetal wastes are removed. The placenta also releases hormones that maintain the state of pregnancy.

| Week | 1 | 2 | 3 | 4 | 5 | 6 | 8 | 16 | 38 |
|------|---|---|---|---|---|---|---|----|----|
| CR length° | < 0.1 cm | < 0.15 cm | 0.3 cm | 0.6 cm | 0.8 cm | 1 cm | 3.5 cm | 14 cm | 26 cm |
| Weight | | | | < 1 g | | | < 5 g | 200 g | 3400 g |

| | Preconception | First Trimester | Second and Third Trimesters |
|---|---|---|---|
| Sperm and egg unite | ◄— Zygote —► | ◄———— Embryonic development ————► | ◄— Fetal development —► |
| Risk from toxic agents | Low | Major structural abnormalities | Physiological defects and minor structural abnormalities |
| Central nervous system | | | |
| Heart | | | |
| Limbs | | | |
| Eyes | | | |
| Ears | | | |
| Palate | | | |
| Teeth | | | |
| External genitalia | | | |

**FIGURE 14-1** ► Harmful effects of toxic agents during pregnancy. Vulnerable periods of fetal development are indicated with purple bars. The purple shading indicates the time of greatest risk to the organ. The most serious damage to the fetus from exposure to toxins is likely to occur during the first 8 weeks after conception, two-thirds of the way through the first trimester. As the white bars in the chart show, however, damage to vital parts of the body—including the eyes, brain, and genitals—can also occur during the later months of pregnancy.

**zygote** The fertilized ovum; the cell resulting from the union of an egg cell (ovum) and sperm until it divides.

**trimesters** Three 13- to 14-week periods into which the normal pregnancy (the length of a normal pregnancy is about 40 weeks, measured from the first day of the woman's last menstrual period) is divided somewhat arbitrarily for purposes of discussion and analysis. Development of the offspring, however, is continuous throughout pregnancy, with no specific physiological markers demarcating the transition from one trimester to the next.

## Early Growth—The First Trimester Is a Very Critical Time

In the formation of the human organism, egg and sperm unite to produce the **zygote** (Fig. 14-1). From this point, the reproductive process occurs very rapidly:

- Within 30 hours—zygote divides in half to form 2 cells.
- Within 4 days—cell number climbs to 128 cells.
- At 14 days—the group of cells is called an embryo.
- Within 35 days—heart is beating, embryo is 1/30 of an inch (8 millimeters) long, eyes and limb buds are clearly visible.
- At 8 weeks—the embryo is known as a fetus.
- At 13 weeks (end of first trimester)—most organs are formed, and the fetus can move.

For purposes of discussion, the duration of pregnancy—normally, 38 to 42 weeks—is commonly divided into three periods, called **trimesters.** Growth begins in the first

**FIGURE 14-2** ▶ The fetus in relationship to the placenta. The placenta is the organ through which nourishment flows to the fetus.

Amniotic fluid

Umbilical cord (fetal circulation)

Placenta (supplies nutrients and oxygen from maternal circulation)

Uterus

trimester with a rapid increase in cell number. This type of growth dominates embryonic and early fetal development. The newly formed cells then begin to grow larger. Further growth is a mix of increases in cell number and cell size. By the end of 13 weeks—the first trimester—most organs are formed and the fetus can move (see Fig. 14-1).

As the embryo or fetus develops, nutritional deficiencies and other insults have the potential to impose damage or risk to organ systems. For example, adverse reactions to medications, high intakes of vitamin A, exposure to radiation, or trauma can alter or arrest the current phase of fetal development, and the effects may last a lifetime (review Fig. 14-1). The most critical time for these potential problems is during the first trimester. Most **spontaneous abortions** —premature terminations of pregnancy that occur naturally—happen at this time. About one-half or more pregnancies end in this way, often so early that a woman does not even realize she was pregnant. (An additional 15% to 20% are lost before normal delivery.) Early spontaneous abortions usually result from a genetic defect or fatal error in fetal development. Smoking, alcohol abuse, use of aspirin and NSAIDs, and illicit drug use raise the risk for spontaneous abortion.

A woman should avoid substances that may harm the developing fetus, especially during the first trimester. This holds true, as well, for the time when a woman is trying to become pregnant. As previously mentioned, she is unlikely to be aware of her pregnancy for at least a few weeks. In addition, the fetus develops so rapidly during the first trimester that, if an essential nutrient is not available, the fetus may be affected even before evidence of the nutrient deficiency appears in the mother.

For this reason, the quality—rather than the quantity—of the woman's nutritional intake is most important during the first trimester. In other words, women should consume the same amount of calories, but the foods chosen should be more nutrient dense. Although some women lose their appetite and feel nauseated during the first trimester, they should be careful to meet nutrient needs as much as possible.

Although a mother's decisions, practices, and precautions during pregnancy contribute to the health of her fetus, she cannot guarantee her fetus good health because some genetic and environmental factors are beyond her control. She and others involved in the pregnancy should not hold an unrealistic illusion of total control.

**spontaneous abortion** Cessation of pregnancy and expulsion of the embryo or nonviable fetus prior to 20 weeks gestation. This is the result of natural causes, such as a genetic defect or developmental problem; also called *miscarriage* .

### Second Trimester

By the beginning of the second trimester, a fetus weighs about 1 ounce. Arms, hands, fingers, legs, feet, and toes are fully formed. The fetus has ears and begins to form

▶ A healthy 1-week-old baby. At birth, a baby usually weighs about 7.5 pounds and is 20 inches long.

tooth sockets in its jawbone. Organs continue to grow and mature, and, with a stethoscope, or Doppler instrument, physicians can detect the fetus's heartbeat. Most bones are distinctly evident through the body. Eventually, the fetus begins to look more like an infant. It may suck its thumb and kick strongly enough to be felt by the mother. As was shown in Figure 14-1, the fetus can still be affected by exposure to toxins, but not to the degree seen in the first trimester.

During the second trimester, the mother's breast weight increases by approximately 30% due to the development of milk-producing cells and the deposition of 2 to 4 pounds of fat for **lactation.** This stored fat serves as a reservoir for the extra calories needed to produce breast milk.

**lactation** The period of milk secretion following pregnancy; typically called *breastfeeding.*

**gestation** The period of intrauterine development of offspring, from conception to birth; in humans, gestation lasts for about 40 weeks after the woman's previous menstrual period.

### Third Trimester

By the beginning of the third trimester, a fetus weighs about 2 to 3 pounds. The third trimester is a crucial time for fetal growth. The fetus will double in length and will increase its weight by three to four times. The fetus takes higher priority than the mother with regard to iron and will deplete the stores of the mother. If the mother is not meeting her iron needs, she can be severely depleted after delivery. An infant born after about 26 weeks of **gestation** has a good chance of survival if cared for in a nursery for high-risk newborns. However, the infant will not contain the stores of minerals (mainly iron and calcium) and fat normally accumulated during the last month of gestation. This and other medical problems, such as a poor ability to suck and swallow, complicate nutritional care for preterm infants.

At 9 months, the fetus usually weighs about 7 to 9 pounds (3 to 4 kilograms) and is about 20 inches (50 centimeters) long. A soft spot on the top of the head indicates where the skull bones (fontanels) are growing together. The bones finally close by the time the baby is about 12 to 18 months of age.

**A** goal of *Healthy People 2010* is to reduce low birth weight and preterm births by one-third.

## 14.3 Success in Pregnancy

The goal of pregnancy is to achieve optimal health for both the baby and the mother. For the mother, a successful pregnancy is one in which her physical and emotional health is protected so that she can return to her prepregnancy health status. For the infant, two widely accepted criteria are (1) a gestation period longer than 37 weeks and (2) a birth weight greater than 5.5 pounds (2.5 kilograms). Sufficient lung development, likely to have occurred by 37 weeks of gestation, is critical to the survival of a newborn. The longer the gestation, the greater the ultimate birth weight and maturation state, leading to fewer medical problems and better quality of life for the infant. Overall, a successful pregnancy is the outcome of a complex interplay between genes, various lifestyle practices, and the environment.

## Infant Birthweight

**Low-birth-weight (LBW)** infants are those weighing less than 5.5 pounds (2.5 kilograms) at birth. Most commonly, LBW is associated with **preterm** birth. Medical costs during the first year of life for LBW infants are higher than those for normal-weight infants. In fact, hospital-related costs of caring for LBW newborns total more than $4 billion per year in the United States. Full-term and preterm infants who weigh less than the expected weight for their duration of gestation, the result of insufficient growth, are described as **small for gestational age (SGA).** Thus, a full-term infant weighing less than 5.5 pounds at birth is SGA but not preterm, whereas a preterm infant born at 30 weeks' gestation is probably LBW without being SGA. Infants who are SGA are more likely than normal-weight infants to have medical complications, including problems with blood glucose control, temperature regulation, growth, and development in the early weeks after birth.

## Prenatal Care and Counseling

Adequate prenatal care is a primary determinant of success in pregnancy. Ideally, women should receive examinations and counseling before becoming pregnant and continue regular prenatal care throughout pregnancy. If prenatal care is inadequate, delayed, or absent, untreated maternal nutritional deficiencies can deprive a developing fetus of needed nutrients. In addition, untreated health conditions, such as anemia, AIDS, hypertension, or diabetes, must be carefully addressed to minimize complications of pregnancy. Treating ongoing infections will also decrease risks of fetal damage. Without prenatal care, a woman is three times more likely to deliver an LBW baby—one who will be 40 times more likely to die during the first 4 weeks of life than a normal-birth-weight infant. According to the Physicians Committee for Responsible Medicine, early and consistent prenatal care could reduce the number of LBW births by 12,600 per year in the United States. Although the ideal time to start prenatal care is before conception, about 20% of women in the United States receive no prenatal care throughout the first trimester—a critical time to positively influence the outcome of pregnancy.

Food habits cannot be predicted from income, education, or lifestyle. Although some women already have good dietary habits, most can benefit from nutritional advice. All should be reminded of habits that may harm the growing fetus, such as severe dieting or fasting. By focusing on appropriate prenatal care, nutrient intake, and health habits, parents give their fetus—and later, their infant—the best chance of thriving. Overall, the chances of producing a healthy baby are maximized with education, an adequate diet, and early and consistent prenatal medical care.

## Effects of Maternal Age

The age of the mother is another factor that determines pregnancy outcome. The ideal age for pregnancy is between 20 and 35 years of age. Outside that age range—at either extreme—complications are more likely to arise. Pregnant teens frequently exhibit a variety of risk factors that can complicate pregnancy and pose a risk to the fetus. For instance, teenagers are more likely than adult women to be underweight at the beginning of pregnancy and to gain too little weight during pregnancy. In addition, their bodies generally lack the maturity needed to carry a fetus safely. Sixteen percent of LBW infants are born to teenage mothers. This is true even if the mothers receive adequate prenatal care. At the other end of the spectrum, advanced maternal

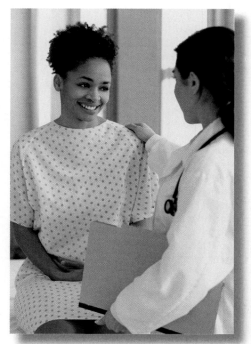

▲ To ensure optimal health and rapid treatment of medical conditions that develop during pregnancy, a pregnant woman should consult with her health-care provider on a regular basis. Ideally, this consultation should begin before she becomes pregnant.

**low birth weight (LBW)** Referring to any infant weighing less than 2.5 kilograms (5.5 pounds) at birth; most commonly results from preterm birth.

**preterm** An infant born before 37 weeks of gestation; also referred to as *premature* .

**small for gestational age (SGA)** Referring to infants who weigh less than the expected weight for their length of gestation. This corresponds to less than 2.5 kilograms (5.5 pounds) in a full-term newborn. A preterm infant who is also SGA will most likely develop some medical complications.

**W**omen with acquired immune deficiency syndrome (AIDS) may pass the virus that causes this disease to the fetus during pregnancy or delivery. About one in three infected newborns will develop AIDS symptoms and die within just a few years. Studies show that these odds of mother-infant transmission can be cut significantly if the woman begins taking the drug azidothymidine (AZT) and other related AIDS medications by the fourteenth week of pregnancy. Providing these medications just before birth is helpful as well. Thus, screening pregnant women for AIDS and providing AZT treatment to those with AIDS are advocated by some experts.

**U**SDA warns pregnant women to thoroughly cook (e.g., microwave) all ready-to-eat meats, including hot dogs and cold cuts, until they are steaming to reduce risk of *Listeria* infections.

age poses special risks for pregnancy. The risks of LBW and preterm delivery increase modestly, but progressively, with maternal age beyond 35 years. Given close monitoring, however, a woman older than 35 years has an excellent chance of producing a healthy infant.

## Closely Spaced and Multiple Births

Siblings born in succession to a mother with less than a year between birth and subsequent conception are more likely to be born with low birth weights than are those farther apart in age. The risks of low birth weight, preterm birth, or small size for gestational age are 30% to 40% higher for infants conceived less than 6 months following a birth compared to those conceived 18 to 23 months following a birth. These poor outcomes are probably linked to a lack of enough time to rebuild nutrient stores depleted by the pregnancy. Similarly, multiple births (i.e., twins) increase the risk for preterm birth.

## Smoking, Medication Use, and Drug Abuse

Smoking, use of some medications, and illicit drug use during pregnancy all lead to harmful effects. Smoking is linked to preterm birth and appears to increase the risk of birth defects, sudden infant death, and childhood cancer. Problem drugs include aspirin (especially when used heavily), hormone ointments, nose drops and related "cold" medications, rectal suppositories, weight-control pills, and medications prescribed for previous illnesses. Illicit drug use is particularly harmful during pregnancy. Many chemicals in recreational drugs cross the placenta and affect the fetus, whose detoxification systems are immature. During organ development, such insults can cause malformations. Marijuana, the most common illegal drug used during the reproductive years, can result in reduced blood flow to the uterus and placenta, leading to poor fetal growth. Low birth weight and higher risk of premature delivery often are seen in infants whose mothers used marijuana during pregnancy. Cocaine use also has devastating consequences for the developing fetus.

## Food Safety

Any foodborne illness during any stage of life is a concern. One type of foodborne illness that poses particular danger for pregnant women is caused by the bacterium *Listeria monocytogenes* (review Chapter 13). Infection with this microorganism typically causes mild flulike symptoms, such as fever, headache, and vomiting, about 7 to 30 days after exposure. However, pregnant women, newborn infants, and people with depressed immune function may suffer more severe symptoms, including spontaneous abortion and serious blood infections. In these high-risk people, 25% of infections may be fatal. Unpasteurized milk, soft cheeses made from raw milk (e.g., brie, Camembert, feta, and blue cheeses), and raw cabbage can be sources of *Listeria* organisms, so it is especially important that pregnant women (and other people at high risk for infection) avoid these products. Experts advise consuming only pasteurized milk products and cooking meat, poultry, and seafood thoroughly to kill this and other foodborne organisms. It is unsafe in pregnancy to eat any raw meats or other raw animal products, uncooked hot dogs, or undercooked poultry. These food safety recommendations are included in the Dietary Guidelines for Americans discussed later in the chapter (Table 14-2 on page 554).

## Nutritional Status

Is attention to good nutrition worth the effort? Yes; evidence shows that the effort is justified. Extra nutrients and calories are used for fetal growth, as well as for the changes the mother's body undergoes to accommodate the fetus. Her uterus and breasts grow, the placenta develops, her total blood volume increases, the heart and kidneys work harder, and stores of body fat increase.

Although it is difficult to predict what degree of poor nutrition will affect each pregnancy, a daily diet containing only 1000 kcal has been shown to greatly restrict fetal growth and development. Increased maternal and infant death rates seen in famine-stricken areas of Africa provide further evidence.

Genetic background can explain little of the observed differences in birth weight between developed and developing countries. Both environmental factors and nutritional factors are important. The worse the nutritional condition of the mother at the beginning of pregnancy, the more valuable a healthy prenatal diet and/or use of prenatal supplements are in improving the course and outcome of her pregnancy.

## Nutrition Assistance for Low-Income Families

A low socioeconomic status is also associated with problems in pregnancy. Typical characteristics of low socioeconomic status include poverty, inadequate health care, poor health practices, lack of education, and unmarried status. In the United States, about 31% of all births are to unwed mothers, many of whom are poor.

Several U.S. government programs provide high-quality health care and foods to reduce infant mortality. These are designed to alleviate the negative impact of poverty and insufficient education and nutrient intake on pregnancy outcome. An example of such a program is the Special Supplemental Nutrition Program for Women, Infants, and Children (WIC). This program offers health assessments and vouchers for foods that supply high-quality protein, calcium, iron, and vitamins A and C to pregnant women, infants, and children (up to age 5 years) from low-income populations. The WIC program is available in all areas of the United States and has a staff trained to help women have healthy babies. More than 8 million women, infants, and young children are benefiting from this program, but many eligible pregnant women are not participating.

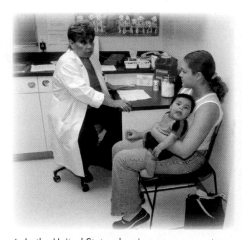

▲ In the United States, low-income pregnant women and their infants (and children) benefit from the nutritional and medical attention provided by the WIC program.

### CONCEPT CHECK

To help ensure the optimal health of both the mother and her offspring, adequate nutrition is vital both before and during pregnancy. In particular, meeting folate needs from a synthetic source starting at least 3 months before pregnancy begins, is effective at preventing a variety of fetal malformations. Organs and body parts in the offspring begin to develop soon after conception. The first trimester is a critical period when inadequate nutrient intake or alcohol and drug use can result in birth defects.

Infants born after 37 weeks of gestation who weigh more than 5.5 pounds (2.5 kilograms) have the fewest medical problems at birth. To reduce infant and maternal medical problems or death, the expectant mother, family, and medical care providers should take the steps necessary to allow the mother to carry the baby in her uterus for the entire 9 months, which in turn contributes to adequate growth. Good nutrition and health practices aid in this goal.

# 14.4 Increased Nutrient Needs to Support Pregnancy

Pregnancy is a time of increased nutrient needs. It is important to recognize the need for individual assessment and counseling of mothers-to-be, as the nutritional and health status of each woman is different. Still, there are some general principles true for most women with regard to increased nutrient needs.

## CRITICAL THINKING

Alexandra wants to have a baby. She has read that it is very important for the woman to be healthy during the pregnancy. However, Jane, her sister, tells her that the time to begin to assess her nutritional and health status is before she becomes pregnant. What additional information should Jane have given Alexandra?

▲ Many women recognize the benefits of remaining active during pregnancy. Healthcare providers typically encourage healthy, well-nourished women to engage in moderate exercise as long as increased calorie and nutrient needs are met.

## Increased Calorie Needs

To support the growth and development of the fetus, pregnant women need to increase their calorie intake. Calorie needs during the first trimester are essentially the same as for the nonpregnant woman. However, during the second and third trimesters, it is necessary for a pregnant woman to consume approximately 350 to 450 kcal more per day than her prepregnancy needs (the upper end of the range is needed in the third trimester).

Rather than seeing this as an opportunity to fill up on sugary desserts or fat-filled snacks, these extra calories should be in the form of nutrient-dense foods. For example, throughout the day, about six whole-wheat crackers, 1 ounce of cheese, and ½ cup of fat-free milk would supply the extra calories (and also some calcium). Although she "eats for two," the pregnant woman must not double her normal calorie intake. The "eating for two" concept refers more appropriately to increased needs for several vitamins and minerals. Micronutrient needs are increased by up to 50% during pregnancy, whereas calorie needs during the second and third trimesters represent only about a 20% increase.

If a woman is active during her pregnancy, she may need to increase her calorie intake by even more than the estimated 350 to 450 kcal per day. Her greater body weight requires more calories for activity. Many women find that they are inactive during the later months, partly because of their increased size, so an extra 350 to 450 kcal in their daily diets is usually enough.

## MAKING DECISIONS

### Staying Active During Pregnancy

While pregnancy is not the time to begin an intense fitness regimen, women can generally take part in most low- or moderate-intensity activities during pregnancy. Walking, cycling, swimming, or light aerobics for 30 minutes or more on most days of the week is generally advised. Such exercise may prevent pregnancy complications and promote an easier delivery. Some research indicates that regular physical activity during pregnancy lowers a woman's risk of developing gestational diabetes by 50% and preeclampsia by 40%. A few types of activities can potentially harm the fetus and should be avoided, especially those with inherent risk of falls and abdominal trauma. Examples of exercises to avoid, especially during the second and third trimesters, include downhill skiing, weightlifting, soccer, basketball, horseback riding, certain calisthenics (e.g., deep knee bends), any contact sports (e.g., hockey), and SCUBA diving.

Women with high-risk pregnancies, such as those experiencing premature labor contractions, may need to restrict their physical activity. To ensure optimal health for both herself and her infant, a pregnant woman should first consult her physician about physical activity and possible limitations.

## Adequate Weight Gain

Key recommendations for weight management during pregnancy and lactation are included in the Dietary Guidelines for Americans (see Table 14-2 on page 554). Adequate weight gain for a mother is one of the best predictors of pregnancy outcome. Her diet should allow for approximately 2 to 4 pounds (0.9 to 1.8 kilograms) of weight gain during the first trimester and then a subsequent weight gain of 0.75 to 1 pound (0.3 to 0.5 kilogram) weekly during the second and third trimesters (Fig. 14-3). A healthy goal for total weight gain for a woman of normal weight (based on BMI; Table 14-1 ) averages about 25 to 35 pounds (11.5 to 16 kilograms). Adolescents and African-American women, who often have smaller babies, are strongly advised to aim for the greater amount. Women carrying twins should gain 35 to 45 pounds, and those carrying triplets should gain 50 pounds (23 kilograms).

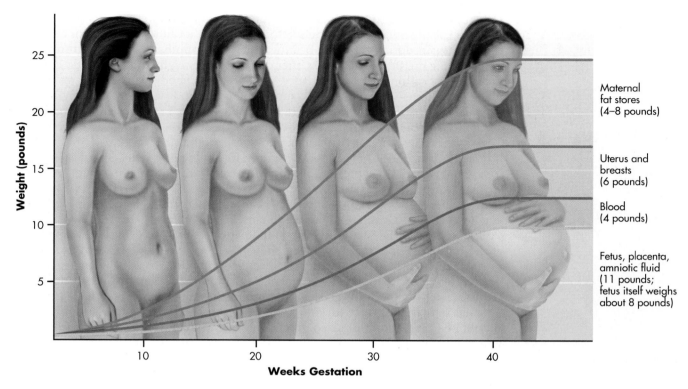

**FIGURE 14-3** ▶ The components of weight gain in pregnancy. A weight gain of 25 to 35 pounds is recommended for most women. The various components total about 25 pounds.

For women who begin pregnancy with a low BMI, the goal increases to 28 to 40 pounds (12.5 to 18 kilograms). The goal decreases to 15 to 25 pounds (7 to 11.5 kilograms) for women at a high BMI. Target weight gain for obese women is 15 pounds (7 kilograms) or more. Figure 14-3 shows why the typical recommendation begins at 25 pounds.

A weight gain of between 25 and 35 pounds for a woman starting pregnancy at normal weight has repeatedly been shown to yield optimal health for both mother and fetus if gestation lasts at least 38 weeks. The weight gain should yield a birth

**TABLE 14-1** Recommended Weight Gain in Pregnancy Based on Prepregnancy Body Mass Index (BMI)

| Prepregnancy BMI Category | Total Weight Gain* | |
| --- | --- | --- |
| | (pounds) | (kilograms) |
| Low (BMI less than 19.8) | 28 to 40 | 12.5 to 18 |
| Normal (BMI 19.8 to 25.9) | 25 to 35 | 11.5 to 16 |
| High (BMI 26 to 29) | 15 to 25 | 7 to 11.5 |
| Obese (BMI greater than 29) | 15 (or more) | 7 (or more) |

*The listed values are for pregnancies with one fetus. Short women (less than 62 inches) should strive for gains at the lower end of the ranges. For women of normal BMI carrying twins, the range is 35 to 45 pounds (16 to 20 kilograms). Adolescents within 2 years of beginning menses and African-American women should strive for gains at the upper end of the ranges.

Reprinted with permission from *Nutrition During Pregnancy and Lactation,* Copyright 1992 by the National Academy of Sciences. Courtesy of the National Academy Press, Washington, DC.

During pregnancy, women in North America are more likely to gain excess weight and make poor food choices than to eat too little.

▲ Following weight gain recommendations during pregnancy helps increase the chances of a successful outcome.

weight of 7.5 pounds (3.5 kilograms). Although some extra weight gain during pregnancy is usually not harmful (about 5 to 10 pounds), it can set the stage for a pattern of weight gain during the child-bearing years if the mother does not return to her approximate prepregnancy weight after delivery. Overweight and obesity do contribute to complications during pregnancy. Excess maternal body weight increases risk for diabetes, hypertension, blood clots, and spontaneous abortions. For the baby, there is a greater chance of birth defects and macrosomia, in which the fetus grows larger than average in utero. Larger infants contribute to a greater need for surgical delivery (i.e., Cesarean sections) among overweight and obese mothers.

Weight gain during pregnancy, especially in the teenage years, should generally follow the pattern in Figure 14-3. Monitoring weekly records of a pregnant woman's weight gain helps assess how much to adjust her food intake. Weight gain is a key issue in prenatal care and a concern of many mothers-to-be. Remember that inadequate weight gain can cause many problems.

If a woman deviates from the desirable pattern, she should make the appropriate adjustment. For example, if a woman begins to gain too much weight during her pregnancy, she should not lose weight to get back on track. Even if a woman gains 35 pounds in the first 7 months of pregnancy, she must still gain more during the last 2 months. She should, however, slow the increase in weight to parallel the rise on the prenatal weight gain chart. In other words, the sources of the unnecessary calories should be found and minimized. Alternately, if a woman has not gained the desired weight by a given point in pregnancy, she shouldn't gain the needed weight rapidly. Instead, she should slowly gain a little more weight than the typical pattern to meet the goal by the end of the pregnancy. A registered dietitian can help make any needed adjustments.

## Increased Protein and Carbohydrate Needs

The RDA for protein increases by an additional 25 grams per day during pregnancy. A cup of milk alone contains 8 grams. Many nonpregnant women already consume protein in excess of their needs and therefore do not need to increase protein intake any further. However, all women should check to make sure they are eating enough protein as well as enough calories, so this protein is not used to meet energy needs.

The RDA for carbohydrate increases to 175 grams daily, primarily to prevent ketosis. Ketone bodies, a by-product of metabolism of fat for energy, are thought to be poorly used by the fetal brain, implying possible slowing of fetal brain development. Carbohydrate intakes of most women, pregnant or not, already exceed the RDA.

## A Word About Lipids

Fat intake should increase proportionally with calorie intake during pregnancy to maintain around 20% to 30% of total calories from fat. Pregnancy is not a time for a low-fat diet, as lipids are a source of extra calories and essential fatty acids needed during pregnancy. Recommendations for the types of lipids during pregnancy are generally the same as for nonpregnant adults. To reduce risk for cardiovascular disease, the American Heart Association recommends no more than 7% of total calories from saturated fat and no more than 1% from *trans* fat. Consumption of dietary cholesterol is not required, but keeping cholesterol intake at a maximum of 300 milligrams per day is also a good goal for maintenance of maternal cardiovascular health.

During pregnancy, it is particularly important to make sure to consume adequate essential fatty acids—linoleic acid (omega-6) and alpha-linolenic acid (omega-3). As you learned in Chapter 5, essential fatty acids cannot be synthesized in the body and must be consumed in the diet. For the developing fetus, essential fatty acids are required for growth, brain development, and eye development. Recommendations are slightly increased by pregnancy: thirteen grams per day of omega-6 fatty acids and

1.4 grams per day of omega-3 fatty acids. These needs can be met by consuming 2 to 4 tablespoons per day of plant oils. Consumption of fish at least two times per week is also helpful in meeting needs for essential fatty acids in the diet. (See the "Nutrition and Your Health" section at the end of this chapter for a discussion of mercury in fish.)

## Increased Vitamin Needs

Vitamin needs generally increase from prepregnancy RDAs/Adequate Intakes by up to 30% for most of the B vitamins and even greater for vitamin B-6 (45%) and folate (50%). Vitamin A needs only increase by 10%, so a specific focus on this vitamin is not needed. And remember, excess amounts of vitamin A are harmful to the developing fetus.

The extra amount of vitamin B-6 and other B vitamins (except folate) needed in the diet is easily met via wise food choices, such as a serving of a typical ready-to-eat breakfast cereal and some animal protein sources. Folate needs, however, often merit specific diet planning and possible vitamin supplementation. The synthesis of DNA, and therefore cell division, requires folate, so this nutrient is especially crucial during pregnancy. Ultimately, both fetal and maternal growth depend on an ample supply of folate. Red blood cell formation, which requires folate, increases during pregnancy. Serious folate-related anemia therefore can result if folate intake is inadequate. The RDA for folate increases during pregnancy to 600 micrograms DFE per day (review Chapter 8 for calculation of DFE). This is a critical goal in the nutritional care of a pregnant woman. Increasing folate intakes to meet 600 micrograms DFE per day for a pregnant woman can be achieved through dietary sources, a supplemental source of folic acid, or a combination of both. Choosing a diet rich in synthetic folic acid, such as from ready-to-eat breakfast cereals or meal replacement bars (look for approximately 50% to 100% of the Daily Value), is especially helpful in meeting folate needs. Recall from Chapter 8 that synthetic folic acid is much more easily absorbed than the various forms of folate found naturally in foods.

## Increased Mineral Needs

Mineral needs generally increase during pregnancy, especially the requirements for iodide and iron. Zinc needs also increase. (Calcium needs do not increase, but still may deserve special attention because many women have deficient intakes.)

Pregnant women need the extra iodide (total of 220 micrograms per day) for prevention of goiter. Typical iodide intakes are enough if the woman uses iodized salt. Animal proteins or a fortified ready-to-eat breakfast cereal in the diet can easily provide enough extra zinc. The extra iron (total of 27 milligrams per day) is needed to synthesize the greater amount of hemoglobin needed during pregnancy and to provide iron stores for the fetus. Women often need a supplemental source of iron, especially if they do not consume iron-fortified foods, such as highly fortified breakfast cereals containing close to 100% of the Daily Value for iron (18 milligrams). Iron supplements decrease appetite and can cause nausea and constipation, so if used, these should be taken between meals or just before going to bed. Milk, coffee, or tea should not be consumed with an iron supplement because these beverages have substances that interfere with iron absorption. Eating foods rich in vitamin C along with nonheme iron-containing foods and iron supplements helps increase iron absorption from those sources. Pregnant women who are not anemic may wait until the second trimester, when pregnancy-related nausea generally lessens, to start iron supplementation if needed.

The consequences of iron-deficiency anemia—especially during the first trimester—can be severe. Negative outcomes include preterm delivery, LBW infants, and increased risk for fetal death in the first weeks after birth.

The Dietary Guidelines for Americans recommend that women who may become pregnant eat foods high in iron and consume adequate amounts of the synthetic form of folate (see Table 14-2 on page 554).

**TABLE 14-2** Key Recommendations from the Latest Dietary Guidelines for Americans, for Women of Childbearing Age Who May Become Pregnant, Pregnant Women, and Breastfeeding Women

| Adequate Nutrients Within Calorie Needs |
|---|
| • *Women of childbearing age who may become pregnant.* Eat foods high in iron from animal products and/or consume iron-rich plant foods or iron-fortified foods with an enhancer of iron absorption, such as vitamin C-rich foods. |
| • *Women of childbearing age who may become pregnant and those in the first few months of pregnancy.* Consume an adequate amount of the synthetic form of the B vitamin folate (called folic acid) daily (from fortified foods or supplements) in addition to food forms of folate found in a varied diet. |

| Weight Management |
|---|
| • *Pregnant women.* Ensure appropriate weight gain as specified by a healthcare provider. |
| • *Breastfeeding women.* Moderate weight reduction is safe and does not compromise weight gain of the nursing infant. |

| Physical Activity |
|---|
| • *Pregnant women.* In the absence of medical complications, incorporate 30 minutes or more of moderate-intensity physical activity on most, if not all, days of the week. Avoid activities with a high risk of falling or abdominal trauma. |
| • *Breastfeeding women.* Be aware that neither acute nor regular exercise adversely affects the mother's ability to successfully breastfeed. |

| Alcoholic Beverages |
|---|
| • Alcoholic beverages should not be consumed by some individuals, including those who cannot restrict their alcohol intake, women of childbearing age who may become pregnant, pregnant and lactating women, children and adolescents, individuals taking medications that may interact with alcohol, and those with specific medical conditions. |

| Food Safety |
|---|
| • *Infants and young children, pregnant women, older adults, and those who are immunocompromised.* Do not eat or drink unpasteurized milk or any products made from unpasteurized milk, raw or partially cooked eggs or foods containing raw eggs, raw or undercooked meat and poultry, raw or undercooked fish or shellfish, unpasteurized juices, and raw sprouts. |
| • *Pregnant women, older adults, and those who are immunocompromised:* Only eat certain deli meats and frankfurters that have been reheated to steaming hot. |

## Use of Prenatal Vitamin and Mineral Supplements

Special supplements formulated for pregnancy are prescribed routinely for pregnant women by most physicians. Some are sold over the counter, while others are dispensed by prescription because of the high synthetic folic acid content (1000 micrograms), which could pose problems for others, such as older people (see Chapter 16). These supplements are high in iron (27 milligrams per pill). There is no evidence that use of such supplements causes significant health problems in pregnancy, aside perhaps from the combined amounts of supplementary and dietary vitamin A (see "Nutrition and Your Health" at the end of this chapter).

Instances when prenatal supplements may especially contribute to a successful pregnancy are with poor women, teenagers, those with a generally deficient diet, women carrying multiple fetuses, those that smoke or use alcohol or illegal drugs, and vegans. In other cases, healthy diets can provide the needed nutrients. When choosing a multivitamin, rely on brands that display the USP symbol on their label, signifying that the supplement meets the content, quality, purity, and safety standards of the

▲ Pregnancy, in particular, is not a time to self-prescribe vitamin and mineral supplements. For example, although vitamin A is a routine component of prenatal vitamins, intakes over three times the RDA for vitamin A have been shown to have toxic effects on the fetus.

U.S. Pharmacopoeia. Also, avoid megadoses of any nutrient. In particular, toxicity of vitamin A is linked with birth defects. High doses of cobalt and vitamin D are also under study for possible ill effects on pregnancy outcome. Skip supplements containing herbs, enzymes, and amino acids. Many of these ingredients have not been evaluated for safety during pregnancy or lactation and may be toxic to the fetus. Furthermore, discard supplements that are past the expiration date, as some ingredients lose potency over time.

## 14.5 Food Plan for Pregnant Women

One dietary approach to support a successful pregnancy is based on MyPyramid. For an active 24-year-old woman, about 2200 kcal are recommended during the first trimester (the same as recommended for such a woman when not pregnant). The plan should include:

- 3 cups of calcium-rich foods from the milk group or use of calcium-fortified foods to make up for any gap between calcium intake and need
- 6 ounce-equivalents from the meat & beans group
- 3 cups from the vegetable group
- 2 cups from the fruit group
- 7 ounce-equivalents from the grain group
- 6 teaspoons of vegetable oil

**A**t **www.mypyramid.gov**, moms-to-be can find individualized dietary information by clicking on the link for MyPyramid for Pregnancy and Breastfeeding. Based on age, height, physical activity, and prepregnancy weight, calorie and food group recommendations are generated for each trimester.

### MAKING DECISIONS

#### Cravings During Pregnancy

It is a common myth that women instinctively know what to eat during pregnancy. Cravings of the last two trimesters are often related to hormonal changes in the mother, or family traditions. Such "instinct" cannot be trusted, however, based on observations that some women crave nonfood items (called **pica**) such as laundry starch, chalk, cigarette ashes, and soil (clay). This practice can be extremely harmful to the mother and the fetus. Overall, though women may have a natural instinct to consume the right foods in pregnancy, humans are so far removed from living by instinct that relying on our cravings to meet nutrient needs is risky. Nutrition advice by experts is more reliable.

**pica** The practice of eating nonfood items, such as dirt, laundry starch, or clay.

Specifically, choices from the milk group should include low-fat or fat-free versions of milk, yogurt, and cheese. These foods supply extra protein, calcium, and carbohydrate, as well as other nutrients. Choices from the meat & beans group should include both animal and vegetable sources. Besides protein, these foods help provide the extra iron and zinc needed. The vegetable and fruit group choices provide a variety of vitamins and minerals. One cup from this combination should be a good vitamin C source, and 1 cup should be a green vegetable or other rich source of folate. Choices from the grain group should focus on whole-grain and enriched foods. One ounce of a whole-grain, ready-to-eat breakfast cereal significantly contributes to meeting many vitamin and mineral needs. Finally, inclusion of plant oils in the diet contributes essential fatty acids. Discretionary calories (up to about 300 kcal) can then be added to allow for weight maintenance.

In the second and third trimesters, about 2600 kcal are recommended for this woman. The plan should now include:

- 3 cups of calcium-rich foods from the milk group or use of calcium-fortified foods
- 6 ½ ounce-equivalents from the meat & beans group
- 3 ½ cups from the vegetable group
- 2 cups from the fruit group

- 8 ounce-equivalents from the grain group
- 7 teaspoons of vegetable oil

Discretionary calories (up to about 400 kcal) can then be added to allow for gradual weight gain. Table 14-3 illustrates one daily menu based on the 2600 kcal plan for pregnancy for women in the second or third trimesters. This menu meets the extra nutrient needs associated with pregnancy. Women who need to consume more than this—and some do for various reasons—should incorporate additional fruits, vegetables, and whole-grain breads and cereals, not poor nutrient sources such as desserts and sugared soft drinks.

### Pregnant Vegetarians

Women who are either lactoovovegetarians or lactovegetarians generally do not face special difficulties in meeting their nutritional needs during pregnancy. Like

▲ A salad each day provides many nutrients for the prenatal diet.

**TABLE 14-3** Sample 2600 kcal Daily Menu That Meets the Nutritional Needs of Most Pregnant and Breastfeeding Women

| | Vitamin B-6 | Folate | Iron | Zinc | Calcium |
|---|:---:|:---:|:---:|:---:|:---:|
| **Breakfast** | | | | | |
| 1 cup Kellogg's Smart Start cereal | ✓ | ✓ | ✓ | ✓ | ✓ |
| 1 cup orange juice | | ✓ | | | |
| 1 cup fat-free milk | ✓ | | | | ✓ |
| **Snack** | | | | | |
| 2 tbsp peanut butter | ✓ | ✓ | ✓ | ✓ | |
| 2 stalks of celery | | ✓ | | | |
| 1 slice whole-wheat toast | | ✓ | ✓ | ✓ | |
| 1 cup plain low-fat yogurt | ✓ | | | | ✓ |
| ½ cup strawberries | | ✓ | | | |
| **Lunch** | | | | | |
| 2 cups spinach salad with 2 tbsp oil and vinegar dressing | | ✓ | | | ✓ |
| ½ tomato | | | | | |
| 1 slice whole-wheat toast | | ✓ | ✓ | ✓ | |
| 1 ½ ounce provolone cheese | ✓ | | | | ✓ |
| **Snack** | | | | | |
| 5 whole-wheat crackers | | ✓ | ✓ | ✓ | |
| 1 cup grape juice | | | | | |
| **Dinner** | | | | | |
| 3 ounces lean hamburger, broiled (with condiments) | ✓ | | ✓ | ✓ | |
| ½ cup baked beans | ✓ | ✓ | ✓ | ✓ | |
| 1 hamburger bun | | ✓ | ✓ | | |
| ½ sliced tomato | | | | | |
| 1 cup cooked broccoli | | ✓ | | | ✓ |
| 1 tsp soft margarine | | | | | |
| Iced tea | | | | | |
| **Snack** | | | | | |
| Granola bar (2 ounces) | | ✓ | ✓ | ✓ | |
| ½ banana | ✓ | | | | |
| Discretionary calories of up to 400 kcal* | | | | | |

*Amount of discretionary calories will vary based on the actual food choices made within each MyPyramid group.

This diet meets nutrient needs for pregnancy and lactation. Lack of a check (✓) indicates a poor source of the nutrient. The vitamin- and mineral-fortified breakfast cereal used in this example makes an important contribution to meeting nutrient needs. Fluids can be added as desired. Total intake of fluids, such as water, should be 10 cups or so per day.

nonvegetarian women, they should be concerned primarily with meeting vitamin B-6, iron, folate, and zinc needs.

On the other hand, for a vegan, careful diet planning during preconception and pregnancy is crucial to ensure sufficient protein, vitamin D (particularly in the absence of sufficient sun exposure), vitamin B-6, iron, calcium, zinc, and especially a supplemental source of vitamin B-12. The basic vegan diet listed in Chapter 6 should be modified to include more grains, beans, nuts, and seeds to supply the necessary extra amounts of some of these nutrients. As mentioned, use of a prenatal multivitamin and mineral supplement also is generally advocated to help fill micronutrient gaps. However, although these are high in iron, this is not true for calcium (200 milligrams per pill). If iron and calcium supplements are used, they should not be taken together, to avoid possible competition for absorption.

## CONCEPT CHECK

Calorie needs increase by an average of about 350 to 450 kcal per day during the second and third trimesters of pregnancy, respectively. Weight gain should be slow and steady up to a total of 25 to 35 pounds for a woman of normal weight (i.e., prepregnancy BMI of 19.8 to 25.9). Protein and certain vitamin and mineral needs increase during pregnancy. Most important to consider are vitamin B-6, folate, iron, iodide, and zinc. A pregnant woman's diet should be varied and generally follow a MyPyramid pattern. A prenatal multivitamin and mineral supplement is commonly prescribed but may not be necessary, depending on one's diet and health status. Taking too many supplements—especially vitamin A—can be hazardous to the fetus.

# 14.6 Physiological Changes of Concern During Pregnancy

During pregnancy, the fetus's needs for oxygen and nutrients, as well as excretion of waste products increase the burden on the mother's lungs, heart, and kidneys. Although a mother's digestive and metabolic systems work efficiently, some discomfort accompanies the changes her body undergoes to accommodate the fetus.

## Heartburn, Constipation, and Hemorrhoids

Hormones (such as progesterone) produced by the placenta relax muscles in the uterus and the gastrointestinal tract. This often causes heartburn as stomach acid refluxes into the esophagus (review Chapter 3). When this occurs, the woman should avoid lying down after eating, eat less fat so that foods pass more quickly from the stomach into the small intestine, and avoid spicy foods she cannot tolerate. She should also consume most liquids between meals to decrease the volume of food in the stomach after meals, and thus relieve some of the pressure that encourages reflux. Women with more severe cases may need antacids or related medications.

Constipation often results as the intestinal muscles relax during pregnancy. It is especially likely to develop late in pregnancy, as the fetus competes with the GI tract for space in the abdominal cavity. To offset these discomforts, a woman should perform regular exercise and consume more fluid, fiber, and dried fruits, such as prunes (dried plums). The Adequate Intake for fiber in pregnancy is 28 grams, slightly more than for the nonpregnant woman. Fluid needs are 10 cups per day. These practices can help prevent constipation and a problem that frequently accompanies it, hemorrhoids. Straining during elimination can lead to hemorrhoids, which are more likely to occur during pregnancy because of other body changes. A re-evaluation of the need for and dose of iron supplementation also should be considered, as high iron intakes are linked to constipation.

## Edema

Placental hormones cause various body tissues to retain fluid during pregnancy. Blood volume also greatly expands during pregnancy. The extra fluid normally causes some swelling (edema). There is no reason to restrict salt severely or use diuretics to limit mild edema. However, the edema may limit physical activity late in pregnancy and occasionally requires a woman to elevate her feet or wear compression stockings to control the symptoms. Overall, edema generally spells trouble only if hypertension and the appearance of extra protein in the urine accompany it (see a following section, "Pregnancy-Induced Hypertension").

## Morning Sickness

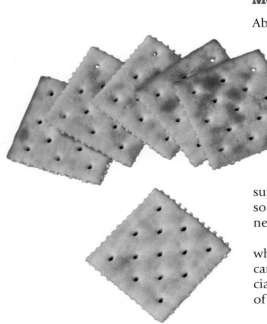

About 70% to 85% of pregnant women experience nausea during the early stages of pregnancy. This nausea may be related to the increased sense of smell induced by pregnancy-related hormones circulating in the bloodstream. Although commonly called "morning sickness," pregnancy-related nausea may occur at any time and persist all day. It is often the first signal to a woman that she is pregnant. To help control mild nausea, pregnant women can try the following: avoiding nauseating foods, such as fried or greasy foods; cooking with good ventilation to dissipate nauseating smells; eating saltine crackers or dry cereal before getting out of bed; avoiding large fluid intakes early in the morning; and eating smaller, more frequent meals. The iron in prenatal supplements triggers nausea in some women, so changing the type of supplement used or postponing use until the second trimester may provide relief in some cases. If a woman thinks her prenatal supplement is related to morning sickness, she should discuss switching to another supplement with her physician.

Overall, if a food sounds good to a pregnant woman with morning sickness, whether it is broccoli, soda crackers, or lemonade, she should eat it and eat when she can, while also striving to follow her prenatal diet. The American College of Obstetricians and Gynecologists recommends the following for the prevention and treatment of nausea and vomiting of pregnancy:

- History of use of a balanced multivitamin and mineral supplement at the time of conception
- Use of megadoses of vitamin B-6 (10–25 milligrams taken 3 to 4 times a day), especially coupled with the antihistamine doxylamine (10 milligrams) with each dose
- Ginger may also be helpful (350 milligrams taken 3 times per day)

Usually, nausea stops after the first trimester; however, in about 10% to 20% of cases, it can continue throughout the entire pregnancy. In cases of serious nausea, the preceding practices offer little relief. Excessive vomiting can cause dangerous dehydration and must be avoided. When vomiting persists (about 0.5% to 2% of pregnancies), medical attention is needed.

▲ A few saltine crackers upon waking or between meals can help lessen pregnancy-related nausea.

## Anemia

To supply fetal needs, the mother's blood volume expands to approximately 150% of normal. The number of red blood cells, however, increases by only 20% to 30%, and this occurs more gradually. As a result, a pregnant woman has a lower ratio of red blood cells to total blood volume in her system. This hemodilution is known as **physiological anemia**. It is a normal response to pregnancy, rather than the result of inadequate nutrient intake. If during pregnancy, however, iron stores and/or dietary iron intake are not sufficient to meet needs, any resulting iron-deficiency anemia

**physiological anemia** The normal increase in blood volume in pregnancy that dilutes the concentration of red blood cells, resulting in anemia; also called *hemodilution*.

requires medical attention. The Dietary Guidelines for Americans recommend that women who may become pregnant eat foods high in iron (Table 14-2).

## Gestational Diabetes

Hormones synthesized by the placenta decrease the efficiency of insulin. This leads to a mild increase in blood glucose, which helps supply calories to the fetus. If the rise in blood glucose becomes excessive, this leads to **gestational diabetes,** often beginning in weeks 20 to 28, particularly in women who have a family history of diabetes or who are obese. Other risk factors include maternal age over 35 and gestational diabetes in a prior pregnancy. In North America, gestational diabetes develops in about 4% of pregnancies; however, it increases to 7% in the Caucasian population. Today, pregnant women often are screened for diabetes at 24 to 28 weeks by checking for elevated blood glucose concentration 1 to 2 hours after consuming 50 to 100 grams of glucose. If gestational diabetes is detected, a special diet that distributes low glycemic load carbohydrates throughout the day needs to be implemented. Sometimes insulin injections or oral medications are also needed. Regular physical activity also helps control blood glucose.

The primary risk of uncontrolled diabetes during pregnancy is that the fetus can grow quite large. This is a result of the oversupply of glucose from maternal circulation coupled with an increased production of insulin by the fetus, which allows fetal tissues to take up an increased amount of building materials for growth. The mother may require a Cesarean section if the size of the fetus is not compatible with a vaginal delivery. Another threat is that the infant may have low blood glucose at birth, because of the tendency to produce extra insulin that began during gestation. Other concerns are the potential for early delivery and increased risk of birth trauma and malformations. Although gestational diabetes often disappears after the infant's birth, it increases the mother's risk of developing diabetes later in life, especially if she fails to maintain a healthy body weight. Studies show that infants of mothers with gestational diabetes may also have higher risks of developing obesity and type 2 diabetes as they grow to adulthood. For all these reasons, proper control of gestational diabetes (and any diabetes present in the mother before pregnancy) is extremely important.

## Pregnancy-Induced Hypertension

**Pregnancy-induced hypertension** is a high-risk disorder that occurs in about 3% to 5% of pregnancies. In its mild forms, it is also known as *preeclampsia* and, in severe forms, as *eclampsia*. Early symptoms include a rise in blood pressure, excess protein in the urine, edema, changes in blood clotting, and nervous system disorders. Very severe effects, including convulsions, can occur in the second and third trimesters. If not controlled, eclampsia eventually damages the liver and kidneys, and mother and fetus may die. The populations most at risk for this disorder are women under age 17 or over age 35, overweight or obese women, and those who have had multiple-birth pregnancies. A family history of pregnancy-induced hypertension in the mother's or father's side of the family, diabetes, African-American race, and a woman's first pregnancy also raise risk. Some research points to dietary inadequacies of vitamin E, vitamin C, calcium, selenium, or zinc as potential causes of this condition.

Pregnancy-induced hypertension resolves once the pregnancy ends, making delivery the most reliable treatment for the mother. However, because the problem often begins before the fetus is ready to be born, physicians in many cases must use treatments to prevent the worsening of the disorder. Bed rest and magnesium sulfate are the most effective treatment methods, although their effectiveness varies. Magnesium likely acts to relax blood vessels, and so leads to a fall in blood pressure. Several other treatments, such as various antiseizure and antihypertensive medications, calcium, and use of antioxidant supplements, are under study.

**gestational diabetes** A high blood glucose concentration that develops during pregnancy and returns to normal after birth; one cause is the placental production of hormones that antagonize the regulation of blood glucose by insulin.

**pregnancy-induced hypertension** A serious disorder that can include high blood pressure, kidney failure, convulsions, and even death of the mother and fetus. Although its exact cause is not known, an adequate diet (especially adequate calcium intake) and prenatal care may prevent this disorder or limit its severity. Mild cases are known as *preeclampsia;* more severe cases are called *eclampsia* (formerly called *toxemia*).

## CRITICAL THINKING

Sandy, 4 months pregnant, has been having heartburn after meals, constipation, and difficult bowel movements. As a student of nutrition, you understand the digestive system and the role of nutrition in health. What remedies might you suggest to Sandy to relieve her problems?

## 14.7 Breastfeeding

Breastfeeding the new infant further fosters his or her health, and so complements the attention given to diet during pregnancy. The American Dietetic Association and the American Academy of Pediatrics recommend breastfeeding exclusively for the first 6 months, with the continued combination of breastfeeding and infant foods until 1 year. The World Health Organization goes beyond that to recommend breastfeeding (with appropriate solid food introduction; see Chapter 15) for at least 2 years. Still, surveys show that only about 70% of North American mothers now begin to breastfeed their infants in the hospital, and at 4 and 6 months only 33% and 20%, respectively, are still breastfeeding their infants. The number falls to 18% at 1 year of age. These statistics refer to Caucasian women; minority women are even less likely to be breastfeeding at these time intervals.

Women who choose to breastfeed usually find it an enjoyable, special time in their lives and their relationship with their new infant. Although bottle feeding with an infant formula is also safe for infants, as discussed in Chapter 15, it does not equal the benefits derived from human milk in all aspects. If a woman doesn't breastfeed her child, breast weight returns to normal soon after birth.

### Ability to Breastfeed

Almost all women are physically capable of breastfeeding their children (see later section "Medical Conditions Precluding Breastfeeding" for exceptions). In most cases, problems encountered in breastfeeding are due to a lack of appropriate information. Anatomical problems in breasts, such as inverted nipples, can be corrected during pregnancy. Breast size generally increases during pregnancy and is no indication of success in breastfeeding. Most women notice a dramatic increase in the size and weight of their breasts by the third or fourth day of breastfeeding. If these changes do not occur, a woman needs to speak with her physician or a lactation consultant.

Breastfed infants must be followed closely over the first days of life to ensure that feeding and weight gain are proceeding normally. Monitoring is especially important with a mother's first child, because the mother will be inexperienced with the technique of breastfeeding. Mothers and healthy infants are commonly discharged from the hospital 1 to 2 days after delivery, whereas 20 years ago they stayed in the hospital for 3 or 4 days or longer. One result of such rapid discharge is a decreased period of infant monitoring by health care professionals. Incidents have been reported of infants developing dehydration and in turn blood clots soon after hospital discharge when breastfeeding did not proceed smoothly. Careful monitoring in this first week by a physician or lactation consultant is advised.

First-time mothers who plan to breastfeed should learn as much as they can about the process early in their pregnancy. Interested women should learn the proper technique, what problems to expect, and how to respond to them. Overall, breastfeeding is a learned skill, and mothers need knowledge to breastfeed safely, especially with the first child.

**M**any of the benefits of breastfeeding can be found in Table 14-4 on page 565 and at **www.4woman.gov./Breastfeeding/index.cfm**, sponsored by the U.S. Surgeon General.

▲ Breastfeeding is the preferred way to feed a young infant.

**H**ealthy People 2010 has set a goal of 75% of women breastfeeding their infants at time of hospital discharge, 50% breastfeeding for 6 months, and 25% still breastfeeding at 1 year.

## Production of Human Milk

During pregnancy, cells in the breast form milk-producing cells called **lobules** (Fig. 14-4). Hormones from the placenta stimulate these changes in the breast. After birth, the mother produces more **prolactin** hormone to maintain the changes in the breast and therefore the ability to produce milk. During pregnancy, breast weight increases by about 1 to 2 pounds.

The hormone prolactin also stimulates the synthesis of milk. Infant suckling stimulates prolactin release from the pituitary gland. Milk synthesis then occurs as an infant nurses. The more the infant suckles, the more milk is produced. Because of this, even twins (and triplets) can be breastfed adequately.

Most protein found in human milk is synthesized by breast tissue. Some proteins also enter the milk directly from the mother's bloodstream. These proteins include immune factors (e.g., antibodies) and enzymes. Fats in human milk come from both the mother's diet and those synthesized by breast tissue. The sugar galactose is synthesized in the breast, whereas glucose enters from the mother's bloodstream. Together, these sugars form lactose, the main carbohydrate in human milk.

## Let-Down Reflex

An important brain-breast connection—commonly called the **let-down reflex**—is necessary for breastfeeding. The brain releases the hormone **oxytocin** to allow the breast tissues to let down (release) the milk from storage sites (Fig. 14-5). It then travels to the nipple area. A tingling sensation signals the let-down reflex shortly before milk flow begins. If the let-down reflex doesn't operate, little milk is available to the infant. The infant then gets frustrated, and this can frustrate the mother.

The let-down reflex is easily inhibited by nervous tension, a lack of confidence, and fatigue. Mothers should be especially aware of the link between tension and

**lobules** Saclike structures in the breast that store milk.

**prolactin** A hormone secreted by the pituitary gland that stimulates the synthesis of milk in the breast.

**let-down reflex** A reflex stimulated by infant suckling that causes the release (ejection) of milk from milk ducts in the mother's breasts; also called *milk ejection reflex*.

**oxytocin** A hormone secreted by the pituitary gland. It causes contraction of the musclelike cells surrounding the ducts of the breasts and the smooth muscle of the uterus.

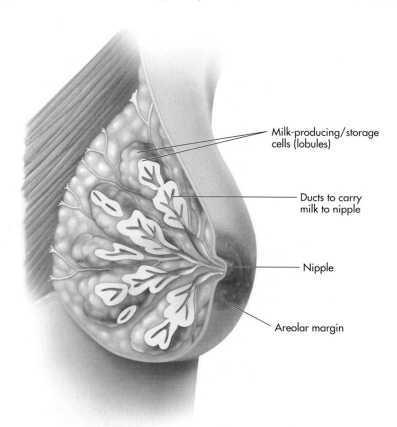

**FIGURE 14-4** ▶ The anatomy of the breast. Many types of cells form a coordinated network to produce and secrete human milk.

Milk-producing/storage cells (lobules)

Ducts to carry milk to nipple

Nipple

Areolar margin

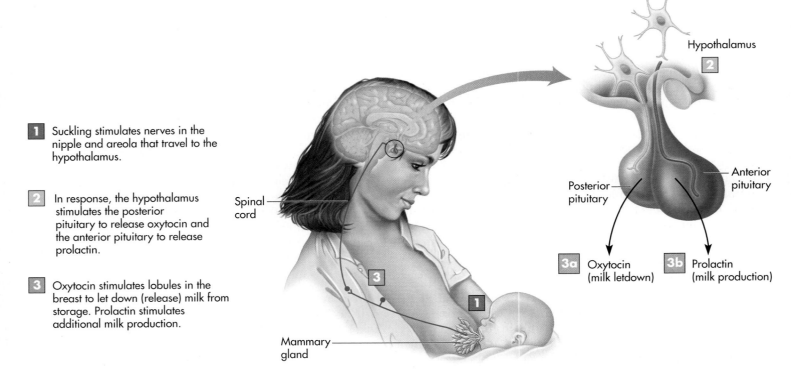

1 Suckling stimulates nerves in the nipple and areola that travel to the hypothalamus.

2 In response, the hypothalamus stimulates the posterior pituitary to release oxytocin and the anterior pituitary to release prolactin.

3 Oxytocin stimulates lobules in the breast to let down (release) milk from storage. Prolactin stimulates additional milk production.

**FIGURE 14-5** ▶ Let-down reflex. Suckling sets into motion the sequence of events that lead to milk let-down, the flow of milk into ducts of the breast.

**D**isposable diapers can absorb so much urine that it is difficult to judge when they are wet. A strip of paper towel laid inside a disposable diaper makes a good wetness indicator. Alternatively, cloth diapers may be used for a day or two to assess whether nursing is supplying sufficient milk.

a weak let-down reflex. They need to find a relaxed environment where they can breastfeed.

After a few weeks, the let-down reflex becomes automatic. The mother's response can be triggered just by thinking about her infant or seeing or hearing another one cry. At first, however, the process can be a bit bewildering. A mother cannot measure the amount of milk the infant takes in, so she may fear that she is not adequately nourishing the infant.

As a general rule, a well-nourished breastfed infant should (1) have six or more wet diapers per day after the second day of life, (2) show a normal weight gain, and (3) pass at least one or two stools per day that look like lumpy mustard. In addition, softening of the breast during the feeding helps indicate that enough milk is being consumed. Parents who sense their infant is not consuming enough milk should consult a physician immediately because dehydration can develop rapidly.

It generally takes 2 to 3 weeks to fully establish the feeding routine: Infant and mother both feel comfortable, the milk supply meets infant demand, and initial nipple soreness disappears. Establishing the breastfeeding routine requires patience, but the rewards are great. The adjustments are easier if supplemental formula feedings are not introduced until breastfeeding is well established, after at least 3 to 4 weeks. Then it is fine if a supplemental bottle or two of infant formula per day is needed.

## Nutritional Qualities of Human Milk

Human milk is different in composition from cow's milk. Unless altered, cow's milk should never be used in infant feeding until the infant is at least 12 months old. Cow's milk is too high in minerals and protein and does not contain enough carbohydrate to meet infant needs. In addition, the major protein in cow's milk is harder for an infant to digest than the major proteins in human milk. The proteins in cow's milk also may spur allergies in the infant. Finally, certain compounds in human milk presently under study show other possible benefits for the infant.

**Colostrum.** At the end of pregnancy, the first fluid made by the human breast is **colostrum.** This thick, yellowish fluid may leak from the breast during late pregnancy and is produced in earnest for a few days to a week after birth. Colostrum contains antibodies and immune system cells, some of which pass unaltered through the infant's immature GI tract into the bloodstream. The first few months of life are the only time when we can readily absorb whole proteins across the GI tract. These immune factors and cells protect the infant from some GI tract diseases and other infectious disorders, compensating for the infant's immature immune system during the first few months of life.

One component of colostrum, the ***Lactobacillus bifidus* factor,** encourages the growth of *Lactobacillus bifidus* bacteria. These bacteria limit the growth of potentially toxic bacteria in the intestine. Overall, breastfeeding promotes the intestinal health of the breastfed infant in this way.

**Mature Milk.** Human milk composition gradually changes until it achieves the normal composition of mature milk several days after delivery. Human milk looks very different from cow's milk. (Table 15-1 in Chapter 15 provides a direct comparison.) Human milk is thin and almost watery in appearance and often has a slightly bluish tinge. Its nutritional qualities, however, are impressive.

Human milk's proteins form a soft, light curd in the infant's stomach and are easy to digest. Some human milk proteins bind iron, reducing the growth of iron-requiring bacteria, some of which can cause diarrhea. Still other proteins offer the important immune protection already noted.

The lipids in human breast milk are high in linoleic acid and cholesterol, needed for brain development. Breast milk also contains long-chain omega-3 fatty acids, such as docosahexaenoic acid (DHA). This polyunsaturated fatty acid is used for the synthesis of tissues in the brain and the rest of the central nervous system and in the retina of the eye.

The fat composition of human milk changes during each feeding. The consistency of milk released initially (fore milk) resembles that of skim milk. It later has a greater fat proportion, similar to whole milk. Finally, the milk released after 10 to 20 minutes (hind milk) is essentially like cream. Babies need to nurse long enough (e.g., a total of 20 or more minutes) to get the calories in the rich hind milk to be satisfied between feedings and to grow well. The overall calorie content of human milk is about the same as that of infant formulas (67 kcal per 100 milliliters).

Human milk composition also allows for adequate fluid status of the infant, provided the baby is exclusively breastfed. A question commonly asked is whether the infant needs additional water, if stressed by hot weather, diarrhea, vomiting, or fever. Providing breastfed infants with up to 4 ounces of water a day from a bottle is fine. However, greater amounts of supplemental water can lead to brain disorders, low blood sodium, and other problems. Thus, extra water should be given only with a physician's guidance.

### Food Plan for Women Who Breastfeed

Nutrient needs for a breastfeeding mother change to some extent from those of the pregnant woman in the second and third trimester (see the inside cover of this book). There is a decrease in folate and iron needs and an increase in the needs for calories, vitamins A, E, and C, riboflavin, copper, chromium, iodide, manganese, selenium, and zinc. Still, these increased needs of the breastfeeding mother will be met by the general diet plan proposed for a woman in the latter stages of pregnancy. Recall that each day of this diet plan includes at least:

- 3 cups of calcium-rich foods such as from the milk group or use of calcium-fortified foods to make up for any gap between calcium intake and need
- 6 ½ ounce-equivalents from the meat & beans group
- 3 ½ cups from the vegetable group
- 2 cups from the fruit group
- 8 ounce-equivalents from the grain group
- 7 teaspoons of vegetable oil

**colostrum** The first fluid secreted by the breast during late pregnancy and the first few days after birth. This thick fluid is rich in immune factors and protein.

***Lactobacillus bifidus* factor** A protective factor secreted in the colostrum that encourages growth of beneficial bacteria in the newborn's intestines.

▲ Breastfeeding promotes the intestinal health of the breastfed infant.

Most substances that the mother ingests are secreted into her milk. For this reason, she should limit intake of or avoid all alcohol and caffeine and check all medications with a pediatrician. Some mothers believe that certain foods, such as garlic and chocolate, flavor the breast milk and upset the infant. If a woman notices a connection between a food she eats and the infant's later fussiness, she could consider avoiding that food. However, she might experiment again with it later, as infants become fussy for other reasons. Some researchers, on the other hand, feel that the passage of flavors from the mother's diet into her milk affords an opportunity for the infant to learn about the flavor of the foods of its family long before solids are introduced. These researchers suspect that bottle-fed infants are missing significant sensory experiences that, until recent times in human history, were common to all infants.

▲ Eating fish at least twice a week will help breastfeeding women ensure that their infants receive important omega-3 fatty acids. It is important, however, to avoid those fish likely contaminated with mercury (swordfish, shark, king mackeral, and tile fish).

Discretionary calories (up to about 400 kcal) can then be added to allow for weight maintenance or gradual weight loss, whichever is needed.

Table 14-3 provided a menu for such a plan. Substituting a soyburger (veggie burger) for the hamburger in that menu would make this a practical guide for a lacto-vegetarian woman as well.

As in pregnancy, a serving of a highly fortified ready-to-eat breakfast cereal (or use of a balanced multivitamin and mineral supplement) is advised to help meet extra nutrient needs. And, as mentioned for pregnant women, breastfeeding mothers should consume fish at least twice a week (or 1 gram per day of omega-3 fatty acids from a fish oil supplement) because the omega-3 fatty acids present in fish are secreted into breast milk and are likely to be important for development of the infant's nervous system.

Milk production requires approximately 800 kcal every day. The Estimated Energy Requirement during lactation is an extra 400 to 500 kcal daily above prepregnancy recommendations. The difference between that needed for milk production and the recommended intake—about 300 kcal—should allow a gradual loss of the extra body fat accumulated during pregnancy, especially if breastfeeding is continued for 6 months or more and the woman performs some physical activity. This shows just one of the natural benefits of following pregnancy with at least several months of breastfeeding.

After giving birth, women are often eager to shed the excess "baby fat." Breastfeeding, however, is no time for crash diets. A gradual weight loss of 1 to 4 pounds per month by the nursing mother is appropriate. At significantly greater rates of weight loss—when calories are restricted to less than about 1500 kcal per day—milk output decreases. A reasonable approach for a breastfeeding mother is to eat a balanced diet that supplies at least 1800 kcal per day; has moderate fat content; and includes a variety of dairy products, fruits, vegetables, and whole grains.

To promote the best possible feeding experience for the infant, there are several other dietary factors to consider. Hydration is especially important during breastfeeding; the woman should drink fluids every time her infant nurses. Drinking about 13 cups of fluids per day encourages ample milk production. Poor health habits, such as smoking cigarettes or drinking more than two alcoholic drinks a day, can decrease milk output. (Even less alcohol can have a deleterious effect on milk output in some women.) To avoid exposure to harmful levels of mercury, precautions concerning fish likely to contain mercury should extend past pregnancy for the breastfeeding mother. Breastfeeding women also may want to avoid eating peanuts or peanut butter, as several studies have shown that peanut allergens pass into breast milk, potentially increasing the infant's risk for peanut allergy. This is most pertinent for those with a family history of food allergies.

## CONCEPT CHECK

Recognition of the importance of breastfeeding has contributed to its greater popularity. Almost all women have the ability to breastfeed. The hormone prolactin stimulates breast tissue to synthesize milk. Infant suckling triggers a let-down reflex, which releases the milk. The more an infant nurses, the more milk is synthesized. Some components of human milk come directly from the mother's bloodstream. The nutrient composition of human milk is different from that of cow's milk and changes as the infant matures. The first fluid produced, colostrum, is rich in immune factors. The mother's diet during breastfeeding is generally similar to that for pregnancy, except for necessary additional fluids.

## Breastfeeding Today

As noted, the vast majority of women are capable of breastfeeding and their infants benefit from it. The many benefits are listed in Table 14-4. Nonetheless, a woman's decision to breastfeed depends on a variety of factors, some of which may make breastfeeding impractical or undesirable for a woman. Mothers who don't want to breastfeed their infants should not feel pressured to do so. Breastfeeding provides distinct advantages, but none so great that a woman who decides to bottle feed should feel she is significantly compromising her infant's well being.

**Advantages of Breastfeeding.**  Just as the milk of all mammals is the perfect nutrition source for the young of that species, human milk is tailored to meet infant nutrient needs for the first 4 to 6 months of life. The possible exceptions are the relative lack of fluoride, iron, and vitamin D. Infant supplements, used under the guidance of a pediatrician, can supply these and are often recommended, especially vitamin D. The American Academy of Pediatrics recommends all infants, including exclusively breast-fed infants, be given 400 IU of vitamin D per day, beginning shortly after birth and continuing until they are consuming that much from food (e.g., at least 2 cups (0.5 liters) of infant formula per day). Some sun exposure also helps in meeting vitamin D needs. Fluoride may be found in the household water supply. If it is not present in adequate amounts or the infant is not receiving tap water, a fluoride supplement should be considered and a dentist consulted. Vitamin B-12 supplements are recommended for the breastfed infant whose mother is a complete vegetarian (vegan).

*Fewer Infections.*  Breastfeeding reduces the infant's overall risk of developing infections. This is partially because an infant can use the antibodies in human milk. Breastfed infants also have fewer ear infections (otitis media) because they do not sleep with a bottle in their mouths. Experts strongly discourage allowing any infants to

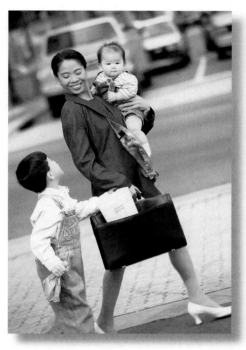

▲ Breastfeeding a baby once returning to work is possible, but requires planning.

**TABLE 14-4**  Advantages of Breastfeeding

| For Infant |
|---|
| • Bacteriologically safe |
| • Always fresh and ready to go |
| • Provides antibodies while infant's immune system is still immature, as well as substances that contribute to maturation of the immune system |
| • Contributes to maturation of gastrointestinal tract via *Lactobacillus bifidus* factor; decreases incidence of diarrhea and respiratory disease |
| • Reduces risk of food allergies and intolerances, as well as some other allergies |
| • Establishes habit of eating in moderation, thus decreasing possibility of obesity later in life by about 20% |
| • Contributes to proper development of jaws and teeth for better speech development |
| • Decreases ear infections |
| • May enhance nervous system development (by providing the fatty acid DHA) and eventual learning ability |
| • May reduce the risk of later developing hypertension and other chronic diseases, such as diabetes |

| For Mother |
|---|
| • Contributes to earlier recovery from pregnancy due to the action of hormones that promote a quicker return of the uterus to its prepregnancy state |
| • Decreases the risk of ovarian and premenopausal breast cancer |
| • Potential for quicker return to prepregnancy weight |
| • Potential for delayed ovulation and therefore reducing chances of pregnancy (short term, however) |

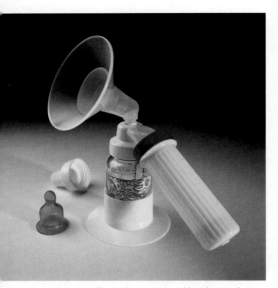

▲ Breast milk can be expressed by the mother using a manual, battery-operated (shown), or electric breast pump. The expressed milk can be stored for times when the mother is not available to breastfeed the infant.

**F**rozen human milk should not be thawed in a microwave. The heat can destroy immune factors in the milk and create hot spots, which may scald the infant's mouth and esophagus.

sleep with a bottle in their mouths, because when that happens, milk can pool in the mouth; back up through the throat; and eventually settle in the ears, creating a growth medium for bacteria. Infant ear infections are a common problem. By avoiding these problems, parents can decrease discomfort for the infant, avoid related trips to the doctor, and prevent possible hearing loss. Tooth decay from nighttime bottles is another likely consequence of sleeping with a bottle in the mouth (see Chapter 15).

*Fewer Allergies and Intolerances.* Breastfeeding also reduces the chances of some allergies, especially in allergy-prone infants (see Chapter 15). The key time to attain this benefit from breastfeeding is during the first 4 to 6 months of an infant's life. A longer commitment than 4 to 6 months is best, but the first few months are most critical. Breastfeeding for even just the first few weeks is beneficial. Another benefit of breastfeeding is that infants are better able to tolerate human milk than formulas. Formulas sometimes must be switched several times until caregivers find the best one for the infant.

*Convenience and Cost.* Breastfeeding frees the mother from the time and expense involved in buying and preparing formula and washing bottles. Human milk is ready to go and sterile. This allows the mother to spend more time with her baby.

**Possible Barriers to Breastfeeding.** Widespread misinformation, the mother's need to return to a job, and social reticence serve as barriers to breastfeeding.

*Misinformation.* Probably the major barriers to breastfeeding are misinformation, such as the idea that one's breasts are too small, and the lack of role models. One positive note has been the widespread increase in the availability of lactation consultants over the past several years. These consultants are a valuable resource for new mothers in the adjustment to breastfeeding. If a woman is interested in breastfeeding, she should find support by talking to women who have experienced it successfully because they can be an invaluable help to the first-time mother. The first-time mother should find a friend she can call on for advice. In almost every community, a group called La Leche League offers classes in breastfeeding and advises women who have problems with it (800-LALECHE or www.lalecheleague.org). Other resources are www.breastfeeding.com, www.breastfeeding.org, and www.nal.usda.gov/wicworks.

*Return to an Outside Job.* Working outside the home can complicate plans to breastfeed. One possibility after a month or two of breastfeeding is for the mother to express and save her own milk. She can use a breast pump or manually express milk into a sterile plastic bottle or nursing bag (used in a disposable bottle system). Saving human milk requires careful sanitation and rapid chilling. It can be stored in the refrigerator for 3–5 days or be frozen for 3–6 months. Thawed milk should be used within 24 hours. There is a knack to learning how to express milk, but the freedom can be worth it, because it allows others to feed the infant the mother's milk. A schedule of expressing milk and using supplemental formula feedings is most successful if begun after 1 to 2 months of exclusive breastfeeding. After 1 month or so, the baby is well adapted to breastfeeding and probably feels enough emotional security and other benefits from nursing to drink both ways.

Some women can juggle both a job and breastfeeding, but others find it too cumbersome and decide to formula-feed. A compromise—balancing some breastfeedings, perhaps early morning and night, with infant formula feedings during the day—is possible. However, too many supplemental infant formula feedings decrease milk production.

*Social Concerns.* Another barrier for some women is embarrassment about nursing a child in public. Historically, our society has stressed modesty and has discouraged public displays of breasts—even for as good a cause as nourishing babies. In the United States, no state or territory has a law prohibiting breastfeeding. However, indecent exposure (including the exposure of women's breasts) has long been a common law or statutory offense. During the 1990s, some individual states, such as Florida and North Carolina, began to clarify the right to breastfeed and to decriminalize public breastfeeding. Since then, several other states have passed similar laws. Women who feel reluctant should be reassured that they do have social support and that breast-feeding can be done discreetly with little breast exposure.

*Medical Conditions Precluding Breastfeeding.* Breastfeeding may be ruled out by certain medical conditions in either the infant or mother. For example, breastfeeding may be detrimental to infants with phenylketonuria. The high concentration of phenylalanine in breast milk may overwhelm the impaired ability of these infants to metabolize this amino acid, leading to production of toxic products.

Certain medications, which pass into the milk and adversely affect the nursing infant, are best avoided while breastfeeding. In addition, a woman in North America or other developed regions of the world who has a serious chronic disease (such as tuberculosis, AIDS, or HIV-positive status) or who is being treated with chemotherapy medications should not breastfeed.

**Environmental Contaminants in Human Milk.** There is some legitimate concern over the levels of various environmental contaminants in human milk. However, the benefits from human milk are well established and the risks from environmental contaminants are still largely theoretical. Thus, it is probably best to continue with what has been shown to work until sufficiently strong research data contradict it. A few measures a woman could take to counteract some known contaminants are to (1) avoid freshwater fish from polluted waters; (2) carefully wash and peel fruits and vegetables; and (3) remove the fatty edges of meat, as pesticides concentrate in fat. In addition, a woman should not try to lose weight rapidly while nursing (more than ¾ to 1 pound per week) because contaminants stored in her fat tissue might then enter her bloodstream and affect her milk. If a woman questions whether her milk is safe, especially if she has lived in an area known to have a high concentration of toxic wastes or environmental pollutants, she should consult her local health department.

## MAKING DECISIONS

### Breast Milk for Preterm Infants

There is no universal answer to whether a woman can breastfeed a preterm infant. In some cases, human milk is the most desirable form of nourishment, depending on infant weight and length of gestation. If so, it must usually be expressed from the breast and fed through a tube until the infant's sucking and swallowing reflex develops. This type of feeding demands great maternal dedication. Fortification of the milk with such nutrients as calcium, phosphorus, sodium, and protein is often necessary to meet the needs of a rapidly growing preterm infant. In other cases, special feeding problems may prevent the use of human milk or necessitate supplementing it with formula. Sometimes total parenteral nutrition (intravenous feeding) is the only option. Working as a team, the pediatrician, neonatal nurses, and registered dietitian must guide the parents in this decision.

▲ If human milk is used to feed the preterm infant, fortification of the milk with certain nutrients is often needed.

## CONCEPT CHECK

Human milk supplies most of an infant's nutritional needs for the first 6 months, although supplementation with vitamin D, iron, and fluoride may be needed. Breastfeeding is often more convenient than formula feeding. Compared with formula-fed infants, breastfed infants have fewer intestinal, respiratory, and ear infections and are less susceptible to some allergies and food intolerances. Despite the advantages of breastfeeding, misinformation, job responsibilities, and social reticence may dissuade a mother from breastfeeding. A combination of breastfeeding and formula feeding is possible when a mother is regularly away from the infant and is not able to express and store her milk for later use. Breastfeeding is not desirable if a mother has certain diseases or must take medication potentially harmful to the infant. The preterm infant, depending on its condition, may benefit from consuming human milk.

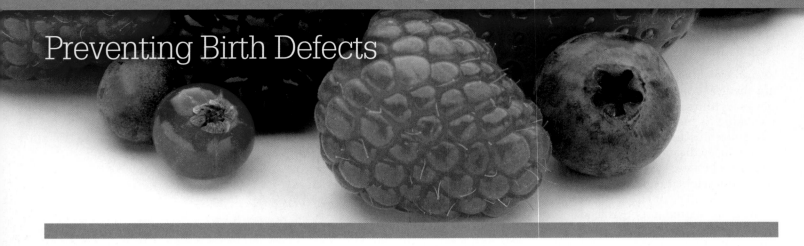

# Preventing Birth Defects

Eating well for a healthy pregnancy not only supplies materials for fetal growth and development, but also helps to direct the amazing process of building a new life. Considering the complexity of the human body and its more than 20,000 genes, it's not surprising that abnormalities of structure, function, or metabolism are sometimes present at birth. Birth defects impact one of every 33 babies born in the United States. In some cases, they are so severe that a baby cannot survive or thrive. Birth defects are the presumed cause of many spontaneous abortions and are at the root of about 20% of infant deaths before one year of age. However, with medical intervention, many babies with birth defects can go on to live healthy and productive lives.

A wide range of physical or mental disabilities results from birth defects. Heart defects are present in approximately 1 of every 100 to 200 newborn babies, accounting for a large proportion of infant deaths. Cleft lip and/or cleft palate are malformations of the lip or roof of the mouth and occur in approximately 1 in 700 to 1000 births. Neural tube defects are malformations of the brain or spinal cord that occur in early stages of pregnancy, during embryonic development. Examples include spina bifida, in which all or part of the spinal cord is exposed, and anencephaly, in which some or all of the brain is missing. Babies born with spina bifida can survive to adulthood, but in many cases, have extreme disabilities. Babies born with anencephaly die soon after birth. Neural tube defects occur in 1 in 1000 births. Down syndrome, a condition in which an extra chromosome

leads to mental retardation and other physical alterations, occurs in about 1 in 800 births. Other common birth defects include musculoskeletal defects, gastrointestinal defects, and metabolic disorders.

What causes a birth defect? About 15%–25% of birth defects are known to be genetic (i.e., inherited or spontaneous mutations of the genetic code). Another 10% are due to environmental influences (e.g., exposure to **teratogens**). The specific cause of the remaining 65%–75% of birth defects is unknown. Although the etiology of birth defects is multifactorial and many elements are beyond human control, good nutrition practices are an important way a mother-to-be can have a positive influence on the outcome of her pregnancy.

## Folic Acid

During the 1980s, researchers in the United Kingdom noticed a relationship between poor dietary habits and a high rate of neural tube defects among children of impoverished women. Subsequent intervention studies demonstrated that administration of a multivitamin supplement during the periconceptional period—the months before conception and during early pregnancy—reduced the recurrence of these birth defects. The specific link between dietary folic acid and neural tube defects was tested and confirmed in several follow-up studies. As you learned in Chapter 8, folate plays a leading role in the synthesis of DNA and the metabolism of amino acids. The rapid cell growth of pregnancy increases needs for folate during pregnancy to 600 micrograms DFE per day. Some women, for genetic reasons,

may have an even higher requirement. Adequate folic acid in the periconceptional period decreases the risk of neural tube defects by about 70% and has also been associated with decreased risk of cleft lip/palate, heart defects, and Down syndrome.

In 1998, the FDA mandated fortification of grain products to provide 140 micrograms of folic acid per 100 grams of grain consumed. In Canada, the level of fortification is 150 micrograms of folate per 100 grams of grain consumed. In general, this increases the average consumption of dietary folic acid by 100 micrograms per day. A well-planned diet can meet the RDA for folic acid, but the U.S. Public Health Service and the March of Dimes recommend that all women of childbearing age take a daily multivitamin and mineral supplement that contains 400 micrograms of folic acid. A physician may recommend prenatal vitamins or a higher dose of folic acid for some women, particularly those who have had a prior pregnancy complicated by a neural tube defect. The Dietary Guidelines for Americans recommend that women who may become pregnant and those in the first few months of pregnancy consume an adequate amount of the synthetic form of folate, folic acid ( Table 14-2 ).

**teratogen** A substance that may cause or increase the risk of a birth defect. Exposure to a teratogen does not always lead to a birth defect; its effects on the fetus depend on the dose, timing, and duration of exposure.

## Iodide

The relationship between folic acid and neural tube defects is a dramatic example of how a nutrient deficiency can negatively impact pregnancy outcome, but it is not the only nutrient of concern. Low iodide status during the first trimester of pregnancy—a critical period of brain development—may lead to cretinism. This is a congenital form of hypothyroidism that leads to diminished physical and mental development if left untreated. When the defect is identified early (by newborn screening tests), cretinism can be prevented by treatment with thyroid hormones. With use of iodized salt, however, iodide deficiencies are rare.

## Antioxidants

A case can be made for antioxidants in the prevention of birth defects as well. Free radicals are constantly generated within the body as a result of normal metabolic processes. An abundance of free radicals results in damage of cells and their DNA, which can lead to gene mutations or tissue malformations. Some research points to free radicals as a source of damage during embryo development and organogenesis. Antioxidant systems within the body act to minimize the damage caused by free radicals, and researchers hypothesize that dietary sources of antioxidants may aid in the prevention of birth defects. At this time, there is insufficient evidence to support supplementation of individual nutrients that participate in antioxidant systems—vitamin E, vitamin C, selenium, zinc, and copper—for the prevention of birth defects. However, use of a balanced multivitamin and mineral supplement while consuming a diet rich in whole grains, legumes, and a variety of fruits and vegetables will provide enough of these nutrients to meet current recommendations.

## Vitamin A

Whereas the needs for most vitamins and minerals increase by about 30% during pregnancy, the requirement for vitamin A increases by only 10%. Studies have shown the teratogenic potential of vitamin A in doses as low as approximately 3000 micrograms RAE per day. This is just over three times the RDA of 770 micrograms RAE/per day for pregnant adult women. Fetal abnormalities resulting from vitamin A toxicity primarily include facial and cardiac defects, but a wide range of defects have been reported. It is rare that food sources of vitamin A would lead to toxicity. Recall from Chapter 8 that preformed vitamin A is found in liver, fish, fish oils, fortified milk and yogurt, and eggs. Carotenoids, found in fruits and vegetables, are precursors of vitamin A that are converted to vitamin A in the small intestine. However, the efficiency of absorption of carotenoids decreases as intake increases. Vitamin A excesses typically arise from high-dose dietary supplements rather than food sources. Typical North American diets supply adequate vitamin A from foods, so supplemental use is not generally necessary. During pregnancy, supplemental preformed vitamin A should not exceed 3000 micrograms RAE per day (15,000 IU per day). Most multivitamins and prenatal vitamins supply less than 1500 micrograms RAE per day. A balanced diet and prudent use of dietary supplements are actions that can sidestep potential problems with vitamin A toxicity.

## Caffeine

Caffeine has been scrutinized for its safety during pregnancy, especially for any link with rate of birth defects. Caffeine decreases the mother's absorption of iron and may reduce blood flow through the placenta. In addition, the fetus is unable to detoxify caffeine. Research shows that as caffeine intake increases, so does the risk of miscarriage or delivering an LBW infant. Heavy caffeine use during pregnancy may also lead to caffeine withdrawal symptoms in the newborn. These risks are reported with caffeine intakes in excess of 500 milligrams, or the equivalent of about 5 cups of coffee per day. Moderate use of caffeine (up to the equivalent of 3 cups of coffee per day), however, is not associated with risk for birth defects. Based on current evidence, drinking no more than three cups of coffee and no more than four cups of caffeinated soft drinks per day during pregnancy (or when

▲ Delivering a healthy baby is more than just luck. Many nutrition- and health-related practices need to be considered.

pregnancy is possible) is advocated. Paying attention to caffeine intake from tea, over-the-counter medicines containing caffeine, and chocolate is also important.

## Aspartame

Phenylalanine, a component of the artificial sweetener, aspartame (NutraSweet® and Equal®), causes concern for some pregnant women. High amounts of phenylalanine in maternal blood disrupt fetal brain development if the mother has a disease known as *phenylketonuria* (see next section). If the mother does not have this condition, however, it is unlikely that the baby will be affected by moderate aspartame use.

For most adults, diet soft drinks are the primary source of artificial sweeteners. Of greater concern than the safety of sweeteners during pregnancy is the quality of foods and beverages consumed. A high intake of diet soft drinks may crowd out healthier beverages, such as water and low-fat milk.

## Obesity and Chronic Health Conditions

Even before becoming pregnant, women of childbearing age should have regular medical checkups to keep an eye on any health conditions that already exist or to identify any developing health problems. In some cases, the condition itself increases risk for birth defects. Obesity, high blood pressure, and uncontrolled diabetes are common health problems known to increase the risk for birth defects, including neural tube defects. In other cases, medications used to control illnesses may pose a risk to the developing fetus. Other health issues, such as seizure disorders and metabolic disorders, could also affect fetal development. A preconception visit with a health professional can help to sort out and make plans to minimize such risks. Once a woman has become pregnant, early and regular prenatal care can aid in the success of a pregnancy.

Women with diabetes are two to three times more likely to give birth to a baby with birth defects compared to women with normal glucose metabolism. Examples of birth defects common in this group include malformations of the spine, legs, and blood vessels of the heart. Some experts speculate that the mechanism by which diabetes increases birth defects is via excessive free radicals, which lead to oxidative damage of DNA during early gestation. Careful control of blood glucose drastically lowers risk for women with diabetes. Optimal blood glucose control can be achieved through a combination of dietary modifications and medications. Given that diabetes is on the rise among women of childbearing age, this elevated rate of birth defects has become an area of heightened awareness.

Another health condition for which maternal nutritional control is of utmost importance is PKU. Recall from Chapter 6 that PKU is an error of metabolism in which the liver lacks the ability to process phenylalanine, leading to an accumulation of this amino acid and its metabolites in body tissues. Babies born to women who have phenylketonuria that is not controlled by diet are at heightened risk for brain defects, such as microcephaly and mental retardation.

## Alcohol

Conclusive evidence shows that repeated consumption of four or more alcoholic drinks at one sitting harms the fetus. Such binge drinking is especially perilous during the first 12 weeks of pregnancy, as this is when critical early developmental events take place in utero. Although scientists don't know whether pregnant women must totally eliminate alcohol use to avoid risk of damage to the fetus, women are advised not to drink any alcohol during pregnancy or when there is a chance pregnancy might occur—until a safe level can be established. The embryo (and, at later stages, the fetus), has no means of detoxifying alcohol.

Women with chronic alcoholism produce children with a recognizable pattern of malformations called **fetal alcohol syndrome (FAS)**. A diagnosis of FAS is based mainly on poor fetal and infant growth, physical deformities (especially of facial features), and mental retardation (Fig. 14-6). The infant is frequently irritable and may develop hyperactivity and a short attention span. Limited hand-eye coordination is common. Defects in vision, hearing, and mental processing often develop over time.

Exactly how alcohol causes these defects is not known. One line of research suggests that alcohol, or products produced by the metabolism of alcohol (e.g., acetaldehyde), cause faulty movement of cells in the brain during early stages of nerve cell development or block the action of certain brain neurotransmitters. In addition, inadequate nutrient intake, reduced nutrient and oxygen transfer across the placenta, cigarette smoking commonly associated with alcohol intake, drug use, and possibly other factors contribute to the overall result.

The Dietary Guidelines for Americans recommend that alcoholic beverages not be consumed by pregnant and lactating women (Table 14-2). For more information about fetal alcohol syndrome visit the website **www.cdc.gov/ncbddd/fas/**.

## Environmental Contaminants

There is little evidence to link birth defects with the amounts of pesticides, herbicides, or other contaminants in foods or public water supplies in North America. However, evaluating such a link can be methodologically difficult and many would argue that regulations concerning contaminants in the food and water supply are too permissive. Thus, it seems prudent to take measures to decrease intake of pesticides and herbicides wherever possible. For fruits and vegetables, peeling, removing outer leaves, and/or thoroughly rinsing and scrubbing with a brush under running water will remove the majority of contaminants. In animal products, pesticides and other contaminants are most likely to accumulate in fatty tissues. Therefore, removing skin, discarding drippings, and trimming visible fat will decrease exposure from meat, poultry, and fish.

For fish, mercury is of particular concern because it can harm the nervous system of the fetus. Thus, FDA warns pregnant women to avoid swordfish, shark, king mackerel, and tile fish because of possible high mercury contamination. Largemouth bass are also implicated. In general, intake of other fish and shellfish should not exceed 12 ounces per week. Canned albacore tuna is a potential mercury source, so it should not be consumed in amounts exceeding 6 ounces per week. As a rule of thumb, consuming a variety of foods minimizes risk of exposure to contaminants from the food supply.

## Summing Up

Although many risk factors for birth defects are beyond our control, a woman

▶ A goal of *Healthy People 2010* is 100% abstinence from alcohol, cigarettes, and illicit drugs by pregnant women.

**fetal alcohol syndrome (FAS)**
A group of irreversible physical and mental abnormalities in the infant that result from the mother's consuming alcohol during pregnancy.

of childbearing potential can make some wise nutrition choices to improve her chances of having a healthy baby without birth defects. A varied and balanced diet, such as the food plan for pregnant women described in this chapter, along with a daily multivitamin and mineral supplement with 400 micrograms of folic acid will ensure adequate nutrient status. It is estimated that daily use of a multivitamin and mineral supplement containing folic acid will decrease the rate of all birth defects by 50%. Discuss use of any other dietary supplements with a physician to be sure that the fetus will not be exposed to toxic levels of vitamin A or other dangerous ingredients. Early and consistent prenatal care can help control obesity and any chronic health conditions that may complicate a pregnancy. Also, avoiding alcohol during pregnancy will eliminate any risk for fetal alcohol syndrome.

Although it seems that advice for a healthy pregnancy is always directed at the mother, fathers-to-be are not off the hook. Health is a family affair, so encouraging healthy eating habits and avoiding smoking and alcohol are important for fathers, too. Less research has been done in the area, but the genetics of the baby are certainly an outcome of both parents. Certainly, inadequate supplies of zinc, folate, and vitamin C affect the quality of sperm, which may impair fertility. Considering that spermatogenesis takes approximately 70 days, the periconceptional period is a time for good nutrition and careful lifestyle practices for the father as well.

▶ In North America, maternal death as a result of childbirth is uncommon—only about 11 deaths in every 100,000 live births. The infant mortality rate, however, is much higher: for each 100,000 live births, about 600 to 700 infants die within the first year. The infant death rate among African-Americans is more than double the rates among Whites and Hispanics in the United States.

▶ Pregnant women should recognize that many cough syrups contain alcohol. Cases have been reported of infants with FAS born to mothers who consumed generous amounts of such cough syrups but no other alcoholic beverages.

**fetal alcohol effects (FAE)** Hyperactivity, attention deficit disorder, poor judgment, sleep disorders, and delayed learning as a result of prenatal exposure to alcohol.

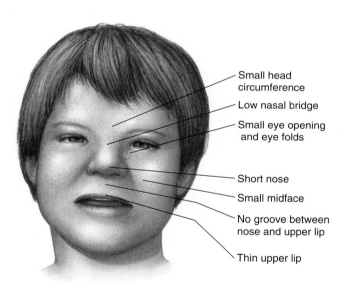

Small head circumference
Low nasal bridge
Small eye opening and eye folds
Short nose
Small midface
No groove between nose and upper lip
Thin upper lip

**FIGURE 14-6** ▶ Fetal alcohol syndrome. The facial features shown are typical of affected children. Additional abnormalities in the brain and other internal organs accompany fetal alcohol syndrome but are not immediately apparent from simply looking at the child. Milder forms of alcohol-induced changes from a lower alcohol exposure to the fetus are known as **fetal alcohol effects.** In this case, behavior problems without physical effects, such as altered facial features, are seen.

## Case Study Preparing for Pregnancy

Lily and her husband have decided that they are ready to prepare for Lily's first pregnancy. She is 25 years old, weighs 135 pounds, and is 67 inches tall. Lily has been reading everything she can find on pregnancy because she knows that her prepregnancy health is important to the success of her pregnancy.

She knows she should avoid alcohol, especially because alcohol is potentially toxic to the growing fetus in the first weeks of pregnancy, and she could become pregnant and not know about it right away. Lily is not a smoker, does not take any medications, and limits her coffee intake to 4 cups a day and soft drink intake to 3 colas per day. Based on her reading, she has decided to breastfeed her infant and has already inquired about childbirth classes. She has modified her diet to include some extra protein, along with more fruits and vegetables. She has also started taking an over-the-counter vitamin and mineral supplement. Lily has always kept in good shape, and she is admittedly worried about gaining too much weight

during pregnancy. Recently, she started a running program 5 days a week, and she plans to continue running throughout her pregnancy.

Answer the following questions, and check your responses in Appendix A.

1. What recommendations do you have regarding Lily's use of dietary supplements?

2. What is Lily doing to prevent neural tube defects? What else could she do?

3. What recommendations would you make regarding Lily's caffeine consumption?

4. Lily is wise to pay attention to her protein intake to prepare for pregnancy and breastfeeding. Should she include fish as a source of protein in her diet? Why or why not?

5. Constipation is a common complaint during pregnancy. What suggestions do you have to help Lily avoid this health concern?

6. What information would you share with Lily about appropriate weight gain during pregnancy?

## Summary

1. Adequate nutrition is vital during pregnancy to ensure the well-being of both the infant and mother. Poor maternal nutrition and use of some medications, especially during the first trimester, can cause birth defects. Growth restriction and altered development can also occur if these insults happen later in pregnancy.

2. Infants born preterm (before 37 weeks gestation) usually have more medical problems at and following birth than normal infants.

3. A woman typically needs an additional 350 to 450 kcal per day during the second and third trimesters of pregnancy to meet her calorie needs. A better measure of meeting energy needs is adequate weight gain. This should occur slowly, reaching a total of 25 to 35 pounds in a woman of healthy weight.

4. Protein, carbohydrate, fiber, vitamin, and mineral needs increase during pregnancy. Following a plan based on MyPyramid is recommended. A supplemental source of iron, in particular, may be needed. Folate nutriture especially should be adequate at the time of conception. Any nutrient supplement use needs to be guided by a physician, as an excess intake of vitamin A and other nutrients during pregnancy can have harmful effects on the fetus.

5. The factors that contribute to poor pregnancy outcome include inadequate health care in general and prenatal care in particular, obesity, teenage pregnancy, smoking, alcohol consumption, illicit drug use (such as cocaine), insufficient carbohydrate intake (less than 175 grams per day), heavy caffeine use, and various infections, such as *listeriosis*.

6. Pregnancy-induced hypertension, gestational diabetes, heartburn, constipation, nausea, vomiting, edema, and anemia are all possible discomforts and complications of pregnancy. Nutrition therapy can help minimize some of these problems.

7. Almost all women are able to breastfeed their infants. The nutrient composition of human milk is different from that of unaltered cow's milk and is much more desirable for the infant. Colostrum, the first fluid produced by the human breast, is rich in immune factors. Mature milk is rich in protein and in lactose. The diet plan recommended for the second and third trimesters of pregnancy is also appropriate for meeting the nutrient needs of the lactating woman, except more fluids in general should be consumed.

8. For the infant, the advantages of breastfeeding over formula feeding are numerous, including fewer intestinal, respiratory, and ear infections and fewer allergies and food intolerances. Moreover, breastfeeding is also less expensive and possibly more convenient for the mother than formula feeding. However, an infant can be adequately nourished with formula if the mother chooses not to breastfeed. Breastfeeding is not desirable if the mother has certain diseases or must take medication potentially harmful to the infant. Likewise, breastfeeding may not be advised for infants with certain medical conditions, including some preterm infants.

## Study Questions

1. Provide three key pieces of advice for parents seeking to maximize their chances of having a healthy infant. Why did you identify those specific factors?

2. Outline current weight-gain recommendations for pregnancy. What is the basis for these recommendations?

3. Identify four key nutrients for which intake should be significantly increased during pregnancy.

4. How is the MyPyramid diet for an average woman adapted to meet the increased nutrient needs of pregnancy?

5. Why does teenage pregnancy receive so much attention these days? At what age do you think pregnancy is ideal? Why?

6. Give three reasons a woman should give serious consideration to breastfeeding her infant.

7. Describe the physiological mechanisms that stimulate milk production and release. How can knowing about these help mothers breastfeed successfully?

8. What guidelines can a woman use to determine whether her breastfed infant is receiving sufficient nourishment?

9. How should the basic food plan suitable for pregnancy be modified during breastfeeding?

10. Where can first-time mothers go for help in establishing successful breastfeeding?

## Check Your Knowledge

Answers to the following multiple choice questions are below.

1. The fetus is most susceptible to damage from nutrient deficiencies; teratogens; and use of certain medications, alcohol, and illicit drugs during
   a. the first trimester.
   b. the second trimester.
   c. the third trimester.
   d. labor and delivery.

2. An infant born at 38 weeks' gestation weighing 5.0 pounds can be described as
   a. preterm.   c. SGA.
   b. LBW.   d. LBW and SGA.

3. If a woman is 5'2 and weighs 150 pounds before becoming pregnant, how much weight should she gain during pregnancy?
   a. 28 to 40 pounds (12.5 to 18 kilograms)
   b. 25 to 35 pounds (11.5 to 16 kilograms)
   c. 15 to 25 pounds (7 to 11.5 kilograms)
   d. As little as possible.

4. Increased carbohydrate needs during pregnancy are set to
   a. prevent ketosis.
   b. alleviate nausea.
   c. prevent pregnancy-induced hypertension.
   d. supply adequate folate.

5. Which of the following is best paired with an iron supplement during pregnancy?
   a. skim milk
   b. orange juice
   c. coffee
   d. tea

6. Obesity during pregnancy is associated with higher rates of
   a. birth defects.
   b. diabetes.
   c. surgical delivery.
   d. All of the above.

7. Consuming one cup of coffee per day is associated with
   a. spontaneous abortions.
   b. LBW.
   c. birth defects.
   d. None of the above.

8. Which of the following may help to alleviate nausea during pregnancy?
   a. postponing meals until the afternoon
   b. drinking large amounts of water
   c. postponing use of iron supplements until the second trimester
   d. All of the above.

9. Which of the following conditions medically prevents a woman from breastfeeding her infant?
   a. breasts are too small
   b. infant has PKU
   c. inverted nipples
   d. None of the above.

10. Physiologically, milk production requires _____ kcals per day.
    a. 300
    b. 500
    c. 800
    d. 1000

Answer Key: 1. a, 2. d, 3. c, 4. a, 5. b, 6. d, 7. d, 8. c, 9. b, 10. c

# Further Readings

1. ADA Reports: Position of the American Dietetic Association: Nutrition and lifestyle for a healthy pregnancy outcome. *Journal of the American Dietetic Association* 108:553, 2008.

   *The key components of a healthy lifestyle during pregnancy include appropriate weight gain; consumption of a variety of foods; appropriate and timely vitamin and mineral intake; avoidance of alcohol, tobacco, and other harmful substances; and safe food handling. Vitamin and mineral supplementation is appropriate for some nutrients, particularly in certain situations, such as for vegans.*

2. ADA Reports: Position of the American Dietetic Association: Promoting and supporting breastfeeding. *Journal of the American Dietetic Association* 105:810, 2005.

   *The American Dietetic Association strongly supports the breastfeeding of infants. This article discusses the benefits from breastfeeding that accrue to the mother and infant, as well as dietary considerations that need to be addressed, such as avoiding consumption of species of fish known to contain high amounts of mercury.*

3. Allen LH: Multiple micronutrients in pregnancy and lactation: An overview. *American Journal of Clinical Nutrition* 81:1206S, 2005.

   *Numerous nutrients contribute to a healthy outcome of pregnancy, including many B vitamins and iron. The author notes in many cases diet changes allow women to meet these needs, but in some cases supplementation is needed, such as for poor women. With respect to diet changes, these should begin before pregnancy so a woman has a healthy status in the first weeks while she is pregnant but still does not know this is the case.*

4. Bodnar LM and others: Periconceptional multivitamin use reduces the risk of preeclampsia. *American Journal of Epidemiology* 164:470, 2006.

   *In the Pregnancy Exposures and Preeclampsia Prevention Study, women who regularly consumed a multivitamin during the periconceptional period had a 45% lower risk of developing preeclampsia during their first pregnancy than those who did not consume multivitamins. The relationship between multivitamin use and disease risk was profoundly affected by prepregnancy body weight: women with BMI less than 25 benefited most from multivitamin use. The mechanism by which multivitamin use may prevent preeclampsia is not known.*

5. Carlson S, Aupperle P: Nutrient requirements and fetal development: Recommendations for best outcomes. *Journal of Family Practice* 56:S1, 2007.

   *Maternal nutrient status before and during pregnancy and during lactation have a long-term impact on infant and child health. Nutrients of particular concern include folic acid, calcium, vitamin D, and omega-3 fatty acids. The importance of essential fatty acids on brain and eye development is highlighted. Although health care professionals should counsel patients to consume a nutrient-rich diet, supplementation may be needed to achieve optimal nutrient status.*

6. Crowther CA and others: Effect of treatment of gestational diabetes mellitus on pregnancy outcomes. *The New England Journal of Medicine* 352:2477, 2005.

   *This study found that treating gestational diabetes when it develops is important to improve the health of the mother, fetus, and ultimately the infant. Diet changes and regular blood glucose monitoring are important parts of the therapy; in some cases insulin injections are also needed to control blood glucose.*

7. Field CJ: The immunological components of human milk and their effect on immune development in infants. *Journal of Nutrition* 135:1, 2005.

   *Human milk contains many factors that improve immune function in the infant. This article reviews a number of these complex factors.*

8. Henriksen T: Nutrition and pregnancy outcome. *Nutrition Reviews* 64:S19, 2006.

   *This article reviews current nutritional practices of pregnant women, which do not conform to what we know to be optimal. The increase in overweight women has been accompanied by a dramatic increase in gestational diabetes and an increase in large babies.*

9. Hulsey TC and others: Maternal prepregnant body mass index and weight gain related to low birth weight in South Carolina. *Southern Medical Journal* 98:411, 2005.

   *A healthy weight at conception and adequate weight gain during pregnancy contributed to a substantial reduction in low-birth-weight infants in this study. For example, women with inadequate weight gains had about a 1.5 to 2 times greater risk of delivering a low-birth-weight infant.*

10. Kelly, AKW: Practical exercise advice during pregnancy. *The Physician and Sports Medicine* 33(6):24, 2005.

    *It is safe for pregnant women to exercise if they are experiencing uncomplicated pregnancies. The author notes that many positive effects of exercise during pregnancy are possible. Most non-weight-bearing exercises (e.g., swimming) and walking are safe for pregnant women. Women should begin with 15 minutes of exercise three times a week and progress as tolerated. The author discusses how to monitor women as they increase their physical activity.*

11. King JC: Maternal obesity, metabolism, and pregnancy outcomes. *Annual Review of Nutrition* 26:271, 2006.

    *Maternal obesity increases risk for complications and adverse outcomes of pregnancy, including gestational diabetes, preeclampsia, birth defects, and large-for-gestational-age births. Evidence is accumulating to support the notion that maternal obesity also negatively impacts chronic disease risk for offspring. The potential mechanisms for these relationships are discussed and practical nutrition advice, based on the 2005 Dietary Guidelines for Americans, is provided.*

12. Lucas RM and others: Future health implications of prenatal and early-life vitamin D status. *Nutrition Reviews* 66:710, 2008.

    *Emerging evidence points to the importance of maternal vitamin D status on the progression of several chronic diseases in the offspring. In addition to its role in bone health, preventive effects of vitamin D on autoimmune disorders, diabetes, cancer, cardiovascular disease, osteoporosis, and psychiatric illness are mediated by the vitamin's involvement in gene expression. Maternal vitamin D supplementation could lead to widespread improvements in public health, but further research is needed to determine appropriate dosage and long-term effects.*

13. Makrides M: Outcomes for mothers and their babies: Do n-3 long-chain polyunsaturated fatty acids and seafoods make a difference? *Journal of the American Dietetic Association* 108: 1622, 2008.

    *Omega-3 fatty acids are important for brain and eye development of the fetus and infant. These fats have been implicated in prevention of preeclampsia, preterm birth, LBW, and SGA, but current evidence does not support supplementation for these purposes. Despite the importance of n-3 fatty acids for fetal development, many women have inadequate intakes of these fats. Available data indicate that pregnant and lactating women should aim to consume at least 200 milligrams per day of omega-3 fatty acids from dietary sources, including oily fish, eggs, and lean red meats.*

14. Moore, VM, Davies, MJ: Diet during pregnancy, neonatal outcomes and later health. *Reproduction, Fertility, and Delivery* 17:341, 2005.

    *Altering the maternal diet before and during pregnancy can induce permanent changes in the* offspring birth size and adult health/life span. Consequences of inadequate maternal nutrition for the offspring depend on the specific time in gestation that they occur. The authors emphasize the importance of improving diet before a woman becomes pregnant in order to protect her health and the health of her offspring.

15. Ramachenderan J and others: Maternal obesity and pregnancy complications: A review. *Australian and New Zealand Journal of Obstetrics and Gynaecology* 48:228, 2008.

   *Obesity in pregnant women leads to a high risk for complications for both the mother and infant and therefore requires strict monitoring by the physician. Effects of obesity on the mother include hypertension, diabetes, clotting disorders, postpartum weight retention, and preterm delivery. For the infant, obesity increases risk of birth defects, macrosomia, birth injuries, and death of the fetus or newborn. The authors suggest that minimal weight gain or even modest weight loss during pregnancy may promote optimal pregnancy outcomes for obese women.*

16. Rosenburg, TJ and others: Maternal obesity and diabetes as risk factors for adverse pregnancy outcomes: Differences among 4 racial/ethnic groups. *American Journal of Public Health* 95:1545, 2005.

   *In this large population-based study, obesity and diabetes were clearly associated with adverse pregnancy outcomes. This highlights the need for women to control these conditions as best as possible during their childbearing years to protect the health of their future infants.*

17. Tamura T, Picciano MF: Folate and human reproduction. *American Journal of Clinical Nutrition* 83:993, 2006.

   *Folate status is important to human reproduction due to its roles in DNA synthesis and metabolism of various amino acids. Folic acid supplementation for the prevention of megaloblastic anemia during pregnancy and neural tube defects represents a major public health advancement. Several other areas of reproductive health are under continued study for relationships with folate status, including placental abruption, preeclampsia, spontaneous abortion, stillbirth, low birth weight, and risk for birth defects other than neural tube defects.*

18. Taylor JS and others: A systematic review of the literature associating breastfeeding with type 2 diabetes and gestational diabetes. *Journal of the American College of Nutrition* 24:320, 2005.

   *Breastfeeding confers health benefits to both mother and child. Breastfed infants have lower rates of obesity, type 1 diabetes, and type 2 diabetes in adulthood compared to formula-fed infants. In addition, mothers who breastfeed have improved glucose tolerance and lower risk for postpartum diabetes compared to nonlactating mothers. Studies show that mothers with diabetes are less likely to breastfeed than their nondiabetic counterparts, but the data reviewed in this article provide evidence that diabetic mothers and their babies could both benefit from breastfeeding.*

19. Wagner, LK: Diagnosis and management of preeclampsia. *American Family Physician* 70:2317, 2004.

   *Preeclampsia is a multisystem disorder of unknown cause. It affects about 5%–7% of pregnancies and is a significant cause of both illness and death in the mother and fetus. Management requires careful monitoring of the mother and fetus once the disorder develops. Magnesium sulfate is the major therapy used, but medications to control related hypertension may also be employed. This article reviews preeclampsia in detail.*

20. Ward EM: Prime the body for pregnancy—preconception care and nutrition for moms-to-be. *Today's Dietitian* 10: 26, 2008.

   *Conception may occur unexpectedly and may go unnoticed for the first several weeks of gestation. For this reason, women of childbearing potential should take steps to ensure a healthy pregnancy before becoming pregnant. The article provides practical guidelines for intakes of key nutrients (e.g., folic acid and iron), supplement use, weight management, physical activity, and caffeine and alcohol consumption.*

## I. Targeting Nutrients Necessary for Pregnant Women

This chapter mentioned that pregnant women may have difficulty meeting their increased needs for folate, vitamin B-6, iron, and zinc. List six foods rich in each of these nutrients next to the appropriate heading. Refer to Chapters 8 and 9 if necessary.

| Nutrient | Foods | Nutrient | Foods |
|---|---|---|---|
| Folate | _____ | Iron | _____ |
| | _____ | | _____ |
| | _____ | | _____ |
| | _____ | | _____ |
| | _____ | | _____ |
| | _____ | | _____ |
| Vitamin B-6 | _____ | Zinc | _____ |
| | _____ | | _____ |
| | _____ | | _____ |
| | _____ | | _____ |
| | _____ | | _____ |
| | _____ | | _____ |

1. Foods rich in more than one of these nutrients would be especially valuable for pregnant women. Write on the line any foods you listed that are good sources of more than one of these critical nutrients.

   _____

2. The needs for folate, vitamin B-6, iron, and zinc increase during pregnancy. For which of these nutrients can pregnant women usually obtain adequate intakes from dietary sources?

   _____

3. Which of these nutrients are commonly taken in supplement form during pregnancy?

   _____

   _____

4. Why might it be hard for pregnant women to meet their increased needs for these nutrients from food alone?

   _____

   _____

# II. Putting Your Knowledge About Nutrition and Pregnancy to Work

A college friend, Angie, tells you that she is newly pregnant. You are aware that she usually likes to eat the following foods for her meals:

## Breakfast

Skips this meal, or eats a granola bar
Coffee

## Lunch

Sweetened yogurt, 1 cup
Small bagel with cream cheese
Occasional piece of fruit
Regular caffeinated soda, 12 ounces

## Snack

Chocolate candy bar

## Dinner

2 slices of pizza, macaroni and cheese, or 2 eggs with 2 slices of toast
Seldom eats a salad or vegetable
Regular caffeinated soda, 12 ounces

## Snacks

Pretzels or chips, 1 ounce
Regular caffeinated soda, 12 ounces

1. Using NutritionCalc Plus software, evaluate Angie's diet for protein, carbohydrate, folate, vitamin B-6, iron, and zinc. How does her intake compare with the recommended amounts for pregnancy?

   _____

   _____

   _____

2. Now redesign her diet and make sure that her intake meets pregnancy needs for protein, carbohydrate, folate, vitamin B-6, and zinc. (Hint: Fortified foods, such as breakfast cereal, are generally nutrient-rich foods, which can more easily help meet one's needs.) Increase the iron content as well, but it still may be below the RDA for pregnancy.

   _____

   _____

   _____

# CHAPTER 15 Nutrition from Infancy Through Adolescence

## Student Learning Outcomes  After studying Chapter 15, you will be able to:

1. Describe the extent to which nutrition affects infant growth and physiological development.

2. Identify diet guidelines to meet the basic nutritional needs for normal growth and development for an infant and discuss

   some do's and don'ts associated with infant feeding.

3. List several challenges parents might face in dealing with childhood eating habits.

4. List the nutrients often found to be lacking in the diets of infants, tod-

   dlers, preschoolers, and teenagers and make recommendations to remedy the problems.

5. Identify common food allergens and suggest several practices that may reduce the risk of developing a food allergy.

## Chapter Outline

Student Learning Outcomes

Refresh Your Memory

15.1 Nutrition and Child Health—An Introduction

15.2 Infant Growth and Nutrition Needs

15.3 Preschool Children: Nutrition Concerns

15.4 School-Age Children: Nutrition Concerns

15.5 Teenage Years: Nutrition Concerns

Nutrition and Your Health: Food Allergies and Intolerances

Case Study: Undernutrition During Infancy

Summary/Study Questions/Check Your Knowledge/Further Readings

Rate Your Plate

As HUMANS GROW THROUGH EARLY YEARS INTO YOUNG ADULTHOOD, OUR NEEDS FOR CALORIES AND NUTRIENTS CHANGE. Infants need more calories, protein, vitamins, and minerals per pound of body weight than young and older adults to support their rapid pace of growth and development. The growth rate of children is slower than that of infants; therefore, children's needs and intake are proportionately less. As the chapter comic suggests, the erratic eating behaviors of young children pose major challenges for parents and other caregivers. In turn, childhood becomes an important time to establish healthful habits, including those related to food choice and physical activity.

Family behaviors exert powerful influences on the child. Thus, education designed to change children's eating behaviors must be directed simultaneously at the main caregivers. Parents and other caregivers usually determine what foods are purchased and how they are prepared. To help children adopt a lifelong healthy dietary intake, a variety of foods should be introduced at home, fastfood and sugared soft drinks should be limited to a few times per week or less, and new foods should be introduced regularly. Maintaining a healthful eating (and physical activity) pattern should continue as children grow into teenagers. In exploring all these stages of life, Chapter 15 looks at the key role nutrients play and how food choices should be tailored to meet changing needs.

## Refresh Your Memory

As you begin your study of nutrition from infancy through adolescence in Chapter 15, you may want to review:

- MyPyramid and the 2005 Dietary Guidelines in Chapter 2
- The immune system in Chapter 3
- Diagnosis and treatment of type 2 diabetes in Chapter 4
- Common sources of saturated fat, cholesterol, and *trans* fat in Chapter 5
- Vegetarianism in Chapter 6

## 15.1 Nutrition and Child Health— an Introduction

Current statistics describing nutrition and overall health among children and adolescents in North America have shown both positive and negative trends. On a positive note, more children are receiving vaccinations than ever before and fewer teenagers are giving birth. In contrast to this good news, the number of children and teenagers with obesity and type 2 diabetes is rising, and physical activity in general is on the decline as more time is spent sitting in front of computer screens and television sets. Low calcium intakes are also receiving much attention, as soft drinks have replaced much of the milk that children and teenagers previously consumed on a daily basis. Fruits, vegetables, and whole grains are also often in short supply in their diets. In this chapter, we will look at these trends and their effects on nutrition and overall health of this age group.

## 15.2 Infant Growth and Nutrition Needs

During infancy, attitudes toward foods and the eating process begin to take shape. If parents and other caregivers practice good nutrition and are flexible, they can lead an infant into lifelong healthful food habits. An infant that starts life in such an environment has a good chance of starting life with the nutrients needed to support brain and body growth spurts, and of developing a willingness to try new foods. However, these physical and psychological advantages alone don't guarantee that a child will thrive.

At what age should an infant be fed solid foods? Which foods are most appropriate for those early stages of solid food introduction? Which foods should not be fed to infants? Why? Chapter 15 provides some answers.

MARVIN © Reprinted with special permission of King Features Syndicate, Inc.

Children also need specific attention focused on them; they need to grow in a stimulating environment, and they need a sense of security. For example, children hospitalized for growth failure gain weight more quickly when more caring stimulation, such as holding and rocking the infant, accompanies needed nutrients.

## The Growing Infant

All babies seem to do is eat and sleep. There's a good reason for this. An infant's birth weight doubles in the first 4 to 6 months and triples within the first year. Never again is growth so rapid. Such rapid growth requires a lot of nourishment and sleep. After the first year, growth is slower; it takes 5 more years to double the weight seen at 1 year. An infant also increases in length in the first year by 50% and then continues to gain height through the teen years. These gains are not necessarily continuous—spurts of growth alternate with plateaus. Height is essentially maximized by age 19, although increases of several inches may occur in the early twenties, especially for boys (Fig. 15-1). Head size in proportion to total height shrinks from one-fourth to one-eighth during the climb from infancy to adulthood.

The human body needs a lot more food to support growth and development than it does to merely maintain its size once growth ceases. When nutrients are missing at critical phases of this process, growth and development may slow or even stop. In

**FIGURE 15-1 ▶** Growth charts for assessment of children in the growing years. The growth of a youngster is plotted to show how the charts are used in health care settings. (a) Growth charts used to assess length (height) and weight in young girls. a certain length (height) and weight correspond to a percentile value, a ranking of the person among 100 peers. This chart shows that at 36 months of age, the girl was at the 75th percentile for length and the 62nd percentile for weight. (b) Growth charts used to assess weight-for-height relationships in boys ages 2 to 20 years. Today, these charts for older children and adolescents typically use BMI for the evaluation. At 6 years of age the boy was at the 85th percentile for BMI.

*Source: Developed by the National Center for Health Statistics in collaboration with the National Center for Disease Prevention and Health Promotion (2000).* www.cdc.gov/growthcharts. *Revised November 21, 2000.*

**undernutrition** Failing health that results from a long-standing dietary intake that is not enough to meet nutritional needs.

**percentile** Classification of a measurement of a unit into divisions of 100 units.

countries of the developing world, about one-third of the children under 5 years of age are short and underweight for their ages. Poor nutrition—called **undernutrition**—is at the heart of the problem. This occurs to a lesser extent in North America. The undernourished children are smaller versions of nutritionally fit children. In poorer countries, when breastfeeding ceases, children are often fed a high-carbohydrate, low-protein diet. This diet supports some growth but does not allow children to attain their full genetic potential. To grow, children must consume adequate amounts of calories, protein, calcium, iron, zinc, and other nutrients.

## Effect of Undernutrition on Growth

As with the fetus in utero, the long-term effects of nutritional problems in infancy and childhood depend on the severity, timing, and duration of the nutritional insult to cell processes.

The single best indicator of a child's nutritional status is growth, particularly weight gain in the short run and length (height) in the long run. Mild zinc deficiencies in North American children have been linked to poor growth. Improving the diets of these children then leads to improved growth. Overall, eating a poor diet as an infant or a child hampers the cell division that occurs at that critical stage. Consuming an adequate diet later usually won't compensate for lost growth, however, as the hormonal and other conditions needed for growth will not likely be present. In addition, growth ceases in girls and boys when the skeleton reaches its final size. This happens as growth plates at the ends of the bones fuse, which begins around 14 years of age in girls and 15 years of age in boys. The final stages of this process end at about 19 years of age in girls and 20 years of age in boys. Furthermore, muscles can increase in diameter later in life but their linear growth is limited by the length of the shorter bone.

For these reasons, a 15-year-old Central American girl who is 4 feet 8 inches tall cannot attain the adult height of a typical North American girl simply by eating better. Girls experience their peak rate of growth right before the onset of the menses. Once the time for growth ceases (in women, this is about 5 years after they start menstruating), a sufficient nutrient intake helps maintain health and weight but cannot make up for lost growth.

## Assessment of Infant Growth and Development

Health professionals assess a child's increases in height and weight by comparing them with typical growth patterns recorded on charts (review Fig. 15-1). The charts contain **percentile** divisions, which represent the typical measurements for 90% to 96% of children. A percentile represents the rank of the person among 100 peers matched for age and gender. If a young boy, for example, is at the 90th percentile of height-for-age, he is shorter than 10% and taller than 89% of children his age. A child at the 50th percentile is considered average. Fifty children will be taller than this child; 49 will be shorter.

Individual growth charts are available for both males and females from the National Center for Health Statistics (as shown in Fig. 15-1). For ages ranging from birth to 36 months, options for growth charts include weight-for-age, length-for-age, weight-for-length, and head circumference-for-age. For males and females who are 2 to 20 years old, growth charts are available to determine weight-for-age and height-for-age; however, the preferred growth chart for children and adolescents is body mass index (BMI)-for-age. For adults, BMI has fixed cutoff points (for example, a BMI of 25 for an adult is considered overweight). As Figure 15-1 shows, this is not true for children, as BMI is both gender- and age-specific.

In 2006, the World Health Organization released a new set of growth standards for children from birth through five years of age to replace the NCHS charts currently in use. The WHO growth charts provide a way to assess the same parameters listed (e.g., height or length, weight, BMI, and head circumference) but they are based on data collected from children from various regions of the world raised under conditions for optimal growth and development: breastfed as infants, followed recommended infant and child feeding practices set forth by WHO, had adequate health care, and mothers did not use tobacco during or after pregnancy. In contrast, the NCHS growth charts are based on data from primarily Caucasian children who were mostly formula-fed during infancy. The new WHO growth standards stress that breastfeeding is the biological norm for infant nutrition. Look for these new growth charts to become more widely available over the next few years.

Infants and children should have their growth assessed during regular health checkups. It takes 1 to 3 years for the genetic potential (in terms of percentile ranking on growth charts) of infant growth to be established. By 3 years of age, a child's measurements, such as length (height)-for-age, should generally track along the established percentile. If the child's growth doesn't keep up with his or her length-for-age percentile, the physician needs to investigate whether a medical or nutritional problem is impeding the predicted growth. Inappropriate weight gain—too little or too much—should also be investigated.

Infants born preterm may catch up in growth in 2 to 3 years. This requires that the child move up in the percentiles. If this occurs—especially in length-for-age—it is usually no cause for alarm. On the other hand, moving up in the percentiles for weight-for-height can be disturbing if the child approaches the 80th to 90th percentiles. A child at the 85th percentile or above for BMI is considered at risk for overweight. At or above the 95th percentile, the child is considered overweight. At the 95th percentile, the diagnosis of obesity can also be established if the physical exam of the child indicates he or she is truly overfat. This is generally the case at this percentile.

▲ The new WHO Growth Standards for Children differ from previous standards in part because they reflect data based upon children from around the world who were raised in conditions for optimal growth and development. Go to http://www.who.int/childgrowth/en/ for more information on the WHO Child Growth Standards.

**C**hildren under 2 to 3 years of age are measured lying on their backs with knees unflexed, so the term *length* is used rather than *height*.

## MAKING DECISIONS

### Head Circumference and Brain Development

The brain grows faster in infancy than at any other time of life. To accommodate this growth, an infant's head circumference must be very large in proportion to the rest of the body. The rapid growth stops at about 18 months of age. In early physical checkups, a health professional usually measures the head circumference as one means of assessing growth, especially brain growth. How nutritional status affects brain development and intelligence quotient (IQ) is difficult to measure because scientists have not determined how to separate the effects of nature from those of nurture. However, several studies have determined that breastfed babies have higher IQs than do babies who were fed with infant formula. At the same time, studies from Central America suggest that IQ after age 5 years relates more closely to the amount of schooling a child receives than to nutritional intake during childhood.

## Adipose Tissue Growth

Since 1970, researchers have speculated that overfeeding during infancy may increase the number of adipose tissue cells. Today, we know that the number of adipose cells can also increase as adulthood obesity develops. Still, if calorie intake is limited during infancy to keep down the number of adipose cells, the growth of other organ systems may also be severely restricted. Special concern revolves around body growth and development, especially brain and nervous system development. In addition, most overweight infants become normal-weight preschoolers without excessive diet restrictions. For these reasons, it's unwise to greatly restrict diet, and especially fat intake in infants. After the first 12 months, fat intake can range from 30% to 40% of calorie intake for ages 1 to 3 years, and 25% to 35% of calorie intake for older children (and teenagers).

▲ Brain growth is faster in infancy than in any other stage of life. Therefore an infant's head needs to be larger in comparison to the body to allow for such growth.

Children older than 2 years are less likely to experience failure to thrive because they can often get food for themselves. Younger children, for the most part, are limited to what caregivers provide.

## Failure to Thrive

Occasionally, an infant doesn't grow much in the first few months. Physical problems that may contribute to restricted growth range from poor oral cavity development, infections, and heart irregularities to constant diarrhea associated with intestinal problems. However, more than half the infants who fail to thrive have no apparent disease. Sometimes the cause is poor infant-parent interaction. This stems from misinformation, lack of a parent role model, too little concern about the child's welfare, or even from exerting too much control over feedings (e.g., maternal anxiety, force feeding). Poverty or food insecurity may also be at the root of infant or child undernutrition. In general, the problems arise from the parents' inexperience, rather than intentional negligence. Consequences of failure to thrive include poor physical growth, impaired mental development, and behavioral problems. When health professionals encounter an infant failing to thrive, the true causes need to be identified and then treated.

### CONCEPT CHECK

Growth occurs rapidly during infancy: Birth weight doubles in about 4 to 6 months and triples within the first year. Undernutrition in childhood can irreversibly inhibit growth and maturation, so that an individual never attains his or her full genetic potential for height. Infant and child growth is assessed by tracking body weight, length (height), and head circumference over time. Body mass index (BMI) is generally used to assess weight-for-height after 2 years of age. It is not desirable for infants to become overweight, although no evidence strongly indicates that overweight infants become overweight adults. However, severe calorie restriction is not recommended for infants because it may slow the growth of organ systems. When infants do not grow properly, their failure to thrive may stem from physical disorders or inadequate care, including inappropriate feeding practices.

▲ Formula-fed infants should remain on formula until 1 year of age.

## Infant Nutritional Needs

Infants' nutritional needs vary as they grow, and these differ from adult needs in both amount and proportion. Initially, human milk or infant formula (generally using heat-treated cow's milk as a base) supplies needed nutrients. Solid foods are not needed until around 6 months. Even after solid foods are added, the basis of an infant's diet for the first year is still human milk or infant formula. Because of the critical importance of adequate nutrition in infancy and the difficulties encountered in feeding some infants, there is more discussion in this chapter on this developmental period than on the later periods of childhood.

**Calories.** Calorie needs (based on Estimated Energy Requirements) in infancy are (89 kcal × weight of infant [kilograms]) + 75 from 0 to 3 months. From 4 to 6 months, such needs are (89 kcal × weight of infant [kilograms]) + 44; from 7 to 12 months it is (89 kcal × weight of infant [kilograms]) − 78. Based on body weight comparisons, at 6 months of age, this amounts to about 700 kcal daily and is two to four times more calories per kilogram of body weight than adults need. Infants need an easy way to get this amount of calories. Either human milk or infant formula is ideal for the first few months. Both are high in fat and supply about 640 kcal per quart of fluid (about 670 kcal per liter; Table 15-1). Later, human milk or infant formula, supplemented by solid foods, can provide even more calories and variety as well for the maturing infant.

The infant's high calorie needs are primarily driven by rapid growth and high metabolic rate. The high metabolic rate is caused in part by the ratio of the infant's body surface to its weight. More body surface allows more heat loss from the skin; the body must use extra calories to replace that heat.

**TABLE 15-1** Composition of Human and Cow's Milk and Infant Formulas per liter. At 3 Months of Age, Infants Typically Consume 0.75 to 1 liter of Human Milk or Formula per Day.

| | Energy (kcal) | Protein (grams) | Fat (grams) | Carbohydrate (grams) | Minerals* (grams) |
|---|---|---|---|---|---|
| **Milk** | | | | | |
| Human milk | 670** | 11 | 45 | 70 | 2 |
| Cow's milk, whole† | 670 | 36 | 36 | 49 | 7 |
| Cow's milk, fat-free† | 360 | 36 | 1 | 51 | 7 |
| **Casein/Whey-Based Formulas** | | | | | |
| Similac | 680 | 14 | 36 | 71 | 3 |
| Enfamil | 670 | 15 | 37 | 69 | 3 |
| Good Start | 670 | 16 | 34 | 73 | 3 |
| **Soybean Protein-Based Formulas** | | | | | |
| ProSobee | 670 | 20 | 35 | 67 | 4 |
| Isomil | 680 | 16 | 36 | 68 | 4 |
| **Transition Formulas/Beverages‡** | | | | | |
| Similac Toddler's Best | 670 | 25 | 33 | 75 | 3 |
| Enfamil Next Step | 670 | 17 | 33 | 74 | 3 |
| Carnation Follow-Up | 670 | 17 | 27 | 88 | 3 |

*Calcium, phosphorus, and other minerals.

**Rough estimate; ranges from 650–700 kcal per liter.

†Not appropriate for infant feeding, based primarily on high protein and mineral content.

‡For use after 6 months of age or later (see label).

**L**ooking at Table 15-1, it is easy to see why fat-free milk products are not recommended for infants—these do not supply adequate fat and calories to meet needs. Fat-free milk (and reduced fat and whole milk as well) also would provide too much protein and minerals if it were used to meet calorie needs.

**Carbohydrate.** Carbohydrate needs in infancy are 60 grams per day at 0 to 6 months and 95 grams per day at 7 to 12 months. These needs are based on the typical intakes of human milk by breastfed infants and their eventual use of solid foods. Both carbohydrate goals are satisfied by usual intakes of infants on a proper diet.

**Protein.** Daily protein needs in infancy are about 9 grams per day for younger infants and about 14 grams per day for older infants. These needs also are based on the typical intakes of human milk by breastfed infants for 0 to 6 months, and then on the needs for growth for older infants. About half of total protein intake should come from essential (indispensable) amino acids. As with carbohydrate, protein needs are easily satisfied by either human milk or infant formula. Protein intake should not greatly exceed this standard. Excess nitrogen and minerals supplied by high-protein diets would exceed the ability of an infant's kidneys to excrete the waste products of protein metabolism, thus putting much stress on overall kidney function.

In North America, infant protein deficiency is unlikely, except in cases of mistakes in formula preparation, such as when an infant's formula is excessively diluted with water. Protein deficiency may also be induced by elimination diets used to detect food **allergies** (hypersensitivities). As foods are eliminated from the diet, infants may not be offered enough protein to compensate for the high-protein sources no longer present (see the "Nutrition and Your Health" section later in this chapter).

**Fat.** Infants need about 30 grams of fat per day. Essential fatty acids should make up about 15% of total fat intake (about 5 grams per day). Both recommendations are again based on the typical intakes of human milk by breastfed infants and the eventual intake of solid foods. Fats are an important part of the infant's diet because they are vital to the development of the nervous system. As a concentrated source of calories, fat also helps resolve the potential problem of the infant's high calorie needs and small stomach capacity. Again, restriction of fat intake is not advised for infants or children under age 2. (Fig. 15-2).

 See the "Nutrition and Your Health: Food Allergies and Intolerances" at the end of this chapter.

**allergy** A hypersensitive immune response that occurs when immune bodies produced by us react with a protein we sense as foreign (an antigen).

**FIGURE 15-2** ▶ The labels on infant foods, like those on adult foods, contain a Nutrition Facts panel. However, the information provided on infant food labels differs from that on adult food labels, especially with respect to total fat, saturated fat, and cholesterol content (see Fig. 2-12 for a comparison). Some cereal brands are fortified with various other micronutrients.

**Serving Size**
Serving sizes for infant foods are based on the average amount eaten at one time by a child under 2 years.

**Total Fat**
Shows the amount of total fat in a serving of the food. Unlike adult food labels, labels on infant foods do not list calories from fat, saturated fat, or cholesterol, since infants and toddlers under 2 years need fat. Parents should not attempt to limit their infant's fat intake.

**Daily Values**
Food labels for infants and children under 4 years list the Daily Value percentages for protein, vitamins, and minerals. Unlike adult food labels, Daily Values for fat, cholesterol, sodium, potassium, carbohydrate, and fiber are not listed.

Arachidonic acid (AA) and docosahexaenoic acid (DHA) are two long-chain fatty acids that have important roles in infant development. The nervous system, especially the brain and eyes, depend on these fatty acids for proper development. During the last trimester, DHA and AA provided by the mother accumulate in the brain and retinas of the eyes in the fetus. Breastfed infants are able to continue to acquire these fatty acids from human milk, especially if their mothers are regularly eating fish. Until recently, no infant formulas sold in the United States included AA or DHA, but many brands are now available with both AA and DHA. These are particularly useful for feeding preterm infants.

**Vitamins of Special Interest.** As noted in Chapter 8, vitamin K is routinely given by injection to all infants at birth. Formula-fed infants receive the rest of the vitamins they need from the formula. Breastfed infants should be given a vitamin D supplement (400 IU per day) until they are weaned to infant formula and are consuming at least 500 milliliters of it per day. Breast-fed infants whose mothers are total vegetarians (vegans) should also receive vitamin B-12 in supplement form.

**Minerals of Special Interest.** Infants are born with some internal stores of iron. However, by the time birth weight doubles (4 to 6 months of age), iron stores are generally depleted if not otherwise part of the diet. If the mother was iron deficient during the pregnancy, these iron stores will be exhausted even sooner. As you will recall from Chapter 9, iron-deficiency anemia can lead to poor mental development in infants. Several studies indicate that iron deficiency anemia during infancy, even if corrected, has a lasting impact in terms of impaired cognition, motor development, and behavioral problems later in life. To maintain a desirable iron status, the American Academy of Pediatrics recommends that formula-fed infants should be given an iron-fortified formula from birth. Low-iron infant formulas are sometimes prescribed to treat infants with various GI tract problems, but otherwise their use is discouraged. In contrast, breastfed infants at about 6 months of age need solid foods to supply extra iron. This need for iron is a major consideration in the decision to introduce solid foods. Some physicians recommend liquid iron supplements from birth or by 1 month of age for breastfed infants, especially if the infant shows evidence of iron deficiency.

To aid in tooth development, fluoride supplements are recommended for breastfed infants after 6 months of age. The same holds true for formula-fed infants if the water supply used in home formula preparation—either tap or bottled water—does not contain fluoride. Formula manufacturers use fluoride-free water in formula preparation. Parents should consult their dentist for advice on meeting their infant's fluoride needs. The American Dental Association does not recommend fluoridated bottled water for use by infants because it creates a risk for enamel fluorosis in teeth during their development before eruption through the gums.

Infants also need adequate amounts of zinc and iodide to support growth. However, when human milk and infant formula are provided in quantities to meet calorie needs, sufficient zinc and iodide are generally supplied.

**Water.** An infant needs about 3 cups (700 to 800 milliliters) of water per day. Infants typically consume enough human milk or formula to supply this amount. In hot climates, however, supplemental water may be necessary. Furthermore, any conditions that lead to water loss—diarrhea, vomiting, fever, or too much sun—can call for supplemental water.

Infants are easily dehydrated, a condition that has serious effects if not remedied. Early signs of dehydration in infants include:

- More than 6 hours without a wet diaper
- Dark yellow or strong-smelling urine
- Unusual lethargy
- Dry mouth and lips
- Absence of tears when crying

Special fluid-replacement formulas containing electrolytes such as sodium and potassium are available in supermarkets and pharmacies to treat mild to moderate dehydration. A physician should guide any use of these products. As dehydration becomes more severe, the infant's eyes and/or the soft spot on the head may appear sunken, hands and feet may be cold and splotchy, and he or she may be excessively

## MAKING DECISIONS

### Extra Fluid for Infants

In some stores, bottled water products marketed specifically for infants may be placed alongside infant formulas and electrolyte-replacement solutions. This placement may give parents and caregivers the mistaken impression that bottled water products are an appropriate feeding supplement or substitute for fluid replacement for infants; they are not and should not be used for such purposes. It is important to remember that excessive fluid can also be harmful, especially to the brain.

tired and fussy. Such severe dehydration can result in rapid loss of kidney function and warrants medical intervention. Hospitalization and intravenous fluid treatment may be necessary for extreme cases or when the infant is unable to keep anything in the stomach.

### CONCEPT CHECK

Most nutrient needs in the first 6 months are met by human milk or infant formula. Breastfed infants need a vitamin D supplement and possibly an iron supplement; formula-fed infants and breastfed infants may need fluoride supplements after 6 months of age. Infants usually receive enough water from the human milk or infant formula they drink.

Overall, it is best to limit supplemental fluids to about 4 ounces (120 milliliters) per day, unless the physician thinks that a greater need exists because of disease or other conditions. In sum, extremes in fluid intake—either too little or too much—can lead to health problems.

## Formula Feeding for Infants

Breastfeeding was covered in detail in Chapter 14. Let's now focus on formula feeding. You'll recall that a major advantage of breastfeeding is the provision of immune protection to the infant. Overall, in areas of the world where high standards for water purity and cleanliness are common, formula feeding is a safe alternative for infants (but generally is not as beneficial as breastfeeding).

**Formula Composition.** Infants cannot tolerate cow's milk as such because of its high protein and mineral content. Cow's milk is perfect for the greater growth needs of calves, but not for human infants. Thus, cow's milk must be altered by formula manufacturers to be safe for infant feeding. Altered forms of cow's milk, known as infant formulas, must conform to strict federal guidelines for nutrient composition and quality. Formulas generally contain lactose and/or sucrose for carbohydrate, heat-treated proteins from cow's milk, and vegetable oils for fat (review Table 15-1). Soy protein–based formulas are available for infants who can't tolerate lactose or the types of proteins found in cow's milk. If the soybean-based formula is not tolerated, the next step is to try a predigested formula in which the proteins have been broken down into small polypeptides and amino acids. A variety of other specialized formulas also are available for specific medical conditions. In any case, it is important to use an iron-fortified formula unless a physician recommends otherwise.

Some transition formulas/beverages have been introduced for older infants and toddlers (review Table 15-1). Some of these products are intended for use after 6 months of age if the infant is consuming solid foods, whereas others are intended for use only by toddlers. These transition products are lower in fat than human milk or standard infant formulas; their iron content is higher than that of cow's milk, and their overall mineral content is generally more like that of human milk than cow's milk. According to the manufacturers, the advantages of these transition formulas/beverages over standard formulas for older infants and toddlers include reduced cost and better flavor. Parents should consult their physician with regard to the use of these products.

**Formula Preparation.** Some infant formulas come in ready-to-feed form. These are poured into a clean bottle and fed immediately. Room-temperature formula is acceptable for many infants. Otherwise, to warm a bottle of formula, a caregiver can run hot water over it or place it briefly in a pan of simmering water. Infant formulas should not be heated in a microwave oven because hot spots may develop, which can burn the infant's mouth and esophagus.

Powdered and concentrated fluid formula preparations are also commonly used. All utensils used to prepare formula should be washed and thoroughly rinsed.

**P**arents should consult a physician when choosing an appropriate infant formula. Not all formula-like products are designed for infant use. A 5-month-old girl was admitted to a hospital in Arkansas with symptoms of heart failure, rickets, inflamed blood vessels, and possible nerve damage after being fed Soy Moo (a soy beverage sold in health stores) since 3 days of age. The symptoms suggest severe vitamin deficiencies.

**B**isphenol A (BPA) is a chemical used in the manufacture of many plastics, including some baby bottles. Human exposure to BPA, mainly through leaching of the chemical from packaging into foods and beverages, is widespread. Concern about exposure stems from animal studies that link BPA with reproductive and developmental defects. However, the consensus among regulatory agencies in the United States and Canada is that current levels of BPA exposure are not harmful, even for infants. For parents who wish to limit exposure, BPA-free baby bottles are available.

Powdered or concentrated formulas should be combined with clean, cold water, exactly following the directions on the formula label. The formula is then warmed, if desired, and fed immediately to the infant. Hot water from the faucet should not be used to make formula, since it poses a risk for high lead content (see Chapter 13). Cold water poses much less risk. For infants up to 6 months of age, pediatricians commonly recommend boiling (and then cooling) the water to be used in formula preparation and sterilizing bottles and utensils by immersion in boiling water.

Refrigerating prepared formula for 1 day is safe. However, formula left over from a feeding should be discarded because it will be contaminated by bacteria and enzymes from the infant's saliva. If well water is used, it should be boiled before making formula for at least the infant's first 3 months of life, and it should be analyzed for excessive concentration of naturally occurring nitrates, which can lead to a severe form of anemia. If nitrates are high in municipal water systems, consumers will be warned (such as in a local newspaper) not to use the water for making infant formula until the concentration falls to a safe amount. The American Dental Association does not recommend that formula be mixed with bottled nursery water, available alongside infant formula in most supermarkets, for risk of eventual tooth discoloration from high fluoride levels.

▲ Careful attention during feeding allows the caregiver to notice the infant's signal as to when the feeding should cease.

## Feeding Technique

Infants swallow a lot of air as they ingest either formula or human milk, so it's important to burp an infant after either 10 minutes of feeding or 1 to 2 ounces (30 to 60 milliliters) has been consumed from a bottle and again at the end of feeding. Spitting up a bit of milk is normal at this time.

When the infant begins acting full, bottle feeding should be stopped, even if some milk is left in the bottle. Common cues that signal that an infant has had enough include turning the head away, being inattentive, falling asleep, and becoming playful. Generally, the infant's appetite is a better guide than standardized recommendations concerning feeding amounts. Breastfeeding infants usually have had enough to eat after about 20 minutes. Although it's difficult to tell how much milk breastfed infants are getting, they also give signs when full. By carefully observing bottle-feeding or breastfeeding infants and responding to their cues appropriately, caregivers not only can be assured that the infants' calorie needs are being met but also can foster a climate of trust and responsiveness.

Once fed, an infant should not be placed on its stomach. Placing the infant on its back is recommended by the American Academy of Pediatrics. The reason that an infant should not be placed on its stomach is because this sleeping position has been linked to sudden infant death syndrome (SIDS). The Back to Sleep campaign, started in 1994 in the United States, has reduced SIDS by 40%.

The Back to Sleep campaign, however, has led to a problem known as flattened head syndrome (clinically known as positional plagiocephaly). Infant skulls are soft and therefore can change in shape. Flattened head syndrome can occur if an excessive amount of an infant's day is spent on his or her back or against a highchair/car seat. In response to this concern, the American Academy of Pediatrics has recommended periodic repositioning of an infant's head while asleep and allowing for supervised time on his or her stomach while awake. In addition, some infants may need to wear specially fitted helmets to correct the shape of their heads.

▲ The Back to Sleep campaign advises that infants be placed on their backs for sleeping.

## Expanding the Infant's Mealtime Choices

By about 6 months of age, the infant is ready to start eating "table food." Initially, table foods add to—rather than replace—formula or human milk. In the first attempts to introduce solid foods, just getting the food into the infant's mouth may prove to be a challenge. By the end of the first year, though, the infant should be eating a variety of meats, vegetables, fruits, and grains so that the diet begins to resemble a balanced pattern, setting the stage for lifelong preferences and dietary habits (Table 15-2).

**TABLE 15-2** Sample Daily Menu for a 1-Year-Old Child*

| | |
|---|---|
| **Breakfast**<br>1 to 2 tbsp applesauce<br>¼ cup Cheerios<br>½ cup whole milk | **Snack**<br>½ ounce cheddar cheese<br>4 wheat crackers<br>½ cup whole milk |
| **Snack**<br>½ hard-cooked egg<br>½ slice wheat toast with ½ tsp margarine<br>½ cup orange juice | **Dinner**<br>1 ounce hamburger (crumbled)<br>1 to 2 tbsp mashed potatoes with ½ tsp margarine<br>1 to 2 tbsp cooked carrots (cut in strips, not coins)<br>½ cup whole milk |
| **Lunch**<br>1 ounce roasted chicken, minced<br>1 to 2 tbsp rice with ½ tsp margarine<br>1 to 2 tbsp cooked peas<br>½ cup whole milk | **Snack**<br>½ banana<br>2 oatmeal cookies (no raisins)<br>½ cup whole milk |

| **Nutritional Analysis** | |
|---|---|
| Total energy (kcal) | 1100 |
| % energy from | |
| Carbohydrate | 40% |
| Protein | 19% |
| Fat | 41% |

*This diet is just a start. A 1-year-old may need more or less food. In those cases, serving sizes should be adjusted. The milk can be fed by cup; some can be put into a bottle if the child has not been fully weaned from the bottle. The juice should be fed in a cup.

Throughout the process of expanding the infant's mealtime choices, it is essential to allow the infant to control the situation—the caregiver must proceed slowly and respond to the infant's cues that he or she is hungry or has had enough to eat.

**Recognizing the Infant's Readiness for Solid Foods.** How does the caregiver know it is time to introduce solid foods? Infant size can serve as a rough indicator of readiness—reaching a weight of at least 13 pounds (6 kilograms) is a preliminary sign of readiness for solid foods. Another physiological cue is frequency of feeding, such as consuming more than 32 ounces (1 liter) of formula daily or breastfeeding more than 8 to 10 times within 24 hours. Underlying these noticeable signals are several important developmental factors:

1. *Nutritional need.* Before the infant is 6 months old, nutritional needs can generally be met with human milk and/or formula. After 6 months of age, however, many infants need the additional calories supplied by solid foods. In terms of individual nutrients, iron stores are exhausted by about 6 months of age. Either solid foods or iron supplements are then needed to supply iron if the child is breastfed or fed a low-iron or iron-free formula. (As previously mentioned, a vitamin D supplement should also be given to breastfed infants.)

2. *Physiological capabilities.* As the infant ages, the ability to digest and metabolize a wider range of food components improves. Before about 3 months of age, an infant's digestive tract cannot readily digest starch. Also, kidney function is limited until about 4 to 6 weeks of age. Until then, waste products from excessive amounts of dietary protein or minerals are difficult to excrete.

3. *Physical ability.* Three physical markers indicate that a child is ready for solid foods: (1) the disappearance of the extrusion reflex (thrusting the tongue forward and pushing food out of the mouth), (2) head and neck control, and (3) the ability to sit up with support. These usually occur around 4 to 6 months of age, but they vary with each infant.

4. *Allergy prevention.* An infant's intestinal tract is "leaky"—whole proteins can readily be absorbed from birth until 4 to 5 months of age. If the infant is exposed too early to some types of proteins—particularly those in cow's milk

and egg whites—the infant may be predisposed to future allergies and other health problems, such as diabetes. For this reason, it is best to minimize the number of different types of proteins in an infant's diet, especially during the first 3 months (see the "Nutrition and Your Health" section on food allergies at the end of this chapter for details).

With these considerations in mind—nutritional need, physiological and physical readiness, and allergy prevention—the American Academy of Pediatrics recommends that solid foods not be introduced until about 6 months of age and that infants receive no unaltered cow's milk before 1 year.

▲ Iron-fortified rice cereal is recommended as the first solid food to be fed to infants.

## MAKING DECISIONS

### Introducing Solid Foods

Parents may believe that the early addition of solid foods will help an infant sleep through the night. Actually, this achievement is a developmental milestone, and the amount of food consumed by the infant is of little relevance to the achievement of a good night's sleep. Before 4 to 6 months of age, infants are not physically mature enough to consume much solid food. Only occasionally does a rapidly growing infant need solid foods to meet calorie and nutrient needs before 6 months of age.

**Foods to Match Needs and Developmental Abilities During the First Year.** If solid foods are introduced before 6 months of age, the primary goal of the food should be to meet iron needs. Therefore, the first solid foods should be iron-fortified cereals. Some pediatricians may recommend lean ground (strained) meats for more absorbable forms of iron. Rice is the best cereal to begin with because it is least likely to cause allergies.

When starting solid foods, it is important to start with a teaspoon serving size of a single-ingredient food item, such as rice cereal, and increase the serving size gradually. Once the new food has been fed for about a week without ill effects, another food can be added to the infant's diet. At first, this can be another type of cereal or perhaps a cooked and strained (or mashed) vegetable, meat, fruit, or egg yolk.

Waiting about 7 days between the introduction of each new food is important because it can take that long for evidence of an allergy or intolerance to develop. Allergy symptoms to look for include diarrhea, vomiting, a rash, or wheezing. If one or more of these symptoms appears, the suspected problem food should be avoided for several weeks and then reintroduced in a small quantity. If the problem continues, a physician should be consulted.

Some foods that commonly cause an allergic response in infants are egg whites, chocolate, nuts, and cow's milk. It is best not to introduce these foods during infancy. Also, it is important to avoid introducing mixed foods until each component of the combination dish has been given separately. Otherwise, if an allergy or intolerance develops, it will be difficult to identify the offending food. Many babies outgrow food allergies during childhood.

Many strained foods for infant feeding are available at the supermarket. Single food items are more desirable than mixed dinners and desserts, which are less nutrient-dense. Most brands have no added salt, but some fruit desserts contain a lot of added sugar.

As an alternative, plain, unseasoned cooked foods—vegetables, fruits, and meats—can be ground up in an inexpensive plastic baby food grinder/mill. Another option is to puree a larger amount of food in a blender, freeze it in ice-cube portions, store in plastic bags, and defrost and warm as needed. Careful attention to cleanliness is necessary. Seasonings that may please the rest of the family should not be added to infant foods made at home. The infant doesn't notice the difference if salt, sugar, or spices are omitted. It is best to introduce infants to a variety of foods, so that at the

▶ **Typical Solid Food Progression, Starting at 6 Months***

| | |
|---|---|
| Week 1 | Rice cereal |
| Week 2 | Add strained carrots |
| Week 3 | Add applesauce |
| Week 4 | Add oat cereal |
| Week 5 | Add cooked egg yolk |
| Week 6 | Add strained chicken |
| Week 7 | Add strained peas |
| Week 8 | Add plums |

*Extending the rice cereal step for a month or so is advised if solid food introduction begins at 4 months of age. Also, if at any point signs of allergy or intolerance develop, substitute another similar food item.

▲ Repeated exposure fosters acceptance of new tastes and textures.

**early childhood caries** Tooth decay that results from formula or juice (and even human milk) bathing the teeth as the child sleeps with a bottle in his or her mouth. The upper teeth are mostly affected as the lower teeth are protected by the tongue; formerly called *nursing bottle syndrome* and *baby bottle tooth decay*.

▲ Early childhood caries. An extreme example of tooth decay probably resulting from frequently putting the child to bed with a bottle. The upper teeth have decayed almost all the way to the gum line.

end of the first year, the infant is consuming many foods—human milk or formula, meats, fruits, vegetables, and grains.

Self-feeding skills require coordination and can develop only if the infant is allowed to practice and experiment. By 6 to 7 months of age, the infant has learned to handle finger foods and transfer objects from one hand to the other with some dexterity. At about this time, teeth also begin to appear. Dry toast, sliced in strips, offers hours of enjoyment. By age 7 to 8 months, infants can push food around on a plate, play with a drinking cup, hold a bottle, and self-feed a cracker or a piece of toast. Through mastery of these manipulations, infants develop confidence and self-esteem. It is important that parents be patient and support these early feeding attempts, even though they appear inefficient.

At 9 to 10 months of age, the infant's desire to explore, experience, and play with foods may hinder feeding. Food is used as a means to explore the environment, and therefore feeding time is often very messy—a bowl of macaroni may end up in the child's hair. Presenting a new food on several consecutive days can aid in an infant's acceptance of that food. Caregivers need to relax and take this phase of infant development in stride. Sloppy, friendly mealtimes make for good memories. By the end of the first year, finger-feeding becomes more efficient and chewing is easier as more teeth erupt. Still, experimentation and unpredictability are to be expected.

To ease the efforts in feeding solid foods, consider the following tips:

- Use a baby-sized spoon; a small spoon with a long handle is best.
- Hold the infant comfortably on the lap, as for breastfeeding or bottle feeding, but a little more upright to ease swallowing. When in this position, the infant expects food.
- Put a small dab of food on the spoon tip and gently place it on the infant's tongue.
- Convey a calm and casual approach to the infant, who needs time to get used to food.
- Expect the infant to take only two or three bites of the first meals.

## Weaning from the Breast or Bottle

Around the age of 6 months, juices can be offered in a sippy cup with a wide, flat bottom. Drinking from a cup rather than from a bottle helps prevent **early childhood caries.** If an infant drinks continuously from a bottle, the carbohydrate-rich fluid bathes the teeth, providing an ideal growth medium for bacteria adhering to the teeth. These bacteria then make acids, which dissolve tooth enamel. To avoid dental caries, infants should not be put to bed with a bottle or placed in an infant seat with a bottle propped up.

By about 10 months of age, infants are learning to self-feed and likewise to drink independently from a cup. As children drink from a cup more frequently, fewer bottle feedings and/or breastfeedings are necessary. The added mobility of crawling and walking should naturally lead to gradual weaning from the bottle or breast. Even so, getting a baby out of the bedtime-bottle habit can be difficult. Determined caregivers can either wince through a few nights of their baby's crying or slowly wean the baby away from the bottle with either a pacifier or water (for a week or so).

## Dietary Guidelines for Infant Feeding

It can be difficult for new parents to make sense of nutrition goals for infants in the face of changing dietary recommendations from health authorities, cultural preferences, and outdated advice from friends and family. In response to various controversies surrounding infant feeding, the American Academy of Pediatrics has issued a number of statements concerning infant diets. The following guidelines are based on these statements:

- *Build to a variety of foods.* For the first months of life, human milk (or infant formula) is all an infant needs. (Vitamin D needs of breastfed infants is an exception.)

When the infant is ready, start adding new foods, one at a time. During the first year, the goal is to teach an infant to enjoy a variety of nutritious foods. A lifetime of healthy eating habits begins with this important first step.

- *Pay attention to your infant's appetite to avoid overfeeding or underfeeding.* Feed infants when they are hungry. Never force an infant to finish an unwanted serving of food. Watch for signs that indicate hunger or fullness. This will reinforce the infant's natural capability to self-regulate food intake.
- *Infants need fat.* Although fat contributes to many adult health problems, it's an essential source of calories for growing infants. Fat also helps the nervous system develop.
- *Choose fruits, vegetables, and grains, but don't overdo high-fiber foods.* During the second half of the first year, infants are fed a variety of fruits and vegetables. However, studies show that by 1 year of age, vegetable consumption is dominated by white potatoes. Continuing to offer choices of green and yellow vegetables during infancy and the toddler years will enhance intake of important vitamins, minerals, and phytochemicals. In terms of fiber, although many adults benefit from high-fiber diets, they are not good for infants. They are bulky, filling, and often low in calories. The natural amounts of fiber and nutrients in fruits, vegetables, and grains are appropriate as part of a healthy infant diet.
- *Infants need sugars in moderation.* Sugars are an additional source of calories for active, rapidly growing infants. Foods such as human milk, fruits, and 100% juices are natural sources of sugars and other nutrients as well. Foods that contain artificial sweeteners should be avoided; they don't provide the calories growing infants need. On the other hand, excessive intake of sugars, particularly from fruit-flavored drinks and soft drinks, contribute to the epidemic of childhood obesity.
- *Infants need sodium in moderation.* Sodium is a necessary mineral found naturally in almost all foods. As part of a healthy diet, infants need sodium for their bodies to work properly. However, average intakes of sodium among infants and toddlers are above the AI. Caregivers should delay introduction of cow's milk (a source of sodium for infants) until 1 year of age and refrain from offering heavily-seasoned and processed foods.
- *Choose foods containing iron, zinc, and calcium.* Infants need good sources of iron, zinc, and calcium for optimum growth in the first 2 years. These minerals are important for healthy blood, optimal growth, and strong bones. Many infant and toddler foods (e.g., cereal, crackers, and biter biscuits) are fortified with these minerals.

In essence, there is no evidence that restrictive diets during infancy have positive effects, whereas their hazards are well documented.

## What Not to Feed an Infant

Following are several foods and practices to avoid when feeding an infant:

- *Honey.* This product may contain spores of *Clostridium botulinum*. The spores can eventually develop into bacteria in the stomach and lead to a foodborne illness known as *botulism*. This can be fatal, especially in children under 1 year old (see Chapter 13).
- *Excessive infant formula or human milk.* After 6 to 8 months, solid foods should play a greater role in satisfying an infant's increasing appetite. The main reason to switch is that solid foods contain considerably more bioavailable iron than do human milk and low-iron formulas. About 24 to 32 ounces (¾ to 1 liters) of human milk or formula daily is ideal after 6 months, with food supplying the rest of the infant's calorie needs.
- *Foods that tend to cause choking.* These foods include hot dogs (unless finely cut into sticks, not coin shapes), candy, whole nuts, grapes, coarsely cut meats, raw carrots, popcorn, and peanut butter. Caregivers should not allow younger children to gobble snack foods during playtime and should supervise all meals.

▲ Early feeding attempts should be encouraged, even though they're messy.

**E**gg whites also should not be fed to children before 1 year of age to help prevent the development of allergies.

▶ **A Summary of Infant Feeding Recommendations**

### Breastfed Infants

- Breastfeed for 6 months or longer, if possible. Then introduce infant formula if and when breastfeeding declines or ceases. (Breast milk can also be pumped and placed in a bottle for later use.)
- Provide a vitamin D supplement (400 IU per day).
- Investigate the need for vitamin B-12, fluoride, and iron supplementation to prevent deficiencies.

### Formula-Fed Infants

- Use infant formula for the first year of life, preferably an iron-fortified type.
- Investigate the need for a fluoride supplement if the water supply is not fluoridated.

### All Infants

- Add iron-fortified cereal at about 6 months of age.
- Provide a variety of basic, soft foods after 6 months of age, advancing to a varied diet.

▲ The older infant enjoys finger-feeding.

- *Cow's milk, especially low-fat or fat-free cow's milk.* The American Academy of Pediatrics strongly urges parents not to give children under age 2 fat-reduced, 1%, or fat-free milk. Before age 2, the amount of this milk needed for calorie needs would supply too many minerals and in turn could overwhelm the kidneys' ability to excrete the excess. The lower fat intake might also harm nervous system development. Beyond 2 years, children can drink fat-reduced, 1%, or fat-free milk, because by this age they are consuming enough solid foods to supply calorie and fat needs.
- *Feeding excessive amounts of apple or pear juice.* The fructose and sorbitol contained in these juices can lead to diarrhea because they are slowly absorbed. Also, if fruit juice or related drink products are replacing formula or milk in the diet, the infant may not be receiving adequate amounts of calcium and other minerals essential for bone growth. Studies have shown a link between excessive amounts of fruit juice and failure to thrive, GI tract complications, obesity, short stature, and poor dental health. Thus, these substances should be used sparingly. Infants over the age of 6 months can usually safely consume up to 6 ounces of juice in the course of a day, with no more than 2 to 4 ounces at a time.

## Inappropriate Infant Feeding Practices

Parents and other caregivers should be aware of a variety of potential health problems related to infant nutrition, so that corrective action can be taken quickly. In some cases, such problems stem from inappropriate feeding practices and inadequate nutrient intakes, including the following:

- Diet providing insufficient iron
- Absence from the diet of an entire food group in MyPyramid as solid foods are introduced and become the main source of nutrients
- Use of cow's milk
- Premature introduction of potential allergy-causing foods, such as egg whites and nuts
- Drinking raw (unpasteurized) milk, which may be contaminated with bacteria or viruses
- Drinking goat's milk, low in folate, iron, vitamin C, and vitamin D
- Failure to begin drinking from a cup by 1 year of age
- Continuing to feed from a bottle past 18 months of age
- Intake of supplemental vitamins or minerals above 100% of the appropriate RDA or other nutrient standard
- Drinking large amounts of fruit juice after 6 months of age, especially as a substitute for infant formula or human milk. (Recall that fruit juice is not to be fed at all before 6 months of age.)

The website of the American Academy of Pediatrics (www.aap.org) can also provide useful information on these and other nutrition-related problems in infancy.

### CONCEPT CHECK

Infant formulas generally contain lactose or sucrose, heat-treated proteins from cow's milk, and vegetable oil. Formulas may or may not be fortified with iron. Sanitation is important in preparing and storing formula. Solid foods should not be added to an infant's diet until the child is both ready for and needs solid food, usually at about 6 months of age. The first solid foods can be iron-fortified infant cereals, with gradual additions of other foods—one at a time each week. Some foods to avoid giving to infants in the first year are honey, cow's milk (particularly fat-reduced, 1%, or fat-free milk), foods that may cause the child to choke, and excessive amounts of fruit juice or related products (e.g., fruit drinks).

# 15.3 Preschool Children: Nutrition Concerns

The rapid growth rate that characterizes infancy tapers off quickly during the subsequent few years. The average annual weight gain is only 4.5 to 6.6 pounds (2 to 3 kilograms), and the average annual height gain is only 3 to 4 inches (7.5 to 10 centimeters) between the ages of 2 and 5. As a toddler's growth rate tapers off, eating behavior changes. For example, the decreased growth rate leads to a decreased appetite, often called "picky eating," compared with infants.

Because of a reduced appetite, planning a diet that meets the nutrient needs of a preschool child poses a special challenge to caregivers. MyPyramid for Preschoolers (ages 2–5), available at www.mypyamid.gov/preschoolers.index.html, offers numerous resources for planning nutritious, age-appropriate meals and snacks. Additional nutrition guidance, starting with pregnancy and extending through the preschool years, is available from the *Start Healthy, Stay Healthy* Resource Center at http://www.gerber.com/Nutrition_Feeding/Start_Healthy_Stay_Healthy.aspx. Choosing nutrient-dense foods is particularly important with children who eat relatively little. This is a good time to emphasize some whole grains, fruits, and vegetables without increasing fat and simple sugar intake. A whole-grain ready-to-eat breakfast cereal with limited fat and sugar is an excellent choice. There is no need to decrease fat or simple sugar intake severely, but fatty and sweet food choices should not overwhelm more nutritious ones.

Excessive sodium intake is a concern for preschool children as well. Caregivers can lower sodium intake by limiting salt added during cooking and at the table; cutting back on use of processed foods (e.g., luncheon meats, hot dogs); rinsing canned beans and vegetables before cooking; and encouraging consumption of fruits, vegetables, and whole grains in place of prepackaged snacks. The preschool years are the best time for a child to start a healthful pattern of living and eating, focusing on regular physical activity and nutritious foods. Parents and other caregivers are role models: If they eat a variety of foods, the children will eat a variety of foods. One possible policy is the one-bite rule: Within reason, children should take at least one bite or taste of the foods presented to them. For snacks, parents should select several possibilities of acceptable choices and allow children to choose one; responsibility for food choice by the child ideally should start early.

## How to Help a Child Choose Nutritious Foods

One way adults can encourage young children to eat nutritious, well-balanced meals is to serve new foods and repeat exposure to them. The dinner hour is a good time for children to experience new foods and to develop food preferences. Preschool children especially tend to be wary of new foods. One reason is that they have more taste buds, and their taste buds are more sensitive than those of adults. In addition, they have a general distrust of unfamiliar foods. If adults can be patient and persevere, children will build good food habits. It may take 8 to 10 exposures to a new food before a child finds it acceptable. Above all, the dinner table should not become a battleground, and using one food as a bribe to eat another—for example, a piece of pie for peas—is strongly discouraged.

Certain food characteristics, such as crisp textures and mild flavors, are appealing to children. Familiarity also plays an important role in food acceptance. In contrast, young children are especially wary of hot-temperature foods and tend to reject them.

Preschoolers eventually develop skill with spoons and forks and can even use dull knives. However, it's still a good idea to serve some finger foods. A goal should be to make mealtime a happy, social time to share and enjoy healthful foods.

## Childhood Feeding Problems

Tensions between parents, or between parents and children, especially during mealtime, often contribute to eating problems. Getting to the root of family problems and

> **Summary of Macronutrient Needs during Childhood**

**Carbohydrates**

- 130 grams per day to supply energy for the central nervous system and prevent ketosis

**Protein**

- 13-19 grams per day (ages 1-3)
- 34-52 grams per day (older children)

**Fat**

- at least 5 grams per day of essential fatty acids
- eventually aim for 20% to 35% of total calorie intake by age 19

▲ Interest in food starts early in life.

creating a more harmonious family atmosphere are important steps toward resolving many childhood feeding problems. In addition, many parents must be educated as to what to expect of a preschool child and what food-related goals to set. Let's consider some typical complaints and concerns of parents, the causes of the problems, and suggestions for correcting them.

**"My Child Won't Eat as Much or as Regularly as He Did as an Infant."** This behavior is typical of preschoolers, because their growth rate slows after infancy; thus, they don't need as much food. Parents often need reminding that a 3-year-old can't be expected to eat as voraciously as an infant or to eat adult-size portions. Table 15-3 shows a general food plan, based on MyPyramid, appropriate for preschool and school-age children. Until about 5 years of age, portion sizes in the vegetables group, fruits group, and meat & beans group should be about 1 tablespoon per year of life, and can be increased as needed. The same advice does not apply to the grains or milk groups, but consuming too much milk can leave the diet short on iron. Luckily, normal-weight children have a built-in feeding mechanism, which adjusts hunger to regulate food intake at each stage of growth. If a child is developing and growing normally and the caregiver is providing a variety of healthful foods, all can be confident of the child's well-being.

A pattern of picky eating is usually just another expression of independence for children, who have a strong desire to establish a self-determined routine. Caregivers should avoid nagging, forcing, and bribing children to encourage eating. Indirectly, these tactics reinforce picky-eating behaviors due to the added attention given to them. Overall, parents should focus on offering a variety of healthy choices, allowing the child to exert some autonomy over the specific type of food and the amount eaten. A child's sudden loss of appetite, however, may be reason for concern, as a poor appetite may be a sign of underlying illness.

Parents should also be reminded that food likes and dislikes change rapidly in childhood and are influenced by food temperature, appearance, texture, and taste. Sometimes children object to having foods mixed, as in stews and casseroles, even if they normally like the ingredients separately.

In addition, parents should recognize that this is an important age for children to explore the world around them. Even good eaters are sometimes more interested in exploring than eating. There's room for occasional indulgences, a skipped meal or

**T**wo-year-olds commonly prefer particular foods, but parents needn't worry about this. A child may switch from one specific food focus (often called a *jag*) to another with equal intensity (older infants may also act this way). If the caregiver continues to offer choices, the child will soon begin to eat a wider variety of foods again, and the specific food focus will disappear as suddenly as it appeared.

**C**hoking is a very preventable hazard for young children. Some suggestions for caregivers include:

- Set a good example at the table by taking small bites and chewing foods thoroughly.
- Have children sit at the table, take their time, and focus on the food during meals and snacks.
- Avoid giving children any foods that are round, firm, sticky, or cut into large chunks. Some examples of foods to avoid are nuts, grapes, raisins, popcorn, peanut butter, and hard pieces of raw fruits or vegetables.

**TABLE 15-3** Food Plans for Children Based on MyPyramid

| Food Group | Serving Size | Approximate Number of Servings [1] | | | | |
|---|---|---|---|---|---|---|
| | | Age 2 [2] | Age 5 [3] | Age 8 [3] | Age 12 [3, 4] | Age 16 [3,4] |
| Grains | ounce | 3 | 5 | 5 | 6–7 | 6–10 |
| Vegetables | cup | 1 | 1.5 | 2 | 2.5–3 | 2.5–3.5 |
| Fruits | cup | 1 | 1.5 | 1.5 | 2 | 2–2.5 |
| Milk | cup | 2 | 2 | 3 | 3 | 3 |
| Meat & Beans | ounce | 2 | 4 | 5 | 5.5–6 | 5.5–7 |
| Oils | teaspoon | 3 | 4 | 5 | 6 | 6–8 |
| Discretionary calories | kcal | up to 165 | up to 170 | up to 130 | up to 265–290 | up to 265–425 |

[1] Log on to www.mypyramid.gov for other ages and other physical activity levels.
[2] Based on less than 30 minutes of physical activity.
[3] Based on 30–60 minutes of physical activity.
[4] The lower amounts refer to girls.

two, or once in a while "less than ideal" choices. It's eating and lifestyle habits over the course of a month (and lifetime) that matter. Children master their eating when adults set a good example, provide opportunities to learn, give support for exploration, and limit inappropriate behavior.

**"My Child Is Always Snacking, Yet She Never Finishes Her Meal."** Children have small stomachs. Offering them six or so small meals succeeds better than limiting them to three meals each day. Sticking to three meals a day offers no special nutritional advantages; it's just a social custom. Snacking is fine, as long as good dental habits are practiced. When we eat isn't nearly as important as what we eat. If nutritious snacks are readily available, these are good to offer at midmorning or midafternoon when the child becomes hungry. Fruits and vegetables (fresh, frozen, or juice) and whole-grain breads and crackers are good snack choices. It is important that these snack choices be planned ahead in order to have healthy choices available. Working parents should make sure their children are provided with nutritious snacks to tide them over until dinnertime.

When a child refuses to eat, it's best not to overreact. Doing so may give the child the idea that not eating is a means of getting attention or manipulating a scene. Most children don't starve themselves to any point approaching physical harm. When children refuse to eat, have them sit at the table for a while; if they still aren't interested in eating, remove the food and wait until the next scheduled meal or snack.

**"My Child Never Eats Vegetables."** Children generally eat enough fruit but not an adequate amount of vegetables. Everyone dislikes certain foods. Again, the one-bite policy can be used, including vegetable servings. It takes time for a child to become enthusiastic about a new food; however, with continual exposure and a positive role model, chances are the child may even grow to like it.

Children cannot and should not be forced to eat. They need to develop independence and identities separate from their parents. As stated earlier, children have to choose for themselves—a practice that should be encouraged. No one food is an essential part of a diet. Hunger is still the best means for getting a child to eat. It may be effective to feed children vegetables at the start of a meal, when they are hungriest. Offer new foods with familiar ones. A platter of raw or lightly cooked carrots, broccoli, green and red peppers, cabbage, and mushrooms eaten as a snack with friends may be accepted. A 4- or 5-year-old child can safely eat raw vegetables without fear of choking. Recall that children often are more sensitive than adults to strong flavors and odors. Nutritious dips, such as Ranch dressing, "sell" vegetables to many children. Vegetables may acquire more appeal when children help prepare them. And, as with any food, it is important to remember that children are entitled to their own likes and dislikes, too.

## Do Children Need a Multivitamin and Mineral Supplement?

Major scientific groups, such as the American Dietetic Association and the American Society for Clinical Nutrition, believe that multivitamin and mineral supplements are generally unnecessary for healthy children; it's better to emphasize good foods. In fact, consuming fortified foods as well as supplements may lead to intakes above the UL for some nutrients, such as vitamin A and zinc. Children's supplements that are made to look like candy may result in accidental overdose, such as for iron. Fortified ready-to-eat breakfast cereals with milk are especially helpful in closing any gap between current micronutrient intake and needs, such as for vitamin E, folate, and vitamin D. Two micronutrients of particular concern are iron and zinc. These may be lacking in children's diets because they consume such small portions of rich sources, such as animal protein foods. In addition, since the 2005 Dietary Guidelines for Americans suggest that children over age 2 years follow a diet low in saturated fat and cholesterol, rich sources of iron and zinc may be lacking in their diets. To compensate, parents can

▲ Milk is a nutrient-dense source of protein, calcium, zinc, and other nutrients to support growth. It is especially challenging to meet calcium needs in childhood without regular dairy product consumption (see Chapter 9 for alternative sources of calcium).

search for a whole-grain breakfast cereal that the child likes that also has about 50% of the Daily Value for iron and 25% of the Daily Value for zinc. (This will supply sufficient amounts of both nutrients because the Daily Values are based on the higher needs of adults.) If that's not possible, especially for a child who is ill, has a very erratic food preference pattern or appetite, or is on a weight-loss diet, the American Academy of Pediatrics states that the child may benefit from a children's multivitamin and mineral supplement not exceeding 100% of Daily Values on the label, especially if these conditions persist. Still, as mentioned many times in this textbook, such a practice does not substitute for an otherwise healthy diet—children included.

If current childhood feeding practices are to become more healthful, the focus should be on whole-grain breads and cereals, fruits, vegetables, and low-fat milk and milk products. Children do not need to be severely restricted but, rather, should modify food habits with small changes. Some easy diet changes to begin with are bagels instead of doughnuts, fat-free frozen yogurt instead of ice cream, fat-reduced or 1% milk instead of whole milk, fruit instead of crackers and cheese for snacks, and airpopped popcorn instead of chips.

## Nutritional Problems in Preschool Children

Three nutrition-related problems found in preschool children are iron-deficiency anemia, constipation, and dental caries. Proper diet can help correct or relieve these conditions. Vegetarian diets can also pose problems. Autism and lead poisoning are additional conditions that can be affected by nutritional status.

**Iron-Deficiency Anemia.**  The best way to prevent iron-deficiency anemia in children is to provide foods that are adequate sources of iron. Iron-fortified breakfast cereals and a few ounces of lean meat are convenient means of increasing iron in a child's diet. The high proportion of heme iron in many animal foods allows the iron to be more readily absorbed than is iron from plant foods. Consuming a vitamin C source along with the less readily absorbed iron in plants and supplements aids absorption.

Childhood iron-deficiency anemia is most likely to appear in children between the ages of 6 and 24 months. It can lead to decreases in both stamina and learning ability because the oxygen supply to cells decreases. Another effect is lowered resistance to disease. Fortunately, childhood anemia is not common today in North America, probably because of children's use of iron-fortified breakfast cereals. Also deserving of credit in the United States is the Special Supplemental Nutrition Program for Women, Infants, and Children (WIC), sponsored by the U.S. federal government. This program emphasizes the importance of iron-fortified formulas and cereals and distributes these foods—along with nutrition education—to low-income parents of infants and preschool children considered to be at nutritional risk.

**Constipation.**  Constipation may be associated with a more serious disease, yet some young children experience constipation unrelated to any medical condition. When presented with a constipated child, a physician first has to rule out a medical cause, such as intestinal blockage. And, although the most common GI tract symptom that reflects intolerance to cow's milk is diarrhea, chronic constipation may also result. Treatment for constipation generally consists of first evacuating the bowels, generally with an enema. The promotion of regular bowel habits then follows, with laxative use as directed by the physician. Several months to years of supportive intervention may be required for effective treatment.

The primary dietary interventions to alleviate constipation include eating more fiber and drinking more fluids. In the initial stages of treatment, providing certain fruit juices (e.g., prune, grape, and apple) and substituting soy milk for cow's milk may relieve constipation. In the long run, however, whole fruits (e.g., plums, peaches, and apricots) are better choices than juices because whole fruits are less concentrated sources of calories. Other foods to emphasize for fiber include vegetables, whole-grain

---

**F**or children who follow a totally vegetarian diet, attention should also focus on protein and vitamin B-12 intake.

**C**hapter 4 noted that it's unlikely that the use of sugar is the cause of hyperactivity or antisocial behavior in most children.

▲ Excessive fruit drink and fruit juice use is another potential problem in preschool (and later adolescent) years. The American Academy of Pediatrics recommends no more than 4 to 6 ounces per day for children 1 to 6 years (and 8 to 12 ounces per day for ages 7 to 18 years). Sweetened soft drinks should also be limited.

▶ **Food and Nutrition Board Fiber Recommendations for Children**

**Young Children**

| | |
|---|---|
| 1–3 years | 19 grams/day |
| 4–8 years | 25 grams/day |

**Boys**

| | |
|---|---|
| 9–13 years | 31 grams/day |
| 14–18 years | 38 grams/day |

**Girls**

| | |
|---|---|
| 9–13 years | 26 grams/day |
| 14–18 years | 26 grams/day |

breads and cereals, and beans. The daily fiber goals for children set by the Food and Nutrition Board vary by age (see margin). Few children meet these goals. Accompanying fluid recommendations are 4 cups (900 milliliters) per day for toddlers and about 5 cups (1200 milliliters) per day for older children.

**Dental Caries.** A proper diet goes a long way in reducing the risk for dental caries in young children. The following tips can help reduce dental problems in children:

- Begin oral hygiene when teeth start to appear.
- Seek early pediatric dental care.
- Drink fluoridated water.
- Use small amounts of fluoridated toothpaste twice daily.
- Snack in moderation.
- Have a dentist apply tooth sealants if needed.
- Avoid sticky, high-sugar snacks, especially between meals.
- If toddlers or preschoolers are chewing gum, sugarless gum is the best choice, as this has been shown to reduce the incidence of dental caries.

**Vegetarianism in Childhood.** Vegetarian diets can pose several risks for young children. These include the possibility of developing iron-deficiency anemia, a deficiency of vitamin B-12, and rickets from a vitamin D deficiency. During the first few years of life, children also may not consume enough calories when following a bulky vegetarian diet. But these known pitfalls are easily avoided by informed diet planning (see the "Nutrition and Your Health: Vegetarian and Plant-Based Diets in Chapter 6). Diets for children who eat totally vegetarian fare should focus on protein, vitamin B-12, iron, and zinc content, with additional emphasis on vitamin D (or regular sun exposure) and calcium. Some of these dietary inadequacies can be compensated for by increasing oils, nuts, seeds, ready-to-eat breakfast cereals, and fortified soy milk in the diet.

**Autism.** Autism spectrum disorder (ASD) is characterized by a range of problems with social interaction, verbal and nonverbal communication, and/or unusual, repetitive, or limited activities and interests. These disorders usually are diagnosed in early childhood and affect an estimated 1 in every 150 children, with higher prevalence in boys than girls. The causes for ASD are not well understood, but there is a definite genetic component.

ASD can both affect and be affected by nutritional status. In addition to developmental and behavioral abnormalities, many children with ASD also experience GI disorders, such as constipation, diarrhea, or reflux disease. Such disorders may impair nutrient intake or absorption. Some autistic children may have feeding problems related to developmental impairments. Also, picky eating behaviors may affect nutrient intake. Thus, careful attention to nutrient-dense food choices is warranted.

There are many nutrient-based theories concerning the causes and treatment of ASD. Nutritional interventions, such as dietary restrictions or nutrient supplements, are commonly employed by families affected by ASD. A widely-used nutritional intervention is the gluten-free, casein-free (GFCF) diet, which eliminates all wheat, barley, rye, and milk products. Proponents of this treatment propose that sensitivities to certain food proteins may have effects on neurotransmitter synthesis, thereby altering nervous system function. Clinical evidence supporting the effectiveness of the GFCF diet is limited, but promising. If the GFCF diet is used, families should enlist the aid of a registered dietitian to ensure dietary adequacy, particularly for protein, calcium, vitamin D, folic acid, and some B-vitamins. Other popular therapies for ASD include supplementation with probiotics, vitamin B-6 (0.6 mg/kg/d), magnesium (6.0 mg/kg/d), and omega-3 fatty acids (not exceeding 800 mg/d). Although sparse, research on these therapies is encouraging. There is evidence of altered absorption or metabolism of nutrients among children with autism, so even

**D**espite a popularly-held belief scientific evidence does not support a causal relationship between mercury in vaccines and autism. Although small risks are inherent with routine vaccinations, the risks of infectious diseases are far worse.

with adequate nutrient intake, availability of some nutrients for metabolic processes may be low. Even though these supplements carry a low risk of adverse effects, caution is warranted to avoid overdoses. Because of the rising incidence of ASD and the lack of curative treatments, nutritional interventions for ASD will continue to be an active area of research.

**Lead Poisoning.** Humans may be exposed to lead from drinking contaminated water, consuming or inhaling lead dust (e.g., from cracked and peeling lead paint), contaminated dietary supplements (e.g., calcium supplements derived from bone meal), or foods stored or prepared in lead-containing containers. In 2006, nearly 40,000 children were diagnosed with lead poisoning in the United States. Young children are particularly susceptible to the damaging effects of lead poisoning, which include long-term intellectual and behavioral impairments as well as increased risk for several chronic diseases in adulthood. Although it does not address the source of exposure, proper nutrition can reduce the risks of lead poisoning for children. Consuming regular meals, moderating fat intake, and ensuring adequate iron and calcium status are dietary practices known to reduce lead absorption. Adequate zinc, thiamin, and vitamin E intakes also reduce the harmful effects of absorbed lead. For lowest lead levels, only cold water should be used for drinking and preparation of formula or food. Letting cold water run from the tap for 2–3 minutes after a long period of inactivity (e.g., overnight) will limit the amount of lead that has accumulated in tap water. If the public water supply contains a high concentration of lead, bottled water is a safer alternative, particularly for formula preparation. Overall, a balanced meal plan that offers a variety of whole grains, lean meats, and low-fat dairy products is especially useful for protecting children from lead poisoning.

## CONCEPT CHECK

The rapid growth rate of an infant's first year slows during the toddler and preschool years (ages 1 to 5). As a child's appetite decreases, adults need to serve nutrient-dense foods and allow the child to decide how much to eat. Sudden shifts in food preferences are to be expected. Snacking is fine if attention is given to the selection of healthful foods and good dental hygiene. Although a children's multivitamin and mineral supplement is usually not needed—a plan following MyPyramid that includes a serving of fortified ready-to-eat breakfast cereal should meet nutrient needs—use of such a supplement is a reasonable practice. Children need plenty of iron-rich food to prevent iron-deficiency anemia, as well as zinc for growth. Adequate mineral status also reduces risk of lead poisoning. Adequate fiber and fluid help prevent constipation. Diets for children who eat totally vegetarian fare should focus on meeting needs for protein, vitamin D (or regular sun exposure), vitamin B-12, calcium, iron, and zinc. Potentially useful, evidence-based nutritional treatments for autism include the gluten-free, casein-free diet, and supplementation with vitamin B-6, magnesium, probiotics, and essential fatty acids.

# 15.4 School-Age Children: Nutrition Concerns

The diets of many school-age students can stand general improvement, particularly with regard to fruit, vegetable, whole-grain, and dairy choices. Drinking minimal amounts of sugared soft drinks is also advised. One survey of U.S. schoolchildren revealed that on the day of the survey, 40% of the children ate no vegetables, except for potatoes or tomato sauce, and 20% ate no fruits. Another study showed that only 2% of about 3300 children 2 to 19 years old had met their recommended servings from all six MyPramid groups. In general, the nutritional concerns and goals applicable to school-age children are the same as those discussed in relation to preschoolers. However, with the added pressures of peers, health messages from the media,

▲ Nutrition education ideally begins in the home as parents and other caregivers provide a healthy, well-balanced diet.

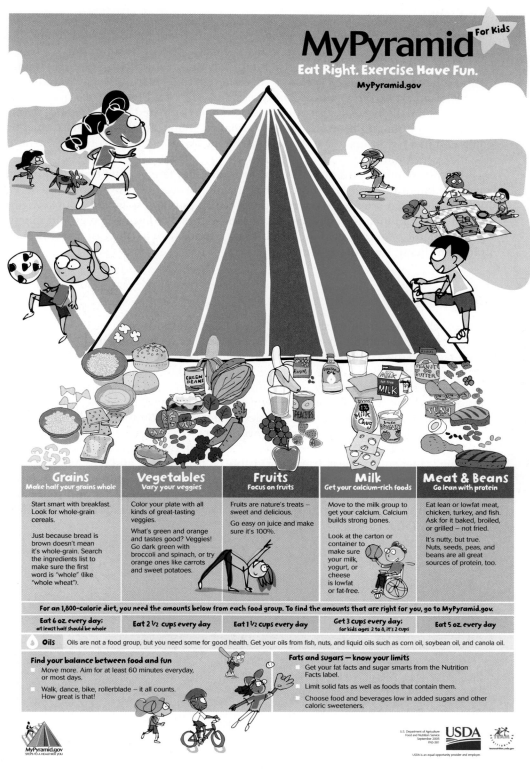

**FIGURE 15-3 ▶** The USDA has tailored MyPyramid for preschoolers (age 2–5) and school-age children (age 6–11; shown). The accompanying websites (**http://mypyramid.gov/ preschoolers/index.html** and **http:// mypyramid.gov/kids/index.html**) promote the early development of healthy eating and exercise habits that will persist as the child matures. An interactive MyPyramid Blast Off Game and meal tracking worksheet appeal to children. For caregivers, the sites contain information and resources to use in modeling and educating children about proper nutrition.

and an increasing desire for independence, these goals may be harder to achieve as children grow older. MyPyramid continues to be a good basis for diet planning, with an emphasis on moderating fat and sugar intake and ensuring adequate iron, zinc, and calcium intake (Fig. 15-3). The only difference is that the number of servings increases as calorie needs increase (review Table 15-3). Now let's look at several nutritional issues of particular concern during the school-age years.

## Breakfast

Once children enter school, their eating patterns become more scheduled, and the consumption of regular meals—especially breakfast—becomes an important focus. A fortified ready-to-eat breakfast cereal is typically the greatest source of iron, vitamin A, and folic acid for children ages 2 to 18. Although there is controversy over the true benefit of breakfast for cognitive ability, children who eat breakfast are more likely to meet their daily needs for vitamins and minerals compared to children not eating breakfast. To influence morning test performance, it appears that breakfast must be eaten within a few hours of a test; the subsequent rise in blood glucose is thought to enhance performance.

Breakfast menus need not be limited to traditional fare. A little imagination can spark the interest of even the most reluctant child. Instead of conventional breakfast foods, parents can offer leftovers from dinner, such as pizza, spaghetti, soups, yogurt topped with trail mix, chili with beans, or sandwiches. For lasting energy and satiety, combine traditional carbohydrate-rich breakfast foods with a source of protein, such as low-fat cheese, nuts, or eggwhites.

## Fat Intake

Diets of school-age children should include a variety of foods from each major group, not necessarily excluding any specific food because of its fat content. Overemphasis on fat-reduced diets during childhood has been linked to an increase in eating disorders and encourages an inappropriate "good food, bad food" attitude.

However, surveys of dietary intake among children show that they are consuming too much saturated fat, most of which comes from whole milk, full-fat dairy products, and fatty meats. Furthermore, few children (or adults) meet recommendations to include two servings of fish per week to ensure adequate intake of omega-3 fats. Emphasizing low-fat dairy products (after age 2), offering broiled or baked fish, choosing leaner cuts of meat, trimming visible fat from meats, and removing the skin from poultry before serving foods will establish heart-healthy eating habits to last a lifetime. Snacks for children should also include only moderate fat and sugar and emphasize fruit, vegetables, whole grain, and dairy choices. Ideas for healthy snacks are found in Table 15-4.

▲ Sweets should be consumed in moderation in childhood, but do not have to be avoided altogether.

## CRITICAL THINKING

Tim refuses to eat breakfast before school. He doesn't like cereal, toast, or any of the other usual breakfast foods. What can Tim's parents do to ensure that he eats nutritious foods before leaving for school?

## MAKING DECISIONS

### Nutrition Education for Children

Children spend the majority of their waking hours in school, so it is a great place to learn about positive, healthy eating habits. A strong emphasis on nutrition in schools can help children understand why healthy diet habits will make them feel more energetic, look better, and work more efficiently. Federally-funded programs such as USDA's Team Nutrition and the CDC's National Bone Health Campaign are a good start, but more changes are needed. School foodservice outlets, including cafeterias and vending machines, must present healthier options for school children. Instruction on food preparation in home economics classes and after-school programs will help children learn to prepare healthy meals and snacks. Increased participation in physical education classes and recreational sports is more likely to improve academic performance than detract from it. However, positive nutrition influences must extend beyond the classroom to change persistent trends toward obesity and chronic diseases. Caregivers and other adult role models need to create safe opportunities for children to be active and must practice what they preach when it comes to healthy habits.

**TABLE 15-4** Twenty Healthy Snack Ideas for School-Age Children

| | Iron | Zinc | Calcium | Vitamin C | Fiber |
|---|---|---|---|---|---|
| Almonds (1 oz) | | | ✓ | | ✓ |
| Applesauce (1/2 cup) | | | | ✓ | ✓ |
| Bean and cheese burrito (1) | ✓ | ✓ | ✓ | | ✓ |
| Cheese (1 oz) and whole-wheat crackers (6) | ✓ | ✓ | ✓ | | ✓ |
| Dried cranberries (1/4 cup) | | | | ✓ | ✓ |
| Frozen fruit pieces (1 cup) | | | | ✓ | ✓ |
| Fruit salad (1 cup) | | | | ✓ | ✓ |
| Fruit smoothie (1 cup) | | | | ✓ | ✓ |
| Hard-boiled egg | ✓ | ✓ | | | |
| Hummus (2 tbsp) with bell pepper rings (1 cup) | | | | ✓ | ✓ |
| Low-fat microwave popcorn (3 tbsp unpopped) | | | | | ✓ |
| Mini-pizzas on whole-grain English muffins (2) | ✓ | ✓ | ✓ | ✓ | ✓ |
| Peanut butter (2 tbsp) and apple slices (1 cup) | | ✓ | | ✓ | ✓ |
| Quick breads, such as banana bread, 1 slice | ✓ | | | | ✓ |
| String cheese (1 stick) | | | ✓ | | |
| Trail mix (1/4 cup) | ✓ | ✓ | | ✓ | ✓ |
| Tuna salad (1/2 cup) in whole-wheat pita pocket | ✓ | ✓ | | | ✓ |
| Whole-grain cereal (1 cup) | ✓ | ✓ | | | ✓ |
| Whole-wheat pasta salad with veggies (1 cup) | ✓ | ✓ | | ✓ | ✓ |
| Yogurt (8 oz) with granola (2 tbsp) | | ✓ | ✓ | | ✓ |

## Type 2 Diabetes

Type 2 diabetes is generally thought to be an adult condition. As reviewed in the "Nutrition and Your Health" section, "Diabetes—When Blood Glucose Regulation Fails" in Chapter 4, it frequently occurs in overweight people older than 40. However, physicians have noted an alarming increase in the frequency of the disease among children (and teenagers). This is primarily due to the rise in obesity in this age group, coupled with minimal physical activity. Up to 85% of children with the disease are overweight at diagnosis. Experts are calling for screening for diabetes in at-risk children every 2 years, starting at age 10 or at the onset of puberty. Besides obesity and a sedentary lifestyle, other risk factors include having a first- or second-degree relative with the disease or belonging to a non-White population. Appropriate diet and lifestyle intervention should be implemented, along with the use of diabetes medications when necessary. A regular intake of low-glycemic-load fruits, vegetables, and whole-grain breads and cereals is especially recommended.

## Early Signs of Cardiovascular Disease

Also paralleling the increase in childhood obesity, early signs of cardiovascular disease have become increasingly prevalent among children and adolescents. It is evident that cardiovascular disease begins early in life. Therefore, lifestyle modifications to delay the progression of the disease are important throughout the lifespan. The American Academy of Pediatrics now recommends that at-risk children first undergo cholesterol screening sometime between the ages of 2 and 10, followed by repeated cholesterol screening every 3 to 5 years. Children are considered "at risk" if they are overweight, have high blood pressure, smoke, or have diabetes; if they have a family history of cardiovascular disease; or if family history is unknown. For children whose cholesterol is elevated, lifestyle approaches, such as weight management through dietary modification and increased physical activity, are the first line of therapy. Following a meal plan that conforms to MyPyramid guidelines would be appropriate for prevention of cardiovascular disease. Some high-risk children may be candidates for cholesterol-lowering medications.

## Overweight and Obesity

In the United States, more than 30% of school-age children are overweight or obese. The number of cases is increasing, especially in minority populations. In the short run, ridicule, embarrassment, possibly depression, and short stature linked to early puberty are the main consequences of such obesity. In the long run, significant health problems associated with obesity, such as cardiovascular disease, type 2 diabetes, and hypertension, usually will appear in adulthood. However, an increase in these health-related complications has been noted in children. Childhood obesity is a serious health threat because about 40% of obese children (and about 80% of obese adolescents) become obese adults. Significant weight gain generally begins between ages 5 and 7, during puberty, or during the teenage years.

Research points to many potential causes of childhood obesity. Recall the nature versus nurture discussion in Chapter 7. Some infants are born with lower metabolic rates; they use calories more efficiently and in turn can more easily produce fat stores. Studies also suggest, though, that this genetic link accounts for only one-third of individual differences in body weight.

Researchers believe that, although diet is an important factor, inactivity is also a contributor to the increase in childhood obesity. Studies show that as children age, physical activity steadily declines. By age 15, only one-third of children are getting the recommended 60 minutes of exercise per day. It doesn't help that physical education classes are now elective in many high schools. Today's generation of children now glues itself to the TV for an average of 24 hours per week; many children spend another 10 hours or so playing computer and video games. The American Academy of Pediatrics recommends a limit of 14 hours of TV and video time per week for children over age 2 (no television is recommended for children younger than 2 years). In addition, excessive snacking, overreliance on fast-food restaurants, parental neglect, the media in general, lack of safe areas to play, and the abundant availability of high-calorie food choices contribute to childhood obesity. Sugared soft drinks are especially implicated.

The initial approach in treating an obese child is to assess how much physical activity he or she engages in. If a child spends much free time in sedentary activities (such as watching television or playing video games), more physical activities should be encouraged. The U.S. federal government and health professionals recommend 60 minutes or more of moderate to intense physical activity per day for children and adolescents. Learning to engage in and enjoy regular physical activity will help children not only to attain a healthy body weight but also to keep a similar body weight later in life. An increase in physical activity won't just happen; parents and other caregivers need to plan for it. Getting the family together for a brisk walk

▲ Regular physical activity is an important part of prevention and treatment of weight problems in childhood. The goal is about 60 minutes of such activity each day. Many children do not meet this goal.

after dinner encourages healthy habits for all involved. Age-appropriate activities for elementary school-age children include walking, dancing, jumping rope, and participation in organized sports that focus on fun rather than intense competition. For middle school-age children, more complex organized sports (e.g., football and basketball) are of interest and some weight training with small weights can also be beneficial.

Moderation in calorie intake is important, especially the limitation of high-calorie foods, such as sugared soft drinks and whole milk. The focus should be on more vitamin and mineral-dense foods and healthy snacks. An emphasis on appropriate portion sizes may help youth learn to curb excessive food intake. Making small changes such as substituting low-fat for whole milk, or canned fruit in its own juice instead of heavy syrup, can moderately cut calories without sacrificing taste or disrupting normal eating patterns. To specifically address the increased burden of overweight and obesity among minority populations, health professionals must become versed in varied cultural food preferences.

Resorting to a weight-loss diet is usually not necessary—it's best to emphasize changing habits that allow for weight maintenance. Children have an advantage over adults in dealing with obesity; their bodies can use stored energy for growth. Thus, if weight gain can be moderated, increases in height and resulting lean body tissue may reduce the percentage of body weight accounted for as stored fat, yielding a more healthful weight-to-height ratio. This is one reason it's desirable to treat obesity in childhood. Further growth can contribute to success. If weight loss is necessary in younger children, it should be gradual, about ½ to 1 pound per week. In some cases, the child should be watched closely to ensure that the rate of growth continues to be normal. The child's calorie intake shouldn't be so low that gains in height diminish. In some cases, medications may be prescribed under a physician's care to reduce food intake (sibutramine [Meridia]) and/or fat absorption (orlistat [Xenical]). For the 3% of American children who are morbidly obese, bariatric surgery may be an option for weight management.

### CONCEPT CHECK

The school-age child is advised to follow MyPyramid and especially moderate choices high in fat and simple sugars. Breakfast is an important meal to refuel the body for a new school day and to help ensure fulfilling nutrient needs for the day. Attention to regular physical activity and healthy diet should help prevent/treat childhood obesity and build a desirable lifestyle pattern for later life.

## 15.5 Teenage Years: Nutrition Concerns

Most girls begin a rapid growth spurt between the ages of 10 and 13, and most boys experience rapid growth between the ages of 12 and 15. Nearly every organ in the body grows during these periods. Most noticeable are increases in height and weight and the development of secondary sexual characteristics. Girls usually begin menstruating (reach **menarche**) during this growth spurt, and they grow very little beyond 2 years after menarche. Early-maturing girls may begin their growth spurt as early as age 7 to 8, whereas early-maturing boys may begin growing by age 9 to 10.

During this adolescent growth spurt, girls gain about 10 inches (25 centimeters) in height, and boys gain about 12 inches (30 centimeters). Girls also tend to accumulate both lean and fat tissue, whereas boys tend to gain mostly lean tissue. This growth spurt provides about 50% of ultimate adult weight and about 15% of ultimate adult height (review Fig. 15-1).

As the growth spurt begins, teenagers begin to eat more. If teens choose nutritious food, they can take advantage of their increased hunger and easily satisfy their nutrient

**T**o get kids involved in exercise, new physical education classes have been introduced into schools. These classes provide lifelong fitness lessons in such activities as rock climbing, in-line skating, and recreational jogging. These classes help promote activity because they take the focus away from teams and competition, which often discourage and embarrass kids who lack athletic talent.

▲ Super-sized portions of foods such as hamburgers and sugared soft drinks served to children are contributing to the obesity and type 2 diabetes epidemics they are experiencing.

**menarche** The onset of menstruation. Menarche usually occurs around age 13, 2 or 3 years after the first signs of puberty start to appear.

**D**rinking soft drinks in place of milk causes many teenagers to have inadequate calcium intake. Over the last 20 years, soft drinks have been replacing milk as the preferred beverage of adolescents. Only half of school-age boys and 20% of girls meet recommendations for calcium intake. This trend has been linked to decreased bone mass and increased bone fractures in this age group.

**A** strictly vegetarian diet must be monitored for adequate energy, protein, iron, vitamin B-12, calcium, and vitamin D (the latter if sun exposure is not sufficient). These nutrients become particularly important in teenagers, as their diets are often already compromised.

▲ An active lifestyle coupled with a healthy diet should be part of the teen years. Both habits contribute to bone development and bone strength.

**A**lcoholism is a significant health problem that may have its roots in the teen years. Smoking—another habit that compromises health—also often begins in teen years. Some of the impetus for smoking is the desire to control body weight—but this is not an advisable method.

needs. As discussed for younger age groups, MyPyramid can provide the basis for meeting these nutrient needs (Table 15-3). Following such a plan will meet carbohydrate needs (130 grams per day) and protein needs (52 grams per day for males and 46 grams per day for females).

## Nutritional Problems and Concerns of Teens

Anorexia nervosa and bulimia nervosa are nutritional concerns of the teen years, as covered in detail in Chapter 11. Other nutritional problems are more common during the teen years. A survey of high school students showed that only a little over 25% had eaten five servings of fruits and vegetables on the previous day, and they are consuming approximately 25% more sodium than recommended. Another concern is that many teenage girls stop drinking milk, so they may not consume enough calcium to allow for maximal mineralization of bones through their early twenties. Inadequate calcium intake during the teenage years sets the stage for development of osteoporosis later in life.

Many teenagers are not meeting their needs for calcium. The Adequate Intake for calcium for both males and females between ages 9 and 18 years is 1300 milligrams per day, compared with only 800 milligrams per day for younger children. Three servings per day from the milk, yogurt, and cheese group are recommended for all teenagers and young adults to meet calcium needs. Figure 2-1 in Chapter 2 shows the stark contrast between milk and typical soft drinks with respect to calcium and other nutrients. If dairy products are not consumed, alternative calcium sources need to be included.

A further concern is iron deficiency. Iron-deficiency anemia sometimes appears in girls after they start menstruating (menarche) and in boys during their growth spurt. About 10% of teenagers have low iron stores or related anemia. Teens who strive to forge an identity by adopting dietary patterns unfamiliar to their families—vegetarianism, for example—may not know enough about the alternate diet pattern to keep from developing health problems, such as iron-deficiency anemia. It's important that teenagers choose good food sources of iron, such as lean meats, whole grains, and enriched cereals. Teenage girls, particularly those with heavy menstrual flows, need to eat good sources of iron (or regularly consume an iron supplement). Iron-deficiency anemia is a highly undesirable condition for a teen. It can produce increased fatigue and decreased ability to concentrate and learn. School and physical performance may suffer.

### MAKING DECISIONS

#### Nutrition and Acne

Acne is a common teen concern—about 80% of teens experience it. Although it's popularly believed that eating nuts, chocolate, and pizza can make acne worse, scientific studies have failed to show a strong link between these dietary factors and acne. Based on the results of observational research, two dietary practices currently under study for possible roles in the development of acne include high glycemic load and consumption of cow's milk. However, sufficient evidence is not currently available to support any drastic dietary changes to control acne. A balanced diet and adequate fluid intake combined with sensible hygiene practices remain the best practices to promote skin health.

Many acne medications, such as Accutane, contain analogs of vitamin A (e.g., 13-cis retinoic acid). Although these treatments can be effective, close supervision by a physician is crucial, as vitamin A analogs can be toxic. Vitamin A itself is no help in treating acne, and excess amounts of vitamin A or related analogs taken during pregnancy can cause birth defects. Thus, girls taking these vitamin A medications should not become pregnant.

## Helping Teens Eat More Nutritious Foods

Teenagers face a variety of challenges. They pursue their independence, experience identity crises, seek peer acceptance, and worry about physical appearance. These factors affect food choice. Advertisers take advantage of this by pushing a vast array of products—candy, gum, soft drinks, and snacks—at the teenage market. Potato chips and French fries make up more than one-third of the vegetable servings consumed by teens. Additionally, many schools offer French fries on a regular basis, and soft drink machines can be found in school hallways and cafeterias, in turn competing with the school lunch. The increased consumption of fast-foods, sugary beverages, and snack foods crowds out nutrient-dense foods, thus limiting intake of calcium, iron, zinc, fat-soluble vitamins, and folate.

Teens often do not think about the long-term benefits of good health. They have a hard time relating today's actions to tomorrow's health outcomes. Many teenagers tend to think they can change habits later; there's no hurry.

Still, healthful teen food habits do not require giving up favorite foods. Small portions of fatty foods can complement larger portions of fat-free and reduced-fat dairy products, lean meats, vegetable proteins, fruits, vegetables, and whole-grain products. An example of this type of meal is a plain hamburger with a garden salad (minimize the amount of regular dressing or use a low-fat variety), small order of French fries or chili, and a medium diet soft drink or reduced-fat or fat-free milk.

## Are Teenage Snacking Practices Harmful?

Teens often obtain one-fourth to one-third of all their calories and major nutrients from snacks. Unfortunately, studies have found just what you might expect—that teens snack mostly on potato and corn chips, cookies, candies, and ice cream. Key reasons for snacking include an opportunity to get out and socialize with friends, accessibility, hunger, and celebration of a special event. Teenagers can obtain many nutrients from snacking. Even fast-food restaurants offer some good food choices. By choosing wisely and eating in moderation, teens can eat at fast-food restaurants occasionally and still consume a very healthful diet. Snacks and fast-food restaurants themselves are not the problem; poor food choices in terms of type and quantity are.

Lack of exercise and poor dietary habits formed during teenage years often continue into adulthood and may increase risk of chronic diseases, such as cardiovascular disease, osteoporosis, and some types of cancer. Getting this message across to teenagers is an important and challenging task for parents.

**O**besity is a growing problem among teenagers, and about 30% of obese teenagers have the metabolic syndrome (Syndrome **X**) discussed in Chapters 4 and 5. If a teen attains ultimate adult height and is still obese, a weight-loss regimen may be necessary. This is especially appropriate after the adolescent growth spurt. Weight loss should be gradual, perhaps 1 pound per week, and generally follow the advice in Chapter 7. Weight loss medications may also be prescribed.

▲ The teenage years are noted for snacking. With reasonable food choices, teenagers can have healthful diets.

### CONCEPT CHECK

A second period of rapid growth occurs during the teen years. Girls generally start this growth spurt earlier than boys. MyPyramid can direct meal planning. Common nutritional problems in these years arise from poor food choices and include inadequate calcium intake in girls and iron-deficiency anemia. Changes occur so rapidly during these years, and in so many areas—psychological, social, and physical—it may be difficult to stress the relevance of nutrition to teenagers. Moderation in fat and sugar intake are important goals to consider when choosing snacks.

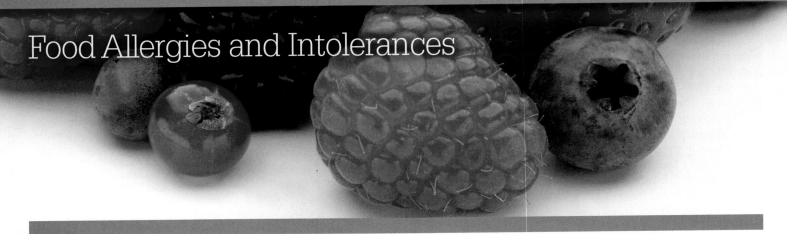

# Food Allergies and Intolerances

Food allergies are on the rise. Between 1997 and 2007, food allergies among children increased by 18%. What used to be a rare medical incident is now the cause for 30,000 emergency room visits and 150 to 200 deaths per year. Today, food allergies affect an estimated 11 million Americans (about 2% of adults and about 8% of children).

Adverse reactions to foods—indicated by sneezing, coughing, nausea, vomiting, diarrhea, hives, and other rashes, are broadly classed as food allergies (also called hypersensitivities) or **food intolerances.** Whereas allergies involve an immune response to a foreign protein (**allergen**), intolerances are caused by an individual's inability to digest a certain food component or by the direct effect of a food component or contaminant on the body. Let's examine each process, first allergies and then intolerances.

## FOOD ALLERGIES: SYMPTOMS AND MECHANISM

Allergic reactions to foods are common (Fig. 15-4) and occur more frequently in females than males. Food allergies occur most often during infancy and young adulthood. Three types of reactions may occur after the ingestion of problem foods by susceptible people:

- *Classic*–itching, reddening skin, asthma, swelling, choking, and a runny nose
- *GI tract*–nausea, vomiting, diarrhea, intestinal gas, bloating, pain, constipation, and indigestion

- *General*–headache, skin reactions, tension and fatigue, tremors, and psychological problems

Any reaction milder than these is a **food sensitivity.**

Allergic reactions vary not only in the body system affected, but also in their duration, ranging from seconds to a few days. A generalized, all-systems reaction

**food intolerance** An adverse reaction to food that does not involve an allergic reaction.

**allergen** A foreign protein, or antigen, that induces excess production of certain immune system antibodies; subsequent exposure to the same protein leads to allergic symptoms. Whereas all allergens are antigens, not all antigens are allergens.

**food sensitivity** A mild reaction to a substance in a food that might be expressed as slight itching or redness of the skin.

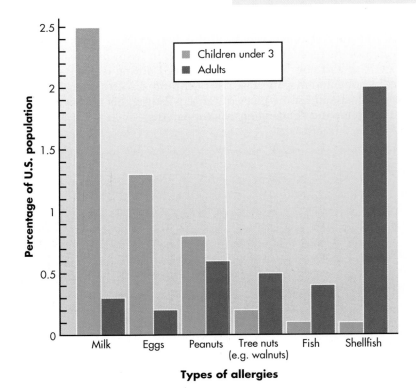

**FIGURE 15-4** ▶ Types of allergies and percentage of U.S. population with those allergies.

*Source: Journal of Allergy and Clinical Immunology (study done by Mount Sinai School of Medicine)* is called **anaphylactic shock.** This severe allergic response results in low blood pressure and distress of the respiratory system and GI tract. It can be fatal. A person who is extremely sensitive to a food may not be able to touch the food or even be in the same room where it is being cooked without reacting to it. Although any food can trigger anaphylactic shock, the most common culprits are peanuts (a legume, not a nut), tree nuts (e.g., walnuts, pecans, etc.), shellfish, milk (look for an ingredient called casein on the label), eggs (look for the ingredient albumin on the label), soybeans, wheat, and fish. Other foods frequently identified with adverse reactions include meat and meat products, fruits, and cheese. For a small number of people, avoiding foods such as peanuts or shellfish is a matter of life and death.

Basically, allergies are an inappropriate response of the immune system. When immune cells identify a harmful foreign protein (**antigen**), they destroy it and produce antibodies to it, so that the next response to the harmful substance will be swift and effective. Almost all food allergies are caused by proteins in foods that act as antigens (also called **allergens**). In these cases, the immune system mistakes the food protein for a harmful substance and mounts an immune response, leading to symptoms such as hives, runny nose, and GI disturbances.

No one is sure why the immune system sometimes overreacts to harmless proteins. The early introduction of solid foods to infants may trigger food allergies. The reasoning is that the infant's GI tract is immature and "leaky," allowing some undigested proteins to be absorbed into the bloodstream. This is beneficial for breastfed infants, who can absorb immune proteins from breast milk. However, if some food proteins are introduced before the GI tract has matured, these antigens may enter the bloodstream and stimulate an immune response.

The hygiene hypothesis offers another interesting explanation: in our "germophobic" society, with the protection of antibiotics, hand sanitizers, and antimicrobial soaps and cleaners, our immune systems aren't vigorously challenged by antigens. As a result, the immune system may become sensitized to innocuous substances, such as food proteins. Recent research supports the hygiene hypothesis. Children who grow up on farms or who have pets, and are thereby exposed to many antigens, have fewer allergies and asthma than children who grow up in more sterile environments.

Whatever the explanation, one thing is clear: food allergies are an important concern for many parents and others who work with children.

### Testing for a Food Allergy

The diagnosis of a food allergy can often be a difficult task (Table 15-5). It requires the participation of a skilled physician. The first step in determining whether a food allergy is present is to record a detailed

**anaphylactic shock** A severe allergic response that results in lowered blood pressure and respiratory and gastrointestinal distress. This can be fatal.

**antigen** Any substance that induces a state of sensitivity and/or resistance to microorganisms or toxic substances after a lag period; substance that stimulates a specific aspect of the immune system.

▶ People with a history of serious allergic reactions and those who have asthma should carry a self-administered form of epinephrine, such as EpiPen, to subside an episode of anaphylactic shock, should it occur.

▶ The American Academy of Allergy, Asthma, and Immunology has a 24-hour toll-free hot line (800-822-2762) to answer questions about food allergies and to help direct people to specialists. Free information on food allergies is available by contacting The Food Allergy & Anaphylaxis Network. The telephone number is (800-929-4040); the website is **www.foodallergy.org.**

▲ Eggs, wheat, milk, peanuts, tree nuts, soybeans, and seafood pose the greatest risk for food allergies in childhood.

**TABLE 15-5** Assessment Strategies for Food Allergies

| History | Include description of symptoms, time between food ingestion and onset of symptoms, duration of symptoms, most recent allergic episode, quantity of food required to produce reaction, suspected foods, and allergic diseases in other family members. |
|---|---|
| Physical examination | Look for signs of an allergic reaction (rash, itching, intestinal bloating, etc.). |
| Elimination diet | Establish a diet lacking the suspected offending foods and stay on it for 1 to 2 weeks or until symptoms clear. |
| Food challenge | Add back small amounts of excluded foods, one at a time, as long as anaphylactic shock is not a possible consequence. |
| Blood test | Determine presence of antibodies in blood that bind to food antigens tested. |
| Skin test | Place a sample of the suspected allergen under the skin and watch for an inflammatory reaction. |

history of symptoms, including the time from ingestion to onset of symptoms, duration of symptoms, most recent reaction, food suspected of causing a reaction, and quantity and nature of food needed to produce a reaction. A family history of allergic diseases can also help, as allergic reactions tend to run in families. A physical examination may reveal evidence of an allergy, such as skin diseases and asthma. Various diagnostic tests can rule out other conditions. The diagnostic first step is to eliminate from the diet—for 1 to 2 weeks—all tested compounds that appear to cause allergic symptoms, plus all other foods suspected of causing an allergy based on the person's food history. The person generally starts out eating foods to which almost no one reacts, such as rice, vegetables, noncitrus fruits, and fresh meats and poultry. If symptoms are still present, the person can more severely restrict the diet or even use special formula diets that are hypoallergenic.

Once a diet is found that causes no symptoms, called an **elimination diet,** foods can be added back one at a time. This type of food challenge is an option only when the culprit foods are known to pose no risk of anaphylactic shock in the person. Doses of ½ to 1 teaspoon (2.5 to 5 milliliters) are given at first. The amount is increased until the dose approximates usual intake. Any reintroduced food that causes significant symptoms to appear is identified as an allergen for the person.

Laboratory tests can also aid in diagnosis of food allergies. Skin testing involves pricking the skin with a small amount of purified food extract and observing any allergic response (e.g., a red eruption at the prick site). These types of tests are easy and safe, even for infants, but they may not clearly diagnose a food allergy. A positive skin-prick test merely indicates that a person has been sensitized to a food; it can't definitively identify if that food is the cause for the symptoms in question. Newer types of blood testing, however, have more diagnostic value. Blood tests estimate the blood concentration of antibodies that bind certain foodborne antigens.

### Living with Food Allergies

Once potential allergens are identified, dietary modifications must be made. In some cases, small amounts of the offending food can be consumed without an observable reaction. Also, some food allergens are destroyed by heating, so cooking may eliminate the allergic response. This is effective primarily for allergies to fruits or vegetables, not for the more common allergies to milk, peanuts, or seafood. For most cases, though, complete avoidance of allergy-causing food ingredients is the safest course of action. This makes careful reading of food labels essential. As of 2006, the Food Allergen Labeling and Consumer Protection Act now requires manufacturers to clearly identify the presence of major food allergens (milk, eggs, fish, shellfish, peanuts, tree nuts, wheat, and soy) on food product labels.

A major challenge when treating a person with a food allergy is to make sure that what remains in the diet can still provide essential nutrients. The small food intake of children permits less leeway in removing offending foods that may contain numerous nutrients. A registered dietitian can help guide the diet-planning process to ensure that the remaining food choices still meet nutrient needs or to guide supplement use, if that is necessary.

About 80% of young children with food allergies outgrow them before 3 years. Parents should be made aware of this and not assume the allergy will be long-lived. Food allergies diagnosed after 3 years of age are often more long-lived, but not always. In these cases, about 33% of people outgrow their food allergies within 3 years. For others, the condition may be prolonged; some food allergies can last a lifetime, such as those for peanuts, tree nuts, and shellfish. Periodic reintroduction of offending foods can be tried every 6 to 12 months or so to see whether the allergic reaction has decreased. If no symptoms appear, tolerance to the food has developed.

Several strategies are under study to ease the dietary restrictions imposed by food allergies. One possibility includes treatment with antibodies that will increase the threshold at which an allergic response occurs. For a person with an allergy to peanuts, for example, this would alleviate some anxiety about severe reactions to trace amounts of peanuts found in foods. Similarly, immunotherapy, which exposes allergic individuals to very small, but progressively larger amounts of food allergens; may help some people build up a tolerance to certain food components. Vaccines are another area of research. Also, scientists are working on genetically engineered foods that do not contain common allergens.

### Preventing Food Allergies

With the rising number of cases of food allergies, many new parents wonder when and how to introduce new foods during infancy and early childhood. It is evident that introducing foods other than human milk or infant formula before 4 months of age is associated with higher risk of allergic diseases. Most experts, including the American Academy of Pediatrics and the American College of Allergy, Asthma, and Immunology, advise waiting to introduce solid foods until after 6 months of age for lowest risk of food allergies.

Any food can contain a potential allergen, but certain foods have been found to have high allergenic potential: peanuts, tree nuts, eggs, cow's milk, fish, and seafood. The exact timing of introduction of these foods is a matter of debate. It is up to the health professional to advise parents individually, taking into account duration of breastfeeding and family history of food and other allergies. A consensus statement from the American College of Allergy, Asthma, and Immunology recommends waiting until 12 months of age to introduce cow's milk, 24 months of age to introduce eggs (whites), and 36 months of age to introduce peanuts, tree nuts, fish, and other seafood.

If an allergy-prone woman is pregnant or breastfeeding, many experts advise that she should avoid offending foods—such as eggs, shellfish, and peanuts—because allergens can cross the placenta during pregnancy. Allergens are also secreted via her milk. She should work with her physician and registered dietitian to make sure

---

**elimination diet** A restrictive diet that systematically tests foods that may cause an allergic response by first eliminating them for 1 to 2 weeks and then adding them back, one at a time.

she still consumes an adequate diet. In addition, when food allergies are common in the family, women are advised to breastfeed their infants exclusively for 6 months. Human milk contains factors that play a role in the maturation of the small intestine. Formula-fed infants, especially those on cow's milk–based formulas, have a greater risk for developing food allergies. Breastfeeding, thus, should continue for as long as possible, preferably to 1 year.

Beyond promotion of exclusive breastfeeding for the first six months of life and delaying introduction of cow's milk until 1 year of age, other preventive practices are still speculative. Postponing introduction of other potential allergens into the infant's diet is prudent, but not proven. Likewise, although we know that allergens do cross the placenta and are secreted in human milk, there is little evidence to support avoidance of common allergens during pregnancy or breastfeeding to prevent allergies.

### Food Intolerances

Food intolerances are adverse reactions to foods that do not involve allergic mechanisms. Generally, larger amounts of an offending food are required to produce the symptoms of an intolerance than to trigger allergic symptoms. Common causes of food intolerances include:

- Constituents of certain foods (e.g., red wine, tomatoes, pineapples) that have a druglike activity, causing physiological effects such as changes in blood pressure
- Certain synthetic compounds added to foods, such as sulfites, food-coloring agents, and monosodium glutamate (MSG)
- Food contaminants, including antibiotics and other chemicals used in the production of livestock and crops, as well as insect parts not removed during processing
- Toxic contaminants, which may be ingested with improperly handled and prepared foods containing *Clostridium botulinum*, *Salmonella* bacteria, or other foodborne microorganisms (see Chapter 13)
- Deficiencies in digestive enzymes, such as lactase (review Chapter 4)

Almost everyone is sensitive to one or more of these causes of food intolerance, many of which produce GI tract symptoms.

Sulfites, added to foods and beverages as antioxidants, cause flushing, spasms of the airway, and a loss of blood pressure in susceptible people. Wine, dehydrated potatoes, dried fruits, gravy, soup mixes, and restaurant salad greens commonly contain sulfites. A reaction to MSG may include an increase in blood pressure, numbness, sweating, vomiting, headache, and facial pressure. MSG is commonly found in restaurant food and many processed foods (e.g., soups). A reaction to tartrazine, a food-coloring additive, includes spasm of the airway, itching, and reddening skin. Tyramine, a derivative of the amino acid tyrosine, is commonly found in "aged" foods, such as cheeses and red wines. This natural food constituent can cause high blood pressure in people taking monoamine oxidase (MAO) inhibitor medications, which may be prescribed for clinical depression.

The basic treatment for food intolerances is to avoid specific offending components. However, total elimination often is not required because people generally are not as sensitive to compounds causing food intolerances as they are to allergens.

---

## Case Study Undernutrition During Infancy

Damon is a 7-month-old boy who has been taken into a clinic for a routine checkup. On examination, he was found to be moderately underweight relative to his age and body length. His physician scheduled a follow-up appointment in 3 months. At the 10-month visit, Damon appeared sluggish and was now even more underweight for his age and length.

A registered dietitian interviewed Damon's 16-year-old mother to collect information on Damon's dietary intake. His intake over the previous 24 hours consisted of two bottles of infant formula, three 8-ounce bottles of Kool-Aid, and a hot dog. However, the mother was still in school, and at night she often left Damon with the neighbor, so that she could go out with friends for a few hours. Thus, she was not aware of all that he ate.

Answer the following questions, and check your responses in Appendix A.

1. Damon's mother did not specify what type of formula he takes. What questions would you ask about his formula?
2. What potential dangers await Damon if his growth continues to lag behind?
3. What foods should Damon's caregivers offer that are appropriate for his age and nutritional needs?
4. What problems might arise from consumption of sugary drinks from a bottle?
5. Does Damon need any vitamin or mineral supplements?

## Summary

1. Growth is rapid during infancy; birth weight doubles in 4 to 6 months, and length increases by 50% in the first year. An adequate diet, especially in terms of calories, as well as the nutrients protein and zinc, is essential to support normal growth. Undernutrition can cause irreversible changes in growth and development. Growth in infants and children can be assessed by measuring body weight, height (or length), and head circumference over time. Growth charts have been revised to include a more valid measurement for determining children's growth, body mass index (BMI).

2. Nutrient needs in the first 6 months can be met by human milk or iron-fortified infant formula. Supplementary vitamin D is needed for breastfed infants, and many infants may need supplemental iron and fluoride. Infant formulas generally contain lactose or sucrose, heat-treated proteins from cow's milk, and vegetable oil. These formulas may or may not be fortified with iron. Sanitation is important when preparing and storing formula.

   Most infants do not need solid foods before 6 months of age. Solid food should not be added to an infant's diet until the nutrients are needed,

the GI tract can digest complex foods, the infant has the physical ability to control tongue thrusting, and the risk of developing food allergies has decreased.

The first solid foods given should be iron-fortified infant cereals or ground meats. Other single foods can be added gradually, at the rate of about one each week. Some foods to avoid giving infants in the first year include honey, cow's milk (especially fat-reduced varieties), foods with added salt or sugar, and foods that may cause choking. Introducing iron-containing solid food at the appropriate time and not offering cow's milk until 1 year of age can generally prevent iron-deficiency anemia in late infancy.

3. A slower growth rate results in decreased appetite among preschool children. With smaller portion sizes and picky eating behaviors, nutrient-dense food offerings are crucial. Choosing iron-rich foods, such as lean red meats, is important at this age. Portion sizes of 1 tablespoon of each food for each year of life is a good starting point for the vegetables, fruits, and meats & beans groups of MyPyramid. Preschoolers also should be given

some leeway in determining serving size and should be encouraged to try new foods.

Obese children and adolescents are more likely to become obese adults and, so, incur greater health risks. Parents can provide healthful food choices, and children should control portion sizes. When controlled early through diet and exercise interventions, the problem of obesity may correct itself as the child continues to grow in height.

4. During the adolescent growth spurt, both boys and girls have increased needs for iron and calcium. Inadequate calcium intake by teenage girls is a major concern because it can set the stage for the development of osteoporosis later in life. Teenagers generally should moderate their intake of high-fat and sugar-rich foods—especially snacks and fast-food, which they often consume in abundance—and perform regular physical activity.

5. The most common food allergies are associated with peanuts, tree nuts, shellfish, milk, eggs, soybeans, wheat, and fish. Food allergies occur most often during infancy and young adulthood.

## Study Questions

1. List two factors that limit "catch-up" growth in adulthood when a nutrient-deficient diet has been consumed throughout childhood.

2. Describe how you would assess whether an 8-month-old infant is consuming a healthful diet.

3. Outline three key factors that help determine when to introduce solid foods into an infant's diet.

4. A 3-month-old infant is taken to a clinic with failure to thrive. What are two possible explanations?

5. List three reasons why preschoolers are noted for "picky" eating. For each, describe an appropriate parent response.

6. What three factors are likely to contribute to obesity in a typical 10-year-old child?

7. Compare the guidelines for infant feeding summarized in Chapter 15 with the 2005 Dietary Guidelines for Americans for children over age 2 and adults discussed in Chapter 2. Which guidelines are similar? Do any contradict each other? If so, why?

8. Describe three pros and cons of snacking. What is the basic advice for healthful snacking from childhood through the teenage years?

9. Which two nutrients are of particular concern in planning diets for teenagers? Why does each deserve to be singled out?

10. List three nutrients of concern for a teenage vegetarian.

# Check Your Knowledge

Answers to the following multiple choice questions are below.

1. Inadequate intake of which of the following results in poor growth?
   a. calories
   b. iron
   c. zinc
   d. All of the above.

2. Using the formulas for Estimated Energy Requirements provided in the text, an 11-month-old girl who weighs 19 pounds needs approximately _____ kcal per day.
   a. 690
   b. 810
   c. 845
   d. 930

3. Introduction of cow's milk should be delayed until 12 months of age because it
   a. contains too much fat.
   b. doesn't contain enough minerals (e.g., calcium and phosphorus) to meet infant needs.
   c. may induce a food allergy.
   d. All of the above.

4. You are trying to introduce an apple and blueberry puree to a seven-month-old infant, but she rejects it. What should you do?
   a. assume she doesn't like apples and blueberries
   b. offer the food again on another day
   c. force a spoonful into her mouth
   d. None of the above.

5. Milk is a nutrient-dense source of all of the following except
   a. protein.
   b. iron.
   c. calcium.
   d. zinc.

6. A gluten-free, casein-free diet may be used to treat
   a. rickets.
   b. anemia.
   c. lead poisoning.
   d. autism.

7. Of the following options, which is preferred to ensure adequate vitamin and mineral intake for a picky eater?
   a. consume a fortified breakfast cereal
   b. promise dessert as a reward for eating meats and vegetables
   c. use a multivitamin and mineral supplement
   d. None of the above.

8. Which of the following is advised for treatment of overweight among school-age children?
   a. eating fewer meals
   b. following a low-carbohydrate eating plan
   c. 60 minutes or more of moderate to intense physical activity
   d. avoiding dairy products

9. The prevailing dietary habits of North American teenagers contribute to all of the following except
   a. acne.
   b. high blood pressure.
   c. low bone mass.
   d. type 2 diabetes.

10. Your friend breaks out in hives and feels nauseous after eating a salad containing mango. She probably has a food
    a. sensitivity.
    b. allergy.
    c. intolerance.
    d. a, b, and c.

Answer key: 1. d, 2. a, 3. c, 4. b, 5. b, 6. d, 7. a, 8. c, 9. a, 10. b

# Further Readings

1. ADA Reports: Position of the American Dietetic Association: Child and adolescent food and nutrition programs. *Journal of the American Dietetic Association* 106:1467, 2006.

   *It is the position of the American Dietetic Association that all children and adolescents, regardless of age, sex, socioeconomic status, racial diversity, ethnic diversity, linguistic diversity, or health status, should have access to food and nutrition programs that ensure the availability of a safe and adequate food supply that promotes optimal physical, cognitive, social, and emotional growth and development.*

2. ADA Reports: Position of the American Dietetic Association: Nutrition guidance for healthy children ages 2 to 11 years. *Journal of the American Dietetic Association* 108:1716, 2008.

   *MyPyramid combined with the Dietary Guidelines for Americans provide an appropriate blueprint for feeding children. Diets of many children are not following this advice and in turn are contributing to the nutritional problems common in childhood and later adulthood.*

3. Bounds W and others: The relationship of dietary and lifestyle factors to bone mineral indexes in children. *Journal of the American Dietetic Association* 105:735, 2005.

   *A primary influence on healthy bone mass parameters in this study was a nutritious diet—one ample in protein, phosphorus, vitamin K, magnesium, zinc, iron, and calories. Height and weight were also positively correlated to bone status.*

4. Council on Sports Medicine and Fitness and Council on School Health. Active healthy living: Prevention of childhood obesity through increased physical activity. *Pediatrics* 117:1834, 2006.

   *In light of the increasingly sedentary lifestyles of today's youth, physical activity should be encouraged during and after school and as part of home life. Benefits of regular physical activity among children and adolescents include physical changes (e.g., improved insulin sensitivity, lowered blood pressure) and psychological improvements (e.g., increased self-esteem, less depression). Specific goals and examples of activities to promote are provided for each age group.*

5. Curtis LT and others: Nutritional and environmental approaches to preventing and treating autism and attention-deficit hyperactivity disorder (ADHD): A review. *Journal of Alternative and Complementary Medicine* 14:79, 2008.

   *This article provides a thorough review of hypothesized environmental and nutritional links to autism and attention-deficit hyperactivity disorder. Adequate evidence does not exist to support a relationship between autism and environmental exposure to mercury. Nutritional interventions of scientific merit in the treatment of autism include avoidance of food allergens and correcting deficiencies of some B vitamins, magnesium, iron, zinc, and omega-3 fatty acids. For treatment of ADHD, some studies show a benefit of eliminating refined sugars and food additives such as coloring agents and preservatives.*

6. Daniels SR and others: Lipid screening and cardiovascular health in childhood. *Pediatrics* 122:198, 2008.

   *In light of the rising incidence of early signs of cardiovascular disease among youth, this clinical report from the American Academy of Pediatrics replaces previous guidelines for cholesterol screening among children and adolescents. Children with risk factors for cardiovascular disease should undergo regular lipid screening starting by age 10. Treatments for dyslipidemia in children include dietary modifications, physical activity, and lipid-lowering medications.*

7. Elder JH: The gluten-free, casein-free diet in autism: An overview with clinical implications. *Nutrition in Clinical Practice* 23:583, 2008.

   *The gluten-free, casein-free (GFCF) diet is a popular but intense treatment for children with autism spectrum disorders. Some researchers hypothesize that intestinal absorption in autistic children is altered (i.e., "leaky gut syndrome"), such that food sensitivities to wheat and dairy proteins develop. Absorbed food proteins may cause inflammation and other effects on the central nervous system. A review of current research on effectiveness of the GFCF diet concludes that it may be useful for alleviating symptoms in some children with autism, but proper dietary planning is essential to prevent nutrient deficiencies.*

8. Fitzgibbon ML, Stolley M: Promoting health in an unhealthful environment: Lifestyle challenges for children and adolescents. *Journal of the American Dietetic Association* 106:518, 2006.

   *This article summarizes the diet and health challenges that youth face. Youth are bombarded with conflicting messages that support the overconsumption of unhealthful foods while at the same time stigmatizing obesity and promoting dieting and unrealistic thinness.*

9. Gadding SS and others: Dietary recommendations for children and adolescents: A guide for practitioners. *Pediatrics* 117:544, 2006.

   *The American Heart Association recognizes that the dietary patterns of children and adolescents put them at risk for cardiovascular diseases in adulthood and even during childhood. Age-appropriate recommendations are provided for total energy intake, dietary fats, added sugars, sodium, and physical activity. In addition, this article provides practical advice for health professionals and schools for encouraging compliance with the guidelines.*

10. Greer FR: Groups compare CDC, WHO growth curves. *American Academy of Pediatrics News* 27 (9):1, 2006.

    *The 2006 World Health Organization (WHO) growth standards have been compared to the Centers for Disease Control and Prevention (CDC) 2000 growth reference. New recommendations for the use of growth curves in the United States more similar to the WHO growth curves are likely. Using the WHO curves for infants 0-2 years of age indicates that fewer U.S. infants would be below the 5th percentile for weight-for-age and more U.S. infants would be above the 95th percentile.*

11. Hellekson K: Report on the diagnosis, evaluation, and treatment of high blood pressure in children and adolescents. *American Family Physician* 71:1014, 2005.

    *Screening for high blood pressure is an important part of regular checkups of children by the child's physician. The latest recommendations for treating high blood pressure includes a diet rich in vegetables, fruit, and low-fat dairy products; low in salt; and moderate in high-calorie foods and drinks. Regular physical activity is also important, as is weight loss if needed.*

12. Kirk S and others: Pediatric obesity epidemic: Treatment options. *Journal of the American Dietetic Association* 105:S44, 2005.

    *Reducing calorie intake and increasing energy expenditure are important for treating pediatric obesity. Medications and obesity-related surgery may also be employed. The authors stress the importance of involving the family to create a supportive environment as part of the overall therapeutic approach.*

13. Koplan JP and others: Preventing childhood obesity: Health in the balance: Executive Summary. *Journal of the American Dietetic Association* 105:131, 2005.

    *Preventing childhood obesity involves a healthy eating pattern and regular physical activity. The goal should be achieving and maintaining a healthy body weight. The authors note that many social factors will have to be altered to facilitate this goal, such as providing more outlets for physical activity.*

14. Kranz S and others: Dietary fiber intake by American preschoolers is associated with more nutrient-dense diets. *Journal of the American Dietetic Association* 105:221, 2005.

    *Children in general would benefit from diets higher in fiber. Improving diet choices will allow for this, including increasing whole-grain, fruit, and vegetable content. The healthier the overall diet, the greater number of fiber-rich foods.*

15. Lee LA, Burks W: Food allergies: Prevalence, molecular characterization, and treatment/prevention strategies. *Annual Review of Nutrition* 26:539, 2006.

    *This article precisely defines food allergies, presents statistics regarding prevalence of various allergies, details what is known about the biological mechanisms behind food allergies, and sets forth recommendations for their treatment and prevention.*

16. Monsen ER: New findings from the Feeding Infants and Toddlers Study. *Journal of the American Dietetic Association* 106:S5, 2006.

    *The Gerber-sponsored Feeding Infants and Toddlers Study (FITS), covered in several articles in this issue, examined usual intakes of nutrients from foods and supplements, as well as other dietary practices, with an emphasis on dietary habits of Hispanic infants and children. Findings of the study confirm that infants and toddlers do not consume enough fruits, vegetables, or fiber, and that intakes of total kilocalories, dietary fats, and sodium are on the rise.*

17. Rao G: Childhood obesity: Highlights of AMA expert committee recommendations. *American Family Physician* 78:56, 2008.

    *This article outlines key recommendations from the American Medical Association's Expert Committee on the Assessment, Prevention, and Treatment of Child and Adolescent Overweight and Obesity. Weight management should be addressed yearly at medical check-ups with all children. In addition, for those children who are overweight or obese (based on BMI for age), additional screening of blood lipids, glucose, and liver and kidney function is warranted. The four-stage approach for treatment of childhood obesity includes reducing consumption of sweetened beverages and fast foods; limiting time spent watching TV, playing video games, and sitting at the computer; participating in 60 minutes or more of physical activity each day; and encouraging family meals.*

18. Shaikh U and others: Vitamin and mineral supplement use by children and adolescents in the 1999-2004 National Health and Nutrition Examination Survey: Relationship with nutrition, food security, physical activity, and health care access. *Archives of Pediatrics and Adolescent Medicine* 163:250, 2009.

    *Although about one-third of children and teenagers use vitamin and mineral supplements, those who take them usually need them least. Young people with poor dietary intake, sedentary lifestyles, and inadequate access to health care are least likely to use dietary supplements. The authors reiterate that a varied and balanced diet is sufficient to meet nutrient needs for most children and teenagers.*

19. Wagner CL and others: Prevention of rickets and vitamin D deficiency in infants, children, and adolescents. *Pediatrics* 122(5): 1142, 2008.

    *Rickets and vitamin D deficiency is of concern for infants as well as older children and adolescents in the United States and is attributable to inadequate vitamin D intake and decreased exposure to sunlight. The American Academy of Pediatrics recommends that all infants and children, including adolescents, have a minimum daily intake of 400 IU of vitamin D beginning soon after birth.*

20. Wiecha JL and others: When children eat what they watch: Impact of television viewing on dietary intake in youth. *Archives of Pediatrics and Adolescent Medicine* 160:436, 2006.

    *This study of children in Boston found that increased television viewing was related to increased consumption of foods advertised during that viewing and increased total calorie intake over time. Each hour increase in television viewing was associated with a general increase of 167 kcal per day.*

## I. Getting Young Bill to Eat

Bill is 3 years old, and his mother is worried about his eating habits. He refuses to eat vegetables, meat, and dinner in general. Some days he eats very little food. He wants to eat snacks most of the time. Mealtime is a battle because Bill says he isn't hungry, and his mother wants him to eat a sit-down lunch and dinner to make sure he gets all the nutrients he needs and to eat everything served on his plate. He drinks five or six glasses of whole milk per day because that is the one food he likes.

When his mother prepares dinner, she makes plenty of vegetables, boiling them until they are soft, hoping this will appeal to Bill. Bill's dad waits to eat his vegetables last, regularly telling the family that he eats them only because he has to. He also regularly complains about how dinner has been prepared. Bill saves his vegetables until last and usually gags when his mother orders him to eat them. Bill has been known to sit at the dinner table for an hour until the war of wills ends. Bill's mother serves casseroles and stews regularly because they are convenient. Bill likes to eat breakfast cereal, fruit, and cheese and regularly requests these foods for snacks. However, his mother tries to deny his requests, so that he will have an appetite for dinner. Bill's mother comes to you and asks you what she should do to get Bill to eat.

### Analysis

1. List four mistakes Bill's parents are making that contribute to Bill's poor eating habits.

   _____

   _____

   _____

   _____

2. List four strategies they might try to promote good eating habits in Bill.

   _____

   _____

   _____

   _____

# II. Evaluating a Teen Lunch

The following are two typical teen lunches and nutritional information for each:

| Meal 1 | Meal 2 |
|---|---|
| 2 pieces cheese pizza | 1 large hamburger sandwich with condiments |
| 1 milk chocolate candy bar | 30 French fries |
| 20 fluid ounces cola | 20 fluid ounces cola |

| | Meal 1 | Meal 2 | Nutrient Needs for Teens |
|---|---|---|---|
| Energy (kcal) | 990 | 1000 | Males: 3000 Females: 2200 |
| Protein | 32 | 20 | Males: 59 Females: 44 |
| Vitamin C (milligrams) | 5 | 18 | Both genders: 45 to 75 |
| Vitamin A (micrograms RAE) | 300 | 10 | Males: 900 Females: 700 |
| Iron (milligrams) | 3 | 4 | Males: 11 Females: 15 |
| Calcium (milligrams) | 545 | 100 | Both genders: 1300 |

1. Keeping in mind that meals should meet about one-third of nutrient needs, what are the shortcomings and excesses of these meals (i.e., given the nutritional information, compare these meals with one-third the RDA for protein, vitamin C, vitamin A, and iron and the Adequate Intake for calcium)?

   _____

   _____

   _____

2. How would you change these meals to improve balance and to meet the nutrient needs above? (Hint: Use NutritionCalc Plus.)

   _____

   _____

   _____

3. Reflect on your food choices as a teenager. Do you think your meal choices were balanced and varied? Why or why not? What could you have done to improve your nutritional habits at that time?

   _____

   _____

   _____

# III. Public Health Efforts to Combat Childhood Obesity

Major public health initiatives aim to counter the rapid rise in childhood obesity and related health conditions. Whether school-based, community-driven, or targeted at families, the overarching goals are to promote healthy eating habits and increased physical activity.

1. Find out what is going on in your area to combat childhood obesity. As a starting point, here are a few examples:

   - *We Can!™* (Ways to Enhance Children's Activity and Nutrition): http://wecan.nhibi.nih.gov
   - **HealthCorps:** http://www.healthcorps.net/
   - **Action for Healthy Kids:** http://www.actionforhealthykids.org
   - **The President's Council on Fitness and Sports:** http://www.fitness.gov/

   _____

   _____

   _____

   _____

Imagine that you have been appointed to develop a public health campaign to decrease childhood obesity in your community.

2. What are the specific needs in your community (e.g., lack of safe space for physical activity, overabundance of fast food outlets)?

   _____

   _____

   _____

   _____

3. Who will be your target audience? Why?

   _____

   _____

   _____

   _____

4. What activities will you undertake to reach your target audience? What will set your program apart from other efforts in your community?

   _____

   _____

   _____

   _____

5. How will you define the success of your program? List two or more measurable objectives for your campaign.

   _____

   _____

   _____

   _____

# CHAPTER 16 Nutrition During Adulthood

## Student Learning Outcomes  After studying Chapter 16, you will be able to:

1. List several hypotheses about the causes of aging.
2. Discuss factors that affect the rate of aging.
3. Describe how physiological changes that occur during adulthood affect nutritional needs.
4. Compare the dietary intake of adults with current recommendations.

5. Make recommendations for dietary changes in the prevention and treatment of nutritional problems in older adults.
6. Identify nutrition-related health issues of the adult years and describe the prevention and treatment options.

7. Compare benefits of moderate alcohol use to risks of alcohol abuse.
8. List several nutritional programs available to help meet nutritional needs of older adults.

## Chapter Outline

Student Learning Outcomes

Refresh Your Memory

16.1  The Graying of North America

16.2  Physiological Changes During Adulthood

16.3  Nutrient Needs During Adulthood

16.4  Factors Related to Food Intake and Nutrient Needs

16.5  Nutrition Implications of Alcohol Consumption

16.6  Ensuring a Healthful Diet for the Adult Years

Nutrition and Your Health: *Nutrition and Cancer*

Case Study: Dietary Assistance for an Older Adult

Summary/Study Questions/Check Your Knowledge/Further Readings

Rate Your Plate

**EATING IS ONE OF OUR GREAT PLEASURES.** Guided by common sense and moderation, eating well is also a means to good health. Most of us want a long, productive life, free of illness. Yet, as the comic in this chapter suggests, many people from early middle age onward suffer from obesity, cardiovascular disease, hypertension and strokes, type 2 diabetes, osteoporosis, and other chronic diseases. We can slow the development of—and in some cases even prevent—these diseases by following a dietary pattern such as that proposed by MyPyramid. The effect of such a diet is most profitable if we begin early and continue throughout adulthood. We serve ourselves best—as individuals and as a nation—by striving to maintain vitality even in the later decades of life. This concept was first explored in Chapter 1 and is discussed again in this chapter, in light of the nutrition needs of adults.

Keep in mind that present day-to-day health practices can significantly influence health during later life. Although genetics does play a role, as discussed in Chapter 3, many of the health problems that occur with age are not inevitable; they result from diet-related disease processes that influence physical health. Much can be learned from healthy older people whose attention to a healthy diet and physical activity—along with a little luck—keeps them active and vibrant well beyond typical retirement years. Successful aging is the goal. Age quickly or slowly—it is partly your choice.

**Refresh Your Memory**

As you begin your study of adult nutrition issues in Chapter 16, you may want to review:

- Implications of the 1994 Dietary Supplement Health and Education Act in Chapter 1
- The effect of genetics on health in Chapter 3
- The various body systems covered in Chapter 3
- The sources of fiber and sugar in Chapter 4
- Definition of healthy body weight in Chapter 7
- The dietary sources of vitamin D, the various B vitamins, and calcium in Chapters 8 and 9
- Recommendations for salt intake in Chapter 9
- The benefits of regular physical activity in Chapter 10

## 16.1 The Graying of North America

Due to advances in health care and sanitation, the demographics of developed countries are shifting so that as a population, we are getting older. In North America, the group constituting those aged 85+ years is the fastest growing segment. Between 1997 and 2050, the population aged 85+ years in the United States is expected to increase from 3.4 million to 19 million. Even more amazing, 1 million or more people in the United States could be over 100 years old in 2050.

This "graying" of North America poses some problems. Although people older than age 65 account for just 13% of the U.S. population, they account for more than 25% of all prescription medications used, 40% of acute hospital stays, and 50% of the federal health budget. Hip fractures alone cost the nation about $12 billion per year. Of older persons, 65% or more have nutrition-related problems, such as cardiovascular disease, type 2 diabetes, hypertension, and osteoporosis.

Is a decline in health inevitable as we age? Which diet and lifestyle interventions have been shown to slow (or reverse) the aging process? Which nutrition problems are typically seen in older adults? How should one compensate for these? Chapter 16 provides some answers.

Postponing these chronic diseases for as long as possible will help control health care costs. Health and independence contribute quality—not just quantity—to life as age advances and lessen the load on an already overburdened healthcare system. Keep in mind that aging is not a disease. Furthermore, diseases that commonly accompany old age—osteoporosis and atherosclerosis, for example—are not an inevitable part of aging. Many can be prevented or managed. Some people do die of old age, not as a direct result of disease.

## 16.2 Physiological Changes During Adulthood

Adulthood, the longest stage of the life cycle, begins when an adolescent completes his or her physical growth. Unlike earlier stages of the life cycle, nutrients are used primarily to maintain the body rather than support physical growth. (Pregnancy is the only time during adulthood when substantial amounts of nutrients are used for growth.) As adults get older, nutrient needs change. For example, vitamin D needs increase for older adults. Based on the needs for various nutrients, the Food and Nutrition Board divided the adult years into four stages: ages 19 to 30, 31 to 50, 51 to 70, and beyond 70 years of age. The intervals encompassing ages 19 through 50 are often referred to as young adulthood, 51 to 70 as middle adulthood, and beyond 70 years of age as older adulthood.

Adulthood is characterized by body maintenance and gradual physical and physiological transitions, often referred to as aging. **Aging** can be defined as the time-dependent physical and physiological changes in body structure and function that occur normally and progressively throughout adulthood as humans mature and become older. One view of aging describes it as a process of slow cell death, beginning soon after fertilization. When we are young, aging is not apparent because the major metabolic activities are geared toward growth and maturation. We produce plenty of active cells to meet physiological needs. During late adolescence and adulthood, the body's major task is to maintain cells. From the beginning of adulthood until age 30 or so, body systems are at their peak efficiency rate. Stature, stamina, strength, endurance, efficiency, and health are at their lifetime highs. Rates of cell synthesis and breakdown are balanced in most tissues. Inevitably, though, cells age and die. After about age 30, the rate of cell breakdown slowly begins to exceed the rate of cell renewal, leading to a gradual decline in organ size and efficiency. Eventually, the body can't adjust to meet all physiological demands, and body functioning begins to decrease (Fig. 16-1). Still, body systems and organs usually retain enough **reserve capacity** to handle normal, everyday demands throughout one's entire lifetime.

▲ As the "baby boom" turns 65 in 2011, the health concerns of an aging population will demand increasing attention.

**aging** Time-dependent physical and physiological changes in body structure and function that occur normally and progressively throughout adulthood as humans mature and become older.

**reserve capacity** The extent to which an organ can preserve essentially normal function despite decreasing cell number or cell activity.

**FIGURE 16-1** ▶ Declines in physiological function seen with aging. The decline in many body functions is especially evident in sedentary people.

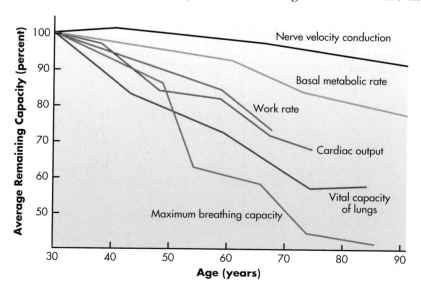

Problems caused by diminished capacity typically don't arise unless severe demands are placed on the aging body. For example, alcohol intake can overtax an aging liver. The stress of shoveling a snow-covered sidewalk can exceed the capacity of the heart and lungs. Coping with an illness also can push an older body beyond its capacity.

The causes of aging remain a mystery. Most likely, the physiological changes of aging are the sum of automatic cellular changes, lifestyle practices, and environmental influences, as listed in Table 16-1. Even with the most supportive environment and healthy lifestyle, cell structure and function inevitably change over time. The eventual death of deteriorating cells is actually beneficial because it likely prevents diseases such as cancer. Unfortunately, there are negative consequences to this natural cell progression because, as more and more cells in an organ die, organ function decreases. For example, **kidney nephrons** are continually lost as we age. In some people, this loss exhausts the kidneys' reserve capacity and ultimately leads to kidney failure. Most people, however, maintain sufficient kidney function throughout life.

The diseases and degenerative processes commonly observed in older people have long been assumed to be unavoidable consequences of aging. Certainly, some of the declines we blame on aging may be inevitable, such as gradual reductions in tissue

**kidney nephrons** The units of kidney cells that filter wastes from the bloodstream and deposit them into the urine.

**glycosylation** The process by which glucose attaches to (glycates) other compounds, such as proteins.

**TABLE 16-1** Current Hypotheses About the Causes of Aging

**Errors occur in copying the genetic blueprint (DNA).**
Once sufficient errors in DNA copying accumulate, a cell can no longer synthesize the major proteins needed to function, and it therefore dies.

**Connective tissue stiffens.**
Parallel protein strands, found mostly in connective tissue, cross-link to each other. This decreases flexibility in key body components.

**Electron-seeking compounds damage cell parts.**
Electron-seeking free radicals can break down cell membranes and proteins. One way to prevent some damage from these compounds is to consume adequate amounts of vitamins E and C, selenium, and carotenoids.

**Hormone function changes.**
The blood concentration of many hormones, such as testosterone in men, falls during the aging process. Replacement of these and other hormones is possible, but the resulting risks and benefits are largely unknown.

**Glycosylation of proteins.**
Blood glucose, when chronically elevated, attaches to (glycates) various blood and body proteins. This decreases protein function and can encourage immune system attack on such altered proteins.

**The immune system loses some efficiency.**
The immune system is most efficient during childhood and young adulthood, but with advancing age, it is less able to recognize and counteract foreign substances, such as viruses, that enter the body. Nutrient deficiencies, particularly of protein, vitamin E, vitamin B-6, and zinc, also hamper immune function.

**Autoimmunity develops.**
Autoimmune reactions occur when white blood cells and other immune system components begin to attack body tissues in addition to foreign proteins. Many diseases, including some forms of arthritis, involve this autoimmune response.

**Death is programmed into the cell.**
Each human cell can divide only about 50 times. Once this number of divisions occurs, the cell automatically succumbs.

**Excess calorie intake speeds body breakdown.**
Experimentally, underfed animals, such as spiders, mice, and rats, live longer. Usual calorie intake must be reduced by about 30% to see this effect. This approach is the only proven way to substantially slow the aging process.

▲ Adopting diet and lifestyle practices that minimize a decline in body function is an investment in your future health. Visit www.nia.nih.gov for a free fact sheet on healthy aging.

and organ cell numbers, graying hair, and reduced lung capacity. However, many of the so-called usual or degenerative age-related changes can, in fact, be minimized, prevented, and/or reversed by healthy lifestyles (e.g., eating nutritious diets, exercising regularly, getting enough sleep) and avoiding adverse environmental factors (e.g., excessive exposure to sunlight and cigarette smoke). These discoveries have led researchers to introduce the concepts of "usual aging" and "successful aging."

## Usual and Successful Aging

Body cells age, no matter what health practices we follow. However, to a considerable extent, you can choose how quickly you age throughout your adult years. *Usual aging* refers to those changes commonly thought to be a typical or expected part of aging, such as increasing body fatness, decreasing lean body mass, rising blood pressure, declining bone mass, and increasingly poor health. Researchers point out that many of these changes really represent an acceleration of the aging process induced by unhealthy lifestyle choices, adverse environmental exposures, and/or chronic disease. For instance, blood pressure does not tend to rise with age among people whose diets are traditionally low in sodium. Also, lean body mass is maintained much better in older people who exercise than in those who don't.

*Successful aging,* on the other hand, describes physical and physiological function declines that occur only because one grows older, not because lifestyle choices, environmental exposures, and chronic disease have aggravated or sped up the rate of aging. Those who are successful agers experience age-related declines at a slower rate and the onset of chronic disease symptoms at a later age than usual agers. Striving to have the greatest number of healthy years and the fewest years of illness is often referred to as **compression of morbidity.** In other words, a person tries to delay the onset of disabilities caused by chronic disease and to compress significant sickness related to aging into the last few years–or months–of life.

## Factors Affecting the Rate of Aging

**Life span** refers to the maximum number of years a human can live. As far as we know, this hasn't changed in recorded time. The longest human life documented to date is 122 years for a woman and 114 years for a man. **Life expectancy,** alternatively, is the time an average person born in a specific year, such as 2009, can expect to live. Life expectancy in North America is about 75 years for men and about 80 years for women, with a span of "healthy years" of about 64. Furthermore, a person who survives to age 80 can expect to live an additional 7 to 10 years.

The rate at which one ages is individual; it is determined by heredity, lifestyle, and environment. With the exception of heredity, most of the factors that influence the rate of aging are directly linked to choices that are under our control.

## Heredity

Heredity defines who you are biochemically and, to some extent, it defines how long you will live (longevity). Living to an old age tends to run in some families. If your parents and grandparents lived a long time, you are likely to have the potential to live to an old age, too. One of the most obvious genetic characteristics influencing longevity is gender. In the case of humans, as well as most other species, females tend to live longer than males.

Another genetic characteristic that can influence longevity is metabolic efficiency. Individuals with a "thrifty metabolism" require fewer calories for metabolic processes and are able to store body fat more easily than those with faster metabolic rates. Throughout history, it was the individuals with thrifty metabolism who tended to live the longest because they efficiently stored fat during times of plenty and thus had the energy stores needed to survive frequent periods of food scarcity. In today's

**K**eep in mind that extending life without delaying onset of chronic disease prolongs suffering in many cases. In addition, the greater number of disabled years is costly to all North Americans. For these reasons, prolonging life without compressing the number of disabled years is called the "failure of success."

**compression of morbidity** Delay of the onset of disabilities caused by chronic disease.

**life span** The potential oldest age a person can reach.

**life expectancy** The average length of life for a given group of people born in a specific year (such as this year).

**B**esides having other long-lived family members, people who live to 100 years generally:

- Do not smoke and do not drink heavily
- Gain little weight in adulthood
- Eat many fruits and vegetables
- Perform daily physical activity
- Challenge their minds
- Have a positive outlook
- Maintain close friendships
- Are (or were) married (especially true for men)
- Have a healthy rate of HDL cholesterol production

environment of labor-saving devices and abundant, energy-dense foods, however, a thrifty metabolism may actually reduce longevity. Accumulation of excessive body fat increases the risk of developing health problems that reduce life expectancy (e.g., heart disease, hypertension, and certain cancers).

As you know, heredity is largely unchangeable. However, heredity is not necessarily destiny—individuals can exert some control over the expression of their genetic potential. Lifestyle and environment both can modify the expression of genetic potential.

## Lifestyle

Lifestyle is one's pattern of living—it includes food choices, exercise patterns, and substance use (e.g., alcohol, drugs, and tobacco). Lifestyle choices can have a major impact on health and longevity, as well as on the expression of genetic potential. If individuals have a family history of premature heart disease, they can adjust their diet, exercise, and tobacco use patterns to slow the progression of the disease, get needed medical care, and possibly extend their lifetime. The converse is true, too. That is, lifestyle choices (e.g., high-fat diet and couch potato mentality) can increase susceptibility to diseases that hasten the rate of aging, ultimately shortening life expectancy, even if a person's genetic potential is for a very long life.

Worldwide, the highest average life expectancy is in Okinawa, a stretch of islands off the coast of Japan: 86 years for women and 78 years for men. Researchers suggest that these statistics are rooted in the traditional diet and lifestyle of inhabitants of Okinawa. The Okinawan diet is based on rice, fish, vegetable protein sources, fruits, vegetables, tea, herbs for seasonings, and small amounts of meat. Alcohol and salt intake is minimal. The low energy density translates into a generally low calorie intake, and BMI averages 21 kg/m². A desire to mimic their weight management success, compression of morbidity, and longevity has given rise to several popular books and websites that promote Okinawan dietary practices.

Followers of the traditional Mediterranean Diet also enjoy some of the lowest recorded rates of chronic disease in the world (See Chapter 2, p. 53). As introduced in Chapter 5, the Mediterranean Diet features the following:

- Olive oil, a source of heart-healthy monounsaturated fat, as the main dietary fat
- Abundant daily intake of fruits, vegetables (especially leafy greens), whole grains, beans, nuts, and seeds
- An emphasis on minimally processed and, wherever possible, seasonally fresh and locally grown foods
- Daily intake of small amounts of cheese and yogurt
- Weekly intake of low to moderate amounts of fish
- Limited use of eggs and red meat
- Regular exercise
- Moderate drinking of wine at mealtime

Common themes among these life-prolonging dietary practices are their focus on unprocessed, fiber-rich foods, healthy sources of fat (e.g., vegetable oils and fish), and lean sources of protein. Besides diet, populations who enjoy extended quality and quantity of life include physical activity as a major part of their daily routines. Compare these lifestyle choices with those of typical North Americans.

## Environment

Some aspects of the environment that exert a powerful influence on the rate of aging are income, education level, health care, shelter, and psychosocial factors. For instance, being able to purchase nutritious foods, quality health care, and safe housing helps decrease the rate of aging. Having the education needed to earn a sufficient income, as well as the knowledge required to select a nutritious diet and make wise lifestyle choices, also can slow the aging process. In addition, the willingness to seek

## CRITICAL THINKING

The "fountain of youth" remains a mystery. Many people believe a source exists that can stop the aging process, allowing youth to remain. However, Neil, a history student, asserts that the fountain of youth is not a place or a particular thing but, rather, a combination of diet and lifestyle. How can he justify this claim?

health care promptly when it is needed, the capacity to follow the instructions of a health-care provider, and the desire to accept the responsibility for one's own health can slow the rate of aging. Likewise, shelter that protects individuals from physical danger, climatic extremes, and solar radiation helps slow the aging process. Allowing people to make at least some decisions for themselves and control their own activities (autonomy) and providing psychosocial support (informational and emotional resources) promote successful aging and psychological well-being. In contrast, aging is likely to accelerate if any or all of the converse (i.e., insufficient income, low education level, lack of health care, inadequate shelter, and/or lack of autonomy and psychosocial support) are true.

### CONCEPT CHECK

Although lifespan has not changed, life expectancy has increased dramatically over the past century. This means an increasing proportion of the North American population is over 65 years of age and will live for decades longer. Avoiding continually rising health care costs and maximizing satisfaction with life require postponing and minimizing chronic illness. Aging begins early in life and is influenced by heredity, lifestyle, and environment. A healthy diet and regular physical activity can play a pivotal role in slowing the aging process.

## 16.3 Nutrient Needs During Adulthood

The challenge of the adult years is to maintain the body, preserve its function, and avoid chronic disease-that is, to age successfully. A healthy diet can help achieve this goal. One blueprint for a healthy diet comes from the 2005 Dietary Guidelines for Americans, discussed in Chapter 2. Its advice can be summarized into three main points:

1. Consume a variety of nutrient-dense foods and beverages from the basic food groups of MyPyramid that result in a diet low in saturated and *trans* fat, cholesterol, added sugars, salt, and alcohol (if used). Foods to emphasize are vegetables, fruits, beans, whole-grain breads and cereals, reduced-fat milk or milk products, and water.
2. Maintain body weight in a healthy range by balancing energy intake with energy expended. Engage in at least 30 minutes of moderate-intensity physical activity, above usual activity, at work or home on most days of the week.
3. Practice safe food handling when preparing food. Clean hands, food contact surfaces, and fruits and vegetables before preparation, and cook foods to a safe temperature to kill microorganisms.

Overall, good nutrition benefits adults in many ways. Meeting nutrient needs delays the onset of certain diseases; improves the management of some existing diseases; speeds recovery from many illnesses; increases mental, physical, and social well-being; and often decreases the need for and length of hospitalization. As you know, American adults are fairly well nourished, although some dietary excesses and inadequacies do exist. For instance, common dietary excesses are calories, fat, sodium, and, for some, alcohol. The diets of adult women tend to fall short of the recommended amounts of vitamins D and E, folate, magnesium, calcium, zinc, and fiber. The diets of adult men tend to be low in the same nutrients, except vitamin D, which does not become problematic until age 50. The iron intake of most women during their childbearing years (19 to 50) is insufficient to meet their needs; however, due to a reduced iron need after **menopause,** older women do get enough iron.

People age 65 and up, particularly those in long-term care facilities and hospitals, are the single largest group at risk of malnutrition. They may become underweight and show signs of numerous micronutrient deficiencies (e.g., vitamins B-6 and B-12

**menopause** Cessation of menses in women, usually beginning at about age 50.

and folate). Friends, relatives, and health care professionals should monitor nutrient intake in all older people, including those who live in long-term care facilities. Family members can play a valuable role in making sure nutrient needs are met by looking for weight maintenance based on regular, healthful meal patterns. To pinpoint those over age 65 at risk of nutrient deficiencies, the American Academy of Family Physicians, the American Dietetic Association, and the National Council on Aging developed the Nutrition Screening Initiative checklist (Fig. 16-2). Older Americans, family members, and health care providers can use the checklist to identify those at nutritional risk *before* health deteriorates significantly. If problems arise in consuming a healthful diet, registered dietitians can offer professional and personalized advice.

## Defining Nutrient Needs

The DRIs for adults are divided by gender into four age groups to reflect how nutrient needs change as adults grow older. These changes in nutrient needs take into consideration aging-related physiological alterations in body composition, metabolism, and organ function.

**Calories.** After age 30 or so, total calorie needs of physically inactive adults fall steadily throughout adulthood. This is caused by a gradual decline in basal metabolism. To

**FIGURE 16-2** ▶ A nutrition checklist for older adults.

*Reprinted with permission by the Nutrition Screening Initiative, a project of the American Academy of Family Physicians, the American Dietetic Association, and the National Council on Aging, Inc., and funded in part by a grant from Ross Products Division, Abbott Laboratories.*

## A Nutrition Test for Older Adults

Here's a nutrition check for anyone over age 65. Circle the number of points for each statement that applies. Then compute the total and check it against the nutritional score.

| Points | |
|---|---|
| 2 | 1. The person has a chronic illness or current condition that has changed the kind or amount of food eaten. |
| 3 | 2. The person eats fewer than two full meals per day. |
| 2 | 3. The person eats few fruits, vegetables, or milk products. |
| 2 | 4. The person drinks 3 or more servings of beer, liquor, or wine almost every day. |
| 2 | 5. The person has tooth or mouth problems that make eating difficult. |
| 4 | 6. The person does not have enough money for food. |
| 1 | 7. The person eats alone most of the time. |
| 1 | 8. The person takes three or more different prescription or over-the-counter drugs each day. |
| 2 | 9. The person has unintentionally lost or gained 10 pounds within the last 6 months. |
| 2 | 10. The person cannot always shop, cook, or feed himself or herself. |
| **Total** | |

### Nutritional score:

**0–2: Good.** Recheck in 6 months.

**3–5: Marginal.** A local agency on aging has information about nutrition programs for the elderly. The National Association of Area Agencies on Aging can assist in finding help; call (800) 677-1116. Recheck in 6 months.

**6 or more: High risk.** A doctor should review this test and suggest how to improve nutritional health.

a considerable extent, adults can exert control over this reduction in calorie need by exercising. Exercise can halt, slow, and even reverse reductions in lean body mass and subsequent declines in calorie need. Also, keeping calorie needs high makes it easier to meet one's nutrient needs and avoid becoming overweight.

**Protein.** The protein intake of adults of all ages in North America tends to exceed current recommended levels. However, some recent studies indicate that consuming protein in amounts slightly higher than the RDA may help preserve muscle and bone mass. Adults who have limited food budgets, have difficulty chewing meat, or are lactose intolerant may not get enough protein. Recall from Chapter 6 that any protein consumed in excess of that needed for the maintenance of body tissue will be broken down and used as energy or stored as fat. The waste products of metabolism of protein must be removed by the kidneys; excessive protein intake may accelerate kidney function decline.

**Fat.** The fat intake of adults of all ages is often at or above the recommendations. It's a good idea for almost all adults to reduce their fat intake because of the strong link between high-fat diets and obesity, heart disease, and certain cancers. In addition, reducing fat intake "frees up" some calories that can be better "spent" on complex carbohydrates.

**Carbohydrates.** The total carbohydrate intake of adults of all ages in North America is often lower than recommended. In addition, many adults need to shift the carbohydrate composition of their diets to emphasize complex carbohydrates while minimizing intake of sugary, simple carbohydrates. A diet rich in complex carbohydrates helps us achieve nutrient needs and stay within calorie bounds because many highly sweetened foods are low in nutrients and high in calories. Substituting foods rich in complex carbohydrates for sweets also makes it easier for the body to control blood glucose levels—a function that becomes less efficient as the increases in body fatness and inactivity associated with usual aging occur. Declines in carbohydrate metabolism are so common that more than 20% of those age 65 years or older have diabetes. A diet rich in fiber helps adults reduce their risk of colon cancer and heart disease, lower their blood cholesterol levels, and avoid constipation. The typical American adult gets slightly more than half the recommended amount of dietary fiber.

**Water.** Many adults, especially those in the later years, fail to consume adequate quantities of water. In fact, many are in a constant state of mild dehydration and at risk of electrolyte imbalances. Low fluid intakes in older adults may be caused by a fading sensitivity to thirst sensations, chronic diseases, and/or conscious reductions in fluid intake in order to reduce the frequency of urination. Some also may have increased fluid output because they are taking certain medications (i.e., diuretics and laxatives), have an **ostomy,** and/or experience an age-related decline in the kidneys' ability to concentrate urine. Dehydration is very dangerous and, among other symptoms, can cause disorientation and mental confusion, constipation, impacted fecal matter, and death.

**Minerals and Vitamins.** Adequate intake of all vitamins and minerals is important throughout the adult years. The micronutrients that need special attention because they tend to be present in less than optimal amounts in the diets of many adults are calcium, vitamin D, iron, zinc, magnesium, folate, and vitamins B-6, B-12, and E. Adults with impaired absorption or who are unable to consume a nutritious diet may benefit from mineral or vitamin supplements matched with their needs. In fact, many nutrition experts recommend a daily balanced multivitamin and mineral supplement

▲ As we age, our nutrient needs change. For example, vitamin D needs are higher for older stages of adulthood.

**ostomy** Surgically created short circuit in intestinal flow where the end point usually opens from the abdominal cavity rather than the anus—for example, a colostomy. Short circuiting the intestinal flow means more water is lost in fecal matter than would be if the intestinal tract were intact.

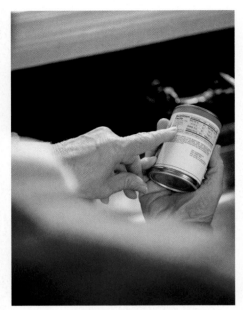

▲ Sodium needs for older adults are 1200 to 1300 milligrams per day. Older adults routinely consume at least this much sodium. Potassium needs are 4700 milligrams per day. Many older adults do not meet this goal.

for older adults, especially for those 70 years of age and older. Supplements or fortified foods can be especially helpful when it comes to meeting vitamin D and vitamin B-12 needs.

*Calcium and Vitamin D* These bone-building nutrients tend to be low in the diets of all adults. They become particularly problematic after age 50. Inadequate intake of these nutrients, coupled with their reduced absorption, the reduced synthesis of vitamin D in the skin, and the kidneys' decreased ability to put vitamin D in its active form, greatly contributes to the development of osteoporosis. Getting enough of these nutrients is a challenge for many older adults because food sources of vitamin D are limited in the North American diet, and the major sources—fatty fish and fortified milk—are not widely consumed by older adults. Plus, with increasing age, lactase production frequently decreases. As you know, one of the richest and most absorbable sources of these nutrients, milk, contains lactose. To get the vitamin D and calcium needed, many with lactose intolerance can consume small amounts of milk at mealtime with no ill effects. Calcium-fortified foods, cheese, yogurt, fish eaten with bones (e.g., canned sardines or salmon), and dark green leafy vegetables can help those with lactose intolerance meet calcium needs—but these foods often do not provide vitamin D. Just 10 to 15 minutes per day of sunlight can make a large difference in vitamin D status.

*Iron* Iron deficiency anemia, the most common type of malnutrition during the adult years, is found most frequently in women in their reproductive years because their diets do not provide enough iron to compensate for the iron lost monthly during menstruation. Other common causes of iron deficiency in adults of all ages include digestive tract injuries that cause bleeding (i.e., bleeding ulcers or hemorrhoids) and the use of medicines, such as aspirin, that cause blood loss. Impaired iron absorption due to age-related declines in stomach acid production may contribute to iron deficiency in older adults.

*Zinc* In addition to less than optimal dietary zinc intake during adulthood, zinc absorption declines as stomach acid production diminishes with age. Poor zinc status may contribute to the taste sensation losses, mental lethargy, and delayed wound healing many elderly adults experience.

*Magnesium* This mineral tends to be low in adults' diets. Inadequate magnesium intakes may contribute to the loss of bone strength, muscular weakness, and mental confusion seen in some elderly adults. It also can lead to sudden death from poor heart rhythm and is linked to cardiovascular disease, osteoporosis, and diabetes. The best source of magnesium is the diet; supplements can cause loose stools and diarrhea.

*Folate and Vitamins B-6 and B-12* Sufficient folate, because of its role in prevention of neural tube defects, are very important to women during the childbearing years. In later years, folate and vitamins B-6 and B-12 are especially important because they are required to clear homocysteine from the bloodstream. Introduced in Chapter 5, elevated blood concentrations of homocysteine are associated with increased risk of the cardiovascular disease, stroke, bone fracture, and neurological decline seen in some elderly people. Vitamin B-12 is a particular problem for the older population because a deficiency may exist even when intake appears to be adequate. As people age, the stomach slows its production of acid and intrinsic factor, which leads to poor absorption of vitamin B-12 and eventually pernicious anemia. Adults age 51 years and older need to meet vitamin B-12 needs with foods or supplements fortified with synthetic vitamin B-12.

*Vitamin E* The dietary intake of most of the population falls short of recommendations for vitamin E. Low vitamin E intake means the body has a reduced supply of antioxidants, which may increase the degree of cell damage caused by free radicals, promote the progression of chronic diseases and cataracts, and speed aging. In addition, low vitamin E levels can lead to declines in physical abilities.

**Carotenoids.** Dietary intakes of certain carotenoids have been shown to have a variety of important anti-aging and health protective effects. Specifically, lutein and zeaxanthin have been linked with the prevention of cataracts and age-related macular degeneration. Diets high in fruit and vegetables, the major sources of carotenoids and other beneficial phytochemicals, are consistently shown to be protective of a wide variety of age-related conditions.

## Are Adults Following Current Dietary Recommendations?

In general, adults in North America are trying to follow many of the diet recommendations described in this chapter. Since the mid-1950s, they have consumed less saturated fat as more people substitute fat-free and low-fat milk for cream and whole milk. However, they eat more cheese, usually a concentrated form of saturated fat. Since 1963, they have eaten less butter, fewer eggs, less animal fat, and more vegetable oils and fish. These changes generally follow the recommendations to reduce the intake of saturated fat and cholesterol in favor of unsaturated fat choices. Animal breeders are raising much leaner cattle and hogs than those produced in 1950, which also helps reduce saturated fat intake.

Other aspects of the average adult diet are less promising. The latest nutrition survey of eating habits in the United States shows that the major contributors of calories to the adult diet are white bread, beef, doughnuts, cakes and cookies, soft drinks, milk, chicken, cheese, alcoholic beverages, salad dressing, mayonnaise, potatoes, and sugars/syrups/jams. If the trend in diets were truly toward decreasing sugar and saturated fat intake, and increasing fiber intake, many of these foods would not appear at the top of the list.

▲ A daily serving of a whole-grain breakfast cereal provides a rich source of vitamins, minerals, and fiber and so contributes to healthy aging.

### CONCEPT CHECK

The 2005 Dietary Guidelines for Americans direct people to eat a variety of foods; maintain healthy weight; choose a diet low in saturated fat, *trans* fat, and cholesterol; choose a diet with plenty of vegetables, fruits, legumes (beans), and whole-grain products; use sugars and salt sparingly; and drink little or no alcohol. Micronutrients of concern for an aging population include calcium, iron, zinc, magnesium, folate, carotenoids, and vitamins D, B-6, B-12, and E.

## 16.4 Factors Related to Food Intake and Nutrient Needs

Diet is one of the main factors directly involved in the development of several health conditions during adulthood. The effects of diet and nutrients on many of these conditions, including atherosclerosis, cancer, constipation, diabetes, diverticular disease, heartburn, hypertension, obesity, and osteoporosis, were discussed in earlier chapters. Still other health problems, including arthritis, Alzheimer's disease, and depression, are not directly diet-related, but nutrition is implicated in their prevention and/or treatment.

An important concept to remember is that an aging body loses resilience–it becomes less able to handle stressors and restore balance (homeostasis). For example, compared to a healthy 30-year-old adult, it takes twice as long for the kidneys of an 80-year-old to remove wastes and restore blood levels to normal after eating excess protein. Similarly, the breakdown of alcohol, drugs, and even nutrient supplements is

**R**esearchers believe that maintaining lean muscle mass may be the most important strategy for successful aging. This is because maintaining lean muscle mass:

- Maintains basal metabolic rate, which helps decrease the risk of obesity
- Keeps body fat low, which helps control blood cholesterol levels and helps avoid the onset of type 2 diabetes
- Maintains body water, which decreases the risk of dehydration and improves body temperature regulation

**sarcopenia** In general, loss of muscle tissue. Among older adults this loss of lean mass greatly increases their risk of illness and death.

**sarcopenic obesity** Loss of muscle mass accompanied by gains in fat mass.

slowed. Consequently, blood levels of these substances rise higher and have a strong and longer effect in older adults than in younger people. Taking steps to avoid stressing the body's capabilities (e.g., avoiding excessive protein intake or megadose dietary supplements) can help preserve optimal physiological function in older adults.

Like those of other age groups, the food choices and nutritional adequacy of adults' diets depend on the interplay of physiological, psychosocial, and economic factors. Alterations in any one of these factors can result in deteriorations in the quality of dietary intake, nutritional status, and health.

## Physiological Factors

The implications of many of the physiological changes that occur during adulthood on dietary intake and nutrient needs are summarized in Table 16-2. Some of the changes listed (e.g., tooth loss, loss in taste and smell perceptions) can influence dietary intake. Other changes (e.g., loss of lean body tissue) can alter nutrient and/or calorie needs. Still other changes (e.g., reduced stomach acidity, diminished kidney function) can cause changes in nutrient utilization. Chronic diseases and the need for medications are additional physiological changes many adults experience that can influence food intake and nutrient needs. The following section details the interactions of several of these factors on nutritional status during adulthood.

**Body Composition.** The primary changes in body composition that occur as the adult years progress are: diminished lean body mass, increased fat stores, and decreased body water. The loss of lean body mass is termed **sarcopenia.** Some muscle cells shrink and others are lost as muscles age; some muscles lose their elasticity as they accumulate fat and collagen. Loss of muscle mass leads to a decrease in basal metabolism, muscle strength, and energy needs. Less muscle mass also leads to lower physical activity, which makes the prognosis for maintaining muscle even worse. Clearly, it is best to avoid this vicious cycle.

Lifestyle greatly determines the rate of muscle mass deterioration. As you might predict, an active lifestyle helps maintain muscle mass, whereas an inactive one encourages its loss. In fact, much of what we associate with old age is due to a lifetime of physical inactivity. Ideally, an active lifestyle should be maintained throughout life and include both aerobic and strength training (see Making Decisions). Physical activity increases muscle strength and mobility, improves balance and decreases the risk of falling, eases daily tasks that require some strength, improves sleep, slows bone loss, and increases joint movement, thus reducing injuries. It also has a positive impact on a person's mental outlook. Strength training (resistance) helps reverse some of the decline in daily function associated with the muscle loss typically seen in older adulthood.

As lean tissue declines with age, body fat often increases, a condition called **sarcopenic obesity.** Much of this increase in body fat results from overeating and limited physical activity, although even athletic men and lean women typically gain some degree of midsection fat after age 50. A small fat gain in adulthood may not compromise health, but large gains are problematic. Recall that obesity can raise blood pressure and blood glucose and make walking and performing daily tasks more difficult.

Decreases in body weight are common in adults age 70 and older. Weight loss is a problem for older people in particular because it increases the risk of nutrition-related illness and death. It may indicate illness, reduced tolerance to medication, or withdrawal from life. The effects of current medication, as well as changes in taste and smell, may inhibit appetite, too. In addition, many older people live alone, a circumstance associated with depressed appetite.

**Skeletal System.** Recall from Chapter 9 that bone loss in women occurs primarily after menopause. Bone loss in men is slow and steady from middle age throughout later life. Many older people may suffer from undiagnosed osteomalacia, a condition

**TABLE 16-2** Typical Physiological Changes of Aging and Recommended Diet and Lifestyle Responses

| Physiological Changes | Recommended Responses |
|---|---|
| Appetite ↓ | • Monitor weight and strive to eat enough to maintain healthy weight.<br>• Use meal replacement products, such as Boost® and Ensure Plus®. |
| Sense of taste and smell ↓ | • Vary the diet.<br>• Experiment with herbs and spices. |
| Chewing ability ↓ | • Work with a dentist to maximize chewing ability.<br>• Modify food consistency as necessary.<br>• Eat calorie-rich snacks. |
| Sense of thirst ↓ | • Consume plenty of fluid each day.<br>• Stay alert for evidence of dehydration (e.g., minimal output or dark-colored urine). |
| Stomach acidity ↓ | • Consume iron-rich foods with a source of vitamin C.<br>• Choose foods fortified with vitamin B-12 or use a supplemental source, containing vitamin B-12. |
| Bowel function ↓ | • Consume enough fiber daily, choosing primarily fruits, vegetables, and whole-grain breads and cereals.<br>• Meet fluid needs. |
| Lactase production ↓ | • Limit milk serving size at each use.<br>• Substitute yogurt or cheese for milk.<br>• Use reduced-lactose or lactose-free products.<br>• Seek nondairy calcium sources. |
| Iron status ↓ | • Include some lean meat and iron-fortified foods in the diet.<br>• Ask physician to monitor blood iron status. |
| Liver function ↓ | • Consume alcohol in moderation, if at all.<br>• Avoid consuming excess vitamin A. |
| Insulin function ↓ | • Maintain healthy body weight.<br>• Perform regular physical activity. |
| Kidney function ↓ | • If necessary, work with physician and registered dietitian to modify protein and other nutrients in diet. |
| Immune function ↓ | • Meet nutrient needs, especially protein, vitamin E, vitamin B-6, and zinc.<br>• Perform regular physical activity. |
| Lung function ↓ | • Avoid tobacco products.<br>• Perform regular physical activity. |
| Vision ↓ | • Regularly consume sources of carotenoids, vitamin C, vitamin E, and zinc (e.g., fruits, vegetables and whole-grain breads and cereals).<br>• Moderate total fat intake.<br>• Wear sunglasses in sunny conditions.<br>• Avoid tobacco products.<br>• Perform regular physical activity (to lessen insulin resistance).<br>• In the case of diagnosed moderate macular degeneration, talk with a physician about following a protocol of zinc, copper, vitamin E, vitamin C, and beta-carotene supplementation. |
| Lean tissue ↓ | • Meet nutrient needs, especially protein and vitamin D.<br>• Perform regular physical activity, including strength training. |
| Cardiovascular function ↓ | • Use diet modifications or physician-prescribed medications to keep blood lipids and blood pressure within desirable ranges.<br>• Stay physically active.<br>• Achieve and maintain a healthy body weight. |
| Bone mass ↓ | • Meet nutrient needs, especially calcium and vitamin D (regular sun exposure helps meet needs for vitamin D).<br>• Perform regular physical activity, especially weight-bearing exercise.<br>• Women should consider use of approved osteoporosis medications at menopause.<br>• Remain at a healthy weight (especially avoid unneeded weight loss). |
| Mental function ↓ | • Meet nutrient needs, especially for vitamin E, vitamin C, vitamin B-6, folate, and vitamin B-12.<br>• Strive for lifelong learning.<br>• Perform regular physical activity.<br>• Obtain adequate sleep. |
| Fat stores ↓ | • Avoid overeating.<br>• Perform regular physical activity. |

Registered dietitians, physicians, and pharmacists can help with any needed adjustments arising from these and other drug-related problems.

▲ Older people benefit from aerobic and strength-training (resistance) exercises. Download a free copy of *Exercise & Physical Activity: Your Everyday Guide* from the National Institute on Aging at **www.nia.nih.gov**.

mainly caused by insufficient vitamin D. Osteoporosis can limit the ability of older people to move about, shop, prepare food, and live normally. Consuming adequate vitamin D, calcium, and protein and not smoking, drinking alcohol moderately or not at all, and engaging in weight-bearing exercises can help preserve bone mass. Medications also can help lessen bone loss.

## MAKING DECISIONS

### Exercise Guidelines for Older Adults

Aerobic Exercise: All adults should engage in moderate intensity aerobic exercise for 30 minutes daily, at least five times per week, or vigorous intensity aerobic exercise for 20 minutes daily for three days weekly. This amount of aerobic activity aids in prevention of chronic diseases. Longer duration of daily exercise may be required for weight loss or weight maintenance. Weight bearing exercises are particularly helpful for preservation of bone mass.

Strength Training: To maintain lean tissue and basal metabolic rate, strength training should include eight to ten different exercises (each with two sets of eight to fifteen repetitions), performed two to three times per week. Exercises that involve the large muscle groups (e.g., arms, back, and legs) and exercises that enhance grip strength should be emphasized. Start slowly, concentrate on breathing, rest between sets, avoid locking joints in the arms and legs, and stop an exercise if it becomes painful.

Flexibility Exercises: To prevent injuries, ten minutes of stretching major muscle and tendons should accompany aerobic or strength exercises.

Balance Exercises: For those over age 65 who are at risk for falling, exercises that improve balance (e.g., yoga, tai chi) are recommended in addition to aerobic, strength, and flexibility exercises.

Having an exercise plan, developed with a health professional to accommodate individual health risks and needs, will enhance success for older adults. Men older than age 40; women older than age 50; those with heart conditions, diabetes, or joint problems; and anyone who has been sedentary should consult a physician before beginning an exercise program.

Learn more at: **www.acsm.org**.

**Digestive System.** The production of HCl, intrinsic factor, and lactase declines with advancing age and, as a result, impairs the absorption of several nutrients. Constipation is the main intestinal problem for older people. To prevent constipation, older people should meet fiber needs, drink enough fluids, and exercise. Fiber medications are generally unnecessary but may be useful when total energy consumption does not allow for enough fiber intake. Because some medications can cause constipation, a physician should be consulted to determine if a laxative or stool softener is needed.

In addition to changes in the GI tract, the functions of the accessory organs decline as we age. For instance, the liver functions less efficiently. A history of significant alcohol consumption or liver disease will cause the liver to function even less efficiently. As liver efficiency declines, its ability to detoxify many substances, including medications, alcohol, and vitamin and mineral supplements, drops. The possibility for vitamin toxicity increases.

The gallbladder also functions less efficiently in later years. Gallstones can block the flow of bile out of the gallbladder into the small intestine, thereby interfering with fat digestion. Obesity is a major risk factor for gallbladder disease, especially in older women. A low-fat diet or surgery to remove the gallbladder may be necessary.

Although pancreatic function may decline with age, this organ has a large reserve capacity. One sign of a failing pancreas is high blood glucose, although this can occur as the result of several conditions. The pancreas may be secreting less insulin, or cells may be resisting insulin action (as is commonly seen in obese people with upper-body fat storage). Where appropriate, improved nutrient intake, regular physical activity, and loss of excess body weight can improve insulin action and blood glucose regulation.

**Nervous System.** A gradual loss of nerve cells that transmit signals may decrease taste and smell perceptions and impair neuromuscular coordination, reasoning, and memory. Both hearing and vision decline with age. Hearing impairment is greatest in those who have been exposed constantly to loud noises, such as urban traffic, aircraft noise, and music. Because they cannot hear well, older people may avoid social contacts, which increases their risk of poor dietary intake.

Declining eyesight, frequently caused by retina degeneration and cataracts, can affect a person's abilities to grocery shop, locate desired foods, read labels for nutritional content, and prepare foods at home. Vision losses also may cause people to curtail social contacts, reduce physical activity, and not practice daily personal health and grooming routines. Macular degeneration, one form of failing eyesight in old age, is quite common, affecting about 1.75 million adults in the U.S. A major risk factor is cigarette smoking. Diets rich in carotenoids help reduce the risk of macular degeneration. The risk of developing cataracts is decreased by consuming a diet rich in fruits and vegetables.

Neuromuscular coordination losses may make it difficult to shop for and prepare food. Physical tasks as simple as opening food packages can become so difficult that individuals restrict dietary intake to foods that require little preparation and depend on others to provide food that is ready to eat. Eating may become difficult, too. Loss of coordination makes it a challenge to grasp cup handles and manipulate eating utensils. As a result, older adults may avoid foods that can be easily spilled (e.g., soups and juices) or that need to be cut (e.g., meats, large vegetable pieces) and restrict food intake to easy-to-eat finger foods. Some may even withdraw from social interaction and eat alone, which can lead to inadequate nutrient intake.

**Immune System.** With age, the immune system often operates less efficiently. Consuming adequate protein, vitamins (especially folate and vitamins A, D, and E), iron, and zinc helps maximize immune system function. Recurrent sicknesses and poor wound healing are warning signs that a deficient diet (especially of protein and zinc) may be hindering the function of the immune system. On the other hand, overnutrition appears to be equally harmful to the immune system. For example, obesity and excessive fat, iron, and zinc intakes can suppress immune function.

**Endocrine System.** As adulthood progresses, the rate of hormone synthesis and release can slow. A decrease in insulin release or sensitivity to insulin, for instance, means that it takes longer for blood glucose levels to return to normal after a meal. Maintaining a healthy weight, exercising regularly, eating a diet low in fat and high in fiber, and avoiding foods with a high glycemic index can enhance the body's ability to use insulin and restore elevated blood glucose levels to normal after a meal.

**Chronic Disease.** The prevalence of obesity, heart disease, osteoporosis, cancer, hypertension, and diabetes rises with age. More than eight, out of every ten, elderly people have one of these chronic and potentially debilitating diseases. Half of all elderly people have at least two chronic conditions. Chronic diseases may have a strong impact on dietary intake. For instance, excessive fatness, heart disease, and osteoporosis may impair physical mobility to the extent that victims are unable to shop for and prepare food. Chronic disease also can influence nutrient and calorie needs. Cancer, for example, boosts both nutrient and calorie needs. Hypertension may indicate a need to lower sodium intake. Nutrient utilization can be affected by chronic disease, too. For instance, diabetes alters the body's ability to utilize glucose. In addition, the effects of heart disease on the kidneys may impair their ability to reabsorb glucose, amino acids, and vitamin C.

▲ Poor dental health contributes to decreased food intake and digestive problems. Serving softer, easier to chew foods and allowing extra time for chewing and swallowing improves food intake.

## MAKING DECISIONS

### Nutrition Interventions for Arthritis

There are over 100 forms of arthritis, a disease that causes the degeneration and roughening of the cartilage that covers and cushions the joints. Such changes in the joints cause them to ache and become inflamed and painful to move. Osteoarthritis, which increases in prevalence with advancing age, is the leading cause of disability among older persons. Rheumatoid arthritis, which is not as common, is more prevalent in younger adults.

Although precise causes or cures are unknown, many unproven "remedies" have been publicized. Unusual diets, food restrictions, and nutrient supplements are some of the more popular treatments. However, no special diet, food, or nutrient has been proven to reliably prevent, relieve, or cure arthritis in humans. As far as supplements go, glucosamine and/or chondroitin have been most extensively studied in relation to arthritis. Many, but not all studies demonstrate these supplements can relieve pain, slow the progression of joint degeneration, or rebuild cartilage. Maintaining a healthy weight, which reduces stress on painful arthritic joints, is the only diet-related treatment known to offer some relief. MyPyramid can be used as a guide in making healthy food choices for weight management.

**Medications.** Older adults are major consumers of medications (prescription and over-the-counter) and nutrient supplements. Half of all people over age 65 take several medicines each day. The rate of supplement use increases throughout adulthood, such that by age 50, approximately half of all adults are using supplements daily. Physiological declines that occur during aging (e.g., reduced body water, reduced liver and kidney function) cause the effects of medications and nutrient supplements to be exaggerated and persist longer in older adults.

Medications can improve health and quality of life, but some also adversely affect nutritional status, particularly of those who are older and/or take many different medications. For instance, some medications depress taste and smell acuity or cause anorexia or nausea that can blunt interest in eating and lead to reduced dietary intake. Some medications alter nutrient needs. Aspirin, for example, increases the likelihood of stomach bleeding, so long-term use may elevate the need for iron, as well as other nutrients. Antibiotics may deplete the body of vitamin K. Some medications may impair nutrient utilization—diuretics and laxatives may cause excessive excretion of water and minerals. Even vitamin and mineral supplements can affect nutritional status. Iron supplements taken in large doses can interfere with the functioning of zinc and copper. Folate supplements can mask vitamin B-12 deficiencies. People who must take medications should eat nutrient-dense foods and avoid any specific food or supplement that interferes with the function of the medication. For example, vitamin K can reduce the action of oral anticoagulants, aged cheese can interfere with certain drugs used to treat hypertension and depression, and grapefruit can interfere with medications such as tranquilizers and those that lower cholesterol levels. A physician or pharmacist should be consulted about any restrictions on food and/or supplements.

## Alternative Medicine and Aging

At least half of adults report using some kind of dietary or herbal supplement. Recall from Chapter 2 that these products are not evaluated by FDA for effectiveness or safety since they fall under the regulation of the 1994 Dietary Supplement Health and Education Act (DSHEA). Purity and quantity of the product in the bottle are also suspect. Table 16-3 reviews some popular herbal remedies used by older adults. Note from the table that these products can pose health risks in certain people. In addition, they may be expensive, ($100 per month or more in some cases) and are not covered by health insurance plans. Use of many herbal products has declined because of expense and questionable benefits. In 2003, sales of ginseng and St. John's wort declined by 30% and 38%, respectively.

A rational approach to the use of herbal products is to use only one product at a time, keep a diary of symptoms, and check with one's physician first before discontinuing a prescribed medication. In addition, FDA advises anyone who experiences adverse side effects from an herbal remedy to contact a physician. Physicians are then encouraged to report such adverse events to FDA, state and local health departments, and consumer protection agencies.

For additional information about herbal remedies, access the following websites. These are regularly updated and cover the herbals listed in Table 16-3, as well as many others.

Alternative Medicine Foundation
www.amfoundation.org/
National Institutes of Health National Center for Complementary and Alternative
    Medicine (NCCAM)
nccam.nih.gov/
American Botanical Council
abc.herbalgram.org/
Complementary and Alternative Medicine Program at Stanford (CAMPS)
camps.stanford.edu/
National Institutes of Health Office of Dietary Supplements
ods.od.nih.gov/
Natural Medicines Comprehensive Database
www.naturaldatabase.com

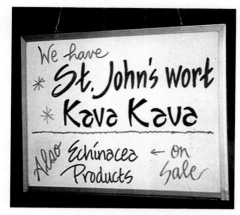

▲ Some herbal products are effective for treating specific medical problems. Follow label instructions carefully. Note potential side effects listed, as well as who should not use the product. The best advice is to only use these substances under strict supervision of a physician.

**TABLE 16-3** A Close Look at Some Popular Herbal Remedies

| Product | Purported Effects | Side Effects | Who Should Especially Seek Physician Guidance Before Use |
|---|---|---|---|
| Black cohosh | • Mild reduction of postmenopausal symptoms (shown to be effective in some but not all women; use should not go beyond 6 months in general) | • Nausea<br>• Fall in blood pressure | • Women who have had breast cancer<br>• Pregnant women<br>• Anyone taking estrogen, hypertension medications, or blood-thinning medications* |
| Cranberry | • Prevention or treatment of urinary tract infections (some evidence of efficacy) | • Use of concentrated tablets may increase risk of kidney stones | • People susceptible to kidney stones<br>• Anyone taking antidepressants or prescription painkillers |
| Echinacea | • Stimulation of the immune system<br>• Prevention or treatment of colds or other infections (mild effect at best) | • Nausea<br>• Skin irritation<br>• Allergic reactions<br>• Minor GI tract upset<br>• Increased urination | • Anyone with an autoimmune disease<br>• Pre- or postsurgical patients<br>• Anyone with allergies to daisies |
| Garlic | • Antibiotic properties<br>• Slight reduction of blood cholesterol or blood pressure in some, but not all, studies | • GI tract upset (e.g., heartburn, flatulence)<br>• Unpleasant odor | • Pre- or postsurgical patients<br>• Perinatal women<br>• People with a history of gallstones<br>• Anyone taking blood-thinning medications or AIDS medications |
| Ginkgo biloba | • Increased circulation<br>• Improvement of memory (especially for people with Alzheimer's disease; low evidence of efficacy) | • Mild headache<br>• GI tract upset<br>• Irritability<br>• Reduced blood clotting<br>• Seizures (if contaminated with toxic ginkgo seeds) | • People with bleeding disorders<br>• Pre- or postsurgical patients<br>• Anyone with allergies to the plant<br>• Concurrent use of feverfew, garlic, ginseng, dong quai, or red clover<br>• Anyone taking diabetes medications, blood-thinning medications, vitamin E supplements, antidepressants, or diuretics |

**TABLE 16-3** *(continued)*

| Product | Purported Effects | Side Effects | Who Should Especially Seek Physician Guidance Before Use |
|---|---|---|---|
| Ginseng | • Increased energy<br>• Stress relief<br>• Decreased weakness and fatigue (efficacy largely unknown) | • Hypertension<br>• Asthma attacks<br>• Irregular heartbeat<br>• Insomnia<br>• Headache<br>• Nervousness<br>• GI tract upset<br>• Reduced blood clotting<br>• Menstrual irregularities and breast tenderness | • Anyone who takes a prescription drug should consult a physician before using<br>• Women on hormone replacement therapy<br>• Women who have had breast cancer<br>• Anyone with chronic GI tract disease<br>• Anyone with uncontrolled hypertension<br>• Anyone taking blood-thinning medications, diabetes medications, antidepressants, or heart failure medications |
| St. John's wort | • Alleviation of depression (mild effect at best) | • Mild GI tract upset<br>• Rash<br>• Tiredness<br>• Restlessness<br>• Increased sensitivity to sunlight | • Anyone who takes a prescription drug<br>• People with UV sensitivity, including that induced by medications or other treatments**<br>• People with bipolar disorder<br>• Anyone recovering from a graft or organ transplant<br>• Anyone taking ritalin, caffeine, HIV medications, heart failure medications, cholesterol-lowering medications, blood-thinning medications, chemotherapy, oral contraceptives, antidepressants, antipsychotic medications, or asthma medications |
| Valerian | • Alleviation of restlessness and other sleeping disorders that stem from nervous conditions<br>• Reduction of anxiety (some evidence of efficacy) | • Impaired attention<br>• Headache<br>• Morning grogginess<br>• Irregular heartbeat<br>• GI tract upset<br>• Disagreeable odor<br>• Withdrawal delerium | • Anyone taking central nervous system depressants***<br>• Anyone who drinks alcohol<br>• People about to operate heavy machinery or drive |

Pregnant or breastfeeding women, children under 2 years of age, anyone over the age of 65 years, and anyone with a chronic disease should never take supplements unless under the guidance of a physician. A concern has been raised with regard to patients who abruptly end alternative medicines at the start of hospital treatments or deny that they are involved in alternative therapy. Interactions between alternative therapies and pharmaceutical drugs can be drastic and include complications such as delirium, clotting abnormalities, and rapid heartbeat, resulting in the need for intensive care. Full disclosure of all prescription and non-prescription treatments aids in prevention of such complications. Experts recommend that, if time permits, patients stop taking herbal products for about a week before a scheduled surgery or otherwise take all original supplement containers to the hospital, so that the anesthesiologist can evaluate what was taken.

*Coumadin, aspirin, Heparin, Lovenox, or Fragmin

**Sulfa medications, anti-inflammatory medications, or acid-reflux medications

***Valium, halcion, seconal

## Psychosocial Factors

Worries about possible embarrassment caused by deteriorating physical capabilities may cause older adults to withdraw from social interaction and eat alone rather than with others. Those who eat alone, regardless of the reason, seldom eat as much or as nutritiously as they should. Both young and old people who eat without companionship tend to feel unmotivated to shop for or prepare foods. Many become apathetic toward life, which over time causes health and nutritional status to decline. As you'll see later in the chapter, several nutrition assistance programs can help older people obtain the food and social support needed for good health.

**Depression** A positive outlook on life and intact support networks help make food and eating interesting and satisfying. In contrast, social isolation, grief, chronic pain and infirmity, or a change in lifestyle can lead to depression, loss of appetite, lack of interest in food, and disability. Depression occurs in about 12% to 30% of nursing home residents and 17% to 37% of older adults who reside outside of nursing homes. Left untreated, depression can lead to a continual decline in appetite, which results in weakness, poor nutrition, mental confusion, and increased feelings of isolation and loneliness (Fig. 16-3). In contrast, some people cope by overeating, which can lead to obesity and its associated problems. Depression may signal an underlying illness and can also impair recovery from existing illnesses or injuries. As many as 15% of cases end in suicide. For these reasons, early detection of depression is important in older adults. Depression is often treatable, but medication alone will not help those experiencing major life changes, such as the death of a spouse. Adequate social support and/or psychological intervention are also essential.

**Alzheimer's Disease.** Alzheimer's disease is an irreversible, abnormal, progressive deterioration of the brain that causes victims to steadily lose the ability to remember, reason, and comprehend. Alzheimer's disease often takes a terrible toll on the mental and eventual physical health of older people. About 4.5 million adults in the U.S. have the disease.

The 10 warning signs of Alzheimer's disease are listed in the margin. No one is sure exactly what causes this disease, but scientists have proposed various causes, including alterations in cell development or protein production in the brain, strokes, altered blood lipoprotein composition, obesity, poor blood glucose regulation (e.g., diabetes), high blood pressure, high blood cholesterol, and high free radical levels.

Early efforts at prevention are key, because the process of cognitive decline begins 10 to 20 years before warning signs appear. Preventive measures for Alzheimer's disease focus on maintaining brain activity through lifelong learning, eating a diet rich in fruits and vegetables, and taking ibuprofen. The role of nutrition in preventing or minimizing the risk of this disease is being investigated. Getting enough antioxidant nutrients, such as vitamin C, vitamin E, and selenium, helps protect the body from the damaging effects of free radicals. Adequate intakes of folate and vitamins B-6 and B-12 are especially important because elevated blood homocysteine is also a risk factor. Dietary fats, too, may play a role in keeping this disease at bay. Individuals with diets rich in omega-3 and omega-6 foods and low in saturated and *trans* fatty acids seem to have a reduced risk of Alzheimer's disease.

The dietary intakes of those with Alzheimer's disease are poor, compared with those of a similar age without this disease. Caregivers of those who have Alzheimer's disease need to monitor the patient's weight to ensure maintenance of a healthy weight and nutritional state. Other tips are serving omega-3 rich fish in meals twice per week and making sure eating habits do not pose a health risk (e.g., holding food in one's mouth or forgetting to swallow). Regular physical activity has also been shown to improve mental status in people afflicted with this disease.

**Economic Factors.** The amount of money available for purchasing food can have a great impact on the types and amounts of food one eats. Unemployment, underemployment,

**T**en Warning Signs of Alzheimer's Disease

1. Recent memory loss that affects job performance
2. Difficulty performing familiar tasks
3. Problems with language
4. Disorientation to time and place
5. Faulty or decreased judgment
6. Problems with abstract thinking
7. Tendency to misplace things
8. Changes in mood or behavior
9. Changes in personality
10. Loss of initiative

Social isolation; perhaps spouse has died.

Loses interest in food: diet deteriorates.

Poor diet leads to weakness; this increases a feeling of isolation and abandonment.

Further isolation can then decrease desire for self-care.

Health declines visibly; weakness remains.

Self-care is seriously hampered.

**FIGURE 16-3** ▶ The decline of health often seen in older adults. A small change leads to a chain of events or "domino effect" that results in poor health. This decline needs to be prevented whenever possible.

▲ Of all the alcohol sources, red wine in moderation is often singled out as the best choice because of the added bonus of the many phytochemicals present (e.g., resveratrol). These are leached out from the grape skins as the red wine is fermented. Dark beer is also a source of phytochemicals.

**ethanol** Chemical term for the form of alcohol found in alcoholic beverages.

retirement, or anything else that limits income makes it difficult to get the best, most healthful foods and can diminish nutritional status and health. Insufficient income is a particular problem among those ages 65 and up and, as a result, they frequently have trouble making sure they remain well nourished. The Commodity Foods Program and Supplemental Nutrition Assistance Program are two federal U.S. programs that can help low-income individuals of all ages procure the foods they need.

### CONCEPT CHECK

Physiological, psychosocial, and economic factors impact the nutritional status of older adults. The following organ systems and functions can decrease as we age: appetite; sense of taste, smell, thirst, hearing, and sight; digestion and absorption; liver, gallbladder, pancreatic, kidney, lung, and heart function; and the immune system. In addition, bone mass and muscle mass gradually decrease, the latter largely because of a deficient diet and inactivity. Appropriate dietary changes, regular physical activity, maintaining social contacts, and participating in nutrition assistance programs can often help reduce the impact of these factors.

## 16.5 Nutrition Implications of Alcohol Consumption

Given the wide spectrum of alcohol use and abuse, knowledge of alcohol consumption and its relationship to overall health is essential to the study of nutrition. Alcoholic beverages contain the chemical form of alcohol known as **ethanol.** Although not a nutrient *per se*, alcohol is a source of calories (about 7 kcal per gram) for approximately half of adults, constituting about 3% of total calories in the average North American diet (Table 16-4). Bear in mind that alcoholic beverages served in bars and restaurants can be 20% to 45% larger than the "standard drinks" described below.

Moderate consumption of alcohol by a person of legal age is an acceptable practice and even has some health benefits. However, only about half of alcohol consumed

**TABLE 16-4** Alcohol, Carbohydrate, and Calorie Content of Alcoholic Beverages*

| Beverage | Amount (fluid ounces) | Alcohol (grams) | Carbohydrates (grams) | Calories (kcal) |
|---|---|---|---|---|
| **Beer** | | | | |
| Regular | 12.0 | 13 | 13 | 146 |
| Light | 12.0 | 11 | 5 | 99 |
| **Distilled Spirits** | | | | |
| Gin, rum, vodka, bourbon, whiskey (80 proof), brandy, cognac | 1.5 | 14 | — | 96 |
| **Wine** | | | | |
| Red | 5 | 14 | 2 | 102 |
| White | 5 | 14 | 1 | 100 |
| Dessert, sweet | 5 | 23 | 17 | 225 |
| Rosé | 5 | 14 | 2 | 100 |
| **Mixed Drinks** | | | | |
| Manhattan | 3.0 | 26 | 3 | 191 |
| Martini | 3.0 | 27 | — | 189 |
| Bourbon and soda | 3.0 | 11 | — | 78 |
| Whiskey sour | 3.0 | 14 | 113 | 144 |

*There is little to no fat or protein contribution to calorie content.
Source: USDA.

▲ One standard drink is universally defined as one 12-oz bottle of beer or wine cooler, one 5-ounce glass of wine, 3 ounces of sherry or liqueur, or 1.5 ounces of 80-proof distilled spirits.

is done so in moderation. Nearly 14 million people in the United States suffer from alcoholism, and another 31.9 million engage in binge drinking. Alcohol by far is the most commonly abused drug.

## How Alcoholic Beverages are Produced

The basis of alcohol production is fermentation, a process by which microorganisms break down simple sugars (e.g., glucose or maltose) to alcohol, carbon dioxide, and water in the absence of oxygen. High-carbohydrate foods especially encourage the growth of yeast, the microorganism responsible for alcohol production. Wine is formed by the fermentation of grape or other fruit juices. Beer is made from malted cereal grain. Distilled spirits (e.g., vodka, gin, whiskey) are made from any number of fruits, vegetables, and grains. Production temperatures, the composition of the food used for fermentation, and aging techniques determine the characteristics of the product.

## Absorption and Metabolism of Alcohol

Alcohol requires no digestion. It is absorbed rapidly from the GI tract by diffusion, making it the most efficiently absorbed of all calorie sources. Once absorbed, alcohol is freely distributed into all the fluid compartments within the body. About 1% to 3% of alcohol is excreted via urine and about 1% to 5% evaporates via the breath, the basis for the breathalyzer test. Most alcohol (90% to 98%), however, is metabolized. The liver is the primary site for alcohol metabolism, and some may also be metabolized by the cells lining the stomach. The main pathway of alcohol metabolism involves the enzymes **alcohol dehydrogenase** and **acetaldehyde dehydrogenase**. Alcohol cannot be stored in the body, so it takes absolute priority over other energy sources for metabolism.

As a person's alcohol consumption exceeds the body's capacity to metabolize it, blood alcohol concentration rises, the brain is exposed to alcohol, and symptoms of intoxication appear (see Table 16-5). Absorption and metabolism of alcohol depend on numerous factors: gender, race, body size, physical condition, meal composition, rate of gastric emptying, the alcohol content of the beverage, use of certain drugs, chronic alcohol abuse, and even how much sleep one has had. Women absorb and metabolize alcohol differently than men. The amount of alcohol metabolized by the cells lining the stomach is greater in men than in women. Women also have less body water in which to dilute the alcohol than do men. Overall, women develop alcohol-related ailments, such as cirrhosis of the liver, more rapidly than men do with the same alcohol-consumption habits.

## Benefits of Moderate Alcohol Use

When used in moderation, alcohol is linked to several health benefits. Benefits of alcohol use are associated with specific intakes of about one drink per day for men and slightly less than one for women. Socialization and relaxation are among the intangible benefits of moderate alcohol use by people of legal drinking age. In terms of physiological benefits, moderate drinkers experience lower risk of developing cardiovascular diseases and type 2 diabetes. Previous consumers of alcohol no longer experience the benefits of alcohol when consumption ceases. See Table 16-6 for additional benefits of alcohol consumption.

## Risks of Alcohol Abuse

Despite the few benefits of regular, moderate use, the risks of **alcohol abuse** are more numerous and harmful. Although it is one of the most preventable health problems, excessive consumption of alcohol contributes significantly to 5 of the 10 leading causes of death in North America: heart failure, certain forms of cancer, **cirrhosis of the liver**, motor vehicle and other accidents, and suicides (review Table 16-6 for

**A**lcohol proof represents twice the volume of alcohol in percentage terms. Thus, 80 proof vodka is 40% alcohol.

**alcohol dehydrogenase** An enzyme used in alcohol (ethanol) metabolism that converts alcohol into acetaldehyde.

**acetaldehyde dehydrogenase** An enzyme used in ethanol metabolism that eventually converts acetaldehyde into carbon dioxide and water.

**alcohol abuse** Excessive alcohol consumption that leads to severe alcohol-related health and other problems, such as recurrent sickness, inability to fulfill major obligations, use in hazardous situations (e.g., driving), related legal problems, or use despite social and interpersonal difficulties.

**cirrhosis** A loss of functioning liver cells, which are replaced by nonfunctioning connective tissue. Any substance that poisons liver cells can lead to cirrhosis. The most common cause is a chronic, excessive alcohol intake. Exposure to certain industrial chemicals also can lead to cirrhosis.

▲ There is no such thing as controlled drinking once a person has alcoholism. Total abstinence is mandatory for recovery.

**TABLE 16-5** Blood Alcohol Concentration and Symptoms

| Concentration* | Sporadic Drinker | Chronic Drinker | Hours for Alcohol to Be Metabolized** |
|---|---|---|---|
| 50 (party high) (0.05%) | Congenial euphoria; decreased tension; noticeable impairment in driving and coordination | No observable effect | 2–3 |
| 75 (0.075%) | Gregarious | Often no effect | 3–4 |
| 80 to 100 (0.08%–0.1%) | Uncoordinated; 0.08% is legally drunk (as in drunk driving) in the United States and Canada. | Minimal signs | 4–6 |
| 125–150 (0.125%–0.15%) | Unrestrained behavior; episodic uncontrolled behavior | Pleasurable euphoria or beginning of uncoordination | 6–10 |
| 200–250 (0.2%–0.25%) | Alertness lost; lethargic | Effort is required to maintain emotional and motor control | 10–24 |
| 300–350 (0.3%–0.35%) | Stupor to coma | Drowsy and slow | 10–24 |
| >500 (>0.5%) | Some will die | Coma | >24 |

*Milligrams of alcohol per 100 milliliters of blood.

**For a social drinker; alcohol metabolism is somewhat faster in chronic alcohol abusers.

Modified from Wyngaarder JB, Smith LH: *Cecil Textbook of Medicine*, fourth edition, Philadelphia, 1988, WB Saunders. Used with permission.

**alcohol dependence** The person experiences repeated alcohol-related difficulties, such as an inability to control use, spending a great deal of time associated with alcohol use, continued use of alcohol despite physical or psychological consequences, persistent desire or unsuccessful efforts to cut down or control alcohol use, and withdrawal symptoms. Tolerance is also seen.

**alcoholism** As defined by the American Medical Association, an illness characterized by significant impairment directly related to persistent and excessive use of alcohol.

## CRITICAL THINKING

For many people, drinking and smoking go hand-in-hand. What risks and diseases could correlate with the combination of these behaviors?

additional health risks). In the United States, about $185 billion is spent annually in terms of lost productivity, premature deaths, direct treatment expenses, and legal fees associated with alcoholism. Overall, alcohol abuse typically reduces a person's life expectancy by 15 years.

Alcoholic beverages have little nutritional value and, thus, nutrient deficiencies are a common result of alcoholism. The protein and vitamin content is extremely low, except in beer, where it is marginal. Iron content varies from drink to drink, with red wine ranking especially high in iron. Typical deficiencies seen in alcoholism arise mostly from poor nutrient intakes, but increased urinary losses and fat malabsorption (linked to poor pancreatic function) are also to blame. Vitamins most susceptible to depletion in alcoholism include vitamins A, D, E, and K; thiamin; niacin; folate; vitamin B-6 and B-12, and vitamin C. Mineral deficiencies of calcium, phosphorus, potassium, magnesium, zinc, and iron are possible. On the other hand, vitamin and mineral toxicity is also of concern. Damage to the GI tract and liver, as well as high levels of some minerals in alcoholic beverages, may lead to toxicity of vitamin A, iron, lead, or cobalt. In nutritional treatment of alcoholism, the immediate aim is eliminating alcohol intake, followed by replenishment of nutrient stores.

**Alcohol dependence** is the most common psychiatric disorder, affecting 13% of the North American population. Studies suggest that about 40% of a person's risk for developing alcoholism comes from genetic factors, although the gene or genes have not been identified. Therefore, people with a family history of alcoholism, particularly children of alcoholics, should be especially aware of their alcohol consumption.

Early diagnosis of **alcoholism** can prevent multiple health problems and save millions in health care costs. Asking a person about the quantity and frequency of alcohol consumption is an important means of detecting abuse and dependence (see the margin note on the CAGE questionnaire on p. 642). Alcoholics may exhibit some or all of the following criteria:

- Physiologic dependence on alcohol with evidence of withdrawal symptoms when intake is interrupted
- Tolerance to the effects of alcohol, prompting greater alcohol intake to achieve the desired effect

**TABLE 16-6** A Summary of Benefits and Risks of Alcohol Use

| | Moderate Use* | Alcohol Abuse** |
|---|---|---|
| Coronary heart disease | Decreased risk of death in those at high risk for coronary heart disease-related death, primarily by increasing HDL-cholesterol in some people, decreasing blood clotting, and relaxing blood vessels | Heart rhythm disturbances, heart muscle damage, increased blood triglycerides, and increased blood clotting |
| Hypertension and stroke | Mild decrease in blood pressure; less ischemic stroke in people with normal blood pressure | Increased blood pressure (hypertension); more ischemic and hemorrhagic stroke |
| Peripheral vascular disease | Decreased risk due to reduced blood clotting | No benefit |
| Blood glucose regulation and type 2 diabetes | Decreased risk of developing type 2 diabetes; decreased risk of death from cardiovascular disease | Hypoglycemia; reduced insulin sensitivity; damage to pancreas (site of insulin production) |
| Bone and joint health | Some increase in bone mineral content in women, linked to estrogen output | Loss of active bone-forming cells and eventual osteoporosis (many nutrient deficiencies also contribute to this problem); increased risk of gout |
| Brain function | Enhanced brain function and decreased risk of dementia by increasing blood circulation in the brain | Brain tissue damage and decreased memory |
| Skeletal muscle health | No benefit | Skeletal muscle damage |
| Cancer | No benefit | Increased risk of oral, esophageal, stomach, liver, lung, colorectal, and breast cancer, to name a few (especially if the diet is deficient in the vitamin folate) |
| Liver function | No benefit | Fatty infiltration and eventual liver cirrhosis, especially if a person is also infected with hepatitis C; iron toxicity |
| GI tract disease | Decreased risk of certain bacterial infections in the stomach | Inflammation of the stomach (and pancreas); absorptive cell damage leading to malabsorption of nutrients |
| Immune system function | No benefit | Reduced function and increased infections |
| Nervous system function | No benefit | Loss of nerve sensation and nervous system control of muscles |
| Sleep disturbances | Some relaxation | Fragmented sleep patterns; worsens sleep apnea |
| Impotence and decreased libido | No benefit | Contributes to the problem in both men and women |
| Drug overdose | No benefit | Contributes to the problem, especially in combination with sedatives |
| Obesity | No benefit | Increased abdominal fat deposition, contributes to weight gain as calories from alcoholic beverages quickly add up |
| Nutrient intake | May supply some B vitamins and iron | Leads to numerous nutrient deficiencies: protein, vitamins, and minerals |
| Alcoholism | No benefit. Due to risk for birth defects, even moderate alcohol use is not advised during pregnancy (see Chapter 14) | Increased risk of developing alcoholism, including the teenage and young adult years |
| Fetal health | No benefit | Variety of toxic effects on the fetus when alcohol is consumed by pregnant women (see Chapter 14) |
| Socialization and relaxation | Provides some benefit to socialization and leads to relaxation by increasing brain neurotransmitter activity | Contributes to violent behavior and agitation |
| Traffic deaths and other violent deaths | No benefit | Contributes to both traffic death and violent death |

*About one drink per day for men and slightly less than one for women.

**The risks from alcohol abuse begin at an intake of more than two to three drinks per day for men or one to two drinks per day for women and all adults age 65 and older. Binge drinking (more than four drinks in a row for women or more than five drinks for men) can be especially harmful.

**T**he CAGE questionnaire is used to identify alcohol abuse. More than one positive response suggests an alcohol problem.

C: Have you ever felt you ought to *cut* down on drinking?

A: Have people *annoyed* you by criticizing your drinking?

G: Have you ever felt bad or *guilty* about your drinking?

E: Have you ever had a drink first thing in the morning to steady your nerves or get rid of a hangover (*eye-opener)?*

**E**thnicity plays an important role in both the probability of and health risks associated with alcohol dependency and abuse. Native Americans suffer the highest rates of unintentional injuries, suicide, homicide, and domestic abuse related to alcohol use. African-American alcoholics are at greater risk than other racial groups for tuberculosis, hepatitis C, HIV/AIDS, and other infectious diseases. Hispanic Americans are at particular risk for cirrhosis-related death.

▲ Alcohol is particularly damaging to the liver. Pictured are (a) healthy liver, (b) liver with cirrhosis. There is no cure for this disease except a liver transplant.

- Evidence of alcohol-associated illnesses such as alcoholic liver disease or irreversible brain damage exhibited by memory loss, inability to concentrate, and decline in intellectual functions
- Continued drinking in defiance of strong medical and social contraindications and disruptions in normal life
- Depression, blackouts, and impairment in social and occupational functioning

Other signs of alcoholism include: alcohol odor on the breath; flushed face and reddened skin; and nervous system disorders, such as tremors. Unexplained work absences, frequent accidents, and falls or injuries of vague origin are possible signs of alcoholism. Laboratory evidence (e.g., impaired liver function, enlarged red blood cells, and elevated triglycerides) are also helpful for diagnosis of alcoholism.

Older adults are uniquely vulnerable to alcoholism, perhaps due to an abundance of free time, social events involving drinking, loneliness, or depression. Common symptoms of alcoholism—trembling hands, slurred speech, sleep problems, memory loss, and unsteady gait—can be easily overlooked as signs of old age. Slower alcohol metabolism and decreased body water allow older adults to become intoxicated from a smaller amount of alcohol than their younger counterparts. Even moderate alcohol consumption can exacerbate some chronic health conditions, such as diabetes and osteoporosis. As well, even small amounts of alcohol can react negatively with various medications used by older persons. The adverse health effects of drinking may be amplified in older adults, so people over the age of 65 should limit alcohol consumption to no more than one drink per day.

Once a diagnosis of alcohol abuse or dependence is established, a physician can arrange appropriate treatment and counseling for the person and family. Treatment of alcoholism often includes the use of certain medications, counseling, and social support. Total abstinence must be the ultimate objective. Alcoholics Anonymous (AA) or other reputable therapy programs can support alcoholics and their families as they recover from this devastating disease.

## MAKING DECISIONS

### Liver Cirrhosis

Alcohol is most damaging to the liver. Cirrhosis develops in up to 20% of cases of alcoholism and is the second leading reason for liver transplants, affecting about 2 million people in the United States. This chronic and usually relentlessly progressive disease is characterized by fatty infiltration of the liver. Fatty liver occurs in response to increased synthesis of fat and decreased use of it for energy by the liver. Eventually, the enlarged fat deposits choke off the blood supply, depriving the liver cells of oxygen and nutrients. Liver cells can accumulate so much fat that they burst and die and are replaced by connective (scar) tissue. At this stage, the liver is deemed cirrhotic. Early stages of alcoholic liver injury are reversible, but advanced stages are not. Once a person has cirrhosis, there is a 50% chance of death within 4 years, a far worse prognosis than many forms of cancer. While no specific level of alcohol consumption guarantees cirrhosis, some evidence suggests that damage is caused by a dose as low as 40 grams per day for men (3 beers) and 20 grams per day for women (1½ beers).

## Guidance Regarding Alcohol Use

No government agencies recommend drinking alcohol. The 2005 Dietary Guidelines for Americans provides the following advice regarding use of alcoholic beverages:

- Those who choose to drink alcoholic beverages should do so sensibly and in moderation—defined as the consumption of up to one drink per day for women and older adults and up to two drinks per day for men.
- Alcoholic beverages should not be consumed by some individuals, including those who cannot restrict their alcohol intake, women of childbearing age who may become pregnant, pregnant and lactating women, children and adolescents,

individuals taking medications that can interact with alcohol, and those with specific medical conditions.

- Alcoholic beverages should be avoided by individuals engaging in activities that require attention, skill, or coordination, such as driving or operating machinery.

As the understanding of the relationship between drinking alcohol and health grows, registered dietitians and other health professionals can promote healthy lifestyles—not by encouraging indiscriminate drinking, but rather by reassuring adults that moderate alcohol consumption may have beneficial health outcomes.

## CONCEPT CHECK

Alcohol is not an essential nutrient but does supply calories for the body. It requires no digestion, and alcohol metabolism takes precedence over metabolism of the other energy-yielding nutrients. Alcohol is primarily metabolized in the liver by alcohol dehydrogenase and acetaldehyde dehydrogenase. A number of individual factors, such as gender, race, and body composition, determine how a person reacts to alcohol. Despite modest benefits of moderate alcohol use, alcoholism interferes with all aspects of family, professional, and social life. Excessive alcohol use increases the risk of hypertension, strokes, heart damage, birth defects, inflammation of the pancreas, brain damage, and malnutrition, to name a few. Treatment of alcoholism often includes the use of certain medications, counseling, and social support.

▲ The limit for alcohol intake for older adults is one drink per day.

*Healthy People 2010* set an important goal regarding alcohol use: Reduce by 25% the proportion of adults who exceed the guidelines for appropriate alcohol use (currently, 73% of those who consume alcohol).

## 16.6 Ensuring a Healthful Diet for the Adult Years

Recommended dietary practices for later years would be to increase the diet's nutrient density and to make sure fiber and fluid intake is adequate. In addition, some protein should come from lean meats to help meet protein, vitamin B-6, vitamin B-12, iron, and zinc needs.

Singles of all ages face logistical problems with food: Purchasing, preparing, storing, and using food with minimal waste are challenging. Economy packages of meats and vegetables are normally too large to be useful for a single person. Many singles live in small dwellings, some without kitchens and freezers. Creating a diet to accommodate a limited budget and facilities and a single appetite requires special considerations. The following are some practical suggestions for diet planning for singles:

- If one owns a freezer, cook large amounts, divide into portions, and freeze.
- Buy only what one uses; small containers may be expensive, but letting food spoil is also costly.
- Ask the grocer to break open a family-sized package of wrapped meat or fresh vegetables and separate it into smaller units.
- Buy only several pieces of fruit—perhaps a ripe one, a medium-ripe one, and an unripe one—so that the fruit can be eaten over a period of several days.
- Keep a box of dry milk handy to add nutrients to recipes for baked foods and other foods for which this addition is acceptable.

Table 16-7 provides more ideas for healthful eating in later years.

Nutritional deficiencies and protein-calorie undernutrition have been identified among some aging populations, particularly those in hospitals, nursing homes, or long-term care facilities. These nutritional problems increase the risk for many diseases, including bed sores (pressure ulcers), and compromise recovery from illness and surgery. Friends, relatives, and health care professionals should monitor nutrient intake in all older people, including those who live in long-term care facilities. Family members can play a valuable role in making sure nutrient needs are met by looking for weight maintenance based on regular, healthful meal patterns. If problems arise in consuming a healthful diet, registered dietitians can offer professional and personalized advice.

*T*o learn more about alcoholism, visit these websites:

National Institute on Alcohol Abuse and Alcoholism; **www.niaaa.nih.gov**

American Society of Addiction Medicine; **asam.org**

American Self-Help Clearinghouse; **mentalhelp.net/selfhelp**.

*A*ppendix C reviews diet planning guidelines issued by the Canadian government for Canadians. In addition, Chapter 1 discussed *Healthy People 2010*, a U.S. federal agenda aimed at disease prevention and health promotion.

**D**etermine:

- **D**isease
- **E**ating poorly
- **T**ooth loss or mouth pain
- **E**conomic hardship
- **R**educed social contact and interaction
- **M**ultiple medications
- **I**nvoluntary weight loss or gain
- **N**eed for assistance with self-care
- **E**lder at an advanced age

**T**o learn about meal programs for senior citizens in your area, call the *Administration on Aging's Elder Care Locator*, (800) 677-1116. For general information on programs for older persons, visit the following websites: *National Institute on Aging*, **www.nia.nih.gov**; *American Geriatrics Society*, **www.americangeriatrics.org/**; and *Administration on Aging*, **www.aoa.gov**.

▲ Great attention to food safety is also important for older adults. Chapter 13 provides advice on this topic, such as washing one's hands and work surface before preparing food.

**TABLE 16-7** Guidelines for Healthful Eating in Later Years

- Eat regularly; small, frequent meals may be best. Use nutrient-dense foods as a basis for menus.

- Use labor-saving devices and some convenience foods, but try to incorporate some fresh foods into daily menus.

- Try new foods, new seasonings, and new ways of preparing foods. Use canned goods in moderation or choose those low in sodium.

- Keep easy-to-prepare foods on hand for times when you feel tired.

- Have a treat occasionally, perhaps an expensive cut of meat or a favorite fresh fruit.

- Eat in a well-lit or sunny area; serve meals attractively; use foods with different flavors, colors, shapes, textures, and smells.

- Arrange kitchen and eating area so that food preparation and clean-up are easier.

- Eat with friends, relatives, or at a senior center when possible.

- Share cooking responsibilities with a neighbor.

- Use community resources for help in shopping and other daily care needs.

- Stay physically active.

- If possible, take a walk before eating to stimulate appetite.

- When necessary, chop, grind, or blend hard-to-chew foods. Softer, protein-rich foods (e.g., shredded meats, eggs) can be substituted for meat when poor dental function limits normal food intake. Prepare soups, stews, cooked whole-grain cereals, and casseroles.

- If your dexterity is limited, cut the food ahead of time, use utensils with deep sides or handles, and obtain more specialized utensils if needed.

Overall, older adults benefit from good nutrition in many ways. As we discussed for younger adults, meeting nutrient needs delays the onset of some diseases; improves the management of some existing diseases; hastens recovery from many illnesses; increases mental, physical, and social well-being; and often decreases the need for and length of hospitalization. A Modified MyPyramid (Fig. 16-4) for Older Adults incorporates the basic nutrition and activity messages of MyPyramid, but emphasizes nutrients of special concern (e.g., calcium, vitamin D, vitamin B-12). A focus on nutrient-dense food choices, plenty of fluids, modified physical activity goals, and use of certain dietary supplements address the unique needs of older adults.

Obtaining enough food may be difficult for some older persons, especially if they are unable to drive and relatives do not live close enough to help with cooking or shopping. For an older person, a request for help may be equated to a loss of independence. Pride, or fear of being victimized by those they hire, may stand in the way of much-needed help. In these cases, friends can be a big help. Special transportation arrangements may also be available through a local transit company or taxi service.

Many eligible older people are missing meals and are poorly nourished because they don't know of available programs to help them. Irregular meal patterns and weight loss, often caused by difficulties in preparing food, are warning signs that undernutrition may be developing. An effort should be made to identify poorly nourished people and inform them of community services.

## Community Nutrition Services for Older People

Health care advice and services for older people can come from clinics, private practitioners, hospitals, and health maintenance organizations. Home health care agencies, adult day-care programs, adult over-night-care programs, and **hospice care** (for the terminally ill) can provide daily care.

The Nutrition Screening Initiative, a nutrition checklist for health care workers, family members, and older persons, can be used as a tool to increase health and nutrition awareness and to plan related education of older persons (Fig. 16-2). The Nutrition Screening Initiative uses the acronym "DETERMINE" (see margin) to help identify older people whose health needs require extra attention.

Nutrition programs for those age 60 and over in the United States include congregate meal programs, which provide lunch at a central location, and home-delivered meals (often known as Meals on Wheels if sponsored by the local private or public agencies). About 2.6 million older adults are served each year. About half of the meals use the home-delivered method.

The U.S. federal government sets specific standards for home-delivered meals and for those served in congregate feeding centers. The meals are designed to provide one-third of RDA/AI. The social aspect often improves appetite and general outlook on life.

Still, congregate meal programs generally provide one meal a day (some provide more) and usually just 5 days per week. Another problem with home-delivered meals is that the one or two meals delivered may never be eaten, and, if not eaten on delivery and left at room temperature, they may become unsafe to eat later. Thus, these programs can help older adults but probably don't meet all their nutritional needs.

In addition to congregate and home-delivered meals, federal commodity distribution is available in some areas of the United States to low-income older people. Older people whose incomes are below the poverty level can benefit from the SNAP program (food stamps) (see Chapter 12 for details on these programs). Food cooperatives and a variety of clubs and religious and social organizations provide additional aid.

**Modified MyPyramid for Older Adults**

2007© TUFTS UNIVERSITY

**FIGURE 16-4** ▶ Modified MyPyramid for Older Adults. Nutrient density is important for aging adults because micronutrient needs remain high despite declining calorie needs.

**hospice care** A program offering care that emphasizes comfort and dignity in death.

## CONCEPT CHECK

A nutrient-dense diet helps meet the unique needs of aging adults. Carefully planned use of multivitamin and mineral supplements can also help, especially for adults 70 years of age and older. Diet planning should be tailored to the individual's physiological, psychosocial, and economic status. In the United States, many nutrition services–such as congregate and home-delivered meals–are available to help the aging population obtain a healthful diet.

# Nutrition and Cancer

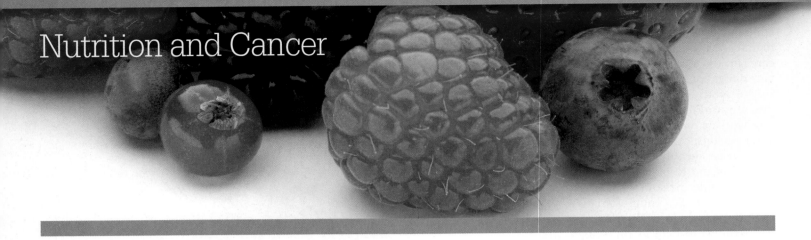

Cancer is the second leading cause of death for North American adults. It is further estimated that more than 1500 people die each day of cancer in the United States. Cancer-related expenses exceed $100 billion each year. The top four cancers, causing more than 50% of cancer deaths, are lung, colorectal, breast, and prostate cancers. Of those, lung cancer in female smokers is the only form increasing on a yearly basis.

Cancer is many diseases; these differ in the types of cells affected and, in some cases, in the factors contributing to cancer development (Fig. 16-5). For example, the factors leading to skin cancer differ from those leading to breast cancer. Similarly, the treatments for the different types of cancer often vary.

Cancer essentially represents abnormal and uncontrollable division of cells that results from mutations in DNA. This initiates the cancer process. The cells then go through a variety of steps (called promotion and progression). A cancer cell is the result. Without effective treatment, cancer then typically leads to death. Most cancers take the form of tumors, although not all tumors are cancers. A **tumor** is spontaneous new tissue growth that serves no physiological purpose. It can be **benign,** like a wart, or **malignant,** like most lung cancers. The terms *malignant tumor* and *malignant neoplasm* are synonymous with cancer.

Whereas benign tumors are only dangerous if their presence interferes with normal body functions, malignant (cancerous) tumors are capable of invading surrounding structures, including blood vessels, the lymph system, and nervous tissue. Cancer can also spread, or **metastasize,** to distant sites via the blood and lymphatic circulation, thereby producing invasive tumors in almost any part of the body. Metastasis then makes the cancer much more difficult to treat. That cancer can spread explains why early detection of cancer is so important. Cancers that can be diagnosed in the early stages are those in the colon, breast, and cervix.

Genetics, environment, lifestyle are potent forces that influence the risk for developing cancer. A genetic predisposition is especially important in development of colon cancer, some types of breast cancer (e.g., mutated BRCA1 or BRCA2 gene) and prostate cancer (35%, 27%, and 42%, respectively). About 30 cancer-susceptibility genes have been identified. However, experts estimate that only 1% to 5% of most cancers can be explained by the inheritance of a cancer gene. Overall, lifestyle and environmental exposures are also critical factors in most forms of cancer, as evidenced by the variation in cancer rates from country to country. In fact, diet likely accounts for 30% to 40% or more of all cancers.

Although we have little control over our genetic risks for cancer, we can exert a great deal of authority when making decisions about lifestyle risks, especially with regard to smoking, alcohol abuse, physical activity, and nutrient intake (food choice). It is well established that one-third of all cancers in North America are due directly to tobacco use. About half of the cancers of the mouth, pharynx, and larynx are associated with heavy use of alcohol. A combination of alcohol use and smoking increases cancer risks even higher.

▲ Cruciferous vegetables such as cabbage and cauliflower are rich in cancer-preventing phytochemicals.

**tumor** Mass of cells; may be cancerous (malignant) or noncancerous (benign).

**benign** Noncancerous; tumors that do not spread.

**malignant** Malicious; in reference to a tumor, the property of spreading locally and to distant sites.

**metastasize** The spreading of disease from one part of the body to another, even to parts of the body that are remote from the site of the original tumor. Cancer cells can spread via blood vessels, the lymphatic system, or direct growth of the tumor.

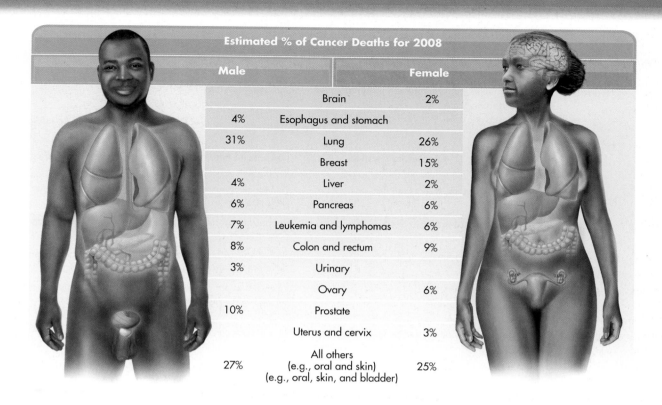

| Estimated % of Cancer Deaths for 2008 | | |
| Male | | Female |
| --- | --- | --- |
| | Brain | 2% |
| 4% | Esophagus and stomach | |
| 31% | Lung | 26% |
| | Breast | 15% |
| 4% | Liver | 2% |
| 6% | Pancreas | 6% |
| 7% | Leukemia and lymphomas | 6% |
| 8% | Colon and rectum | 9% |
| 3% | Urinary | |
| | Ovary | 6% |
| 10% | Prostate | |
| | Uterus and cervix | 3% |
| 27% | All others (e.g., oral and skin) (e.g., oral, skin, and bladder) | 25% |

**FIGURE 16-5** ▶ Cancer is many diseases. Numerous types of cells and organs are its target. About one-third of all cancers arise from smoking (primarily lung cancer).

## A Closer Look at Diet and Cancer

Some food constituents may contribute to cancer development, whereas others have a protective effect (Table 16-8). First the association between fat/calorie intake and cancer risk is discussed, and then some of the food constituents that may reduce the risk for cancer are presented.

### Contribution of Calorie and Fat Intakes to Cancer Risk

An excess calorie intake, leading eventually to obesity, is related to all major forms of cancer, except lung cancer. This is the main diet-cancer risk factor. This includes cancer of the breast (especially in postmenopausal women), pancreas, kidney, gallbladder, colon, **endometrium,** and prostate gland. The link probably occurs between adipose tissue and the synthesis of estrogen. High concentrations of circulating estrogen in the blood over time promote cancer. Excess insulin output resulting from an obese, insulin-resistant state is also implicated.

The National Cancer Institute (NCI) also believes there is sufficient evidence for a link between dietary fat and cancer to encourage North Americans to reduce fat intake. It recommends initially decreasing dietary fat to about 30% of total calorie intake and eventually to 20% or less of total calories if the person is at high risk and can follow such a dietary pattern.

Some scientists, however, believe that the NCI has overreacted to the fat and cancer issue. Although epidemiological evidence does link fat and certain forms of cancer, the evidence is not strong. A stronger link exists between cancer and excess calories in the diet. In animal experiments, restricting total calorie intake to about 70% of usual intake results in about a 40% reduction in tumor development, regardless of the amount of fat in the diet. Calorie restriction is the most effective technique for preventing cancer in laboratory animals.

Unfortunately, it is difficult for humans to reduce dietary calories to 70% of usual intake. So while the data obtained from laboratory animal studies are interesting, nutritionists do not see any practical way to make recommendations on the basis of these studies. In addition, once cancer is present, calorie restriction is no longer helpful.

### Cancer-Inhibiting Food Constituents

Many single nutrients may have cancer-inhibiting properties. These anticarcinogens include antioxidants and certain phytochemicals (review Table 16-8).

The antioxidant activity of vitamin C and vitamin E helps to prevent formation of **nitrosamines** in the GI tract, thus preventing formation of a potent carcinogen. Vitamin E also helps protect unsaturated fatty acids from damage by free radicals. Overall, carotenoids, vitamin E, vitamin C, and selenium function as or contribute to antioxidant protection

**endometrium** The membrane that lines the inside of the uterus. It increases in thickness during the menstrual cycle until ovulation occurs. The surface layers are shed during menstruation if conception does not take place.

**nitrosamine** A carcinogen formed from nitrates and breakdown products of amino acids; can lead to stomach cancer.

**TABLE 16-8** Some Food Constituents Suspected of Having a Role in Cancer

| Constituent | Dietary Sources | Action |
| --- | --- | --- |
| **Possibly Protective\*** | | |
| Vitamin A | Liver, fortified milk, fruits, vegetables | Encourages normal cell development. |
| Vitamin D | Fortified milk | Increases production of a protein that suppresses cell growth, such as in the colon. |
| Vitamin E | Whole grains, vegetable oils, green leafy vegetables | Prevents formation of nitrosamines; general antioxidant properties. |
| Vitamin C | Fruits, vegetables | Can block conversion of nitrites and nitrates to potent carcinogens; likely has general antioxidant properties. |
| Folate | Fruits, vegetables, whole grains | Encourages normal cell development; especially reduces the risk of colon cancer. |
| Selenium | Meats, whole grains | Part of antioxidant system that inhibits tumor growth and kills developing cancer cells. |
| Carotenoids, such as lycopene | Fruits, vegetables | Likely act as antioxidants; some of these possibly influence cell metabolism. Lycopene in particular may reduce the risk of prostate cancer. |
| Flavonoids, indoles, phenols, and other phytochemicals | Vegetables, especially cabbage, cauliflower, broccoli, brussels sprouts, garlic, onions, tea | May reduce cancer in the stomach and other organs. |
| Calcium | Milk products, green vegetables | Slows cell division in the colon, binds bile acids and free fatty acids, thus reducing colon cancer risk. |
| Omega-3 fatty acids | Cold-water fish, such as salmon and tuna | May inhibit tumor growth. |
| Soy products | Tofu, soy milk, tempeh, soy nuts | Phytic acid present possibly binds carcinogens in the intestinal tract; the genistein component possibly reduces growth and metastasis of malignant cells. |
| Conjugated linoleic acid | Milk products, meats | May inhibit tumor development and act as an antioxidant. |
| Fiber-rich foods | Fruits, vegetables, whole-grain breads and cereals, beans, nuts | Colon and rectal cancer risk may be decreased by accelerating intestinal transit or binding carcinogens such that they are excreted. |
| **Possibly Carcinogenic** | | |
| Excessive calorie intake | All macronutrients can contribute | Excess fat mass leading to obesity; linked to increased synthesis of estrogen and other sex hormones, which in excess may themselves increase the risk for cancer. Resulting excess insulin output from creation of an insulin-resistant state is also implicated. |
| Total fat | Meats, high-fat milk and milk products, animal fats and vegetable oils | The strongest evidence is for excessive saturated and polyunsaturated fat intake. Saturated fat is linked to an increased risk of prostate cancer. |
| High glycemic load carbohydrates | Cookies, cakes, sugared soft drinks, candy | Insulin surges associated with these foods may increase tumor growth, such as in the colon. |
| Alcohol | Beer, wine, liquor | Contributes to cancers of the throat, liver, bladder, breast, and colon (especially if the person does not consume enough folate). |
| Nitrites, nitrates | Cured meats, especially ham, bacon, and sausages | Under very high temperatures will bind to amino acid derivatives to form nitrosamines, potent carcinogens. |
| Multi-ring compounds: Aflatoxin | Formed when mold is present on peanuts or grains | May alter DNA structure and inhibit its ability to properly respond to physiologic controls; aflatoxin in particular is linked to liver cancer. |
| Benzo(a)pyrene and other heterocyclic amines | Charcoal-broiled foods, especially meats | Linked to stomach and colon cancer. To limit this risk, trim fat from meat before cooking, cut barbecuing time by partially cooking meat (such as in a microwave oven), and don't consume blackened parts. |

\*Many of the actions listed for these possibly protective agents are speculative and have been verified only by experimental animal studies. The best evidence supports obtaining these nutrients and other food constituents from foods. The U.S. Preventive Services Task Force (USPSTF) supports this statement, noting there is no clear evidence that nutrient supplements provide the same benefits.

for the body. Some of these antioxidant systems help prevent DNA mutations by electron-seeking compounds, the main way that cancer develops in the first place.

In addition, phytochemicals from fruits and vegetables, and even tea, block cancer development in some types of cells. Numerous studies suggest that fruit and vegetable intake reduces the risk of nearly all types of cancer. These foods are normally rich in carotenoids, vitamin C, and vitamin E. Adequate vitamin D intake is suspected of reducing breast, colon, prostate, and other forms of cancer. Calcium is also linked to a decreased risk for developing colon cancer. In sum, a diet that follows MyPyramid, so that fruits, vegetables, whole grains, low-fat and fat-free dairy products, and some plant oils are eaten daily, is aimed at cancer prevention. It is likely that all of these foods have a "cocktail" effect, and that no one particular food can make as strong a claim.

### Nutrition Concerns during Cancer Treatment

Nutrition concerns during cancer treatment may vary depending on the site of the cancer, but the overall goals of medical nutrition therapy are to minimize weight loss and prevent nutrient deficiencies. Weight loss, particularly loss of muscle mass, is a major concern during cancer treatment because poor nutrition status can limit recovery from illness. Common effects of cancer and/or cancer treatments include fatigue, mouth sores, dry mouth, taste abnormalities, nausea, and diarrhea– all of which can lead to poor food intake.

During cancer treatment, the best food to eat is any food the patient can tolerate. Food choices vary based on each patient's individual symptoms, but cool, non-acidic liquids and soft, mildly-flavored foods are generally well-accepted. Small, frequent meals and foods with high nutrient density and calorie density should be emphasized to meet calorie and protein needs. Often, liquid nutritional supplements are needed. Because immunity may be suppressed during cancer treatment, safe food handling practices also are extremely important (review Chapter 13).

## The Bottom Line

Given the toll of cancer treatment and lack of a definitive cure, efforts at prevention are key. A variety of dietary changes will reduce your risk for cancer. Start by making sure that your diet is moderate in calorie and fat content and that you consume many fruits and vegetables, whole-grain breads and cereals, beans, some fish, and low-fat or fat-free milk products. In addition, remain physically active; avoid obesity; consume alcohol in moderation (if at all); and limit intake of animal fat and salt-cured, smoked, and nitrate-cured foods.

Remember also that if a cancer is left untreated, it can spread quickly throughout the body. When this happens, it is much more likely to lead to death. Thus early detection is critical. Aids to early detection include the following warning signs (acronym is CAUTION):

- A change in bowel or bladder habits
- A sore that does not heal
- Unusual bleeding or discharge
- A thickening or lump in the breast or elsewhere
- Indigestion or difficulty in swallowing
- An obvious change in a wart or mole
- A nagging cough or hoarseness

Unexplained weight loss is an additional warning sign.

There are still other ways to detect cancer early. Colonoscopy examinations for middle-age and older adults, PSA (prostate-specific antigen) tests for middle-age and older men, and Papanicolaou tests (Pap smears) and regular breast examinations (and mammograms starting about age 40) for women are recommended by the American Cancer Society. Finally, to learn still more about cancer, review these sources of credible cancer information on the Internet:

American Cancer Society
www.cancer.org
National Cancer Institute
www.cancer.gov
Oncolink
cancer.med.upenn.edu
Harvard University Center
for Cancer Prevention
www.yourdiseaserisk.harvard.edu

▶ **American Institute for Cancer Research Diet and Health Guidelines for Cancer Prevention**

1. Choose a diet rich in a variety of plant-based foods.
2. Eat plenty of vegetables and fruits.
3. Maintain a healthy weight and be physically active.
4. Drink alcohol only in moderation, if at all.
5. Select foods low in fat and salt.
6. Prepare and store food safely.

*And always remember …*

Do not use tobacco in any form.

## Case Study Dietary Assistance for an Older Adult

Frances is a 78-year-old woman who suffers from macular degeneration, osteoporosis, and arthritis. Since her husband died a year ago, she has moved from their family house to a small one-bedroom apartment. Her eyesight is progressively getting worse, making it hard to go to the grocery store or even to cook (for fear of burning herself). She is often lonely; her only son lives 1 hour away and works two jobs, but he visits her as often as he can. Frances has lost her appetite and, as a result, often skips meals during the week. She has resorted to eating mostly cold foods, simple to prepare but seriously limiting diet variety and palatability in her diet. She is slowly losing weight as a result of her dietary changes and loss of appetite.

Her typical diet usually consists of a breakfast that may include 1 slice of wheat toast with margarine, honey, and cinnamon, and 1 cup of hot tea. If she has lunch, she normally has ½ can of peaches, half of a turkey and cheese sandwich, and ½ glass of water. For dinner, she might have half of a tuna fish sandwich made with mayonnaise and 1 cup of iced tea. She usually includes one or two cookies at bedtime.

*Answer the following questions, and check your responses in Appendix A.*

1. What nutrients are likely to be inadequate in her current diet?
2. What potential effects will Frances' poor dietary pattern have on her health status?
3. Which physiological changes of aging will add to the effects of her poor diet (review Table 16-2)?
4. What services are available in the community that could help Frances improve her diet and possibly increase her appetite?

5. What other convenience foods could be included in her diet to make it more healthful and more varied?

## Summary

1. Although maximum life span hasn't changed, life expectancy has increased dramatically over the past century. For many societies, this means that an increasing proportion of the population is over 65 years of age. As health care costs rise, the goal of delaying disease becomes ever important.

2. During adulthood, nutrients are used primarily to maintain the body rather than support physical growth. As adults get older, nutrient needs change. Adulthood is characterized by body maintenance and gradual physiological transitions, often referred to as "aging." The physiologic changes of aging are the sum of cellular changes, lifestyle practices, and environmental influences. Many of these changes can be minimized, prevented, and/or reversed by healthy lifestyles. Usual aging refers to the age-related physical and physiological changes that are commonly thought to be typical of aging. Successful aging describes the declines in physical and physiological function that occur because one grows older. Striving to have the greatest number of healthy years and the fewest of illness is referred to as compression of morbidity. The rate at which one ages is individual; it is determined by heredity, lifestyle, and environment.

3. A healthy diet based on MyPyramid and the 2005 Dietary Guidelines for Americans can help to preserve body function, avoid chronic disease, and age successfully. These guidelines recommend that individuals eat a variety of foods; balance the food eaten with physical activity to maintain or improve weight; choose a diet with plenty of whole grains, vegetables, and fruits; choose a diet low in saturated fat, *trans* fat, and cholesterol; limit sugars and salt; and moderate alcoholic beverage intake. Regular physical activity is also important, as is safe food preparation. American adults are fairly well nourished, although common dietary excesses are calories, fat, sodium, and for some, alcohol.

Common dietary inadequacies include vitamins D and E, folate, magnesium, calcium, zinc, and fiber. People ages 65 and older, particularly those in long-term care facilities and hospitals, are at risk for malnutrition. The Nutrition Screening Initiative checklist can help identify older adults at risk of nutrient deficiencies. The DRIs for adults are divided by gender and age to reflect how nutrient needs change as adults grow older. These changes in nutrient needs take into consideration the aging-related physiological alterations in body composition, metabolism, and organ function.

4. The food choices and nutritional adequacy of adults' diets depend on physiological, psychosocial, and economic factors. Alterations in any of these factors can result in deteriorations in the quality of dietary intake, nutritional status, and health. Physiological factors include changes in body composition body systems, and chronic diseases that influence dietary intake and

alter nutrient needs and/or nutrient utilization. Of particular concern is sarcopenia, or loss of muscle mass that frequently accompanies aging. The use of medications and supplements can improve health and quality of life, but some also adversely affect nutritional status. Herbal products should be used with caution. Psychosocial influences on nutritional status include changes in lifestyle and social interaction and the presence of mental health issues, such as depression and Alzheimer's disease. Economic factors may also have a great impact on the types and amounts of food one eats.

5. Alcohol use is a complex issue because it involves psychological, social, economic, health, legal, and family issues. Alcohol is metabolized in the liver and other tissues. The benefits of alcohol use are associated with low to moderate alcohol consumption. These benefits include the pleasurable and social aspects of alcohol use, a reduction in various forms of cardiovascular disease, increase in insulin sensitivity, and protection against some harmful stomach bacteria. Alcohol has the potential to worsen health has well. Excessive consumption of alcohol contributes significantly to five of the ten leading causes of death in North America. Alcohol increases the risk of developing certain forms of heart damage, inflammation of the pancreas, GI tract damage, vitamin and mineral deficiencies, cirrhosis of the liver, certain forms of cancer, hypertension, and hemorrhagic stroke—to name a few.

If alcohol is consumed, it should be consumed in moderation with meals. Women are advised to drink no more than one drink per day, as are adults 65 years and older; men are advised to limit intake to two drinks per day.

6. Diet plans for adults should be based on nutrient-dense foods and need to be individualized for existing health problems, physical abilities, presence of drug-nutrient interactions, possible depression, and economic constraints. A balanced multivitamin and mineral supplement can be used to help meet needs, especially for adults age 70 years and older. Most communities have congregate or home-delivered meal systems, food stamps, and other provisions to provide nutrition aid for those who qualify.

## Study Questions

1. List three important points made by the 2005 Dietary Guidelines for Americans for the general population and give an example of why each one may be difficult for older adults to implement. What are some suggestions for overcoming these barriers?

2. What is the difference between life span and life expectancy?

3. List five general guidelines for cancer prevention.

4. Describe two hypotheses proposed to explain the causes of aging, and note evidence for each in your daily life experiences.

5. List four organ systems that can decline in function in later years, along with a diet/lifestyle response to help cope with the decline.

6. Defend the recommendation for regular physical activity during older adulthood, including some resistance activity (weight training).

7. How might the nutritional needs of older people differ from those of younger people? How are their needs similar? Be specific.

8. What three resources in a community are widely available to aid older adults in maintaining nutritional health?

9. Describe some warning signs of depression and note a possible nutritional implication as this problem advances.

10. List four warning signs of undernutrition in older people that are part of the acronym DETERMINE. Briefly justify the inclusion of each.

## Check Your Knowledge

Answers to the following multiple choice questions are below.

1. Among the older population of the United States, the age of the fastest growing segment is _____ years.
   a. 65
   b. 74
   c. 79
   d. 85+

2. The diets of adults tend to be low in ____.
   a. vitamin E
   b. calcium
   c. fiber
   d. All of the above.

3. The reason the incidence of obesity increases with age is that
   a. the basal metabolic rate decreases with age.
   b. physical activity often decreases with age.
   c. energy intake exceeds energy expenditure.
   d. All of the above.

4. The immune system becomes less efficient with age, so it is especially important to consume adequate _____ and _____, nutrients that contribute to immune function.
   a. vitamin A, vitamin B-6
   b. protein, zinc
   c. zinc, iodide
   d. vitamin A, vitamin K

5. Which of the following does not describe a physiological change of aging?

a. decreases in digestion and absorption capacity
b. reduction in lean body mass
c. lower basal metabolism
d. increase in taste sensitivity

6. To maintain optimal nutritional status and healthy weight, the diet of an older person should have a ____ nutrient density and be _____ in energy content.
a. low, high
b. low, low
c. high, moderate
d. high, high

7. Nutrition programs such as congregate meals or home-delivered meals provide which of the following?

a. an improved nutritional status
b. a social atmosphere
c. an economical meal for low-income elderly
d. All of the above.

8. During aging, the needs for vitamins and minerals
a. continually fluctuate.
b. greatly decrease.
c. somewhat increase in some cases.
d. greatly increase.

9. Alcohol is digested in the
a. stomach.
b. small intestine.

c. liver.
d. None of the above; alcohol requires no digestion.

10. Alcohol is most damaging to the
a. brain cells because alcohol can be used as an energy source even before glucose.
b. kidney cells because this is where alcohol is excreted.
c. cells of the gastrointestinal tract because they are in direct contact with ingested alcohol.
d. liver cells where alcohol is metabolized.

Answers: 1.d, 2.d, 3.d, 4.b, 5.d, 6.c, 7.d, 8.c, 9.c, 10.d

## Further Readings

1. ADA Reports: Position of the American Dietetic Association: Nutrition across the spectrum of aging. *Journal of the American Dietetic Association* 105:616, 2005.

   *Behaviors such as a healthful diet, being physically active, and not using tobacco in any form are three keys to healthful aging. The American Dietetic Association supports these practices, as well as encourages older adults to seek medical and nutritional care to treat ongoing health problems, such as diabetes and hypertension.*

2. Brannon CA: Alcohol: Functional food or addictive drug? *Today's Dietitian,* 10(12):8, 2008.

   *Alcohol has a long history as a functional and medicinal agent, but potential for abuse is high. This article describes the process of ethanol production, health benefits, and risks of alcohol use. A moderate intake of one to two drinks per day, particularly red wine at mealtimes, appears to be beneficial.*

3. Brannon CA: Perimenopause: Nutritional management. *Today's Dietitian* 8(10):10, 2006.

   *For most women, perimenopause begins in the mid-40s to early 50s. The most significant change during perimenopause is fluctuating levels of estrogen and progesterone. This article reviews several nutrition-related symptoms of this stage of the female life cycle and offers suggestions of several functional foods that contain components that may decrease these unpleasant symptoms.*

4. DeKosky ST and others: Ginkgo biloba for prevention of dementia. *Journal of the American Medical Association* 300: 2253, 2008.

   *Due to its purported antioxidant effects, ginkgo biloba is popularly used for prevention or treat-ment of Alzheimer's disease. This large-scale clinical trial compared the effects of ginkgo biloba (120 mg twice per day) to placebo in more than 3000 older adults. The trial showed no effect of ginkgo biloba for preventing or delaying all-cause or Alzheimer's-type dementia.*

5. Dickerson LM, Gibson MV: Management of hypertension in older persons. *American Family Physician* 71: 469, 2005.

   *Hypertension is a too common result of the aging process, especially elevated systolic blood pressure. The authors suggest older people try to combat this trend by following a healthy diet low in sodium and alcohol (if consumed), as well as performing regular physical activity. Typical medications used to treat hypertension in the population are also reviewed.*

6. DiMaria-Ghalili RA, Amella E: Nutrition in older adults. *American Journal of Nursing* 105(3): 40, 2005.

   *Malnutrition in older persons is important to prevent, as it is a bigger risk than being overweight to the health of this population. Risk factors that contribute to this state of malnutrition include a poor diet, as well as limited income, isolation, chronic illness, and various physiological changes that result from aging. These in turn can be addressed by appropriate lifestyle interventions reviewed in the article.*

7. Getting smart about Alzheimer's. *Tufts University Health & Nutrition Letter* 23(3):1, 2005.

   *As many as 4.5 million Americans suffer from Alzheimer's disease. Consuming a diet rich in brightly colored fruits and vegetables contains many phytochemicals that may prevent the disease. Consuming fish on a regular basis is also important, as well as avoiding obesity, exercising regularly, and keeping mentally active. Meeting B vitamin needs is also crucial, as many contribute to brain health, such as niacin.*

8. Grieger L: Dietary tips for baby boomers: Ageless advice for an aging generation. *Today's Dietitian,* 10(3): 38, 2008.

   *This article summarizes evidence-based guidelines for healthful aging. Maintaining a healthy weight is considered to be the most important strategy for reducing chronic disease risk, thus improving quality of life in one's older years. Dietary practices that support and complement this advice include replacing calorie-rich, processed foods with nutrient-dense, unprocessed foods. Plant foods are emphasized because they are low in calories, yet high in vitamins, minerals, fiber, and phytochemicals. Fish is advocated as a source of omega-3 fatty acids.*

9. Kushi LH and others: American Cancer Society guidelines on nutrition and physical activity for cancer prevention: Reducing the risk of cancer with healthy food choices and physical activity. *CA: A Cancer Journal for Clinicians* 56: 254, 2006.

   *Four general guidelines are presented as lifestyle modifications to reduce cancer risk. Maintenance of a healthy body weight is supported by a wealth of research. As far as food choices, a diet low in red and processed meats and rich in fruits, vegetables, and whole grains is advocated as a strategy for reducing cancer risk. Regular physical activity is also important to include. Alcohol should be consumed in moderation, if at all. ACS emphasizes the importance of a supportive social environment for incorporating such changes into a healthy lifestyle.*

10. Litchford MD: Declining nutritional status in older adults. *Today's Dietitian*, 6(7): 12, 2004.

   *The most common causes of declining nutritional status in older adults are poor food choices, failing cognitive status, oral health problems, loss of appetite, and dehydration. Implementing an action plan to treat these problems is important; a registered dietitian can help develop such a plan.*

11. Liu RH: Potential synergy of phytochemicals in cancer prevention: Mechanism of action. *Journal of Nutrition* 134:347S, 2004.

   *No single antioxidant can replace the combination of natural phytochemicals in fruits and vegetables to achieve the health benefits. Antioxidants or bioactive compounds are best acquired through whole-food consumption, not from dietary supplements. Consumption of 5–10 servings daily of a wide variety of fruits and vegetables is an appropriate strategy for significantly reducing the risk of chronic diseases, such as cancer, and to meet nutrient requirements for optimum health.*

12. Manini TM and others: Daily activity energy expenditure and mortality among older adults. *Journal of the American Medical Association* 296:171, 2006.

   *Energy expended in free-living activity by healthy older adults (aged 70–82 years) was strongly associated with lower risk of mortality. This study of 302 high-functioning, community-dwelling older adults suggests that any activity may increase survival.*

13. Newton KM and others: Treatment of vasomotor symptoms of menopause with black cohosh, multibotanicals, soy, hormone therapy, or placebo: A randomized trial. *Annals of Internal Medicine* 145:869, 2006.

   *Herbal supplements are frequently used to treat vasomotor symptoms of menopause (e.g., hot flashes), so this 1-year randomized study was conducted. Herbal supplements and hormone therapy were compared to a placebo in 351 women, age 45 to 55 years, in menopausal transition or postmenopausal with two or more vasomotor symptoms per day. Vasomotor symptoms or symptom intensity did not differ between the herbal interventions, including black cohosh, or placebo except for those receiving a multibotanical plus soy supplement whose symptoms were worse than with the placebo. Hormone therapy (estrogen with or without progesterone) did result in a decrease in vasomotor symptoms compared to the placebo.*

14. Petersen RC and others: Vitamin E and donepezil for the treatment of mild cognitive impairment. *The New England Journal of Medicine* 352:2379, 2005.

   *Megadose vitamin E therapy did not slow development of mild cognitive impairment in this study. This result questions earlier studies that showed a modest, but short-lived effect of such therapy. The medication donepezil was somewhat effective, but even this therapy only led to a modest benefit.*

15. Pierce JP and others: Greater survival after breast cancer in physically active women with high vegetable-fruit intake regardless of obesity. *Journal of Clinical Oncology* 25: 2345, 2007.

   *Among breast cancer survivors, women who engaged in regular physical activity (minimum of 30 minutes per day on 6 days per week) and consumed at least 5 servings per day of fruits and/or vegetables experienced half the risk of cancer recurrence as survivors who were not following these lifestyle practices.*

16. Redman LM and others: Effect of calorie restriction in non-obese humans on physiological, psychological and behavioral outcomes. *Physiology & Behavior* 94: 643, 2008.

   *Calorie restriction extends the life span and retards related chronic diseases of rats, mice, fish, flies, and other species. This may be due to a reduction in metabolic rate and oxidative stress, improved insulin sensitivity, and/or altered nervous system and hormonal activities. Although prospective, long-term studies of calorie restriction in humans are not feasible, evidence from epidemiological studies and short-term clinical trials indicate that calorie restriction decreases risk for diabetes and cardiovascular disease and improves biomarkers of aging without inducing disordered eating behaviors, constant feelings of hunger, depression, or cognitive decline. The authors point out, however, that the ability to adhere to a calorie-restricted diet will be low in an obesogenic environment. Research continues for an "anti-aging" pill that mimics the effects of calorie restriction in humans.*

17. Rhone M, Basu A: Phytochemicals and age-related eye disease. *Nutrition Reviews* 66: 465, 2008.

   *Age-related eye diseases, such as age-related macular degeneration and cataracts, are the leading causes of blindness in older adults. Nutrition interventions to prevent and/or treat eye disease are reviewed. Evidence supports the efficacy of lutein and zeaxanthin for protection against age-related eye disease. Other phytochemicals, such as flavonoids, are promising for the promotion of eye health, but more research is needed before supplementation can be recommended for this purpose. A healthy diet that supports weight management and emphasizes fruits and vegetables is currently the best practice for protecting the health of aging eyes.*

18. Riediger ND and others: A systemic review of the roles of n-3 fatty acids in health and disease. *Journal of the American Dietetic Association* 109: 668, 2009.

   *Omega-3 fatty acids, abundant in fish, fish oils, some plant oils, and now fortified foods (e.g., eggs, spreads), have been implicated in the prevention and treatment of many diseases. Of interest for aging adults, omega-3 fatty acids have been shown to improve cardiovascular risk, cancer risk, and several mental health disorders (including depression and Alzheimer's disease). Complaints regarding consumption of fish oils include nausea and fishy burps. Megadose supplements may lead to excessive bleeding. Avoiding shark, swordfish, king mackerel, tilefish, and any fish harvested from contaminated waters can reduce the risk of consuming environmental toxins, including mercury. Typical North American diets are deficient in these healthy fats, but increased availability of fortified foods will support adequate consumption of omega-3 fatty acids.*

19. Stenholm S and others: Sarcopenic obesity—definition, etiology and consequences. *Current Opinions in Clinical Nutrition and Metabolic Care* 11: 693, 2008.

   *Older adults suffer from loss of muscle mass accompanied by gains in fat mass. Such body composition changes dramatically increase risks for disease and disability. The authors review potential causes for sarcopenic obesity, including changes in diet, physical activity, hormone levels, and inflammation.*

20. Trichopoulou A and others: Modified Mediterranean diet and survival: EPIC-elderly prospective cohort study. *British Medical Journal* 330:991, 2005.

   *A diet characterized by high intakes of vegetables, legumes, fruits, cereals, and unsaturated fats; moderate amounts of fish and alcohol; and low-to-moderate amounts of dairy products and meats lessened the risk of developing cardiovascular disease in people in this study. Total mortality was also reduced, especially so in people who closely adhered to this diet pattern.*

# I. Am I Aging Healthfully?

*Take Control of Your Aging* by Dr. William B. Malarkey (Wooster Book Co., Wooster OH, 1999) includes a plan that incorporates various diet and lifestyle factors associated with successful aging. Indicate the degree to which you are following such a plan (or alternatively fill this out with a parent or another older relative in mind).

**Physical:** Do you eat a well-balanced diet, exercise on a regular basis, remain free of illness, abstain from smoking, refrain from drinking alcohol excessively, and experience refreshing sleep?

_____
_____
_____

**Intellectual:** Are you analytical, do you read regularly, do you learn new things each day, do you engage your mental ability at work (or at school), and do you often reflect on your life?

_____
_____
_____

**Emotional:** Are you at peace, do you like who you are, are you optimistic, and do you laugh and relax regularly?

_____
_____
_____

**Relational:** Are you a good listener, do you feel supported by friends, do you attend social functions, do you talk with family members often, and do you feel close to coworkers (or fellow students)?

_____
_____
_____

**Spiritual:** Do you appreciate nature, give to or serve others, meditate or seek religious worship, and feel life has meaning?

_____
_____
_____

The more of these factors that you include in your life, the more well-rounded your plan is for maintaining overall health. Any one of the five areas in which you are not achieving success should show you characteristics to work on in the future.

## II. Helping Older Adults Eat Better

During their lifetimes, most people usually eat meals with families or loved ones. As people reach their older ages, many of them are faced with living and eating alone. In a study of the diets of 4400 older adults in the United States, one man in every five living alone and over age 55 ate poorly. One of four women between the ages of 55 and 64 years followed a low-quality diet. These poor diets can contribute to deteriorating mental and physical health. Consider the following example of the living situation of an older adult.

Neal, a 70-year-old man, lives alone in a home in a local suburban area. His wife died one year ago. He doesn't have many friends; his wife was his primary confidante. His neighbors across the street and next door are friendly, and Neal used to help them with yard projects in his spare time. Neal's health has been good, but he has had trouble with his teeth recently. His diet has been poor, and in the past 3 months his physical and mental vigor have deteriorated. He has been slowly lapsing into a depression and, so, keeps the shades drawn and rarely leaves his house. Neal keeps very little food in the house because his wife did most of the cooking and shopping, and he just isn't that interested in food.

If you were one of Neal's relatives and learned of Neal's situation, what six things could you do or suggest to help improve his nutritional status and mental outlook? Look back into this chapter to get some ideas.

1. _____

2. _____

3. _____

4. _____

5. _____

6. _____

## CASE STUDY SOLUTIONS

### Chapter 1: Eating Habits in College

1. The most positive aspect of Andy's diet is that it contains good sources of protein from animal products also rich in zinc and iron. Alternating his hamburger and fries for lunch with pizza or tacos is a move in the right direction.

2.a. On the downside, Andy's diet is low in dairy products, fruits, and vegetables. This will result in a low intake of calcium, several of the vitamins and the phytochemical (plant-based) substances discussed in Chapter 1. His diet is also low in fiber because fast-food restaurants primarily use refined grain products, rather than whole-grain products and have few fruit and vegetable choices on the menu. Most of the beverages are soft drinks loaded with sugar. Many menu items, especially fries and chicken nuggets, are high in fat.

2.b. Most super-sized options apply to foods rich in fat (French fries) and sugar (soft drinks) resulting in excessive amounts of these two components.

2.c. He could choose a low-fat granola bar instead of the candy bar for breakfast, or he could take the time to eat a bowl of whole-grain breakfast cereal with low-fat or fat-free milk to increase fiber and calcium (in the latter case) intake. Overall, Andy could improve his intake of fruits, vegetables, and dairy products by focusing on variety in food choice and balance among the food groups.

2.d. Andy could alternate between tacos and bean burritos to gain the benefits of plant proteins in a diet. When choosing pizza, he can replace high-fat toppings (e.g., pepperoni), with veggies (e.g., green peppers and onions). Many sub shops and delis offer several low-fat sandwiches, emphasizing lean meats such as turkey and vegetable toppings. For his beverages, Andy could order milk at least half of the time at his restaurant visits and substitute diet soft drinks for the regular variety. This would help moderate his sugar intake.

### Chapter 2: Dietary Supplements

1. Whitney should be cautious about taking any supplement, especially one advertised as a "recent breakthrough." As you have read, dietary supplements are not closely regulated by FDA.

2. A general statement such as "increases energy" would be considered a structure/function claim and therefore does not require prior approval by FDA with regard to product labeling.

3. FDA will not have evaluated either the safety or effectiveness of such a product, and even harmful dietary supplements are difficult for FDA to recall.

4. There is a chance that the supplement, if effective, would contain little or none of the purported active ingredients.

5. Unfortunately, Whitney will find out all of this the hard way and will be out $60.

6. Whitney's hard-earned money would be better spent on a medical checkup at the Student Health Center. Consumers need to be cautious about nutrition information, especially regarding dietary supplements marketed as cure-alls and breakthroughs. Let the buyer beware!

## Chapter 3: Gastroesophageal Reflux Disease

1. Overeating at mealtimes appears to bring on Caitlin's regular bouts of heartburn. Other factors that encourage relaxation of the sphincter and/or irritate the esophagus are smoking; being overweight; and consumption of chili powder, onions, garlic, peppermint, caffeine, alcohol, and chocolate.
2. Typical dietary advice includes consuming smaller, more frequent meals low in fat, not overeating at mealtimes, waiting about 2 hours after meals before lying down, and elevating the head of the bed about 6 inches (review Table 3-4). These recommendations reduce the risk of stomach contents forcing their way back up the esophagus. Other helpful advice includes stopping smoking if practiced, losing excess weight if overweight, and limiting the intake of the items listed in the solution to question 1.
3. If dietary advice does not control symptoms, the primary medication used to control GERD inhibits acid production in the stomach (see earlier discussion on the proton pump inhibitors such as omeprazole [Prilosec] also used to treat peptic ulcers). If this and other medical therapy fails to control the problem, surgery to strengthen the lower esophageal sphincter is possible.
4. Caitlin's GERD can be treated, but most likely will be a lifelong condition. Even surgery will generally not cure the problem. Lifetime diet and lifestyle management, and most likely medications, will still be needed to manage the problem.
5. Lifelong management of GERD is important because long-standing GERD increases the risk of esophageal cancer.

## Chapter 4: Problems with Milk Intake

1. Myeshia suspected that she was sensitive to milk because she developed bloating and gas when she consumed milk during one meal.
2. The disaccharide, lactose, is the most likely cause of Myeshia's symptoms.
3. When the enzyme lactase is missing or in short supply in the small intestine, undigested lactose travels to the large intestine and is fermented by bacteria there. The fermentation of lactose by bacteria produces abdominal gas, bloating, and pain. Diarrhea can also occur because the presence of lactose in the colon draws water from the blood vessels into the large intestine.
4. Lactose maldigestion is a normal pattern of physiology that often begins to develop at about ages 3 to 5 years in populations that do not rely on milk and other dairy foods as a main food source. When significant symptoms develop after lactose intake it is then called lactose intolerance.
5. The primary form of lactose maldigestion is estimated to occur in about 75% of the world's population. Most lactose maldigesters are African-Americans (like Myeshia), Asian-Americans, and Latino/Hispanic Americans. The occurrence of lactose maldigestion also increases as people age.
6. The active bacteria cultures in yogurt digest the lactose when these bacteria are broken apart in the small intestine and release their lactase.
7. Many products, such as low-lactose milk and lactase pills, are available to enable lactose maldigesters to tolerate milk.
8. Many lactose maldigesters can consume moderate amounts of lactose with minimal or no intestinal discomfort because of the eventual lactose breakdown by bacteria in the large intestine.
9. In North America and Western Europe, milk and other dairy products are important sources of calcium and vitamin D. These are important for maintaining bone health.

10. Secondary lactose maldigestion occurs when a condition (e.g., long-standing diarrhea from a viral infection), results in a significant decline in lactase production.

## Chapter 5: Planning a Heart-Healthy Diet

1. Jackie's approach to lowering blood cholesterol does not incorporate the best choices. She has excluded a great deal of fat in her diet, perhaps more than necessary, and has failed to include some key food groups that have cholesterol-lowering components.
2. Lowering fat as drastically as she has is not really necessary, especially for a physically active 21-year-old female.
3. Jackie could allow a more liberal amount of fat in her diet by including more monounsaturated fats. Canola oil and olive oil, as well as fats found in nuts and avocados are rich sources of monounsaturated fats. These fats do not increase blood cholesterol. In addition she should include good sources of omega-3 fatty acids such as fatty fish, walnuts, flaxseeds, or soybean oil. One option is to use a canola oil-and-vinegar dressing on her salad, rather than lemon juice.
4. She has excluded a great deal of fat in her diet by merely replacing it with refined carbohydrates.
5. To make a shift to a more heart-healthy diet, Jackie would need to include at least 2 cups of fruit and 3 cups of vegetables a day, along with more whole-grain products. She should use whole-wheat bread instead of white bread for her sandwiches and eat a breakfast cereal that has at least 3 grams of fiber per serving.
6. Taking a brisk walk each morning is an excellent way to guarantee at least 30 minutes of activity on most days of the week. Exercise has been shown to increase concentration of HDL-cholesterol in the blood and decrease risk of cardiovascular disease.

## Chapter 6: Planning a Vegetarian Diet

1. Studies show that the incidence of and the death rates from some chronic diseases, such as certain cardiovascular diseases, hypertension, many forms of cancer, type 2 diabetes, and obesity, are lower for vegetarians than for nonvegetarians.
2. Many components of a healthy vegetarian diet—whole grains, nuts, soy products, beans, 2 to 4 servings of fruits, and 3 to 5 servings of vegetables per day— are missing. With so few fruits and vegetables, his diet is also low in the many phytochemicals under study for numerous health benefits.
3. Protein appears to be low in the diet because Jordan has not replaced meat with a good plant source of protein. Vitamin B-12, iron, and zinc are also missing from the foods he is choosing. His diet seems to be adequate in calcium and riboflavin because he is including dairy products (milkshake and cheese).
4. Some of Jordan's food choices are high in fat (Danish pastry, milkshake, cookies) and sugar (fruit punch).
5. A healthy vegetarian diet includes whole grains, nuts, soy products, beans, 2 to 4 servings of fruits, and 3 to 5 servings of vegetables per day. It is apparent that he has not yet learned to implement the concept of complementary proteins, so the quality of protein in his diet is low. Meals that combine legumes or vegetables with grains or nuts (see Fig. 6-13) will provide the needed amounts of all amino acids.

## Chapter 7: Choosing a Weight-Loss Program

1. Joe's weight has been climbing, so he has been experiencing positive energy balance.
2. When Joe is not working, his activity level is low. His time watching TV and studying does not use much energy. Joe should try to find time for physical activity after work and on weekends.

3. Balancing calorie intake with energy expenditure is the main key to weight loss and weight maintenance. Changes that Joe could make to his diet include a decrease in high-fat and -calorie items in his take-out meals. He should include more fruits, vegetables, and whole grains in his meals. A whole-grain cereal with fruit would be a healthy and convenient substitute for his pastry for breakfast. A grilled chicken sandwich or a taco salad would be a nutritious change for lunch. Grilled chicken or chili with a baked potato or salad would be healthier choices for dinner. Table 7-3 includes many ideas for food substitutions that will lower calories.

4. Joe will be wasting his money if he buys the product seen in the infomercial. Unfortunately, regulation of the supplement industry is woefully lacking. In the future, if there is a meaningful breakthrough in weight loss and weight control, health authorities such as the Surgeon General's Office or the National Institutes of Health will make North Americans aware of that fact.

5. The characteristics of a sound weight-loss diet are shown in Figure 7-15. These characteristics include a slow and steady rate of loss, flexibility relative to your habits and tastes, nutritional adequacy, behavior modification, physical activity, and maintenance of overall health.

## Chapter 8: Choosing a Dietary Supplement

1. The maintenance dose of two to three tablets per day poses no risk *per se* because this dose of Nutramega does not exceed the Tolerable Upper Intake levels for vitamin A, vitamin C, niacin, or vitamin B-6.

2. a. **Vitamin A**
      33% (0.33) times the Daily Value of 1000 micrograms RAE equals 330 micrograms RAE per tablet. Sixteen tablets would yield 5280 micrograms RAE. The Upper Level is 3000 micrograms RAE for preformed vitamin A. Seventy-five percent of the vitamin A is preformed vitamin A, so this yields 3960 micrograms RAE of preformed vitamin A (5280 × 0.75 = 3960), or 1.3 times the Upper Level (3960/3000 = 1.3).

   b. **Vitamin C**
      700% (7) times the Daily Value of 60 milligrams equals 420 milligrams per tablet. 16 tablets would yield 6720 milligrams. The Upper Level is 2000 milligrams. This would then yield 3.4 times the Upper Level (6720/2000 = 3.4).

   c. **Niacin**
      200% (2) times the Daily Value of 20 milligrams equals 40 milligrams per tablet. 16 tablets would yield 640 milligrams. The Upper Level is 35 milligrams. This would then yield 18.3 times the Upper Level (640/35 = 18.3).

   d. **Vitamin B-6**
      100% (1) times the Daily Value of 2 milligrams equals 2 milligrams per tablet. 16 tablets would yield 32 milligrams. This is less than the Upper Level of 100 milligrams.

   e. The suggested use of Nutramega "at the first sign of feeling ill" poses some health risks for Amy. Taking two to three tablets every 3 hours would mean taking at least 16 tablets per day. This dosage would provide an intake of vitamin A, vitamin C, and niacin well in excess of the Upper Levels for these nutrients.

3. Nutramega is expensive compared to the cost of the typical multivitamin and mineral supplement (a 1-month supply would cost about $2 compared to about $50 for Nutramega).

4. Overall, Amy is smart to be concerned about meeting her nutrient needs, but the stress she is under does not increase nutrient needs.

5. A healthy diet as suggested by MyPyramid should be Amy's primary focus. Taking a balanced multivitamin and mineral supplement is also a reasonable practice.

## Chapter 9: Giving Up Milk

1.  Factors contributing to her potential risk of osteoporosis include a poor dietary intake of calcium and vitamin D. Her diet also is low in protein, an important nutrient for the synthesis of connective tissue important in the skeletal system.
2.  Ashley is increasing her chances of developing osteoporosis later in life because of her current high-risk lifestyle. Her new smoking habit and her low level of daily physical activity increase her risk of developing osteoporosis.
3.  Ashley should rethink her rationale for avoiding milk. Fat-free milk is low in calories and provides much calcium. Dairy products such as milk do not lead to weight gain *per se*. There are even some studies suggesting that a regular intake of dairy products rich in calcium may aid in weight loss when on an otherwise calorie-restricted diet.
4.  Ashley needs to find some reliable sources of calcium and vitamin D. These could include calcium-fortified juices, calcium-fortified bread and snack bars, and calcium-fortified chewable chocolate candies. Tofu (made with calcium) is another potential source, as well as calcium-fortified soy milk. Tofu and soy milk are also good sources of high-quality plant protein. Meeting the Adequate Intake of 1000 milligrams of calcium per day for her age would not be that hard if she were to make an effort to use these calcium-rich foods and/or incorporate other rich sources.
5.  To decrease her risk of osteoporosis and several other chronic diseases, Ashley should stop smoking. In addition, including at least 30 minutes of physical activity on most days of the week will decrease her risk of osteoporosis and help her maintain a healthy weight.

## Chapter 10: Planning a Training Diet

1.  Michael is correct in following a high-carbohydrate diet.
2.  In his effort to minimize his fat intake, he is probably not consuming enough calories, protein, iron, and calcium to support his training routine. He has fallen into the bagel, pasta, and pretzel routine that sports nutritionists warn is not conducive to peak performance. Low protein, iron, and overall calories may contribute to fatigue.
3.  Michael's performance would improve if he also had a high-protein source at each meal. He could include milk with breakfast and possibly some low-fat yogurt or low-fat cheese at lunch. He should have a carbohydrate/protein snack before his workout, such as half a sandwich with fruit and some water. The sandwich and fruit will help provide him with fuel to support his vigorous training. In the evenings, he could substitute oil and vinegar dressing for the fat-free dressing on his salad and cheese and crackers for the pretzels to improve protein intake.
4.  During his workouts, he could consume a sports drink to meet fluid needs and supply some carbohydrate, or he could consume water, along with a few fig cookies or other high-carbohydrate food.
5.  Overall, it is important for Michael to fuel his body before, during, and after workouts.

## Chapter 11: Eating Disorders—Steps to Recovery

1.  Sarah has the characteristics to be diagnosed with anorexia nervosa.
2.  Sarah's disordered eating habits began when she became self-conscious about her body when her peers teased her about being overweight. She began exercising each day and was successful at losing weight. Her disordered eating then began with restricting her food intake more. She enjoyed the self-control she had over her body.

3. Sarah has the following physical symptoms of anorexia nervosa: she refuses to maintain a healthy weight-for-height, is at a weight below 85% of that expected, has a distorted view of her appearance, and has had no menstrual periods for over 3 consecutive months.

4. Her treatment would most likely consist of moderate bed rest to promote weight gain and an intake of 1000 to 1600 kcal initially, then increased by increments of about 100 to 200 kcal every few days until an acceptable rate of weight gain is achieved. The goal is to achieve a body weight that is at least 90% of an expected weight for her height, such as a BMI of at least 19.

5. Several nutrient deficiencies are likely in this case. Deficiencies of calcium and iron are probably most likely. The physician would likely prescribe a multivitamin and mineral supplement, along with an additional supplement of calcium as needed to make sure intake is in the range of 1200 to 1500 milligrams per day. Additional iron may be needed if Sarah is anemic. This overall practice will correct vitamin and mineral deficiencies that exist. The calcium in particular will contribute to bone maintenance.

6. Sarah would need to be hospitalized initially, due to her low BMI of 13.8.

7. A team of health professionals, most likely consisting of a physician, registered dietitian, and psychologist, would provide therapy. Sarah's cooperation would be the most important element for therapy to be successful. She needs to realize that she has a problem and that she needs help. She must be willing to accept the assistance these professionals are willing to offer. The team, especially the psychologist, may use cognitive behavior therapy to help Sarah improve her self-image.

8. Sarah's outlook for recovery is not good unless she realizes she has a problem. Even if she is willing to accept the therapy and counseling, a relapse is likely to occur. Only 50% of anorexia nervosa patients have been found to recover fully from the disease. Sarah's disordered eating habits have been in place for about 6 years, so her problem is deep-rooted. The chances of recovery are greater if a vigorous treatment program is reinforced with close follow-up.

## Chapter 12: Undernutrition During Childhood

1. Jamal should not be surprised that the children in the village were often sick and listless. The living conditions and recent natural disaster have added to the already poor conditions in this village. We know that children are especially susceptible to the effects of poverty and undernutrition.

2. Based on the reports that the children do not get enough to eat and on the outward signs of the children's health, protein, vitamin A, iron, iodide, and zinc are likely to be deficient in the diets of these children.

3. Protein, vitamin A, iron, iodide, and zinc deficiencies contribute to poor growth and stunting because of their essential functions in the body. One or more of these deficiencies is likely present in many children in the village.

4. Protein, vitamin A, iron, iodide, and zinc deficiencies may also contribute to depressed immune function, which can cause diarrhea and illness. These deficiencies are particularly risky in children.

5. The diets of these children are most likely also marginal in caloric content. A low-calorie intake during childhood will further depress the growth and overall health compromised by the protein and micronutrient deficiencies. Recall from Chapter 6 that protein-calorie malnutrition (PCM) is a form of undernutrition caused by an extremely deficient intake of calories or protein and generally is accompanied by an illness.

6. The recent storm will hopefully cause the Philippine government to send food and medicines to the village, which will be a short-term solution to some of their nutrition and health needs.

7. Poverty and undernutrition occur at much lower rates in the United States and other developed countries. Childhood nutrition concerns in developed countries are more likely to be the increasing incidence of overweight and obesity. As we discussed in Chapter 7, maintaining a healthy weight requires the proper balance of calories in and calories out. In Chapter 15 we will learn that overweight children are becoming more common because the typical number of calories they consume per day has increased at the same time that calorie expenditure in physical activity has decreased.

## Chapter 13: Preventing Foodborne Illnesses at Gatherings

1. Nicole likely contracted *Clostridium perfringens*, based on the fact that she had diarrhea but did not vomit and the symptoms occurred about 8 hours after consuming the contaminated food (review Table 13-3).
2. Spores of *Clostridium perfringens* are typically present in meat. Thorough cooking will kill any of the live bacteria present, but the product may still contain spores. These can later develop into bacteria if the food is kept in a warm setting for a few hours. The beef in the empanadas was likely the bearer of the spores, and they likely germinated and produced a toxin as the beef sat in the car and on the buffet table.
3. Consuming food at large gatherings is risky for several reasons. First, foods for these events are typically cooked ahead of time and not consumed right away. Unfortunately, the foods end up remaining in the "danger zone" between 41°F and 135°F. Hot foods should be kept hot and cold foods cold. Unfortunately, proper refrigeration or heating equipment is not always available at these events. In addition, many people handle foods and serving utensils at large gatherings. It is important for anyone handling food or serving utensils to thoroughly wash their hands before and after handling food and to avoid coughing or sneezing over foods. Also, when returning to the "buffet" table, always use a clean plate to avoid cross-contamination. Finally, the focus at these events is usually on having fun and socializing and not on food safety.
4. The main precaution that was ignored was keeping the food out of the "danger zone." Overall, it is risky to leave perishable items such as meat, fish, poultry, eggs, and dairy products at room temperature for more than 1 to 2 hours.
5. Ideally, the cooked food should have remained at room temperature for no longer than 1 hour. Thus, soon after Nicole and her husband took it out of the oven, it should have been separated into a few smaller pans to speed cooling and then refrigerated because they knew it was not going to be served within 1 to 2 hours. Before leaving, they could have recombined the dish into one clean pan. Once they arrived at the party, the dish should have been refrigerated again, and then thoroughly reheated when it was time to eat.

## Chapter 14: Preparing for Pregnancy

1. Lily's use of an over-the-counter vitamin and mineral supplement provides ample synthetic folic acid and can help fill some gaps between dietary intakes and requirements for various nutrients. Still, she should discuss this supplement use with her physician and would eventually benefit more from a prenatal supplement, as this will have more iron than the over-the-counter supplement. She should be sure not to exceed 100% of the Daily Value for preformed vitamin A because toxicities of this vitamin could cause birth defects. Lily is wise to avoid use of herbal supplements during pregnancy unless her physician approves of them.

2. Folate deficiency is known to be linked to neural tube defects. The synthetic folic acid in vitamin and mineral supplements is well absorbed and will certainly help to meet her needs for this nutrient. Consuming more fruits and vegetables—especially green leafy vegetables—is also a wise choice. A fortified, ready-to-eat breakfast cereal also contributes to vitamins and mineral intake. Her physician may recommend a prenatal supplement instead of the over-the-counter supplement.

3. Many experts would say that she is consuming too much caffeine and would be wise to cut down coffee and caffeine-containing soft drinks to a total of three servings or fewer per day.

4. If Lily likes fish, she could include two servings of fish per week in her diet plan for pregnancy and breastfeeding. Fish are a good source of protein and also supply healthy fats, including omega-3 fatty acids, linked to brain and eye development in the fetus. However, Lily should avoid some types of fish that may have high mercury content, which can harm the nervous system of the developing fetus. Fish that typically have high levels of mercury include swordfish, shark, king mackerel, tile fish, largemouth bass, and canned albacore tuna.

5. The additional fruits and vegetables Lily is consuming will provide some fiber to help prevent constipation. Other ideas to increase her fiber intake include consuming a variety of whole grains and incorporating beans and legumes into her diet plan. Lily should also increase her fluid intake and be sure to maintain regular exercise, such as walking.

6. Lily expressed concern about her weight gain during pregnancy. Research clearly shows that adequate weight gain during pregnancy is critical for growth and development of the fetus. Inadequate weight gain contributes to risk for delivering a low-birth-weight or small-for-gestational-age baby. On the other hand, excessive weight gain during pregnancy can present problems as well. Excessive weight gain may promote long-term health problems and complicate the pregnancy with gestational diabetes or large-for-gestational age babies. At her pre-pregnancy weight and height, Lily's BMI ($21$ kg/m²) is within the normal range, so she should aim to gain 25–35 pounds during the entire pregnancy. During the second and third trimesters, consuming an extra 350–450 kilocalories per day of nutrient-dense foods will help her to meet this goal. Regular, moderate exercise is also recommended throughout pregnancy. However, pregnancy is not a time to begin a vigorous exercise routine. Walking or riding a stationary bike are good activities to regulate weight gain. Lily should be reassured that her choice to breastfeed her baby will help her to lose those extra pounds after the baby is born.

## Chapter 15: Undernutrition During Infancy

1. Ask if the formula is iron-fortified. Also, verify that Damon's caregivers are appropriately preparing his formula—adding the correct amount of powder or concentrated liquid to water. Be sure that Damon's caregivers plan to continue giving him formula until 1 year of age.

2. The scenario described puts Damon at risk for failure to thrive, likely due to his caregiver's lack of knowledge about appropriate infant feeding practices. His diet is probably lacking in total calories as well as calcium, iron, and zinc. Inadequacies may lead to stunted growth, cognitive problems, behavioral problems, and weak bones.

3. In addition to an iron-fortified infant formula, Damon should be eating fortified infant cereals, pureed fruits, vegetables, and meats, and even some table foods that are soft and cut into small pieces. After six months of age, solid foods help to meet increased nutrient demands. Processed foods, such as the hot dog described in the scenario, are usually high in sodium, fat, or sugars. These are not ideal for meeting Damon's nutritional needs. Allowing Damon to self-feed to some extent will help him to develop motor skills and build confidence.

Potentially allergenic foods, such as seafood, egg whites, cow's milk, peanuts, and tree nuts, should not be offered until Damon is older.

4.  Infants should not be drinking sugary beverages such as colas or fruit-flavored drinks, as these items lack the nutrient density essential to meeting Damon's needs. His caregivers should provide him no more than 4 to 6 ounces of 100% fruit juice. To prevent early childhood caries and develop self-feeding skills, Damon should be learning to drink from a cup rather than a bottle.

5.  The combination of an appropriately-prepared, iron-fortified infant formula and a variety of solid foods should provide Damon all the nutrients he needs. However, if he is anemic, he may need an iron supplement.

## Chapter 16: Dietary Assistance for an Older Adult

1.  Frances' typical diet is low in many nutrients, including protein, calcium, iron, zinc, and vitamins B-12 and D.

2.  Her poor diet will cause a more rapid decline in her lean tissue and bone mass, as well as decrease her iron status, vision, and mental function.

3.  Physiological changes that will exacerbate the effects of her poor diet include increases in fat stores and decreases in her appetite; sense of taste, smell and thirst; chewing ability; bowel function; lactase production; iron status; liver, kidney, lung, cardiovascular, and immune function; vision; lean tissue; bone mass; and mental function. Review Table 16-2 for the recommended responses to these changes.

4.  Frances could contact a local government office that offers congregate meal programs at a central location. She could inquire about location and availability of transportation to the site. This would give her social contact with other older persons, probably an important element missing in her life. This could help alleviate her loneliness. She could also request Meals on Wheels (if available) to provide one hot meal per day. One hot meal per day prepared for her may be what she needs to help stimulate her appetite. She could also have groceries delivered to her home if her budget could withstand the extra cost.

5.  Other convenience foods that could be added to her diet include milk; assorted nuts; peanut butter; breakfast cereals; canned chicken or deli meats; yogurt; sliced cheese; cottage cheese; calcium-fortified orange juice; canned or frozen fruits and vegetables; and some fresh fruits and vegetables that do not require preparation, such as prewashed lettuce and bananas. A further possibility is a nutrition bar or a liquid nutritional supplement, such as a can of Ensure® Plus. The resulting increase in her nutrient intake would help prevent disease in the future and increase her sense of well-being.

# APPENDIX B  Daily Values Used in Food Labels

The Daily Values Used on Food Labels in the United States, with a Comparison to the Latest RDAs and Other Nutrient Standards*

| Dietary Constituent | Unit of Measure | Current Daily Values for People Over 4 Years of Age | RDA or Other Current Dietary Standard Males 19 Years Old | Females 19 Years Old |
|---|---|---|---|---|
| Total Fat[†] | g | <65 | — | — |
| Saturated fatty acids[†] | " | <20 | — | — |
| Protein[†] | " | 50 | 56 | 46 |
| Cholesterol[§] | mg | <300 | — | — |
| Carbohydrate[†] | g | 300 | 130 | 130 |
| Fiber | " | 25 | 38 | 25 |
| Vitamin A | µg Retinol activity equivalents | 1000 | 900 | 700 |
| Vitamin D | International units | 400 | 200 | 200 |
| Vitamin E | " | 30 | 22–33 | 22–33 |
| Vitamin K | µg | 80 | 120 | 90 |
| Vitamin C | mg | 60 | 90 | 75 |
| Folate | µg | 400 | 400 | 400 |
| Thiamin | mg | 1.5 | 1.20 | 1.10 |
| Riboflavin | " | 1.7 | 1.30 | 1.10 |
| Niacin | " | 20 | 16 | 14 |
| Vitamin B-6 | " | 2 | 1.30 | 1.30 |
| Vitamin B-12 | µg | 6 | 2.40 | 2.40 |
| Biotin | mg | 0.3 | 0.03 | 0.03 |
| Pantothenic acid | " | 10 | 5 | 5 |
| Calcium | " | 1000 | 1000 | 1000 |
| Phosphorus | " | 1000 | 700 | 700 |
| Iodide | µg | 150 | 150 | 150 |
| Iron | mg | 18 | 8 | 18 |
| Magnesium | " | 400 | 400 | 310 |
| Copper | " | 2 | 0.9 | 0.9 |
| Zinc | " | 15 | 11 | 8 |
| Sodium[‡] | " | <2400 | 1500 | 1500 |
| Potassium[‡] | " | 3500 | 4700 | 4700 |
| Chloride[‡] | " | 3400 | 2300 | 2300 |
| Manganese | " | 2 | 2.3 | 1.8 |
| Selenium | µg | 70 | 55 | 55 |
| Chromium | " | 120 | 35 | 25 |
| Molybdenum | " | 75 | 45 | 45 |

Abbreviations: g = gram, mg = milligram, µg = microgram

*Daily Values are generally set at the highest nutrient recommendation in a specific age and gender category. Many Daily Values exceed current nutrient standards. This is in part because aspects of the Daily Values were originally developed in the early 1970s using estimates of nutrient needs published in 1968. The Daily Values have yet to be updated to reflect the current state of knowledge.

[†]These Daily Values are based on a 2000 kcal diet, instead of RDAs, with a caloric distribution of 30% from fat (and one-third of this total from saturated fat), 60% from carbohydrate, and 10% from protein.

[‡]The considerably higher Daily Values for sodium and chloride are there to allow for more diet flexibility, but the extra amounts are not needed to maintain health.

[§]Based on recommendations of U.S. federal agencies.

The information in this appendix includes advice on dietary patterns, as well as regulations that apply to food labeling. Previous **Recommended Nutrient Intakes (RNIs)** for nutrients have been replaced by the Dietary Reference Intakes (DRIs) that apply to Canadian and U.S. citizens. These are listed on the inside cover. Both Canadian and American scientists worked on the various DRI committees, coming up with a set of harmonized Dietary Reference Intakes for both countries.

## SUMMARY OF THE NUTRITION RECOMMENDATIONS FOR CANADIANS

The Canadian federal department responsible for helping Canadians maintain and improve their health is Health Canada. The Office of Nutrition Policy and Promotion is within the Health Products and Food Branch of Health Canada and focuses on nutrition. Health Canada's National Dietary Guidance programs have been in existence since the 1930s and have always relied on scientific and other related evidence. Since 1977, a pattern of eating that meets nutrient needs and reduces the risk of chronic diseases has been promoted. In the 1990s, dietary guidance included *Canada's Guidelines for Healthy Eating* and *Food Guide to Healthy Eating* as well as *Nutrition for a Healthy Pregnancy* and *Nutrition for Healthy Term Infants*. The *Recommended Nutrient Intake* (RNI), a Canadian version of the RDA, was published in 1990.

In 1995, the U.S. Institutes of Medicine (IOM) brought together Canadian and American scientists to work on various committees, which came up with a set of harmonized Dietary Reference Intakes for both countries. The DRIs replaced the previous RNIs, and a new set of recommendations (EAR, AI, RDA, UL) similar to those in the United States were adopted in Canada. This led to a review and subsequent revision of *Canada's Food Guide to Healthy Eating* and *Guidelines for Healthy Eating*.

The revised *Canada's Food Guide* (Fig. C-1) was released in early 2007. The basic message to Canadians is to "Eat Well" with *Canada's Food Guide*. Learning more about *Canada's Food Guide* will help Canadians know how much food they need, what types of foods are better for them, and the importance of physical activity in their day.

In addition, if Canadians have the amount and type of food recommended and follow the tips included in *Canada's Food Guide*, this will help them:

- Meet their needs for vitamins, minerals, and other nutrients.
- Reduce their risk of obesity, type 2 diabetes, heart disease, certain types of cancer, and osteoporosis.
- Contribute to their overall health and vitality.

*Canada's Food Guide* places foods into four groups: vegetables and fruits; grain products; milk and alternatives; and meat and alternatives. *Canada's Food Guide* also includes information on the recommended number of Food Guide Servings per day, examples of what is one Food Guide Serving and how to make each Food Guide Serving count within each food group (Fig. C-2) and at each meal (Fig. C-3). Recommendations are also included about the types and amounts of oils and fats to consume, along with guidance to enjoy a variety of foods and to satisfy your thirst with water. Similar to the MyPyramid recommendations, *Canada's Food Guide* emphasizes the combination of eating well and being active every day (Fig. C-4). The new Canadian Nutrition Facts label is also highlighted in *Canada's Food Guide* with the message to "Read the label." Finally, specific nutrition advice for different ages and stages is included (Fig. C-5). Another similarity to the U.S. MyPyramid is the availability of "My Food Guide," a web-based interactive tool that will help you personalize the information found in *Canada's Food Guide*. Check out "My Food Guide" at http://www.hc-sc.gc.ca/fn-an/food-guide-aliment/myguide-monguide/index-eng.php.

**Recommended Nutrient Intake (RNI)**
The Canadian version of RDA published in 1990.

▶ Excellent World Wide Web resources for Canadians are Health Canada (www.hc-sc.gc.ca), Dietitians of Canada (www.dietitians.ca), and the Institute of Nutrition, Metabolism, and Diabetes (www.cihr-irsc.gc.ca).

▶ A downloadable copy of *Canada's Food Guide* is available at http://www.hc-sc.gc.ca/fn-an/food-guide-ailment/index-eng.php.

**FIGURE C-1** ▶ Eating Well with Canada's Food Guide.

# Recommended Number of *Food Guide Servings* per Day

| | Children | | | Teens | | Adults | | | |
|---|---|---|---|---|---|---|---|---|---|
| **Age in Years** | 2-3 | 4-8 | 9-13 | 14-18 | | 19-50 | | 51+ | |
| **Sex** | Girls and Boys | | | Females | Males | Females | Males | Females | Males |
| **Vegetables and Fruit** | 4 | 5 | 6 | 7 | 8 | 7-8 | 8-10 | 7 | 7 |
| **Grain Products** | 3 | 4 | 6 | 6 | 7 | 6-7 | 8 | 6 | 7 |
| **Milk and Alternatives** | 2 | 2 | 3-4 | 3-4 | 3-4 | 2 | 2 | 3 | 3 |
| **Meat and Alternatives** | 1 | 1 | 1-2 | 2 | 3 | 2 | 3 | 2 | 3 |

The chart above shows how many Food Guide Servings you need from each of the four food groups every day.

**Having the amount and type of food recommended and following the tips in *Canada's Food Guide* will help:**

• Meet your needs for vitamins, minerals and other nutrients.

• Reduce your risk of obesity, type 2 diabetes, heart disease, certain types of cancer and osteoporosis.

• Contribute to your overall health and vitality.

**FIGURE C-2** ► Information about Food Guide Servings from *Canada's Food Guide*.

## What is One Food Guide Serving?
### Look at the examples below.

**Fresh, frozen or canned vegetables**
125 mL (½ cup)

**Leafy vegetables**
Cooked: 125 mL (½ cup)
Raw: 250 mL (1 cup)

**Fresh, frozen or canned fruits**
1 fruit or 125 mL (½ cup)

**100% Juice**
125 mL (½ cup)

**Bread**
1 slice (35 g)

**Bagel**
½ bagel (45 g)

**Flat breads**
½ pita or ½ tortilla (35 g)

**Cooked rice, bulgur or quinoa**
125 mL (½ cup)

**Cereal**
Cold: 30 g
Hot: 175 mL (¾ cup)

**Cooked pasta or couscous**
125 mL (½ cup)

**Milk or powdered milk (reconstituted)**
250 mL (1 cup)

**Canned milk (evaporated)**
125 mL (½ cup)

**Fortified soy beverage**
250 mL (1 cup)

**Yogurt**
175 g
(¾ cup)

**Kefir**
175 g
(¾ cup)

**Cheese**
50 g (1 ½ oz.)

**Cooked fish, shellfish, poultry, lean meat**
75 g (2 ½ oz.)/125 mL (½ cup)

**Cooked legumes**
175 mL (¾ cup)

**Tofu**
150 g or
175 mL (¾ cup)

**Eggs**
2 eggs

**Peanut or nut butters**
30 mL (2 Tbsp)

**Shelled nuts and seeds**
60 mL (¼ cup)

**Oils and Fats**
- Include a small amount – 30 to 45 mL (2 to 3 Tbsp) – of unsaturated fat each day. This includes oil used for cooking, salad dressings, margarine and mayonnaise.
- Use vegetable oils such as canola, olive and soybean.
- Choose soft margarines that are low in saturated and trans fats.
- Limit butter, hard margarine, lard and shortening.

**FIGURE C-2** ▶ (continued)

## *Make each Food Guide Serving count...*
### *wherever you are – at home, at school, at work or when eating out!*

▸ **Eat at least one dark green and one orange vegetable each day.**
- Go for dark green vegetables such as broccoli, romaine lettuce and spinach.
- Go for orange vegetables such as carrots, sweet potatoes and winter squash.

▸ **Choose vegetables and fruit prepared with little or no added fat, sugar or salt.**
- Enjoy vegetables steamed, baked or stir-fried instead of deep-fried.

▸ **Have vegetables and fruit more often than juice.**

▸ **Make at least half of your grain products whole grain each day.**
- Eat a variety of whole grains such as barley, brown rice, oats, quinoa and wild rice.
- Enjoy whole grain breads, oatmeal or whole wheat pasta.

▸ **Choose grain products that are lower in fat, sugar or salt.**
- Compare the Nutrition Facts table on labels to make wise choices.
- Enjoy the true taste of grain products. When adding sauces or spreads, use small amounts.

▸ **Drink skim, 1%, or 2% milk each day.**
- Have 500 mL (2 cups) of milk every day for adequate vitamin D.
- Drink fortified soy beverages if you do not drink milk.

▸ **Select lower fat milk alternatives.**
- Compare the Nutrition Facts table on yogurts or cheeses to make wise choices.

▸ **Have meat alternatives such as beans, lentils and tofu often.**

▸ **Eat at least two Food Guide Servings of fish each week.***
- Choose fish such as char, herring, mackerel, salmon, sardines and trout.

▸ **Select lean meat and alternatives prepared with little or no added fat or salt.**
- Trim the visible fat from meats. Remove the skin on poultry.
- Use cooking methods such as roasting, baking or poaching that require little or no added fat.
- If you eat luncheon meats, sausages or prepackaged meats, choose those lower in salt (sodium) and fat.

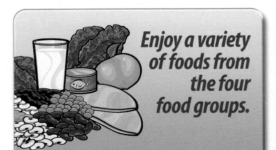

*Enjoy a variety of foods from the four food groups.*

*Satisfy your thirst with water!*

Drink water regularly. It's a calorie-free way to quench your thirst. Drink more water in hot weather or when you are very active.

* Health Canada provides advice for limiting exposure to mercury from certain types of fish. Refer to www.healthcanada.gc.ca for the latest information.

**FIGURE C-2** ▸ *(continued)*

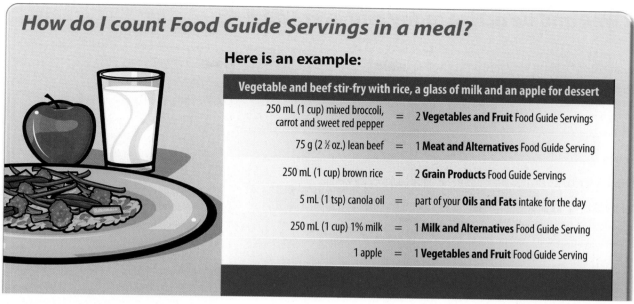

## How do I count Food Guide Servings in a meal?

### Here is an example:

| Vegetable and beef stir-fry with rice, a glass of milk and an apple for dessert | | |
|---|---|---|
| 250 mL (1 cup) mixed broccoli, carrot and sweet red pepper | = | 2 **Vegetables and Fruit** Food Guide Servings |
| 75 g (2 ½ oz.) lean beef | = | 1 **Meat and Alternatives** Food Guide Serving |
| 250 mL (1 cup) brown rice | = | 2 **Grain Products** Food Guide Servings |
| 5 mL (1 tsp) canola oil | = | part of your **Oils and Fats** intake for the day |
| 250 mL (1 cup) 1% milk | = | 1 **Milk and Alternatives** Food Guide Serving |
| 1 apple | = | 1 **Vegetables and Fruit** Food Guide Serving |

**FIGURE C-3** ▶ How to count Food Guide Servings in a meal.

### Nutrition Labels

New labeling requirements were published on January 1, 2003. The new regulations require most food labels to carry a mandatory Nutrition Facts table listing Calories and 13 key nutrients.

## How to Read the Canadian Nutrition Label

The Regulations provide for the optional declaration of the number of Calories both from fat and from saturates plus *trans*. Recommendations on the % of Calories from fat apply to the total diet rather than to an individual food. Therefore, inclusion of the % of Calories from fat in the Nutrition Facts table may be confusing and is not permitted.

The Nutrition Facts table provides information on saturated and *trans* fatty acids, shown to raise serum cholesterol levels. The declaration of the other groups of fatty acids, monounsaturates, omega-3, and omega-6 polyunsaturates, is optional unless claims are made, in which case all three must be declared.

Potassium is not included as a mandatory nutrient of the Nutrition Facts table because it is not considered to be a nutrient of general public health importance. The declaration of potassium, however, is mandatory when a claim is made for the sodium or salt content of a food that contains an added potassium salt.

Daily Value is a comparison standard comprised of
(a) vitamin or mineral amounts referred to in the definition of a recommended daily intake for that vitamin or mineral
(b) nutrient amounts referred to in the definition of reference standard for that nutrient

Serving size is stipulated for various foods.

The amount of vitamins and minerals is expressed as a percentage of the Daily Value per serving of stated size.

### Nutrition Facts
Per 1 cup (264g)

| Amount | % Daily Value |
|---|---|
| **Calories** 260 | |
| **Fat** 13g | 20% |
| Saturated Fat 3g + *Trans* Fat 2g | 25% |
| **Cholesterol** 30mg | |
| **Sodium** 660mg | 28% |
| **Carbohydrate** 31g | 10% |
| Fibre 0g | 0% |
| Sugars 5g | |
| **Protein** 5g | |
| Vitamin A 4%   Vitamin C 2% | |
| Calcium 15%   Iron 4% | |

g = gram
mg = milligram

# Eat well and be active today and every day!

## The benefits of eating well and being active include:

- Better overall health.
- Lower risk of disease.
- A healthy body weight.
- Feeling and looking better.
- More energy.
- Stronger muscles and bones.

## Be active

To be active every day is a step towards better health and a healthy body weight.

*Canada's Physical Activity Guide* recommends building 30 to 60 minutes of moderate physical activity into daily life for adults and at least 90 minutes a day for children and youth. You don't have to do it all at once. Add it up in periods of at least 10 minutes at a time for adults and five minutes at a time for children and youth.

*Start slowly and build up.*

## Eat well

Another important step towards better health and a healthy body weight is to follow *Canada's Food Guide* by:

- Eating the recommended amount and type of food each day.
- Limiting foods and beverages high in calories, fat, sugar or salt (sodium) such as cakes and pastries, chocolate and candies, cookies and granola bars, doughnuts and muffins, ice cream and frozen desserts, French fries, potato chips, nachos and other salty snacks, alcohol, fruit flavoured drinks, soft drinks, sports and energy drinks, and sweetened hot or cold drinks.

## Read the label

- Compare the Nutrition Facts table on food labels to choose products that contain less fat, saturated fat, trans fat, sugar and sodium.
- Keep in mind that the calories and nutrients listed are for the amount of food found at the top of the Nutrition Facts table.

## Limit trans fat

When a Nutrition Facts table is not available, ask for nutrition information to choose foods lower in trans and saturated fats.

### Nutrition Facts
Per 0 mL (0 g)

| Amount | % Daily Value |
|---|---|
| **Calories** 0 | |
| **Fat** 0 g | 0 % |
| Saturates 0 g | 0 % |
| + Trans 0 g | |
| **Cholesterol** 0 mg | |
| **Sodium** 0 mg | 0 % |
| **Carbohydrate** 0 g | 0 % |
| Fibre 0 g | 0 % |
| Sugars 0 g | |
| **Protein** 0 g | |

| | | | |
|---|---|---|---|
| Vitamin A | 0 % | Vitamin C | 0 % |
| Calcium | 0 % | Iron | 0 % |

## Take a step today...

- ✓ Have breakfast every day. It may help control your hunger later in the day.
- ✓ Walk wherever you can – get off the bus early, use the stairs.
- ✓ Benefit from eating vegetables and fruit at all meals and as snacks.
- ✓ Spend less time being inactive such as watching TV or playing computer games.
- ✓ Request nutrition information about menu items when eating out to help you make healthier choices.
- ✓ Enjoy eating with family and friends!
- ✓ Take time to eat and savour every bite!

## For more information, interactive tools, or additional copies visit Canada's Food Guide on-line at:
### www.healthcanada.gc.ca/foodguide

### or contact:
Publications
Health Canada
Ottawa, Ontario K1A 0K9
**E-Mail:** publications@hc-sc.gc.ca
**Tel.:** 1-866-225-0709
**Fax:** (613) 941-5366
**TTY:** 1-800-267-1245

Également disponible en français sous le titre : Bien manger avec le Guide alimentaire canadien

This publication can be made available on request on diskette, large print, audio-cassette and braille.

**FIGURE C-4** ▶ Recommendations to eat well and be active from *Canada's Food Guide*.

# *Advice for different ages and stages...*

## Children

Following *Canada's Food Guide* helps children grow and thrive.

Young children have small appetites and need calories for growth and development.

- Serve small nutritious meals and snacks each day.

- Do not restrict nutritious foods because of their fat content. Offer a variety of foods from the four food groups.

- Most of all... be a good role model.

## Women of childbearing age

All women who could become pregnant and those who are pregnant or breastfeeding need a multivitamin containing **folic acid** every day. Pregnant women need to ensure that their multivitamin also contains **iron**. A health care professional can help you find the multivitamin that's right for you.

Pregnant and breastfeeding women need more calories. Include an extra 2 to 3 Food Guide Servings each day.

**Here are two examples:**
- Have fruit and yogurt for a snack, or

- Have an extra slice of toast at breakfast and an extra glass of milk at supper.

## Men and women over 50

The need for **vitamin D** increases after the age of 50.

In addition to following *Canada's Food Guide*, everyone over the age of 50 should take a daily vitamin D supplement of 10 μg (400 IU).

**FIGURE C-5** ▶ Advice for different ages and stages from *Canada's Food Guide.*

The new regulations make nutrition labeling mandatory on most food labels using a new format. The regulations also update requirements for nutrient content claims and permit, for the first time in Canada, diet-related health claims for foods.

## Templates for Canadian "Nutrition Facts" Tables

### Bilingual Label

**Nutrition Facts**
**Valeur nutritive**
Per 125 mL (87 g) / 0par 125 mL (87 g)

| Amount<br>Teneur | % Daily Value<br>% valeur quotidienne |
|---|---|
| **Calories / Calories** 80 | |
| **Fat / Lipids** 0.5 g | **1** % |
| Saturated / saturés     0 g<br>+ *Trans* / trans     0 g | **0** % |
| **Cholesterol / Cholestérol** 0 mg | |
| **Sodium / Sodium** 0 mg | **0** % |
| **Carbohydrate / Glucides** 18 g | **6** % |
| Fibre / Fibres 2 g | **8** % |
| Sugars / Sucres 2 g | |
| **Protein / Protéines** 3 g | |
| Vitamin A / Vitamine A | 2 % |
| Vitamin C / Vitamine C | 10 % |
| Calcium / Calcium | 0 % |
| Iron / Fer | 2 % |

### English Label

**Nutrition  Facts**
Per 125 mL (87 g)

| Amount | % Daily Value |
|---|---|
| **Calories** 80 | |
| **Fat** 0.5 g | **1** % |
| Saturated 0 g<br>+ *Trans* 0 g | **0** % |
| **Cholesterol** 0 mg | |
| **Sodium** 0 mg | **0** % |
| **Carbohydrate** 18 g | **6** % |
| Fibre 2 g | **8** % |
| Sugars 2 g | |
| **Protein** 3 g | |
| Vitamin A  2 % | Vitamin C 10 % |
| Calcium    0 % | Iron         2 % |

### French Label

**Valeur nutritive**
par 125 mL (87 g)

| Teneur | % valeur quotidienne |
|---|---|
| **Calories** 80 | |
| **Lipids** 0,5 g | **1** % |
| saturés 0 g<br>+ trans 0 g | **0** % |
| **Cholestérol** 0 mg | |
| **Sodium** 0 mg | **0** % |
| **Glucides** 18 g | **6** % |
| Fibres 2 g | **8** % |
| Sucres 2 g | |
| **Protéines** 3 g | |
| Vitamine A  2 % | Vitamine C 10 % |
| Calcium    0 % | Fer         2 % |

g = gram
mg = milligram

## New Canadian Nutrition Facts Label for Children Under Two Years of Age

**Nutrition  Facts**
Per 1 jar (126 mL)

| | Amount |
|---|---|
| **Calories** | 110 |
| **Fat** | 0g |
| **Sodium** | 10 mg |
| **Carbohydrate** | 27g |
| Fibre | 4g |
| Sugars | 18g |
| **Protein** | 0g |
| **% Daily Value** | |
| Vitamin A  6% | Vitamin C 45% |
| Calcium    2% | Iron         2% |

g = gram
mg = milligram

## Recommended Daily Intakes and Reference Standards

The following are the Recommended Daily Intakes and Reference Standards used on Nutrition Labels for persons 2 years of age and older.* † ‡

| Dietary Constituent | Amount | Dietary Constituent | Amount |
|---|---|---|---|
| Fat | **65 g** | Folacin | 220 µg |
| The sum of saturated fatty acids and *trans* fatty acids | **20 g** | Vitamin B$_{12}$ | 2 µg |
| Cholesterol | **300 mg** | Pantothenic acid or pantothenate | 7 mg |
| Carbohydrate | **300 g** | Vitamin K | **80 mg** |
| Fibre | **25 g** | Biotin | **30 µg** |
| Sodium | **2400 mg** | Calcium | 1100 mg |
| Chloride | **3400 µg** | Phosphorus | 1100 mg |
| Potassium | **3500 mg** | Magnesium | 250 mg |
| Vitamin A | 1000 RE | Iron | 14 mg |
| Vitamin D | 5 µg | Zinc | 9 mg |
| Vitamin E | 10 mg | Iodide | 160 µg |
| Vitamin C | 60 mg | Selenium | **50 µg** |
| Thiamin, thiamine or vitamin B$_1$ | 1.3 mg | Copper | **2 mg** |
| Riboflavin or vitamin B$_2$ | 1.6 mg | Manganese | **2 mg** |
| Niacin | 23 NE | Chromium | **120 µg** |
| Vitamin B$_6$ | 1.8 mg | Molybdenum | **75 µg** |

*RE = retinol equivalents
†NE = niacin equivalents
‡Together these constitute the Daily Values used on the Canadian Nutrition Facts Label. Reference Standards are bolded.

## Approved Nutrient Content Claims for Canada

The following is a sample of approved nutrient content claims for food labels (for the complete list of regulations see the website http://gazette.gc.ca/archives/p1/2005/2005-05-07/html/reg4-eng.html).

### Energy

- *Free of energy:* The food provides less than 5 Calories or 21 kilojoules per reference amount and serving of stated size.
- *Low in energy:* The food provides 40 Calories or 167 kilojoules or less per reference amount and serving of stated size.
- *Reduced in energy:* The food is processed, formulated, reformulated, or otherwise modified so that it provides at least 25% less energy per reference amount of a similar food.
- *Lower in energy:* The food provides at least 25% less energy per reference amount of a similar food.

- *Source of energy:* The food provides at least 100 Calories or 420 kilojoules per reference amount and serving of stated size.
- *More energy:* The food provides at least 25% more energy, totalling at least 100 more Calories or 420 more kilojoules per reference amount of a similar food.

### Protein

- *Low in protein:* The food contains no more than 1 gram of protein per 100 grams of the food.
- *Source of protein:* The food has a protein rating of 20 or more, as determined by official method

FO-1, *Determination of Protein Rating,* October 15, 1981, (*a*) per reasonable daily intake; or (*b*) per 30 grams combined with 125 milliliters of milk, if the food is a breakfast cereal.
- *Excellent source of protein:* The food has a protein rating of 40 or more, as determined by official method FO-1, *Determination of Protein Rating,* October 15, 1981, (*a*) per reasonable daily intake; or (*b*) per 30 grams combined with 125 milliliters of milk, if the food is a breakfast cereal.
- *More protein:* The food (*a*) has a protein rating of 20 or more, as determined by official method

FO-1, *Determination of Protein Rating,* October 15, 1981, (i) per reasonable daily intake, or (ii) per 30 grams combined with 125 milliliters of milk, if the food is a breakfast cereal; and (*b*) contains at least 25% more protein, totalling at least 7 grams more, per reasonable daily intake compared to the reference food of the same food group or the similar reference food.

## Fat

- *Free of fat:* The food contains less than 0.5 grams of fat per reference amount and serving of stated size.
- *Low in fat:* The food contains 3 grams or less of fat per reference amount and serving of stated size and, if the reference amount is 30 grams or 30 milliliters or less, per 50 grams.
- *Reduced in fat:* The food is processed, formulated, reformulated, or otherwise modified so that it contains at least 25% less fat than the reference amount of a similar food.
- *Lower in fat:* The food contains at least 25% less fat per reference amount of the food, than the reference amount of the reference food of the same food group.
- *100% fat-free:* The food (*a*) contains less than 0.5 grams of fat per 100 grams; (*b*) contains no added fat.
- *No added fat:* The food contains no added fats or oils set out in Division 9, or added butter or ghee, or ingredients that contain added fats or oils, or butter or ghee.
- *Free of saturated fatty acids:* The food contains less than 0.2 grams saturated fatty acids and less than 0.2 grams *trans* fatty acids per reference amount and serving of stated size.
- *Low in saturated fatty acids:* (1) The food contains 2 grams or less of saturated fatty acids and *trans* fatty acids combined per reference amount and serving of stated size. (2) The food provides 15% or less energy from the sum of saturated fatty acids and *trans* fatty acids.
- *Reduced in saturated fatty acids:* The food is processed, formulated, reformulated, or otherwise modified without increasing the content of *trans* fatty acids, so that it contains at least 25% less saturated fatty acids per reference amount of the food than the reference amount of the similar reference food.
- *Lower in saturated fatty acids:* The food contains at least 25% less saturated fatty acids and the content of *trans* fatty acids is not higher per reference amount of the food, than the reference amount of the reference food of the same food group.
- *Free of trans fatty acids:* The food contains less than 0.2 grams of *trans* fatty acids per reference amount and serving of stated size.
- *Reduced in trans fatty acids:* The food is processed, formulated, reformulated, or otherwise modified without increasing the content of saturated fatty acids, so that it contains at least 25% less *trans* fatty acids per reference amount of the food than the reference amount of the similar reference food.
- *Lower in trans fatty acids:* The food contains at least 25% less *trans* fatty acids and the content of saturated fatty acids is not higher per reference amount of the food compared to the reference amount of a similar food.
- *Source of omega-3 polyunsaturated fatty acids:* The food contains 0.3 grams or more of omega-3 polyunsaturated fatty acids per reference amount and serving of stated size.
- *Source of omega-6 polyunsaturated fatty acids:* The food contains 2 grams or more of omega-6 polyunsaturated fatty acids per reference amount and serving of stated size.

## Cholesterol

- *Free of cholesterol:* The food contains less than 2 milligrams of cholesterol per reference amount and serving of stated size.
- *Low in cholesterol:* The food contains 20 milligrams or less of cholesterol per reference amount and serving of stated size (if the reference amount is 30 grams or 30 milliliters or less, per 50 grams).
- *Reduced in cholesterol:* The food is processed, formulated, reformulated, or otherwise modified so that it contains at least 25% less cholesterol per reference amount of a similar food.
- *Lower in cholesterol:* The food contains at least 25% less cholesterol per reference amount of a similar food.

## Sodium or Salt

- *Free of sodium or salt:* The food contains less than 5 milligrams of sodium per reference amount and serving of stated size.
- *Low in sodium or salt:* The food contains 140 milligrams or less of sodium per reference amount and serving of stated size.
- *Reduced in sodium or salt:* The food is processed, formulated, reformulated, or otherwise modified so that it contains at least 25% less sodium per reference amount of a similar food.
- *Lower in sodium or salt:* The food contains at least 25% less sodium per reference amount of the food.
- *No added sodium or salt:* The food contains no added salt, other sodium salts, or ingredients that contain sodium that functionally substitute for added salt.
- *Lightly salted:* The food contains at least 50% less added sodium than the sodium added to a similar reference food.

## Sugars

- *Free of sugars:* The food contains less than 0.5 milligrams of sugars per reference amount and serving of stated size.
- *Reduced in sugars:* The food is processed, formulated, reformulated, or otherwise modified so that it contains at least 25% less sugars, totalling at least 5 grams less, per reference amount of the food.

- *Lower in sugars:* The food contains at least 25% less sugars, totalling at least 5 grams less, per reference amount of the food.
- *No added sugars:* The food contains no added sugars, no ingredients containing added sugars or ingredients that contain sugars that functionally substitute for added sugars.

## Fibre

- *Source of fibre:* The food contains 2 grams or more (*a*) of fibre per reference amount and serving of stated size, if no fibre or fibre source is identified in the statement or claim; or (*b*) of each identified fibre or fibre from an identified fibre source per reference amount and serving of stated size, if a fibre or fibre source is identified in the statement or claim.
- *High source of fibre:* The food contains 4 grams or more (*a*) of fibre per reference amount and serving of stated size, if no fibre or fibre source is identified in the statement or claim; or (*b*) of each identified fibre or fibre from an identified fibre source per reference amount and serving of stated size, if a fibre or fibre source is identified in the statement or claim.
- *Very high source of fibre:* The food contains 6 grams or more (*a*) of fibre per reference amount and serving of stated size, if no fibre or fibre source is identified in the statement or claim; or (*b*) of each identified fibre or fibre from an identified fibre source per reference amount and serving of stated size, if a fibre or fibre source is identified in the statement or claim.
- *More fibre:* The food contains at least 25% more fibre, totalling at least 1 gram more, if no fibre or fibre source is identified in the statement or claim, or at least 25% more of an identified fibre or fibre from an identified fibre source, totalling at least 1 gram more, if a fibre or fibre source is identified in the statement or claim compared to reference amount of a similar food.

## Light and Lean

- *Light in energy or fat:* The food meets the conditions set out for the subject "reduced in energy" or "reduced in fat."
- *Lean:* The food (*a*) is meat or poultry that has not been ground, a marine or fresh water animal or a product of any of these; and (*b*) contains 10% or less fat.
- *Extra lean:* The food (*a*) is meat or poultry that has not been ground, a marine or fresh water animal or a product of any of these; and (*b*) contains 7.5% or less fat.

## Approved Health Claims for Nutrition Labels

If a manufacturer follows specific guidelines addressing both the nutrients noted in the claim as well as guidelines pertaining to other nutrients in a food, the following health claims can be made.

- A healthy diet containing foods high in potassium and low in sodium may reduce the risk of high blood pressure, a risk factor for stroke and heart disease.
- A healthy diet with adequate calcium and vitamin D, and regular physical activity, help to achieve strong bones and may reduce the risk of osteoporosis.
- A healthy diet low in saturated and *trans* fats may reduce the risk of heart disease.
- A healthy diet rich in a variety of vegetables and fruit may help reduce the risk of some types of cancer.
- Foods very low in starch and fermentable sugars can make the following health claims:
  - Won't cause cavities;
  - Does not promote tooth decay;
  - Does not promote dental caries; or is
  - Non-cariogenic.

## THE EXCHANGE SYSTEM

**Exchange System** A system for classifying foods into numerous lists based on the foods' macronutrient composition and establishing serving sizes, so that one serving of each food on a list contains the same amount of carbohydrate, protein, fat, and calorie content.

**exchange** The serving size of a food on a specific exchange list.

The **Exchange System** is a valuable tool for roughly estimating the calorie, protein, carbohydrate, and fat content of a food or meal. This tool organizes many details of the nutrient composition of foods into a manageable framework. By using the Exchange System, you can plan daily menus to fall roughly within specific percentages of macronutrients without having to look up or memorize the nutrient values of numerous foods, so the time you spend now becoming familiar with the Exchange System will pay off in the future.

In the Exchange System, individual foods are placed into three broad groups: carbohydrate, meat and meat substitutes, and fat. Within these groups are lists that contain foods of similar macronutrient composition: various types of milk, fruit, vegetables, starch, other carbohydrates, meat and meat substitutes, and fat. These lists are designed so that, when the proper serving size is observed, each food on a list provides about the same amount of carbohydrate, protein, fat, and calories. This equality allows the exchange of foods on each list, hence the term *Exchange System*.

The Exchange System was originally developed for planning diabetic diets. Diabetes is easier to control if the person's diet has about the same composition day after day. If a certain number of **exchanges** from each of the various lists is eaten each day, that regularity is easier to achieve. However, because the Exchange System provides a quick way to estimate the calorie, carbohydrate, protein, and fat content in any food or meal, it is a valuable menu-planning tool for people without diabetes, as well.

### Becoming Familiar with the Exchange System

To use the Exchange System, you must know which foods are on each list and the serving sizes for each food.

Table D-1 gives the serving sizes for foods on each exchange list, as well as the carbohydrate, protein, fat, and calorie content per exchange. The meat and milk lists are divided into subclasses, which vary in fat content and, hence, in the amount of calories they provide. Foods on the meat and fat lists contain essentially no carbohydrate; those on the fruit and fat lists lack appreciable amounts of protein; and those on the vegetable, fruit, and other carbohydrates lists contain essentially no fat. You need to study Table D-1 and Figure D-1 to become familiar with the exchange lists, the sizes of the exchanges (that is, serving sizes) on each list, and the amounts of carbohydrate, protein, fat, and calories per exchange.

Before you can turn a group of exchanges into a daily meal plan, you must be aware of which foods are on each exchange list (Fig. D-1). The entire U.S. Exchange System (2003) is presented in Appendix D, which you should consult frequently while exploring the system to discover its various peculiarities. For example, the starch list includes not only bread, dry cereal, cooked cereal, rice, and pasta, but also baked beans, corn on the cob, and potatoes. These foods are not identical to those composing the bread, cereal, rice, and pasta group in MyPyramid. The Exchange System is not concerned with the origin of a food, whether animal or vegetable. It is primarily concerned with the macronutrients carbohydrate, protein, and fat in each food on a specific list. For example, the carbohydrate composition of potatoes resembles that of bread more than that of broccoli, although potatoes are vegetables. In addition, several foods on the meat and meat substitutes list are not meats. The list of other carbohydrates includes jam, angel food cake, fat-free frozen yogurt, and foods such as frosted cake that count as both other carbohydrate exchanges and fat exchanges. Bacon appears in the fat list, rather than the high-fat meat category.

**TABLE D-1**   Nutrient Composition of Exchange System Lists (2003 Edition)

| Groups/Lists | Household Measures* | Carbohydrate (g) | Protein (g) | Fat (g) | Energy (kcal) |
|---|---|---|---|---|---|
| **Carbohydrate Group** | | | | | |
| Starch | 1 slice, ¾ cup raw, or ½ cup cooked | 15 | 3 | 1 or less† | 80 |
| Fruit | 1 small/medium piece | 15 | — | — | 60 |
| Milk | 1 cup | | | | |
| Fat-free/very low-fat | | 12 | 8 | 0–3† | 90 |
| Reduced-fat | | 12 | 8 | 5 | 120 |
| Whole | | 12 | 8 | 8 | 150 |
| Other carbohydrates | Varies | 15 | Varies | Varies | Varies |
| Nonstarchy vegetables | 1 cup raw or ½ cup cooked | 5 | 2 | — | 25 |
| **Meat and Meat Substitutes Group** | 1 ounce | | | | |
| Very lean | | — | 7 | 0–1 | 35 |
| Lean | | — | 7 | 3 | 55 |
| Medium-fat | | — | 7 | 5 | 75 |
| High-fat | | — | 7 | 8 | 100 |
| **Fat Group** | 1 teaspoon | — | — | 5 | 45 |

*An estimate; see exchange lists for actual amounts.
†Calculated as 1 gram for purposes of calorie contribution.

Starch exchange choices

Meat and meat substitutes exchange choices

Vegetable exchange choices

Fruit exchange choices

Milk exchange choices

Fat exchange choices

**FIGURE D-1** ▶ Foods arranged according to the Exchange System lists.

**TABLE D-2**   Possible Exchange Patterns That Yield 55% of Calories as Carbohydrate, 30% as Fat, and 15% as Protein

| Exchange List | kcal/Day | | | | | | |
|---|---|---|---|---|---|---|---|
| | 1200* | 1600* | 2000 | 2400 | 2800 | 3200 | 3600 |
| Milk (reduced-fat) | 2 | 2 | 2 | 2 | 2 | 2 | 2 |
| Vegetable | 3 | 3 | 3 | 4 | 4 | 4 | 4 |
| Fruit | 3 | 4 | 5 | 6 | 8 | 9 | 9 |
| Starch | 5 | 8 | 11 | 13 | 15 | 18 | 21 |
| Meat (lean) | 4 | 4 | 4 | 5 | 6 | 7 | 8 |
| Fat | 2 | 4 | 6 | 8 | 10 | 11 | 13 |

This is just one set of options. More meat could be included if less milk were used, for example.

*Calorie intakes of 1200 and 1600 kcal contain 20% of calories as protein and 50% of calories as carbohydrate to allow for greater flexibility in diet planning.

Free foods (essentially calorie-free) include bouillon, diet soda, coffee, tea, dill pickles, and vinegar, as well as herbs and spices. Most vegetables, such as cabbage, celery, mushrooms, lettuce, and zucchini, also can be considered free foods; their minimal energy contribution need not count in the calculations when they are eaten in moderation (1 to 2 servings per meal or snack).

## Using the Exchange System to Develop Daily Menus

Now let's use the Exchange System to plan a 1-day menu. Let's target a calorie content of 2000 kcal, with 55% derived from carbohydrates (1100 kcal), 15% from protein (300 kcal), and 30% from fat (600 kcal). This can be translated into 2 reduced-fat milk exchanges, 3 vegetable exchanges, 5 fruit exchanges, 11 starch exchanges, 4 lean meat exchanges, and 6 fat exchanges (Table D-2). This is only one of many possible combinations; the Exchange System offers great flexibility.

Table D-3 arbitrarily separates these exchanges into breakfast, lunch, dinner, and a snack. Breakfast includes 1 reduced-fat milk exchange, 2 fruit exchanges, 2 starch exchanges, and 1 fat exchange. This total corresponds to ¾ cup of a ready-to-eat breakfast cereal, 1 cup of reduced-fat milk, 1 slice of bread with 1 teaspoon margarine, and 1 cup of orange juice.

Lunch consists of 2 fat exchanges, 4 starch exchanges, 1 vegetable exchange, 1 reduced-fat milk exchange, and 2 fruit exchanges. This translates into one slice of bacon with 1 teaspoon mayonnaise on two slices of bread, with tomato—in other words, a bacon and tomato sandwich. You can also add lettuce to the sandwich. This can be considered a free vegetable choice. Add to this meal a 9-inch banana (1 exchange = 1 small banana), 1 cup of reduced-fat milk, and 6 graham crackers (2½ inches by 2½ inches). Later add a snack of ¾ ounce of pretzels for another starch exchange.

Dinner consists of 4 lean meat exchanges, 1 fruit exchange, 2 vegetable exchanges, 1 fat exchange, and 2 starch exchanges. This total corresponds to a 4-ounce broiled steak (meat only, no bone), 1 medium baked potato (1 exchange = 1 small baked potato) with 1 teaspoon of margarine, 1 cup of broccoli, and 1 kiwi fruit. Coffee (if desired) is not counted, because it contains no appreciable calories.

Finally, we have a snack containing 2 starch exchanges and 2 fat exchanges. This translates into 1 bagel with 2 tablespoons of regular cream cheese.

This 1-day menu is only one of many possible with the exchange lists. Apple juice could replace the orange juice; two apples could be exchanged for the banana. The choices are endless. An exchange diet is much easier to plan if you use individual foods, as was done here; however, the Exchange System tables list some combination foods to help you. Using combination foods, such as pizza or lasagna, however, makes it more difficult to calculate the number of exchanges in a serving. For instance,

**TABLE D-3**  Sample 1-Day 2000-kcal Menu Based on the Exchange System Plan*

**Breakfast**

| | |
|---|---|
| 1 reduced-fat milk exchange | 1 cup reduced-fat milk (some on cereal) |
| 2 fruit exchanges | 1 cup orange juice |
| 2 starch exchanges | ¾ cup ready-to-eat breakfast cereal, 1 piece whole-wheat toast |
| 1 fat exchange | 1 teaspoon soft margarine on toast |

**Lunch**

| | |
|---|---|
| 4 starch exchanges | 2 slices whole-wheat bread, 6 graham crackers (2½ inches by 2½ inches) |
| 2 fat exchanges | 1 slice bacon, 1 teaspoon mayonnaise |
| 1 vegetable exchange | 1 sliced tomato |
| 2 fruit exchanges | 1 banana (9 inches) |
| 1 reduced-fat milk exchange | 1 cup reduced-fat milk |

**Snack**

| | |
|---|---|
| 1 starch exchange | ¾ ounce pretzels |

**Dinner**

| | |
|---|---|
| 4 lean meat exchanges | 4 ounces lean steak (well trimmed) |
| 2 starch exchanges | 1 medium baked potato |
| 1 fat exchange | 1 tsp soft margarine |
| 2 vegetable exchanges | 1 cup cooked broccoli |
| 1 fruit exchange | 1 kiwi fruit |
| | Coffee (if desired) |

**Snack**

| | |
|---|---|
| 2 starch exchanges | 1 bagel |
| 2 fat exchanges | 2 tablespoons regular cream cheese |

*The target plan was a 2000 kcal intake, with 55% of calories from carbohydrate, 15% from protein, and 30% from fat. Computer analysis indicates that this menu yielded 2040 kcal, with 53% of calories from carbohydrate, 16% from protein, and 31% from fat—in close agreement with the targeted goals.

lasagna typically has meat exchanges, vegetable exchanges, and starch exchanges. With practice, you will be able to tackle such complex foods (Fig. D-2). For now, using individual foods makes learning the Exchange System much easier. Finally, you might want to prove to yourself that the food choices listed in Table D-3 really meet the Exchange plan. This demonstration will give you practice turning exchanges into food servings.

**FIGURE D-2** ▶ Record the Exchange System pattern you have chosen in the left-hand column. Then distribute the exchanges throughout the day, noting the food to be used and the serving size.

| Exchange List | Total Exchanges to be Consumed Daily | Exchanges Consumed at Each Meal | | |
|---|---|---|---|---|
| | | Breakfast | Lunch | Dinner |
| MILK | | | | |
| VEGETABLE | | | | |
| FRUIT | | | | |
| STARCH | | | | |
| MEAT AND SUBSTITUTES | | | | |
| FAT | | | | |

# EXCHANGE SYSTEM LISTS

The exchange lists are the basis of a meal planning system designed by a committee of the American Diabetes Association and the American Dietetic Association. While designed primarily for people with diabetes and others who must follow special diets, the exchange lists are based on principles of good nutrition that apply to everyone. © 2003 by the American Diabetes Association and the American Dietetic Association.

## MILK EXCHANGE LIST

### Fat-Free and Low-Fat Milk

(12 g carbohydrate, 8 g protein, 0–3 g fat, 90 kcal)

| | |
|---|---|
| 1 cup | fat-free, ½%, and 1% milk, and buttermilk |
| ⅓ cup | powdered (fat-free dry, before adding liquid) |
| ½ cup | canned, evaporated fat-free milk |
| 1 cup | buttermilk made from fat-free or low-fat milk |
| 1 cup | soy milk (low-fat or fat-free) |
| ⅔ cup (6 oz) | yogurt made from fat-free milk (plain, unflavored) |
| ⅔ cup (6 oz) | yogurt, fat-free, flavored, sweetened with nonnutritive sweetener and fructose |

### Reduced-Fat Milk

(12 g carbohydrate, 8 g protein, 5 g fat, 120 kcal)

| | |
|---|---|
| 1 cup | 2% milk |
| 1 cup | soy milk |
| ¾ cup | yogurt plain, low-fat (added milk solids) |
| 1 cup | sweet acidophilus milk |

### Whole Milk

(12 g carbohydrate, 8 g protein, 8 g fat, 150 kcal)

| | |
|---|---|
| 1 cup | whole milk |
| ½ cup | evaporated whole milk |
| 1 cup | goat's milk |
| 1 cup | kefir |
| 1 cup | yogurt, plain (made from whole milk) |

## NON-STARCHY VEGETABLE EXCHANGE LIST

(5 g carbohydrate, 2 g protein, 0 g fat, 25 kcal)
1 vegetable exchange equals: ½ cup cooked vegetables or vegetable juice or 1 cup raw vegetables

| | | |
|---|---|---|
| artichoke | cucumber | peppers (all varieties) |
| artichoke hearts | eggplant | radishes |
| asparagus | green onions or scallions | salad greens (all varieties) |
| beans (green, wax, Italian) | greens (e.g., collard) | sauerkraut |
| bean sprouts | kohlrabi | spinach |
| beets | leeks | squash (summer) |
| broccoli | mixed vegetables (without corn, peas, or pasta) | tomato (fresh, canned, sauce) |
| brussels sprouts | | tomato/vegetable juice |
| cabbage | mushrooms | turnips |
| carrots | okra | water chestnuts |
| cauliflower | onions | watercress |
| celery | pea pods | zucchini |

## FRUIT EXCHANGE LIST

### Fruit

(15 g carbohydrate, 0 g protein, 0 g fat, 60 kcal)
1 fruit exchange equals:

| | | | |
|---|---|---|---|
| 1 (4 oz) | apple, unpeeled (small) | ½ cup | applesauce (unsweetened) |
| 4 rings | apple, dried | 4 (5½ oz) | apricots, fresh |

| | |
|---|---|
| 8 halves | apricots, dried |
| ½ cup | apricots, canned |
| 1 (4 oz) | banana (small) |
| ¾ cup | blackberries |
| ¾ cup | blueberries |
| ⅓ melon (11 oz) | cantaloupe (small) |
| 1 cup cubes | cantaloupe |
| 12 (3 oz) | cherries |
| ½ cup | cherries, canned |
| 3 | dates |
| 2 (3½ oz) | figs, fresh (large) |
| 1½ | figs, dried |
| ½ cup | fruit cocktail |
| ½ (11 oz) | grapefruit (large) |
| ¾ cup | grapefruit sections, canned |
| 17 (3 oz) | grapes (small) |
| 1 slice (10 oz) | honeydew melon (or 1 cup cubes) |
| 1 (3½ oz) | kiwi |
| ¾ cup | mandarin orange sections |
| ½ (5½ oz) | mango (or ½ cup) |
| 1 (5 oz) | nectarine (small) |
| 1 (6½ oz) | orange (small) |
| ½ (8 oz) | papaya (or 1 cup cubes) |
| 1 (4 oz) | peach, fresh (medium) |

| | |
|---|---|
| ½ cup | peaches, canned |
| 1 (4 oz) | pear, fresh |
| ½ cup | pear, canned |
| ¾ cup | pineapple, fresh |
| ½ cup | pineapple, canned |
| 2 (5 oz) | plums (small) |
| ½ cup | plums, canned |
| 3 | plums dried (prunes) |
| 2 tbsp | raisins |
| 1 cup | raspberries |
| 1¼ cup | strawberries (raw, whole) |
| 2 (8 oz) | tangerines (small) |
| 1 slice (13½ oz) | watermelon (or 1¼ cups cubes) |

### Fruit Juice

| | |
|---|---|
| ½ cup | apple juice/cider |
| ⅓ cup | cranberry juice cocktail |
| 1 cup | cranberry juice cocktail, reduced-calorie |
| ⅓ cup | fruit juice blends, 100% juice |
| ⅓ cup | grape juice |
| ½ cup | grapefruit juice |
| ½ cup | orange juice |
| ½ cup | pineapple juice |
| ⅓ cup | prune juice |

## STARCH EXCHANGE LIST

(15 g carbohydrate, 3 g protein, 0–1 g fat, 80 kcal)
1 starch exchange equals:

### Bread

| | |
|---|---|
| ¼ (1 oz) | bagel |
| 2 slices (1½ oz) | bread, reduced-calorie |
| 1 slice (1 oz) | bread, white, whole-wheat, pumpernickel, or rye |
| 4 (⅔ oz) | bread sticks, crisp, 4 inch × ½ inch |
| ½ | English muffin |
| ½ (1 oz) | hot dog or hamburger bun |
| ¼ | naan, 8 inch × 2 inch |
| 1 | pancake, 4 inch across × ¼ inch thick |
| ½ | pita, 6 inches across |
| 1 slice (1 oz) | raisin bread, unfrosted |
| 1 (1 oz) | roll, plain (small) |
| 1 | tortilla, corn, 6 inches across |
| 1 | tortilla, flour, 6 inches across |
| ⅓ | tortilla, flour, 10 inches across |
| 1 | waffle, 4 inches square or across, reduced-fat |

### Cereals and Grains

| | |
|---|---|
| ½ cup | bran cereal |
| ½ cup | bulgur |
| ½ cup | cereal, cooked |
| ¾ cup | cereal, unsweetened, ready-to-eat |
| 3 tbsp | cornmeal (dry) |
| ⅓ cup | couscous |
| 3 tbsp | flour (dry) |
| ¼ cup | granola, low-fat |
| ¼ cup | Grape-Nuts® |
| ½ cup | grits |
| ½ cup | kasha |
| ⅓ cup | millet |
| ¼ cup | muesli |
| ½ cup | oats |
| ⅓ cup | pasta |
| 1½ cups | puffed cereal |
| ⅓ cup | rice, white or brown |
| ½ cup | Shredded Wheat |
| ½ cup | sugar-frosted cereal |
| 3 tbsp | wheat germ |

## Starchy Vegetables

| | |
|---|---|
| ⅓ cup | baked beans |
| ½ cup | corn |
| ½ (5 oz) | corn on the cob (large) |
| 1 cup | mixed vegetables with corn, peas, or pasta |
| ½ cup | peas, green |
| ½ cup | plantain |
| ½ cup or ½ medium (3 oz) | potato, boiled |
| ¼ large (3 oz) | potato, baked with skin |
| ½ cup | potato, mashed |
| 1 cup | squash, winter (acorn, butternut, pumpkin) |
| ½ cup | yam, sweet potato, plain |

## Crackers and Snacks

| | |
|---|---|
| 8 | animal crackers |
| 3 | graham crackers, 2½-inch square |
| ¾ oz | matzoh |
| 4 slices | melba toast |
| 24 | oyster crackers |
| 3 cups | popcorn (popped, no fat added or low-fat microwave) |
| ¾ oz | pretzels |
| 2 | rice cakes, 4 inches across |
| 6 | saltine-type crackers |
| 15–20 (¾ oz) | snack chips, fat-free (tortilla, potato) |
| 2–5 (¾ oz) | whole-wheat crackers, no fat added |

## Dried Beans, Peas, and Lentils

### (Counts as 1 starch exchange plus 1 very lean meat exchange)

| | |
|---|---|
| ½ cup | beans and peas (garbanzo, pinto, kidney, white, split, black-eyed) |
| ½ cup | lentils |
| ⅔ cup | lima beans |
| 3 tbsp | miso |

## Starchy Foods Prepared with Fat

### (Counts as 1 starch exchange, plus 1 fat exchange)

| | |
|---|---|
| 1 | biscuit, 2½ inches across |
| ½ cup | chow mein noodles |
| 1 piece (2 oz) | corn bread, 2-inch cube |
| 6 | crackers, round butter type |
| 1 cup | croutons |
| 1 cup (2 oz) | French-fried potatoes (oven-baked) (see also the fast-foods list) |
| ¼ cup | granola |
| ⅓ cup | hummus |
| ⅕ (1 oz) | muffin, 5 oz |
| 3 cups | popcorn, microwaved |
| 3 | sandwich crackers, cheese or peanut butter filling |
| 9–13 (3/4 oz) | snack chips (potato, tortilla) |
| ⅓ cup | stuffing, bread (prepared) |
| 2 | taco shells, 6 inches across |
| 1 | waffle, 4-inch square or across |
| 4–6 (1 oz) | whole-wheat crackers, fat added |

# SWEETS, DESSERTS AND OTHER CARBOHYDRATES EXCHANGE LIST

One exchange equals 15 g carbohydrate, or 1 starch, or 1 fruit, or 1 milk.

## Exchanges per Serving

| | | |
|---|---|---|
| ¹⁄₁₂ cake (about 2 oz) | angel food cake, unfrosted | 2 carbohydrates |
| 2-inch square (about 1 oz) | brownie, unfrosted (small) | 1 carbohydrate, 1 fat |
| 2-inch square (about 1 oz) | cake, unfrosted | 1 carbohydrate, 1 fat |
| 2-inch square (about 2 oz) | cake, frosted | 2 carbohydrates, 1 fat |
| 2 | cookies, fat-free (small) | 1 carbohydrate |
| 2 (about ⅔ oz) | cookies or sandwich cookies with creme filling (small) | 1 carbohydrate, 1 fat |
| ¼ cup | cranberry sauce, jellied | 1½ carbohydrates |
| 1 (about 2 oz) | cupcake, frosted (small) | 2 carbohydrates, 1 fat |
| 1 (1½ oz) | doughnut, plain cake (medium) | 1½ carbohydrates, 2 fats |
| 3¾ inches across (2 oz) | doughnuts, glazed | 2 carbohydrates, 2 fats |
| 1 bar (1⅓ oz) | Energy, sport, or breakfast bar | 2 carbohydrates, 1 fat |
| 1 bar (2 oz) | Energy, sport, or breakfast bar | 3 carbohydrates, 1 fat |
| ½ cup (3½ oz) | fruit cobbler | 3 carbohydrates, 1 fat |
| 1 bar (3 oz) | fruit juice bars, frozen, 100% juice | 1 carbohydrate |

| | | |
|---|---|---|
| 1 roll (¾ oz) | fruit snacks, chewy (puréed fruit concentrate) | 1 carbohydrate |
| 1½ tbsp | fruit spread, 100% fruit | 1 carbohydrate |
| ½ cup | gelatin, regular | 1 carbohydrate |
| 3 | gingersnaps | 1 carbohydrate |
| 1 bar (1 oz) | granola or snack bar (regular and low-fat) | 1½ carbohydrates |
| 1 tbsp | honey | 1 carbohydrate |
| ½ cup | ice cream, low-fat | 1½ carbohydrates |
| ½ cup | ice cream | 1 carbohydrate, 2 fats |
| ½ cup | ice cream, light | 1 carbohydrate, 1 fat |
| ½ cup | ice cream, fat-free, no sugar added | 1 carbohydrate |
| 1 tbsp | jam or jelly, regular | 1 carbohydrate |
| 1 cup | milk, chocolate, whole | 2 carbohydrates, 1 fat |
| ⅙ pie | pie, fruit, 2 crusts (8 inches across) | 3 carbohydrates, 2 fats |
| ⅛ pie | pie, pumpkin or custard (8 inches across) | 2 carbohydrates, 2 fats |
| ½ cup | pudding, regular (made with reduced-fat milk) | 2 carbohydrates |
| ½ cup | pudding, sugar-free (made with fat-free milk) | 1 carbohydrate |
| 1 can (10–11 oz) | reduced-calorie meal replacement (shake) | 1½ carbohydrates, 0–1 fat |
| 1 cup | rice milk, low-fat or fat-free, plain | 1 carbohydrate |
| 1 cup | rice milk, low-fat, flavored | 1½ carbohydrates |
| ¼ cup | salad dressing, fat-free | 1 carbohydrate |
| ½ cup | sherbet, sorbet | 2 carbohydrates |
| ½ cup | spaghetti or pasta sauce, canned | 1 carbohydrate, 1 fat |
| 1 cup (8 oz) | sports drinks | 1 carbohydrate |
| 1 tbsp | sugar | 1 carbohydrate |
| 1 (2½ oz) | sweet roll or Danish | 2½ carbohydrates, 2 fats |
| 2 tbsp | syrup, light | 1 carbohydrate |
| 1 tbsp | syrup, regular | 1 carbohydrate |
| 5 | vanilla wafers | 1 carbohydrate, 1 fat |
| ⅓ cup | yogurt, frozen, fat-free | 1 carbohydrate |
| 1 cup | yogurt, low-fat with fruit | 3 carbohydrates, 0–1 fat |

## MEAT AND MEAT SUBSTITUTES EXCHANGE LIST

### Very Lean Meat and Substitutes List

(0 g carbohydrate, 7 g protein, 0–1 g fat, and 35 kcal)
One very lean meat exchange equals:

**Poultry**

1 oz   chicken or turkey (white meat, no skin), Cornish hen (no skin)

**Fish**

1 oz   fresh or frozen cod, flounder, haddock, halibut, trout; tuna, fresh or canned in water

**Shellfish**

1 oz   clams, crab, lobster, scallops, shrimp, imitation shellfish

**Game**

1 oz   duck or pheasant (no skin), venison, buffalo, ostrich

**Cheese with 1 g or less fat per oz**

¼ cup   fat-free or low-fat cottage cheese
1 oz   fat-free cheese

**Other**

1 oz   processed sandwich meats with 1 g or less fat per oz, such as deli thin, shaved meats, chipped beef, turkey, ham

¼ cup   egg substitute, plain
2   egg whites
1 oz   hot dogs with 1 g or less fat per oz
1 oz   kidney (high in cholesterol)
1 oz   sausage with 1 g or less fat per oz

**Counts as one very lean meat and one starch exchange:**

½ cup   dried beans, peas, lentils (cooked)

## Lean Meat and Substitutes List

(0 g carbohydrate, 7 g protein, 3 g fat, and 55 kcal)
One lean meat exchange equals:

**Beef**

1 oz     USDA Select or Choice grades of lean beef trimmed of fat, such as round, sirloin, and flank steak; tenderloin; roast (rib, chuck, rump); steak (T-bone, porterhouse, cubed), ground round

**Pork**

1 oz     lean pork, such as fresh ham; canned, cured, or boiled ham; Canadian bacon; tenderloin, center loin chop

**Lamb**

1 oz     roast, chop, leg

**Veal**

1 oz     lean chop, roast

**Poultry**

1 oz     chicken, turkey (dark meat, no skin), chicken white meat (with skin), domestic duck or goose (well drained of fat, no skin)

**Fish**

| | |
|---|---|
| 1 oz | herring (uncreamed or smoked) |
| 6 | oysters (medium) |
| 1 oz | salmon (fresh or canned), catfish |
| 2 | sardines (canned, medium) |
| 1 oz | tuna (canned in oil, drained) |

**Game**

1 oz     goose (no skin), rabbit

**Cheese**

| | |
|---|---|
| ¼ cup | 4.5%–fat cottage cheese |
| 2 tbsp | grated Parmesan |
| 1 oz | cheeses with 3 g or less fat per oz |

**Other**

| | |
|---|---|
| 1½ oz | hot dogs with 3 g or less fat per oz |
| 1 oz | processed sandwich meat with 3 g or less fat per oz, such as turkey pastrami or kielbasa |
| 1 oz | liver, heart (high in cholesterol) |

## Medium-Fat Meat and Substitutes List

(0 g carbohydrate, 7 g protein, 5 g fat, and 75 kcal)
One medium-fat meat exchange equals:

**Beef**

1 oz     most beef products (ground beef; meatloaf; corned beef; short ribs; prime grades of meat trimmed of fat, such as prime rib)

**Pork**

1 oz     top loin, chop, Boston butt, cutlet

**Fish**

1 oz     any fried fish product

**Cheese (with 5 g or less fat per oz)**

| | |
|---|---|
| 1 oz | feta |
| 1 oz | mozzarella |
| ¼ cup (2 oz) | ricotta |

**Lamb**

1 oz     rib roast, ground

**Veal**

1 oz     cutlet (ground or cubed, unbreaded)

**Poultry**

1 oz     chicken dark meat (with skin), ground turkey or ground chicken, fried chicken (with skin)

**Other**

| | |
|---|---|
| 1 | egg (high in cholesterol, limit to 3 per week) |
| 1 oz | sausage with 5 g or less fat per oz |
| ¼ cup | tempeh |
| 4 oz (½ cup) | tofu |

## High-Fat Meat and Substitutes List

(0 g carbohydrate, 7 g protein, 8 g fat, and 100 kcal)
One high-fat meat exchange equals:

**Pork**

1 oz     spareribs, ground pork, pork sausage

**Cheese**

1 oz     all regular cheeses, such as American, cheddar, Monterey Jack, Swiss

**Other**

| | |
|---|---|
| 1 oz | processed sandwich meats with 8 g or less fat per oz, such as bologna, pimento loaf, salami |
| 1 oz | sausage, such as bratwurst, Italian, knockwurst, Polish, smoked |
| 1 | hot dog (turkey or chicken) (10 per pound) |
| 3 slices | bacon (20 slices per pound) |

**Counts as one high-fat meat plus one fat exchange:**

1     hot dog (beef, pork, or combination) (10 per pound)

# FAT EXCHANGE LIST

## Monounsaturated Fats List

(5 g fat and 45 kcal)
One exchange equals:

| | | | |
|---|---|---|---|
| 2 tbsp (1 oz) | avocado (medium) | 6 nuts | mixed (50% peanuts) |
| 1 tsp | oil (canola, olive, peanut) | 10 nuts | peanuts |
| | olives: | 4 halves | pecans |
| 8 | ripe, black (large) | ½ tbsp | peanut butter, smooth or crunchy |
| 10 | green, stuffed (large) | 1 tbsp | sesame seeds |
| 6 nuts | almonds, cashews | 2 tsp | tahini or sesame paste |

## Polyunsaturated Fats List

(5 g fat and 45 kcal)
One exchange equals:

| | | | |
|---|---|---|---|
| | margarine: | | salad dressing: |
| 1 tsp | stick, tub, or squeeze | 1 tbsp | regular |
| 1 tbsp | lower-fat (30% to 50% vegetable oil) | 2 tbsp | reduced-fat |
| | mayonnaise: | | Miracle Whip Salad Dressing®: |
| 1 tsp | regular | 2 tsp | regular |
| 1 tbsp | reduced-fat | 1 tbsp | reduced-fat |
| 4 halves | nuts, walnuts, English | 1 tbsp | seeds: pumpkin, sunflower |
| 1 tsp | oil (corn, safflower, soybean) | | |

## Saturated Fats List

(5 g fat and 45 kcal)
One exchange equals:

| | | | |
|---|---|---|---|
| 1 slice | bacon, cooked (20 slices per pound) | | butter: |
| 1 tsp | bacon, grease | 1 tsp | stick |
| 2 tbsp (½ oz) | chitterlings, boiled | 2 tsp | whipped |
| | cream cheese: | 1 tbsp | reduced-fat |
| 1 tbsp (½ oz) | regular | | sour cream: |
| 2 tbsp (1 oz) | reduced-fat | 2 tbsp | regular |
| 1 tsp | shortening or lard | 3 tbsp | reduced-fat |

# FREE FOODS LIST

A *free food* is any food or drink that contains less than 20 kcal or less than 5 g of carbohydrate per serving. Foods with a serving size listed should be limited to three servings per day. Foods listed without a serving size can be eaten as often as you like.

## Fat-Free or Reduced-Fat Foods

| | | | |
|---|---|---|---|
| 1 tbsp (½ oz) | cream cheese, fat-free | 1 tsp | Miracle Whip®, reduced-fat nonstick cooking spray |
| 1 tbsp | creamers, nondairy, liquid | | |
| 2 tsp | creamers, nondairy, powdered | 1 tbsp | salad dressing, fat-free nonstick cooking spray |
| 1 tbsp | mayonnaise, fat-free | | |
| 1 tsp | mayonnaise, reduced-fat | 1 tbsp | salad dressing, fat-free or low-fat, Italian |
| 4 tbsp | margarine, fat-free | 2 tbsp | salad dressing, fat-free, Italian |
| 1 tsp | margarine, reduced-fat | 1 tbsp | sour cream, fat-free, reduced-fat |
| 1 tbsp | Miracle Whip®, fat-free | 1 tbsp | whipped topping, regular |
| | | 2 tbsp | whipped topping, light or fat-free |

## Sugar-Free Foods

| | | | |
|---|---|---|---|
| 1 candy | candy, hard, sugar-free; gelatin dessert, sugar-free; gelatin, unflavored; gum, sugar-free | 2 tsp | jam or jelly, light sugar substitutes* |
| | | 2 tbsp | syrup, sugar-free |

## Drinks

bouillon, broth, consommé
bouillon or broth, low-sodium
carbonated or mineral water
club soda
1 tbsp  cocoa powder, unsweetened

coffee
diet soft drinks, sugar-free
drink mixes, sugar-free
tea
tonic water, sugar-free

## Condiments

| | | | |
|---|---|---|---|
| 1 tbsp | catsup | 2 slices | pickles, sweet (bread and butter) |
| | horseradish | ¾ oz | pickles, sweet (gherkin) |
| | lemon juice | ¼ cup | salsa |
| | lime juice | 1 tbsp | soy sauce, regular or light |
| | mustard | 1 tbsp | taco sauce |
| 1 tbsp | pickle relish | | vinegar |
| 1½ | pickles, dill (medium) | 2 tbsp | yogurt |

## Seasonings

flavoring extracts
garlic
herbs, fresh or dried
pimento

spices
Tabasco® or hot pepper sauce
wine, used in cooking
Worcestershire sauce

# COMBINATION FOODS LIST

| | Entrées | Exchanges per Serving |
|---|---|---|
| 1 cup (8 oz) | tuna noodle casserole, lasagna, spaghetti with meatballs, chili with beans, macaroni and cheese | 2 carbohydrates, 2 medium-fat meats |
| 2 cups (16 oz) | chow mein (without noodles or rice) | 1 carbohydrate, 2 lean meats |
| ½ cup (3½ oz) | tuna or chicken salad | ½ carbohydrate, 2 lean meats, 1 fat |
| | **Frozen Entrées and Meals** | |
| generally 14–17 oz | dinner-type meal | 3 carbohydrates, 3 medium-fat meats, 3 fats |
| 3 oz | meatless burger, soy-based | ½ carbohydrate, 2 lean meats |
| 3 oz | meatless burger, vegetable and starch-based | 1 carbohydrate, 1 lean meat |
| ¼ of 12-inch (6 oz) | pizza, cheese, thin crust | 2 carbohydrates, 2 medium-fat meats, 1 fat |
| ¼ of 12-inch (6 oz) | pizza, meat topping, thin crust | 2 carbohydrates, 2 medium-fat meats, 2 fats |
| 1 (7 oz) | pot pie | 2½ carbohydrates, 1 medium-fat meat, 3 fats |
| 8–11 oz | entrée or meal with less than 340 kcal | 2–3 carbohydrates, 1–2 lean meats |
| | **Soups** | |
| 1 cup | bean | 1 carbohydrate, 1 very lean meat |
| 1 cup (8 oz) | cream (made with water) | 1 carbohydrate, 1 fat |
| 6 oz prepared | instant | 1 carbohydrate |
| 8 oz prepared | instant with beans/lentils | 2½ carbohydrates, 1 very lean meat |
| ½ cup (4 oz) | split pea (made with water) | 1 carbohydrate |
| 1 cup (8 oz) | tomato (made with water) | 1 carbohydrate |
| 1 cup (8 oz) | vegetable beef, chicken noodle, or other broth-type | 1 carbohydrate |

## Fast-Foods

| | | Exchanges per Serving |
|---|---|---|
| 1 (5–7 oz) | burritos with beef | 3 carbohydrates, 1 medium-fat meat, 1 fat |
| 6 | chicken nuggets | 1 carbohydrate, 2 medium-fat meats, 1 fat |
| 1 each | chicken breast and wing, breaded and fried | 1 carbohydrate, 4 medium-fat meats, 2 fats |
| 1 | chicken sandwich, grilled | 2 carbohydrates, 3 very lean meats |
| 6 (5 oz) | chicken wings, hot | 1 carbohydrate, 3 medium-fat meats, 4 fats |
| 1 | fish sandwich/tartar sauce | 3 carbohydrates, 1 medium-fat meat, 3 fats |
| 1 medium serving (5 oz) | French fries | 4 carbohydrates, 4 fats |
| 1 | hamburger (regular) | 2 carbohydrates, 2 medium-fat meats |
| 1 | hamburger (large) | 2 carbohydrates, 3 medium-fat meats, 1 fat |
| 1 | hot dog with bun | 1 carbohydrate, 1 high-fat meat, 1 fat |
| 1 | individual pan pizza | 5 carbohydrates, 3 medium-fat meats, 3 fats |
| ¼ 12-inch (about 6 oz) | pizza, cheese, thin crust | 2½ carbohydrates, 2 medium-fat meats |
| ¼ 12-inch (about 6 oz) | pizza, meat, thin crust | 2½ carbohydrates, 2 medium-fat meats, 1 fat |
| 1 (5 oz) | soft-serve cone (small) | 2½ carbohydrates, 1 fat |
| 1 sub (6 inches) | submarine sandwich | 3 carbohydrates, 1 vegetable, 2 medium-fat meats, 1 fat |
| 1 (3–3½ oz) | taco, hard or soft shell | 1 carbohydrate, 1 medium-fat meat, 1 fat |

Although it may seem overwhelming at first, it is easy to track the foods you eat. One tip is to record foods and beverages consumed as soon as possible after consumption.

I. **Fill in the food record form that follows.** Appendix E contains a blank copy (see the completed example in Table E-1). Then, to estimate the nutrient values of the foods you are eating, consult food labels and use the NutritionCalc Plus software (CD or online) available with this book. If these resources do not have the serving size you need, adjust the value. If you drink ½ cup of orange juice, for example, but a table has values only for 1 cup, halve all values before you record them. Then, consider pooling all the same food to save time; if you drink a cup of 1% milk three times throughout the day, enter your milk consumption only once as 3 cups. As you record your intake for use on the nutrient analysis form that follows, consider the following tips:
   - Measure and record the amounts of foods eaten in portion sizes of cups, teaspoons, tablespoons, ounces, slices, or inches (or convert metric units to these units).
   - Record brand names of all food products, such as "Quick Quaker Oats."
   - Measure and record all those little extras, such as gravies, salad dressings, taco sauces, pickles, jelly, sugar, catsup, and margarine.
   - For beverages
     - List the type of milk, such as whole, fat-free, 1%, evaporated, chocolate, or reconstituted dry.
     - Indicate whether fruit juice is fresh, frozen, or canned.
     - Indicate type for other beverages, such as fruit drink, fruit-flavored drink, Kool-Aid, and hot chocolate made with water or milk.
   - For fruits
     - Indicate whether fresh, frozen, dried, or canned.
     - If whole, record number eaten and size with approximate measurements (such as 1 apple—3 in. in diameter).
     - Indicate whether processed in water, light syrup, or heavy syrup.
   - For vegetables
     - Indicate whether fresh, frozen, dried, or canned.
     - Record as portion of cup, teaspoon, or tablespoon, or as pieces (such as carrot sticks—4 in. long, ½ in. thick).
     - Record preparation method.
   - For cereals
     - Record cooked cereals in portions of tablespoon or cup (a level measurement after cooking).
     - Record dry cereal in level portions of tablespoon or cup.
     - If margarine, milk, sugar, fruit, or something else is added, measure and record amount and type.
   - For breads
     - Indicate whether whole wheat, rye, white, and so on.
     - Measure and record number and size of portion (biscuit—2 in. across, 1 in. thick; slice of homemade rye bread—3 in. by 4 in., ¼ in. thick).
     - Sandwiches: list all ingredients (lettuce, mayonnaise, tomato, and so on).

- For meat, fish, poultry, and cheese
  - Give size (length, width, thickness) in inches or weight in ounces after cooking for meat, fish, and poultry (such as cooked hamburger patty—3 in. across, ½ in. thick).
  - Give size (length, width, thickness) in inches or weight in ounces for cheese.
  - Record measurements only for the cooked, edible part—without bone or fat left on the plate.
  - Describe how meat, poultry, or fish was prepared.
- For eggs
  - Record as soft or hard cooked, fried, scrambled, poached, or omelet.
  - If milk, butter, or drippings are used, specify types and amount.
- For desserts
  - List commercial brand or "homemade" or "bakery" under brand.
  - Purchased candies, cookies, and cakes: specify kind and size.
  - Measure and record portion size of cakes, pies, and cookies by specifying thickness, diameter, and width or length, depending on the item.

**TABLE E-1**  One Day's Food Record—This Activity Can Help You Understand More About Your Food Habits

| Time | Minutes Spent Eating | M or S* | H† (0–3) | Activity While Eating | Place of Eating | Food and Quantity | Others Present | Reason for Choice |
|---|---|---|---|---|---|---|---|---|
| 7:10 a.m. | 15 | M | 2 | Standing, fixing lunch | Kitchen | Orange juice, 1 cup<br>Crispix, 1 cup<br>Non-fat milk, ½ cup<br>Sugar, 2 tsp<br>Black coffee | — | Health<br>Habit<br>Health<br><br>Taste<br>Habit |
| 10:00 a.m. | 4 | S | 1 | Sitting, taking notes | Classroom | Diet cola, 12 oz | Class | Weight control |
| 12:15 p.m. | 40 | M | 2 | Sitting, talking | Student union | Chicken sandwich with lettuce and mayonnaise (3 oz chicken, 2 slices of white bread, 2 tsp mayonnaise)<br>Pear, 1 medium<br>Non-fat milk, 1 cup | Friends | Taste<br><br><br><br>Health<br>Health |
| 2:30 p.m. | 10 | S | 1 | Sitting, studying | Library | Regular cola, 12 oz | Friend | Hunger |
| 6:30 p.m. | 35 | M | 3 | Sitting, talking | Kitchen | Pork chop, 1<br>Baked potato, 1<br>Margarine, 2 tbsp<br>Lettuce and tomato salad, 1 cup<br>Ranch dressing, 2 tbsp<br>Peas, ½ cup<br>Whole milk, 1 cup<br>Cherry pie, 1 piece<br>Iced tea, 12 oz | Boyfriend | Convenience<br>Health<br>Taste<br>Health<br><br>Taste<br><br>Health<br>Habit<br>Taste<br>Health |
| 9:10 p.m. | 10 | S | 2 | Sitting, studying | Living room | Apple, 1 medium<br>Glass mineral water, 1 | — | Weight control<br>Weight control |

*M or S: Meal or snack
†H: Degree of hunger (0 = none; 3 = maximum)

| Time | Minutes Spent Eating | M or S* | H† (0–3) | Activity While Eating | Place of Eating | Food and Quantity | Others Present | Reason for Choice |
|------|----------------------|---------|----------|------------------------|-----------------|--------------------|----------------|--------------------|
|  |  |  |  |  |  |  |  |  |
|  |  |  |  |  |  |  |  |  |
|  |  |  |  |  |  |  |  |  |
|  |  |  |  |  |  |  |  |  |
|  |  |  |  |  |  |  |  |  |
|  |  |  |  |  |  |  |  |  |
|  |  |  |  |  |  |  |  |  |
|  |  |  |  |  |  |  |  |  |

*M or S: Meal or snack
†H: Degree of hunger (0 = none; 3 = maximum)

II. **Now complete the nutrient analysis form as shown, using your food record.**
   A blank copy of this form for your use is on pages A-41 and A-42. NutritionCalc
   Plus will create such a table for you if you enter all food eaten.

Nutrient Analysis Form (Sample)

| Name | Quantity | kcal | Protein (g) | Carbohydrates (g) | Fiber (g) | Total fat (g) | Monounsaturated fat (g) | Polyunsaturated fat (g) | Saturated fat (g) | Cholesterol (g) | Calcium (mg) | Iron (mg) |
|---|---|---|---|---|---|---|---|---|---|---|---|---|
| Egg bagel, 3.5-in. diameter | 1 ea. | 180 | 7.45 | 34.7 | 0.748 | 1.00 | 0.286 | 0.400 | 0.171 | 44.0 | 20.0 | 2.10 |
| Jelly | 1 tbsp | 49.0 | 0.018 | 12.7 | — | 0.018 | 0.005 | 0.005 | 0.005 | — | 2.00 | 0.120 |
| Orange juice, prepared fresh or frozen | 1½ cup | 165 | 2.52 | 40.2 | 1.49 | 0.210 | 0.037 | 0.045 | 0.025 | — | 33.0 | 0.411 |
| Cheeseburger, McDonald's | 2 ea. | 636 | 30.2 | 57.0 | 0.460 | 32.0 | 12.2 | 2.18 | 13.3 | 80.0 | 338 | 5.68 |
| French fries, McDonald's | 1 order | 220 | 3.00 | 26.1 | 4.19 | 11.5 | 4.37 | 0.570 | 4.61 | 8.57 | 9.10 | 0.605 |
| Cola beverage, regular | 1½ cup | 151 | — | 38.5 | — | — | — | — | — | — | 9.00 | 0.120 |
| Pork loin chop, broiled, lean | 4 oz | 261 | 36.2 | — | — | 11.9 | 5.35 | 1.43 | 4.09 | 112 | 5.67 | 1.04 |
| Baked potato with skin | 1 ea. | 220 | 4.65 | 51.0 | 3.90 | 0.200 | 0.004 | 0.087 | 0.052 | — | 20.0 | 2.75 |
| Peas, frozen, cooked | ½ cup | 63.0 | 4.12 | 11.4 | 3.61 | 0.220 | 0.019 | 0.103 | 0.039 | — | 19.0 | 1.25 |
| Margarine, regular or soft, 80% fat | 20 g | 143 | 0.160 | 0.100 | — | 16.1 | 5.70 | 6.92 | 2.76 | — | 5.29 | — |
| Iceberg lettuce, chopped | 2 cup | 14.6 | 1.13 | 2.34 | 1.68 | 0.212 | 0.008 | 0.112 | 0.028 | — | 21.2 | 0.560 |
| French dressing | 2 oz | 300 | 0.318 | 3.63 | 0.431 | 32.0 | 14.2 | 12.4 | 4.94 | — | 7.10 | 0.227 |
| Reduced-fat (i.e., 2%) milk | 1 cup | 121 | 8.12 | 11.7 | — | 4.78 | 1.35 | 0.170 | 2.92 | 22.0 | 297 | 0.120 |
| Graham crackers | 2 ea. | 60.0 | 1.04 | 10.8 | 1.40 | 1.46 | 0.600 | 0.400 | 0.400 | — | 6.00 | 0.367 |
| Totals | | 2584 | 99.0 | 300 | 17.9 | 112 | 44.1 | 24.8 | 33.4 | 266 | 792 | 15.4 |
| RDA or related nutrient standard* | | 2900 | 58 | 130 | 38 | | | | | | 1000 | 8 |
| % of nutrient needs | | 89 | 170 | 230 | 47 | | | | | | 79 | 193 |

Abbreviations: g = grams, mg = milligrams, µg = micrograms

*Values from inside cover. The values listed are for a male age 19 years. The number of kcal is a rough estimate. It is better to base energy needs on actual energy output.

†In RAE units. Table values generally are in RE units because the food values have not been updated to reflect the latest vitamin A standards. RAE equals SRE for foods with preformed vitamin A, such as for the pork chop, but RAE are only about half the RE listed for foods with provitamin A carotenoids, such as for the peas (see Chapter 8 for details).

‡Amounts refer to actual folate content, rather than dietary folate equivalents (DFE). This difference is important to consider if the food contains added synthetic folic acid as part of enrichment or fortification. Any such folic acid is absorbed about twice as much as the folate present naturally in foods. So the total contribution of folate in the food in comparison to human needs will be greater than if all the folate was naturally in the food product. Nutrient analysis tables have yet to be updated to reflect the dietary folate equivalents of products (see Chapter 8 for more details).

Nutrient Analysis Form (Sample) Cont'd

| Magnesium (mg) | Phosphorus (mg) | Potassium (mg) | Sodium (mg) | Zinc (mg) | Vitamin A (RE) | Vitamin C (mg) | Vitamin E (mg) | Thiamin (mg) | Riboflavin (mg) | Niacin (mg) | Vitamin B-6 (mg) | Folate (µg) | Vitamin B-12 (µg) |
|---|---|---|---|---|---|---|---|---|---|---|---|---|---|
| 18.0 | 61.0 | 65.0 | 300 | 0.612 | 7.00 | — | 1.80 | 2.58 | 0.197 | 2.40 | 0.030 | 16.3 | 0.065 |
| 0.720 | 1.00 | 16.0 | 4.00 | — | 0.200 | 0.710 | 0.016 | 0.002 | 0.005 | 0.036 | 0.005 | 2.00 | — |
| 36.0 | 60.0 | 711 | 3.00 | 0.192 | 28.5 | 145 | 0.714 | 0.300 | 0.060 | 0.750 | 0.165 | 163 | |
| 45.8 | 410 | 314 | 1460 | 5.20 | 134 | 4.10 | 0.560 | 0.600 | 0.480 | 8.66 | 0.230 | 42.0 | 1.82 |
| 26.7 | 101 | 564 | 109 | 0.320 | 5.00 | 12.5 | 0.203 | 0.122 | 0.020 | 2.26 | 0.218 | 19.0 | 0.027 |
| 3.00 | 46.0 | 4.00 | 15.0 | 0.049 | — | — | — | — | — | — | — | — | — |
| 34.0 | 277 | 476 | 88.2 | 2.54 | 3.15 | 0.454 | 0.405 | 1.30 | 0.350 | 6.28 | 0.535 | 6.77 | 0.839 |
| 55.0 | 115 | 844 | 16.0 | 0.650 | — | 26.1 | 0.100 | 0.216 | 0.067 | 3.32 | 0.701 | 22.2 | — |
| 23.0 | 72.0 | 134 | 70.0 | 0.750 | 53.4 | 7.90 | 0.400 | 0.226 | 0.140 | 1.18 | 0.090 | 46.9 | — |
| 0.467 | 4.06 | 7.54 | 216 | 0.041 | 199 | 0.028 | 2.19 | 0.002 | 0.006 | 0.004 | 0.002 | 0.211 | 0.017 |
| 10.1 | 22.4 | 177 | 10.1 | 0.246 | 37.0 | 4.36 | 0.120 | 0.052 | 0.034 | 0.210 | 0.044 | 62.8 | — |
| 5.81 | 3.63 | 7.03 | 666 | 0.045 | 0.023 | — | 15.9 | — | — | — | 0.006 | — | — |
| 33.0 | 232 | 377 | 122 | 0.963 | 140 | 2.32 | 0.080 | 0.095 | 0.403 | 0.210 | 0.105 | 12.0 | 0.888 |
| 6.00 | 20.0 | 36.0 | 86.0 | 0.113 | — | — | — | 0.020 | 0.030 | 0.600 | 0.011 | 1.80 | — |
| 298 | 1425 | 3732 | 3165 | 11.7 | 607 | 204 | 22.5 | 5.52 | 1.79 | 25.9 | 2.14 | 395 | 3.65 |
| 400 | 700 | 4700 | 1500 | 11 | 900[†] | 90 | 15 | 1.2 | 1.3 | 16 | 1.3 | 400[‡] | 2.4 |
| 75 | 204 | 80 | 210 | 106 | 67 | 226 | 150 | 450 | 138 | 162 | 160 | 99 | 152 |

Nutrient Analysis Form

| Name | Quantity | kcal | Protein (g) | Carbohydrates (g) | Fiber (g) | Total fat (g) | Monounsaturated fat (g) | Polyunsaturated fat (g) | Saturated fat (g) | Cholesterol (g) | Calcium (mg) | Iron (mg) |
|------|----------|------|-------------|-------------------|-----------|---------------|-------------------------|-------------------------|-------------------|-----------------|--------------|-----------|
| | | | | | | | | | | | | |
| | | | | | | | | | | | | |
| | | | | | | | | | | | | |
| | | | | | | | | | | | | |
| | | | | | | | | | | | | |
| | | | | | | | | | | | | |
| | | | | | | | | | | | | |
| | | | | | | | | | | | | |
| | | | | | | | | | | | | |
| | | | | | | | | | | | | |
| | | | | | | | | | | | | |
| | | | | | | | | | | | | |
| | | | | | | | | | | | | |
| | | | | | | | | | | | | |
| | | | | | | | | | | | | |
| | | | | | | | | | | | | |
| | | | | | | | | | | | | |
| | | | | | | | | | | | | |
| | | | | | | | | | | | | |
| | | | | | | | | | | | | |
| | | | | | | | | | | | | |
| | | | | | | | | | | | | |
| Totals | | | | | | | | | | | | |
| RDA or related nutrient standard* | | | | | | | | | | | | |
| % of nutrient needs | | | | | | | | | | | | |

*Values from inside cover. The number of kcals is a rough estimate. It is better to base energy needs on actual energy output.

†Use RAE values.

‡Use DFE values.

Nutrient Analysis Form cont'd

| Magnesium (mg) | Phosphorous (mg) | Potassium (mg) | Sodium (mg) | Zinc (mg) | Vitamin A (RE) | Vitamin C (mg) | Vitamin E (mg) | Thiamin (mg) | Riboflavin (mg) | Niacin (mg) | Vitamin B-6 (mg) | Folate (μg) | Vitamin B-12 (μg) |
|---|---|---|---|---|---|---|---|---|---|---|---|---|---|
| | | | | | | | | | | | | | |
| | | | | | | | | | | | | | |
| | | | | | | | | | | | | | |
| | | | | | | | | | | | | | |
| | | | | | | | | | | | | | |
| | | | | | | | | | | | | | |
| | | | | | | | | | | | | | |
| | | | | | | | | | | | | | |
| | | | | | | | | | | | | | |
| | | | | | | | | | | | | | |
| | | | | | | | | | | | | | |
| | | | | | | | | | | | | | |
| | | | | | | | | | | | | | |
| | | | | | | | | | | | | | |
| | | | | | | | | | | | | | |
| | | | | | | | | | | | | | |
| | | | | | | | | | | | | | |
| | | | | | | | | | | | | | |
| | | | | | | | | | | | | | |
| | | | | | | | | | | | | | |
| | | | | | | | | | | | | | |
| | | | | | | | | | | | | | |
| | | | | | | | | | | | | | |
| | | | | | | | | | | | | | |
| | | | | | | | | | | | | | |
| | | | | | | | | | | | | | |

III. **Complete the following table as you summarize your dietary intake.**

Percentage of kcal from Protein, Fat, Carbohydrate, and Alcohol

**Intake**

| Protein (P): | ____g/day × 4 kcal per gram | = (P)____kcal per day |
| Fat (F): | ____g/day × 9 kcal per gram | = (F)____kcal per day |
| Carbohydrate (C): | ____g/day × 4 kcal per gram | = (C)____kcal per day |
| Alcohol (A): | | = (A)____kcal per day* |
| | Total kcal (T)/day | = (T)____kcal per day |

Percentage of kcal from protein:

$\frac{(P)}{(T)} \times 100 =$ ____%

Percentage of kcal from fat:

$\frac{(F)}{(T)} \times 100 =$ ____%

Percentage of kcal from carbohydrate:

$\frac{(C)}{(T)} \times 100 =$ ____%

Percentage of kcal from alcohol:

$\frac{(A)}{(T)} \times 100 =$ ____%

Note: The four percentages can total 99, 100, or 101, depending on the way in which figures were rounded off earlier.

*To calculate how many kcal in a beverage are from alcohol, first look up the beverage using the Nutrition Calc software. Then determine how many kcal are from carbohydrate (multiply carbohydrate grams times 4), fat (fat grams times 9), and protein (protein grams times 4). The remaining kcal are from alcohol.

IV. **Use the table on the following page to again record your food intake for one day, placing each food item in the correct category of MyPyramid, with the correct number of servings (see Chapter 2).** A food such as toast with soft margarine contributes to two categories—namely, to the grains group and to the oils group. You can expect that many food choices will contribute to more than one group. Indicate the number of servings from MyPyramid that each food yields.

Indicate the Number of Servings from MyPyramid That Each Food Yields

| Food or Beverage | Amount Eaten | Milk | Meat & Beans | Fruits | Vegetables | Grains | Oils |
|---|---|---|---|---|---|---|---|
| | | | | | | | |
| | | | | | | | |
| | | | | | | | |
| | | | | | | | |
| | | | | | | | |
| | | | | | | | |
| | | | | | | | |
| | | | | | | | |
| | | | | | | | |
| | | | | | | | |
| | | | | | | | |
| | | | | | | | |
| | | | | | | | |
| | | | | | | | |
| | | | | | | | |
| | | | | | | | |
| | | | | | | | |
| | | | | | | | |
| | | | | | | | |
| | | | | | | | |
| | | | | | | | |
| | | | | | | | |
| | | | | | | | |
| | | | | | | | |
| | | | | | | | |
| | | | | | | | |
| | | | | | | | |
| | | | | | | | |
| | | | | | | | |
| | | | | | | | |
| | | | | | | | |
| | | | | | | | |
| Group totals | | | | | | | |
| Recommended servings from www.mypyramid.gov | | | | | | | |
| Overages/Shortages in numbers of servings | | | | | | | |

V. **Evaluation.** Are there weaknesses suggested in your nutrient intake that correspond to missing servings in MyPyramid? Consider adjusting your food choices to meet MyPyramid recommendations to improve your nutrient intake.

VI. **For the same day you keep your food record, also keep a 24-hour record of your activities.** Include sleeping, sitting, and walking, as well as the obvious forms of exercise. Calculate your energy expenditure for these activities using Table 7-4 in Chapter 7 or the diet analysis software available with this book. Try to substitute a similar activity if your particular activity is not listed. Calculate the total kcal you used for the day (total for column 3). Following is an example of an activity record. A blank form follows for your use. Ask your professor whether you are to turn in the form or the activity printout from NutritionCalc Plus.

Weight (kg)*: 70 kg

| Activity | Time (Minutes): Convert to Hours | Energy Cost | | |
| --- | --- | --- | --- | --- |
| | | Column 1 kcal/kg/hr (from Table 7-4) | Column 2 (Column 1 × Time) | Column 3 (Column 2 × Weight in kg) |
| Brisk walking | (60 min) 1 hr | 4.4 | (× 1) = 4.4 | (× 70) = 308 |

*lb/2.2

Weight (kg)*:

| Activity | Time (Minutes): Convert to Hours | Energy Cost | | |
| --- | --- | --- | --- | --- |
| | | Column 1 kcal/kg/hr (from Table 7-4) | Column 2 (Column 1 × Time) | Column 3 (Column 2 × Weight in kg) |
| | | | | |
| | | | | |
| | | | | |
| | | | | |
| | | | | |
| | | | | |
| | | | | |
| | | | | |
| | | | | |
| | | | | |
| Total kcal used (from adding all of column 3) | | | | |

*lb/2.2

## AMINO ACIDS

**Histidine (His)**
(essential)

**Tryptophan (Trp)**
(essential)

**Glycine (Gly)**

**Methionine (Met)**
(essential)

**Leucine (Leu)**
(essential)

**Alanine (Ala)**

**Arginine (Arg)**
(essential in infancy)

**Lysine (Lys)**
(essential)

**Proline (Pro)**

**Glutamic Acid (Glu)**

**Aspartic Acid (Asp)**

**Serine (Ser)**

**Phenylalanine (Phe)**
(essential)

**Isoleucine (Ile)**
(essential)

**Tyrosine (Tyr)**

**Glutamine (Gln)**

**Asparagine (Asn)**

**Threonine (Thr)**
(essential)

**Valine (Val)**
(essential)

**Cysteine (Cys)**

# VITAMINS

**Vitamin A: retinol**

**Beta-carotene**

**Vitamin E**

**Vitamin K**

Carbon #1

Carbon #25

**7-dehydrocholesterol**

Carbon #25

Carbon #1

**1,25-dihydroxy-vitamin D₃ (calcitriol)**

**Active vitamin D (calcitriol) and its precursor 7-dehydrocholesterol**

**Thiamin**

**Niacin (nicotinic acid and nicotinamide)**

Nicotinic acid

Nicotinamide

**Riboflavin**

Pyridoxine

Pyridoxal

Pyridoxamine

**Vitamin B-6 (a general name for three compounds—pyridoxine, pyridoxal, and pyridoxamine)**

**Biotin**

**Pantothenic acid**

**Folate (folic acid form)**

**Vitamin C (ascorbic acid)**

**Vitamin B-12 (cyanocobalamin)** The arrows in this diagram indicate that the spare electrons on the nitrogens are attracted to the cobalt atom.

**Ketone Bodies**

O
‖
CH₃ — C — CH₃
Acetone

CO₂

O         O
‖         ‖
CH₃ — C — CH₂ — C — OH
Acetoacetic Acid

2H⁺

OH              O
|               ‖
CH₃ — CH — CH₂ — C — OH
ß-Hydroxybutyric Acid

Point of cleavage to yield
ADP and energy release

Triphosphate

OH
|
HO — P = O
|
O
|
HO — P = O
|
O
|
HO — P = O
|
O

Adenine

NH₂
|
C
N⁄ ⁛ \N
H — C        C — H
‖        ‖
N        N
|
C — N⁄ ⁛
H — C
N

Ribose
(a sugar)

CH₂
|
C   H        H   C
|   |        |   \H
H C            C
|            |
OH           OH

**Adenosine Triphosphate
(ATP)**

# APPENDIX G  Metropolitan Life Insurance Company
## Height-Weight Table and Determination of Frame Size

1983 Metropolitan Life Insurance Company Height-Weight Table* †

| Women | | | | | Men | | | | |
|---|---|---|---|---|---|---|---|---|---|
| Height | | Frame | | | Height | | Frame | | |
| Ft. | In. | Small | Medium | Large | Ft. | In. | Small | Medium | Large |
| 4 | 10 | 102–111 | 109–121 | 118–131 | 5 | 2 | 128–134 | 131–141 | 138–150 |
| 4 | 11 | 103–113 | 111–123 | 120–134 | 5 | 3 | 130–136 | 133–143 | 140–153 |
| 5 | 0 | 104–115 | 113–126 | 122–137 | 5 | 4 | 132–138 | 135–145 | 142–156 |
| 5 | 1 | 106–118 | 115–129 | 125–140 | 5 | 5 | 134–140 | 137–148 | 144–160 |
| 5 | 2 | 108–121 | 118–132 | 128–143 | 5 | 6 | 136–142 | 139–151 | 146–164 |
| 5 | 3 | 111–124 | 121–135 | 131–147 | 5 | 7 | 138–145 | 142–154 | 149–168 |
| 5 | 4 | 114–127 | 124–138 | 134–151 | 5 | 8 | 140–148 | 145–157 | 152–172 |
| 5 | 5 | 117–130 | 127–141 | 137–155 | 5 | 9 | 142–151 | 148–160 | 155–176 |
| 5 | 6 | 120–133 | 130–144 | 140–159 | 5 | 10 | 144–154 | 151–163 | 158–180 |
| 5 | 7 | 123–136 | 133–147 | 143–163 | 5 | 11 | 146–157 | 154–166 | 161–184 |
| 5 | 8 | 126–139 | 136–150 | 146–167 | 6 | 0 | 149–160 | 157–170 | 164–188 |
| 5 | 9 | 129–142 | 139–153 | 149–170 | 6 | 1 | 152–164 | 160–174 | 168–192 |
| 5 | 10 | 132–145 | 142–156 | 152–173 | 6 | 2 | 155–168 | 164–178 | 172–197 |
| 5 | 11 | 135–148 | 145–159 | 155–176 | 6 | 3 | 158–172 | 167–182 | 176–202 |
| 6 | 0 | 138–151 | 148–162 | 158–179 | 6 | 4 | 162–176 | 171–187 | 181–207 |

*Based on a weight-height mortality study conducted by the Society of Actuaries and the Association of Life Insurance Medical Directors of America, Metropolitan Life Insurance Medical Directors of America, Metropolitan Life Insurance Company, revised 1983.
†Weights in pounds (lb) at ages 25 to 59 based on lowest mortality. Height includes 1-in. heel. Weight for women includes 3 lb for indoor clothing. Weight for men includes 5 lb for indoor clothing.
Reprinted courtesy of Metropolitan Life Insurance Company, *Statistical Bulletin*.

Permission granted courtesy of Metropolitan Life Insurance Company, *Statistical Bulletin*.

## USING THE METROPOLITAN LIFE INSURANCE TABLE TO ESTIMATE HEALTHY WEIGHT

The Metropolitan Life Insurance table is a common method for estimating healthy weight. The table lists, for any height, the weight that is associated with a maximum life span. The table does not tell the healthiest weight for a living person; it lists the weight associated with longevity.

There are many criticisms of this table. These stem from the inclusion of some people and the exclusion of others. For example, only policyholders of life insurance are included. In addition, smokers are included, but anyone over the age of 60 is excluded. Weight is only measured at the time of purchase of insurance, and there is no follow-up. All of these factors contribute to the fact that this table is to be used only as a rough screening tool; not meeting the exact recommendations should not be cause for alarm.

To diagnose overweight or obesity using the table, calculate the percentage of the Metropolitan Life Insurance table weight. Use the midpoint of a weight range for a specific height.

Equation: $\dfrac{(\text{Current wt.} - \text{wt. from table})}{\text{Weight from table}} \times 100$

Example:     $$\frac{140 - 120}{120} \times 100 = 17\% \text{ over standard}$$

Overweight can be defined as weighing at least 10% more than the weight listed on the table. Determination of obesity is 20% more than that listed on the table. Moreover, this measure of obesity comes in degrees. Whereas mild obesity carries little health risk, severe obesity raises overall health risk twelvefold.

| Degrees of Obesity | |
|---|---|
| **% Over Healthy Body Weight** | **Form of Obesity** |
| 20–40% | Mild |
| 41–99% | Moderate |
| 100%+ | Severe |

## DETERMINING FRAME SIZE

### Method 1

Height is recorded without shoes.

Wrist circumference is measured just beyond (toward the hand) the bony (styloid) process at the wrist joint on the right arm, using a tape measure.

The following formula is used:

$$r = \frac{\text{Height (cm)}}{\text{Wrist circumference (cm)}}$$

Frame size can be determined as follows:[†]

| Males | Females |
|---|---|
| $r > 10.4$ small | $r > 11$ small |
| $r = 9.6{-}10.4$ medium | $r = 10.1{-}11$ medium |
| $r < 9.6$ large | $r < 10.1$ large |

[†]From Grant JP: *Handbook of Total Parenteral Nutrition*. Philadelphia: WB Saunders, 1980.

### Method 2

The person's right arm is extended forward, perpendicular to the body, with the arm bent so the angle at the elbow forms 90 degrees, with the fingers pointing up and the palm turned away from the body. The greatest breadth across the elbow joint is measured with a sliding caliper along the axis of the upper arm, on the two prominent bones on either side of the elbow. This is recorded as the elbow breadth. The following tables give elbow breadth measurements for medium-framed men and women of various heights. Measurements lower than those listed indicate a small frame size; higher measurements indicate a large frame size.[‡]

| Men | | Women | |
|---|---|---|---|
| **Height in 1″ Heels** | **Elbow Breadth** | **Height in 1″ Heels** | **Elbow Breadth** |
| 5′2″–5′3″ | 2½–2⅞″ | 4′10″–4′11″ | 2¼–2½″ |
| 5′4″–5′7″ | 2⅝–2⅞″ | 5′0″–5′3″ | 2¼–2½″ |
| 5′8″–5′11″ | 2¾–3″ | 5′4″–5′7″ | 2⅜–2⅝″ |
| 6′0″–6′3″ | 2¾–3¼″ | 5′8″–5′11″ | 2⅜–2⅝″ |
| 6′4″ and over | 2⅞–3¾″ | 6′0″ and over | 2½–2¾″ |

[‡]From Metropolitan Life Insurance Co., 1983.

Consider the following reliable sources of food and nutrition information:

## Journals That Regularly Cover Nutrition Topics

*American Family Physician\**
*American Journal of Clinical Nutrition*
*American Journal of Epidemiology*
*American Journal of Medicine*
*American Journal of Nursing*
*American Journal of Obstetrics and Gynecology*
*American Journal of Physiology*
*American Journal of Public Health*
*American Scientist*
*Annals of Internal Medicine*
*Annual Review of Medicine*
*Annual Review of Nutrition*
*Archives of Disease in Childhood*
*Archives of Internal Medicine*
*British Journal of Nutrition*
*BMJ (British Medical Journal)*
*Canadian Journal of Dietetic Practice and Research*
*Cancer*
*Cancer Research*
*Circulation*
*Diabetes*
*Diabetes Care*
*Disease-a-Month*
*FASEB Journal*
*FDA Consumer\**
*Food and Chemical Toxicology*
*Food Engineering*
*Food Technology*
*Gastroenterology*
*Geriatrics*
*Gut*
*Journal of the American College of Nutrition\**
*Journal of the American Dietetic Association\**
*Journal of the American Geriatrics Society*
*JAMA (Journal of the American Medical Association)*
*Journal of Applied Physiology*
*Journal of Clinical Investigation*
*Journal of Food Science*
*JNCI (Journal of the National Cancer Institute)*
*Journal of Nutrition*
*Journal of Nutrition Education and Behavior\**
*Journal of Nutrition for the Elderly*
*Journal of Pediatrics*
*Lancet*
*Mayo Clinic Proceedings*
*Medicine & Science in Sports & Exercise*
*Nature*
*The New England Journal of Medicine*
*Nutrition*
*Nutrition Reviews*
*Nutrition Today\**
*Pediatrics*
*The Physician and Sports Medicine*
*Postgraduate Medicine\**
*Proceedings of the Nutrition Society*
*Science*
*Science News\**
*Scientific American\**

The majority of these journals are available in college and university libraries or in a specialty library on campus, such as one designated for health services or home economics. As indicated, a few journals will be filed under their abbreviations, rather than the first word in their full name. A reference librarian can help you locate any of these sources. The journals with an asterisk (*) are ones you may find especially interesting and useful because of the number of nutrition articles presented each month or the less technical nature of the presentation.

## Magazines for the Consumer That cover Nutrition Topics

*Better Homes and Gardens*
*Good Housekeeping*

*Health*
*Men's Health*

*Parents*
*Self*

## Textbooks and Other Sources for Advanced Study of Nutrition Topics

Bowman BA, Russell RM: *Present knowledge in nutrition.* Vol. I and II. 9th ed. Washington DC: International Life Sciences Institute, 2006.

Brody T: *Nutritional biochemistry.* 2nd ed. San Diego: Academic Press, 1999.

Gropper SS, Smith JL: *Advanced nutrition and human metabolism.* 5th ed. Florence, KY: Wadsworth, Cengage 2009.

Mahan LK, Escott-Stump S: *Krause's food, and nutrition, therapy.* 12th ed. St. Louis: W.B. Saunders, 2008.

Murray RK and others: *Harper's illustrated biochemistry.* 27th ed. New York: McGraw-Hill, 2006.

Schils ME, Shike M, Ross AC, Caballero B, Cousins RJ: *Modern nutrition in health and disease.* 10th ed. Philadelphia: Lippincott, Williams & Wilkins, 2005.

Stipanuk MH: *Biochemical, physiological, & molecular aspects of human nutrition.* 2nd ed. Philadelphia: Elsevier Health Sciences, 2006.

*Newsletters That Cover Nutrition Issues on a Regular Basis*

*American Institute for Cancer Research e.Newsletter*
American Institute for Cancer Research
www.aicr.org

*Consumer Health Digest*
National Council Against Health Fraud
www.ncahf.org

*Dairy Council Digest*
National Dairy Council
www.nationaldairycouncil.org

*Diabetes E-News* (and others)
American Diabetes Association
www.diabetes.org

*Environmental Nutrition*
www.environmentalnutrition.com

*Harvard Health Letter* (and others)
Harvard Medical School
www.health.harvard.edu/newsletters

*Health and Nutrition Letter*
Tufts University
www.healthletter.tufts.edu

*In-Touch*
Heinz Infant Nutrition Institute
www.hini.org

*Mayo Clinic House call*
Mayo Clinic
www.mayoclinic.com

*Nutrition Action Healthletter*
Center for Science in the Public Interest
www.cspinet.org

*Nutrition Research Update*
Egg Nutrition Center
www.enc-online.org

*Soy Connection*
United Soybean Board
www.soyconnection.com

*U-Mail: Everyday Nutrition Solutions You Can Use*
National Cattlemen's Beef Association
www.beefnutrition.org

*Wellness Letter*
University of California at Berkeley
www.wellnessletter.com

*Professional Organizations*

American Academy of Pediatrics
141 Northwest Point Boulevard
Elk Grove Village, IL 60007-1098
www.aap.org

American Cancer Society
1599 Clifton Road, NE
Atlanta, GA 30329
www.cancer.org

American College of Sports Medicine
PO Box 1440
Indianapolis, IN 46206-1440
www.acsm.org

American Dental Association
211 East Chicago Avenue
Chicago, IL 60611-2678
www.ada.org

American Diabetes Association
1701 North Beauregard Street
Alexandria, VA 22311
www.diabetes.org

American Dietetic Association
120 South Riverside Plaza #2000
Chicago, IL 60606-6995
www.eatright.org

American Geriatrics Society
350 Fifth Avenue #801
New York, NY 10118
www.americangeriatrics.org

American Heart Association
7272 Greenville Avenue
Dallas, TX 75231
www.americanheart.org

American Medical Association
515 North State Street
Chicago, IL 60610
www.ama-assn.org

American Public Health Association
800 I Street, NW
Washington, DC 20001-3710
www.apha.org

American Society for Nutrition
9650 Rockville Pike #L-4500
Bethesda, MD 20814
http://www.asnutrition.org/

Canadian Council of Food and Nutrition
2810 Matheson Boulevard
East, 1st Floor
Mississaugo, Ontario L4W 4X7
http://www.ccfn.ca/

Canadian Diabetes Association
1400-522 University Avenue
Toronto, ON M5G 2R5
www.diabetes.ca

Canadian Society for Nutritional Sciences
Department of Family Relations and Applied Nutrition
University of Guelph
Guelph ON N1G 2W7
www.nutritionalsciences.ca

Dietitians of Canada
480 University Avenue #604
Toronto, ON M5G 1V2
www.dietitians.ca

Environmental Working Group
1436 U Street, NW #100
Washington, DC 20009
www.ewg.org

Food and Nutrition Board
Institute of Medicine
The National Academies
500 Fifth Street, NW
Washington, DC 20001
www.iom.edu/cMs/3788.aspx

Institute of Food Technologists
525 West Van Buren #1000
Chicago, IL 60607
www.ift.org

National Council on Aging
1901 L Street, NW, 4th floor
Washington, DC 20036
www.ncoa.org

National Osteoporosis Foundation
1232 22nd Street, NW
Washington, DC 20037-1202
www.nof.org

Society for Nutrition Education
9100 Purdue Road, Suite 200
Indianapolis, IN 46268
www.sne.org

*Professional Organizations with a Commitment to Nutrition Issues*

Bread for the World Institute
50 F Street, NW #500
Washington, DC 20001
www.bread.org

Food Research and Action Center
1875 Connecticut Avenue, NW #540
Washington, DC 20009
www.frac.org

Institute for Food and Development Policy
398 60th Street
Oakland, CA 94618
www.foodfirst.org

La Leche League International
PO Box 4079
Schaumburg, IL 60168-4079
www.llli.org

March of Dimes
1275 Mamaroneck Avenue
White Plains, NY 10605
www.marchofdimes.com

National Council Against Health Fraud
119 Foster Street
Peabody, MA 01960
www.ncahf.org

National WIC Association
2001 S Street, NW #580
Washington, DC 20009
www.nwica.org

Overeaters Anonymous
PO Box 44020
Rio Rancho, NM 87174-4020
www.oa.org

Oxfam America
226 Causeway Street, 5th floor
Boston, MA 02114-2206
www.oxfamamerica.org

*Local Resources for Advice on Nutrition Issues*

Registered dietitians (RDs or in Canada also RDNs) in health care, city, county, or state agencies, as well as in private practice
Cooperative extension agents in county extension offices
Nutrition faculty affiliated with departments of food and nutrition, home economics, and dietetics

*Government Agencies Concerned with Nutrition Issues or That Distribute Nutrition Information*

*United States*

Agricultural Research Service
United States Department of Agriculture
Jamie L. Whitten Building
1400 Independence Avenue, SW
Washington, DC 20250
www.ars.usda.gov

Federal Citizen Information Center
31201 Bryan Circle
Pueblo, CO 81001
www.pueblo.gsa.gov

Food and Drug Administration
10903 New Hampshire Avenue
Silver Spring, MD 20993
www.fda.gov

Food Safety & Inspection Service
United States Department of Agriculture
331-E Jamie L. Whitten Building
1400 Independence Avenue, SW
Washington, DC 20250-3700
www.fsis.usda.gov

MyPyramid
USDA Center for Nutrition Policy and Promotion
3101 Park Center Drive #1034
Alexandria, VA 22302-1594
www.mypyramid.gov

National Agricultural Library
Abraham Lincoln Building
10301 Baltimore Avenue
Beltsville, MD 20705-2351
www.nal.usda.gov

National Cancer Institute
6116 Executive Boulevard #3036A
Bethesda, MD 20892-8322
www.cancer.gov

National Center for Health Statistics
1600 Clifton Road
Atlanta, GA 30333
www.cdc.gov/nchs

National Heart, Lung, and Blood Institute
Building 31, Room 5A48
31 Center Drive, MSC 2486
Bethesda, MD 20892
www.nhlbi.nih.gov

National Institute on Aging
Building 31, Room 5C27
31 Center Drive, MSC 2292
Bethesda, MD 20892
www.nia.nih.gov

U.S. Government Printing Office
710 North Capitol Street, NW
Washington, DC 20401
www.gpo.gov

*Canada*

Canadian Food Inspection Agency
1400 Merivale Road
Ottawa, Ontario K1A 0Y9
www.inspection.gc.ca

Health Canada
Brooke Claxton Building
Ottawa, Ontario K1A 0K9
www.hc-sc.gc.ca

*United Nations*

Food and Agriculture Organization
Liaison Office with North America
2175 K Street, NW #500
Washington, DC 20037
www.fao.org

World Health Organization
Avenue Appia 20
1211 Geneva 27
Switzerland
www.who.int

*Trade Organizations and Companies That Distribute Nutrition Information*

Abbott Nutrition
625 Cleveland Avenue
Columbus, OH 43215-1724
www.abbottnutrition.com

American Institute of Baking
1213 Bakers Way
PO Box 3999
Manhattan, Kansas 66505-3999
www.aibonline.org

American Meat Institute
1150 Connecticut Avenue, NW, 12th floor
Washington, DC 20036
www.meatami.com

Beech-Nut Nutrition
13023 Tesson Ferry Road
St. Louis, MO 63128
www.beechnut.com

Campbell Soup Company
1 Campbell Place
Camden, NJ 08103-1701
www.campbellsoup.com

Dannon Company
100 Hillside Avenue, 3rd Floor
White Plains, NY 10603
www.dannon.com

Del Monte Foods
One Market Plaza #11
PO Box 193575
San Francisco, CA 94105
www.delmonte.com

DSM Nutritional Products
45 Waterview Boulevard
Parsippany, NJ 07054-1298
www.nutraaccess.com

General Mills/Pillsbury
PO Box 9452
Minneapolis, MN 55440
www.generalmills.com

Gerber Products Company
445 State Street
Fremont, MI 49413-0001
www.gerber.com

H.J. Heinz
90 Sheppard Avenue East #400
Toronto, ON M2N 7K5
www.heinzbaby.com

Idaho Potato Commission
661 South Rivershore Lane
Eagle, ID 83616
www.idahopotatoes.com

Kellogg Company
One Kellogg Square
Battle Creek, MI 49016
www.kelloggs.com/us/

Kraft Foods Global
Three Lakes Drive
Northfield, IL 60093
www.kraftfoods.com

Mead Johnson Nutritionals
2400 West Lloyd Expressway
Evansville, IN 47721-0001
www.meadjohnson.com

National Dairy Council
10255 West Higgins Road #900
Des Plaines, IL 60018
www.nationaldairycouncil.org

NutraSweet Company
222 Merchandise Mart Plaza
Chicago, IL 60654
www.nutrasweet.com

Sunkist Growers
14130 Riverside Drive
Sherman Oaks, CA 91423
www.sunkist.com

## METRIC-ENGLISH CONVERSIONS

### Length

| English (USA) | Metric |
|---|---|
| inch (in) | = 2.54 cm, 25.4 mm |
| foot (ft) | = 0.30 m, 30.48 cm |
| yard (yd) | = 0.91 m, 91.4 cm |
| mile (statute) (5280 ft) | = 1.61 km, 1609 m |
| mile (nautical) | |
| (6077 ft, 1.15 statute mi) | = 1.85 km, 1850 m |

| Metric | English (USA) |
|---|---|
| millimeter (mm) | = 0.039 in (thickness of a dime) |
| centimeter (cm) | = 0.39 in |
| meter (m) | = 3.28 ft, 39.37 in |
| kilometer (km) | = 0.62 mi, 1091 yd, 3273 ft |

### Weight

| English (USA) | Metric |
|---|---|
| grain | = 64.80 mg |
| ounce (oz) | = 28.35 g |
| pound (lb) | = 453.60 g, 0.45 kg |
| ton (short—2000 lb) | = 0.91 metric ton (907 kg) |

| Metric | English (USA) |
|---|---|
| milligram (mg) | = 0.002 grain (0.000035 oz) |
| gram (g) | = 0.04 oz ($^1/_{28}$ of an oz) |
| kilogram (kg) | = 35.27 oz, 2.20 lb |
| metric ton (1000 kg) | = 1.10 tons |

### Volume

| English (USA) | Metric |
|---|---|
| cubic inch | = 16.39 cc |
| cubic foot | = 0.03 m$^3$ |
| cubic yard | = 0.765 m$^3$ |
| teaspoon (tsp) | = 5 ml |
| tablespoon (tbsp) | = 15 ml |
| fluid ounce | = 0.03 liter (30 ml)* |
| cup (c) | = 237 ml |
| pint (pt) | = 0.47 liter |
| quart (qt) | = 0.95 liter |
| gallon (gal) | = 3.79 liters |

| Metric | English (USA) |
|---|---|
| milliliter (ml) | = 0.03 oz |
| liter (L) | = 2.12 pt |
| liter | = 1.06 qt |
| liter | = 0.27 gal |

1 liter ÷ 1000 = 1 milliliter or 1 cubic centimeter ($10^{-3}$ liter)
1 liter ÷ 1,000,000 = 1 microliter ($10^{-6}$ liter)
*Note: 1 ml = 1 cc

## METRIC AND OTHER COMMON UNITS

| Unit/Abbreviation | Other Equivalent Measure |
|---|---|
| milligram/mg | $^1/_{1000}$ of a gram |
| microgram/µg | $^1/_{1,000,000}$ of a gram |
| deciliter/dl | $^1/_{10}$ of a liter (about ½ cup) |
| milliliter/ml | $^1/_{1000}$ of a liter (5 ml is about 1 tsp) |
| International Unit/IU | Crude measure of vitamin activity generally based on growth rate seen in animals |

## FAHRENHEIT-CELSIUS CONVERSION SCALE

To convert temperature scales:
Fahrenheit to Celsius °C = (°F − 32) × 5/9
Celsius to Fahrenheit °F = 9/5 (°C) + 32

## HOUSEHOLD UNITS

| 3 teaspoons | = 1 tablespoon | = 15 grams |
|---|---|---|
| 4 tablespoons | = ¼ cup | = 60 grams |
| 5$^1/_3$ tablespoons | = $^1/_3$ cup | = 80 grams |
| 8 tablespoons | = ½ cup | = 120 grams |
| 10$^2/_3$ tablespoons | = $^2/_3$ cup | = 160 grams |
| 16 tablespoons | = 1 cup | = 240 grams |
| 1 tablespoon | = ½ fluid ounce | = 15 milliliters |
| 1 cup | = 8 fluid ounces | = 15 milliliters |
| 1 cup | = ½ pint | = 240 grams |
| 2 cups | = 1 pint | = 480 grams |
| 4 cups | = 1 quart | = 960 grams = 1 liter |
| 2 pints | = 1 quart | = 960 grams = 1 liter |
| 4 quarts | = 1 gallon | = 3840 grams = 4 liters |

**absorption** The process by which substances are taken up from the GI tract and enter the bloodstream or the lymph.

**absorptive cells** The intestinal cells that line the villi; these cells participate in nutrient absorption.

**Acceptable Daily Intake (ADI)** Estimate of the amount of a sweetener that an individual can safely consume daily over a lifetime. ADIs are given as mg per kg of body weight per day.

**acesulfame K** Alternative sweetener that yields no energy.

**acetaldehyde dehydrogenase** An enzyme used in ethanol metabolism that eventually converts acetaldehyde into carbon dioxide and water.

**acquired immune deficiency syndrome (AIDS)** A disorder in which a virus (human immunodeficiency virus [HIV]) infects specific types of immune system cells. This leaves the person with reduced immune function and, in turn, defenseless against numerous infectious agents; typically contributes to the person's death.

**additives** Substances added to foods, such as preservatives.

**adenosine diphosphate (ADP)** A breakdown product of ATP. ADP is synthesized into ATP using energy from foodstuffs and a phosphate group (abbreviated $P_i$).

**adenosine triphosphate (ATP)** The main energy currency for cells. ATP energy is used to promote ion pumping, enzyme activity, and muscular contraction.

**Adequate Intake (AI)** Nutrient intake amount set for any nutrient for which insufficient research is available to establish an RDA. AIs are based on estimates of intakes that appear to maintain a defined nutritional state in a specific life stage.

**adipose tissue** A group of fat storing cells.

**adjustable gastric banding** A restrictive procedure in which the opening from the esophagus to the stomach is reduced by a hollow gastric band.

**aerobic** Requiring oxygen.

**aging** Time-dependent physical and physiological changes in body structure and function that occur normally and progressively throughout adulthood as humans mature and become older.

**air displacement** A method for estimating body composition that makes use of the volume of space taken up by a body inside a small chamber.

**alcohol** Ethyl alcohol or ethanol ($CH_3CH_2OH$) is the compound in alcoholic beverages.

**alcohol abuse** Excessive alcohol consumption that leads to severe alcohol-related health and other problems, such as recurrent sickness, inability to fulfill major obligations, use in hazardous situations (e.g., driving), related legal problems, or use despite social and interpersonal difficulties.

**alcohol dehydrogenase** An enzyme used in alcohol (ethanol) metabolism that converts alcohol into acetaldehyde.

**alcohol dependence** The person experiences repeated alcohol-related difficulties, such as an inability to control use, spending a great deal of time associated with alcohol use, continued use of alcohol despite physical or psychological consequences, persistent desire or unsuccessful efforts to cut down or control alcohol use, and withdrawal symptoms. Tolerance is also seen.

**alcoholism** As defined by the American Medical Association, an illness characterized by significant impairment directly related to persistent and excessive use of alcohol.

**aldosterone** A hormone produced by the adrenal glands that acts on the kidneys to conserve sodium (and therefore water).

**allergen** A foreign protein, or antigen, that induces excess production of certain immune system antibodies; subsequent exposure to the same protein leads to allergic symptoms. Whereas all allergens are antigens, not all antigens are allergens.

**allergy** A hypersensitive immune response that occurs when immune bodies produced by us react with a protein we sense as foreign (an antigen).

**alpha-linolenic acid** An essential omega-3 fatty acid with 18 carbons and three double bonds.

**amino acid** The building block for proteins containing a central carbon atom with nitrogen and other atoms attached.

**amniotic fluid** Fluid contained in a sac within the uterus. This fluid surrounds and protects the fetus during development.

**amphetamine** A group of medications that induce stimulation of the central nervous system and have other effects in the body. Abuse is linked to physical and psychological dependence.

**amylase** Starch-digesting enzyme produced by the salivary glands or pancreas.

**amylopectin** A digestible branched-chain type of starch composed of glucose units.

**amylose** A digestible straight-chain type of starch composed of glucose units.

**anaerobic** Not requiring oxygen.

**anal sphincters** A group of two sphincters (inner and outer) that help control expulsion of feces from the body.

**analog** A chemical compound that differs slightly from another, usually natural, compound. Analogs generally contain extra or altered chemical groups and may have similar or opposite metabolic effects compared with the native compound. Also spelled *analogue*.

**anaphylactic shock** A severe allergic response that results in lowered blood pressure and respiratory and gastrointestinal distress. This can be fatal.

**anemia** Generally refers to a decreased oxygen-carrying capacity of the blood. This can be caused by many factors, such as iron deficiency or blood loss.

**animal model** Use of animals to study disease to understand more about human disease.

**anorexia nervosa** An eating disorder involving a psychological loss or denial of appetite, followed by self-starvation; related in part to a distorted body image and to various social pressures commonly associated with puberty.

**anthropometric assessment** Measurement of body weight and the lengths, circumferences, and thicknesses of parts of the body.

**antibody** Blood protein (immunoglobulin) that binds foreign proteins found in the body. This helps to prevent and control infections.

**antidiuretic hormone** A hormone that is secreted by the pituitary gland and that acts on the kidneys to decrease water excretion.

**antigen** Any substance that induces a state of sensitivity and/or resistance to microorganisms or toxic substances after a lag period; foreign substance that stimulates a specific aspect of the immune system.

**antioxidant** Generally a compound that stops the damaging effects of reactive substances seeking an electron (i.e., oxidizing agents). This prevents breakdown (oxidizing) of substances in foods or the body, particularly lipids.

**anus** Last portion of the GI tract; serves as an outlet for that organ.

**appetite** The primarily psychological (external) influences that encourage us to find and eat food, often in the absence of obvious hunger.

**arachidonic acid** An omega-6 fatty acid made from linoleic acid with 20 carbon atoms and 4 carbon-carbon double bonds.

**artery** A blood vessel that carries blood away from the heart.

**aseptic processing** A method by which food and container are separately and simultaneously sterilized; it allows manufacturers to produce boxes of milk that can be stored at room temperature.

**aspartame** Alternative sweetener made of 2 amino acids and methanol; about 200 times sweeter than sucrose.

**atherosclerosis** A buildup of fatty material (plaque) in the arteries, including those surrounding the heart.

**atom** Smallest combining unit of an element, such as iron or calcium. Atoms consist of protons, neutrons, and electrons.

**bacteria** Single-cell microorganisms; some produce poisonous substances, which cause illness in humans. Bacteria can be carried by water, animals, and people. They survive on skin, clothes, and hair and thrive in foods at room temperature. Some can live without oxygen and survive by means of spore formation.

**bariatrics** The medical specialty focusing on the treatment of obesity.

**basal metabolism** The minimal amount of calories the body uses to support itself in a fasting state when resting (e.g., 12 hours for both) and awake in a warm, quiet environment. It amounts to roughly 1 kcal per kilogram per hour for men and 0.9 kcal per kilogram per hour for women; these values are often referred to as *basal metabolic rate (BMR)*.

**benign** Noncancerous; tumors that do not spread.

**beriberi** The thiamin deficiency disorder characterized by muscle weakness, loss of appetite, nerve degeneration, and sometimes edema.

**BHA, BHT** Butylated hydroxyanisole and butylated hydroxytoluene—two common synthetic antioxidants added to foods.

**bile** A liver secretion stored in the gallbladder and released through the common bile duct into the first segment of the small intestine. It is essential for the digestion and absorption of fat.

**binge-eating disorder** An eating disorder characterized by recurrent binge eating and feelings of loss of control over eating that have lasted at least 6 months. Binge episodes can be triggered by frustration, anger, depression, anxiety, permission to eat forbidden foods, and excessive hunger.

**bioavailability** The degree to which an ingested nutrient is absorbed and thus is available to the body.

**biochemical assessment** Measurement of biochemical functions (e.g., concentrations of nutrient by-products or enzyme activities in the blood or urine) related to a nutrient's function.

**bioelectrical impedance** The method to estimate total body fat that uses a low-energy electrical current. The more fat storage a person has, the more impedance (resistance) to electrical flow will be exhibited.

**biological pest management** Control of agricultural pests by using natural predators, parasites, or pathogens. For example, ladybugs can be used to control an aphid infestation.

**biotechnology** A collection of processes that involves the use of biological systems for altering and, ideally, improving the characteristics of plants, animals, and other forms of life.

**bisphosphonates** Compounds primarily composed of carbon and phosphorus that bind to bone mineral and in turn reduce bone breakdown. Examples are alendronate (Fosamax), risedronate (Actonel), and ibandronate (Boniva).

**body mass index (BMI)** Weight (in kilograms) divided by height (in meters) squared; a value of 25 and above indicates overweight and a value of 30 and above indicates obesity.

**bolus** A moistened mass of food swallowed from the oral cavity into the pharynx.

**bomb colorimeter** An instrument used to determine the calorie content of a food.

**bond** A linkage between two atoms formed by the sharing of electrons, or attractions.

**bone mass** Total mineral substance (such as calcium or phosphorus) in a cross section of bone, generally expressed as grams per centimeter of length.

**bone mineral density** Total mineral content of bone at a specific bone site divided by the width of the bone at that site, generally expressed as grams per cubic centimeter.

**branched-chain amino acids** Amino acids with a branching carbon backbone; these are leucine, isoleucine, and valine. All are essential amino acids.

**brown adipose tissue** A specialized form of adipose tissue that produces large amounts of heat by metabolizing energy-yielding nutrients without synthesizing much useful energy for the body. The unused energy is released as heat.

**buffers** Compounds that cause a solution to resist changes in acid-base conditions.

**bulimia nervosa** An eating disorder in which large quantities of food are eaten at one time (binge eating) and then purged from the body by vomiting, or misuse of laxatives, diuretics, or enemas. Alternate means to counteract the binge behavior are fasting and excessive exercise.

**capillary** A microscopic blood vessel that connects the smallest arteries and veins; site of nutrient, oxygen, and waste exchange between body cells and the blood.

**capillary bed** Network of one-cell thick vessels that create a junction between arterial and venous circulation. It is here that gas and nutrient exchange occurs between body cells and the blood.

**carbohydrate** A compound containing carbon, hydrogen, and oxygen atoms. Most are known as *sugars, starches,* and *fibers.*

**carbohydrate loading** A process in which a high carbohydrate intake is consumed for 6 days before an athletic event while tapering exercise duration in an attempt to increase muscle glycogen stores.

**carbon skeleton** Amino acid structure that remains after the amino group ($-NH_2$) has been removed.

**cardiovascular system** The body system consisting of the heart, blood vessels, and blood. This system transports nutrients, waste products, gases, and hormones throughout the body and plays an important role in immune responses and regulation of body temperature.

**carotenoids** Pigment materials in fruits and vegetables that range in color from yellow to orange to red; three of the various carotenoids yield vitamin A. Many are antioxidants.

**case-control study** A study in which individuals who have a disease or condition, such as lung cancer, are compared with individuals who do not have the condition.

**celiac disease** Immunological or allergic reaction to the protein gluten in certain grains, such as wheat and rye. The effect is to destroy the intestinal enterocytes, resulting in a much reduced surface area due to flattening of the villi. Elimination of wheat, rye, and certain other grains from the diet restores the intestinal surface.

**cell** The structural basis of plant and animal organization. In animals it is bounded by a cell membrane. Cells contain both genetic material and systems for synthesizing energy-yielding compounds. Cells have the ability to take up compounds from and excrete compounds into their surroundings.

**cell-mediated immunity** A process in which certain white blood cells come in contact with the invading cells to destroy them.

**cell nucleus** An organelle bound by its own double membrane and containing chromosomes, the genetic information for cell protein synthesis and cell replication.

**cellulose** An undigestible nonfermentable straight-chain polysaccharide made of glucose molecules.

**cerebrovascular accident (CVA)** Death of part of the brain tissue due typically to a blood clot. Also termed a *stroke.*

**chain-breaking** Breaking the link between two or more behaviors that encourage overeating, such as snacking while watching television.

**chemical reaction** An interaction between two chemicals that changes both chemicals.

**cholecystokinin (CCK)** A hormone that participates in enzyme release from the pancreas, bile release from the gallbladder, and hunger regulation.

**cholesterol** A waxy lipid found in all body cells. It has a structure containing multiple chemical rings that is found only in foods that contain animal products.

**chromosome** A single, large DNA molecule and its associated proteins; contains many genes to store and transmit genetic information.

**chylomicron** Lipoprotein made of dietary fats surrounded by a shell of cholesterol, phospholipids, and protein. Chylomicrons are formed in the absorptive cells of the small intestine after fat absorption and travel through the lymphatic system to the bloodstream.

**chyme** A mixture of stomach secretions and partially digested food.

**cirrhosis** A loss of functioning liver cells, which are replaced by nonfunctioning connective tissue. Any substance that poisons liver cells can lead to cirrhosis. The most common cause is a chronic, excessive alcohol intake. Exposure to certain industrial chemicals also can lead to cirrhosis.

*cis* **fatty acid** A form of an unsaturated fatty acid that has the hydrogens lying on the same side of the carbon-carbon double bond.

**clinical assessment** Examination of general appearance of skin, eyes, and tongue; evidence of rapid hair loss; sense of touch; and ability to cough and walk.

**coagulation** Blood clotting; essentially a transition of blood from a liquid cell suspension into a solid, gel-like form.

**coenzyme** A compound that combines with an inactive enzyme to form a catalytically active form. In this manner, coenzymes aid in enzyme function.

**cofactor** A mineral or other substance that binds to a specific region on a protein, such as an enzyme, and is necessary for the protein's function.

**cognitive behavior therapy** Psychological therapy in which the person's assumptions about dieting, body weight, and related issues are confronted. New ways of thinking are explored and then practiced by the person. In this way, an individual can learn new ways to control disordered eating behaviors and related life stress.

**cognitive restructuring** Changing one's frame of mind regarding eating—for example, instead of using a difficult day as an excuse to overeat, substituting other pleasures for rewards, such as a relaxing walk with a friend.

**colostrum** The first fluid secreted by the breast during late pregnancy and the first few days after birth. This thick fluid is rich in immune factors and protein.

**Community-supported agriculture (CSA)** Farms that are supported by a community of growers and consumers who provide mutual support and share the risks and benefits of food production, usually including a system of weekly delivery or pick-up of vegetables and fruit, sometimes dairy products and meat.

**complementary proteins** Two food protein sources that make up for each other's inadequate supply of specific essential amino acids; together they yield a sufficient amount of all nine and, so provide high-quality (complete) protein for the diet.

**complex carbohydrate** Carbohydrate composed of many monosaccharide molecules. Examples include glycogen, starch, and fiber.

**compound** A group of different types of atoms bonded together in definite proportion.

**compression of morbidity** Delay of the onset of disabilities caused by chronic disease.

**connective tissue** Protein tissue that holds different structures in the body together. Some structures are made up of connective tissue—notably, tendons and cartilage. Connective tissue also forms part of bone and the nonmuscular structures of arteries and veins.

**constipation** A condition characterized by infrequent bowel movements.

**contingency management** Forming a plan of action to respond to a situation in which overeating is likely, such as when snacks are within arm's reach at a party.

**control group** Participants in an experiment who are not given the treatment being tested.

**cortical bone** Dense, compact bone that comprises the outer surface and shafts of bone; also called compact bone.

**creatine** An organic (i.e., carbon-containing) molecule in muscle cells that serves as a part of a high-energy compound (termed creatine phosphate or phosphocreatine) capable of synthesizing ATP from ADP.

**cretinism** The stunting of body growth and poor mental development in the offspring that results from inadequate maternal intake of iodide during pregnancy.

**cystic fibrosis** Inherited disease that can cause overproduction of mucus. Mucus can block the pancreatic duct, decreasing enzyme output.

**cytoplasm** The fluid and organelles (except the nucleus) in a cell.

**Delaney Clause** A clause to the 1958 Food Additives Amendment of the Pure Food and Drug Act in the United States that prevents the intentional (direct) addition to foods of a compound shown to cause cancer in laboratory animals or humans.

**dementia** A general loss or decrease in mental function.

**denaturation** Alteration of a protein's three-dimensional structure, usually because of treatment by heat, enzymes, acid or alkaline solutions, or agitation.

**dental caries** Erosions in the surface of a tooth caused by acids made by bacteria as they metabolize sugars.

**deoxyribonucleic acid (DNA)** The site of hereditary information in cells; DNA directs the synthesis of cell proteins.

**diastolic blood pressure** The pressure in the arterial blood vessels when the heart is between beats.

**dietary assessment** Estimation of typical food choices relying mostly on the recounting of one's usual intake or a record of one's previous days' intake.

**dietary fiber** Fiber found in food.

**Dietary Guidelines for Americans** General goals for nutrient intakes and diet composition set by the USDA and the U.S. Department of Health and Human Services.

**Dietary Reference Intakes (DRIs)** Term used to encompass nutrient recommendations made by the Food and Nutrition Board of the National Academy of Sciences. These include RDAs, EARs, AIs, EERs, and ULs.

**digestion** The process by which large ingested molecules are mechanically and chemically broken down to produce basic nutrients that can be absorbed across the wall of the GI tract.

**digestive system** The body system consisting of the gastrointestinal tract and accessory structures such as the liver, gallbladder, and pancreas. This system performs the mechanical and chemical processes of digestion, absorption of nutrients, and elimination of wastes.

**diglyceride** A breakdown product of a triglyceride consisting of two fatty acids bonded to a glycerol backbone.

**direct calorimetry** A method of determining a body's energy use by measuring heat released from the body. An insulated chamber is usually used.

**disaccharide** Class of sugars formed by the chemical bonding of two monosaccharides.

**discretionary calories** The calories allowed in a diet after the person has met overall nutrition needs. This generally small amount of calories gives individuals the flexibility to consume some foods and beverages that may contain alcohol (e.g., beer and wine), added sugars (e.g., soft drinks, candy, and desserts), or added fats that are part of moderate- or high-fat foods (e.g., many snack foods).

**disordered eating** Mild and short-term changes in eating patterns that occur in relation to a stressful event, an illness, or a desire to modify one's diet for a variety of health and personal appearance reasons.

**diuretic** A substance that increases the volume of urine.

**diverticula** Pouches that protrude through the exterior wall of the large intestine.

**diverticulitis** An inflammation of the diverticula caused by acids produced by bacterial metabolism inside the diverticula.

**diverticulosis** The condition of having many diverticula in the large intestine.

**docosahexaenoic acid (DHA)** An omega-3 fatty acid with 22 carbons and six carbon-carbon double bonds. It is present in large amounts in fatty fish and is slowly synthesized in the body from alpha-linolenic acid. DHA is especially present in the retina and brain.

**double-blind study** An experimental design in which neither the participants nor the researchers are aware of each participant's assignment (test or placebo) or the outcome of the study until it is completed. An independent third party holds the code and the data until the study has been completed.

**dual energy X-ray absorptiometry (DEXA)** A highly accurate method of measuring body composition and bone mass and density using multiple low-energy X–rays.

**early childhood caries** Tooth decay that results from formula or juice (and even human milk) bathing the teeth as the child sleeps with a bottle in his or her mouth. The upper teeth are mostly affected as the lower teeth are protected by the tongue; formerly called *nursing bottle syndrome* and *baby bottle tooth decay.*

**eating disorder** Severe alterations in eating patterns linked to physiological changes. The alterations are associated with food restriction, binge eating, purging, and fluctuations in weight. They also involve a number of emotional and cognitive changes that affect the way a person perceives and experiences his or her body.

**edema** The buildup of excess fluid in extracellular spaces.

**eicosapentaenoic acid (EPA)** An omega-3 fatty acid with 20 carbons and five carbon-carbon double bonds. It is present in large amounts in fatty fish and is slowly synthesized in the body from alpha-linolenic acid.

**electrolytes** Substances that separate into ions in water and, in turn, are able to conduct an electrical current. These include sodium, chloride, and potassium.

**element** A substance that cannot be separated into simpler substances by chemical processes. Common elements in nutrition include carbon, oxygen, hydrogen, nitrogen, calcium, phosphorus, and iron.

**elimination diet** A restrictive diet that systematically tests foods that may cause an allergic response by first eliminating them for 1 to 2 weeks and then adding them back, one at a time.

**embryo** In humans, the developing offspring in utero from about the beginning of the third week to the end of the eighth week after conception.

**emulsifier** A compound that can suspend fat in water by isolating individual fat droplets, using a shell of water molecules or other substances to prevent the fat from coalescing.

**endocrine gland** A hormone-producing gland.

**endocrine system** The body system consisting of the various glands and the hormones these glands secrete. This system has major regulatory functions in the body, such as reproduction and cell metabolism.

**endometrium** The membrane that lines the inside of the uterus. It increases in thickness during the menstrual cycle until ovulation occurs. The surface layers are shed during menstruation if conception does not take place.

**endoplasmic reticulum (ER)** An organelle in the cytoplasm composed of a network of canals running through the cytoplasm. Part of the endoplasmic reticulum contains ribosomes.

**endorphins** Natural body tranquilizers that may be involved in the feeding response and function in pain reduction.

**energy balance** The state in which energy intake, in the form of food and beverages, matches the energy expended, primarily through basal metabolism and physical activity.

**energy density** A comparison of the calorie (kcal) content of a food with the weight of the food. An energy-dense food is high in calories but weighs very little (e.g., potato chips), whereas a food low in energy density has few calories but weighs a lot, such as an orange.

**enterohepatic circulation** A continual recycling of compounds between the small intestine and the liver; bile acids are one example of a recycled compound.

**environmental assessment** Includes details about living conditions, education level, and the ability of the person to purchase, transport, and cook food. The person's weekly budget for food purchases is also a key factor to consider.

**enzyme** A compound that speeds the rate of a chemical reaction but is not altered by the reaction. Almost all enzymes are proteins (some are made of genetic material).

**epidemiology** The study of how disease rates vary among different population groups.

**epiglottis** The flap that folds down over the trachea during swallowing.

**epinephrine** A hormone also known as *adrenaline;* it is released by the adrenal glands (located on each kidney) and various nerve endings in the body. It acts to increase glycogen breakdown in the liver, among other functions.

**epithelial cells** The cells that line the outside of the body and the inside of all external passages within it, such as the GI tract.

**epithelial tissue** The surface cells that line the outside of the body and all external passages within it.

**ergogenic** Work-producing. An ergogenic aid is a mechanical, nutritional, psychological, pharmacological, or physiological substance or treatment intended to directly improve exercise performance.

**erythrocytes** Mature red blood cells. These have no nucleus and a life span of about 120 days; they contain hemoglobin, which transports oxygen and carbon dioxide.

**erythropoietin** A hormone secreted mostly by the kidneys that enhances red blood cell synthesis and stimulates red blood cell release from bone marrow.

**esophagus** A tube in the GI tract that connects the pharynx with the stomach.

**essential amino acids** The amino acids that cannot be synthesized by humans in sufficient amounts or at all and therefore must be included in the diet; there are nine essential amino acids. These are also called *indispensable amino acids.*

**essential fatty acids** Fatty acids that must be supplied by the diet to maintain health. Currently, only linoleic acid and alpha-linolenic acid are classified as essential.

**essential nutrient** In nutritional terms, a substance that, when left out of a diet, leads to signs of poor health. The body either can't produce this nutrient or can't produce enough of it to meet its needs. Then, if added back to a diet before permanent damage occurs, the affected aspects of health are restored.

**Estimated Energy Requirement (EER)** Estimate of the energy (kcal) intake needed to match the energy use of an average person in a specific life stage.

**ethanol** Chemical term for the form of alcohol found in alcoholic beverages.

**extracellular fluid** Fluid present outside the cells; represents about one-third of body fluid.

**extracellular space** The space outside cells; represents one-third of body fluid.

**famine** An extreme shortage of food, which leads to massive starvation in a population; often associated with crop failures, war, and political unrest.

**fasting hypoglycemia** Low blood glucose that follows about a day of fasting.

**fat-soluble vitamins** Vitamins that dissolve in fat and such substances as ether and benzene but not readily in water. These vitamins are A, D, E, and K.

**fatty acid** Major part of most lipids; primarily composed of a chain of carbons flanked by hydrogen.

**female athlete triad** A condition characterized by disordered eating, lack of menstrual periods (amenorrhea), and osteoporosis.

**fermentation** The conversion of carbohydrates to alcohols, acids, and carbon dioxide without the use of oxygen.

**fetal alcohol effects (FAE)** Hyperactivity, attention deficit disorder, poor judgment, sleep disorders, and delayed learning as a result of prenatal exposure to alcohol.

**fetal alcohol syndrome (FAS)** A group of irreversible physical and mental abnormalities in the infant that result from the mother's consuming alcohol during pregnancy.

**fetus** The developing human life form from 8 weeks after conception until birth.

**fiber** Substances in plant foods not digested by the processes that take place in the human stomach or small intestine. These add bulk to feces. Fiber naturally found in foods is also called dietary fiber.

**food insecure** Condition in which the quality, variety, and/or desirability of the diet is reduced and there is difficulty at times providing enough food for everyone in the household.

**food insecurity** A condition of anxiety regarding running out of either food or money to buy more food.

**food intolerance** An adverse reaction to food that does not involve an allergic reaction.

**food sensitivity** A mild reaction to a substance in a food that might be expressed as slight itching or redness of the skin.

**foodborne illness** Sickness caused by the ingestion of food containing harmful substances.

**fructose** A six-carbon monosaccharide that usually exists in a ring form; found in fruits and honey; also known as *fruit sugar*.

**fruitarian** A person who primarily eats fruits, nuts, honey, and vegetable oils.

**functional fiber** Fiber added to foods that has been shown to provide health benefits.

**functional foods** Foods that provide health benefits beyond those supplied by the traditional nutrients they contain. For example, a tomato contains the phytochemical lycopene, so it can be called a functional food.

**fungi** Simple parasitic life forms, including molds, mildews, yeasts, and mushrooms. They live on dead or decaying organic matter. Fungi can grow as single cells, like yeast, or as a multicellular colony, as seen with molds.

**galactose** A six-carbon monosaccharide that usually exists in a ring form; closely related to glucose.

**gallbladder** An organ attached to the underside of the liver; site of bile storage, concentration, and eventual secretion.

**gastroesophageal reflux disease (GERD)** Disease that results from stomach acid backing up into the esophagus. The acid irritates the lining of the esophagus, causing pain.

**gastrointestinal (GI) tract** The main sites in the body used for digestion and absorption of nutrients. It consists of the mouth, esophagus, stomach, small intestine, large intestine, rectum, and anus. Also called the digestive tract.

**gastroplasty** Gastric bypass surgery performed on the stomach to limit its volume to approximately 30 milliliters. Also referred to as stomach stapling.

**gender and development (GAD) approach** Understanding the roles and responsibilities of both men and women in the process of sustainable development.

**gene** A specific segment on a chromosome. Genes provide the blueprint for the production of cell proteins.

**gene expression** Use of DNA information on a gene to produce a protein. Thought to be a major determination of cell development.

**generally recognized as safe (GRAS)** A list of food additives that in 1958 were considered safe for consumption. Manufacturers were allowed to continue to use these additives, without special clearance, when needed for food products. FDA bears responsibility for proving they are not safe, but can remove unsafe products from the list.

**genetic engineering** Manipulation of the genetic makeup of any organism with recombinant DNA technology.

**genetically modified organism (GMO)** Any organism created by genetic engineering.

**gestation** The period of intrauterine development of offspring, from conception to birth; in humans, gestation lasts for about 40 weeks after the woman's previous menstrual period.

**gestational diabetes** A high blood glucose concentration that develops during pregnancy and returns to normal after birth; one cause is the placental production of hormones that antagonize the regulation of blood glucose by insulin.

**ghrelin** A hormone made by the stomach that increases the desire to eat.

**glucagon** A hormone made by the pancreas that stimulates the breakdown of glycogen in the liver into glucose; this ends up increasing blood glucose. Glucagon also performs other functions.

**glucose** A six-carbon sugar that exists in a ring form; found as such in blood, and in table sugar bound to fructose; also known as *dextrose*, it is one of the simple sugars.

**glycemic index (GI)** The blood glucose response of a given food, compared to a standard (typically, glucose or white bread). Glycemic index is influenced by starch structure; fiber content; food processing; physical structure; and macronutrients in the meal, such as fat.

**glycemic load (GL)** The amount of carbohydrate in a serving of food multiplied by the glycemic index of that carbohydrate. The result is then divided by 100.

**glycerol** A three-carbon alcohol used to form triglycerides.

**glycogen** A carbohydrate made of multiple units of glucose with a highly branched structure. It is the storage form of glucose in humans and is synthesized (and stored) in the liver and muscles.

**glycosylation** The process by which glucose attaches to (glycates) other compounds, such as proteins.

**goiter** An enlargement of the thyroid gland; this is often caused by insufficient iodide in the diet.

**Golgi complex** The cell organelle near the nucleus that processes newly synthesized protein for secretion or distribution to other organelles.

**green revolution** This refers to increases in crop yields that accompanied the introduction of new agricultural technologies in less-developed countries, beginning in the 1960s. The key technologies were high-yielding, disease-resistant strains of rice, wheat, and corn; greater use of fertilizer and water; and improved cultivation practices.

**gruels** A thin mixture of grains or legumes in milk or water.

**gums** A viscous fiber containing chains of galactose, glucuronic acid, and other monosaccharides; characteristically found in exudates from plant stems.

**H2 blocker** Medication, such as cimetidine (Tagamet®), that blocks the increase of stomach acid production caused by histamine.

**heart attack** Rapid fall in heart function caused by reduced blood flow through the heart's blood vessels. Often part of the heart dies in the process. Technically called a myocardial infarction.

**heat cramps** A frequent complication of heat exhaustion. They usually occur in people who have experienced large sweat losses from exercising for several hours in a hot climate and have consumed a large volume of water. The cramps occur in skeletal muscles and consist of contractions for 1 to 3 minutes at a time.

**heat exhaustion** The first stage of heat-related illness that occurs because of depletion of blood volume from fluid loss by the body. This increases body temperature and can lead to headache, dizziness, muscle weakness, and visual disturbances, among other effects.

**heatstroke** Heatstroke can occur when internal body temperature reaches 104°F. Sweating generally ceases if left untreated, and blood circulation is greatly reduced. Nervous system damage may ensue, and death is likely. Often the skin of individuals who suffer heatstroke is hot and dry.

**helminth** Parasitic worm that can contaminate food, water, feces, animals, and other substances.

**hematocrit** The percentage of blood made up of red blood cells.

**heme iron** Iron provided from animal tissues in the form of hemoglobin and myoglobin. Approximately 40% of the iron in meat is heme iron; it is readily absorbed.

**hemicellulose** A nonfermentable fiber containing xylose, galactose, glucose, and other monosaccharides bonded together.

**hemochromatosis** A disorder of iron metabolism characterized by increased iron absorption and deposition in the liver and heart tissue. This eventually poisons the cells in those organs.

**hemoglobin** The iron-containing part of the red blood cell that carries oxygen to the cells and some carbon dioxide away from the cells. The heme iron portion is also responsible for the red color of blood.

**hemolysis** Destruction of red blood cells. The red blood cell membrane breaks down, allowing cell contents to leak into the fluid portion of the blood.

**hemorrhage** An escape of blood from blood vessels.

**hemorrhagic stroke** Damage to part of the brain resulting from rupture of a blood vessel and subsequent bleeding within or over the internal surface of the brain.

**hemorrhoid** A pronounced swelling of a large vein, particularly veins found in the anal region.

**high-density lipoprotein (HDL)** The lipoprotein in the blood that picks up cholesterol from dying cells and other sources and transfers it to the other lipoproteins in the bloodstream, as well as directly to the liver; low HDL increases the risk for cardiovascular disease.

**high-quality (complete) proteins** Dietary proteins that contain ample amounts of all nine essential amino acids.

**histamine** A breakdown product of the amino acid histidine that stimulates acid secretion by the stomach and has other effects on the body, such as contraction of smooth muscles, increased nasal secretions, relaxation of blood vessels, and changes in relaxation of airways.

**hormone** A compound secreted into the bloodstream by one type of cell that acts to control the function of another type of cell. For example, certain cells in the pancreas produce insulin, which in turn acts on muscle and other types of cells to promote uptake of nutrients from the blood.

**hospice care** A facility offering care that emphasizes comfort and dignity in death.

**human immunodeficiency virus (HIV)** The virus that leads to acquired immune deficiency syndrome (AIDS).

**hunger** The primarily physiological (internal) drive to find and eat food, mostly regulated by innate caue to eating.

**hydrogenation** The addition of hydrogen to a carbon-carbon double bond, producing a single carbon-carbon bond with two hydrogens attached to each carbon. Hydrogenation of unsaturated fatty acids in a vegetable oil increases its hardness, so this process is used to convert liquid oils into more solid fats, used in making margarine and shortening. *Trans* fatty acids are a by-product of hydrogenation of vegetable oils.

**hyperglycemia** High blood glucose, above 125 milligrams per 100 milliliters of blood.

**hypoglycemia** Low blood glucose, below 40 to 50 milligrams per 100 milliliters of blood.

**hypothalamus** A region at the base of the brain that contains cells that play a role in the regulation of hunger, respiration, body temperature, and other body functions.

**hypotheses** Tentative explanations by a scientist to explain a phenomenon.

**identical twins** Two offspring that develop from a single ovum and sperm and, consequently, have the same genetic makeup.

**ileocecal sphincter** The ring of smooth muscle between the end of the small intestine and the large intestine.

**immune system** The body system consisting of white blood cells, lymph glands and vessels, and various other body tissues. The immune system provides defense against foreign invaders, primarily due to the action of various types of white blood cells.

**immunoglobulins** Proteins found in the blood that bind to specific antigens; also called antibodies. The five major classes of immunoglobulins play different roles in antibody-mediated immunity.

**incidental food additives** Additives that appear in food products indirectly, from environmental contamination of food ingredients or during the manufacturing process.

**indirect calorimetry** A method to measure energy use by the body by measuring oxygen uptake. Formulas are then used to convert this gas exchange value into energy use.

**infrastructure** The basic framework of a system of organization. For a society, this includes roads, bridges, telephones, and other basic technologies.

**inorganic** Any substance lacking carbon atoms bonded to hydrogen atoms in the chemical structure.

**insulin** A hormone produced by the pancreas. Among other processes, insulin increases the synthesis of glycogen in the liver and the movement of glucose from the bloodstream into body cells.

**intentional food additives** Additives knowingly (directly) incorporated into food products by manufacturers.

**international unit (IU)** A crude measure of vitamin activity, often based on the growth rate of animals in response to the vitamin. Today IUs have largely been replaced by more precise milligram or microgram measures.

**intracellular fluid** Fluid contained within a cell; it represents about two-thirds of body fluid.

**intrinsic factor** A protein-like compound produced by the stomach that enhances vitamin B-12 absorption.

**ion** An atom with an unequal number of electrons and protons. Negative ions have more electrons than protons; positive ions have more protons than electrons.

**irradiation** A process in which radiation energy is applied to foods, creating compounds (free radicals) within the food that destroy cell membranes, break down DNA, link proteins together, limit enzyme activity, and alter a variety of other proteins and cell functions of microorganisms that can lead to food spoilage. This process does not make the food radioactive.

**isomers** Different chemical structures for compounds that share the same chemical formula.

**ketone bodies** Partial breakdown products of fat that contain three or four carbons.

**ketosis** The condition of having a high concentration of ketone bodies and related breakdown products in the bloodstream and tissues.

**kidney nephrons** The units of kidney cells that filter wastes from the bloodstream and deposit them into the urine.

**kilocalorie (kcal)** Heat energy needed to raise the temperature of 1000 grams (1 L) of water 1 degree Celsius; also written as *Calories.*

**kwashiorkor** A disease occurring primarily in young children who have an existing disease and consume a marginal amount of calories and insufficient protein in relation to needs. The child generally suffers from infections and exhibits edema, poor growth, weakness, and an increased susceptibility to further illness.

**lactase** An enzyme made by absorptive cells of the small intestine; this enzyme digests lactose to glucose and galactose.

**lactation** The period of milk secretion following pregnancy; typically called *breast-feeding.*

**lactic acid** A three-carbon acid formed during anaerobic cell metabolism; a partial breakdown product of glucose; also called *lactate.*

*Lactobacillus bifidus* factor A protective factor secreted in the colostrum that encourages growth of beneficial bacteria in the newborn's intestines.

**lactoovovegetarian** A person who consumes plant products, dairy products, and eggs.

**lactose intolerance** A condition in which symptoms such as abdominal gas and bloating appear as a result of severe lactose maldigestion.

**lactose maldigestion (primary and secondary)** Primary lactose maldigestion occurs when production of the enzyme lactase declines for no apparent reason. Secondary lactose maldigestion occurs when a specific cause, such as long-standing diarrhea, results in a decline in lactase production. When significant symptoms develop after lactose intake, it is then called lactose intolerance.

**lactose** Glucose bonded to galactose; also known as *milk sugar.*

**lactovegetarian** A person who consumes plant products and dairy products.

**lanugo** Down-like hair that appears after a person has lost much body fat through semi-starvation. The hair stands erect and traps air, acting as insulation for the body to compensate for the relative lack of body fat, which usually functions as insulation.

**laxative** A medication or other substance that stimulates evacuation of the intestinal tract.

**lean body mass** Body weight minus fat storage weight equals lean body mass. This includes organs such as the brain, muscles, and liver, as well as bone and blood and other body fluids.

**lecithin** A group of phospholipid compounds that are major components of cell membranes.

**leptin** A hormone made by adipose tissue in proportion to total fat stores in the body that influences long-term regulation of fat mass. Leptin also influences reproductive functions, as well as other body processes, such as release of the hormone insulin.

**let-down reflex** A reflex stimulated by infant suckling that causes the release (ejection) of milk from milk ducts in the mother's breasts; also called *milk ejection reflex.*

**life expectancy** The average length of life for a given group of people born in a specific year (such as this year).

**life span** The potential oldest age a person can reach.

**lignins** A nonfermentable fiber made up of a multiringed alcohol (noncarbohydrate) structure.

**limiting amino acid** The essential amino acid in lowest concentration in a food or diet relative to body needs.

**linoleic acid** An essential omega-6 fatty acid with 18 carbons and two double bonds.

**lipase** Fat-digesting enzyme produced by the salivary glands, stomach, and pancreas.

**lipid** A compound containing much carbon and hydrogen, little oxygen, and sometimes other atoms. Lipids do not dissolve in water, and include fats, oils, and cholesterol.

**lipoprotein** A compound found in the bloodstream containing a core of lipids with a shell composed of protein, phospholipid, and cholesterol.

**lipoprotein lipase** An enzyme attached to the cells that form the inner lining of blood vessels; it breaks down triglycerides into free fatty acids and glycerol.

**lobules** Saclike structures in the breast that store milk.

**locavore** Someone who eats food grown or produced locally or within a certain radius such as 50, 100, or 500 miles.

**long-chain fatty acid** A fatty acid that contains 12 or more carbons.

**low birth weight (LBW)** Referring to any infant weighing less than 2.5 kilograms (5.5 pounds) at birth; most commonly results from preterm birth.

**low-density lipoprotein (LDL)** The lipoprotein in the blood containing primarily cholesterol; elevated LDL is strongly linked to cardiovascular disease risk.

**lower esophageal sphincter** A circular muscle that constricts the opening of the esophagus to the stomach. Also called the *gastroesophageal sphincter.*

**lower-body obesity** The type of obesity in which fat storage is primarily located in the buttocks and thigh area. Also known as gynoid or gynecoid obesity.

**lower-quality (incomplete) proteins** Dietary proteins that are low in or lack one or more essential amino acids.

**lymph** A clear fluid that flows through lymph vessels; carries most forms of fat after their absorption by the small intestine.

**lymphatic system** A system of vessels and lymph that accepts fluid surrounding cells and large particles, such as products of fat absorption. Lymph eventually passes into the bloodstream from the lymphatic system.

**lysosome** A cellular organelle that contains digestive enzymes for use inside the cell for turnover of cell parts.

**lysozyme** An enzyme produced by a variety of cells; it can destroy bacteria by rupturing their cell membranes.

**macronutrient** A nutrient needed in gram quantities in a diet.

**macular degeneration** A painless condition leading to disruption of the central part of the retina (in the eye) and, in turn, blurred vision.

**major mineral** A mineral vital to health that is required in the diet in amounts greater than 100 milligrams per day.

**malignant** Malicious; in reference to a tumor, the property of spreading locally and to distant sites.

**malnutrition** Failing health that results from long-standing dietary practices that do not coincide with nutritional needs.

**maltase** An enzyme made by absorptive cells of the small intestine; this enzyme digests maltose to two glucoses.

**maltose** Glucose bonded to glucose.

**marasmus** A disease resulting from consuming a grossly insufficient amount of protein and calories; one of the diseases classed as protein-calorie malnutrition. Victims have little or no fat stores, little muscle mass, and poor strength. Death from infections is common.

**megadose** Intake of a nutrient beyond estimates of needs to prevent a deficiency or what would be found in a balanced diet; 2 to 10 times human needs is a starting point for such a pharmacological dosage.

**megaloblast** A large, immature red blood cell that results from the particular cell's inability to divide normally.

**megaloblastic anemia** Anemia characterized by the presence of abnormally large red blood cells.

**menarche** The onset of menstruation. Menarche usually occurs around age 13, 2 or 3 years after the first signs of puberty start to appear.

**menopause** The cessation of the menstrual cycle in women, usually beginning at about 50 years of age.

**metabolic syndrome** A condition in which a person has poor blood glucose regulation, hypertension, increased blood triglycerides, and other health problems. This condition is usually accompanied by obesity, lack of physical activity, and a diet high in refined carbohydrates. Also called Syndrome X.

**metabolism** Chemical processes in the body by which energy is provided in useful forms and vital activities are sustained.

**metastasize** The spreading of disease from one part of the body to another, even to parts of the body that are remote from the site of the original tumor. Cancer cells can spread via blood vessels, the lymphatic system, or direct growth of the tumor.

**methyl group** $CH_3$

**micronutrient** A nutrient needed in milligram or microgram quantities in a diet.

**microorganism** Bacteria, virus, or other organism invisible to the naked eye, some of which cause diseases. Also called *microbes.*

**mineral** Element used in the body to promote chemical reactions and to form body structures.

**mitochondria** The main sites of energy production in a cell. They also contain the pathway for oxidizing fat for fuel, among other metabolic pathways.

**monoglyceride** A breakdown product of a triglyceride consisting of one fatty acid attached to a glycerol backbone.

**monosaccharide** Simple sugar, such as glucose, that is not broken down further during digestion.

**monounsaturated fatty acid** A fatty acid containing one carbon-carbon double bond.

**motility** Generally, the ability to move spontaneously. It also refers to movement of food through the GI tract.

**mottling** The discoloration or marking of the surface of teeth from fluorosis.

**mucilages** A viscous fiber consisting of chains of galactose, mannose, and other monosaccharides; characteristically found in seaweed.

**mucus** A thick fluid secreted by many cells throughout the body. It contains a compound that has both carbohydrate and protein parts. It acts as a lubricant and means of protection for cells.

**muscle tissue** A type of tissue adapted to contract to cause movement.

**myelin sheath** A lipid and protein combination (lipoprotein) that covers nerve fibers.

**myocardial infarction** Death of part of the heart muscle. Also termed a *heart attack.*

**myoglobin** Iron-containing protein that binds oxygen in muscle tissue.

**negative energy balance** The state in which energy intake is less than energy expended, resulting in weight loss.

**negative protein balance** A state in which protein intake is less than related protein losses, such as often seen during acute illness.

**neotame** General-purpose, non-nutritive sweetener that is approximately 7000 to 13,000 times sweeter than table sugar. It has a chemical structure similar to aspartame's. Neotame is heat stable and can be used as a tabletop sweetener, as well as in cooking applications. It is not broken down to its amino acid components in the body after consumption.

**nervous system** The body system consisting of the brain, spinal cord, nerves, and sensory receptors. This system detects sensations, directs movements, and controls physiological and intellectual functions.

**nervous tissue** Tissue composed of highly branched, elongated cells, which transport nerve impulses from one part of the body to another.

**neural tube defect** A defect in the formation of the neural tube occurring during early fetal development. This type of defect results in various nervous system disorders, such as spina bifida. Folate deficiency in the pregnant woman increases the risk that the fetus will develop this disorder.

**neuron** The structural and functional unit of the nervous system. Consists of a **cell body, dendrites,** and an **axon.**

**neuropeptide Y** A chemical substance made in the hypothalamus that stimulates food intake. The hormone leptin inhibits neuropeptide Y production.

**neurotransmitter** A compound made by a nerve cell that allows for communication between it and other cells.

**night blindness** A vitamin A deficiency condition in which the retina (in the eye) cannot adjust to low amounts of light.

**night eating syndrome** Eating a lot of food in the late evening and nocturnal awakenings with ingestion of food.

**nitrosamine** A carcinogen formed from nitrates and breakdown products of amino acids; can lead to stomach cancer.

**non-specific immunity** Defenses that stop the invasion of pathogens; requires no previous encounter with a pathogen.

**nonessential amino acids** Amino acids that can be synthesized by a healthy body in sufficient amounts; there are 11 nonessential amino acids. These are also called *dispensable amino acids.*

**nonfermentable fiber** A fiber that is not easily metabolized by intestinal bacteria.

**nonheme iron** Iron provided from plant sources and animal tissues other than in the forms of hemoglobin and myoglobin. Nonheme iron is less efficiently absorbed than heme iron; absorption is closely dependent on body needs.

**norepinephrine** A neurotransmitter from nerve endings and a hormone from the adrenal gland. It is released in times of stress and is involved in hunger regulation, blood glucose regulation, and other body processes.

**NSAIDs** Nonsteroidal anti-inflammatory drugs; includes aspirin, ibuprofen (Advil®), and naproxen (Aleve®).

**nutrient density** The ratio derived by dividing a food's nutrient content by its calorie content. When the food's contribution to our nutrient need for that nutrient exceeds its contribution to our calorie need, the food is considered to have a favorable nutrient density.

**nutrients** Chemical substances in food that contribute to health, many of which are essential parts of a diet. Nutrients nourish us by providing calories to fulfill energy needs, materials for building body parts, and factors to regulate necessary chemical processes in the body.

**nutrigenomics** Study of how food impacts health through its interaction with our genes and its subsequent effect on gene expression.

**nutritional state** The nutritional health of a person as determined by anthropometric measurements (height, weight, circumferences, and so on), biochemical measurements of nutrients or their by-products in blood and urine, a clinical (physical) examination, a dietary analysis, and economic evaluation; also called nutritional status.

**oleic acid** An omega-9 fatty acid with 18 carbons and one double bond.

**omega-3 (ω-3) fatty acid** An unsaturated fatty acid with the first double bond on the third carbon from the methyl end ( $CH_3$).

**omega-6 (ω-6) fatty acid** An unsaturated fatty acid with the first double bond on the sixth carbon from the methyl end ( $CH_3$).

**organ** A group of tissues designed to perform a specific function—for example, the heart, which contains muscle tissue, nerve tissue, and so on.

**organ system** A collection of organs that work together to perform an overall function.

**organelles** Compartments, particles, or filaments that perform specialized functions within a cell.

**organic** Any substance that contains carbon atoms bonded to hydrogen atoms in the chemical structure.

**osmosis** The passage of a solvent such as water through a semipermeable membrane from a less concentrated compartment to a more concentrated compartment.

**osteomalacia** Adult form of rickets. The weakening of the bones seen in this disease is caused by low calcium content. A reduction in the amount of the vitamin D hormone in the body is one cause.

**osteoporosis** Decreased bone mass related to the effects of aging, genetic background, and poor diet in both genders, and hormonal changes at menopause in women.

**ostomy** Surgically created short circuit in intestinal flow where the end point usually opens from the abdominal cavity rather than the anus—for example, a colostomy. Short circuiting the intestinal flow means more water is lost in fecal matter than would be if the intestinal tract were intact.

**overnutrition** A state in which nutritional intake greatly exceeds the body's needs.

**ovum** The egg cell from which a fetus eventually develops if the egg is fertilized by a sperm cell.

**oxalic acid (oxalate)** An organic acid found in spinach, rhubarb, and other leafy green vegetables that can depress the absorption of certain minerals present in the food, such as calcium.

**oxidize** In the most basic sense, the loss of an electron or gain of an oxygen by a chemical substance. This change typically alters the shape and/or function of the substance.

**oxytocin** A hormone secreted by the pituitary gland. It causes contraction of the musclelike cells surrounding the ducts of the breasts and the smooth muscle of the uterus.

**parasite** An organism that lives in or on another organism and derives nourishment from it.

**parathyroid hormone (PTH)** A hormone made by the parathyroid glands that increases synthesis of the vitamin D hormone and aids calcium release from bone and calcium conservation by the kidneys, among other functions.

**pasteurizing** The process of heating food products to kill pathogenic microorganisms and reduce the total number of bacteria.

**pectin** A viscous fiber containing chains of galacturonic acid and other monosaccharides; characteristically found between plant cell walls.

**pepsin** A protein-digesting enzyme produced by the stomach.

**peptide bond** A chemical bond formed between amino acids in a protein.

**percentile** Classification of a measurement of a unit into divisions of 100 units.

**peristalsis** A coordinated muscular contraction used to propel food down the gastrointestinal tract.

**pernicious anemia** The anemia that results from a lack of vitamin B-12 absorption; it is pernicious because of associated nerve degeneration that can result in eventual paralysis and death.

**peroxisome** A cell organelle that destroys toxic products within the cell.

**pH** A measure of relative acidity or alkalinity of a solution. The pH scale is 0 to 14. A pH below 7 is acidic; a pH above 7 is alkaline.

**phagocytes** Cells that engulf substances; include neutrophils and macrophages.

**phagocytosis** A process in which a cell forms an indentation, and particles or fluids entering the indentation are then engulfed by the cell.

**pharynx** The organ of the digestive tract and respiratory tract located at the back of the oral and nasal cavities, commonly known as the throat.

**phenylketonuria (PKU)** Disease caused by a defect in the liver's ability to metabolize the amino acid phenylalanine into the amino acid tyrosine; untreated, toxic by-products of phenylalanine build up in the body and lead to mental retardation.

**phosphocreatine (PCr)** A high-energy compound that can be used to re-form ATP. It is used primarily during bursts of activity, such as lifting and jumping.

**phospholipid** Any of a class of fat-related substances that contain phosphorus, fatty acids, and a nitrogen-containing component. Phospholipids are an essential part of every cell.

**photosynthesis** Process by which plants use energy from the sun to synthesize energy-yielding compounds, such as glucose.

**physical fitness** The ability to perform moderate to vigorous activity without undue fatigue.

**physiological anemia** The normal increase in blood volume in pregnancy that dilutes the concentration of red blood cells, resulting in anemia; also called *hemodilution*.

**phytic acid (phytate)** A constituent of plant fibers that binds positive ions to its multiple phosphate groups.

**phytochemical** A chemical found in plants. Some phytochemicals may contribute to a reduced risk of cancer or cardiovascular disease in people who consume them regularly.

**pica** The practice of eating nonfood items, such as dirt, laundry starch, or clay.

**placebo** Generally a fake medicine or treatment used to disguise the treatments given to the participants in an experiment.

**placenta** An organ that forms in the uterus in pregnant women. Through this organ, oxygen and nutrients from the mother's blood are transferred to the fetus, and fetal wastes are removed. The placenta also releases hormones that maintain the state of pregnancy.

**plaque** A cholesterol-rich substance deposited in the blood vessels; it contains various white blood cells, smooth muscle cells, various proteins, cholesterol and other lipids, and eventually calcium.

**plasma** The fluid, extracellular portion of the circulating blood. This includes the blood serum plus all blood-clotting factors. In contrast, **serum** is the fluid that remains after clotting factors have been removed from plasma.

**polypeptide** A group of amino acids bonded together, from 50 to 2000 or more.

**polysaccharide** Class of complex carbohydrates containing many glucose units, from 10 to 1000 or more.

**polyunsaturated fatty acid** A fatty acid containing two or more carbon-carbon double bonds.

**pool** The amount of a nutrient stored within the body that can be mobilized when needed.

**portal circulation** The portion of the circulatory system that uses a large vein (portal vein) to carry nutrient-rich blood from capillaries in the intestines and portions of the stomach to the liver.

**portal vein** Large vein leaving from the intestine and stomach and connecting to the liver.

**positive energy balance** The state in which energy intake is greater than energy expended, generally resulting in weight gain.

**positive protein balance** A state in which protein intake exceeds related protein losses, as is needed during times of growth.

**prebiotic** Substance that stimulates bacterial growth in the large intestines.

**pregnancy-induced hypertension** A serious disorder that can include high blood pressure, kidney failure, convulsions, and even death of the mother and fetus. Although its exact cause is not known, an adequate diet (especially adequate calcium intake) and prenatal care may prevent this disorder or limit its severity. Mild cases are known as *preeclampsia*; more severe cases are called *eclampsia* (formerly called *toxemia* ).

**preservatives** Compounds that extend the shelf life of foods by inhibiting microbial growth or minimizing the destructive effect of oxygen and metals.

**preterm** An infant born before 37 weeks of gestation; also referred to as *premature* .

**probiotic** Product that contains specific types of bacteria. Use is intended to colonize the large intestine with the specific bacteria in the product. An example is yogurt.

**prolactin** A hormone secreted by the pituitary gland that stimulates the synthesis of milk in the breast.

**prostate gland** A solid, chestnut-shaped organ surrounding the first part of the urinary tract in the male. The prostate gland secretes substances into the semen.

**protease** Protein-digesting enzyme produced by the stomach, small intestine, and pancreas.

**protein equilibrium** A state in which protein intake is equal to related protein losses; the person is said to be in protein balance.

**protein turnover** The process by which cells break down old proteins and resynthesize new proteins. In this way the cell will have the proteins it needs to function at that time.

**protein-calorie malnutrition (PCM)** A condition resulting from regularly consuming insufficient amounts of calories and protein. The deficiency eventually results in body wasting, primarily of lean tissue, and an increased susceptibility to infections.

**protein** Food and body compounds made of amino acids; proteins contain carbon, hydrogen, oxygen, nitrogen, and sometimes other atoms, in a specific configuration. Proteins contain the form of nitrogen most easily used by the human body.

**proton pump inhibitor** A medication that inhibits the ability of gastric cells to secrete hydrogen ions. Low doses of this class of medications are also available without prescription (e.g., omeprazole [Prilosec]).

**protozoa** One-celled animals that are more complex than bacteria. Disease-causing protozoa can be spread through food and water.

**provitamin/precursor** A substance that can be made into a vitamin, if the body needs it.

**pyloric sphincter** The ring of smooth muscle between the stomach and the small intestine.

**pyruvic acid** A three-carbon compound formed during glucose metabolism; also called *pyruvate*.

**radiation** Literally, energy that is emitted from a center in all directions. Various forms of radiation energy include X-rays and ultra-violet rays from the sun.

**rancid** Containing products of decomposed fatty acids that have an unpleasant flavor and odor.

**reactive hypoglycemia** Low blood glucose that follows a meal high in simple sugars, with corresponding symptoms of irritability, headache, nervousness, sweating, and confusion; also called *postprandial hypoglycemia*.

**receptor** A site in a cell at which compounds (such as hormones) bind. Cells that contain receptors for a specific compound are partially controlled by that compound.

**recombinant DNA technology** A test tube technology that rearranges DNA sequences in an organism by cutting the DNA, adding or deleting a DNA sequence, and rejoining DNA molecules with a series of enzymes.

**Recommended Dietary Allowance (RDA)** Nutrient intake amount sufficient to meet the needs of 97% to 98% of the individuals in a specific life stage.

**rectum** Terminal portion of the large intestine.

**registered dietitian (R.D.)** A person who has completed a baccalaureate degree program approved by the American Dietetic Association, performed at least 900 hours of supervised professional practice, and passed a registration examination.

**relapse prevention** A series of strategies used to help prevent and cope with weight-control lapses, such as recognizing high-risk situations and deciding beforehand on appropriate responses.

**reserve capacity** The extent to which an organ can preserve essentially normal function despite decreasing cell number or cell activity.

**resting metabolism** The amount of calories the body uses when the person has not eaten in 4 hours and is resting (e.g., 15 to 30 minutes) and awake in a warm, quiet environment. It is roughly 6% higher than basal metabolism due to the less strict criteria for the test; often referred to as *resting metabolic rate (RMR)*.

**retinoids** Chemical forms of preformed vitamin A; one source is animal foods.

**ribonucleic acid (RNA)** The single-stranded nucleic acid involved in the transcription of genetic information and translation of that information into protein structure.

**ribosomes** Cytoplasmic particles that mediate the linking together of amino acids to form proteins; may exist freely in the cytoplasm or attached to endoplasmic reticulum.

**rickets** A disease characterized by poor mineralization of newly synthesized bones because of low calcium content. This deficiency disease arises in infants and children from insufficient amounts of the vitamin D hormone in the body.

**saccharin** Alternative sweetener that yields no energy to the body; 300 times sweeter than sucrose.

**saliva** Watery fluid, produced by the salivary glands in the mouth, that contains lubricants, enzymes, and other substances.

**salivary amylase** A starch-digesting enzyme produced by salivary glands.

**salt** Compound of sodium and chloride in a 40:60 ratio.

**sarcopenia** In general, loss of muscle tissue. Among older adults this loss of lean mass greatly increases their risk of illness and death.

**sarcopenic obesity** Loss of muscle mass accompanied by gains in fat mass.

**satiety** A state in which there is no longer a desire to eat; a feeling of satisfaction.

**saturated fatty acid** A fatty acid containing no carbon-carbon double bonds.

**scavenger cells** Specific form of white blood cells that can bury themselves in the artery wall and accumulate LDL. As these cells take up LDL, they contribute to the development of atherosclerosis.

**scurvy** The deficiency disease that results after a few weeks to months of consuming a diet that lacks vitamin C; pinpoint sites of bleeding on the skin are an early sign.

**secretory vesicles** Membrane-bound vesicles produced by the Golgi apparatus; contains protein and other compounds to be secreted by the cell.

**self-monitoring** Tracking foods eaten and conditions affecting eating; actions are usually recorded in a diary, along with location, time, and state of mind. This is a tool to help people understand more about their eating habits.

**sequestrants** Compounds that bind free metal ions. By so doing, they reduce the ability of ions to cause rancidity in foods containing fat.

**serotonin** A neurotransmitter synthesized from the amino acid tryptophan that affects mood (sense of calmness), behavior, and appetite, and induces sleep.

**set point** Often refers to the close regulation of body weight. It is not known what cells control this set point or how it functions in weight regulation. There is evidence, however, that mechanisms exist that help regulate weight.

**sickle cell disease (sickle cell anemia)** An illness that results from a malformation of the red blood cell because of an incorrect structure in part of its hemoglobin protein chains. The disease can lead to episodes of severe bone and joint pain, abdominal pain, headache, convulsions, paralysis, and even death.

**simple sugar** Monosaccharide or disaccharide in the diet.

**small for gestational age (SGA)** Referring to infants who weigh less than the expected weight for their length of gestation. This corresponds to less than 2.5 kilograms (5.5 pounds) in a full-term newborn. A preterm infant who is also SGA will most likely develop some medical complications.

**solvent** A liquid substance in which other substances dissolve.

**sorbitol** Alcohol derivative of glucose that yields about 3 kcal/g but is slowly absorbed from the small intestine; used in some sugarless gums and dietetic foods.

**specific immunity** Function of lymphocytes directed at specific antigens.

**spontaneous abortion** Cessation of pregnancy and expulsion of the embryo or nonviable fetus prior to 20 weeks gestation. This is the result of natural causes, such as a genetic defect or developmental problem; also called *miscarriage*.

**spores** Dormant reproductive cells capable of turning into adult organisms without the help of another cell. Various bacteria and fungi form spores.

**starch** A carbohydrate made of multiple units of glucose attached together in a form the body can digest; also known as *complex carbohydrate*.

**sterol** A compound containing a multi-ring (steroid) structure and a hydroxyl group (–OH). Cholesterol is a typical example.

**stimulus control** Altering the environment to minimize the stimuli for eating—for example, removing foods from sight and storing them in kitchen cabinets.

**stress fracture** A fracture that occurs from repeated jarring of a bone. Common sites include bones of the foot.

**stroke** A decrease or loss in blood flow to the brain that results from a blood clot or other change in arteries in the brain. This in turn causes the death of brain tissue. Also called a *cerebrovascular accident*.

**subclinical** Stage of a disease or disorder not severe enough to produce symptoms that can be detected or diagnosed.

**sucralose** Alternative sweetener that has chlorines in place of 3 hydroxyl (–OH) groups on sucrose; 600 times sweeter than sucrose.

**sucrase** An enzyme made by absorptive cells of the small intestine; this enzyme digests sucrose to glucose and fructose.

**sucrose** Fructose bonded to glucose; table sugar.

**sugar** A simple carbohydrate with the chemical composition $(CH_2O)_n$. The basic unit of all sugars is glucose, a six-carbon ring structure. The primary sugar in the diet is sucrose, which is made up of glucose and fructose.

**sustainable agriculture** Agricultural system that provides a secure living for farm families; maintains the natural environment and resources; supports the rural community; and offers respect and fair treatment to all involved, from farm workers to consumers to the animals raised for food.

**sustainable development** Economic growth that will simultaneously reduce poverty, protect the environment, and preserve natural capital.

**symptom** A change in health status noted by the person with the problem, such as stomach pain.

**synapse** The space between one neuron and another neuron (or cell).

**systolic blood pressure** The pressure in the arterial blood vessels associated with the pumping of blood from the heart.

**teratogen** A substance that may cause or increase the risk of a birth defect. Exposure to a teratogen does not always lead to a birth defect;

its effects on the fetus depend on the dose, timing, and duration of exposure.

**tetany** A body condition marked by sharp contraction of muscles and failure to relax afterward; usually caused by abnormal calcium metabolism.

**theory** An explanation for a phenomenon that has numerous lines of evidence to support it.

**thermic effect of food (TEF)** The increase in metabolism that occurs during the digestion, absorption, and metabolism of energy-yielding nutrients. This represents 5% to 10% of calories consumed.

**thermogenesis** This term encompasses the ability of humans to regulate body temperature within narrow limits (thermoregulation). Two visible examples of thermogenesis are fidgeting and shivering when cold.

**thyroid hormones** Hormones produced by the thyroid gland that among their functions increase the rate of overall metabolism in the body.

**tissues** Collections of cells adapted to perform a specific function.

**tocopherols** The chemical name for some forms of vitamin E. The alpha form is the most potent.

**Tolerable Upper Intake Level (UL)** Maximum chronic daily intake level of a nutrient that is unlikely to cause adverse health effects in almost all people in a specific life stage.

**total fiber** Combination of dietary fiber and functional fiber in a food. Also just called *fiber*.

**total parenteral nutrition** The intravenous feeding of all necessary nutrients, including the most basic forms of protein, carbohydrates, lipids, vitamins, minerals, and electrolytes.

**toxins** Poisonous compounds produced by an organism that can cause disease.

**trabecular bone** The spongy, inner matrix of bone, found primarily in the spine, pelvis, and ends of bones; also called spongy or cancellous bone.

**trace mineral** A mineral vital to health that is required in the diet in amounts less than 100 milligrams per day.

***trans* fatty acids** A form of an unsaturated fatty acid, usually a monounsaturated one when found in food, in which the hydrogens on both carbons forming that double bond lie on opposite sides of that bond, rather than on the same side, as in most natural fats. Stick margarine, shortenings, and deep fat-fried foods in general are rich sources.

**transcription** Information on DNA needed to make a protein is copied onto RNA.

**transgenic** Organism that contains genes originally present in another organism.

**translation** The information contained in RNA is used to determine the amino acids in a protein.

**triglyceride** The major form of lipid in the body and in food. It is composed of three fatty acids bonded to glycerol.

**trimesters** Three 13- to 14-week periods into which the normal pregnancy (the length of a normal pregnancy is about 40 weeks, measured from the first day of the woman's last menstrual period) is divided somewhat arbitrarily for purposes of discussion and analysis. Development of the offspring, however, is continuous throughout pregnancy, with no specific physiological markers demarcating the transition from one trimester to the next.

**trypsin** A protein-digesting enzyme secreted by the pancreas to act in the small intestine.

**tumor** Mass of cells; may be cancerous (malignant) or noncancerous (benign).

**type 1 diabetes** A form of diabetes prone to ketosis and that requires insulin therapy.

**type 2 diabetes** A form of diabetes characterized by insulin resistance and often associated with obesity. Insulin therapy can be used but is often not required.

**ulcer** Erosion of the tissue lining, usually in the stomach (gastric ulcer) or the upper small intestine (duodenal ulcer). As a group these are generally referred to as peptic ulcers.

**umami** A brothy, meaty, savory flavor in some foods. Monosodium glutamate enhances this flavor when added to foods.

**undernutrition** Failing health that results from a long-standing dietary intake that is not enough to meet nutritional needs.

**underwater weighing** A method of estimating total body fat by weighing the individual on a standard scale and then weighing him or her again submerged in water. The difference between the two weights is used to estimate total body volume.

**underweight** A body mass index below 18.5. The cutoff is less precise than for obesity because this condition has been less studied.

**unsaturated fatty acid** A fatty acid containing one or more carbon-carbon double bonds.

**upper-body obesity** The type of obesity in which fat is stored primarily in the abdominal area; defined as a waist circumference more than 40 inches (102 centimeters) in men and more than 35 inches (89 centimeters) in women; closely associated with a high risk for cardiovascular disease, hypertension, and type 2 diabetes. Also known as android obesity.

**urea** Nitrogenous waste product of protein metabolism; major source of nitrogen in the urine.

**urea** Nitrogenous waste product of protein metabolism; major source of nitrogen in the urine, chemically

**ureter** Tube that transports urine from the kidney to the urinary bladder.

**urethra** Tube that transports urine from the urinary bladder to the outside of the body.

**urinary system** The body system consisting of the kidneys, urinary bladder, and the ducts that carry urine. This system removes waste products from the circulatory system and regulates blood acid-base balance, overall chemical balance, and water balance in the body.

**vegan** A person who eats only plant foods.

**vein** A blood vessel that carries blood to the heart.

**very-low-calorie diet (VLCD)** Known also as *protein-sparing modified fast (PSMF)*, this diet allows a person 400 to 800 kcal per day, often in liquid form. Of this, 120 to 480 kcal is carbohydrate, and the rest is mostly high-quality protein.

**very-low-density lipoprotein (VLDL)** The lipoprotein created in the liver that carries cholesterol and lipids that have been taken up or newly synthesized by the liver.

**villi** (singular, **villus**) The fingerlike protrusions into the small intestine that participate in digestion and absorption of food.

**virus** The smallest known type of infectious agent, many of which cause disease in humans.

A virus is essentially a piece of genetic material surrounded by a coat of protein. They do not metabolize, grow, or move by themselves. They reproduce only with the aid of a living cellular host.

**viscous fiber** A fiber that is readily fermented by bacteria in the large intestine.

**vitamin** Compound needed in small amounts in the diet to help regulate and support chemical reactions and processes in the body.

**water** The universal solvent; chemically, $H_2O$. The body is composed of about 60% water. Water (fluid) needs are about 9 (women) or 13 (men) cups per day; needs are greater if one exercises heavily.

**water-soluble vitamins** Vitamins that dissolve in water. These vitamins are the B vitamins and vitamin C.

**white blood cells** One of the formed elements of the circulating blood system; also called *leukocytes*. White blood cells are able to squeeze through intracellular spaces and migrate. They phagocytize bacteria, fungi, and viruses, as well as detoxify proteins that may result from allergic reactions, cellular injury, and other immune system cells.

**whole grains** Grains containing the entire seed of the plant, including the bran, germ, and endosperm (starchy interior). Examples are whole-wheat and brown rice.

**xerophthalmia** Literally "dry eye." This is a cause of blindness that results from a vitamin A deficiency. A lack of mucus production by the eye, which leaves it at a greater risk of damage from surface dirt and bacteria.

**xylitol** Alcohol derivative of the 5-carbon monosaccharide xylose.

**zygote** The fertilized ovum; the cell resulting from the union of an egg cell (ovum) and sperm until it divides.

# PHOTO CREDITS

Getty Images RF; p. 293: © PhotoDisc/OS49 RF; Fig 8-1: A Colour Atlas and Text of Nutritional Disorders by Dr. Donald D. McLaren/Mosby-Wolfe Europe Ltd.; Fig 8-2: National Eye Institute, National Institute of Health; p. 295: Getty Images RF; p. 297: Kevin Sanchez/Cole Group/Getty Images RF; p. 298: © Royalty Free/Corbis; Fig 8-6: Jeffrey L. Rotman/Corbis; p. 301: © Gregg Kidd and Joanne Scott; p. 303: C Squared Studios/Getty Images RF; p. 305: Visuals Unlimited; p. 306: © Royalty Free/Corbis; p. 310: D. Fischer and Pl. Lyos/Cole Group/Getty Images RF; Fig 8-18(top): A Colour Atlas and Text of Nutritional Disorders by Dr. Donald D. McLaren/Mosby-Wolfe Europe Ltd.; (bottom): Dr. P. Marazzi/Science Photo Library/Photo Researchers, Inc.; Fig 8-20(left): Dr. M.A. Ansary/Photo Researchers, Inc.; (right): © Lester V. Bergman/Corbis; p. 314: Getty Images/Jonelle Weaver RF; p. 318: © Corbis/Vol. 130 RF; p. 320: C Squared Studios/Getty Images RF; Fig 8-26(top): Michael Abbey/Photo Researchers, Inc.; (bottom): Biophoto Associates/SPL/Photo Researchers, Inc.; p. 323: Photodisc/PunchStock RF; p. 324: © Peter Cade/Getty Images RF; p. 325: Royalty Free/Corbis; p. 327: David Buffington/Getty Images RF; Fig 8-31(both): Dr. P. Marazzi/Photo Researchers, Inc.; p. 330(top): Royalty Free/Corbis; (bottom): Michael Matisse/Getty Images RF; p. 331: C Squared Studios/Getty Images RF; p. 334: © Digital Vision RF; p. 336: © The Ohio State University Communications Photo Service, Jodi Miller; p. 337: © PhotoDisc/Vol. 67 RF; Fig 8-38(salad): © PhotoDisc/OS49 RF; (orange juice): © Corbis/Vol. 83 RF; p. 338: Photodisc Collection/Getty Images RF; p. 339: Adam Crowley/Getty Images RF; p. 344: © Image Source/PunchStock RF

## Chapter 9

Opener: © Photodisc Collection/Getty Images RF; p. 350, 352: © Royalty-Free/Corbis; p. 354: Getty Images; p. 355: © Corbis/Vol. 83 RF; p. 357, 358, 359: MHHE Image Library; p. 360: © Corbis/Vol. 43 RF; p. 362: C Squared Studios/Getty Images RF; p. 364: © Stockdisc/PunchStock RF; p. 365: MHHE Image Library; p. 367: McGraw-Hill Companies, Inc./Andrew Resek, photographer; p. 369: © Corbis/Vol. 43 RF; p. 372(top): © Corbis/RF website; (bottom): Michael Lamotte/Cole Group/Getty Images RF; p. 374: © Royalty Free/Corbis; p. 375: Courtesy National Cattlemen's Beef Associations; p. 378(top): Keith Brofsky/Getty Images RF; (bottom): Photo courtesy of Harold H. Sandstead, M.D.; p. 379: © Corbis/Vol. 130 RF; p. 381: © Corbis/Vol. 43 RF; p. 382: A Colour Atlas and Text of Nutritional Disorders by Dr. Donald D. McLaren/Mosby-Wolfe Europe Ltd.; p. 384: Courtesy of Fishery Products International, Denver, MA; p. 386(top): © Paul Casamassimo, DDS, MS; (bottom): © PhotoDisc/Vol. 02 RF; p. 387(top): © Corbis/RF website; (bottom): C Squared Studios/Getty Images RF; Fig 9-23: Ryan McVay/Getty Images RF; p. 392(left): © PhotoDisc/Vol. 40 RF; (right): Rob Melnychuk/Getty Images RF; p. 393: Ryan McVay/Getty Images RF; p. 396: Yoav Levy/Phototake; p. 398: © Royalty Free/Corbis; p. 399: © Royalty Free/Corbis

## Chapter 10

Opener: © Getty Images; p. 409: The McGraw-Hill Companies, Inc./Lars A. Niki, photographer; p. 411: JupiterImages RF; p. 412: © Getty Images/Vol. 67 RF; p. 413: © PhotoDisc/Sports Metaphors RF; p. 414: Royalty Free/Corbis; p. 416: JupiterImages RF; p. 417: © Corbis/Vol. 20 RF; p. 418: © James Mulligan; p. 419: © Corbis/RF website; p. 422(top): © IngramPublishing/SuperStock RF; (bottom): Royalty Free/Corbis; p. 423(top): © Gordon Wardlaw; (bottom): RF/

Corbis; p. 425: © PhotoDisc/Vol. 51 RF; p. 426: © Corbis/Vol. 103 RF; p. 428(top): © Getty Images/Vol. 1/Photolink RF; (bottom): © John A. Rizzo/Getty Images RF; p. 429: PhotoDisc/Vol. 51 RF; p. 434(top): © Corbis/Vol. 20 RF; (bottom): Royalty Free/Corbis; p. 438: JupiterImages RF

## Chapter 11

Opener: © Corbis/Vol. 75 RF; p. 447: © The McGraw-Hill Companies, Inc./Lars A. Niki, photographer; p. 448: © Photodisc website RF; p. 449: © Royalty Free/Corbis; p. 450: Mark Andersen/Getty Images RF; p. 451: Ryan McVay/Getty Images RF; p. 452: © PhotoDisc website RF; Fig 11-1(potato): The McGraw-Hill Companies, Inc./Christopher Kerrigan, photographer; (steak): RF Comstock Images; (healthy man & woman): RF/Getty Images; p. 455: © Tom Stewart Photography/Corbis; p. 456: JupiterImages RF; p. 457: © Brand X Pictures/PunchStock RF; Fig 11-3: © Paul Casamassimo, DDS, MS; p. 458: Royalty Free/Corbis; p. 459: © PhotoDisc website RF; p. 460: Jack Star/PhotoLink/Getty Images RF; p. 461: © BananaStock/PunchStock RF; Fig 11-4: © Photodisc/Vol. 45 RF; p. 463: The McGraw-Hill Companies, Inc./Lars A. Niki, photographer; p. 464: © PhotoDisc website RF; p. 465: © PhotoDisc/Vol. 95 RF; p. 466: © Corbis/RF website; p. 467: © BananaStock/PunchStock RF; p. 471: © Digital Vision/PunchStock RF

## Chapter 12

Opener: © Dr. Parvinder Sethi; p. 474: © Corbis/RF website; p. 478: USDA photo by Peter Manzelli; p. 480: © Royalty Free/Corbis; p. 481: © PhotoDisc/Vol. 25 RF; p. 483: The McGraw-Hill Companies, Inc./Barry Barker, photographer; p. 484: Getty Images/Digital Vision RF; p. 485: The McGraw-Hill Companies, Inc./Barry Barker, photographer; p. 486(both): © The Ohio State University Communications Photo Service; p. 487: © Corbis/RF website; p. 489: © Corbis/Vol. 25 RF; p. 491: MHHE Image Library; p. 494: © Corbis/Vol. 609 RF; p. 495: © The Ohio State University Communications Photo Service, Jodi Miller; Fig 12-7(top,left): © Corbis/RF website; (all others): AP Wide World Photos; p. 498: Corbis/RF website; p. 499: John Wang/Getty Images RF

## Chapter 13

Opener: Creatas Images/JupiterImages RF; p. 507: Royalty Free/Corbis; p. 508: © The Ohio State University Communications Photo Service; p. 511: © John A. Rizzo/Getty Images RF; Table 13-3 (egg): © Photodisc/Getty Images RF; (chicken): © I. Rozenbaum/F. Cirou/Photo Alto RF; (hamburger): © John A. Rizzo/Getty Images RF; (washing hands): © Comstock Images/PictureQuest RF; (whisk/bowl): Michael Lamotte/Cole Group/Getty Images RF; (ladel): © Ingram Publishing/Fotosearch RF; (cheese): Digital Vision/Getty Images RF; (beans): Photo provided by Jarden Home Brands, marketers of Ball[[reg]] and Kerr[[reg]] fresh preserving products. Jarden Home Brands is a division of Jarden Corporation (NYSE: JAH); (oysters): © I. Rozenbaum/F. Cirou/Photo Alto RF; (steak): © Foodcollection/Getty Images RF; p. 514(top): Royalty Free/Corbis; (bottom): © Image Source/Corbis RF; Table 13-5(bacon): © Ingram Publishing/Alamy RF; (fish): © Image Source/Corbis RF; (beef): © I. Rozenbaum/F. Cirou/Photo Alto RF; (hamburger): © The Ohio State University Communications Photo Service; (tap water): © Don Farrall/Getty Images RF; (glass of water): © John A. Rizzo/Getty Images RF; p. 517: © Corbis/Vol. 83 RF; p. 518: © Corbis/Vol. 192

RF; p. 520: Bob Montesciaros/Cole Group/Getty Images RF; p. 521(top): Rob Melnychuk/Getty Images RF; (bottom): © The Ohio State University Communications Photo Service; p. 522: © Image Source/Corbis RF; p. 523: © Corbis/Vol. 43 RF; p. 525: © The Ohio State University Communications Photo Service; p. 526: © PhotoDisc website RF; p. 527(top): © Corbis/Vol. 49 RF; (bottom): © Comstock Images/PictureQuest RF; (USDA label): USDA; p. 528: C Squared Studios/Getty Images RF; p. 529: McGraw-Hill Companies, Inc./Christopher Kerrigan, photographer; p. 530: © Iconotec.com RF; p. 532(food safety logo): USDA; p. 532: © Greg Wolff; p. 533: © PhotoDisc/Vol. 48 RF; p. 535: © PhotoDisc/Vol. 58 RF; p. 538: Jess Alford/Getty Images RF; p. 539(top): Digital Vision/Getty Images RF; (bottom): David Buffington/Getty Images RF

## Chapter 14

Opener: Royalty Free/Corbis; p. 543: © BananaStock/PunchStock RF; p. 546: © Gordon Wardlaw, photographer Greg Wolff; p. 547: Blend Images/Getty Images RF; p. 549: USDA; p. 550: Keith Brofsky/Getty Images RF; p. 554: Photodisc Collection/Getty Images RF; p. 556: © Corbis/RF website; p. 558: © Corbis/Vol. 83 RF; p. 560: Getty Images; p. 563: Scott T. Baxter/Getty Images RF; p. 564: © PhotoDisc/Vol. 192 RF; p. 565: © PhotoDisc/EP039 RF; p. 566: Spike Mafford/Getty Images RF; p. 567: © Corbis/Vol. 52 RF; p. 569: Getty Images RF; p. 572: © Digital Vision/PunchStock RF; p. 577: Andersen Ross/Getty Images RF

## Chapter 15

Opener: Comstock/Febienne Dudognon RF; p. 583(top): World Health Organization; (bottom): © PhotoDisc/Vol. 113 RF; p. 584: © Corbis/Vol. 135 RF; p. 589(top): © PhotoDisc/Vol. 58 RF; (bottom): Corbis/PictureQuest RF; p. 591: © PhotoDisc/Vol. 113 RF; p. 592(top): Corbis/PictureQuest RF; (bottom): © Paul Casamassimo, DDS, MS; p. 593: © Corbis/Vol. 9 RF; p. 594: © Corbis/Vol. 552 RF; p. 595: Joanne Scott; p. 597: USDA Photo by Ken Hammond; p. 598: Ablestock/Alamy RF; p. 600: Blend Images/Alamy RF; p. 602: © Corbis/Vol. 552 RF; p. 603: C Squared Studios/Getty Images RF; p. 604: Gregg Kidd and Joanne Scott; p. 605: Corbis/RF website; p. 606: © PhotoDisc/Vol. 95 RF; p. 607: © Corbis/Vol. 124 RF; p. 609: © Gregg Kidd and Joanne Scott; p. 611: © PhotoDisc/Vol. 61 RF; p. 615: The McGraw-Hill Companies, Inc./Jill Braaten, photographer

## Chapter 16

Opener: Dynamic Graphics/JupiterImages RF; p. 621: © Corbis/RF website; p. 622: © Corbis/RF website; p. 627: © Digital Vision/PunchStock RF; p. 628: Steve Mason/Getty Images RF; p. 629: Mitch Hrdlicka/Getty Images RF; p. 632(top): © PhotoDisc Vol. 15 RF; (bottom): © Stockbyte/Punchstock RF; p. 635: © Gordon Wardlaw; p. 638(top): PhotoDisc/Vol. 20 RF; (bottom): © Corbis/Vol. 192 RF; p. 639: © PhotoDisc website RF; p. 642(both): Arthur Glauberman/Photo Researchers, Inc.; p. 643: PhotoDisc/Vol. 48 RF; p. 644: © RF/Corbis; p. 646: PhotoDisc/OS49 RF; p. 650: © PhotoDisc website RF; p. 654: © RF/Corbis; p. 655: © PhotoDisc/SS45 RF

## Appendix

(grapes): © Burke Triolo Productions/Getty Images; Fig D-1(all): Greg Kidd & Joanne Scott

# INDEX

## A

Absorption
- of alcohol, 639
- energy for, 247
- GI tract and, 96, 105
- of lipids, 180–81
- processes of, 103
- of proteins, 219–21
- in small intestine, 100

Absorptive cells, 100, 101–2, 103, 141, 143
Academy for Eating Disorders, 464
Acceptable Daily Intake (ADI) guideline, 137, 138
Acesulfame-K, 137, 138
Acetaldehyde dehydrogenase, 639
Acetycholine, 330
Acid, 99
Acid groups, 167
Acid reflux. *See* Heartburn
Acid-base balance (pH), 107, 222
Acne, 606
Acquired immune deficiency syndrome (AIDS)
- alcohol and, 642
- breastfeeding and, 567
- defined, 484
- nutrition and, 489
- pregnancy and, 542, 547, 548
- undernutrition and, 483
- vitamins and, 327
- worldwide impact of, 487–90

Acrylamide, 524
Active absorption, 103
Additives, 515–21
Adenosine diphosphate (ADP), 412, 414
Adenosine triphosphate (ATP), 86, 412–16
Adequate Intakes (AIs), 60–63, 148, 190
Adipose tissue, 21, 22, 107, 156
- bioelectrical impedance and, 255
- brown, 249
- cancer and, 647
- growth and infants, 583
- heartburn and, 115
- high insulin output and, 144
- triglycerides and, 188
- water and, 348
- weight loss and, 261

Adjustable gastric banding, 272
Administration on Aging, 644
Administration on Aging's Elder Care Locator, 644
Adrenaline. *See* Epinephrine
Adulthood, nutrition for
- alcohol and, 638–43
- case study on dietary assistance for older adult, 650
- demographics of, 620
- ensuring healthful, 643–45
- factors related to food intake/nutrient needs, 629–38
- introduction to, 619

- nutrient needs, 625–29
- physiological changes and, 621–25

Advanced glycation endproducts (AGEs), 154
Aerobic exercise, 632
Aerobic, defined, 85
African Americans, 17, 140, 155, 360, 391, 392, 478, 571
Age-related nutrition needs. *See* Adulthood, nutrition for; Infants; Preschool children, nutrition for; School-age children, nutrition for; Teenage years, nutrition for
Aging, 621
Agriculture/Agrifood Canada, 17
AIDS. *See* Acquired immune deficiency syndrome (AIDS)
Air displacement, 254
Alcohol, 6, 14, 17, 24, 25, 54
- absorption in stomach, 105
- antidiuretic hormone and, 353
- athlete fluid needs and, 425
- breastfeeding and, 564
- cancer and, 646, 648
- critical thinking about, 109
- diabetes and, 156
- Dietary Guidelines for Americans and, 52, 55, 57
- eating disorders and, 450, 460
- energy balance and, 247
- hypertension and, 5, 17, 392
- improving diets and, 18, 19
- magnesium and, 370–71
- maltose and, 130
- Mediterranean diet and, 54, 193
- nutrition implications of consumption of, 638–43
- osteoporosis and, 398
- percentages of calories advocated and, 16
- pregnancy and, 543, 545, 554, 570, 571
- in prevention of birth defects, 570
- state of nutritional health and, 45
- stomach and, 100
- teenage years and, 606
- ulcers and, 114
- upper-body obesity and, 257
- vitamins and, 309, 312, 319, 324
- warning signs/symptoms of alcohol poisoning, 26

Alcohol abuse, 639
Alcohol dehydrogenase, 639
Alcohol dependence, 640
Alcoholism, 639, 640, 641, 642
Aldosterone, 353
Allergens, 608
Allergies, 219, 585, 590–91, 608–11
Alliance of Genetic Support Groups, 110
Alpha-linolenic acid, 169, 173, 185, 187. *See also* Omega-3 fatty acids
Alternative medicine, 634–36
Alternative Medicine Foundation, 635
Alternative sweeteners, 134, 135, 137–38
Alzheimer's disease, 6, 108, 637

American Academy of Allergy, Asthma, and Immunology, 608
American Academy of Family Physicians, 626
American Academy of Pediatrics, 300, 510, 560, 589, 591, 592, 594, 598, 604, 610
American Botanical Council, 635
American Cancer Society, 55, 649
American College of Allergy, Asthma, and Immunology, 610
American College of Obstetricians and Gynecologists, 558
American College of Sports Medicine (ACSM), 409, 425, 431, 462
American Council on Exercise, 431
American Council on Science and Health, 73
American Dental Association (ADA), 587
American Diabetes Association, 137
American Dietetic Association, 36, 560, 597, 626
American Geriatrics Society, 644
American Heart Association (AHA)
- on antioxidant supplements, 198
- on cardiovascular/heart disease, 190–91, 199
- Dietary Guidelines and, 55
- on eating fish, 186
- on fat intake, 173, 552
- on fish oil supplements, 187
- on soy protein, 232
- on trans fats, 178
- on vitamin E supplements, 302

American Institute for Cancer Research, 231, 232
American Medical Association (AMA), 137
American Recovery and Reinvestment Act of 2009, 478, 480, 481
American Self-Help Clearinghouse, 643
American Society for Clinical Nutrition, 597
American Society of Addiction Medicine, 643
Amino acids, 10, 13. *See also* Essential amino acids; Nonessential amino acids; Protein(s)
- bond to form proteins, 213
- classification of, 212
- Dietary Supplement Health and Education Act (DSHEA) of 1994 and, 71
- genetics and, 108, 109
- glutamine, 433
- introduction to, 211–13
- metabolism of, 224
- neurotransmitters and, 222
- proteins and, 215
- small intestine and, 103
- supplements of, 227
- vitamin-like compounds and, 332

Amniotic fluid, 351
Amphetamines, 270
Amylase, 99, 139, 140
Amylopectin, 130, 131

Amylose, 130, 131
"Ana" role model, 454
Anabolic steroids, 433
Anaerobic, defined, 85
Anal sphincters, 105
Analog, 295
Anaphylactic shock, 608–9, 610
Anemia. *See also* Iron-deficiency anemia
    nutrient needs for adulthood and, 628
    pregnancy and, 547, 558–59
    in preschool children, 598
    sanitation and, 487
    teenage years and, 606
    undernutrition and, 475, 476
Anencephaly, 321, 322
Angular cheilitis, 312
Animal models, 63
Anisakis, 515
Anorexia nervosa
    athletes and, 463
    characteristics of persons with, 449
    closer look at, 450–55
    overview of, 447–50
    thoughts of an anorexic woman, 465–66
Antacids, 114, 115
Anthropometric assessment, 43–44
Antibodies, 95
Antidiuretic hormone, 353
Antigens, 95, 608
Antioxidants, 198, 328, 424, 517, 569, 647, 649
Anus, 105
Anxiety disorders, 112, 448
Appetite, 20, 21, 22, 40
Arachidonic acid (AA), 186, 586
Ariboflavinosis, 476
Arteries, 89, 90
Arthritis, 634
Artificial sweeteners. *See* Alternative sweeteners
Aseptic processing, 510
Asian Americans, 140, 155, 478
Aspartame, 137, 569
Atherosclerosis, 184, 197, 199, 232, 391, 392
Athletes, dietary advice for, 418–25
Atoms, 9, 14
Attention deficit hyperactivity disorder
    (ADHD), 150
Autism spectrum disorder (ASD), 599–600
*Avidin*, 521

**B**

B vitamins. *See also names of individual B vitamins*
    assessing diet and, 17
    cardiovascular disease and, 199
    Dietary Guidelines for Americans and, 56
    intakes of, 308–10
    intrinsic factor and, 100
    listing of, 308
    MyPyramid and, 50, 52
    nutrient needs for adulthood and, 628
    pregnancy and, 553, 558
    toxicity of, 292
    underconsumption of, 54
    undernutrition and, 41
    vegetarian diets and, 234–35
    as water-soluble, 308
    white blood cells and, 96

*B. cereus*, 508
*Bacillus*, 511
Back to Sleep campaign, 589
Bacteria. *See also names of types of bacteria*
    absorption of carbohydrates and, 141
    dental caries and, 151, 152
    diarrhea and, 116
    food safety and, 506, 508, 510–14
    large intestine and, 104
    ulcers and, 112
Bariatrics, 272
Basal metabolism, 248, 249, 260
Behavior modification, 267–69
Behavioral disorders, 187
Benecol, 200
Benign tumors, 646
Beriberi, 310, 475, 476
Beta-carotene, 65, 297, 298, 336
Beverage Guidance System, 353–54
BHA (butylated hydroxyanisole), 177
BHT (butylated hydroxytoluene), 177
Bicarbonate, 99, 106
*Bifidobacteria*, 104
Bile, 99, 106, 116
Bile acids, 180, 181
Bile duct, 106
Binge-eating disorder, 26, 447, 448, 458–61.
    *See also* Bulimia nervosa
Bioavailability, 308, 357–58
Biochemical assessment, 43–44
Bioelectrical impedance, 254–55, 256
Biological pest management, 528
Biotechnology, 492–95
Biotin, 105, 291, 308, 316–17, 332
Birth defects, preventing, 568–71
Bisphenol A (BPA), 588
Bisphosphonates, 397
Bladder, 106, 107
Blockers, 113
Blood circulation, 90
Blood clots/clotting
    aspirin and, 199
    calcium and, 365
    copper and, 384
    essential fatty acids and, 186
    pregnancy and, 552
    proteins and, 211
    vitamin K and, 305–6, 307
Blood donations, 377, 378
Blood doping, 424, 434
Blood glucose, 5, 7, 138, 153. *See also* Glucose;
    Hyperglycemia
    alcohol and, 641
    chromium and, 387
    diabetes and, 153, 154, 155, 156
    metabolic syndrome and, 157, 158
    physical fitness and, 414, 415
    plant foods and, 232–33
    proteins and, 223
Blood pressure, 10, 107, 198, 391–93. *See also*
    Hypertension
BodPod, 254, 256
Body mass index (BMI), 252–53, 452, 551
Bolus, 99, 100
Bomb calorimeter, 14, 247
Bonds, 7, 8
Bone mass, 395–96, 397

Bone mineral density, 395
*Botulism*, 593
Branched-chain amino acids (BCAA), 211, 433
Breast cancer, 109, 232, 233, 646, 647, 649
Breastfeeding
    ability to breastfeed, 560
    advantages of, 565–66
    allergy prevention and, 611
    barriers to, 566–67
    fatty acids and, 586
    feeding technique and, 589
    food plan for, 563–64
    minerals and, 587
    MyPyramid and, 555
    nutritional needs and, 556
    nutritional qualities of human milk,
        562–63
    physical activity and, 554
    production of human milk, 561
    recommendations for, 594
    undernutrition in developing world and,
        484, 487
    vitamins and, 299, 326, 586
    weight management and, 260–61, 554
Brown adipose tissue, 249
Brown sugar, 136
Buffers, 222
*Bulimia—A Guide to Recovery* (Hall and
    Cohn), 466
Bulimia nervosa, 447–50, 455–59, 463,
    464, 466
Bureau of Alcohol, Tobacco, Firearms and
    Explosives (ATF), 509

**C**

Cadmium, 524
Caffeine, 416, 425, 433, 522–23, 543, 564, 569
Calcium
    assessing diet and, 17
    athletes and need for, 424–25
    caffeine and, 523
    cancer and, 649
    constipation and, 115
    daily intake of, 13
    fatty acids and, 189
    on food labels, 66
    functions of, 365
    health benefits of, 365–66
    high-protein diets and, 227
    hypertension and, 392
    for infants, 593
    limitations of nutritional assessment
        and, 44
    as mineral, 11
    MyPyramid and, 52
    nutrient needs for adulthood and, 628
    osteoporosis and, 394, 398
    overnutrition and, 42
    skeletal system and, 107
    sodium and, 361
    soft drinks and, 41
    sources/needs, 366–67
    storage of nutrients, 107
    summary of, 373
    supplements, 336, 367–68
    teenage years and, 606

ulcers and, 112
underconsumption of, 54
upper level for, 368
vegetarian diets and, 235
vitamin D and, 299
Calories, 14–15, 17, 24–25. *See also* Bomb
    calorimeter; Kilocalorie (kcal); Weight
    control
    athletes and need for, 418–19
    breastfeeding and, 564
    cancer and, 647, 648
    in carbohydrates, 126, 133
    Dietary Guidelines for Americans and, 54
    discretionary, 45–46, 47
    energy density and, 39
    food labels and, 66, 68
    health diets and, 36
    for infants, 584
    MyPyramid and, 48–49
    nutrient density and, 39
    nutrient needs for adulthood and, 626–27
    overconsumption of, 54
    overnutrition and, 42
    pregnancy and, 550, 555–56
    proteins and, 11
    school-age children and, 605
    student athletes and, 26–27
    weight control and, 263–65
*Campylobacter*, 511, 512
Canada, 24, 72, 137, 177, 178, 227, 568.
    *See also* Health Canada
Canadian Ministries of Health, 55
Cancer, 5, 6, 7, 20. *See also individual types
    of cancer*
    adult nutritional needs and, 633
    alcohol and, 641
    American Institute for Cancer Research diet/
        health guidelines for prevention of, 232
    caffeine and, 523
    diet and, 146
    DNA code and, 215
    estrogen replacement and, 397
    excess body fat and, 255
    excess weight and, 243
    food additives and, 520
    genetics and, 109, 110–11
    minerals and, 365, 381
    nitrates/nitrites and, 517
    nutrition and, 646–49
    obesity and, 109
    osteoporosis and, 396
    pesticides and, 526
    phytochemicals and, 12, 37
    plant proteins and, 210
    poor diet/sedentary lifestyle as risk factors
        for, 5
    proteins and, 11
    rectal bleeding and, 116
    safety of water and, 356
    smoking and, 18
    trans fats and, 168
    vegetables/fruits and, 37
    vegetarian diets and, 231, 232–33
    vitamins and, 295, 299, 300, 322, 328
Capillaries, 89, 91, 103
Capillary beds, 221
Carbohydrate loading, 421

Carbohydrates. *See also* Fiber; Hyperglycemia;
    Hypoglycemia; Metabolic syndrome;
    Sugars
    absorption of, 139, 140–41
    animal sources of, 130
    athletes and need for, 419–22
    calculating calories for, 15
    cancer and, 648
    during childhood, 595
    as class of nutrient, 7, 8
    complex, 7, 130–31
    daily intake of, 13
    dental caries and, 151–52
    Dietary Guidelines for Americans and, 58
    digestion of, 139–40
    eating well in college and, 25
    for endurance exercise, 428, 429–30
    on food labels, 66
    in foods, 132–38
    forms/characteristics of simple/
        complex, 129
    as fuel for muscles, 414–16
    glycemic index/load and, 144–45
    and health concerns related to diabetes,
        153–56
    for infants, 585
    introduction to, 126–27
    as less fattening than fats/oils, 125–26
    nutrient needs for adulthood and, 627
    as percentage of calories advocated, 16
    polysaccharide as class of complex, 7
    pregnancy and, 552
    proteins and, 11, 221
    recommendations for intake of, 147–48
    satiety and, 175
    simple, 127–30
    from simple sugars vs. starches, 16–17
    small intestine and, 100
    as source of calories, 14
    storage of, 107
    student athletes and, 27
    variety in diet and, 37
Carbon skeletons, 224, 226
Cardiovascular system, 87–90. *See also*
    Cardiovascular/heart disease
Cardiovascular/heart disease, 5, 11, 12, 18, 37
    adult nutritional needs and, 633
    AHA on, 190–91
    alcohol and, 641
    atherosclerosis and, 184
    beta-carotene supplements and, 65
    blood pressure and, 391
    caffeine and, 523
    carotenoids and, 295
    case study on heart healthy diet, 201
    as cause of death, 6
    cholesterol and, 10
    copper and, 384
    deaths from, 18
    diabetes and, 155
    diet and, 146
    Dietary Guidelines for Americans and, 55
    eating fish and, 186
    estrogen replacement and, 397
    excess body fat and, 255
    excess weight and, 243
    fiber and, 147, 148

fish oil and, 187
    genetics and, 108, 109
    high-density lipoproteins (HDL) and, 184
    high-protein diets and, 227
    increased interest in health/fitness/nutrition
        and, 7
    kidneys and, 107
    lack of physical activity/poor diet and, 6
    lifestyle patterns and, 18
    lipids and, 165, 196–200
    magnesium and, 370
    medications for, 200
    metabolic syndrome and, 157, 158
    NSAIDs and, 112
    poor diet/sedentary lifestyle as risk factors
        for, 5
    risk factors for, 198, 199
    school-age children and, 604
    trans fats and, 178
    upper-body obesity and, 257
    vegetarian diets and, 231, 232
    vitamins and, 300, 302
Carnitine, 331
Carotenoids, 294, 295, 298, 629
Carpenter, Karen, 454
Case-control studies, 63
Catalase enzyme, 86
Cecum ascending colon, 104
Celiac disease, 117
Cell nucleus, 85, 86
Cell-mediated immunity, 96
Cells, 7, 126, 142. *See also* Neurons
    absorptive, 100, 101–2, 103, 140
    cell (plasma) membrane, 83–85, 94, 103
    cholesterol and, 190
    essential fatty acids and, 10
    genetics and, 13, 108
    intestinal, 95
    levels of organization of human body
        and, 83
    metabolism of, 86
    organelles of, 83–86
    pareital, 101
    scavenger, 184
    vitamins and, 295
Cellulose, 130, 131, 132, 133
Center for Excellence for Nutritional
    Genomics, 110
Centers for Disease Control Division of
    Nutrition and Physical Activity, 431
Centrioles, 84
Cerebrovascular accident (CVA). *See* Stroke
Chain-breaking, 267
Chemical reactions, 11
Child and Adult Care Food Program, 479
Chloride, 11, 364, 373
Cholecystokinin (CCK), 21, 22, 219
Cholesterol, 5, 18, 19, 44. *See also* Lipids
    assessing diet and, 17
    bile and, 99, 180
    calcium and, 365–66
    cardiovascular disease and, 10, 198
    chemical forms of, 171
    chylomicrons and, 182
    as component of cell membrane, 84
    content of foods, 174
    definitions for nutrient claims on, 175

Cholesterol—*Cont.*
　　diabetes and, 155
　　fat intake and, 192
　　fiber and, 147
　　on food labels, 66, 68
　　in foods, 172–73
　　free, 184
　　gallstones and, 116
　　genetics and, 109
　　good/bad in bloodstream, 184
　　*Healthy People 2010* on reducing, 199
　　lipids and, 167, 183
　　lipoproteins and, 182, 183, 184
　　medications for, 200
　　metabolic syndrome and, 157, 158
　　overconsumption of, 54
　　plant proteins and, 210
　　roles of, 190
　　saturated fat and, 10
　　as sterol, 170
　　suggestions to minimize, 16
　　tips for avoiding too much, 194
　　vegetarian diets and, 231
Choline, 308, 330–31
Chromium, 387, 389
Chromosomes, 85
Chronic diseases, 5, 6
Chronic, defined, 5
Chylomicrons, 182–83
Chyme, 100, 101, 106, 219
*Ciguatera*, 508
Circulatory system, 89
Cirrhosis, 639, 642
Cis form, of fatty acids, 177
Clinical assessment, 43–44
*Clostridia*, 104
*Clostridium botulinum*, 136, 508, 511, 513, 514,
　　534, 593, 611
*Clostridium perfringens*, 513, 514, 533, 534
Coagulation, 305
Coenzymes, 290, 308
Cofactors, 356
Cognitive behavioral therapy, 116, 455, 458
Cognitive restructuring, 267
College students
　　eating well in college, 24–28
　　vegetarian diets of, 231
Colon, 104
Colon cancer, 647, 649
　　alcohol and, 146
　　fiber and, 146
　　genetics and, 109
　　meat and, 227
　　obesity and, 146
　　plant foods and, 232
　　proteins and, 11
　　smoking and, 146
　　sugars and, 146
Colostrum, 563
Commodity Supplemental Food Program, 479
Community-supported agriculture (CSA),
　　291, 530
Complementary and Alternative Medicine
　　Program at Stanford (CAMPS), 635
Complementary proteins, 217
Compounds, 14
Compression of morbidity, 623

Congregate Meals for the Elderly, 479
Conjugated linoleic acid (CLA), 12, 168
Connective tissue, 87
Constipation, 115, 146, 557, 598–99
Contingency management, 267
Control groups, 63
Copper, 42, 96, 384–85, 389
Coronary artery bypass graft (CABG), 200
Coronary artery disease (CAD)/Coronary heart
　　disease (CHD). *See* Cardiovascular/heart
　　disease
Cortical bone, 394–95
Cox-2 inhibitors, 112
Creatine, 413, 433
Cretinism, 383
*Cryptosporidium*, 356, 508, 515
Cyclamate, 137
*Cyclospora cayetanensis*, 515
Cystic fibrosis, 117, 189, 293, 299
Cytoplasm, 85

# D

Daily Values (DVs)
　　for fiber, 148
　　on food labels, 66, 67
　　nutrient standards/recommendations and,
　　　61, 62
　　Nutrition Facts panels and, 70
　　of vitamin A, 297
DASH diet, 56
Death, causes of, 6
Debting, 457
Decker, Joe, 410
Defensive eating, 247
Delaney Clause, 517, 520
Dementia, 313
Denaturation, 215, 219
Dental caries, 150, 151–52, 599
Deoxyribonucleic acid (DNA), 85, 110, 214–15
　　cancer and, 646
　　epigenetics and, 108
　　folate and, 320, 322, 324
　　sustainable agriculture and, 493–94
　　vitamins and, 295, 298, 302, 325
Depression, 21, 187, 448, 456, 635–36
Descending colon, 104
Dextrose, 5, 7. *See also* Glucose
Diabetes, 5, 6, 11. *See also* Diabetes, type 1;
　　Diabetes, type 2
　　adult nutritional needs and, 633
　　alternative sweeteners and, 138
　　aspirin and, 199
　　cardiovascular disease and, 198
　　Exchange System and, 70
　　fiber and, 147, 148
　　genetics and, 108, 109
　　gestational, 153
　　and health concerns related to carbohydrate
　　　intake, 153–56
　　insulin and, 143, 144
　　kidneys and, 107
　　magnesium and, 370
　　metabolic syndrome and, 157, 158
　　obesity and, 109
　　plant foods and, 232–33
　　prediabetes, 155

　　pregnancy and, 542, 547, 552, 559
　　in prevention of birth defects, 570
　　sodium and, 360
　　sugar alcohols and, 136
　　sugar and, 150
　　symptoms of, 153–54
Diabetes, type 1, 5, 153, 154–55. *See also*
　　Diabetes
　　complications from, 155
　　eating disorders and, 450
　　genetics and, 109
　　insulin and, 143
Diabetes, type 2. *See also* Diabetes
　　compared to Type 1 diabetes, 153
　　defined, 5, 153
　　described, 155–56
　　Dietary Guidelines and, 55
　　excess body fat and, 255
　　excess weight and, 243
　　genetics and, 108, 109
　　insulin and, 144
　　metabolic syndrome and, 158
　　school-age children and, 603
　　soft drinks and, 150
　　upper-body obesity and, 257
　　vegetarian diets and, 231, 233
Diarrhea, 116, 136, 140, 141
Diastolic blood pressure, 198
Diet(s). *See also* Mediterranean Diet; Vegetarian/
　　vegan diets
　　current state of North American, 16–18
　　elimination, 610
　　fad, 82, 98, 115, 243–44, 261, 275–77
　　food groups and, 37–38
　　improving, 18–20
　　lack of physical activity and poor, 6
　　low-fat diets, 175–76
　　variety in, 36–37, 46, 50
Dietary Approaches to Stop Hypertension
　　(DASH), 392–93
Dietary assessment, 43–44
Dietary Guidelines for Americans, 54–60, 70.
　　*See also* Dietary Guidelines for Americans
　　(2005)
　　on alcohol, 570
　　defined, 52
　　on folate, 568
　　high-protein diets and, 227
　　key recommendations of, 56–58
　　practical use of, 55
　　pregnancy and, 548, 550, 553, 554, 559
　　recommendations for weight control,
　　　269–70
　　recommended diet changes, 59
　　on trans fats, 178
　　vegetables/fruits and, 290
Dietary Guidelines for Americans (2005), 52,
　　54, 55, 59, 71, 148. *See also* Dietary
　　Guidelines for Americans
　　adulthood nutrient needs and, 625
　　on alcohol, 642–43
　　definition of whole grain, 147
　　on fat intake, 190, 191
　　on folate, 324
　　on food safety, 532
　　on iron, 328
　　on nutrition for children, 597

on physical activity, 410
on plant-based diets, 231
on sodium, 360
on vitamin B-12, 327
on weight management, 262, 265
Dietary guidelines, for Japanese, 18
*Dietary Reference Intakes,* 9
Dietary Reference Intakes (DRIs), 60, 61, 62, 63
Dietary Supplement Health and Education Act (DSHEA) of 1994, 71, 335, 634
Dietary supplements. *See also* Alternative medicine; Erogenic aids; Herbal remedies; Supplement Facts labels
    adult use of, 634
    amino acid, 227
    antioxidant supplements and cardiovascular disease, 198
    athletes and, 424
    beta-carotene, 65, 295
    calcium, 235, 367–68
    case study on, 73
    cautions about, 71–73
    on choosing, 337, 339
    chromium, 387
    conjugated linoleic acid as, 168
    Dietary Guidelines for Americans and, 55
    Dietary Supplement Health and Education Act (DSHEA) of 1994, 71
    facts labels, 72
    fiber as, 134
    fish oil capsules, 187
    of folate, 323, 324, 543
    health problems and, 17
    labels for herbal, 66
    mineral, 289–90, 358–59
    overnutrition and, 42
    phytochemicals and, 12, 37
    pregnancy and, 549
    prenatal vitamin/mineral, 554–55
    to reduce intestinal gas, 141
    sales of, 335
    Stevia as, 138
    storage of, in body, 107
    student athletes and, 27
    top, 336
    vitamin, 289–90, 293, 294, 319
    who needs, 335–37
Digestion, 98, 99, 100, 112–17, 219–21, 247. *See also* Digestive system
Digestive system, 96–106. *See also* Digestion
    adult nutritional needs and, 632–33
    basic function of, 87
    circulatory system and, 89
    components/functions of, 88
    lipids and, 179–81
    as organ system, 83
    as serving immune system, 87
    stomach, 104
Digestive tract. *See* Gastrointestinal (GI) tract
Diglyceride, 169
Dioxin, 524
Direct calorimetry, 250
Disaccharides, 7, 127, 128–30, 134–35, 139, 140–41
Discretionary calories, 45–46, 47
Disordered eating, 447
Diuretics, 362

Diverticula, 146
Diverticulitis, 146
Diverticulosis, 112
DNA. *See* Deoxyribonucleic acid (DNA)
Docosahexaenoic acid (DHA), 13, 186, 563, 586
Dopamine, 222
Double-blind studies, 63, 65, 66
Down syndrome, 568
Drug use/abuse, 107, 543, 545, 548, 570, 641
Drugs. *See* Medication(s)
Dual energy X-ray absorptiometry (DEXA), 257, 396–97
Duodenum, 101, 112

## E

*E. coli,* 508, 510, 511, 514, 532, 534
Early childhood caries, 592
Eating disorders. *See also* Anorexia nervosa; Bulimia nervosa
    binge-eating disorder, 458–61
    case study on, 467
    contacts for further information on, 464
    defined, 447
    eating well in college and, 26
    female athlete triad, 462–63
    food as more than source of nutrients and, 447
    introduction to, 445
    main types of, 447
    night eating syndrome, 461–62
    from ordered to disordered eating habits, 446–47, 448
    passion for thinness and, 449
    polycystic ovary syndrome and, 464
    prevention of, 463–64
Eclampsia, 559
Edema, 222, 310, 349, 558
Eicosapentaenoic acid (EPA), 186
Electrolytes, 11, 27, 349, 427, 431
Electronic Benefit Transfer (EBT) cards, 478
Elements, 7, 10
Elimination diet, 610
Embryo, 543
Emergency Food Assistance Program (TEFAP), 479
Emulsifiers, 173, 174, 190, 518
Endocrine gland, 93–94
Endocrine system, 88, 89, 93–94, 633
Endometrium, 647
Endoplasmic reticulum (ER), 86
Endorphins, 21, 22, 447
Energy balance, 245–50
Energy bars, 408, 429, 430, 432
Energy density, 39–40, 41
Energy sources, 14–16
Enterohepatic circulation, 106, 107
Environmental assessment, 43–44
Environmental Protection Agency (EPA), 355, 356, 509, 525, 526, 527
Enzymes, 10, 84–85. *See also* Lipase
    catalase, 86
    complex carbohydrates and, 130
    copper and, 384
    digestion and, 98, 99, 139, 140
    food intolerances and, 611

lysozyme, 95
    model of enzyme action, 98
    proteins and, 10, 211
    small intestine and, 100
    stomach and, 100, 101
Ephedra, 72
Epidemiology, 63
Epigenetics, 108
Epigenome, 108
Epiglottis, 99, 100
Epinephrine, 93, 94, 143
Epithelial cells, 295
Epithelial tissue, 87
Erogenic aids, 432–34
Erythrocytes, 320
Erythropoietin, 107
*Escherichia,* 511, 512
Esophagus, 98, 99, 112, 114, 115
Esophageal cancer, 114
Essential amino acids, 212, 213, 216
Essential fatty acids (EFAs), 10, 169, 185–88. *See also* Omega-3 fatty acids; Omega-6 fatty acids
Essential nutrients, 5
Estimated Energy Requirements (EERs), 60, 61, 62, 250–51
Estrogen, 115, 257, 462, 647
Estrogen replacement, 397
Ethanol, 638
Exchange System, 70
Exercise. *See* Physical activity
*Exercise & Physical Activity: Your Everyday Guide,* 632
Exercise bulimia, 26
Extracellular fluid, 348–49, 359, 364
Extracellular space, 221

## F

"Face the Fats" campaign, 178
Facilitated diffusion, 102–3
Family tree, 110, 111
Famine, 475–77, 490
Fasting hypoglycemia, 157
Fat(s). *See also* Fatty acids; Lipids; Monounsaturated fatty acids; Oils; Polyunsaturated fatty acids; Saturated fatty acids; Trans fatty acids; Unsaturated fatty acids
    animal vs. plant sources of, 17
    calculating calories for, 15
    calories and, 17
    cancer and, 647, 648
    carbohydrates and, 125–26, 142
    during childhood, 595
    daily intake of, 13
    definitions for nutrient claims on, 175
    diabetes and, 154
    Dietary Guidelines for Americans and, 58
    endurance exercise and, 429
    on food labels, 66, 68
    food sources of, 173
    for infants, 585–86
    lymphatic system and digestion/absorption of, 91
    metabolic syndrome and, 158
    as percentage of calories advocated, 16

Fat(s)—*Cont.*
  physical fitness and, 416–17
  proteins and, 221
  satiety and, 175
  for school-age children, 602
  small intestine and, 100, 103
  as source of calories, 14
  sources of, from MyPyramid, 172
  storage of, 107
  student athletes and, 27
  tips for avoiding too much, 194
Fat-soluble vitamins, defined, 290
Fatty acids, 9, 167–69. *See also* Essential fatty
      acids (EFAs); Lipids; Saturated fatty
      acids; Trans fatty acids; Triglycerides;
      Unsaturated fatty acids
  dietary fats and, 182
  large intestine and, 104
  physical fitness and, 416
  saturated/unsaturated, 10
  sources of, 178
FDA. *See* U.S. Food and Drug
      Administration (FDA)
Feces, 105, 115
Female athlete triad, 462–63
Fermentation, 130
Fetal alcohol effects (FAE), 571
Fetal alcohol syndrome (FAS), 570, 571
Fetus, 298, 543–46, 641
Fiber, 8, 127, 131–32. *See also* Cellulose
  assessing diet and, 17
  biles acids and viscous, 180
  carbohydrates and, 7, 126, 131–32,
      133–34
  for children, 598–99
  classification, 131
  colon cancer and, 146
  constipation and, 115
  dietary supplements and, 336
  diverticula and, 146
  energy density and, 39
  fermentable, 141
  on food labels, 66, 68
  health diets and, 36
  hemorrhoids and, 116
  how much is needed, 148
  improving diets and, 19
  large intestine and, 104
  minerals and, 358
  MyPyramid and, 51, 52
  net carbs and, 144
  nutrients and, 9
  on Nutrition Facts labels, 149
  pregnancy and, 557
  problems with high-fiber diets, 148–50
  putting fiber to work, 146–47
  satiety and, 21
  soluble vs. insoluble, 131–32
  sources of, 149
  underconsumption of, 54
  weight control and, 264
"Finding Your Way to a Healthier You," 54
Flattened head syndrome, 589
Fluid balance, 221–22
Fluoridated water, 152, 385–86
Fluoride, 385–86, 389, 565, 587
Fogle, Jared, 275

Folate
  as B vitamin, 308
  dietary folate equivalents (DFEs), 323, 324
  FDA and, 335
  functions of, 320–21
  nutrient needs for adulthood and, 628
  pregnancy and, 542, 543, 553, 554, 571
  sources/needs, 322–24
  summary of, 333
  upper level for, 325
Folic acid, 291, 568
Food Additives Amendment (1958), 520
Food Allergen Labeling and Consumer
      Protection Act, 610
Food Allergy & Anaphylaxis Network, 608
Food and Agriculture Organization
      (FAO), 486
Food and Nutrition Board (FNB), 60, 126,
      147, 227
  on energy needs, 250
  on fat intake, 166, 192
  on fiber for children, 599
  on intake of protein/carbohydrates/fat, 16
  on protein, 209, 211, 226, 422
  on sugar, 150
  on trans fats, 167, 178
  on vitamins, 302, 336
Food choices
  in college, 24
  what affects, 22–23
Food combinations, 98
Food Distribution Program on Indian
      Reservations, 479
Food groups
  balanced diet and, 37–38
  Dietary Guidelines for Americans and, 56
  MyPyramid and, 45, 47, 48
Food insecure, 474
Food insecurity, 475, 480, 482, 584
Food intolerances, 608, 611
Food labels. *See also* Nutrition Facts labels/panels
  allergies and, 610
  calcium on, 367
  calories and, 14
  cholesterol and, 175
  definitions for nutrient claims on, 68
  diet planning and, 66–70
  exceptions to, 66–67
  fats on, 174, 175
  fiber on, 131, 148
  for food packages, 67
  health claims on, 69–70
  net carbs on, 144
  on sodium, 360
  sugar alcohols on, 136
  sugars on, 127
  trans fats on, 178
  weight control and, 264
Food sensitivities, 608
Food spending, 23
Food Stamp Program. *See* Supplemental
      Nutrition Assistance Program (SNAP)
Foodborne illness, 506–15, 531–35
Free radicals, 302, 304, 569
Freshman fifteen, 24, 25
Fructooligosaccharides, 104–5
Fructose, 128, 140, 141

Fruitarians, 233
Fruits/vegetables
  cancer and, 37, 649
  children and, 597
  eating well in college and, 24, 27
  energy density and, 39
  5 to 9 a-day, 17
  fructose in fruits, 128
  fruits as source of carbohydrate, 127
  MyPyramid and, 48
  organic, 526
  potassium in, 362
  root vegetables as high in amylopectin
      starch, 130
  vitamins and, 290, 292
Functional fiber, 132
Functional foods, 37, 134
Fungi, 506

## G

Galactose, 128, 141
Gallbladder, 106, 180, 233, 632, 647.
      *See also* Gallstones
Gallstones, 116–17, 255
Gamma hydroxybutyric acid (GHB), 434
Gastrin, 100, 219
Gastroesophageal reflux disease (GERD), 113,
      114, 115, 117
Gastroesophageal sphincter. *See* Lower
      esophageal sphincter
Gastrointestinal (GI) tract, 21, 91, 96, 97–99,
      105, 641
Gastroplasty, 272, 273
Gatorade Sport Science Institute, 431
Gemfibrozil, 200
Gender and development (GAD) approach to
      sustainable development, 492
Gene expression, 85, 295
Generally recognized as safe (GRAS), 519
Genes, 13, 85, 86, 108. *See also*
      Deoxyribonucleic acid (DNA); Genetics
Genetic engineering, 493–95
Genetic Information Nondiscrimination Act
      (GINA), 110
Genetically modified organism (GMO),
      493–95, 523
Genetics. *See also* Genes
  birth defects and, 568
  cancer and, 646
  diabetes and, 154
  eating disorders and, 449–50
  emerging field of nutrigenomics, 108–9
  genetic testing, 110–11
  hypertension and, 5
  metabolic syndrome and, 157
  nutritional diseases with genetic link,
      109–10
  physiological changes in adulthood and,
      623–24
  pregnancy and, 549
  protein synthesis and, 215
  ulcers and, 113
  weight control and, 258–61
Genogram, 110, 111
Genome, 108
Genotyping, 110

GERD. *See* Gastroesophageal reflux disease (GERD)
Gestation, 546
Gestational diabetes, 153, 559
Ghrelin, 21, 22
Glands, 93–94
Glossitis, 312
Glucagon, 94, 106, 143
Glucose. *See also* Blood glucose
    absorption of carbohydrates and, 141
    beriberi and, 310
    carbohydrates and, 7, 13, 127, 130, 140, 142–43, 144, 147
    defined, 5
    dextrose, 5, 7
    diabetes and, 5
    disaccharides and, 128–30
    fiber and, 147
    glycemic index/load and, 144
    insulin and, 94
    metabolism and, 86
    model of enzyme action and, 98
    monosaccharide, 7, 128
    photosynthesis and, 127
    physical fitness and, 414–15
    polysaccharides and, 130
    regulating, 142–43
    small intestine and, 103
    storage of, 107
    sugar alcohols and, 136
    vitamin-like compounds and, 332
Glucose tolerance test, 154
Glutamine, 433
Gluten-free, casein-free (GFCF) diet, 599
Glycated hemoglobin, 154
Glycemic index (GI), 144–45
Glycemic load (GL), 144–45, 257, 264
Glycerol, 167, 169, 170, 180, 182, 183, 184
Glycogen, 107, 126, 130, 131, 414, 415
Glycosylation, 622
Goiter, 383, 475, 476
Golgi complex, 86
Goodman, Erika, 453
Green revolution, 485–86
Growth hormone, 94, 433
Gruels, 228
*Guinness Book of World Records*, 410
Gums, 131, 134

## H

H₂ blockers, 113, 114
Harvard University Center for Cancer Prevention, 649
Hazard, 519
Hazard Analysis Critical Control Point (HACCP), 509
Health Canada, 17, 60
Health Claims Report Card, 69
*Healthy People 2010*, 17, 18
    on alcohol, 643
    on breastfeeding, 560
    on cholesterol, 199
    on coronary heart disease, 197
    on food security, 482
    on physical activity, 409
    on pregnancy, 542, 546, 570

    on saturated fats, 191
    on weight control, 261
*Healthy People 2020*, 17
Heart, 88
Heart attacks, 44, 45, 186, 197. *See also* Cardiovascular/heart disease
Heart disease. *See* Cardiovascular/heart disease
Heartburn, 114–15, 557. *See also* Gastroesophageal reflux disease (GERD)
Heat cramps, 426–27
Heat exhaustion, 426
Heatstroke, 427
Heimlich maneuver, 99
*Helicobacter pylori (H. pylori)*, 65, 112, 113
Helminth, 515
Heme iron, 374
Hemicellulose, 131, 132, 133
Hemochromatosis, 377–78
Hemoglobin, 374
Hemolysis, 302
Hemolytic uremic syndrome (HUS), 511
Hemorrhage, 304
Hemorrhagic stroke, 186, 187
Hemorrhoids, 115–16, 146, 557
Hemtocrit, 375
Henrich, Christy, 462–63
Hepatitis A virus, 508, 514
Herbal remedies, 71, 72, 116, 543, 635–36
Herbal teas, 521
High-density lipoprotein (HDL), 182, 183, 184, 199
High-fructose corn syrup, 128, 135, 136
High-quality (complete) proteins, 216
Hispanics, 17, 140, 155, 478, 496, 571
Histamine, 113
Home-Delivered Meals, 479
Homelessness, 481–82
Homocysteine, 109, 199, 331
Honey, 136
Hookworm disease, 487
Hormones, 21, 22. *See also* Cholecystokinin (CCK); Epinephrine; Estrogen; Gastrin; Glucagon; Growth hormone; Insulin; Norepinephrine; Parathyroid hormone (PTH); Progesterone; Prolactin; Testosterone; Thyroid hormones
    aldosterone, 353
    antidiuretic, 353
    cardiovascular system and, 89
    cholesterol and, 190
    diabetes and, 155
    digestion and, 96–97, 99
    endocrine system and, 93–94
    erythropoietin, 107
    gastrin, 100
    glucagon, 106
    glucose and, 143
    heartburn and, 115
    kidneys and, 107
    pancreas and, 106
    polycystic ovary syndrome and, 464
    proteins and, 211, 222
    vitamin D and, 298–99
Hospice care, 645
Human genome, 108
Human immunodeficiency virus (HIV), 327, 484, 488, 542, 567, 642. *See also*

Acquired immune deficiency syndrome (AIDS)
Hunger, 20, 22, 474–75, 477, 483. *See also* Undernutrition
Hydrochloric acid (HCL), 101
Hydrogenation, 177–78
Hyperactivity, 150
Hyperglycemia, 143, 144, 153, 155
Hypertension, 5, 391. *See also* Blood pressure
    adult nutritional needs and, 633
    alcohol and, 641
    aspirin and, 199
    calcium and, 365
    cardiovascular disease and, 198
    as cause of death, 6
    causes of, 391–92
    Dietary Guidelines for Americans and, 55
    ethnic groups and, 17
    excess body fat and, 255
    excess weight and, 243
    genetics and, 108
    kidneys and, 107
    lifestyle and, 18, 393
    magnesium and, 370
    metabolic syndrome and, 157, 158
    poor diet/sedentary lifestyle as risk factors for, 5
    pregnancy and, 542, 547, 552, 559
    preventing, 393
    in prevention of birth defects, 570
    sodium and, 360–61
    upper-body obesity and, 257
    vegetarian diets and, 231
Hypoglycemia, 143, 153, 156–57
Hypothalamus, 20, 21
Hypotheses, 63, 64, 65

## I

I PLEDGE program, 296
Identical twins, 258
Ileocecal sphincter, 103
Ileum, 101
Immune system, 87, 88, 95–96
    adult nutritional needs and, 633
    alcohol and, 641
    cardiovascular system and, 89
    copper and, 384
    diabetes and, 154
    lymphatic system and, 90
    proteins and, 222–23
    vitamin C and, 328
Immunoglobulins, 95, 96
Incidental food additives, 519
Indirect calorimetry, 250
Infants, 580, 581–82, 584–88
    adipose tissue growth and, 583
    assessment of growth/development of, 582–83
    carbohydrates for, 585
    dietary guidelines for feeding, 592–93
    expanding mealtime choices for, 589–92
    failure to thrive and, 584
    fat intake for, 585–86
    feeding technique for, 589
    formula feeding for, 588–89

Infants—*Cont.*
  head circumference/brain development
    of, 583
  inappropriate feeding practices for, 594
  milk for, 585
  protein for, 585
  undernutrition and, 582, 611
  weaning from breast/bottle, 592
  what not to feed, 593–94
Influenza, 6
Infrastructure, 483
Inorganic substances, 11
Inositol, 331
Input traits, 493
Inside MyPyramid, 46–47
Institute of Medicine, 62. *See also* Food and
    Nutrition Board (FNB)
Insulin, 143, 144
  amino acids and, 222
  cancer and, 647
  cholesterol and, 147
  diabetes and, 154, 155, 156
  metabolic syndrome and, 157
  pancreas and, 106
  positive protein balance and, 225
Insulin resistance, 157
Integumentary system, 88
Intentional food additives, 519
Interagency Council on Homelessness, 481
International units (IUs), 298
Interventions, 454
Intestinal cells, 95
Intoxication, 510–11
Intracellular fluid, 348–49, 362
Intrinsic factor, 100, 325, 326
Iodide, 382, 383–84, 389, 475, 553, 569
Ions, 14
Iron. *See also* Iron-deficiency anemia
  absorption/distribution of, 374–75
  assessing diet and, 17
  athletes and need for, 424
  constipation and, 115
  copper and, 384
  on food labels, 66
  functions of, 375
  for infants, 587, 593
  malnutrition and, 475
  nutrient needs for adulthood and, 628
  nutritional status and, 42
  overnutrition and, 42
  pregnancy and, 553, 554
  preschool children and, 598
  semistarvation and, 477
  sources/needs, 375–77
  storage of, in body, 107
  summary of, 389
  teenage years and, 606
  underconsumption of, 54
  undernutrition and, 41
  upper level for, 377–78
  vitamin C and, 328
  white blood cells and, 96
Iron-deficiency anemia
  anorexia nervosa and, 452
  athletes and, 27, 424
  functions of iron and, 375
  infants and, 558, 587

iron sources/needs and, 377
pregnancy and, 553, 558
preschool children and, 598, 599
teenage years and, 606
undernutrition and, 476, 498
Irradiation, 510
Irritable bowel syndrome, 116
Isomers, 304
Isotretinoin (Accutane), 296

**J**

Japanese dietary guidelines, 18
Jejunum, 101

**K**

Ketone bodies, 142
Ketosis, 142, 154, 155, 156
Keys, Ansel, 477
Kidney disease, 6, 11, 18
Kidney nephrons, 622
Kidneys, 106, 107, 155, 227, 232, 350–51, 647
Kilocalorie (kcal), 5, 7, 14. *See also* Calories
Kwashiorkor, 228–29, 475

**L**

La Leche League, 566
Labels. *See* Food labels; Supplement Facts labels
Lactase, 140
Lactation, 546
Lacteals, 91
Lactic acid, 414, 416
*Lactobacilli*, 104
*Lactobacillus bifidus* factor, 563
Lactoovovegetarians, 233
Lactose, 128–29
Lactose maldigestion/intolerance, 112, 140
Lactovegetarians, 233
Lanugo, 452
Large intestine, 103–5, 115, 131, 141, 146
Larynx, 100
Laxatives, 115
Lead, 524
Lead poisoning, 600
Lean body mass, 248
Lecithin, 99, 170, 171, 173, 189–90, 331
Leptin, 21, 22, 259
Let-down reflex, 561–62
Leukocytes, 96
Life expectancy, 623
Life span, 623
Lifestyle, 5, 18, 19, 24, 45, 49, 624
Lignins, 131, 133
Limiting amino acids, 212
Lind, James, 328
Linoleic acid, 169, 173, 185. *See also* Omega-6
    fatty acids
Lipase, 99, 179
Lipectomy, 273
Lipids, 7, 165. *See also* Cholesterol; Fat(s);
    Fatty acids; Phospholipids; Sterols;
    Triglycerides
  cardiovascular disease and, 196–200
  carried in bloodstream, 181–85
  as class of nutrient, 7, 8, 9–10

common properties of, 166
concept map, 195
fats/oils in foods, 172–79
in human breast milk, 563
main types of, 166–71
making lipids available for body use, 179–81
medications to lower blood, 199–200
pregnancy and, 552–53
recommendations for fat intake, 190–94
types of, 10
Lipoic acid, 332
Lipoprotein lipase, 183, 184, 260
Lipoproteins, 182, 183–84
*Listeria*, 511, 514
*Listeria monocytogenes*, 513, 548
Liver
  as accessory organ of digestive system, 106
  alcohol and, 641, 642
  glucose and, 143
  glycogen in, 126
  glycopen in, 130
  high insulin output and, 144
  large intestine and, 105
  lipids and, 183–84
  monosaccharides and, 128
  portal circulation and, 89
  small intestine and, 103
  storage of carbohydrates in, 107
  storage of vitamins/minerals in, 107
Liver disease, 6
Lobules, 561
Locally grown foods, 529–30
Locavores, 529–30
LOHAS (Lifestyle of Health and
    Sustainability), 529
Long-chain fatty acids, 168
Low birth weight (LBW), 547, 548–49
Low bone density, 44
Low-density lipoprotein (LDL), 182, 183, 184,
    197–98, 199
Lower esophageal sphincter, 99, 101
Lower-body obesity, 257, 258
Lower-quality (incomplete) proteins, 216
Lung cancer, 19, 65, 295, 302, 336, 646
Lung diseases, as cause of death, 6
Lymph, 88, 90, 91
Lymph vessels, 91, 103
Lymphatic system, 87–91, 181, 182
Lysosomes, 86
Lysozyme enzyme, 95, 96

**M**

Macrocytic anemia. *See* Megaloblastic anemia
Macronutrients, 8, 20, 22
Macular degeneration, 294, 295
Magnesium
  assessing diet and, 17
  diabetes and, 154, 156
  fatty acids and, 189
  hypertension and, 392
  MyPyramid and, 50
  nutrient needs for adulthood and, 628
  sources/needs, 370–71
  summary of, 373
  underconsumption of, 54
  upper level for, 372

Major minerals, 11, 357
Malignant tumors, 646
Malnutrition, 40, 41, 228–30, 473, 475, 497. *See also* Undernutrition
Maltase, 140
Maltose, 128–30
Manganese, 387, 389
Maple syrup, 136
Marasmus, 228, 229–30, 475
March of Dimes, 568
MarketMaker, 530
Medication(s)
    for acne, 295–96, 606
    AIDS and, 489, 548
    breastfeeding and, 564, 567
    cancer drug, methotrexate/folate, 322
    for cholesterol/triglycerides, 200
    eating disorders and, 455, 458, 461, 462
    health promotion/disease prevention and, 19
    for hypertension, 393
    to lower blood lipids, 199–200
    older adults and, 634
    pregnancy and, 543, 548
    statin drugs, 200
    for weight loss, 270–71
Mediterranean Diet, 52–54, 193, 277, 624
Megadoses, 71, 291
Megaloblast, 320
Megaloblastic anemia, 320–21
Menarche, 605
Menopause, 184, 625
Mercury, 524, 564, 570, 599
Metabolic syndrome, 157–58, 199, 607
Metabolism, 12, 85, 86, 93
    of alcohol, 639
    of amino acids, 224
    basal, 248, 249, 260
    energy for basal, 247
    galactose/glucose and, 128
    genetics and, 109
    glucose and, 142
    resting, 248
    thyroid hormones and, 94
Metastasis, 646
Methyl groups, 167
Metric system, 4, 15–16
Metropolitan Life Insurance Company tables, 452
Micelles, 181
Micronutrients, 8
Microorganisms, 65
Milk intake, case study on problems with, 159
Millennium Declaration, 485
Minerals, 7, 11, 347. *See also* Dietary supplements; *names of individual minerals*
    AIDS and, 489
    alcohol and, 640
    assessing diet and, 17
    athletes and need for, 423–25
    breastfeeding and, 563
    cancer and, 647–48
    for children, 597–98
    daily intake of, 13
    Dietary Supplement Health and Education Act (DSHEA) of 1994 and, 71

fiber and, 150
functions of classes of nutrients and, 8
hypertension and, 392–93
immune system and, 95
for infants, 586
large intestine and, 104
major vs. trace, 9, 11
malnutrition and, 475
MyPyramid and, 51, 52
nutrient density and, 39
nutrient needs for adulthood and, 625, 627–29
overnutrition and, 42
overview of, 356–59
in plant foods, 218
pregnancy and, 543, 553, 557, 559, 571
in prevention of birth defects, 569
semistarvation and, 477
storage of, in body, 107
student athletes and, 27
sugar and, 150
supplements, megadoses of, 71
toxicity of, 358–59
trace, 372, 374, 390
urinary system and, 106
vegetarian diets and, 26, 224–35
Mitochondria, 85
Moderation, 17, 38–39, 46, 50
Molybdenum, 388, 389
Monoglycerides, 169, 179, 181, 182–83
Monosaccharides, 7, 127, 128, 134–35, 140–41, 143
Monounsaturated fatty acids
    American Heart Association on, 178
    chemical forms of, 168
    defined, 167
    in foods, 173
    hydrogenation and, 177
    in oils, 169
    sources of, 170
Morning sickness, 558
Motility, 96, 98
Mottling, 385
Mouth, 97–99, 139
Mucilages, 131, 134
Mucosa, 100
Mucus, 99, 100, 113
    digestive system and, 98, 99, 101, 106
    large intestine and, 104
    vitamin A and, 294
Muscle tissue, 87
Muscles, 126, 130
Muscular system, 88
Mushroom toxins, 521
Myelin sheath, 93
Myocardial infarction, 196. *See also* Heart attacks
Myoglobin, 374
MyPyramid
    anatomy of, 46
    breastfeeding and, 555
    calorie guidelines, 251
    for children, 596
    Dietary Guidelines for Americans and, 55, 56, 59
    essential fatty acids and, 187
    food groups and, 38, 47, 48

meal planning with, 49–52, 70
nutrient needs for adulthood and, 625
for older adults, 644, 645
on plant-based diets, 231
pregnancy and, 555
for preschoolers, 595, 601
recommendations for intake of carbohydrates and, 148
for school-age children, 601
sources of carbohydrates, 134
sources of fats, 171
sources of protein, 217
sources of vitamins/minerals and, 297, 304, 311, 319, 324, 329, 330, 334, 363, 367, 371, 376, 380, 390
titled "Steps to a Healthier You," 45
vegetarian diets and, 234
vs. food label portion sizes, 66
weight and, 261, 264
MyPyramid Plan, 46
MyPyramid Tracker, 47, 52, 264

# N

National Academy of Sciences, 55
National Bone Health Campaign, 602
National Cancer Institute (NCI), 110, 647, 649
National Center for Health Statistics (NCHS), 582–83
National Cholesterol Education Program (NCEP), 192, 199–200
National Collegiate Athletic Association, 419
National Council Against Health Fraud, 73
National Council on Aging, 626
National Dairy Council, 398
National Eating Disorders Association, 464
National Farm to School Program, 530
National Health and Nutrition Examination Survey (NHANES), 17
National Human Genome Research Institute, 110
National Institute of Mental Health, 464
National Institute on Aging, 632, 644
National Institute on Alcohol Abuse and Alcoholism, 643
National Institutes of Health National Center for Complementary and Alternative Medicine (NCCAM), 635
National Institutes of Health Office of Dietary Supplements, 635
National Institutes of Health State-of-the-Science Conference, 336
National Institutes of Health, Office of Dietary Supplements, 73
National Law Center on Homelessness and Poverty, 481
National Marine Fisheries Service/NOAA Fisheries, 509
National Osteoporosis Foundation, 398
National Sanitation Foundation, 356
National School Lunch Program, 479, 480
National Weight Control Registry, 268
Native Americans, 116, 155, 478, 642
Natural Medicines Comprehensive Database, 635
Natural opioids, 447

NCAA's Committee on Competitive Safeguards and Medical Aspects of Sports, 432
Near-infrared reactance, 257
Negative energy balance, 246
Negative protein balance, 225
Neotame, 137, 138
Nervous system, 88, 89, 91–93, 142, 147, 633, 641
Nervous tissue, 87
Net carbs, 144
Neural tube defects, 320–22
Neurons, 92
Neuropeptide Y, 21, 22
Neurotransmitters. *See also* Serotonin
    acetylcholine, 330
    amino acids and, 222
    calcium and, 365
    carbohydrates and, 150
    eating disorders and, 447
    medications for weight loss and, 270
    nervous system and, 92–93
    vitamin B-6 and, 318
New American Plate, The, 231, 232
*New England Journal of Medicine,* 277
Niacin
    as B vitamin, 308
    introduction to, 312–13
    proteins and, 223
    sources/needs, 313, 314–15
    summary of, 332
    synthesis of, 290–91
    upper level for, 314
Nicotinic acid, 200
Night blindness, 294
Night eating syndrome, 447, 461–62
Nitrates/nitrites, 517, 648
Nitrosamine, 647
Nonessential amino acids, 212, 213, 216
Nonfermentable fiber, 131, 132
Nonheme iron, 374
Non-specific immunity, 95
Nonsteroidal anti-inflammatory drugs (NSAIDS), 112, 113, 545
Norepinephrine, 93, 94, 222
Norovirus, 508, 514
NSAIDS. *See* Nonsteroidal anti-inflammatory drugs (NSAIDS)
Nuclear envelope, 84
Nucleolus, 84
Nurture vs. nature, 109
Nutrient density, 39, 40
Nutrients, 4–5, 13
    classes/sources of, 7–12
    Dietary Guidelines for Americans and, 56
    MyPyramid food group, 50
    nutrient density of foods, 39
    organization of body and, 87
    standards/recommendations, 60–62
    storage capacity of, 107
    student athletes and, 26–27
Nutrigenomics, 108–9
Nutrition
    defined, 4
    states of nutritional health, 40–42
    why study, 5–7
Nutrition claims, evaluating, 71

Nutrition Education and Labeling Act (NELA), 68
Nutrition Facts labels/panels. *See also* Food labels
    dietary fiber on, 131, 132
    fats on, 174, 176
    folate on, 324
    for infants, 586
    on reading, 149
    recommendations for intake of carbohydrates, 147
Nutrition Screening Initiative, 645
Nutritional assessment, 42–45
Nutritional state, 40, 41
Nutritive sweeteners, 134–36

## O

Obesity. *See also* Eating disorders; Weight; Weight control; Weight loss
    adult nutritional needs and, 633
    alcohol and, 641
    body mass index and, 252
    calcium and, 366
    cancer and, 109, 647
    cardiovascular disease and, 199
    colon cancer and, 146
    defined, 5
    diabetes and, 109, 155, 156
    Dietary Guidelines for Americans and, 55, 62
    as epidemic, 269
    fiber and, 146–47
    genetics and, 109
    heartburn and, 115
    hemorrhoids and, 115
    hypertension and, 5, 391–92
    hypothalamus and, 20
    leptin levels and, 21
    lifestyle patterns and, 18
    metabolic syndrome and, 157, 158
    nature vs. nurture and, 258–61
    overnutrition and, 42
    physical activity and, 249
    in prevention of birth defects, 570
    sarcopenic, 630
    school-age children and, 604–5
    as second leading cause of preventable death, 6
    treatment of severe, 271–74
    trends, 245
    upper-body/lower-body, 257
    using body fat distribution to evaluate, 257–58
    vegetarian diets and, 231, 233
Oils, 14, 49, 52, 54, 169, 303. *See also* Fat(s); Lipids
Oldways, 52
Oleic acid, 169
Olestra, 177, 189
Omega-3 fatty acids
    breastfeeding and, 564
    defined, 168
    essential fatty acids and, 185, 186–87
    flax seeds/walnuts and, 187
    Food and Nutrition Board on, 192
    in human breast milk, 563
    lipid types and, 169

pregnancy and, 552–53
    vegetarian diets and, 235
Omega-6 fatty acids, 169, 185, 192, 552–53
Oncolink, 649
Organ systems, 82, 83, 87, 88
Organelles, 83–86
Organic compounds, 11
Organic foods, 68, 526, 527, 528–29
Organic Foods Production Act of 1990, 528
Organic substances, 11
Organic Trade Association, 528
Organization of body, 87
Organs, 82, 83, 87, 97
Orlistat class of medication, 270–71, 293
Ornish, Dean, 193, 199, 277
Osmosis, 349, 350
Osteomalacia, 299
Osteoporosis
    adult nutritional needs and, 633
    case study on giving up milk, 399
    defined, 5
    diet/lifestyle factors and, 396
    eating disorders and, 453, 462
    genetics and, 108
    nutritional needs and, 6
    preventing, 394–98
Ostomy, 627
Overnutrition, 40, 41, 42
Ovum, 543
Oxalic acid (oxalate), 357, 358, 521
Oxidize, 197
Oxygenated/deoxygenated blood, 88
Oxytocin, 561

## P

Pancreas
    as accessory organ of digestive system, 106
    adulthood and, 632–33
    bicarbonate and, 99
    cystic fibrosis and, 117
    diabetes and, 154, 156
    digestion of carbohydrates and, 139, 140
    digestive enzymes and, 98
    glucose and, 143
    high insulin output and, 144
Pancreatic cancer, 157, 647
Pantothenic acid, 308, 315–16, 332
Parasites, 506, 508, 515
Parathyroid hormone (PTH), 299
Pareital cells, 101
Parkinson's disease, 6
Passive diffusion, 102
Pasteurizing, 506, 508
Pauling, Linus, 328
Peace Corps, 491
Peak bone mass, 395
Pectin, 131, 132, 134
Pedometers, 266
Pellagra, 313, 314, 475, 476
Pepsin, 219
Peptic ulcer, 112, 113
Peptide bonds, 213
Percentages, 15–16
Percentile, 582
Percutaneous transluminal coronary angioplasty (PTCA), 200

Peristalsis, 99, 100, 101, 115
Pernicious anemia, 325–26, 327
Peroxisomes, 86
Personalized nutrition, 110
Pesticides, 525–27, 570
Ph, defined, 107
Phagocytes, 96
Phagocytosis, 96, 103
Pharynx, 99, 100
Phenylalanine, 213, 569
Phenylketonuria (PKU), 137, 138, 213, 542, 567, 569
Phosphocreatine (PCr), 413–14, 415, 417
Phospholipids
    cell membranes and, 84, 189–90
    choline and, 330–31
    chylomicrons and, 182
    digestion, 180
    in foods, 173
    as lipid, 167, 170
Phosphorus
    daily intake of, 13
    introduction to, 368
    as mineral, 11
    osteoporosis and, 398
    sources/needs, 369
    summary of, 373
    upper level for, 370
    vitamin D and, 299
Photosynthesis, 127
Physical activity. *See also* Physical fitness
    for adults, 632
    benefits of, 409
    carbohydrates and, 134
    cardiovascular disease and, 199
    for children, 604–5
    constipation and, 115
    diabetes and, 155, 156
    Dietary Guidelines for Americans and, 54, 57
    eating disorders and, 456, 457
    eating well in college and, 24, 25
    energy and, 247, 248–49, 252
    exercise bulimia, 26
    gallstones and, 117
    glucose for muscle use and, 130
    health diets and, 36
    hypertension and, 392
    improving diets and, 19
    Mediterranean Diet Pyramid and, 54
    metabolic syndrome and, 157, 158
    MyPyramid and, 46, 47, 48
    osteoporosis and, 398
    planning, 410
    poor diet and lack of, 6
    pregnancy and, 550, 554
    protein to meet energy needs for, 223
    state of nutritional health and, 45
    student athletes, 26–27
    weight and, 263, 265–66, 275
Physical Activity Guidelines for Americans (2008), 60
Physical fitness. *See also* Athletes, dietary advice for; Physical activity
    aerobic activity, 411
    case study on planning a training diet, 434
    defined, 408

designing fitness program, 411
endurance exercise, 428–31
energy bars and, 429–30
energy sources for exercising muscles, 412–18
ergogenic aids to enhance athletic performance, 432–34
fluid needs for athletes, 425–27
guidelines for achieving/maintaining, 410–12
heart rate training chart, 412
introduction to, 407
relationship between nutrition and, 408–10
sports drinks and, 427
training effect, 416
*Physician and Sports-medicine* journal, 431
Physicians Committee for Responsible Medicine, 547
Physiological anemia, 558
Physiology, 3, 82–83
Phytic acid (phytate), 358
Phytochemicals
    alcohol and, 638
    cancer and, 647, 649
    defined, 12
    dietary supplements and, 336
    food sources of, 12
    as functional foods, 37
    MyPyramid and, 51
    in plant foods, 218
    tips for boosting, in diet, 38
    variety in diet and, 37, 38
    vegetarian diets and, 232
Phytosterols, 200
Pica, 555
Pinocytosis, 103
Placebos, 63
Placenta, 543
Plaque, 196
Plasma, 88
Pneumonia, 6
Polychlorinated biphenyls (PCBs), 524
Polycystic ovary syndrome (PCOS), 464
Polypeptides, 214–15
Polysaccharides, 7, 130, 131
Polyunsaturated fatty acids
    American Heart Association on, 178
    amount in diets, 192–93
    essential fatty acids and, 185
    hydrogenation and, 177, 178
    lipid types and, 167, 168, 169
    rancidity and, 176–77
    sources of, 170
Pool, 224
Population, 483–84
Population Services International, 484
Portal circulation, 89, 90
Portal vein, 89, 91, 103, 105, 106
Portion sizes, 38–39, 49, 50, 52, 66, 172, 247, 268
Positive energy balance, 245
Positive protein balance, 225
Potassium
    assessing diet and, 17
    Dietary Guidelines for Americans and, 57
    electrolytes and, 11
    hypertension and, 392

large intestine and, 104
    as mineral, 11
    nervous system and, 92
    sources/needs, 362–64
    summary of, 373
    underconsumption of, 54
Poverty, 480–81, 482–83, 487, 584
Prebiotics, 104, 132
Preeclampsia, 559
Pregnancy
    AIDS and, 489
    calcium and, 365
    case study on preparing for, 572
    excess body fat and, 255
    folate and, 322, 324
    food plan for, 555–57
    gestational diabetes, 153
    introduction to nutrition/health and, 541–42
    iodide and, 383
    isotretinoin (Accutane) and, 296
    maternal death/infant mortality rates, 571
    nutrient needs for, 549–55
    physiological changes of concern during, 557–60
    planning for, 542–43
    prenatal growth/development, 543–46
    preventing birth defects, 568–71
    success in, 546–49
    undernutrition and, 496
    vitamins and, 298, 304, 319
    weight control and, 260
Pregnancy-induced hypertension, 559
Premature infants. *See* Preterm infants
Preschool children, nutrition for, 594
    childhood feeding problems, 595–97
    helping children choose nutritious foods, 595
    introduction to, 595
    problems of, 598–600
    vitamins/minerals and, 597–98
Preservatives, 515
Preterm infants, 230, 547
Probiotics, 104, 105, 116
Progesterone, 115, 257
Prolactin, 561
Prostate cancer
    genetics and, 109
    nutrition and, 646, 647, 649
    plant foods and, 232
    selenium and, 381
    vitamins and, 295, 302
Prostate gland, 295
Protease, 99
Protein equilibrium, 225
Protein sparing, 142
Protein turnover, 221
Protein(s). *See also* Amino acids
    amino acids bond to form, 213
    amount needed, 225–26
    animal vs. plant sources of, 16
    athletes and need for, 419–23
    calculating calories for, 15
    carbohydrates and, 142
    cell membranes and, 84–85
    during childhood, 595
    chylomicrons and, 182

Protein(s)—*Cont.*
as class of nutrient, 7, 8, 10–11
collagen and vitamin C, 328
concept map, 223
daily intake of, 13
deficiency, 228–30
defined, 7
denaturation of, 215–16
digestion/absorption of, 219–21
elements of, 10
enzymes as, 10
food labels and, 66–67
in foods, 216–19
functions of, 221–24
genetics and, 108
high-protein diets, 226–27
immune system and, 95
for infants, 585
introduction to, 210–13
nutrient density and, 39
nutrient needs for adulthood and, 627
organization of, 215
as percentage of calories advocated, 16
physical fitness and, 417
plant sources of, 209–10, 218–19, 232, 233
pregnancy and, 552
satiety and, 175
small intestine and, 100
as source of calories, 14
storage of, 107
student athletes and, 27
supplements, 227
synthesis, 214–15
vegetarian diets and, 26
white blood cells and, 96
Protein-calorie malnutrition (PCM), 228, 475
Protein-energy malnutrition (PEM). *See*
Protein-calorie malnutrition (PCM)
Protein-sparing modified fast (PSMF).
*See* Very-low-calorie diet (VLCD)
Proton pump inhibitors (PPIs), 113, 114–15
Protozoa, 515
Provitamin/precursor, 294
Pyloric sphincter, 100, 101
Pyruvic acid, 414

**Q**

Quackwatch: Your Guide to Quackery, Health
Fraud, and Intelligent Decisions, 73

**R**

Radiation, 510
Rancidity, 176–77
Rating of Perceived Exertion scale (RPE),
412, 413
Reactive hypoglycemia, 156–57
Receptors, 94
Recombinant DNA technology, 493
Recommended Dietary Allowances (RDAs)
for carbohydrates, 147
compared to other dietary reference
intakes, 63
for fat intake, 190
on food labels, 66
food sources of carbohydrate and, 133

introduction to, 60–61
for protein, 225–26
using, 62
for vitamins, 297, 298, 303, 310, 312, 314,
319, 323, 327, 330
weight loss/carbohydrates and, 142
Rectum, 105
Registered dietitians (R.D.s), 72, 73
Relapse prevention, 267–68
Reproductive system, 88
Research. *See* Scientific method
Reserve capacity, 621
Respiratory system, 88, 89
Resting metabolism, 248
Retinoids, 294
Retinol activity equivalents (RAEs), 297, 298
Retinol equivalent (RE), 297
Rheumatoid arthritis, 186–87
Riboflavin, 308, 312, 313, 332
Ribonucleic acid (RNA), 85, 86, 214–15
Ribosomes, 85
Rickets, 299, 300, 475, 476
Risk factors, 5, 199
RNA. *See* Ribonucleic acid (RNA)

**S**

Saccharin, 137
Safe Water Drinking Act, 356
Safety, 519
Safety, food, 508. *See also* Foodborne illness
agencies responsible for, 509
Dietary Guidelines for Americans and,
55, 58
environmental contaminants and, 524–27
food additives and, 515–21
food preservation, 510
food production and, 527–30
introduction to, 505–6
microorganisms and, 510–15
naturally occurring substances and, 521–23
pregnancy and, 548, 554
*Safrole*, 521
Saliva, 99
Salivary amylase, 98, 99
*Salmonella*, 508, 510, 511, 512, 531, 532,
534, 611
Salt/sodium
defined, 17
Dietary Guidelines for Americans and,
52, 57
electrolytes and, 11
on food labels, 66, 68
hypertension and, 5, 17, 392
improving diets and, 18
for infants, 593
iodide and, 383
large intestine and, 104
as major mineral, 359–62
as mineral, 11
nervous system and, 92
osteoporosis and, 398
overconsumption of, 54
preschool children and, 595
sources/needs, 360–61
summary of, 373
upper level for, 361–62

Sanitation, 486–87
Sarcopenia, 630
Sarcopenic obesity, 630
Satiety, 20–21, 175, 223–24
Saturated fatty acids. *See also* Lipids
American Heart Association on, 178
animal fats and, 173, 190
assessing diet and, 17
dairy products and, 176
defined, 10
on food labels, 66
free cholesterol and, 184
*Healthy People 2010* on, 191
hydrogenation and, 177
improving diets and, 18, 19
limitations of nutritional assessment
and, 44
lipid types and, 10, 167, 168, 169
metabolic syndrome and, 158
overconsumption of, 54
rancidity and, 176
sources of, 170
suggestions to minimize, 16
tips for avoiding too much, 194
vegetarian diets and, 231
weight control and, 264
Scavenger cells, 184
School Breakfast Program, 478–79, 480
School-age children, nutrition for, 601–4
Scientific method, 62–66
*Scombroid*, 508
Scurvy, 63, 328, 475, 476
Secretory vesicles, 86
Sedentary lifestyle, 49
Selenium, 381–82, 389
Self-monitoring, 267
Sequestrants, 515, 519
Serotonin
amino acids and, 222
carbohydrates and, 150
defined, 22
eating disorders and, 447, 455
hunger/appetite and, 22
satiety and, 21
Set point, 259–60
*Shigella*, 512
Sibutramine class of medication, 270, 271
Sickle cell disease/anemia, 215
Sigmoid colon, 104
Simple sugars, 7
Skeletal system, 88, 107, 630, 632, 641
Skin, 95
Sleep, 19, 641
Small for gestational age (SGA), 547
Small intestine
absorption of carbohydrates and, 141
absorption of fluid, 105
bacteria and, 104
bile and, 106
described, 100–103
digestion of carbohydrates and, 139, 140
fiber and, 131
lactose maldigestion and, 140
lymph vessels in, 91
organization of, 102
parts of, 101

peptic ulcers and, 113
ulcers and, 112
Smoking
aspirin and, 199
beta-carotene and, 295, 336
breastfeeding and, 564
cancer and, 18, 646
cardiovascular/heart disease and, 18, 198
colon cancer and, 146
kidney disease and, 18
as leading cause of preventable death, 6
osteoporosis and, 394, 398
pregnancy and, 545, 548, 570, 571
state of nutritional health and, 45
teenage years and, 606
ulcers and, 112, 113, 114
upper-body obesity and, 257
vitamins and, 17, 302, 304, 330
Sodium. *See* Salt/sodium
Sodium bicarbonate (baking soda), 433
Solvents, 11, 348
Sorbitol, 136
Special Supplemental Nutrition Program for
Women, Infants, and Children (WIC),
479–80, 549, 598
Specific immunity, 96
Sphingolipids, 12
Spina bifida, 320–22, 568
Spontaneous abortions, 545, 548, 552
Spores, 506
Sports drinks, 427
*Staphylococcus*, 511, 531, 534
*Staphylococcus aureus*, 512
Starch, 7
Starches, 17, 127, 130, 131, 133. *See also*
Carbohydrates
*Start Healthy, Stay Healthy Resource Center*, 595
Start Today (MyPyramid), 47
Statins, 200
Sterols, 167, 170, 171, 200
Stevia, 138
Stimulus control, 267
Stomach, 101, 104, 105, 112, 113
Stress, 19, 21, 112, 113, 116
Stress fractures, 425
Stroke
alcohol and, 392, 641
aspirin and, 199
as cause of death, 6
cerebrovascular accident defined as, 196
defined, 6
diet and, 393
estrogen replacement and, 397
excess weight and, 243
fiber and, 147
as form of cardiovascular disease, 196
hemorrhagic, 186, 187
increased interest in health/fitness/nutrition
and, 7
metabolic syndrome and, 158
NSAIDs and, 112
vitamins and, 300, 302
Subclinical deficiency, 41
Subclinical, defined, 41
Sucralose, 137
Sucrase, 140
Sucrose, 128–29, 134, 135, 136, 152

Sudden infant death syndrome (SIDS), 589
Sugar alcohols, 136, 137, 144
Sugars. *See also* Carbohydrates; Nutritive
sweeteners; Simple sugars; Sucrose
calories and, 17
carbohydrates and, 7, 17, 127
colon cancer and, 146
defined, 127
dental caries and, 151–52
diabetes and, 155, 156
on food labels, 66, 68
hyperactivity and, 126, 150
for infants, 593
model of enzyme action and, 98
names of sugars used in foods, 136
on Nutrition Facts labels, 149
problems with high-sugar diets, 150–51
suggestions for reducing intake of
simple, 151
Suicide, 6
Sulfur, 372, 373
Summer Food Service Program, 479
Superfoods, 12
Supplement Facts labels, 72, 338
Supplemental Nutrition Assistance Program
(SNAP), 478, 479, 480, 481, 645
Supplements. *See* Dietary supplements
Sustainable agriculture, 492–95, 528, 529
Sustainable development, 492
Swallowing, 100
Symptoms, 41, 45
Synapses, 92
Syndrome X, 607. *See also* Metabolic syndrome
Synthetic chemicals, 519
Systolic blood pressure, 198

**T**

Tagatose, 137, 138
Take Control, 200
Tapeworms, 515
Taurine, 332
Team Nutrition, 602
Teenage years, nutrition for, 605–7
Teratogens, 568
Testosterone, 257
Tetany, 365
*Tetrodotoxin*, 521
Theory, 63
Thermic effect of food (TEF), 249
Thermogenesis, 247, 249
Thiamin, 308, 310–12, 332
*Thiaminase*, 521
Thyroid hormones, 94, 222, 383
Tissues, 82, 83, 87
Tocopherols, 303
Tolerable Upper Intake Levels (Upper Levels/
ULs), 60, 61, 62, 63
Total fiber, 132
Total parenteral nutrition, 187
Total-body electrical conductance (TOBEC), 257
Toxicity, 519
Toxicology, 519
Toxins, 507
*Toxoplasma gondii*, 515
Trabecular bone, 394–95
Trace minerals, 11, 357

Trachea, 100
Trans fatty acids. *See also* Lipids
assessing diet and, 17
defined, 10
diabetes and, 154
eating fish and, 187
on food labels, 66
free cholesterol and, 184
hydrogenation and, 177–79
improving diets and, 18, 19
lipid types and, 167, 168, 169
metabolic syndrome and, 158
overconsumption of, 54
rancidity and, 176
sources of, 170
suggestions to minimize, 16
tips for avoiding too much, 194
weight control and, 264
Transcription, 85
Transgenic organism, 493
Translation, 85
Transverse colon, 104
Tretinoin (Retin-A), 295
*Trichinella spiralis*, 515
Triglycerides. *See also* Lipids
absorption of lipids and, 181
broader roles for, 188–89
cardiovascular disease and, 199
chemical forms of, 171
chylomicrons and, 182, 183
defined, 9
described, 169
diabetes and, 155, 156
digestion of lipids and, 179
fats/oils in foods and, 172
fatty acids and, 167
high insulin output and, 144
lipid types and, 167
lipoproteins and, 184
medications for, 200
metabolic syndrome and, 157, 158
omega-3 fatty acids and, 186, 187
Trimesters, 544–46
Trypsin, 219
Tumors, 646
Tyrosine, 213, 222

**U**

U.S. Centers for Disease Control and
Prevention (CDC), 260, 507, 509, 602
U.S. Department of Agriculture (USDA)
Dietary Guidelines for Americans, 52, 54
food safety and, 509, 517, 532, 534, 548
MyPyramid and, 45, 47
on organic food, 528
on pesticides, 526
Team Nutrition of, 602
weight-loss diets and, 275
U.S. Department of Health and Human Services
(HHS), 17, 52, 54, 60
U.S. Food and Drug Administration (FDA)
alternative medicine and, 634–35
alternative sweeteners and, 138
on bottled water, 355
on caffeine, 523
on diet, 146, 147

U.S. Food and Drug Administration
　(FDA)—*Cont.*
　dietary supplements and, 71, 72, 187, 335,
　　336, 338
　erogenic aids and, 432
　on food additives, 515
　food labeling and, 66, 69
　food safety and, 509, 519, 520
　on genetic engineering, 493, 523
　on iron, 377
　on irradiation, 510
　isotretinoin (Accutane) and, 296
　on lead, 368
　on medical therapies for cardiovascular
　　disease, 200
　on medication for bulimia
　　nervosa, 458
　medications for weight loss and,
　　270–71
　on mercury, 570
　net carbs and, 144
　on pesticides, 526–27
　on preventing foodborne illness, 531,
　　532, 533
　safety of sweeteners determined by, 137
　on sodium, 360, 361
　on trans fats, 178
　vegetarian diets and, 232
　on vitamins, 298, 302, 325, 568
　website for, 73
U.S. Public Health Service, 568
U.S. Surgeon General, 55
Ulcers, 65, 112–14
Ultraviolet B (UVB) rays, 298, 299
Umami, 97, 98
Undernutrition. *See also* Malnutrition
　case study on, during infancy, 611
　case study on, in childhood, 499
　crisis of world hunger, 474–78
　at critical life stages, 496–98
　defined, 41, 475, 582
　described, 40, 41, 42
　in developing world, 482–91
　effects of hunger, 477
　infants and, 582, 584
　introduction to problem of, 473
　nutrient-deficiency diseases
　　accompanying, 476
　reducing, in developing world, 490–92
　in United States, 478–82
Underwater weighing, 254, 256, 257
Underweight, 274
United Nations, 483, 484, 485–86, 489,
　　492, 496
Unsaturated fatty acids, 10, 173, 177, 184
Upper Levels. *See* Tolerable Upper Intake Levels
　　(Upper Levels/ULs)
Upper-body obesity, 257, 258
Urea, 87, 106, 224, 227, 350
Ureter, 106, 107
Urethane, 524
Urethra, 106, 107
Urinary system, 88, 89, 106–7
USDA. *See* U.S. Department of Agriculture
　　(USDA)
USP (United States Pharmacopeia) label, 336,
　　359, 368

**V**

Vegans, 193, 233. *See also* Vegetarian/
　vegan diets
Vegetables. *See* Fruits/vegetables
Vegetarian/vegan diets, 231–36
　atherosclerosis and, 199
　athletes and, 424
　case study on, 236
　children and, 598, 599
　college students and, 26
　fat intake and, 193
　pregnancy and, 556–57
　proteins and, 209–10
　in teenage years, 606
　vitamin B-12 and, 326
Veins, 89, 90
Very-low-calorie diet (VLCD), 272
Very-low-density lipoprotein (VLDL), 182,
　　183, 184
*Vibrio*, 508, 511, 513
Villi, 100, 101
Virus, 506
Viruses, 508, 514
Viscous/soluble fibers, 131, 132, 147
Vitamin A
　as fat-soluble, 11, 293
　on food labels, 66
　functions of, 294–96
　overnutrition and, 42
　in prevention of birth defects, 569
　sources/needs, 296–98
　storage of, in body, 107
　summary of, 307
　supplements, 6
　synthesis of, 290
　toxicity and, 292, 337
　white blood cells and, 96
Vitamin B-12
　as B vitamin, 308
　folate and, 325
　functions of, 325–26
　sources/needs, 326–27
　summary of, 333
Vitamin B-6
　as B vitamin, 308
　functions of, 317–18
　sources/needs, 318–19
　summary of, 333
　upper level for, 319–20
Vitamin C
　assessing diet and, 17
　cancer and, 647
　Dietary Guidelines for Americans
　　and, 56
　on food labels, 66
　functions of, 328
　high doses of, 330
　introduction to, 327
　rancidity and, 177
　scurvy and, 63
　sources/needs, 328–30
　summary of, 333
　toxicity, 292
　underconsumption of, 54
　undernutrition and, 41
　upper level for, 330

as water-soluble, 308
white blood cells and, 96
Vitamin D
　assessing diet and, 17
　breastfeeding and, 565
　dietary supplements and, 336
　as fat-soluble, 293
　functions of, 299–300
　for infants, 586
　introduction to, 298–99
　kidneys and, 107
　new benefits/concerns about, 300
　nutrient needs for adulthood and, 628
　nutrients and, 8
　osteoporosis and, 396, 398
　sources/needs, 300
　summary of, 307
　synthesis of, 290
　underconsumption of, 54
　upper level for, 300–301
Vitamin E
　assessing diet and, 17
　cancer and, 647
　cardiovascular disease and, 198
　as dietary supplement, 301, 302
　as fat-soluble, 293
　as food additive, 520
　functions of, 302
　MyPyramid and, 50, 52
　natural vs. synthetic form of, 291
　nutrient needs for adulthood and, 628–29
　rancidity and, 177
　selenium and, 381
　sources/needs, 303–4
　summary of, 307
　toxicity, 292
　underconsumption of, 54
　upper level for, 304–5
Vitamin K
　fats and, 189
　as fat-soluble, 293
　food additives and, 520
　functions of, 305–6
　for infants, 586
　large intestine and, 105
　sources/needs, 305–6
　summary of, 307
　synthesis of, 291
　upper level for, 307
Vitamin-like compounds, 331–32, 334
Vitamins. *See also* Dietary supplements; *names
　　of individual vitamins;* Vitamin-like
　　compounds
　AIDS and, 489
　alcohol and, 640
　assessing diet and, 17
　athletes and need for, 423–25
　breastfeeding and, 563
　cancer and, 647–48
　for children, 597–98
　as class of nutrient, 7, 11
　daily intake of, 13
　defined, 7, 290
　Dietary Supplement Health and Education
　　Act (DSHEA) of 1994 and, 71
　digestive system and, 96
　fats and, 189

functions of classes of nutrients and, 8
immune system and, 95
for infants, 586
interactions with minerals, 358
introduction to, 289–90
large intestine and, 104
malnutrition and, 475
MyPyramid and, 51
nutrient density and, 39
nutrient needs for adulthood and, 625, 627–29
overnutrition and, 42
in plant foods, 218
pregnancy and, 543, 553, 557, 559, 571
in prevention of birth defects, 569
semistarvation and, 477
storage of, in body, 107
student athletes and, 27
sugar and, 150
supplements, megadoses of, 71
tips for preserving vitamin content of food, 293
toxicity and, 292, 337
urinary system and, 106
vegetarian diets and, 26, 234–35
as vital dietary components, 290–93
water-soluble, 308
water-soluble vs. fat-soluble, 9, 11

# W

Wal-Mart, 530
War and political/civil unrest, 484–85, 486
Water
beverage consumption guidelines and, 353–54
body temperature regulation and, 349
bottled, 355, 356
as class of nutrient, 7, 8, 11–12
consuming too much, 355, 427
content of foods, 351
defined, 7
endocrine system and balance of, 93
energy density and, 39
fluoridated, 152
functions of, 350, 351
hard vs. soft, 353

health promotion/disease prevention and, 19
how much is needed, 351–52
for infants, 587–88
intake/output, 352
intracellular/extracellular fluid and, 348–49, 350
introduction to, 347, 348
large intestine and, 104, 105
nutrient needs for adulthood and, 627
proportions of, in human body, 13
safety issues, 355–56
sanitation and supply of, 487
satiety and, 21
sodium and, 359
student athletes and, 27
thirst, 353
waste products and, 350–51
Water-soluble vitamins, 290, 332–33
Weight. *See also* Obesity; Weight control; Weight loss
breastfeeding and, 564
cancer and, 243
cardiovascular disease and, 243
Dietary Guidelines for Americans and management of, 56
eating well in college and, 24
food insecurity and, 480
gallstones and, 116
hypertension and, 243
pregnancy and, 543, 550–52, 554
state of nutritional health and, 45
stroke and, 243
sugar and, 150
treatment of overweight/obesity, 261–63
type 2 diabetes and, 243
Weight control. *See also* Obesity; Weight loss
behavior modification for, 267–69
calories and, 263–65
case study on choosing weight-loss program, 278
determination of energy use by body and, 250–51
energy and, 245–50, 254–58
estimation of healthy weight, 251–52
physical activity and, 265–66
popular diets and, 275–77

professional help for, 269–74
treatment of underweight, 274
Weight cycling/"yo-yo" dieting, 276
Weight loss. *See also* Obesity; Weight control
athletes and, 419
carbohydrates and, 142
eating well in college and, 25
protein to meet energy needs for, 223–24
Weight-Control Information Network (WIN), 263
White blood cells, 96
Whole Foods Market, Inc., 530
Whole grains, 131, 147, 148
World Bank, 491
World Health Organization (WHO), 55, 137, 150, 487, 532, 560, 582–83

# X

Xerophthalmia, 294, 476
Xylitol, 136

# Y

*Yersinia enterocolitica*, 513

# Z

Zinc
colds and, 381
daily intake of, 13
functions of, 379
immune system and, 95
infants and, 582, 593
introduction to, 378–79
malnutrition and, 475
MyPyramid and, 50, 52
nutrient needs for adulthood and, 628
pregnancy and, 553
semistarvation and, 477
sources/needs, 379–80
summary of, 389
upper level for, 381
white blood cells and, 96
Zygote, 544

# A

## Dietary Reference Intakes (DRIs): Recommended Intakes for Individuals, Vitamins
Food and Nutrition Board, Institute of Medicine, National Academies

| Life Stage Group | Vitamin A (μg/d)[a] | Vitamin C (mg/d) | Vitamin D (μg/d)[b,c] | Vitamin E (mg/d)[d] | Vitamin K (μg/d) | Thiamin (mg/d) | Riboflavin (mg/d) | Niacin (mg/d)[e] | Vitamin $B_6$ (mg/d) | Folate (μg/d)[f] | Vitamin B-12 (μg/d) | Pantothenic Acid (mg/d) | Biotin (μg/d) | Choline (mg/d)[g] |
|---|---|---|---|---|---|---|---|---|---|---|---|---|---|---|
| **Infants** | | | | | | | | | | | | | | |
| 0–6 mo | 400* | 40* | 5* | 4* | 2.0* | 0.2* | 0.3* | 2* | 0.1* | 65* | 0.4* | 1.7* | 5* | 125* |
| 7–12 mo | 500* | 50* | 5* | 5* | 2.5* | 0.3* | 0.4* | 4* | 0.3* | 80* | 0.5* | 1.8* | 6* | 150* |
| **Children** | | | | | | | | | | | | | | |
| 1–3 y | 300 | 15 | 5* | 6 | 30* | 0.5 | 0.5 | 6 | 0.5 | 150 | 0.9 | 2* | 8* | 200* |
| 4–8 y | 400 | 25 | 5* | 7 | 55* | 0.6 | 0.6 | 8 | 0.6 | 200 | 1.2 | 3* | 12* | 250* |
| **Males** | | | | | | | | | | | | | | |
| 9–13 y | 600 | 45 | 5* | 11 | 60* | 0.9 | 0.9 | 12 | 1.0 | 300 | 1.8 | 4* | 20* | 375* |
| 14–18 y | 900 | 75 | 5* | 15 | 75* | 1.2 | 1.3 | 16 | 1.3 | 400 | 2.4 | 5* | 25* | 550* |
| 19–30 y | 900 | 90 | 5* | 15 | 120* | 1.2 | 1.3 | 16 | 1.3 | 400 | 2.4 | 5* | 30* | 550* |
| 31–50 y | 900 | 90 | 5* | 15 | 120* | 1.2 | 1.3 | 16 | 1.3 | 400 | 2.4 | 5* | 30* | 550* |
| 51–70 y | 900 | 90 | 10* | 15 | 120* | 1.2 | 1.3 | 16 | 1.7 | 400 | 2.4[h] | 5* | 30* | 550* |
| >70 y | 900 | 90 | 15* | 15 | 120* | 1.2 | 1.3 | 16 | 1.7 | 400 | 2.4[h] | 5* | 30* | 550* |
| **Females** | | | | | | | | | | | | | | |
| 9–13 y | 600 | 45 | 5* | 11 | 60* | 0.9 | 0.9 | 12 | 1.0 | 300 | 1.8 | 4* | 20* | 375* |
| 14–18 y | 700 | 65 | 5* | 15 | 75* | 1.0 | 1.0 | 14 | 1.2 | 400[i] | 2.4 | 5* | 25* | 400* |
| 19–30 y | 700 | 75 | 5* | 15 | 90* | 1.1 | 1.1 | 14 | 1.3 | 400[i] | 2.4 | 5* | 30* | 425* |
| 31–50 y | 700 | 75 | 5* | 15 | 90* | 1.1 | 1.1 | 14 | 1.3 | 400[i] | 2.4 | 5* | 30* | 425* |
| 51–70 y | 700 | 75 | 10* | 15 | 90* | 1.1 | 1.1 | 14 | 1.5 | 400 | 2.4[h] | 5* | 30* | 425* |
| >70 y | 700 | 75 | 15* | 15 | 90* | 1.1 | 1.1 | 14 | 1.5 | 400 | 2.4[h] | 5* | 30* | 425* |
| **Pregnancy** | | | | | | | | | | | | | | |
| ≤18 y | 750 | 80 | 5* | 15 | 75* | 1.4 | 1.4 | 18 | 1.9 | 600[j] | 2.6 | 6* | 30* | 450* |
| 19–30 y | 770 | 85 | 5* | 15 | 90* | 1.4 | 1.4 | 18 | 1.9 | 600[j] | 2.6 | 6* | 30* | 450* |
| 31–50 y | 770 | 85 | 5* | 15 | 90* | 1.4 | 1.4 | 18 | 1.9 | 600[j] | 2.6 | 6* | 30* | 450* |
| **Lactation** | | | | | | | | | | | | | | |
| ≤18 y | 1,200 | 115 | 5* | 19 | 75* | 1.4 | 1.6 | 17 | 2.0 | 500 | 2.8 | 7* | 35* | 550* |
| 19–30 y | 1,300 | 120 | 5* | 19 | 90* | 1.4 | 1.6 | 17 | 2.0 | 500 | 2.8 | 7* | 35* | 550* |
| 31–50 y | 1,300 | 120 | 5* | 19 | 90* | 1.4 | 1.6 | 17 | 2.0 | 500 | 2.8 | 7* | 35* | 550* |

mg = milligram, μg = microgram

**NOTE:** This table (taken from the DRI reports, see www.nap.edu) presents Recommended Dietary Allowances (RDAs) in **bold type** and Adequate Intakes (AIs) in ordinary type followed by an asterisk (*). RDAs and AIs may both be used as goals for individual intake. RDAs are set to meet the needs of almost all (97 to 98 percent) individuals in a group. For healthy breastfed infants, the AI is the mean intake. The AI for other life stage and gender groups is believed to cover needs of all individuals in the group, but lack of data or uncertainty in the data prevent being able to specify with confidence the percentage of individuals covered by this intake.

[a] As retinol activity equivalents (RAEs). 1 RAE = 1 μg retinol, 12 μg β-carotene, 24 μg α-carotene, or 24 μg β-cryptoxanthin. To calculate RAEs from REs of provitamin A carotenoids in foods, divide the REs by 2. For preformed vitamin A in foods or supplements and for provitamin A carotenoids in supplements, 1 RE = 1 RAE.

[b] cholecalciferol. 1 μg cholecalciferol = 40 IU vitamin D.

[c] In the absence of adequate exposure to sunlight.

[d] As α-tocopherol. α-Tocopherol includes *RRR*-α-tocopherol, the only form of α-tocopherol that occurs naturally in foods, and the 2R-stereoisomeric forms of α-tocopherol (*RRR*-, *RSR*-, *RRS*-, and *RSS*-α-tocopherol) that occur in fortified foods and supplements. It does not include the 2S-stereoisomeric forms of α-tocopherol (*SRR*-, *SSR*-, *SRS*-, and *SSS*-α-tocopherol), also found in fortified foods and supplements.

[e] As niacin equivalents (NE). 1 mg of niacin = 60 mg of tryptophan; 0–6 months = preformed niacin (not NE).

[f] As dietary folate equivalents (DFE). 1 DFE = 1 μg food folate = 0.6 μg of folic acid from fortified food or as a supplement consumed with food = 0.5 μg of a supplement taken on an empty stomach.

[g] Although AIs have been set for choline, there are few data to assess whether a dietary supply of choline is needed at all stages of the life cycle, and it may be that the choline requirement can be met by endogenous synthesis at some of these stages.

[h] Because 10 to 30 percent of older people may malabsorb food-bound B-12, it is advisable for those older than 50 years to meet their RDA mainly by consuming foods fortified with B-12 or a supplement containing B-12.

[i] In view of evidence linking folate intake with neural tube defects in the fetus, it is recommended that all women capable of becoming pregnant consume 400 μg from supplements or fortified foods in addition to intake of food folate from a varied diet.

[j] It is assumed that women will continue consuming 400 μg from supplements or fortified food until their pregnancy is confirmed and they enter prenatal care, which ordinarily occurs after the end of the periconceptional period—the critical time for formation of the neural tube.

Adapted from the Dietary Reference Intakes series, National Academies Press. Copyright 1997, 1998, 2000, 2001, by the National Academy of Sciences. The full reports are available from the National Academies Press at www.nap.edu.

**Dietary Reference Intakes (DRIs): Recommended Intakes for Individuals, Elements**
Food and Nutrition Board, Institute of Medicine, National Academies

| Life Stage Group | Calcium (mg/d) | Chromium (µg/d) | Copper (µg/d) | Fluoride (mg/d) | Iodine (µg/d) | Iron (mg/d) | Magnesium (mg/d) | Manganese (mg/d) | Molybdenum (µg/d) | Phosphorus (mg/d) | Selenium (µg/d) | Zinc (mg/d) |
|---|---|---|---|---|---|---|---|---|---|---|---|---|
| **Infants** | | | | | | | | | | | | |
| 0–6 mo | 210* | 0.2* | 200* | 0.01* | 110* | 0.27* | 30* | 0.003* | 2* | 100* | 15* | 2* |
| 7–12 mo | 270* | 5.5* | 220* | 0.5* | 130* | 11 | 75* | 0.6* | 3* | 275* | 20* | 3 |
| **Children** | | | | | | | | | | | | |
| 1–3 y | 500* | 11* | 340 | 0.7* | 90 | 7 | 80 | 1.2* | 17 | 460 | 20 | 3 |
| 4–8 y | 800* | 15* | 440 | 1* | 90 | 10 | 130 | 1.5* | 22 | 500 | 30 | 5 |
| **Males** | | | | | | | | | | | | |
| 9–13 y | 1,300* | 25* | 700 | 2* | 120 | 8 | 240 | 1.9* | 34 | 1,250 | 40 | 8 |
| 14–18 y | 1,300* | 35* | 890 | 3* | 150 | 11 | 410 | 2.2* | 43 | 1,250 | 55 | 11 |
| 19–30 y | 1,000* | 35* | 900 | 4* | 150 | 8 | 400 | 2.3* | 45 | 700 | 55 | 11 |
| 31–50 y | 1,000* | 35* | 900 | 4* | 150 | 8 | 420 | 2.3* | 45 | 700 | 55 | 11 |
| 51–70 y | 1,200* | 30* | 900 | 4* | 150 | 8 | 420 | 2.3* | 45 | 700 | 55 | 11 |
| >70 y | 1,200* | 30* | 900 | 4* | 150 | 8 | 420 | 2.3* | 45 | 700 | 55 | 11 |
| **Females** | | | | | | | | | | | | |
| 9–13 y | 1,300* | 21* | 700 | 2* | 120 | 8 | 240 | 1.6* | 34 | 1,250 | 40 | 8 |
| 14–18 y | 1,300* | 24* | 890 | 3* | 150 | 15 | 360 | 1.6* | 43 | 1,250 | 55 | 9 |
| 19–30 y | 1,000* | 25* | 900 | 3* | 150 | 18 | 310 | 1.8* | 45 | 700 | 55 | 8 |
| 31–50 y | 1,000* | 25* | 900 | 3* | 150 | 18 | 320 | 1.8* | 45 | 700 | 55 | 8 |
| 51–70 y | 1,200* | 20* | 900 | 3* | 150 | 8 | 320 | 1.8* | 45 | 700 | 55 | 8 |
| >70 y | 1,200* | 20* | 900 | 3* | 150 | 8 | 320 | 1.8* | 45 | 700 | 55 | 8 |
| **Pregnancy** | | | | | | | | | | | | |
| ≤18 y | 1,300* | 29* | 1,000 | 3* | 220 | 27 | 400 | 2.0* | 50 | 1,250 | 60 | 12 |
| 19–30 y | 1,000* | 30* | 1,000 | 3* | 220 | 27 | 350 | 2.0* | 50 | 700 | 60 | 11 |
| 31–50 y | 1,000* | 30* | 1,000 | 3* | 220 | 27 | 360 | 2.0* | 50 | 700 | 60 | 11 |
| **Lactation** | | | | | | | | | | | | |
| ≤18 y | 1,300* | 44* | 1,300 | 3* | 290 | 10 | 360 | 2.6* | 50 | 1,250 | 70 | 13 |
| 19–30 y | 1,000* | 45* | 1,300 | 3* | 290 | 9 | 310 | 2.6* | 50 | 700 | 70 | 12 |
| 31–50 y | 1,000* | 45* | 1,300 | 3* | 290 | 9 | 320 | 2.6* | 50 | 700 | 70 | 12 |

**NOTE:** This table presents Recommended Dietary Allowances (RDAs) in **bold type** and Adequate Intakes (AIs) in ordinary type followed by an asterisk (*). RDAs and AIs may both be used as goals for individual intake. RDAs are set to meet the needs of almost all (97 to 98 percent) individuals in a group. For healthy breastfed infants, the AI is the mean intake. The AI for other life stage and gender groups is believed to cover needs of all individuals in the group, but lack of data or uncertainty in the data prevent being able to specify with confidence the percentage of individuals covered by this intake.

**SOURCES:** Dietary Reference Intakes for Calcium, Phosphorus, Magnesium, Vitamin D, and Fluoride (1997); Dietary Reference Intakes for Thiamin, Riboflavin, Niacin, Vitamin B-6, Folate, Vitamin B-12, Pantothenic Acid, Biotin, and Choline (1998); Dietary Reference Intakes for Vitamin C, Vitamin E, Selenium, and Carotenoids (2000); and Dietary Reference Intakes for Vitamin A, Vitamin K, Arsenic, Boron, Chromium, Copper, Iodine, Iron, Manganese, Molybdenum, Nickel, Silicon, Vanadium, and Zinc (2001). These reports may be accessed via www.nap.edu.

Adapted from the Dietary Reference Intake series, National Academies Press. Copyright 1997, 1998, 2000, 2001, by the National Academy of Sciences. The full reports are available from the National Academies Press at www.nap.edu.

B

## Dietary Reference Intakes (DRIs): Recommended Intakes for Individuals, Macronutrients
Food and Nutrition Board, Institute of Medicine, National Academies

| Life Stage Group | Carbohydrate (g/d) | Total Fiber (g/d) | Fat (g/d) | Linoleic Acid (g/d) | α-Linolenic Acid (g/d) | Protein[a] (g/d) |
|---|---|---|---|---|---|---|
| **Infants** | | | | | | |
| 0–6 mo | 60* | ND | 31* | 4.4* | 0.5* | 9.1* |
| 7–12 mo | 95* | ND | 30* | 4.6* | 0.5* | 13.5 |
| **Children** | | | | | | |
| 1–3 y | 130 | 19* | ND[b] | 7* | 0.7* | 13 |
| 4–8 y | 130 | 25* | ND | 10* | 0.9* | 19 |
| **Males** | | | | | | |
| 9–13 y | 130 | 31* | ND | 12* | 1.2* | 34 |
| 14–18 y | 130 | 38* | ND | 16* | 1.6* | 52 |
| 19–30 y | 130 | 38* | ND | 17* | 1.6* | 56 |
| 31–50 y | 130 | 38* | ND | 17* | 1.6* | 56 |
| 51–70 y | 130 | 30* | ND | 14* | 1.6* | 56 |
| >70 y | 130 | 30* | ND | 14* | 1.6* | 56 |
| **Females** | | | | | | |
| 9–13 y | 130 | 26* | ND | 10* | 1.0* | 34 |
| 14–18 y | 130 | 26* | ND | 11* | 1.1* | 46 |
| 19–30 y | 130 | 25* | ND | 12* | 1.1* | 46 |
| 31–50 y | 130 | 25* | ND | 12* | 1.1* | 46 |
| 51–70 y | 130 | 21* | ND | 11* | 1.1* | 46 |
| >70 y | 130 | 21* | ND | 11* | 1.1* | 46 |
| **Pregnancy** | | | | | | |
| 14–18 y | 175 | 28* | ND | 13* | 1.4* | 71 |
| 19–30 y | 175 | 28* | ND | 13* | 1.4* | 71 |
| 31–50 y | 175 | 28* | ND | 13* | 1.4* | 71 |
| **Lactation** | | | | | | |
| 14–18 y | 210 | 29* | ND | 13* | 1.3* | 71 |
| 19–30 y | 210 | 29* | ND | 13* | 1.3* | 71 |
| 31–50 y | 210 | 29* | ND | 13* | 1.3* | 71 |

**NOTE:** This table presents Recommended Dietary Allowances (RDAs) in **bold type** and Adequate Intakes (AIs) in ordinary type followed by an asterisk (*). RDAs and AIs may both be used as goals for individual intake. RDAs are set to meet the needs of almost all (97 to 98 percent) individuals in a group. For healthy breastfed infants, the AI is the mean intake. The AI for other life stage and gender groups is believed to cover needs of all individuals in the group, but lack of data or uncertainty in the data prevent being able to specify with confidence the percentage of individuals covered by this intake.

[a] Based on 0.8g protein/kg body weight for reference body weight.

[b] ND = not determinable at this time

**SOURCES:** Dietary Reference Intakes for Energy, Carbohydrate, Fiber, Fat, Fatty Acids, Cholesterol, Protein, and Amino Acids (2002). This report may be accessed via www.nap.edu.

Adapted from the Dietary Reference Intake series, National Academies Press. Copyright 1997, 1998, 2000, 2001, by the National Academy of Sciences. The full reports are available from the National Academies Press at www.nap.edu.

C

## Dietary Reference Intakes (DRIs): Recommended Intakes for Individuals, Electrolytes and Water

Food and Nutrition Board, Institute of Medicine, National Academies

| Life Stage Group | Sodium (mg/d) | Potassium (mg/d) | Chloride (mg/d) | Water (L/d) |
|---|---|---|---|---|
| **Infants** | | | | |
| 0–6 mo | 120* | 400* | 180* | 0.7* |
| 7–12 mo | 370* | 700* | 570* | 0.8* |
| **Children** | | | | |
| 1–3 y | 1,000* | 3,000* | 1,500* | 1.3* |
| 4–8 y | 1,200* | 3,800* | 1,900* | 1.7* |
| **Males** | | | | |
| 9–13 y | 1,500* | 4,500* | 2,300* | 2.4* |
| 14–18 y | 1,500* | 4,700* | 2,300* | 3.3* |
| 19–30 y | 1,500* | 4,700* | 2,300* | 3.7* |
| 31–50 y | 1,500* | 4,700* | 2,300* | 3.7* |
| 51–70 y | 1,300* | 4,700* | 2,000* | 3.7* |
| > 70 y | 1,200* | 4,700* | 1,800* | 3.7* |
| **Females** | | | | |
| 9–13 y | 1,500* | 4,500* | 2,300* | 2.1* |
| 14–18 y | 1,500* | 4,700* | 2,300* | 2.3* |
| 19–30 y | 1,500* | 4,700* | 2,300* | 2.7* |
| 31–50 y | 1,500* | 4,700* | 2,300* | 2.7* |
| 51–70 y | 1,300* | 4,700* | 2,000* | 2.7* |
| > 70 y | 1,200* | 4,700* | 1,800* | 2.7* |
| **Pregnancy** | | | | |
| 14–18 y | 1,500* | 4,700* | 2,300* | 3.0* |
| 19–50 y | 1,500* | 4,700* | 2,300* | 3.0* |
| **Lactation** | | | | |
| 14–18 y | 1,500* | 5,100* | 2,300* | 3.8* |
| 19–50 y | 1,500* | 5,100* | 2,300* | 3.8* |

**NOTE:** The table is adapted from the DRI reports. See www.nap.edu. Adequate Intakes (AIs) are followed by an asterisk (*). These may be used as a goal for individual intake. For healthy breastfed infants, the AI is the average intake. The AI for other life stage and gender groups is believed to cover the needs of all individuals in the group, but lack of data prevent being able to specify with confidence the percentage of individuals covered by this intake; therefore, no Recommended Dietary Allowance (RDA) was set.

**SOURCE:** *Dietary Reference Intakes for Water, Potassium, Sodium, Chloride, and Sulfate.* This report may be accessed via www.nap.edu.

## Acceptable Macronutrient Distribution Ranges

| Macronutrient | Range (percent of energy) | | |
|---|---|---|---|
| | Children, 1–3 y | Children, 4–18 y | Adults |
| Fat | 30–40 | 25–35 | 20–35 |
| *omega*-6 polyunsaturated fats (linoleic acid) | 5–10 | 5–10 | 5–10 |
| *omega*-3 polyunsaturated fats[a] (α-linolenic acid) | 0.6–1.2 | 0.6–1.2 | 0.6–1.2 |
| Carbohydrate | 45–65 | 45–65 | 45–65 |
| Protein | 5–20 | 10–30 | 10–35 |

[a]Approximately 10% of the total can come from longer-chain n-3 fatty acids.

**SOURCE:** *Dietary Reference Intakes for Energy, Carbohydrate, Fiber, Fat, Fatty Acids, Cholesterol, Protein, and Amino Acids (2002).* The report may be accessed via www.nap.edu.

Adapted from the Dietary Reference Intakes series, National Academies Press. Copyright 1997, 1998, 2000, 2001, by the National Academy of Sciences. The full reports are available from the National Academies Press at www.nap.edu.

**E**

## Dietary Reference Intakes (DRIs): Tolerable Upper Intake Levels (UL[a]), Vitamins
Food and Nutrition Board, Institute of Medicine, National Academies

| Life Stage Group | Vitamin A (μg/d)[b] | Vitamin C (mg/d) | Vitamin D (μg/d) | Vitamin E (mg/d)[c,d] | Vitamin K | Thiamin | Riboflavin | Niacin (mg/d)[d] | Vitamin B-6 (mg/d) | Folate (μg/d)[d] | Vitamin B-12 | Pantothenic Acid | Biotin | Choline (g/d) | Carotenoids[e] |
|---|---|---|---|---|---|---|---|---|---|---|---|---|---|---|---|
| **Infants** | | | | | | | | | | | | | | | |
| 0–6 mo | 600 | ND | 25 | ND | ND | ND | ND | ND | ND | ND | ND | ND | ND | ND | ND |
| 7–12 mo | 600 | ND | 25 | ND | ND | ND | ND | ND | ND | ND | ND | ND | ND | ND | ND |
| **Children** | | | | | | | | | | | | | | | |
| 1–3 y | 600 | 400 | 50 | 200 | ND | ND | ND | 10 | 30 | 300 | ND | ND | ND | 1.0 | ND |
| 4–8 y | 900 | 650 | 50 | 300 | ND | ND | ND | 15 | 40 | 400 | ND | ND | ND | 1.0 | ND |
| **Males, Females** | | | | | | | | | | | | | | | |
| 9–13 y | 1,700 | 1,200 | 50 | 600 | ND | ND | ND | 20 | 60 | 600 | ND | ND | ND | 2.0 | ND |
| 14–18 y | 2,800 | 1,800 | 50 | 800 | ND | ND | ND | 30 | 80 | 800 | ND | ND | ND | 3.0 | ND |
| 19–70 y | 3,000 | 2,000 | 50 | 1,000 | ND | ND | ND | 35 | 100 | 1,000 | ND | ND | ND | 3.5 | ND |
| >70 y | 3,000 | 2,000 | 50 | 1,000 | ND | ND | ND | 35 | 100 | 1,000 | ND | ND | ND | 3.5 | ND |
| **Pregnancy** | | | | | | | | | | | | | | | |
| ≤18 y | 2,800 | 1,800 | 50 | 800 | ND | ND | ND | 30 | 80 | 800 | ND | ND | ND | 3.0 | ND |
| 19–50 y | 3,000 | 2,000 | 50 | 1,000 | ND | ND | ND | 35 | 100 | 1,000 | ND | ND | ND | 3.5 | ND |
| **Lactation** | | | | | | | | | | | | | | | |
| ≤18 y | 2,800 | 1,800 | 50 | 800 | ND | ND | ND | 30 | 80 | 800 | ND | ND | ND | 3.0 | ND |
| 19–50 y | 3,000 | 2,000 | 50 | 1,000 | ND | ND | ND | 35 | 100 | 1,000 | ND | ND | ND | 3.5 | ND |

[a]UL = The maximum level of daily nutrient intake likely to pose no risk of adverse effects. Unless otherwise specified, the UL represents total intake from food, water, and supplements. Due to lack of suitable data, ULs could not be established for vitamin K, thiamin, riboflavin, vitamin B-12, pantothenic acid, biotin, or carotenoids. In the absence of ULs, extra caution may be warranted in consuming levels above recommended intakes.

[b]As preformed vitamin A only.

[c]As α-tocopherol; applies to any form of supplemental α-tocopherol.

[d]The ULs for vitamin E, niacin, and folate apply to synthetic forms obtained from supplements, fortified foods, or a combination of the two.

[e]β-Carotene supplements are advised only to serve as a provitamin A source for individuals at risk of vitamin A deficiency.

[f]ND = Not determinable due to lack of data of adverse effects in this age group and concern with regard to lack of ability to handle excess amounts. Source of intake should be from food only to prevent high levels of intake.

**SOURCES:** Dietary Reference Intakes for Calcium, Phosphorus, Magnesium, Vitamin D, and Fluoride (1997); Dietary Reference Intakes for Thiamin, Riboflavin, Niacin, Vitamin B-6, Folate, Vitamin B-12, Pantothenic Acid, Biotin, and Choline (1998); Dietary Reference Intakes for Vitamin C, Vitamin E, Selenium, and Carotenoids (2000); and Dietary Reference Intakes for Vitamin A, Vitamin K, Arsenic, Boron, Chromium, Copper, Iodine, Iron, Manganese, Molybdenum, Nickel, Silicon, Vanadium, and Zinc (2001). These reports may be accessed via www.nap.edu.

Adapted from the Dietary Reference Intakes series, National Academies Press. Copyright 1997, 1998, 2000, 2001, by the National Academy of Sciences. The full reports are available from the National Academies Press at www.nap.edu.